Essentials of
Pharmacology

BASIC PRINCIPLES AND GENERAL CONCEPTS

Essentials of
Pharmacology

BASIC PRINCIPLES AND GENERAL CONCEPTS
Fourth Edition

DR. V.N. SHARMA
M.B.B.S., M.Sc. (Med.), Ph.D., FAMS

Professor Emeritus of Pharmacology
SMS Medical College, Jaipur

Technical Advisor
Lal Bahadur Shastri College of Pharmacy, Jaipur

Chairman, Ethics Committee
SMS Medical College, Jaipur
Monilek Hospital, Jaipur and
Fortis Escorts Hospital, Jaipur

Formerly
Professor and Head, Dept. of Pharmacology
SMS Medical College, Jaipur;
Professor and Head, Dept. of Pharmacology
and
Principal, Medical Colleges and Controller of
Associated Group of Hospitals,
Jodhpur and Bikaner (Rajasthan)

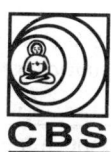

CBS

CBS PUBLISHERS & DISTRIBUTORS PVT. LTD.
NEW DELHI • BENGALURU • CHENNAI • KOCHI • MUMBAI • PUNE

ISBN: 978-81-239-2341-3

First Edition: 1999
Second Edition: 2003
Reprint: 2004, 2005
Third Edition: 2007
Reprint: 2007, 2009
Fouth Edition: 2013
Reprint: 2015

Published by:
Satish Kumar Jain for CBS Publishers & Distributors Pvt. Ltd.,
4819/XI Prahlad Street, 24 Ansari Road, Daryaganj, New Delhi - 110002
delhi@cbspd.com, cbspubs@airtelmail.in • www.cbspd.com
Ph.: 23289259, 23266861, 23266867 • Fax: 011-23243014

Corporate Office: 204 FIE, Industrial Area, Patparganj, Delhi - 110 092
Ph: 49344934 • Fax: 011-49344935
E-mail: publishing@cbspd.com • publicity@cbspd.com

Branches:
• *Bengaluru:* 2975, 17th Cross, K.R. Road, Bansankari 2nd Stage, Bengaluru - 70
  Ph: +91-80-26771678/79 • Fax: +91-80-26771680
  E-mail: cbsbng@gmail.com, bangalore@cbspd.com
• *Chennai:* No. 7, Subbaraya Street, Shenoy Nagar, Chennai - 600030
  Ph: +91-44-26681266, 26680620 • Fax: +91-44-42032115 • E-mail: chennai@cbspd.com
• *Kochi:* 36/14, Kalluvilakam, Lissie Hospital Road, Kochi - 682018
  Ph: +91-484-4059061-65 • Fax: +91-484-4059065 • E-mail: cochin@cbspd.com
• *Mumbai:* 83-C, Dr. E. Moses Road, Worli, Mumbai - 400018
  Ph: +91-9833017933, 022-24902340/41 • E-mail: mumbai@cbspd.com
• *Pune:* Bhuruk Prestige, Sr. No. 52/12/2+1+3/2,
  Narhe, Haveli (Near Katraj-Dehu Road Bypass), Pune - 411041
  Ph: +91-20-64704058/59, 32342277 • E-mail: pune@cbspd.com

Representatives:
• Hyderabad: 0-9885175004 • Kolkata: 0-9831437309, 0-9051152362
• Nagpur: 0-9021734563 • Patna: 0-9334159340 • Vijayawada: 0-9000660880

Printed at:
India Binding House, Noida (UP)

Dedicated
to the memory
of my wife
Saroj Sharma

Preface to the Fourth Edition

Some readers have suggested that it will be useful if chapters on Pharmacovigilance and Stem Cell: Basics & Potential uses are included in the new forthcoming fourth edition. I welcome this suggestion with thanks. An attempt has been made to highlight the following additional chapters (22 & 23) as relevant to the students of pharmacology.

Pharmacovigilance is an important pharmacological science. It plays an important role in the rational use of medicines by providing information about adverse drug reactions (ADRs). Challenges are posed by the ever increasing range and potency of medicines, all of which carry an inevitable and sometimes unpredictable potential for harm. For all medicines there is a trade-off between benefits and the potential for harm. Pharmacovigilance makes an important contribution to the health of the nation.

Stem cells, directed to differentiate into specific cell types, offer the possibility to treat a myriad of diseased states. Elucidation and exploitation of stem cell has the potential to revolutionise treatment of several diseases. Stem cell research is an emerging field with clinical implications focused on repair, replacement or regeneration of cells to salvage impaired organ functions. The promise of stem cell therapies is an exciting one. Through intensive research, stem cell therapeutics can be nurtured safely. The ICMR guidelines on stem cells hold significance.

Overview of **Pharmionics, Pharmacoepidemiology** and **Pharmacoeconomics** have been added in the appendices.

V.N. Sharma

Preface to the First Edition

Pharmacology has become a broad and deep discipline. A single text—even a long one—cannot adequately cover every aspect of the subject. An attempt to summarize the present understanding of pharmacology in a comprehensive book for the serious student of this subject is a formidable undertaking.

This book is an attempt to provide pharmacological knowledge to the medical, dentistry and pharmacy students and also others concerned with health services. The objectives in this text are to provide a basic understanding as well as to present the essential material giving step-by-step easy to understand explanation for the scientific basis of drug therapy, at a level that the students of these disciplines can handle.

The heavily burdened students may find this book of a size that is manageable. Of course, it was rather difficult to decide as to how much detail should be included in this book. Throughout, the goal has been that the text is geared to medical, dental and pharmacy and other health science students. However, only the users of this book can tell to what extent these goals have been met.

The text is organised in a sequence that builds new information on informations already assimilated, for example early presentation of general aspects of pharmacology, followed by autonomic pharmacology prepares students to understand especially the drugs affecting central nervous system and cardiorenal system.

The coverage in each chapter includes pharmacokinetics, drug effects, mode of action, rationale of clinical applications, preparations, dosages, relevant drug interactions, contraindications and adverse effects.

The text incorporates short sets of key points, set off in outlined boxes which summarize important points wherever special emphasis is needed; and the terms associated with the subject.

Each chapter opens with a list of the contents of the chapter at a glance. It indicates knowledge that should be acquired after reading the chapter itself. At the end of each chapter, study questions are given. It is a series of questions designed to provide a check to see if the contents stated in the beginning of the chapter have been mastered. After answering the questions, it is suggested that students should re-read the contents to determine whether they have met the goals.

To cater for graduate students and teachers, fairly extensive list of references has been included at the end of each chapter which will be useful as guide to further reading.

Readers and users are invited to send their reactions and suggestions to me so that plans can be formulated for subsequent edition. Comments will be welcome.

V.N. Sharma

Acknowledgements

I am deeply grateful to:

- Dr. Rakesh Gupta, Ph.D., Professor, L.B.S. College of Pharmacy, Jaipur for contributing Chapters 13 and 20. He also went through the entire manuscript and gave valuable suggestions.
- Dr. (Ms.) Alpana Ram, Ph.D., Associate Professor, G.G.D. University, Bilaspur for contributing Chapters 14 and 15.
- Dr. (Ms.) Sobhna Singh, Ph.D., Associate Professor, M.J.P. Rohilkhand University, Bareilly for drawing figures in the text.
- Dr. Manoj Dixit, Ph.D., Associate Professor, L.B.S. College of Pharmacy, Jaipur for contributing Chapter 18.
- Dr. (Ms.) Reema Dheer, Ph.D., Associate Professor, L.B.S. College of Pharmacy, Jaipur for contributing Chapter 19.
- Dr. Sudhir Mehta, M.D., MAMS, Professor Medicine, S.M.S. Medical College and Hospital, Jaipur for contributing Chapter 23.
- Ms. Deepa Gupta, Associate Professor, L.B.S. College of Pharmacy, Jaipur for contributing Overviews of pharmacoepidemiology and pharmacoeconomics, as appendices 10 and 11.
- Shri Vinod Sain, L.B..S. College of Pharmacy, Jaipur for his significant contribution in computer related operations.
- Shri B.M. Singh and Shri Kuldeep, CBS Publishers & Distributors Pvt. Ltd., for the pains taken by them in excellent arrangement of the text.
- CBS Publishers & Distributors Pvt. Ltd., for the editorial support and publishing this book on priority basis in spite of their busy schedule.

Much of any merit this book may have is due to the generosity of those mentioned above who have, with such good grace given their time and energy. They have given invaluable help and advice in the preparation of this edition.

Errors are my own.

V.N. Sharma

Contents

General Pharmacology

SCOPE OF PHARMACOLOGY

Pharmacology may be defined as the study of drugs. The word pharmacology has been derived from two Greek words—pharmakon (drug) and logos (study). This "science of drugs" includes knowledge of all the aspects of drugs. It includes their origin, source, physical and chemical properties, preparations, doses, routes of administration, pharmacological actions, absorption, distribution, biotransformation, excretion, therapeutic uses, mode (mechanism) of action, precautions, contraindications, interactions, adverse effects and their treatment.

There are two main branches of pharmacology:

1. *Pharmacokinetics:* It is concerned with the absorption, distribution, metabolism (biotransformation) and excretion of drugs (ADME). Pharmacokinetics is what the body does to the drug. This knowledge is essential to obtain the right effect of the right intensity, at the right time, for right duration, with least risk of unpleasantness or harm.
2. *Pharmacodynamics:* It is concerned with the biochemical and physiological effects of drugs and their mode of action, it includes the dose-effect relationship, factors modifying drug effects and dosage, and drug toxicity. Pharmacodynamics is what drugs do to the body. This knowledge is essential to choose a drug to obtain the desired effect with proper dosage.

A good knowledge of pharmacology (both pharmacokinetics and pharmacodynamics) is therefore necessary to use drugs safely and efficiently.

The scope of pharmacology is rapidly expanding in the field of clinical pharmacology, neuropharmacology, cardiovascular pharmacology, renal pharmacology, biochemical pharmacology, molecular pharmacology, immunopharmacology, pharmacoeconomics, behavioral pharmacology and pharmacovigilance.

The expanded scope provides a rational basis for the therapeutic use of drugs.

Rational use of drugs is based on rule of right: the right drug given to the right patient at the right time with the right dosages. They should also fulfill such criteria: safety, affordability, need and efficacy.

The other terms generally used in pharmacology are:

Clinical pharmacology: It is the study of drug action in human beings.

Chemotherapy is concerned with drugs used in the treatment of bacterial, viral and parasitic diseases. The chemotherapeutic agents destroy the infecting organisms without damaging the host tissues.

Therapeutics includes any measure which is taken in the treatment of disease. It is a broad term which includes physiotherapy, radiotherapy, psychotherapy as well as pharmacotherapy (therapy with drugs). Pharmacotherapeutics is concerned with the application of drugs to produce the desired effect, whether this is for the treatment of disease or for prophylactic purpose.

Immunopharmacology deals with the study of immunological aspects of drug action. It also includes effects of drugs on immune response.

Pharmacogenetics is concerned with variations in drug response due to genetic factors, e.g. primaquine-induced haemolysis in G-6PD deficient individuals.

Pharmacometrics deals with identification and comparative evaluation, both qualitative and quantitative, of drug activity.

Pharmacovigilance: Watchfulness about drugs for promoting drug safety, identification to reporting adverse drug reaction and other relevant aspects.

Pharmacy is the science and art of preparing a drug or combination. Pharmacy is concerned with collection, preparation, synthesis of new compounds and standardization.

Pharmacoeconomics is concerned with cost - effectiveness analysis (how to get a given objective at the minimum cost) and cost - utility analysis. Cost - minimization analysis finds the least costly programme among those shown to be of equal benefit when both quantity and quality of life be measured.

Pharmacognosy (pharmakon means drug, gnosis means knowledge) is the study of the sources of drugs obtained from plants and animals.

Drug: World Health Organization Scientific Group has defined a drug as "any substance or product that is used or intended to be used to modify or explore physiological systems or pathological states for the benefit of the recipient."

Drug is a single chemical substance that forms the active ingredient of a medicine, which latter may contain many other substances to deliver the drug in a stable form, acceptable and convenient to the patient. The terms drug and medicine are used more or less interchangeably.

In brief, a drug (word derived from French word drogue meaning 'dry herb') is a chemical substance which is used for the diagnosis, prevention and cure of disease.

Orphan drugs: When a drug is not developed because the developer will not recover the costs, then it is known as orphan drug. These are meant for diagnosis, prevention or treatment of rare diseases.

Dose: It is defined as the quantity of drug which is sufficient to diagnose, prevent or treat a disease.

Dosage: It is the schedule of dose, frequency and duration of administration of a drug.

Toxicology is the aspect of pharmacology that deals with the adverse effects of drugs.

Drug therapeutic index (margin of safety) indicates the relationship between the dosage that produces an undesirable effect and the dosage that produces a desirable therapeutic effect. The greater the ratio of these dosages, the safer the drug and the higher its therapeutic index.

$$TI = \frac{\text{Maximum non-toxic dose}}{\text{Minimum effective dose}}$$

Therapeutic index (LD_{50}/ED_{50}) provides a very crude measurement of the safety of any drug as used in practice. Its main limitations are:

- It is based on animal toxicity data which may not reflect forms of toxicity that are important clinically.
- It takes no account of idiosyncratic toxic reactions.

Certain safety factor (CSF)

It is the ratio derived from the extremes of the refractive quantal response curves i.e. by finding out the ratio between the dose effective in 99% of the subjects (ED_{99}) and the dose which is lethal to 1% of the subjects LD_1 :

$$CSF = \frac{LD_1}{ED_{99}}$$

A CSF value of less than 1 means an overlap between the ED_{99} and LD_1, indicating that the drug is unsafe for therapeutic use.

An alternative **standard safety margin (SSM)**:

It is expressed as the percentage by which the drug has to be increased to match the LD_1 dose. Thus, the greater the percentage of SSM, safer is the drug.

$$\frac{LD_1 - ED_{99} \times 100}{ED_{99}}$$

e.g. $(200 - 150) \times 100 / 150 = 33.34$ means that to match LD_1 (200 mg), the ED_{99} (150 mg) has to be increased to 33.34%.

Sources of information about drugs

Text books and journals provide information about the established and investigational drugs. However, they do not include details about trade names, standards of purity, methods of storage and other aspects which are needed for legal point of view. Such information about drugs is given in Pharmacopoeias and Formulary (collectively known as Drug Compendia).

DRUG COMPENDIA

The Pharmacopoeias are a class of drug compendia. The term pharmacopoeia is derived from two Greek words—pharmakon (means drug) and poiein (means make). Pharmacopoeia is a book which contains the formula or other standards required for the preparation and testing of drugs to ensure uniform purity and potency. The description about drugs or preparations given in pharmacopoeia is known as the monograph. It describes the drug, its purity, method of identification, storage instruction, dose range, and method of standardization. Most of the nations have their own pharmacopoeia, viz. Indian Pharmacopoeia (IP), the British Pharmacopoeia (BP), the United States Pharmacopoeia (USP), European Pharmacopoeia, etc.

There is also an International Pharmacopoeia published by the WHO in many languages which is meant mainly for use by nations who do not have their own Pharmacopoeia. The pharmacopoeias are revised periodically.

Besides Pharmacopoeias, National Formulary is published. This gives information about drugs. There are also other concise books (compendia) which provide authoritative information about drugs.

Previously New and Non-Official remedies, after that New and Non-Official drugs and now "new drugs" publication lists many new natural and synthetic drugs of therapeutic value which may become official in future. Drugs and substances included in the current Pharmacopoeia and National Formulary are known as official; those which were included once but not included in the current edition are designated as unofficial and those which were never included in these books are known as non-official.

DRUG CLASSIFICATION

As most drugs have a variety of actions, often not easily interrelated, a rigid system for drug classification is not really possible. A complication increasingly encountered is that many drugs possess actions that would permit their categorization in several groups e.g. lignocaine is used as a local anaesthetic but it is also used intravenously as an antiarrhythmic agent.

Drugs can be grouped or classified either according to (1) their actions or effects, or (2) on the basis of their chemistry.

1. The principal classes of drugs are enumerated according to the system which they affect.
2. The drugs can also be classified in a physicochemical sense:
   - Those that are charged or uncharged according to environmental pH (electrolytes).
   - Those that are incapable of assuming a charge whatever the environmental pH (unchanged nonpolar substances).
   - Those that are permanently charged whatever the environmental pH (charged, polar substances).

Drugs that are charged or uncharged according

to environmental pH: Usually most molecules are present partly in ionized and partly in unionized state. The degree of ionization influences lipid solubility and hence diffusibility. Ionisable groups in a drug molecule tend either to lose a hydrogen ion (acidic groups) or to add a hydrogen ion (basic groups). The extent to which a molecule has this tendency to ionize is given by the dissociation (or ionization) constant (Ka), usually expressed as the pKa i.e. the negative logarithm of the Ka (just as pH is the negative logarithm of the hydrogen ion concentration). When pH of a solution is the same as pKa of a drug within it, then the drug is 50% ionized and 50% unionized. If the pH is decreased from the pKa value by one unit, an acid becomes 91% unionized and a base becomes 91% ionized. If pH is increased for the pKa value by one unit, an acid becomes 91% ionized and a base becomes 91% unionized and so on. For example, aspirin, which is a moderately strong acid (pKa 3.5) is 99% unionized at pH 1.5 (gastric lumen) and 99% ionized at pH 5.5 (urine). Aspirin in stomach is unionized and so lipid soluble, ought to be readily absorbed, but because of constant gastric emptying only little of a swallowed drug enters this way. Such aspirin that enters gastric epithelial cells (pH 7.4) will ionize and localize there; this ion trapping harms gastric mucosa.

In the more alkaline environment of the small intestine, although aspirin is ionized and less lipid soluble, the vastly greater absorbing surface is capable of taking up most of the drug. Once inside the body, as it is almost completely ionized at body pH, the drug remains in extracellular fluid. The elimination of aspirin is promoted if the urine pH is high as it renders aspirin ionized and lipid insoluble so that the drug does not re-enter tubular cells. In case of salicylate overdose, alkalinisation of urine is helpful.

The converse occurs with basic drugs e.g. pethidine.

There is a wide range of pH in the gut (pH 1.5 in stomach, 6.8 in upper and 7.6 in lower intestine). But the pH inside the body is maintained within a limited range, pH 7.4 ± 0.04 so that only drugs that are substantially unionized at this pH will be lipid soluble.

Urine pH varies between extremes of 4.6 and 8.2; thus the amount of drug reabsorbed from the renal tubular lumen by passive diffusion can be very much affected by the prevailing urine pH.

Drugs that are incapable of assuming a charge include digoxin, chloramphenicol. They do not have ionisable groups so unaffected by environmental pH, are lipid soluble and so diffuse readily across tissue boundaries. These drugs are also referred to as nonpolar.

Drugs that are permanently charged carry groups whose ionization is so strong that they remain charged at all values of the body pH. Such compounds are called polar, as their groups are either negatively charged (acidic, e.g. heparin) or positively charged (basic, e.g. tubocurarine, suxamethonium) and they have very limited capacity to cross cell membranes.

It is a common practice to classify drugs according to (1) chemical structure of drug, (2) disease for which they are used, (3) organ system on which the drugs have pharmacological effects, (4) generation and so on.

All drugs have their own chemical structures, e.g. sulpha drugs (sulphonamides) having the basic nucleus, p-aminobenzenesulphonamide are known as sulphonamides.

Steroids have cyclopentanoperhydrophenanthrene nucleus with the side chain R at C-17 of D ring. Depending solely on the type of substituent R at C-17, steroids are classified into sterols (e.g., cholesterol), sex hormones (e.g., oestrone etc.), cardiac glycosides (e.g., digitoxin), bile acids (e.g., cholic acid) etc.

Drugs used for the treatment of various diseases such as malaria, epilepsy, tuberculosis, hypertension etc. may be grouped by adding the prefix anti-. For example, antimalarial, antiepileptic, antitubercular, antihypertensive agents.

Some drugs are also classified as first, second, third and fourth generation drugs, e.g., cephalosporins. Cefazolin etc. belong to first generation; cefuroxime, cefaclor etc. belong to the second generation; cefotaxime, ceftazidime etc. belong to the third generation, and now cefepime has been added as a fourth generation cephalosporin.

H_1-receptor antagonists (antihistamines) can be grouped as first generation and second generation agents.

Drugs can be categorized according to the organ systems, e.g., drugs acting on cardiovascular system, nervous system, ophthalmic drugs, agents acting on skin, gastrointestinal system etc.

STUDY QUESTIONS

1. Define pharmacology and its two main branches—pharmacokinetics and pharmacodynamics.
2. What do you mean by drug? Classify drugs in a physicochemical sense.
3. What is a dosage? Define dose.
4. Identify therapeutics and pharmacotherapeutics.
5. Why pharmacopoeias are important?
6. Why is the study of pharmacology essential?

GUIDE TO FURTHER READING

Benet, B.B., et al. Noncompartmental determination of the steady-state volume of distribution. J. Pharm. Sci., 68:1071-1074; 1979.

Roberts, M.S., et al. Models of hepatic elimination: comparison of stochastic models to describe residence time distributions and to predict the influence of drug distribution, enzyme heterogeneity, and systemic recycling on hepatic elimination. J. Pharmacokinet. Biopharm., 16:41-83; 1988.

SOURCES, NATURE AND NOMENCLATURE OF DRUGS

SOURCES OF DRUGS

Although there are a few inorganic drugs, for example lithium salts, the majority of drugs are organic compounds and can be derived from several sources.

The following are the sources of drugs:

Naturally occurring compounds: These are extracted from plants and animals and are probably the oldest type of drugs.

The examples of drugs from plant or vegetable sources are atropine, digitalis, morphine, reserpine, ephedrine, emetine, etc. The drugs obtained from animal sources are heparin, insulin, thyroxine, etc.

Modified natural drugs: Some natural drugs can be modified in order to produce better and more efficacious drugs, e.g. porcine insulin can be modified so that it is closer to the human insulin, and semisynthetic penicillins are an important group of drugs in the treatment of infections.

Plants act as sources of active molecules. In many cases, the molecules isolated from plant extracts have been further modified chemically to improve activity or reduce toxicity. The Chinese product artemisinin has been converted to less toxic Artmether. Taxol isolated from Taxus brevifolia or the pacific Yew Tree has been converted to derivatives which are better absorbed. In all the cases, the discovery of these new derivatives was made possible, only due to the fact, that the original plants had shown activity even if it was low and hence was only a lead.

Mineral sources: Iron, iodine, sulphur, calcium, aluminium and magnesium salts are obtained from mineral sources.

Microbial sources: Antibiotics are derived from microbial sources.

Synthetic sources: Drugs produced purely by synthetic means have many advantages over natural drugs and have become one of the principal sources of drugs. They are cheaper and more certain in supply. It is possible to synthesize 'tailor-make' drugs by using structure-activity relationships.

Genetic engineering: This is the newest and most modern method by which drugs can be made. Human insulin can be made by incorporating the necessary gene into *Escherichia coli*, a gram-negative rod.

Genetic engineering has provided an ample opportunity to have an unlimited supply of biological molecules which would have been otherwise impossible to produce from natural sources.

Molecular biology has accelerated the understanding of the genes and structure of many proteins which sustain our well being and physiological functions. Pathways and mechanisms of processing biologically active peptides have been deduced from the sequence of peptides and their corresponding genes.

Many molecules of human origin including lymphokines, erythropoietin, factor VIII, albumin, interferons, interleukins, antibodies, enzymes, vaccines etc. are now produced by genetic engineering.

Human insulin was the first recombinant protein

to be commercialized. The amino acid sequences of both polypeptide chains A and B of insulin molecule are known and these are chemically synthesized and separately fused to the C-terminal of region Beta-galactosidase gene with a strong promoter. The insulin chain A and B are separately produced and assembled into biologically active insulin.

The products developed through genetic engineering are given in Table 1.1.

Table 1.1. List of products of recombination DNA in use

Product	Therapeutic Use(s)
Insulin	Diabetes
Tissue Plasminogen Activator	Thrombolysis
Streptokinase, Urokinase	Thrombolysis
Growth Hormone	Dwarfism
Erythropoietin	Anaemia
Soluble CD4	AIDS
Calcitonin	Osteoporosis
Antibodies	Cancer, Septic shock Immunosuppression
Interferons	Virus infections, Cancer therapy, AIDS
Epidermal growth factor	Wound healing
Fibroblast growth factor	Venous stasis
Interleukin-2	Cancer therapy
Interleukin-4	Cancer therapy
Relaxin	Facilitation of childbirth
Alpha1-antitrypsin	Emphysema
Tumour necrosis factor	Cancer therapy
Lung surfactant protein	Respiratory distress syndrome
Granulocyte macrophage	Cancer therapy
Colony Stimulating Factor	Bone marrow transplant
Vaccines	Hepatitis Herpes

NATURE OF DRUGS

The majority of drugs used today are of synthetic origin. They are prepared from interaction of various chemicals.

The drugs from plant origin contain active principles. The active principles of the crude drugs are pharmacologically active substances obtained from plant material, such as alkaloids, glycosides, oils, resins and tannins.

The active principles of crude drugs obtained from plant material possess pharmacological activity. The aim of isolating active principles are:
- Identification of the active ingredient(s)
- Analysis of pharmacokinetics and pharmacodynamics of the individual ingredients
- Ensuring a precise dosage in their use
- The possibility of chemical synthesis and derivatives of the original constituent with improved therapeutic usefulness may be obtained.

Alkaloids

The term is derived from 'vegetable alkali' (alk = alkali; oid = like). Alkaloids may be defined as organic nitrogenous substances of plant origin exhibiting well defined actions. They have significant pharmacological activity and are restricted to the plant kingdom. These are naturally occurring basic compounds.

Alkaloids possess carbon, hydrogen and nitrogen and in most cases elemental oxygen. They form their crystalline salts with acids like hydrochloric acid, sulphuric acid, citric acid, and tartaric acid. The free alkaloids are insoluble or slightly soluble in water but their salts are freely soluble.

Alkaloids have well marked pharmacological activities like morphine, codeine (analgesic), emetine (antiamoebic), atropine (anticholinergic), reserpine (antihypertensive), quinine (antimalarial), vinblastine, vincristine (anticancer), quinidine (cardiac depressant), caffeine (CNS stimulant), ergometrine (oxytocic), pilocarpine (antiglaucoma), tubocurarine (skeletal muscle relaxant), papaverine (smooth muscle relaxant).

Alkaloids can be classified as:
1. True alkaloids e.g. colchicine, quinine, emetine, morphine, etc. These are derived from amino acids and contain nitrogen in a heterocyclic ring.
2. Protoalkaloids do not have amino acid nitrogen in a heterocyclic ring, e.g. ephedrine, mescaline.
3. Pseudoalkaloids are not derived from amino acid precursors e.g. steroidal alkaloids (coniceine) and purines (caffeine).

Glycosides

Glycosides are compounds which upon hydrolysis give rise to one or more sugars (glycones) and a compound which is not a sugar (aglycone or genin). Most of the glycosides are colourless, crystalline compounds. Anthracene glycosides are red or orange coloured and flavone glycosides are yellowish in colour. These are soluble in water and alcohol but insoluble in other organic solvents like ether, chloroform etc.

On the basis of the nature of sugars the glycosides are called glucosides, fructosides, etc.

Pharmacological classification of glycosides depends on their activity, e.g. cardiac glycosides exhibit their action on heart. Glycosides possessing bitter taste are called bitter glycosides, e.g. glycosides of gentianceae.

Glycosides are used for the treatment of various diseases. Digitalis and strophanthus contain cardiac glycosides which are cardiotonic drugs. Anthraquinone glycosides present in senna, rhubarb, cascara and aloe possess laxative action.

Gums (e.g., gum acacia, gum tragacanth) are colloidal exudates of plants which swell or form mucilage in water. They are used as emulsifying or suspending agents.

Tannin

Tannin (tannic acid) is a mixture of esters of gallic acid with glucose. Tannic acid is astringent and is used as haemostatic.

Fats, Oils and Waxes

Fixed oils and fats are esters of glycerol with higher long-chain fatty acids.

Fats are solid or semisolid at 15.5-16.5°C while oils occur as liquid at this temperature. These compounds are obtained from plants (arachis oil, castor oil) or animals (lard, cod liver oil). There is no chemical difference in fats and oils. The fatty acids may be saturated e.g. palmitic acid, stearic acid, or unsaturated e.g. oleic acid.

Fats and oils have certain common characteristics. They are greasy substances and insoluble in water, sparingly soluble in alcohol, and freely soluble in ether, chloroform and benzene. Their specific gravity is less than water and therefore they float on the surface of water. When a drop of fats or oils is placed on a paper, they form a permanent translucent stain on it and due to this property they are called fixed oils.

Fatty acids are used to treat skin lesions (linolenic and linoleic acids), wounds, burns, sunburns, eczema, emollient, laxative (castor oil), in the preparation of ointments, liniments and suppositories and in the manufacture of soaps.

Waxes are the esters of higher straight-chain fatty acids. Waxes may be of plant origin such as carnauba wax or of animal origin such as Beeswax, Wool-fat (lanolin), etc. In many ways, waxes are identical to fats but more difficult to saponify.

Volatile oils or essential oils are flavouring compounds. All the volatile oils are of vegetable origin. These are colourless liquids and are lighter than water. They are immiscible with water, but the water shaken with an essential oil possesses its flavour due to slight solubility of the oil. Volatile oils are freely soluble in alcohol, ether, chloroform, acetone, etc.

Each volatile oil differs widely in chemical composition. Some of them possess high percentage of a particular compound e.g. eugenol in clove oil (85%), menthol in peppermint oil (70%).

Volatile oils differ from fixed oils in various ways.

- The former oils are evaporated at room temperature. As they are not glyceryl esters of fatty acids they cannot be saponified with alkalies.
- Volatile oils can act as counterirritant, carminative, antiseptic, expectorant, spasmolytic and anthelmintic.
- A volatile oil may contain hydrocarbons which are usually devoid of aroma.
- Volatile oils on exposure to air and light, are oxidized and resins are formed.

Resins

Resins are amorphous, brittle, translucent, hard solids. On heating they are softened and then melt, insoluble in water but dissolve in organic solvents such as alcohol, ether and chloroform.

Resin-containing drugs possess purgative (podophyllum, colocynth), hydragogue (jalap), counterirritant (turpentine) actions. Externally resins

Oils

Mineral Oils	Fixed oils	Essential oils (Volatile oils)
These are petroleum products, no food value, do not become rancid, e.g., liquid paraffin (purgative), hard and soft paraffin as vehicle for ointment	These are nonvolatile, have food value, form soap with alkalies, become rancid after prolonged exposure, e.g., castor oil (purgative), arachis oil (demulcent), groundnut oil, coconut oil (food value)	These are volatile, have aroma but no food value. They do not form soap with alkalies, do not become rancid, mainly used as carminatives, astringents and flavouring agents, e.g., clove oil, pippermint oil

are used as mild antiseptic in the form of cerates, ointments and plasters. They are employed in the preparation of emulsions.

DRUG NOMENCLATURE

A drug can have a variety of names:

Chemical name: This is the full name according to convention for naming chemical compounds. Such names are usually too lengthy and complicated to use. The IUPAC names are cumbersome and very technical; it requires a thorough knowledge of chemistry to understand these. Above all, it is almost impossible to remember them.

Examples :
- Atenolol. 4-[2-Hydroxy-3-[(1-methyl ethyl) amino] propoxy] benzene acetamide.
- Ciprofloxacin. 1-Cyclopropyl-6-fluoro-1,4-di-hydro-4-oxo-7-(1-piperazinyl)-3-quino-line-carboxylic acid.

Approved or official name: It is also known as the generic name; it allows different products with the same ingredient to be identified as such. Unfortunately some compounds have different approved names in different countries, e.g. adrenaline in United Kingdom is known as epinephrine in America.

Generic names are internationally accepted common names of the drugs. The naming usually follows the style of a prototypical agent. For example, Propranolol is the prototypical agent among beta-blockers. The drugs which followed were named Metoprolol, Atenolol, Sotalol, etc. Similarly Cimetidine, Ranitidine, and Famotidine, etc. for H_2-receptor antagonists.

Proprietary name (trade name): It is unique to particular manufacturer. It is a name given to a formulation (medicine) by its manufacturing or marketing company. It serves the purpose of establishing the identity of the product in the market and hence helps in promoting and selling.

STUDY QUESTIONS

1. Describe the different sources of drugs, giving proper examples.
2. Which is considered the newest and most modern source of drugs?
3. What do you mean by 'active principles' of a drug. Define and give examples of alkaloids and glycosides.
4. Why chemical name is generally not acceptable? Which nomenclature you would prefer and why between approved (generic name) name and proprietary or trade name?
5. Define alkaloids. Give examples of alkaloids of medicinal value with their uses.
6. What are glycosides? Name cardiac glycosides. What are their uses?
7. Describe (i) fixed and volatile oils, (ii) resins, and (iii) waxes.

GUIDE TO FURTHER READING

Allan, F.M. Standardization of Drug Names. JAMA, 1974; 299 : 541.

Bloom, B.S., Weirz, D.J., and Pauley, M.D. Cost and price of comparable branded and generic pharmaceuticals. JAMA. 1986, 256 : 2523-2530.

"Drugs of the Future through Genetic Engineering". American Pharmacy, NS21, 1981; 111 : 20.

Gal, J. Stereoisomerism and drug nomenclature. Clin Pharmacol Ther 1988, 44 : 251-253.

Hendeles, L., Hockhaus, G., et al. Genetic and alternative brand-name pharmaceutical equivalents, select with caution. Am J Hosp Pharm 1993, 50 : 323-329.

Huskisson, E.C. Trade names or proper names? — A problem for the prescriber. Br Med J 1973; 4 : 225.

Miller, I.C. Doctors, drugs and names. JAMA 1961; 177 : 27.

Storm, B.L. Generic drug substituted revisited. N Engl J Med 1987, 316 : 1456-1462.

Trout, M.E. and Lee A.M. Genetic substitution: A boon or a bane to the physician and the consumer? In Drug Therapeutics: Concepts for physicians. (Melmon, K.L., ed.). Elsevier North-Holland, Inc., New York, 1981.

Turner, P. Brand names for drugs. Lancet 1976; 2 : 797.

Vere, D. Brand names for drugs. Lancet 1976; 2 : 911.

Webb, V.J. Non-proprietary names. Br Med J 1968; 1 : 484.

DOSAGE FORMS

A dosage form of a drug is a product designed for the use by the patient.

Drug substances are administered as part of a formulation in combination with one or more nonmedical agents (referred to as pharmaceutical ingredients). Through the selective use of these ingredients, the dosage forms of various types result. The pharmaceutical ingredients solubilise, suspend, thicken, dilute, emulsify, stabilize, preserve, colour the medicinal agents into efficacious and appealing dosage forms.

Dosage forms are needed for the following reasons:

- For providing safe and convenient delivery of accurate dosages.
- For the protection of a drug substance from the destructive influences of atmospheric oxygen or moisture.
- For the protection of a drug substance from the destructive influence of gastric HCl after oral use, e.g. enteric coated tablets.
- To conceal the bitter obnoxious taste or odour of a drug substance, e.g. capsules, coated tablets, flavoured syrups.
- To provide drugs for topical application e.g. ointments, eye drops, ear and nasal preparations.
- To provide drugs for insertion in body's orifices, e.g. rectal and vaginal suppositories.
- To provide liquid dosage forms as solutions (when substance is soluble in desired vehicle).
- To provide liquid suspensions of substances that may be insoluble or unstable in the desired vehicle.
- To provide various controlled release tablets, capsules and suspensions for extended drug action.
- To provide preparations for parenteral administrations.

THERAPEUTIC CONSIDERATIONS

The difference in drug absorption between dosage forms is a function of the formulation itself and the route of administration. An individual drug substance may be formulated into multiple dosage forms which result in different drug absorption rates, and times of onset, peak, and duration of effect. For example, absorption of nitroglycerin is very rapid and hence very rapid onset of action when administered by sublingual and buccal dosage forms, whereas the onset of action is slow when nitroglycerin is swallowed or applied topically in the form of ointment and topical disc.

The various dosage forms can be broadly classified into solid, semisolid and liquid dosage forms.

SOLID DOSAGE FORMS

These include compressed tablets, enteric coated tablets, hypodermic tablets (which completely dissolve in water for injection), pellets (formed by compression of certain steroid hormones for implantation subcutaneously to form a depot from which the hormone is slowly released), cachets for powders, pills, capsules, spansules.

Tablets are solid dosage forms containing drug substances with or without suitable diluents, disintegrants, coatings, colourants and other pharmaceutical aids prepared by compression or molding methods.

Compressed tablets

Sugar-coated tablets

They contain a thin sugar coating which may be coloured and are useful in masking the objectionable taste or odour and in protecting materials sensitive to oxidation.

Film coated tablets

They are covered by thin layer of film of water soluble material as hydroxypropyl cellulose, hydroxypropyl methyl cellulose, ethyl cellulose, etc.

Enteric coated tablets

These tablets are coated with substances like cellulose acetate phthalate, polyvinyl acetate phthalate that resist solution in gastric fluid but disintegrate in the intestine.

Multiple compressed tablets

These are made by more than one compression. They are of 2 types:
1. *Layered tablets:* Such tablets are prepared by compressing additional tablet granulation on a previously compressed granulation. Multiple layers may be produced by repeating the operation.
2. *Compression coated/press coated tablets:* They contain a compressed core tablet around which another layer of granulation is compressed.

Effervescent tablets

These tablets are prepared by compressing the active ingredients with mixtures of organic acids such as citric acid or tartaric acid and sodium bicarbonate. When added to water they rapidly dissolve with the release of carbon dioxide.

Buccal and sublingual tablets

These are intended to be held in the mouth where they release their drug contents for absorption directly through the oral mucosa. Buccal tablets are held between the cheek and teeth and sublingual tablets are kept beneath the tongue.

Chewable tablets

They are intended to be chewed in the mouth prior to swallowing.

Lozenges

These are compressed or molded tablets containing drug incorporated in a flavoured hard candy sugar base. They are intended to exert local effect in the mouth or throat.

Dental cones

They are small-sized tablets designed to be placed in the empty socket after tooth extraction to prevent the multiplication of bacteria or reduce bleeding. They provide a slow release of an antibacterial compound, astringent or a coagulant.

Implantation tablets (depot tablets)

These are designed for subcutaneous implantation to provide prolonged drug effects.

Vaginal tablets

Vaginal tablets or inserts are ovoid or pear-shaped tablets designed to undergo slow dissolution and drug release in the vaginal cavity. They contain anti-bacterial agents/antiseptics or astringents to treat vaginal infections or steroids for systemic absorption.

Dispensing tablets

These tablets are intended to be added to a given volume of water to produce a solution of a particular concentration. They are supplied primarily as a convenience for compounding and should never be dispensed as a dosage form.

Hypodermic tablets

They are soft, readily soluble tablets which were originally used for the preparation of injectable solutions. These are of little use now.

Capsules

Capsules are solid dosage forms in which the drug substance is enclosed in either a hard or soft shell made up of a suitable form of gelatin.

Gelatin is a heterogeneous mixture of water soluble proteins of high average molecular weight obtained by treating specific animal tissues like skin, tendons, ligaments and bones with hot water. Gelatin is not found in nature, but derived from collagen by hydrolytic action.

Gelatin is used to prepare capsules and as a nutrient.

SEMISOLID DOSAGE FORMS

These are mainly meant for external use and are exemplified by ointments, pastes, jellies, etc. Liniments are liquid preparation applied to skin by rubbing. Lotions are liquid preparation applied to skin without rubbing.

LIQUID DOSAGE FORMS

Monophasic products are represented by true or colloidal solutions and by solubilised preparations.

Biphasic products are exemplified by emulsions and suspensions and consist of two phases. In emulsions both the phases are liquids, while in suspension the continuous phase is liquid and the disperse phase consists of finely divided solids.

PARENTERAL PRODUCTS

The dosage forms of parenteral products must possess the following characteristics:

- Freedom from living microbes.
- Freedom from microbial products such as toxins, pyrogens.
- Freedom from physical contaminants such as particulate matter, fibres, etc.
- Freedom from chemical contaminants.
- Matching osmotic qualities with respect to body fluids.
- Matching specific gravity with respect to some body fluids.

Table 1.2 shows the primary dosage forms and the route of administration.

STUDY QUESTIONS

1. Define dosage form and give some examples of solid, liquid and semiliquid dosage forms.
2. Describe the characteristics which the parenteral products must possess.
3. What are the various pharmaceutic ingredients used in the preparation of dosage form? What are their functions?
4. Give reasons why substances are rarely administered alone but in combination with nonmedical agents (pharmaceutic ingredients).

Table 1.2. Primary dosage forms and the route of administration

Primary dosage form	Route
Tablets, capsules, solutions, syrups, elixirs, suspensions, magmas, gels, powders	Oral
Tablets, troches or lozenges	Sublingual
Solutions, suspensions	Parenteral
Ointments, creams, pastes, plasters, powders, aerosols, lotions, transdermal patches, discs, solutions	Epicutaneous/ Transdermal
Ointments	Conjunctival
Solutions, suspensions	Intraocular/ intra-aural
Solutions, sprays, inhalants, ointment	Intranasal
Aerosols	Intrarespiratory
Solutions, ointments, suppositories	Rectal
Solutions, ointments, emulsions, tablets, inserts, suppositories	Vaginal

5. State briefly the therapeutic considerations for designing the dosage form. How an individual drug substance may be formulated into multiple dosage forms which result in different drug absorption, onset and duration of action?
6. Define emulsion. What are different types of emulsions?
7. How are tablets manufactured? Why are liquid preparations better than capsules and other solid dosage forms for oral administration?
8. Define (i) enteric coated tablets, (ii) depot tablets, (iii) hypodermic tablets, and (iv) various non-medicinal agents used as pharmaceutical aids.
9. Describe the characteristics which must be possessed by the dosage forms of parenteral products.

GUIDE TO FURTHER READING

Jones, T.M. The influence of excipients on the design and manufacture of tablets and capsules. Drug and Cosmetic Industry, 1979; 124 No. 3; 40.

Turco, S., and King, R.E. Sterile dosage forms: Their Preparations and Clinical Applications, 2nd Ed. Philadelphia, Lea & Febiger, 1979.

Vidt, D.G. Use and Abuse of Intravenous Solutions. JAMA, 1975; 232:533.

ROUTES OF DRUG ADMINISTRATION

Drugs can be applied locally (topically), administered orally and by injection.

It is important to know the route of administration because it determines (1) onset, (2) duration, (3) intensity, and (4) degree of localization of drug action.

The absorption of a drug depends on the selection of the appropriate route of administration. The selection depends on (a) drug factors (physical and chemical properties) and (b) patient factors (desired site and speed of response).

The routes of administration can be (A) Routes for local effect, and (B) Systemic effect.

ROUTES FOR LOCAL EFFECTS

Topical application

Drugs are applied to the skin for local action, for example, antiseptics, antifungal, local anaesthetics, antiinflammatory agents, skin emollients, and protectants.

These are administered as ointments, creams, pastes, lotions, aerosol sprays and solid dry powders.

Drugs are also applied topically to the mucous membranes of ear, nose and eye. The preparations for ear, nose and eye are generally applied for local action only, as they are not absorbed to any great extent after such application. However, nasal preparations may be absorbed and systemic effects are produced.

The topical ocular drug delivery system needs emphasis. The conventional dosage forms such as solutions, suspensions and ointments are relatively inefficient. With these forms there is 1-10% ocular bioavailability. This lower bioavailability is because of (i) constant lacrimal secretion and (ii) nasolacrimal drainage. This leads to frequent instillation of concentrated medication to achieve the desired therapeutic effect. The systemic absorption of the drug drained through the nasolacrimal duct may produce side effects, hence sustained release formulations for eye are needed. For this reason, ophthalmic inserts have been introduced. The insert is flexible multilayered structure which has a drug in its core surrounded on each side by a layer of copolymer membranes. The drug diffuses through the membranes at a constant rate which is controlled by the composition of the polymer, thickness of membranes and solubility of the drug. The devices are sterile. There are no preservatives. The novel ophthalmic drug delivery systems are designed to prolong the presence of a drug in the tear pool by erodible and non-erodible inserts. The erodible films permit greater ocular bioavailability of drug but do not confer the same duration of drug release as the non-erodible 'ocusert'. The non-erodible insert 'ocusert' permits continuous delivery of medication 24 hours a day for 7 days. The device is inserted into the lower conjunctiva. An insert containing pilocarpine has been found useful in the treatment of glaucoma. The medication is released at the predetermined and predictable rates. This improves bioavailability, by eliminating drug loss via drainage of the solution. It also eliminates frequent dosing, and ensures night time medication. However, its drawback is that the device must be removed at the end of the dosing period (7 days).

The topical application on mucous membranes also include mouth, pharynx, larynx, urethra, bladder, gastrointestinal tract, bronchi etc.

The advantage of local application is that the action is limited to the area of application. The disadvantage is that if drug is absorbed, systemic effects may be produced.

Injections in body cavities

The routes for localized actions also include injections in deeper tissues into body cavities, joints, and subarachnoid space.

Intraarterial injection

It is given so that high concentration of drug reaches the site e.g. in the treatment of malignant tumour.

Oral administration

Drugs which act locally in the GIT (neither absorbed nor destroyed) are given orally for local action, e.g. antacids, purgatives, anthelmintics.

Inhalation

Proper technique of inhalation is employed to produce only local effect of certain drugs e.g. in bronchial asthma.

Local injections in eye

Subconjunctival injection

Drug is injected underneath the conjunctiva and is absorbed into the blood stream by the episcleral and conjunctival vessels by simple diffusion. This route is employed for giving antibiotics for the treatment of intraocular infections. Mydriatics and cycloplegics may also be given by this route to achieve prompt and maximum effect of these drugs.

Intracameral injection

Drug is injected directly into the anterior chamber e.g. certain antibiotics or directly into the vitreous chamber e.g. amphotericin B, gentamicin sulphate.

Retrobulbar injection

It is given for getting drugs e.g. antibiotics, vasodilators, steroids into the posterior segment of the globe and to affect the nerves and other structures in that space.

ROUTES FOR SYSTEMIC ACTION

It can be either enteral (oral) or parenteral (by injection).

Enteral

Oral route (drug swallowed)

Compared to the other routes, the oral route is the most common, convenient, safe and economical.

Advantages :
- Self medication
- Relatively safe
- Economical
- Convenient

Disadvantages :
- Slow onset of action
- Irritant and unpalatable can not be given
- Not possible to administer in unconscious patient
- Not possible to administer in non-cooperative patient
- Not possible to administer in presence of vomiting
- Some drugs are destroyed by gastric hydrochloric acid, e.g., penicillin
- Some drugs are destroyed by digestive enzymes e.g., insulin
- Some drugs undergo rapid hepatic first-pass metabolism when given orally, e.g., nitroglycerin, lidocaine
- Presence of food interferes with absorption
- Presence of other drugs interfere with absorption

The advantages of oral route outweigh the disadvantages because the situations where oral route is not possible are only few.

The most popular dosage forms applicable for oral route of administration are tablets, capsules, suspensions and various solutions.

Sublingual route

When drugs are absorbed from the gastrointestinal tract, they will have to pass via the portal vein to the liver before reaching the general circulation (Fig. 1.1). This may be important as many drugs are metabolized (broken down or altered) as they pass through the liver so that only a portion of the drug which is absorbed actually reaches its site of action. This removal of the drug as it passes through the liver is called the first-pass effect.

Currently the buccal or sublingual (beneath the tongue) administration of drugs is employed for a few drugs, viz. nitroglycerin, isoprenaline, isosorbide and certain steroid hormones. The dose of nitroglycerin is very small (400 microgram); if it is

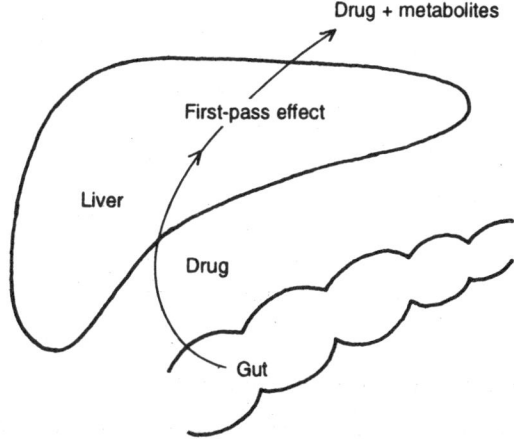

Fig. 1.1. First-pass metabolism of a drug by the liver.

swallowed it will be so much diluted in the gastrointestinal tract that insufficient drug absorption will occur. Moreover this drug is rapidly destroyed in the liver which reduces the chances of reaching the site of action.

Advantages
- Rapid onset of action
- Not destroyed by gastric juice
- Bypass the first-pass biotransformation

Disadvantages
- Not suitable for administration of large volume
- Not suitable for drugs of low lipid/water partition coefficient

Drug that exhibit first-pass metabolism:

In intestinal mucosa	*In liver*
l-dopa	nitroglycerin
chlorpromazine	isosorbide dinitrate
testosterone	morphine
progestogen	pethidine
Alpha-methyldopa	xylocaine,
	imipramine
	amitriptyline
	propranolol

Rectal administration

The rectum and the colon can absorb many soluble drugs.

Advantages
- This route may be employed when oral route can not be used in the presence of vomiting, in unconscious and non-cooperative patients
- This route may be used for some drugs which are inactivated by gastric hydrochloric acid or digestive enzymes
- First-pass biotransformation is avoided

Disadvantages
- Inconvenience of administration
- Slow and uncertain absorption of drugs
- Many drugs cause irritation of rectal mucosa

Vaginal route (vaginal pessaries)

Drugs may be administered locally in the vagina in the form of pessaries e.g. antifungal vaginal pessaries.

Parenteral route (by injection)

The word parenteral is derived from Greek words— para meaning beside, and enteron meaning intestine. The drug may be given parenterally at various sites and to various depths.

This route is employed in case of drugs which are poorly absorbed from gastrointestinal tract (GIT) or destroyed in GIT. It is also the route of choice when rapid absorption of drug is essential as in emergencies. It is a useful route in uncooperative and unconscious patients. The negative side of this route is that there is no retreat once the drug is injected. Strict sterility requirements have to be met for all injections. The administration is carried out by competent personnel.

The following are the usual parenteral routes of administration of drugs:

Intramuscular injections (I.M.)

The injection is given deep into the skeletal muscles.

Advantages
- Rapid onset of action
- Uniform absorption
- Suitable for moderate volume, oily vehicles and some irritating substances

Disadvantages
- Painful
- Self medication not possible

Intravenous injections (I.V.)

Advantages
- Immediate effect
- Large volumes can be administered
- Irritant drugs can be given when diluted
- Valuable in emergency
- 100% bioavailability
- Drug administration can be stopped if adverse effect develops

Disadvantages
- Necessity of strict aseptic measures
- Self medication not possible
- Increased risk of adverse effects
- Expensive
- Not suitable for oily solution or insoluble substance

- Danger of infection
- Preparations for i.v. injections are limited to aqueous solutions of drugs

Subcutaneous (hypodermic, SC) injections

The drug is injected into the subcutaneous tissue.

Advantages
- Slow and sustained absorption
- Self medication
- Suitable for some suspensions
- Suitable for implantation of solid pellets

Disadvantages
- Not suitable for administration of large volumes, the volume injected is 1ml or less.
- Painful and necrosis if irritating drug is injected subcutaneously. Only nonirritant drugs can be given by this route.

The following are the less commonly used parenteral routes of drug administration:

- Intradermal injections: The drug is injected between the epidermis and dermis of the skin, in volume of about a tenth of a millilitre for diagnostic purpose, as in tuberculin and allergy testing. The volume injected is 0.1-0.2 ml.
- Intraperitoneal injections are not given because of producing infection and adhesions. These dangers are too great to warrant this route in humans.
- Intraarterial injections of certain anticancer drugs may be given in the treatment of localized cancers.
- Intrathecal injection of spinal anaesthetics is given in the subarachnoid space.
- Intramedullary injection may be given into bone marrow.
- Intracardiac injection is indicated in an emergency only.
- Intraarticular injection may be given for treating local conditions e.g. hydrocortisone acetate in rheumatoid arthritis. The drug reaches directly into the synovial fluid that lubricates the articulating ends of bones in a joint. However, utmost aseptic precautions are essential.
- Jet injection (hypospray): The drug is introduced with the help of a syringe through a microfine orifice by means of a high velocity jet. It is painless as needle is not used. This is suitable for mass inoculation as thousands of persons can be injected in few hours.

The dosage forms applicable for parenteral routes of administration are:

Injectable preparations are sterile solutions or suspensions in a suitable vehicle. Drugs in solution act faster. A drug in suspension is slowly absorbed and produces prolonged drug action. This is referred to as a depot or repository injection which is mainly limited to intramuscular type of injection. The drug is slowly released into the systemic circulation. If more sustained action is desired at a constant rate over a period of several weeks, this may be achieved by subcutaneous implantation of compressed tablets, called pellets.

OTHER ROUTES FOR SYSTEMIC EFFECTS

Inhalation route

This route of administration provides rapid absorption. The rich capillary area of the alveoli of the lungs, which in man covers about a thousand square feet, provides an excellent absorbing surface for volatile drugs, gases, nonvolatile drugs in the form of aerosol mists of very minute particles of liquids or solids.

Pulmonary (inhalation) route

The size of aerosol particles determine the speed at which they are swept along by inhaled air and hence the size of the particles, more than 100 micron in diameter are trapped in the oropharyngeal cavity, whereas those having diameter between 10 and 60 micron will be deposited on the epithelium of the tracheobronchial, particles, less than 2 micron in diameter can reach the alveoli and are most efficient in producing systemic effects.

Advantages
- Desired local site of action
- Rapid onset of action
- Avoid first-pass biotransformation

Disadvantages
- Poor ability to regulate the dose
- Irritation of pulmonary epithelium
- Cumbersome method of administration

Topical route for systemic effect

The transdermal delivery system in the form of disc or patch releases slowly the drug for percutaneous absorption. Drugs which penetrate skin through pores, sweat glands, hair follicles and sebaceous glands enter general circulation through blood capillaries present just below the epidermal cells. Nitroglycerin, scopolamine, clonidine are among the few drugs applied topically for producing systemic action. Nitroglycerin is also available as an ointment applied topically for systemic action.

Topical routes for systemic effect is mostly through transdermal delivery system.

Transdermal administration

A transdermal device is a laminated structure consisting of 4 layers, as shown in Fig 1.2. It consists of (i) an impermeable backing membrane (mechanical system); (ii) an adjacent polymer layer, which serves as the drug reservoir; (iii) a microporous membrane filled with a non polar material, e.g., paraffin; and (iv) an adhesive film to make close contact with the skin and maintain the device in the desired position.

The transdermal device is a membrane controlled system across the skin. It is designed to support the passage of drug from skin's surface, through its various layers, and into the systemic circulation physically, these systems are sophisticated patches.

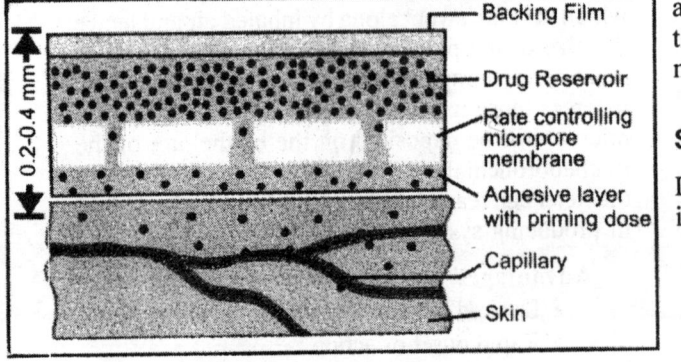

Fig. 1.2. Transdermal device.

The potential benefits are:
- Avoidance of first-pass biotransformation
- A method of continuous administration of drug to maintain a steady concentration (zero-order kinetic)
- Less variability in plasma levels
- Constant plasma levels
- Prolonged duration of action
- Dosing frequency reduced (1,3,7 days)
- Minimal adverse effects
- Improved patient compliance

Only a small number of drugs can be used by this route. The desirable molecular weight should be <1000 and should have adequate lipophilicity and hydrophilicity.

Irritant drugs are avoided. Mass of drug needs to be more than 10mg/24 hours. Drugs that can be used are:

Fentanyl, nitroglycerin, hyoscine, clonidine, oestradiol, and nicotine.

Disadvantages
- Limited to potent drugs as skin is a good barrier and large amounts of drug can not penetrate.
- Maximum daily dose - few mg/day.
- Can not be used for very hydrophilic and very lipophilic drugs.
- Difficult to deliver ionized drugs.
- Limited to drugs with low molecular weight.
- Tolerance can be induced as a result of constant plasma levels.

Currently, patches are used in several therapeutic areas, including pain management, smoking cessation, treatment of heart disease, hormone replacement, and management of motion sickness.

SPECIAL DRUG DELIVERY SYSTEMS

Different approaches to improve drug delivery include:
- Pro-drugs
- Mini pump
- Drug-antibody conjugate
- Biologically erodable microspheres
- Packaging in liposomes

Prodrug (inactive)

There are some drugs which are inert until they are chemically altered within the body. Such agents are called **pro-drugs.**

Purposes of using a pro-drug:

- To modify absorption and distribution
- To modify duration of action
- To reduce adverse effects
- To overcome difficulties encountered in pharmaceutical formulation procedure

Example : Dipivefrine is the pro-drug of adrenaline and it has about 17 times the penetration than adrenaline due to high lipid/water partition coefficient.

Prednisone, l-dopa enalapril, talampicillin are also pro-drugs.

Mini-pump

Its implantation in diabetics provides a control system for auto-insulin injection depending on the blood glucose level.

Drug-antibody conjugate

There is an interesting possibility to attach a drug to an antibody directed against a tumour - specific antigen. But it is too early to predict their success.

Biologically erodable microspheres

Microspheres of biologically erodable polymers can be engineered to be adhered to mucosal epithelium in the gut. Such microspheres can be loaded with drugs to increase absorption. However, this system is yet to be used clinically.

Packaging in liposomes

Liposomes are minute vesicles made by using certain phospholipids. They are filled with non-lipid soluble drug and are mainly taken up by reticuloendothelial cells especially in liver and also concentrate in malignant tumours. It allows selectivity of drug delivery.

Liposomes have also been used for amphotericin in the treatment of systemic mycoses to render it less neurotoxic and better tolerated.

STUDY QUESTIONS

1. What are the different routes of administration of drugs? Discuss the merits and demerits of enteral and parenteral routes.
2. What are the advantages of sublingual route of administration?
3. Explain inhalation route of administration.
4. What are the advantages of topical application of drugs?
5. Why is it necessary to learn routes of administration? What factors are determined by route of administration?
6. What are special drug delivery systems?
7. What is transdermal drug delivery system? What may be the advantages?

GUIDE TO FURTHER READING

Routes of administration and absorption

Benet, L.Z. Effect of route of administration and distribution on drug action. J. Pharmacokinet. Biopharm, 1978; 6:559.

Burstein, N.L. and Anderson, J.A. Review: Corneal penetration and ocular bioavailability of drugs. J. Ocul Pharmacol, 1985; 1:309.

Brodie, B.B. Physiochemical factors in drug absorption. In Absorption and Distribution of Drugs. Binns, T.B. (editor). The Williams & Wilkins Co., Baltimore, 1964, pp. 16-48.

"Drug Delivery Systems". Pharm. Tech. Aster Publishing Corp., Springfield, OR, 1983.

Flynn, G.L. Considerations in Controlled-Release Drug Delivery Systems. Pharm. Tech., 1982; 6:33.

Havner, W.H. Pharmacokinetics: Routes of administration. In Ocular Pharmacology, St. Louis, 1981, The CV Mosby Co.

Lee, V.H.L. Review: New directions in the optimization of ocular drug delivery. J. Ocul. Pharmacol., 1990; 6:157.

Schoenwalas, R.D. Ocular pharmacokinetics/ pharmacodynamics. In Mitra A.K. (editor). Ophthalmic drug delivery systems, Marcel Dekker, New York, 1993.

Schwartz, J.B. and Ando, H.Y. New Drug Delivery Systems: Controlled release. Am. Druggist, 1983; 188:43.

Singer, S.J. and Nicolson, G.L. The fluid-mosaic model of the structure of membranes. Science, 1972; 175:720.

QUANTITATIVE ASPECT OF DRUG ACTION

Quantitative action

It is important that a drug has a desired qualitative action, but the right amount of action is also required, for which the dose has to be precisely adjusted. If it is too little, it will be ineffective, and if too much, then it will produce adverse effects. Certain characteristics of the dose-response relationships are given below:

Dose-response relationships

The desired response may change as the dose is changed. The change in response with alteration of dose is defined by the shape of the dose-response curve, dose plotted on horizontal and response on the vertical axis.

Quantal dose-response curve

It relates to the frequency with which a specified dose of a drug produces a specific response, e.g. 30% decrease in blood pressure among the patients in a clinical trial.

The smallest amount of a drug that will produce a quantal response is not the same for all members of a population. If the frequency of response is plotted against the minimum dose necessary to produce the response the result is often as the following Gaussian frequency distribution curve.

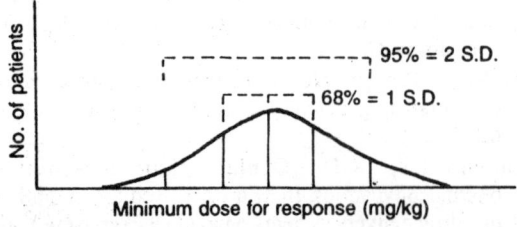

The quantal-response curve is a cumulative graph of the frequency distribution curve.

Graded dose-response curve

The pharmacologic effect increases as the dose is increased to a single subject or isolated tissue.

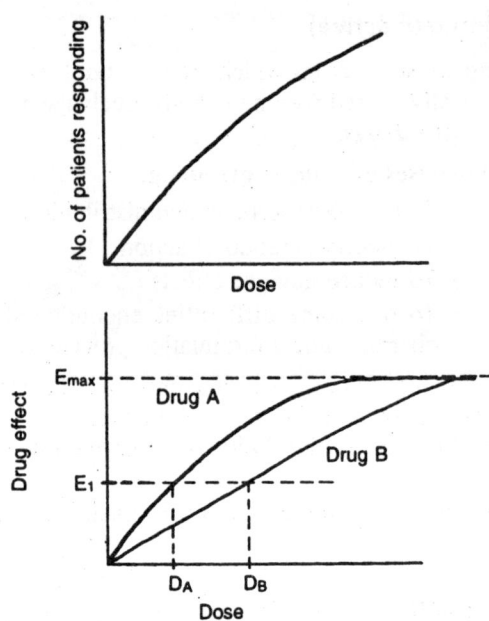

Graded dose-response curves for two drugs. A and B. E_{max} (maximum effect) i.e. efficacy is same for both the drugs, but they differ in potency (doses of drug A and drug B needed to produce the drug effect E_1).

However, at certain dose, the resulting effect will reach a maximum level (ceiling effect).

Log dose-response curve

This causes the hyperbolic graded dose-response curve to become sigmoidal. One advantage of plotting on a logarithmic scale is that potencies usually show dose-response curves that are parallel.

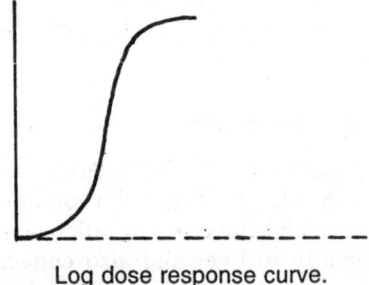

Log dose response curve.

Action vs Effect

Action is the alteration of condition, that brings about the effect. Action precedes effect.

Potency versus efficacy (Fig. 1.3A & B)

Efficacy and potency are different terms. They are often used confusingly.

Efficacy is the maximum effect (E_{max}) of the drug. It is indicated by the height of the log dose-response curve. Efficacy is usually more important than potency in selecting drugs for clinical use.

Potency is a comparative measure which refers to the different doses of two drugs that are needed to produce the same effect. Meaningful comparisons of potency can be made only when the drugs being compared have log dose-response curves.

The difference in weight of drug that has to be administered is of no clinical significance unless it is very large.

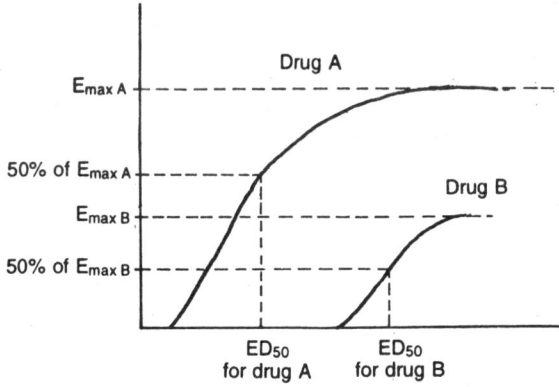

Fig. 1.3A. Log dose-response curves for two drugs A and B. E_{max} is maximum effect, ED_{50} is the smallest dose showing an effect which is half of the E_{max}. The height of the curve (E_{max}) indicates efficacy and the ED_{50} determines the potency.

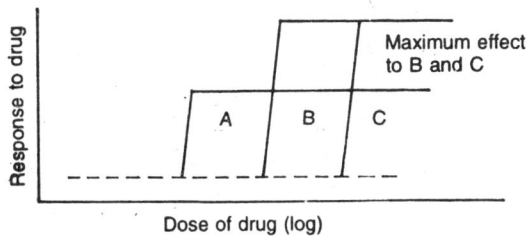

Fig. 1.3B. Maximum effect is a measure of the drugs' efficacy. B is more potent than C but both have the same efficacy; B and C have a greater efficacy than A.

Acquired and natural tolerance

Tolerance is said to have developed when it becomes necessary to increase the dose of a drug to obtain an effect previously obtained with a smaller dose. Acquired tolerance is due to reduced efficacy at receptor sites or due to increased metabolism (due to enzyme induction). Cross-tolerance occurs between drugs of similar chemical structure and sometimes between those of dissimilar structure. Natural tolerance is not induced by the drug but is due to inherent genetic factors.

Biological assay and standardization

Biological assay or bioassay is the process by which the activity of a substance is measured on living material. The activity is expressed relative to that of a standard preparation of the same substance. Bioassay is used when physical or chemical methods are not practicable.

Biological standardization is a specialized form of bioassay. It involves matching of material of unknown potency with an international or national standard with the objective of providing a reliable preparation for therapeutic use and research.

International standards are available for all drugs which can be used as reference standards with known potencies.

Bioassay methods are employed for the following:

- To estimate biologically active constituents e.g. histamine, serotonin, acetylcholine in a tissue extract or body fluids.
- For biological standardization of agents which cannot be obtained in pure form, e.g. certain hormones and heparin.
- To measure the pharmacological activity of a new or chemically unknown drug.
- To find ED_{50} or LD_{50}.

The design of bioassay

The design of bioassays is aimed at:

1. minimizing variation
2. avoiding errors resulting from variation
3. estimation of the limits of error of the assay result

There are several experimental designs developed so that there is maximum efficiency and reliability of bioassays.

Type of bioassays

- **Quantal assays (Direct end point assay)** : 'All or none' response is measured and then their potency compared, e.g. digitalis induced 'cardiac arrest' in guinea pigs; insulin induced 'hypoglycaemic convulsions' in mice; 'head drop' assay for d-tubocurarine in rabbits and calculation of 'LD50' of drugs in mice or rats.

- **Graded response assays** : The response to varying doses of a drug are graded and measured, e.g. bioassay of histamine on guinea pig ileum and bioassay of acetylcholine on frog rectus abdominus muscle.

The following methods may be employed:

Matching assay

If the test sample is too small, the concentration of the unknown which matches in its response with the known dose of the standard is found by trial and error.

Bracketing assay

If the test sample is too small, the observed response with the test drug is bracketed between the one higher and one lower response of the standard.

Interpolation method

The curve of the standard is taken first, then 2-3 responses of the unknown test drug are taken which fall in between the linear portion of the curve of the standard drug. Then by interpolation of these responses at the dose axis, the concentration of the unknown test solution can be found.

Multiple point assay

- 3 point assay (2 + 1 dose assay)
- 4 point assay (2 + 2 dose assay)
- 6 point assay (3 + 3 dose assay)

Here 3 concentrations of the standard and 3 concentrations of the test substance are used in 6 sets of experiments using 6 doses in each set i.e., $6 \times 6 = 36$ doses.

A newly emerging discipline pharmacoeconomics seeks to measure drug effect in social and economic terms. It is beyond the realm of bioassay. This discipline is important in guiding Govt. decisions on drug prescribing and health care policies.

Therapeutic index (TI) and margin of safety

Ehrlich introduced the concept of the therapeutic index as the maximum tolerated dose divided by the minimum curative dose. But the index is not calculated in this way since there are no single such doses that may be applicable to all individuals. The therapeutic index can be calculated in animals by obtaining the ratio LD_{50} / ED_{50} i.e. the minimum dose that is lethal or toxic in 50% animals (LD_{50}) divided by the minimum dose that has the desired effect in 50% of animals (ED_{50}). The therapeutic index concept is useful in comparing the usefulness of one drug with another i.e. safety in relation to efficacy.

$$TI = \frac{LD_{50}}{ED_{50}}$$

Therapeutic index may be misleading if the log dose-response curves for effectiveness and toxicity have different slopes i.e. are not parallel. Hence standard margin of safety may be more useful:

$$\frac{LD_1}{ED_{99}} - 1 \times 100$$

ED_{99} is the dose effective in 99% of the population. It must be increased to cause toxic effects in 1% of population e.g. if 100 mg of a drug causes toxicity in 1% population and 10 mg is effective in 99%, the standard margin of safety is 900. The dose effective in 99% must be increased 900% to be toxic to 1% population.

STUDY QUESTIONS

1. Qualitative action of a drug is important but quantitative action is all the more important. Why?
2. What do you mean by dose-response curve? What is its importance?
3. Define potency and efficacy of a drug. How do they differ? Which is more important clinically?
4. What is therapeutic index? How is it calculated? What is its importance?

5. Define bioassay and drug standardization. What is reference standard of drugs?
6. Explain onset, duration and intensity of drug action.
7. What are the characteristics of dose-response relationships?

GUIDE TO FURTHER READING

Harris, E.L., Fitzgerald, J.D. (eds), 1970. The Principles and Practice of Clinical Trials. Churchill Livingstone, Edinburgh.

Laska, E.M., et al., 1987. Statistical methods and the applications of bioassay. Annu. Rev. Pharmacol., 27:385-397.

Miller, J.N., 1982. Developments in non-isotopic immunoassay. Nature, 295:xiii.

Myerscough, P.R., Schild, H.O., 1958. Quantitative assays of oxytocic drugs on the human post-partum uterus. Br. J. Pharmacol., 13:207.

ABSORPTION OF DRUGS

Absorption of drugs is the entry of drugs into the blood via mucous membrane of gut, or respiratory tract or from the site of injection. It is the process of transfer of drugs from site of administration to the blood.

Its knowledge is important to determine dose and frequency of administration.

Whatever the route of administration, the drug usually must cross one or several semipermeable biological membranes before reaching the site of action.

BIOLOGICAL MEMBRANE

The biological membrane is composed chiefly of lipids and proteins. The schematic illustration of biological membrane is given in Fig. 1.4A and the routes by which solutes can traverse cell membranes are shown in Fig. 1.4B.

Plasma (cell) membrane is an exceedingly thin structure that separates the internal components of a cell from the external environment. The membrane measures from 4.5 nm at the phospholipid bilayer regions up to 10 nm in regions where membrane proteins are present. This is a bilayer (about 100 Å thick; 1 Å = 0.1 nm) of lipid molecules. The polar groups are at the two surfaces. The nonpolar chains

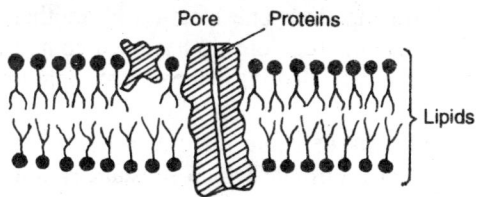

Fig. 1.4A. Schematic illustration of biological membrane.

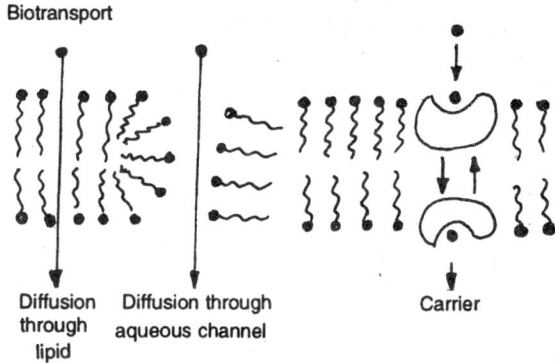

Fig. 1.4B. Routes by which solutes can traverse cell membranes.

are embedded in the matrix with adsorbed extrinsic and intrinsic protein molecules.

The phospholipid molecules are arranged in two parallel rows forming a phospholipid bilayer. A phospholipid molecule consists of a polar phosphate containing 'head' that mixes with water (hydrophilic) and nonpolar fatty acid 'tails' that do not mix with water (hydrophobic). The molecules are oriented in the bilayer so that 'heads' face outward on either side and the 'tails' face each other in the membrane's interior. The phospholipid layer is dynamic since the phospholipid molecules can move sideways and exchange places in their own row. The bilayer is also self-sealing. If a needle is pushed through it and pulled out, the puncture site will seal automatically.

The plasma membrane proteins are classified into 2 categories—integral and peripheral. Integral proteins are embedded in the phospholipid bilayer among the fatty acid 'tails'. Some of these lie at or near the inner and outer membrane surfaces, others penetrate the membrane completely.

Since the phospholipid bilayer is somewhat fluid and flexible and the integral proteins have been observed moving from one location to another in the membrane, the relationship has been compared to iceberg (proteins) floating in the sea (phospholipid bilayer).

The subunits of some integral proteins form minute channels through which substances can be transferred into or out of the cell. Other integral proteins are bound to branching chains of carbohydrates. These integral proteins together provide receptor sites that enable a cell to recognize other cells of its own kind, to recognize and respond to foreign cells that may be potentially dangerous, and to recognize and attach to hormones, and nutrients.

Peripheral proteins are loosely bound to membrane surface and easily separated from it. Far less is known about these than the integral proteins and their functions are not yet fully known. They may serve as enzymes.

The currently accepted model of plasma membrane structure is known as the fluid mosaic model. A mosaic is a pattern of many small pieces fitted together. According to this concept, the membrane is a mosaic of proteins which move laterally in the phospholipid bilayer. Newer concept views proteins as globular molecules dispersed throughout the lipid and in some instances extending from one side of the membrane to the other.

The presence of cholesterol molecules makes the membrane less flexible and less permeable. Glycolipids mediate cell-to-cell recognition and communication, participate in cellular growth and development and may serve as infection sites for bacteria and viruses.

BIOTRANSPORT OF DRUGS

The following mechanisms are involved in the transfer of chemicals across biologic barriers which are called transport processes or transport mechanisms (biotransport):

1. Passive transport
   (a) Simple diffusion
   (b) Filtration
2. Specialized transport
   (a) Active transport
   (b) Facilitated diffusion
   (c) Pinocytosis

Passive transport processes

Simple diffusion

Diffusion is movement till equilibrium is reached. Cell membranes consist of a bimolecular layer of lipoid material interspersed with minute water-filled pores and bound on both sides by protein. The size of these pores varies in different membranes (4-40 Å). Lipid soluble substances readily penetrate the lipoid sheet. Small water soluble polar materials pass through the pores, some of which are charged, and some are not. The passage of a drug across the cell membrane is, therefore, strongly influenced by its lipid solubility, molecular size, degree of ionization and solubility of its ionized and non-ionized forms.

Lipid soluble substances and both nonpolar and polar substances, as long as the last named two possess sufficient lipid solubility, move across the membrane by a process of passive diffusion. Hydrostatic and osmotic differences are involved in the passage through the pores by the further passive process of filtration. Water soluble molecules in solution must be small enough to pass through the pores, and this is a common route for many small, water soluble, polar and non-polar substances, most inorganic ions are also sufficiently small. The filtration proceeds until the concentration of the drug is the same on both sides of the membrane.

Many drugs are the salts of weak bases and strong acids. Salts are highly ionized and hydrophilic but are poorly soluble in lipids. The free base is non-ionized and therefore lipophilic. Cell membranes contain lipids and thus lipophilic drugs tend to pass through them more easily than hydrophilic ones.

Filtration

Filtration is movement of solvents (such as water) and solutes (such as glucose) across a selectively permeable membrane, as a result of gravity or hydrostatic (water) pressure from an area of higher to lower pressure.

Specialized transport

Active transport

It involves movement of substances, usually ions, across a selectively permeable membrane from a region of lower to higher concentration by an interaction with an integral proteins in the membrane, the process requires energy expenditure from the splitting of ATP.

Facilitated diffusion

It involves diffusion of larger molecules across a selectively permeable membrane with the assistance of integral proteins in the membrane that serve as carriers.

Pinocytosis

It is movement of large molecules and particles through plasma membranes in which the membrane surrounds the substance, encloses it, and brings it into the cell. It is a rare mechanism for drugs. Examples include phagocytosis ("cell eating"), pinocytosis ("cell drinking") and receptor-mediated endocytosis. Exocytosis is export of substances from the cell by reverse endocytosis.

Table 1.3 shows comparison among simple diffusion, facilitated diffusion and active transport.

The **biotransport process** explains the transfer of drugs across the biologic membrane but not the movement over any great distance. The circulatory system is the common pathway for carrying drugs from the inner side of the membrane to any tissue or organ.

Hence there are two separate process for drugs to reach the site of action (i) the movement of drugs into the blood stream from its site of administration. This is absorption; and (ii) distribution, i.e., movement of drug into the tissues.

SITES OF DRUG ABSORPTION

Absorption may take place at the following sites:
- The alimentary tract.
- By subcutaneous or intramuscular injection (intravenous injection circumvents the factors involved in absorption).
- Via mucous membranes.
- Via the skin.

Factors that affect absorption

- *Route of administration* via the skin (ointment, etc.), mucous membranes (mouth, rectum, bladder, conjunctiva), gastrointestinal (oral), respiratory tract (inhalation) or by injection, e.g. absorption is faster from I.M. injection than after oral administration.
- *Concentration :* Absorption is faster from high concentration of drug than dilute solution.
- *Physical state :* Crystalloids are better absorbed than colloids. The finer the particle size, more rapid the rate of absorption.
- *Area of absorbing surface :* Greater area helps in absorption.
- *Vascularity and blood flow :* Good circulation of blood at the site is helpful.
- *Solubility and binding :* Highly lipid soluble drugs are unionized which are rapidly absorbed from the gut. Absorption is directly related to solubility, being far more rapid from solution than solid form.
- *Motility of gut :* Rapid motility impedes absorption due to less contact time.

Table 1.3. Comparison among simple diffusion, facilitated diffusion and active transport

Simple diffusion	Facilitated diffusion	Active transport
(a) Down concentration gradient	Down concentration gradient	'Uphill' (transports against concentration gradient)
(b) Nonspecific	Specific	Specific i.e. selective for the chemical structure of a drug
(c) Energy expenditure not required	Not required	Energy dependent; the metabolic energy is often generated by the enzyme known as Na^+-K^+-ATPase
(d) Not saturable	Saturable	Saturable process i.e. increasing concentration gradient will not increase rate of influx
(e) No carrier involved	Carrier mediated	Carrier mediated
(f) For lipid soluble drugs	Nondiffusible substances	Lipid insoluble drugs
(g) Most drugs	Glucose movement into cells	Glucose absorption from gut

• *Ionization* : Highly ionized drugs are not or poorly absorbed from the gut. Ionization is a property of all electrolytes—both weak and strong. Ionization of drug is an important factor in passive transfer of drugs; unionized are lipid soluble, so readily diffusible.

In any solution of drugs, there will be a mixture of salt and free base, the ratio of which will depend on the pH and the property of the compound known as its pKa; pKa is the pH at which there are equal concentrations of base and salt.

$$pH = pKa + log_{10} \frac{[base]}{[salt]}$$

The lower the pKa, the higher will be the proportion of base at a given pH; compounds with a low pKa are better absorbed than those with a high one.

The pKa of a drug cannot be altered, the pH can be changed within certain limits. For example, as the pH of eye drops is raised, the degree of ionization of a weak base will be reduced thus improving corneal epithelial absorption.

The concept of pKa is derived from the Henderson-Hasselbalch equation:

$$pKa = pH + log \frac{\text{conc. of ionized drug}}{\text{conc. of non-ionized drug}}$$
... (for bases)

$$pKa = pH + log \frac{\text{conc. of non-ionized drug}}{\text{conc. of ionized drug}}$$
... (for acids)

The point of 50% dissociation is known as the pKa, the negative logarithm of the acidic dissociation constant. This is related to the environmental pH. So the degree of ionization depends on 2 factors: the pKa of the drug and the ambient pH. pKa is equal to pH when a substance is 50% ionized and 50% non-ionized. The concept is important to explain clinically important facts, for example, aspirin (pKa 3.5) is well absorbed from stomach, weak bases like quinine (pKa 8.4) are absorbed in intestines.

• *Presence of other substances* : Vitamin C facilitates iron absorption, calcium binds to tetracycline and prevents its absorption, liquid paraffin prevents absorption of vitamin D.

• *Other factors* : Disease or injury e.g. permeability of blood-brain barrier increases in inflammation.

In many cases, it is advantageous to prolong the duration of drug action because frequency of administration will be reduced, patient will not have to be disturbed in the night, and patient compliance is improved.

Prolongation of drug action

The duration of drug action can be prolonged:

• By prolonging absorption: oral—sustained release tablet or capsule; parenteral—procaine penicillin oily solution.
• By increasing plasma protein binding e.g. sulphamethoxypyridazine.
• By retarding rate of metabolism e.g. addition of ethinyl group to oestradiol makes it longer acting for use as oral contraceptive.
• By retarding renal excretion e.g. probenecid prolongs duration of action of penicillin and ampicillin.

STUDY QUESTIONS

1. Describe cell membrane. Draw a diagram and label different parts of its structure.
2. What are the different sites of absorption of drugs?
3. What are the different ways by which the biotransport of drug takes place across the biological membranes?
4. List in a tabulated form the differences between passive and active processes of biotransport of drugs.
5. What do you mean by endocytosis and exocytosis?
6. Explain the factors that affect absorption of drugs.
7. What do you understand by the term pKa?

GUIDE TO FURTHER READING

Routes of administration and absorption

Benet, L.Z. Effect of route of administration and distribution on drug action. J. Pharmacokinet. Biopharm, 1978; 6:559.

Burstein, N.L. and Anderson, J.A. Review: Corneal penetration and ocular bioavailability of drugs. J. Ocul Pharmacol, 1985; 1:309.

Brodie, B.B. Physiochemical factors in drug absorption. In Absorption and Distribution of Drugs. Binns, T.B. (editor). The Williams & Wilkins Co, Baltimore, 1964, pp. 16-48.

"Drug Delivery Systems". Pharm. Tech. Aster Publishing Corp., Springfield, OR, 1983.

Flynn, G.L. Considerations in controlled-release drug delivery systems. Pharm. Tech., 1982; 6:33.

Havner, W.H. Pharmacokinetics: Routes of administration. In Ocular Pharmacology, St. Louis, 1981, The CV Mosby Co.

Lee, V.H.L. Review: New directions in the optimization of ocular drug delivery. J. Ocul Pharmacol, 1990; 6:157.

Schoenwald, R.D. Ocular pharmacokinetics/pharmacodynamics. In Metra A.K. (editor). Ophthalmic Drug Delivery Systems, Marcel Dekker, New York, 1993.

Schwartz, J.B. and Ando, H.Y. New drug delivery systems: Controlled release. Am. Druggist, 1983; 188:43.

Singer, S.J. and Nicolson, G.L. The fluid-mosaic model of the structure of membranes. Science, 1972; 175:720.

BIOAVAILABILITY AND THERAPEUTIC EFFECTS OF DRUGS

Definition and differences in chemical equivalence and bioequivalence

After a drug is administered, it is absorbed systemically. When the minimum effective concentration (MEC) is reached at the receptor, a pharmacologic response is initiated. The time from drug administration to the MEC is known as the onset time. As long as the drug concentration remains above the MEC, pharmacologic activity is observed. The duration of activity is the time for which the drug concentration remains above the MEC. As the drug concentration increases, other receptors may combine with the drug to exert an adverse response. This drug concentration is the minimum toxic concentration (MTC). The drug concentration range between the MEC and MTC is the therapeutic window, as shown in Fig. 1.5.

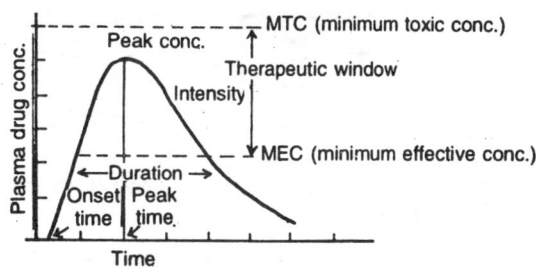

Fig. 1.5. Onset, duration and therapeutic window.

BIOAVAILABILITY

Bioavailability is defined as the fraction of unchanged drug reaching the systemic circulation following administration by any route. It is a measurement of the rate and the extent at which the absorption occurs.

Drug products are pharmaceutical equivalent if they contain same active ingredient and are similar in concentration, dosage form and routes of administration. They are considered to be bioequivalent when the rates and extents of bioavailability of the active ingredient in the two products are not significantly different.

Bioavailability of parenteral and oral products

- I.V. inj: Bioavailability is 100%. All the drug is available for biological activity.
- I.M. inj: Bioavailability is less than I.V. but more than S.C. inj. (I.M./S.C. less than 100% due to local binding of the drug).
- Oral: Less than parenteral.

Differences may be seen primarily among oral dosage forms of poorly soluble, slowly absorbed drugs or other physical characteristics of the drug that are not rigidly controlled in formulation and manufacture of the preparation.

Therefore, oral formulations of a drug from different manufactures may have same amount of drug (chemically equivalent), but may not yield same blood levels (biologically inequivalent). This difference is due to the formulation factors which affect bioavailability (Fig. 1.6).

Besides the drug, tablets or capsules contain a large number of excipients which may affect disintegration of the dosage form, and dissolution of the drug. The solid dosage form (tablet/capsule) has drug plus diluents, binders, lubricants, stabilizing agents,

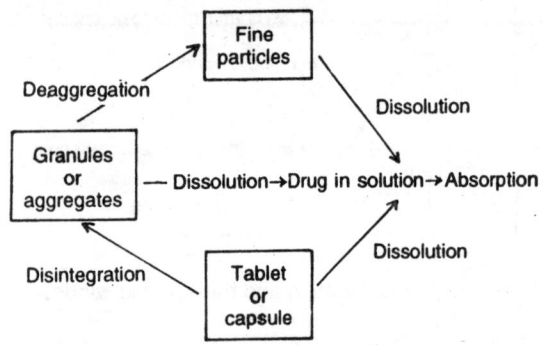

Fig. 1.6. Influence of formulation factors.

etc. Variations may be due to differences in disintegration (break into individual particles of active drug is determined by dosage form), and dissolution rates (rate of dissolution is determined by solubility, crystal form, size and other physical properties and the pH). After dissolution the process of absorption commences and the drug reaches in blood. The variations (differences) in bioavailability may manifest in rate as well as an extent of absorption.

Variation in drug bioavailability is not a characteristic solely of the drug preparation, since variations in enzyme activity of the gut wall or the liver, gastric pH or intestinal motility will all affect it. So bioavailability of a particular preparation can be considered in a given individual on a particular occasion. Then it also does not take into account the time course, e.g. drug A may be absorbed in 30 minutes and drug B in 6 hours.

FACTORS INFLUENCING ABSORPTION AND BIOAVAILABILITY

- Pharmaceutical factors
- Pharmacological factors

Pharmaceutical factors which affect disintegration and dissolution

(i) Particle size: A drug dissolves more rapidly when its surface area is increased by decreasing particle size.

(ii) Salt form: Salts of weakly acidic drugs are highly water soluble. Free acidic drug is precipitated from these salts which has faster dissolution rate and hence enhanced bioavailability.

(iii) Crystal form: Amorphous forms have faster dissolution rate compared to the crystalline forms.

(iv) Water of hydration: Many drugs combine with water, these are called hydrates. Amorphous forms have faster dissolution rate and better availability than the hydrous forms of these drugs.

(v) Nature of excipients/adjuvants: Certain inert substances such as starch, lactose etc. are added as a filling material (when drug content is too small) or as a binding agent. Some of these substances are wetting agents e.g. polysorbate-80 which enhances solvent penetration in drug particles resulting in faster dissolution and more rapid absorption.

(vi) Nonionized lipid soluble drugs are better absorbed whereas strongly acidic or basic drugs are highly ionized drugs which show reduced availability.

Pharmacological factors

(i) Gastric emptying and gastrointestinal motility: Factors that accelerate gastric emptying increase bioavailability as they permit drugs to reach the large absorptive area of small intestine sooner.

(ii) Gastrointestinal diseases: In gastroenteritis, there is decreased absorption of drugs.

(iii) Food and other substances: Generally, gastrointestinal absorption is favoured by an empty stomach. However, the absorption of some antifungal drugs e.g., griseofulvin is increased by giving it with a fatty diet; bioavailability of phenytoin is increased if given after meals due to better dissolution (due to food induced bile secretion).

(iv) First-pass effect: First-pass effect means the drug degradation occurring before the drug enters the systemic circulation resulting in decreased bioavailability.

(v) Drug-drug interactions: It can also affect bioavailability e.g., liquid paraffin decreases the bioavailability of Vitamin A.

(vi) Pharmacogenetic factors: Variations in bioavailability exist among humans due to pharmacogenetic reasons. For example, slow acetylators of INH show increased bioavailability (Americans Whites, Scandinavians); fast acetylators (Eskimos, Japanese, Chinese) show reduced bioavailability.

(vii) Miscellaneous factors, include route of administration, area of absorbing surface, state of circulation at the site of absorption.

The bioavailability of certain drugs is shown in Table 1.4.

Table 1.4. Bioavailability of certain drugs

Drugs	Bioavailability
Aminoglycosides, heparin, tubocurarine	None
Morphine	Poor (about 20%)
Aspirin, digoxin	Moderate (about 60%)
Atenolol, pethidine, ampicillin, propranolol, nifedipine, ranitidine, chloroquine, clonidine, diazepam, phenytoin, metronidazole, trimethoprim, warfarin, valproic acid, amoxycillin, sulphamethoxazole	Marked (about 95%)

Absolute bioavailability is the availability of the drug from a dosage form as compared to the availability of the drug after I.V. administration. It is calculated as the ratio of the AUC (Area Under Curve) for the dosage form given orally to the AUC obtained after I.V. drug administration. An absolute bioavailability of 0.08 or 80% indicates that only 80% of the drug was systemically available from the dosage form.

Relative bioavailability is the availability of the drug from a dosage form as compared to a reference standard. It is calculated as the ratio of the AUC for the dosage form to the AUC for the reference dosage form. A relative bioavailability of 1 (or 100%) implies that drug bioavailability from both dosage forms was the same, but it does not indicate the completeness of systemic drug absorption.

Methods for measuring bioavailability

Plasma drug concentration versus time curve measures the bioavailability of a drug from a drug product.

The time for peak plasma drug concentration

(T_{max}) indicates the rate of systemic drug absorption. If two oral drug products contain same amount of active drug but different excipients, the dosage form which gives faster rate of absorption will have shorter T_{max}.

The peak plasma drug concentration (C_{max}) is the plasma drug concentration at T_{max}. It indicates the intensity of the response. C_{max} should be within the therapeutic window.

For estimating the bioavailability, the drug is administered intravenously and its concentration in plasma measured at intervals. The same procedure is followed after giving the drug in same dose by the oral route. The plasma concentration-time curves following intravenous and oral administration of the same doses are plotted. Area under the curve (AUC) is measured for each type of administration (Figs. 1.7A and 1.7B).

The area of the peaks can be determined by following geometrical methods:

Lines are drawn to the two sides of the peak so that they intersect both with each other and the base line. Take the area of the peak as that of the triangle abc, i.e.

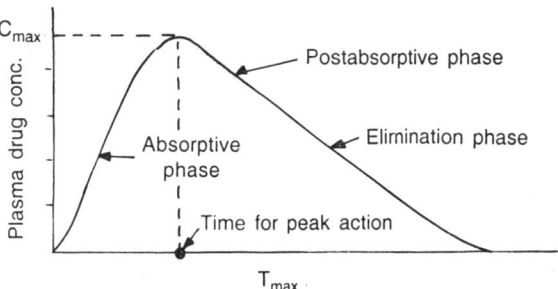

Fig. 1.7A. Bioavailability.

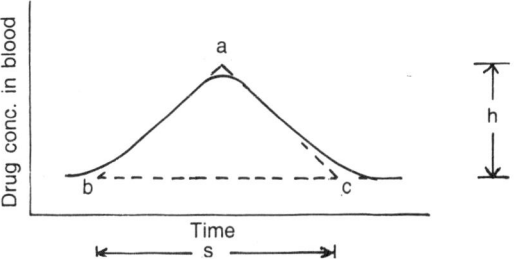

Fig. 1.7B. Bioavailability.

$$AUC = \frac{h \times s}{2}$$

The other formula is :

AUC = Peak height × Width of peak at half peak point

In case the drug cannot be given intravenously, relative bioavailability can be determined by comparing the area under curve (AUC) of the test drug with the AUC of a standard drug preparation of the same drug, both given orally under same condition.

The bioavailability parameters C_{max}, T_{max} and AUC for each drug product should not differ by more than 20%.

Monitoring of plasma concentration of drugs

It is useful for:

- Drugs with low safety margin e.g. digoxin, anticonvulsants, antiarrhythmics.
- If individual variations are large e.g. lithium, antidepressants.
- Aminoglycosides if used in the presence of renal failure.
- In cases of poisoning.
- To check patient compliance.

Monitoring is of no value for:

- Drugs activated in the body e.g. levodopa.
- 'Hit and Run' drugs whose effects last much longer than the drug itself, e.g. reserpine, MAOIs, guanethidine.
- Irreversible anticholinesterases.

STUDY QUESTIONS

1. What is the difference between chemical equivalence and bio-equivalence?
2. Describe the factors which influence bioavailability.
3. Discuss conditions when monitoring of drug plasma concentration is (a) not useful (b) useful.
4. Describe methods for measuring bioavailability.

GUIDE TO FURTHER READING

Burstein N.L., Anderson J.A. Review: Corneal penetration and ocular bioavailability of drugs. J Ocul Pharmacol 1:309, 1985.

Chodos, D.J. and Disanto, A.R. Basics of bioavailability, Kalamazoo, The Upjohn Company, 1973.

Evans W.E., Schentag, J.J., and Jusko, W.J. (eds). Applied Pharmacokinetics. Principles of Therapeutic Drug Monitoring, 3rd ed. Applied Therapeutics. Inc., Vancouver, WA. 1992.

Schoenwald, R. The control of drug bioavailability from ophthalmic dosage forms. In Smolen V.F., Ball L.A., editors. Controlled drug bioavailability, vol 3, New York, 1995, John Wiley & Sons, p. 257.

Skelly, J.P. Bioavailability and Bioequivalence. J. Clin. Pharmacol. 1976; 16:539.

Ueda, C.T. Concepts in Clinical Pharmacology. Essentials of Bioavailability and Bioequivalence. The Upjohn Company, Kalamazoo, 1979, pp. 11.

DISTRIBUTION OF DRUGS IN THE BODY

After absorption, drugs enter the blood stream and are carried round the body. The drug may be in simple solution in the plasma, but many drugs are poorly soluble and are partially bound to plasma proteins. It is important to realize that the fraction of the drug which is bound to protein is inactive and only the free unbound form has pharmacological activity.

The drug exists in plasma in two forms:

- Free form which is pharmacologically active
- Protein bound (pharmacologically inactive)

All drugs do not bind to plasma proteins, some drugs do. The ratio between free and bound forms is fixed for a drug.

The proteins that are involved in the binding of drugs are:

- Plasma albumin: most important, mainly for acidic drugs
- Alpha 1 acid glyoproteins, mostly for basic drugs

Effect of protein binding on drugs distribution and action

- Bound drug is inactive but acts as a temporary store of drug. When free form is decreased, the drug is gradually released from the bound form.
- It is not subjected to glomerular filtration, hence, delays its excretion.
- Many drugs can compete for the same binding site and may produce drug interactions by displacing the other drugs (displacement drug

interaction) and thereby increasing its activity or toxicity.

- Drug which are strongly protein-bound (>90%) have long plasma half-life, hence they are longer acting.
- Causes prolonged low levels of free drug - slowly released from bound reservoir.
- Delays its metabolism.
- Decreases its entry into CNS.

Table 1.5 shows drugs more than 90% bound to plasma proteins.

Table 1.5. Drugs >90% bound to plasma proteins

Basic Drugs	Acidic Drugs
Amitriptyline	Acetylsalicyclic acid
Chlorpromazine	Cloxacilin
Diazepam	Naproxen
Flurazepam	Penicillin
Imipramine	Phenytoin
Lidocaine	Tolbutamide
Lorazepam	Warfarin.
Nifedipine	
Nortriptyline	
Propranolol	
Quinidine	
Verapamil	

Table 1.6 shows conditions capable of altering plasma proteins

Table 1.6. Conditions capable of altering plasma protein

	Albumin	Alpha-1 acid Glycoprotein
Decreased plasma protein	Burns Chronic liver diseases Nephrotic syndrome Chronic renal failure Trauma	Nephrotic syndrome
Increased plasma proteins	Hypothyroidism	Myocardial infarction Renal failure Rheumatoid arthritis, trauma

Factors that determine blood concentration

- *Dose :* Larger the dose, the higher the concentration achieved.

- *Route of administration :* Intravenous injection produces a rapid rise in blood concentration whereas oral administration gives a slow rise and a lower peak concentration. Intramuscular injection rates lie between the two.
- *Distribution of the drug :* This is another important factor in determining the plasma concentration of a drug and also its activity and therapeutic usefulness.

Most of the absorbed drug reaches the interstitial fluid compartment called extracellular fluid space due to wide intercapillary gaps in the body. Plasma protein bound drug does not pass into this compartment. This passage is also restricted in brain (blood-brain barrier) and placenta.

Drugs cross the cell membrane and enter different tissues in the body (intracellular fluid compartment). The distribution in different tissues varies, depending on the characteristics of the tissues. The distribution of drugs in tissues determine the pharmacological activity. The volume of distribution (V_d) of the drug may be low (5 L for heparin) or high (13000 L for chloroquine). Drugs with very low V_d are chiefly confined to plasma and those with high V_d are concentrated in tissues. But V_d does not indicate which tissue. The more widely a drug diffuses, the lower will be the concentration produced by a given dose.

- *The rate of elimination :* The faster the body metabolizes or excretes a drug, the more rapidly blood level will fall.

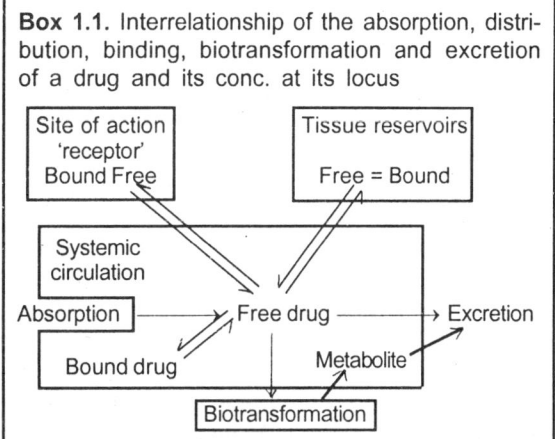

Box 1.1. Interrelationship of the absorption, distribution, binding, biotransformation and excretion of a drug and its conc. at its locus

The movement of drug proceeds until an equilibrium is established between unbound drug in plasma and tissue fluids.

Drugs that are confined to plasma or are distributed to extracellular fluid (ECF) and total body water (TBW) :

- Confined to plasma: e.g. heparin (high molecular weight), mannitol.
- Confined to ECF: polar drugs e.g., tubo-curarine, aminoglycosides.
- Confined to TBW: e.g. ethyl alcohol, diazepam, phenobarbitone, phenytoin.

Storage of drugs

The drugs may be stored in plasma proteins and other tissues.

There is selective concentration of certain drugs in some tissues:

Adipose tissue	Thiopentone
Bone and teeth	Tetracycline, heavy metals
Brain	Chlorpromazine
Kidney	Digoxin, chloroquine
Liver	Tetracycline, chloroquine, emetine
Retina	Chloroquine
Skeletal muscle, heart	Digoxin, emetine, chloroquine, tetracycline
Thyroid	Iodine

PHYSIOLOGICAL BARRIERS TO DRUG DISTRIBUTION

Blood-brain barrier

The endothelial cells of brain capillaries are very tightly joined unlike most capillaries of the body. In addition, brain capillaries are also enveloped by glial cells which are less permeable. This constitutes the blood-brain barrier. As a result of these barriers, only lipid soluble, nonionized form of drugs penetrate more easily to the brain as compared to the water soluble ionized form of drugs. For example, lipid soluble drugs such as volatile anaesthetics, thiopental, morphine, l-dopa, amphetamine, ephedrine, diazepam, propranolol, etc. can pass through the blood brain barrier. The polar drugs such as dopamine, streptomycin, d-tubocurarine, neostigmine, etc. fail to penetrate the blood-brain barrier.

Inflammatory conditions like cerebral meningitis exhibit increased permeability.

There are certain areas which are relatively permeable and do not constitute the part of blood-brain barrier :

- Pituitary gland
- Vomiting centre and chemoreceptor trigger zone (CTZ).
- Pineal body
- Median eminence
- Area postrema near the floor of IV ventricle i.e. vomiting center and chemoreceptor trigger zone where substances diffuse with same ease into the tissue spaces. This is very important because these areas of the brain have sensory organs that respond to different changes in the body fluids.

In the CNS, besides the blood-brain barrier, there is another barrier known as blood-cerebrospinal barrier (Blood-CSF barrier) which is located in choroid plexus. Lipid soluble nonionized forms of drugs only can pass through this barrier as in the case with blood-brain barrier.

But CSF-Brain barrier consists of epithelial cells lining the ventricles which are not connected by occluding zonulae. Therefore, this barrier permits passage of drugs from CSF to brain cells.

Drugs like penicillin which is less lipid soluble penetrates poorly through blood-brain barrier but when given by intrathecal route it can cross CSF - brain barrier and reach into the brain to treat conditions, like brain abscess.

Blood - Tissue Barriers

The capillary wall forms the blood-tissue barrier. This consists of an endothelial cell layer and a basement membrane enveloping the latter. The endothelial cells are 'welded' to each other by tight junctions such that no clefts, gaps, or pores remain that would permit drugs to pass unimpeded from the blood into interstitial fluid.

Redistribution of certain drugs

It is also possible that initial prompt high concentration is achieved in brain with thiopentone, then withdrawn and redistributed to other tissues e.g. muscle and fats, leading to termination of response.

Repeated doses saturate muscles and fat and therefore show longer action than the first dose.

STUDY QUESTIONS

1. Which factors determine concentration of a drug in blood?
2. What are the sites and process of drug distribution in the body?
3. What is the significance or effect, if a drug is highly bound to blood proteins?
4. Which fraction (free or bound) is active?
5. What is the effect of redistribution of certain drugs? Give example.
6. Indicate which particular drugs are selectively stored in certain tissues.
7. Name certain drugs which are highly protein bound (> 90%). Why such drugs have long plasma half-life, low 'efficacy' and less efficient tissue distribution?

GUIDE TO FURTHER READING

Curry, S.H., 1980. Drug Disposition and Pharmacokinetics. Blackwell, Oxford.

de Leve, L.D., et al., 1983. Clinical significance of plasma binding of basic drugs. In Lamble J.W. (ed). Drug Metabolism and Distribution. Elsevier, London.

Gibaldi, M., 1984. Biopharmaceutics and Clinical Pharmacokinetics. Lea & Febiger, Philadelphia.

Jusko, W.J., et al., 1976. Plasma and tissue protein binding of drugs in pharmacokinetics. Drug Metab Rev, 5: 43-140.

Lamble, J.W. (ed), 1983. Drug Metabolism and Distribution. Elsevier, Amsterdam.

BIOTRANSFORMATION (METABOLISM) OF DRUGS

It is chemical alteration of drug in the body, to change nonpolar (lipid soluble) compounds polar (lipid insoluble) so that the metabolites are not reabsorbed in the renal tubules and are excreted.

The term detoxify means inactivation of drug and excretion of its less toxic metabolites. This old term is discarded as the chemical reactions in the body can sometimes yield metabolites of greater toxicity or activity than the parent drug.

Metabolism is a wider term which refers to the total fate of the drug including absorption, distribution, biotransformation and excretion.

Therefore, the two terms detoxification and metabolism should not be interchangeably used with biotransformation. These terms are still loosely used for biotransformation, though not correctly.

Sites of biotransformation

Liver is the most important site, other tissues involved are kidney, plasma, intestines, skin, lungs and spleen.

For the majority of drugs, biotransformation is mediated through the hepatic microsomal systems. Fragments of the hepatic endoplasmic reticulum, in which are located the enzyme systems frequently involved with metabolism of many drugs, are usually called microsomes.

Microsomal enzymes catalyze a few conjugations and most of oxidation, reduction and hydrolysis of the majority of drugs. All the remainder of conjugations and some oxidation, reduction and hydrolysis reactions of a small number of drugs are catalyzed by nonmicrosomal systems, primarily in the liver but also in plasma and other tissues.

Some drugs are excreted largely unchanged but the majority are metabolized via extremely complex routes, the number of metabolites sometimes exceeding a hundred.

Results of biotransformation

Biotransformations may result in inactivation, activation, or change in activity. If the metabolite is active, further biotransformation, or excretion in the urine terminates its activity.

Inactivation (active → inactive; detoxification)

Most of the drugs are active and the metabolites produced are inactive.

Active metabolite from active drug

Phenylbutazone	Oxyphenbutazone
Chloral hydrate	Trichloroethanol
Chloroquine	Hydrochloroquine

Amitriptyline	Nortriptyline
Diazepam	Oxazepam
Propranolol	4-OH-propranolol

Activation of inactive drug (prodrug)

Prednisone	Prednisolone
Levodopa	Dopamine
Proguanil	Proguanil triazine
Bacampicillin	Ampicillin

Prodrugs are compounds which have no in vitro activity but are activated by enzymes to produce new compounds which are active in vivo.

Active drug → toxic metabolite

INH	Acetylhydrazine
Enflurane	Difluoromethoxydifluoroacetic acid and fluoride ion
Halothane	Trifluoroacetic acid
Sulphonamides	Acetyl derivatives

Different ways of biotransformations of metabolism

Biotransformation of drugs involves Phase I non-synthetic reactions; and Phase II synthetic reactions, conjugate reactions.

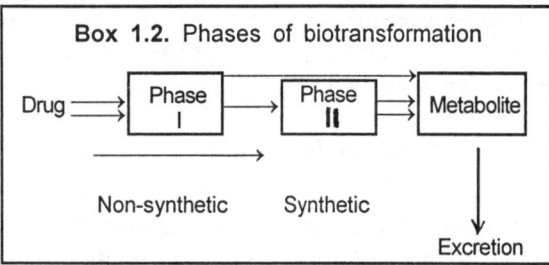

Phase I reactions (nonsynthetic)

The enzymes, often referred as 'microsomal' enzymes, are present in the endoplasmic reticulum (microsomes) of the liver. They are responsible for the metabolic reactions. Phase I metabolites, if polar, are excreted promptly, and if not sufficiently polar, they undergo phase II reactions and become water soluble which are excreted.

The following are the significant groups of reactions in Phase I:

Oxidation

Oxidation is the most common metabolic reaction which involves addition of O_2 or removal of hydrogen from the drug.

Microsomal oxidation : The smooth endoplasmic reticulum of cells in many organs, specially the liver, contains membrane-associated enzymes which are responsible for drug oxidation. The primary components of this enzyme system are cytochrome P-450 reductase and cytochrome 450. This enzyme system has been termed a mixed function oxygenase.

Examples of microsomal oxidation :

Carbon oxidation-hydroxyl-ation of aliphatic or aromatic groups	Phenytoin, Pentobarbital
Sulphoxide formulation	Chlorpromazine
Deamination	Amphetamine
N- or O-dealkylation	Diazepam, Codeine
Desulfuration	Thiobarbital

Nonmicrosomal oxidation : Soluble enzymes in mitochondria of cells can metabolize few compounds e.g.

- Xanthine oxidase converts hypoxanthine to xanthine and xanthine to uric acid.
- Alcohol dehydrogenase and aldehyde dehydrogenase oxidize alcohol to acetal-dehyde and acetate respectively.
- Monoamine oxidase oxidizes catecholamines and 5-HT.
- Tyrosine hydroxylase hydroxylates tyrosine to dopa.

Reduction

Reduction occurs in both the microsomal and nonmicrosomal metabolizing system. It is less common than oxidation.

Examples :

Microsomal reduction	Chloramphenicol
Nonmicrosomal reduction	Chloral hydrate, Naloxone

Hydrolysis

Nonmicrosomal hydrolases include:

- Nonspecific esterases for drugs such as procaine, acetylcholine, succinylcholine.

- Amidases for drugs such as procainamide.
- Peptidases e.g. proinsulin.

Microsomal hydrolases have also been identified.
- Cyclization i.e. formation of ring from straight chain compound—proguanil.
- Decyclization i.e. opening of the ring of cyclic drug molecule—barbiturates.

Phase II reactions (synthetic reactions, conjugate reactions)

It is a process by which a drug or its metabolite is coupled (conjugated) enzymatically with an endogenous substance usually a carbohydrate or an amino acid or a derivative of these, resulting almost invariably in inactivation of the parent drug. Nearly all conjugates are inert and water soluble and pass in urine or bile.

The following are the common conjugate reactions (Phase II):

The enzymes involved in the conjugation reactions are called transferases.

Reaction	Drug substrates
Glucuronidation	Morphine, salicylates, digoxin, diazepam, acetaminophen
Sulphation	Acetaminophen, methyldopa
Glycine	Nicotinic acid
Acetylation	Sulphonamides, INH, dapsone
Methylation	Adrenaline, histamine
Glutathione	Paracetamol, ethacrynic acid
Glutamine	PAS

FACTORS WHICH MODIFY BIOTRANSFORMATION

- *Genetics* : Hydrolysis of succinylcholine and acetylation of INH are genetically determined.
- *Chemical properties of drug* i.e. some drugs are enzyme inducers and some are enzyme inhibitors, e.g. phenobarbital stimulates the metabolism of diphenylhydantoin.
- *Dosages* : Toxic dosages can reduced enzymes required for detoxification.
- *Route of administration :* The metabolism is affected by first-pass effect.
- *Diet* : The stores of glycine are depleted due to starvation. This affects glycine conjugation.

- *Age* : In neonates the ability to metabolize drugs such as chloramphenicol is deficient.
- *Organ dysfunction* : In the presence of liver and kidney dysfunction the ability to metabolize and excrete drugs is impaired respectively.
- *Environmental factors* (smoking, food additives) also influence the metabolism of drugs.

The biotransformation may occur in following phases:

- A drug may undergo complete metabolism in phase I and the metabolite excreted. Another drug may not sufficiently metabolize in phase I, undergoes metabolism in phase II and the metabolite is excreted. Certain drugs may be metabolized directly in phase II and the conjugate (inert) is excreted as metabolite. Thus simultaneous and or sequential metabolism of a drug by phase I and phase II reactions may occur. Multiple reactions may occur e.g. chloramphenicol may be reduced and then conjugated.
- In few cases phase II reaction may precede phase I reaction, e.g. INH undergoes metabolism in phase II (acetylation) and N acetyl INH then undergoes phase I (hydrolysis) metabolic process.

STUDY QUESTIONS

1. Define biotransformation.
2. What biotransformation may lead to?
3. Define prodrugs. Give examples.
4. How biotransformation occurs? What are nonsynthetic or Phase I reactions involved in biotransformation? Give suitable examples.
5. What are the sites of biotransformation? Explain synthetic reactions (phase II reactions, conjugate reactions) involved in the biotransformation of drugs? Give appropriate examples.
6. What are the factors which modify biotransformation?

GUIDE FOR FURTHER READING

Correia, M.A. and Ortiz de Montellano, P. Inhibitors of cytochrome P-450 and possibilities for their application. In Frontiers in Biotransformation, Vol 8, Ruckpaul, K (editor). Taylor & Francis, 1993.

Kroemer, H.K. and Klotz, U. Glucuronidation of drugs. A re-evaluation of the pharmacological significance of the conjugates and modulating factors. Clin Pharmacokinet, 1992; 23:292.

La Du BN, Mondel G, Way EL (editor). Fundamentals of drug metabolism and drug disposition. Williams & Wilkins, 1971.

Nelson, D.R., et al. The P450 superfamily: Update on new sequences, gene mapping, accession numbers, early trivial names of enzymes, and nomenclature. DNA Cell Biol, 1993; 12:1.

Vessell, E.S. Genetic and environmental factors causing variation in drug response. Mutation Res, 1991; 247:241.

Wrighton, S.A., and Stevens, J.C. The human hepatic cytochromes P450 involved in drug metabolism. Crit Rev Toxicol, 1992, 22:1-21.

EXCRETION OF DRUGS

EXCRETION AND ELIMINATION

Excretion is passage out of the systemically absorbed drug or its metabolites. Elimination is breakdown (metabolism) plus excretion.

Drug may be excreted unchanged or after biotransformation.

Routes of excretion

The kidney is the most important organ for excretion of drugs. Colon (unabsorbed portion or from bile, excretion through faeces); lungs (volatile drugs, alcohol, general anaesthetics, paraldehyde); saliva, sweat, breast milk and skin are minor routes of excretion.

Importance of knowing routes of excretion

The route of excretion of drugs determines dose and frequency of administration. Clearance is a measure of drug elimination. It is the volume of plasma cleared of the drug in unit time, expressed as ml/minute.

Kinetics and excretion

Kinetics of clearance follows either first order kinetics or zero-order kinetics.

First order kinetics

Majority of drugs follow exponential (first order)

kinetics. Rate of elimination is directly proportional to drug concentration or a constant fraction of the drug present in the body is eliminated in unit time. The rate of elimination decreases as the mass of the drug available decreases. In this system, log-plasma-concentration-time curve is linear. After a single dose about 97% clearance occurs by the end of 5 half-lives or by the elimination rate constant (k) which is equal to $0.693/t_{1/2}$ interval. A steady-state level is reached when intake equals the elimination.

1 $t_{1/2}$	50% drug eliminated
2 $t_{1/2}$	75% (50 + 25) drug eliminated
3 $t_{1/2}$	87.5% (50 + 25 + 12.5) drug eliminated
4 $t_{1/2}$	93.75% (50 + 25 + 12.5 + 6.25) drug eliminated

Zero-order kinetics (saturable or dose-dependent elimination)

Fixed quantity, not a portion, is eliminated per unit e.g. alcohol. The rate of elimination is constant, independent of the mass of drug present.

Few drugs such as alcohol, phenytoin, salicylates follow Zero-order or saturation kinetics where the rate is constant and independent of the mass of drug present. Such drugs saturate eliminating mechanisms and handled by zero-order kinetics. The plasma $t_{1/2}$ is not constant and rises with increasing plasma concentration.

Mixed-order Kinetics

It is a dose dependent kinetics where smaller doses are handled by first-order kinetics but as the plasma concentration reaches higher value (due to increase in dose, the rate of drug elimination becomes zero order because the metabolizing enzymes or the elimination process get saturated at higher concentration). Some drugs such as phenytoin, digoxin, warfarin, dicumarol, tolbutamide and aspirin (higher doses) obey mixed-order elimination kinetics.

In general, the more polar, ionized, less lipid soluble compounds, or drugs metabolized to this form, are poorly reabsorbed and therefore excreted. Excretion in urine involves 3 processes:

1. Glomerular filtration. Water soluble and polar compounds are unable to diffuse back into circulation and are excreted.
2. Active tubular secretion (in the proximal renal tubules). Drugs such as organic acids e.g.

penicillin, bases, quinine are transported by these systems.

3. Passive tubular reabsorption (in the proximal and distal tubules).

It is the nonionized form of weak acids and bases that undergo reabsorption, which depends primarily on the permeability of the tubular epithelium.

The excretion rate of a compound from the kidneys may be assisted, if necessary, by increasing the formation of urine (with diuretics) and by decreasing its reabsorption by appropriate changes of urinary pH. If urine is made more alkaline the weak acids like aspirin and barbiturates are more ionized and less readily reabsorbed. The reverse occurs if the urine is made more acidic. In the case of weak bases, like pethidine and amphetamine alkalinisation and acidification of the urine have the opposite effects, decreasing and increasing excretion, respectively. Strong acids and strong bases remain ionized at all pH ranges of urine and are therefore not reabsorbed. Drugs that are highly water soluble such as penicillins, mannitol, aminoglycosides are not reabsorbed irrespective of pH of the urine.

Lipid solubility and plasma protein binding and kidney dysfunction decrease renal excretion, whereas ionization in renal tubules increases excretion.

Those drugs which remain unabsorbed after oral administration, and metabolites which enter the bile, are excreted in the faeces.

Lungs are involved in the elimination of gaseous general anaesthetics.

Excretion of drugs via the mother's milk is not appreciable per se, but is of considerable importance as a potential source of adverse effects in the nursing infant.

The metabolites of some drugs are not excreted but deposited in certain tissues, e.g. when adrenaline is oxidized to adrenochrome, it can be deposited in conjunctiva and corneal epithelium.

STUDY QUESTIONS

1. Why is it important to know the routes of excretion as well as the rate of excretion of drugs? What is the clinical significance?
2. Which are the usual routes of excretion?
3. What is the difference between elimination and excretion of a drug?
4. Define first-order and zero-order kinetics. Give examples.
5. How rate of excretion determines the steady state?
6. Can the excretion of drugs via mothers' milk be injurious to the nursing infant? Give examples.

GUIDE TO FURTHER READING

Benet, L.Z., et al. Pharmacokinetics: The dynamics of drug absorption, distribution, and elimination. In Goodman and Gilman's The Pharmacological Basis of Therapeutics, 8th ed. Gilman, A.G., et al. (editors). Pergamon, 1990.

Curry, S.H., 1980. Drug Disposition and Pharmacokinetics. Blackwell, Oxford.

Gibson, G., et al., 1986. Introduction to Drug Metabolism. Chapman & Hall, London.

Holford, N.H.G., et al. Understanding the dose-effect relationship. Clin Pharmacokinet, 1981; 6:429.

Jusko, W.J., et al., 1976. Plasma and tissue protein binding of drugs in pharmacokinetics. Drug Metab Reb 5:43.

Lamble, J.W. (ed), 1983. Drug Metabolism and Distribution. Elsevier, Amsterdam.

Levine, R.R., et al. Mechanisms of drug absorption and excretion. Passage of drugs out and into the gastrointestinal tract. Ann Rev Pharmacol., 4:69, 1964.

Milne, M.D., et al. Nonionic diffusion and excretion of weak acids and bases. Am. J. Med., 24:709, 1958.

Pardridge, W.M., et al., 1988. Recent advances in blood-brain barrier transport. Annu Rev Pharmacol Toxicol 28:25-39.

Testa, B., et al. Drug Metabolism: Chemical and Biological Aspects. Marcel Dekker, 1979.

FACTORS MODIFYING DOSAGE AND DRUG ACTION

FACTORS INFLUENCING DOSING

The blood level and therapeutic effectiveness depend on dose of drug within the body, distribution, route of administration and speed of elimination.

Half-life, steady state

Half-life

Half-life of a drug can serve as a general guide to dosage schedule. The dose interval is decided by plasma half-life ($t_{1/2}$).

The speed of elimination is the main factor in deciding the duration of action.

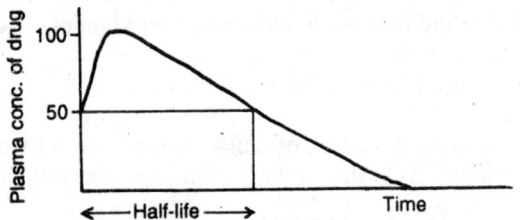

Fig. 1.8. The plasma level of a drug after a single I.V. injection. The plasma half-life ($t_{1/2}$) is the time taken for the plasma concentration to drop by 50 percent.

Half-life ($t_{1/2}$) is the time in which a measure (concentration or effect) declines by 50% (Fig. 1.8).

Half-life is measured in 3 ways, viz. (a) plasma $t_{1/2}$; (b) biological effect $t_{1/2}$ (effect declines by one half); and (c) biological half-life (time in which the total amount of drug in the body after equilibrium of plasma with other compartments (fat, muscle, etc.) is halved. The plasma and biological half-life are close and parallel.

The duration of $t_{1/2}$ is determined by (a) rate of clearance i.e. duration is shorter if the elimination is faster; (b) $t_{1/2}$ is increased by plasma protein binding. Drug is almost completely eliminated after 5 $t_{1/2}$ time. It is true in most of the cases. However, the activity of a drug may continue due to the presence of active metabolites. In some cases the activity may continue for a long time if effects are irreversible ('Hit and run' drugs) e.g. reserpine, organophosphorus compounds. Pathological states (renal or hepatic dysfunction) may increase $t_{1/2}$.

Drug with short plasma $t_{1/2}$ are given at 4, 6 or 8 hourly intervals, while drugs with long half-life (more than 12 hours) have slow rate of clearance, are cumulative in nature and take long time to reach the steady-state level, e.g. digitoxin ($t_{1/2}$ 6.7 days) will take about a month to achieve the steady state.

Rapidly excreted drug with short $t_{1/2}$ requires frequent dosages to maintain constant concentration in the body. Slowly excreted drug with long half-life can be given less often.

Steady-state level

During the time of absorption, the drug concentration in plasma rises, during the time of distribution, the concentration declines rapidly, and during the time of elimination (elimination phase) there is a steady decline.

During the initial period, the intake of the drug is higher than elimination, but when the intake equals the elimination, a steady-state level of plasma concentration is reached. This state is reached after 5 $t_{1/2}$ in case of drug which follow first-order kinetics. The maintenance dose is equivalent to daily clearance of the drug.

Penicillin G has $t_{1/2}$ less than 1 hour as it is rapidly excreted by kidneys, so steady state will be reached in about 5 hours; digoxin $t_{1/2}$ is 36 hours, so steady state is reached at $36 \times 5 = 180$ hours when maintenance doses are given. In order to hasten to achieve steady state with more slowly excreted drugs such as digoxin, a large loading dose may be given followed by smaller maintenance doses.

The approximate half-lives of certain drugs are given below:

Less than 2 hours	Aspirin, benzyl penicillin, amoxicillin, ampicillin, cephalosporins, cloxacillin, rifampicin, gentamicin, heparin, levo-dopa, lignocaine, nitroglycerin
2 to 5 hours	Erythromycin, ethambutol, INH, paracetamol, propranolol, prednisolone, salbutamol, streptomycin, tubocurarine
5 to 10 hours	Sulphonamides, tetracyclines, quini-dine, clonidine, chlordiazepoxide, tolbutamide, nifedipine
10 to 24 hours	Lorazepam, lithium, imipramine, desi-pramine, valproic acid
24 to 36 hours	Nitrazepam, phenytoin, chlorpromazine, diazoxide
More than 36 hours	Digoxin, diazepam, thyroxin, phenobarbitone

DOSING SCHEDULES

- The drugs having very short half-life e.g. norepinephrine 1-2 min.; dopamine 3-5 min.; oxytocin 3-5 min. are usually given by a constant I.V. infusion to maintain their steady state plasma concentration.

- The drugs having a short half-life i.e. between 30 min. to 2 hours, e.g. cephalexin less than 1 hour; benzylpenicillin less than one hour; paracetamol 2 hours, can be given every 6 to 8 hourly by doubling the dose. Giving such drugs every half-life is obviously inconvenient.

- The drugs having half-life between 4 to 12 hours are usually administered at every half-life interval.
- The drugs having half-life 12-24 hours are given at 12 hourly interval. If the half-life of the drug is 24 hours, half of the therapeutic dose is given at every half of the half-life. For example if the dose is 100mg then $100 \times 12/24 = 50$ mg is to be given at 12 hourly interval.
- Drugs having longer half-life usually have high volume of distribution (640L) e.g., digoxin 40 hrs., desipramine 20-60 hrs. (30-60L) diazepam about 40 hours (50-70L), digitoxin about 168 hours (38L) and chloroquine 40 hours (130L) these usually have slow rate of clearance and are cumulative in nature. Usually 5 half-lives are needed to reach the steady state plasma concentration so several days will be required to achieve the desired therapeutic effect for such drugs. Hence, in such cases an initial loading dose (priming dose) is administered then followed by a maintenance dose to maintain the already attained steady state-plasma concentration.

Example : If the desired plasma concentration of digoxin for therapeutic effect is 1-2 µg/L and its apparent volume of distribution (Vd) is 640L then its loading dose will be 1-2 µg × 640 = 640 to 1280 µg or 0.64 to 1.28 mg, the average 0.9 mg will be administered.

The maintenance dose is usually half of the loading dose given every half-life i.e. 0.45 mg every 40 hours. However, it is inconvenient hence the dose is scaled down to every 24 hours $0.45 \times 24/40 = 0.27$ mg. i.e. 0.27mg is required. In practice it is given 0.25 mg every 24 hours and as it is a cumulative drug, it is given 5 days a week.

FACTORS MODIFYING DRUG ACTION AND DOSAGE REGIME

Factors that determine relationship between dose and drug effects are given below.

Pharmacokinetic consideration (Fig. 1.9)

Age

Smaller dosages for the children and the aged are usually necessary as both categories are hyperactive.

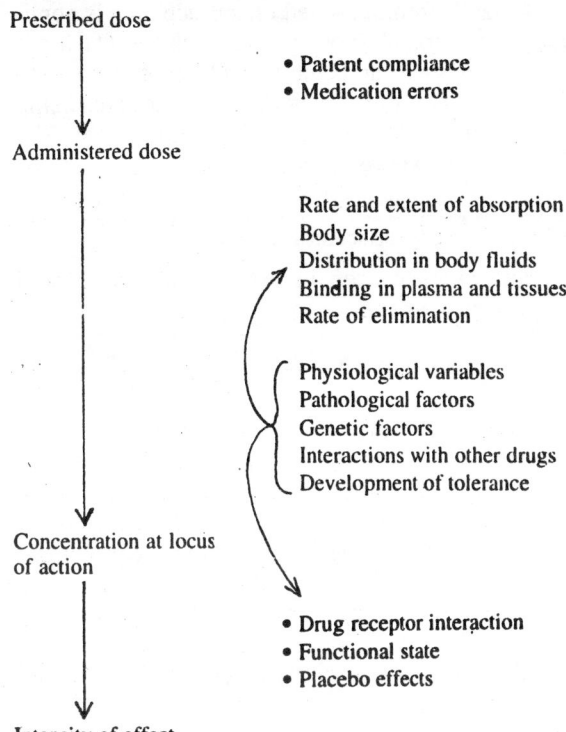

Fig. 1.9. Relationship between prescribed dose and drug effect.

The dose in children may be calculated by employing the following formulae:

Young's formula (2-12 years) :

$$\frac{Age}{Age + 12} \times AD = child's\ dose$$

Clark's formula :

$$\frac{Weight\ in\ kg}{70} \times AD = child's\ dose$$

Cowling's rule :

$$\frac{Age\ at\ next\ birth\ day}{24} \times AD = child's\ dose$$

Dilling's formula :

$$\frac{Age}{20} \times AD = child's\ dose$$

Fried's formula :

$$\frac{Age\ in\ months}{150} \times AD = infant's\ dose$$

Gatzel's formula based on surface area is applicable for all infants, young children and adults. More accurate dosage can be obtained by relating dose to the surface area of the patient, the surface area being derived from the patient's height and weight. The dose is then expressed as:

$$\frac{\text{Body surface area in m}^2 \text{ of child}}{1.7 \text{ (average body surface area in adult)}} \times AD = \text{child's dose}$$

The surface area in m² may be calculated employing Mosteller's formula:

$$\text{Surface area (m}^2) = \sqrt{\frac{\text{height (cm)} \times \text{weight (kg)}}{3600}}$$

However, a child is not a small adult. One should be very careful in calculating the dose particularly in immature newborn. Many drug metabolizing enzymes are inadequate in infants and particularly in immature infants so the drug effect may be prolonged or may produce adverse effects. Similarly in old age the drug metabolizing enzymes may be insufficient and therefore less should be given. There are also certain ailments where the dose is not calculated according to the age but based on the severity of the diseases, for example, diabetes mellitus and diphtheria etc.

Body weight

The average dose is for adults weighing about 70 kg; in obesity this dose may be less.

Sex

Care should be taken during pregnancy and lactation. Drugs like morphine cross placental barrier and depress foetal respiration.

Time and place

Hypnotics are more effective at night. At high altitude due to low barometric pressure body's capacity to oxidize drugs is reduced. The absorption is quicker when the drug is taken on empty stomach.

Route of administration

More dose with oral route than parenteral; same drug may produce different effects by different routes, e.g. magnesium sulphate, castor oil; magnesium sulphate is purgative orally, I.V. injection produces CNS depression, topically reduces swelling. Castor oil topically is soothing and orally purgative.

Physiological variables

Changes in water and electrolyte balance, and acid base states may modify drug effects. Phenylbutazone by increasing sodium and water retention antagonises guanethidine effect. Thiazide diuretics and other drugs causing hypokalaemia will result in increased digitalis toxicity.

Pathological states

Liver disease interferes with detoxification and kidney disease interferes with excretion, for example, morphine is given in smaller doses to patients suffering from liver diseases as it is inactivated in liver. Dose of phenobarbitone should be reduced in renal insufficiency since it is mainly excreted by kidneys.

Genetic factors

Plasma cholinesterase deficiency results in prolonged paralysis with suxamethonium; Glucose-6-phosphate dehydrogenase (G-6-PD) deficiency results in acute haemolysis with aspirin, sulphonamides, primaquine, chloroquine.

Drug allergy or hypersensitivity
(Discussed elsewhere in this Chapter)

Drug abuse and drug dependence
(Discussed elsewhere in this Chapter)

Tolerance

True tolerance can be natural as well as acquired. The natural tolerance may be species and racial tolerance, e.g. rabbit can tolerate large amount of atropine (species tolerance); instillation of ephedrine in eye does not promptly dilate pupil in blacks (racial tolerance).

The acquired tolerance is produced by the repeated administration of certain drugs e.g. morphine, barbiturates. Larger doses have to be used to produce the previous effect. True tolerance is due to (1) rapid detoxification which may be congenital or acquired e.g. barbiturates, (2) cellular or adaptational e.g. morphine, nicotine. True acquired tolerance includes tissue tolerance which means that tolerance develops to certain actions of drugs, e.g. tolerance develops to euphoriant effect of morphine but the pupillary constriction and constipating effect on the gastrointestinal tract do not develop tolerance. It also includes cross tolerance which means that drugs belonging to the same chemical group show tolerance, e.g. if tolerance develops to the effect of glyceryl trinitrate, that individual will also show tolerance to pentaerythritol tetranitrate.

Pseudotolerance develops due to poor absorption. It is observed only with certain orally administered drugs. This type of tolerance will not be observed, if some other route of administration is adopted.

Tachyphylaxis is acute tolerance. The response decreases on repeated administration of certain drugs at short intervals of time, e.g. ephedrine's action in asthma and on blood pressure. It is due to very slow disappearance of the drug from its combination with receptors.

Drug resistance or bacterial resistance

It affects drug action and dosage.

Cumulation

Digitalis glycosides, salicylates are cumulative drugs, hence the subsequent doses are reduced.

Drug combinations

Additive (simple summation of effect) : The effect of 2 or more drugs having same effect when given together produce an effect that is equal in magnitude to the sum of the effects when the drugs are given individually e.g. aspirin and paracetamol.

Drug AB = Drug A + Drug B   (1 + 1 = 2)

Supra-additive :

Synergism : Presence of one drug increases intensity or duration of action of other drug e.g. codeine + aspirin. The total effect is greater than the sum of their individual effects.

Drug AB > Drug A + Drug B   (1 + 1 = > 2)

Potentiation : One drug may be inert but when combined with another effective drug, the effect is more than that of the effective drug, for example, ammonium chloride and mercurial diuretic.

Drug AB > Drug A + Drug B   (0 + 1 = > 1)

Some consider synergism and potentiation same.

Antagonism between drugs (opposing actions) :

Drug AB < Drug A + Drug B

1. *Pharmacologic antagonism* : Antagonism occurs when an antagonist prevents an agonist from interacting with its receptors to produce an effect.

It can be either of the following:

- *Competitive antagonism* : Competitive antagonist competes with agonist in a reversible manner for the same receptor site. The log dose-response curve is shifted to the right indicating that higher concentration of agonist is necessary to achieve the same response as when the antagonist is absent e.g. acetylcholine and atropine (reversible).

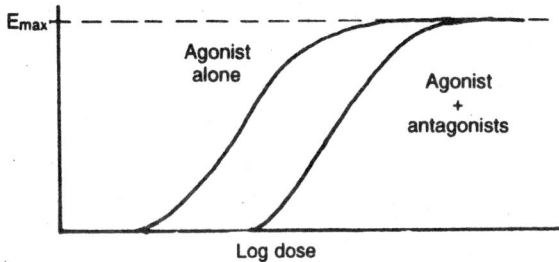

Competitive antagonism results in parallel shift.

- *Noncompetitive antagonism* : Antagonist binds irreversibly to the receptor site. The action of the antagonist cannot be overcome no matter how much agonist is given. There is a nonparallel shift of the log dose-response curve with a lower E_{max}. For example, adrenaline and phenoxybenzamine (irreversible).

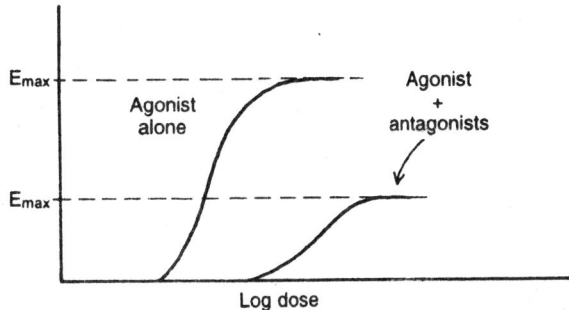

Noncompetitive antagonism results in nonparallel shift with a lower E_{max} (maximum effect).

2. Physical e.g. vitamin A and liquid paraffin.
3. Chemical neutralization e.g. antacids and gastric HCl.
4. Physiological (antagonists act on different receptor sites) e.g. histamine and adrenaline.
5. Antagonism due to drug interactions.

Psychological factors

Emotional and attitudinal factors modify therapeutic response in a patient.

Factors influencing dosage and drug action have been summarized below.

STUDY QUESTIONS

1. What is half-life? How does it serve as a general guide to dosage schedules. Give approximate half-lives of certain drugs.
2. What do you mean by steady-state level?
3. Calculate a dose of drug A for a child of 10 years, if the adult dose is 500 mg.
4. Give different formulae to calculate the dose for a child.
5. Give a formula to calculate the dose for an infant (6 months old).
6. Which is the most accurate formula for calculating the dose for all (infant to the adult)?
7. Name a few conditions where the dose is not dependent on age.
8. How do routes of administration, physiological and pathological factors influence drug action?
9. How do genetic factors, drug allergy and drug dependence affect drug action?
10. Discuss drug combinations producing synergism and potentiation.
11. Explain placebo.
12. Define drug tolerance. What are the different types of tolerance?
13. Give examples of certain drugs which have cumulative effects. How will cumulation affect drug action?
14. What determines onset, duration and intensity of drug effect?
15. Which factors influence blood level and therapeutic effectiveness?

GUIDE TO FURTHER READING

La Du B.N., et al. Fundamentals of Drug Metabolism and Drug Disposition. Williams & Wilkins, 1971.

Klotz, U., et al. The effects of age and liver disease on the disposition and elimination of diazepam in adult man. J. Clin. Invest., 55:347-359; 1975.

Vessell, E.S., et al. Genetic and environmental factors causing variation in drug response. Mutation Res., 1991; 247:241.

Wood, A.J.J., et al. Ethnic differences in drug disposition and responsiveness. Clin Pharmacokinet, 1991; 20:350.

Zanger, U.M., et al. Absence of hepatic cytochrome P450 causes genetically deficient debrisoquin oxidation in man. Biochemistry, 1988; 27:5447.

Zhou, H.H., et al. Racial differences in drug response: Altered sensitivity to and clearance of propranolol in men of Chinese descent as compared with American males. N. Engl. J. Med., 1989; 320:565.

DRUG INTERACTIONS (DIs)

When two or more drugs are given together or close to each other they may act
- Independent of each other
- Interact

Factors influencing dosage and drug action (summarized)

Biological factors	Modified drug effects	Modified drug effects
- Age, body weight	After repeated administration of a single drug:	After concurrent administration of two different drugs:
- Tolerance		
- Surface area	- tolerance	- additive effect
- Time and place of administration	- resistance	- synergism
- Psychological and emotional factors	- allergy	- potentiation
- Genetic factors	- cumulation	- antagonism
- Metabolic disturbances and pathological state		

Drug interaction is a phenomenon of two or more drugs interacting in such a way that effectiveness or toxicity of one or more drugs is altered.

The concept of drug interaction has been extended to include (besides drug-drug interactions) situation in which :

- Food or dietary items influence the activity of a drug.
- Environmental chemicals or smoking influences the activity of a drug.
- Drug-disease interactions where a drug causes undesired effects with certain disease states.
- Drug-laboratory test interaction where a drug causes alteration of laboratory test results.

Drug interactions may be useful in some cases and harmful in many cases.

The knowledge of drug interactions is essential for safe drug therapy.

The problem of drug interactions is increasing. The factors which contribute to the occurrence of drug interactions are:

- Multiple pharmacological effects: Most drugs can influence many physiological systems; two concomitantly administered drugs will affect some of the same systems.
- Polypharmacy employing potent drugs, and particularly if large doses are used.
- Multiple physicians: One may prescribe antihistamine and other may prescribe anti-anxiety agent resulting in excessive depressant effect.
- Concurrent use of prescription and non-prescription drugs.
- Drug abuse: Many patients may be taking drugs such as barbiturates, narcotics, amphetamine.

Sites and mechanism of drug interactions

- In vitro interactions
- In vivo interactions

In vitro interactions

When drugs are added to an I.V. drip or mixed in syringe, problem may arise. Some examples:

Penicillins	Tetracycline	Precipitate
Penicillins	Gentamicin	Inactivated
Gentamicin	Heparin	Precipitate
Gentamicin	Carbenicillin	Inactivated
Hydrocortisone	Tetracycline	Precipitate
Dextrose solution	Penicillin	Inactivated
(sterilized by auto-	Ampicillin	Inactivated
claving has low pH)	Heparin	Inactivated
	Erythromycin	Inactivated
	Hydrocortisone	Inactivated

In vivo interactions

Two important types:
1. Pharmacokinetic interactions i.e. alteration in the delivery of drugs to their site of action.
2. Pharmacodynamic interactions i.e. responsiveness of the target organ or system modified by other agents.

Pharmacokinetic drug interactions

Interactions at site of absorption

- Direct interaction in the gut: Tetracyclines complex with Ca^{++}, Mg^{++} salts (antacid mixture), tetracyclines and iron salts are bound in unabsorbed complex.
- Gut motility: Anticholinergics reduce gastric and intestinal motility, so stay of drugs in stomach is prolonged. Purgatives reduce the time spent in small intestine.
- pH of gut contents: Antacids raise gastric pH, so acidic drugs are more ionized and hence more slowly absorbed.
- Alteration of gut flora: Antimicrobials may potentiate oral anticoagulants by reducing bacterial synthesis of vitamin K in the large gut.
- Relatively specific defects in absorption occur, e.g. phenytoin impairs absorption of folic acid.

interaction during distribution

Displacement interaction (competition for plasma protein binding) : Drugs with greater binding affinity or capacity cause displacement from tissues and plasma binding sites of those drugs which are less strongly bound. Some examples:

Strongly bound	Drug displaced	Effect of interaction
Phenylbutazone	Warfarin	Haemorrhage
Phenylbutazone	Tolbutamide	↑ Hypoglycaemia
Sulphonamides	Tolbutamide	↑ Hypoglycaemia
Salicylates	Methotrexate	↑ Activity and toxicity of methotrexate

Interaction during metabolism

The biotransformation occurs largely in liver, executed by the mixed function oxidase enzymes :

Enzyme inducers : Drugs whose metabolism is increased resulting in reduced activity

Cigarette	Paracetamol, benzodiazepines
Phenytoin	Digitoxin, quinidine, beta-blockers, doxycycline
Rifampin	Oral contraceptives, corticosteroids, tolbutamide, calcium channel blockers, β-adrenoceptor blockers, phenytoin
Barbiturates	Corticosteroids, beta-adrenoceptor blockers, calcium channel blockers, oestradiol, phenytoin

Enzyme inhibitors : Drugs whose metabolism is inhibited resulting in increased activity :

Action on hepatic microsomal enzymes :

Chloramphenicol	Phenytoin, tolbutamide
Sodium valproate	Phenobarbitone, phenytoin

Action on xanthine oxidase :

Allopurinol	6-Mercaptopurine

Action on monoamine oxidase :

MAO inhibitors	Tricyclic antidepressants

Action on aldehyde dehydrogenase :

Disulfiram	Alcohol, phenytoin
Metronidazole	Warfarin, some benzodiazepines

Angiotensin-converting enzyme :

Enalapril	Angiotensin I, bradykinin

Interaction during excretion

Primary drug	Competing drug	Result
Penicillins	Probenecid	Prolonged action of penicillins
Salicylate	Probenecid	Salicylate toxicity
Indomethacin	Probenecid	Indomethacin toxicity
Lithium	Thiazide	Lithium toxicity
Digoxin	Spironolactone	Digoxin toxicity
Methotrexate	Salicylate	Increased methotrexate levels
Methotrexate	Sulphonamide	Increased methotrexate levels

Interference with passive diffusion: Alteration of urinary pH influences ionization of drugs and their excretion. Basic drugs are better excreted in acidic urine (e.g. excretion of amphetamine is increased by giving ammonium chloride and acidic drugs are better excreted in alkaline urine (e.g., enhanced excretion of aspirin occurs if sodium bicarbonate is given).

Table 1.7 shows types of pharmacokinetic interactions.

Table 1.7. Types of pharmacokinetic interactions

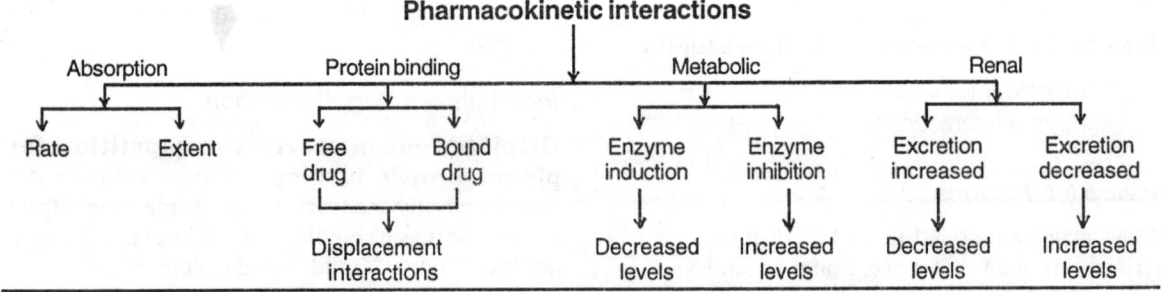

Pharmacodynamic drug interactions

Competition at receptor site

- Atropine blocks cholinergic drugs.
- Phenoxybenzamine blocks alpha-adrenergic receptors.
- Propranolol blocks beta-adrenergic receptors.
- Naloxone is a specific antagonist to morphine.

Inhibition of neuronal uptake

- Tricyclic antidepressants nullify guanethidine action.
- Mutual antagonism or potentiation of drugs acting on same site or influencing same physiological system
- Potentiation of CNS depression by ethanol, hypnotics and antihistamines.

Influence of electrolytes

Drugs causing hypokalaemia such as thiazide diuretics and digitalis results in increased digitalis toxicity. Phenylbutazone by increasing sodium and water retention antagonizes guanethidine action.

Other factors influencing drug interaction

Genetic differences : Toxic hepatitis due to INH is more frequent in rapid acetylators. Lupus erythematosus-like syndrome by hydralazine occurs only in slow acetylators.

Drug-patient interactions : In newborn and in geriatric patients, certain drugs may prove real hazard.

Disease induced changes in plasma binding : The binding of phenytoin is altered in chronic renal failure, unbound drug increased 4-fold.

Examples of some important drug interactions

Useful interactions

- Sulphamethoxazole + Trimethoprim
- Levodopa and Carbidopa
- Disulfiram and alcohol in the treatment of chronic alcoholism.
- Probenecid increases penicillin levels.

Interactions leading to ineffective therapy

Imipramine, Phenylbutazone	Guanethidine	Loss of B.P. control
Barbiturates	Warfarin	Loss of anti-coagulant effect
Oral iron salt	Tetracycline	Mutual loss of effect
Thiazides	Tolbutamide	Control of blood sugar more difficult

Interactions leading to harmful effects

Phenylbutazone	Tolbutamide	Hypoglycaemia
Dicumarol	Phenytoin	↑ Phenytoin effect
Phenobarbitone	Phenytoin	↓ Phenytoin effect
Phenylbutazone	Warfarin	Haemorrhage
Diuretics	Digitalis	↑ Digitalis toxicity
Anticoagulants	Aspirin	Haemorrhage
Sulphonylureas	Aspirin	↑ Hypoglycaemia

Drug-vitamin interactions

- Clofibrate and colchicine decrease absorption of Vitamin B_{12}.
- Alcohol decreases absorption of vitamin B_{12} and also folic acid.
- Liquid paraffin interferes with absorption of vitamins A, D, E and K.
- Vitamin C enhances excretion of tetracyclines, hydralazine enhances vitamin B_6 excretion.
- Phenytoin stimulates folic acid, vitamin D and vitamin K metabolism. The long-term use of phenytoin may lead to lowered serum folic acid levels resulting in megaloblastic anaemia.
- Folic acid increases rate of metabolism of phenytoin, resulting in reduction in blood level of phenytoin.
- Oral contraceptives result in deficiency of folic acid, vitamins B_6, B_{12} and C.

Effect of smoking : Due to the action of polycyclic hydrocarbons that are present in cigarette smoke, there is increased hepatic enzyme activity in individuals who are heavy smokers. Among the drugs whose metabolism is increased and so the therapeutic activity is likely to be reduced are chlorpromazine diazepam, propoxyphene, theophylline, pentazocine, and tricyclic antidepressants.

It should be noted that if the patient stops smoking and is still taking medication, the dosage that had been adequate is now likely to be excessive and will have to be reduced.

In contrast, a significant risk of toxicity exists when oral contraceptives are used by women who smoke, as it has been noted that smoking markedly increases the risk of serious cardiovascular effects e.g. myocardial infarction (MI) especially in women over 35 years of age.

Food-drug interactions

Tetra-cyclines	Milk	Non-absorbable tetracycline complex with Ca in milk and milk products
Iron salts	Eggs, milk	Absorption of iron is decreased due to the insoluble chelate formation
Bishydroxy-coumarin	Food rich in vitamin K, citrus fruits, egg yolk, leafy green vegetables, fish, potato chips	Decreased prothrombin time

Charcoal broiling - when meat is charcoal broiled, polycyclic hydrocarbons are formed and deposited on the meat. It will increase the rate of metabolism of theophylline.

Environmental factors - DDT and related materials may increase the activity of liver enzymes and thus increase the rate of metabolism of other drugs.

Herb - Drug Interactions

Data is limited. Few examples indicate that as with any other drug, there is possibility of herb-drug interactions.

Concomitant use of shankapushpi and phenytoin can reduce blood levels of phenytoin.

If liquorice is used concomitantly with oral or topical corticosteroids, there is potentiation of the effect of corticosteroids.

Mania has resulted in patients of depression who mix antidepressant with panax ginseng.

Drug - disease interactions

- **D isease states** - Impaired renal and hepatic function are the most important conditions that may alter drug activity.
- If there is renal impairment and the usual dose of a drug that is excreted by the kidney is given, there can be an increased and prolonged effect, since it is not being excreted at the normal rate.
- When there is hepatic damage, drugs which are metabolized in the liver may be metabolized at a slower rate and exhibit a prolonged effect.

How to minimise DIs

The occurrence of drug interactions can be minimized if :
1. Careful history from the patient is taken.
2. Multiple drug therapy (polypharmacy) is avoided.
3. By giving proper instructions of possible dangers if the patient changes or adds other drugs without consulting physician.

STUDY QUESTIONS

1. Define drug interaction (DI).
2. Why is the knowledge of DIs essential?
3. Is the problem of DIs increasing? If so, why?
4. Give suitable examples of in vitro DIs.
5. Give suitable examples of DIs at the following pharmacokinetic sites:
   (a) Intestinal absorption
   (b) Distribution and storage sites
   (c) Liver (main site for the biotransformation)
   (d) Excretion site
6. Give appropriate examples of pharmacodynamic drug interactions at receptor site.
7. Describe factors which influence drug interactions.
8. Give examples of some useful drug interactions.
9. Give examples of interactions leading to (a) ineffective therapy and (b) harmful effects.
10. Give examples of food-drug interactions.
11. What steps will minimize the occurrence of drug interactions?

GUIDE TO FURTHER READING

Cluff, L.E., Petrie, J.C. Clinical Effects of Interaction Between Drugs. Excerpta Medica, 1974.

Jankel, C.A. and Speedie, S.M. Detecting drug interactions. A review of the literature. Ann Pharmacother, 1990; 24:982.

Lam, Y.W.F., Shepherd A.M.A. Drug interactions in hypertensive patients. Pharmacokinetic, pharmacodynamic and genetic considerations. Clin Pharmacokinet, 1990; 18:295.

Peck, C.C. Understanding consequences of concurrent therapies. JAMA, 1993, 269:1550-1552.

Rizack, M.A. (Editor). The Medical Letter Handbook of Adverse Interactions. The Medical Letter, 1993.

Smith, N.T., Miller, R.D. and Corbascio, A.N. Drug Interactions in Anesthesia, Lea & Febiger, 1981.

ADVERSE DRUG REACTIONS (ADRs)

Adverse drug reactions (ADRs) are of great concern to the general public, physicians, pharmacists, drug regulatory authorities and the pharmaceutical industry. Any drug, no matter how trivial its therapeutic actions may be, has the potential to do harm. ADR-monitoring and reporting programme in a hospital encourages ADR-surveillance.

WHO defines ADR as "any response to a drug which is noxious and unintended and which occurs at doses normally used in man for prophylaxis, diagnosis or therapy of disease or for modification of a physiological function".

Rawlins and Thomson in 1977 classified ADRs into type A and type B.

The prominent difference between type A and type B reaction are summarized in Table 1.8.

Types of adverse effects

- *Side effects* are due to the actions on organ systems other than on the desired system in therapeutic doses and usually do not necessitate stopping of treatment. Phenobarbitone when used as an antiepileptic produces drowsiness as a side effect, atropine induces dryness of mouth as a side effect when used for abdominal colic.

Table 1.8. Differences between type A and type B adverse Drug Reactions

Type A	Type B
Qualitatively normal but augmented response to drugs	Bizarre effects
Predictable	Unpredictable on the basis of known pharmacology of drug
Effects are dose dependent	Effects are unrelated to dose
Relatively common	Comparatively rare
Do not generally cause serious illness	Can cause serious illness
Resolve when the dose is reduced	Serious illness warrants complete withdrawal of drug
Some examples of Type A reactions :	*Some examples of Type B reactions :*
Analgesic nephropathy Chloroquine retinopathy Chlorpromazine induced parkinsonism	Pharmacogenetics (unusual attributes of the patient interacts with the drug including inherited abnormalities)
	Hypersensitivity (e.g. anaphylaxis, allergic skin rashes, photoallergy, acute angioedema, hypersensitivity mediated blood dyscrasias, Stevens-Johnson syndrome.

In most cases the side effects are not desirable but in few cases the side effect may be desirable, e.g. reserpine in the patient suffering from hypertension is benefited by some of its side effects such as bradycardia, calmness and laxative effects.

- *Toxic effects* (overdosage effects) are due to the exaggerated undesirable pharmacological effects related to the amount of drug in the body (toxic dose, therapeutic dose in intolerant person or prolonged use of cumulative drugs).

- *Pharmacogenetic effects* (Genetic anomalies) are responsible for many quantitative or qualitative abnormalities in the effects of drugs. These abnormalities usually result in adverse drug reactions (ADRs).

Examples:
- Succinylcholine apnoea due to deficiency of the enzyme pseudocholinesterase
- Slow and rapid acetylation of INH
- Resistance to warfarin
- Primaquine induced haemolysis in patients with deficiency of glucose 6-phosphate dehydrogenase.
- *Idiosyncrasy* is a drug reaction that is qualitatively different from the usual effects and can not be attributed to drug allergy. It may be due to genetic variation. In some cases the genetic basis is not yet clear for the idiosyncratic reactions, for example, aplastic anaemia caused by chloramphenicol.

Certain pharmacogenetic effects are given in Table 1.9.

Table 1.9. Some pharmacogenetic examples

Condition	Aberrant enzyme	Drugs producing abnormal response
Glucose 6-phosphate dehydrogenase	G6-PD	Sulphonamides, sulphones, quinine, quinidine, aspirin chloramphenicol
Slow inactivation of INH	Isoniazid acetylase in liver	INH, dapsone, hydralazine
Succinylcholine sensitivity	Pseudo ChE in plasma	Succinylcholine
Malignant hyperthermia with muscular rigidity	Unknown	Halothane, ether succinylcholine
Warfarin resistance	? altered receptor or enzyme in liver with increased affinity for vitamin K	Warfarin

It may be that many reactions now classified as idiosyncratic or even allergic will eventually be recognized as pharmacogenetic disorders or acquired enzyme deficiencies.
- *Hypersensitivity* (allergic) reactions may be due to drug itself or its metabolite which show abnormal symptoms (unrelated to pharmacological actions) and are not dose-related. They are classified as types I, II, III (all immediate types) and IV (delayed on the basis of mechanism involved).

Chemical allergy is an adverse reaction that results from previous sensitization to a particular chemical or to one that is structurally similar. Such reactions are mediated by the immune system. The terms hypersensitivity and drug allergy often are used to describe the allergic state.

Type I	Mild: urticaria, angioneurotic oedema Severe: anaphylaxis
Type II	(Cytotoxic): Thrombocytopenia, haemolytic anaemia, agranulocytosis
Type III	Drug fever, serum sickness
Type IV	T cell mediated delayed reaction: dermatitis, aplastic anaemia, hepatitis

The features of allergic reactions are:
- No relation to pharmacological action
- Not dose-related
- Reaction only on reexposure
- Reactions are reversible and seen in few patients

- *Special toxicities* such as teratogenicity (abnormal development of foetus) and oncogenicity (cancer producing activity).
- *Iatrogenic diseases* (drug induced) e.g. peptic ulcer with aspirin and phenylbutazone; parkinsonism after phenothiazines and reserpine; deafness after streptomycin.
- *Secondary effects*, e.g. superinfection and vitamin deficiency due to prolonged antibiotic therapy. These are indirect consequence of pharmacological action.

How to minimize adverse effects

To minimize the problem of adverse reactions to drugs:
- Good knowledge of drugs is essential.
- Drugs should not be over prescribed. The incidence of adverse reactions increases with the number of drugs prescribed.
- Drugs must not be used indiscriminately.
- Reactions should be recognized early, and necessary remedial steps taken.

Some important adverse effects

Some important adverse drug reaction are given in Table 1.10.

Table 1.10. Important adverse drug reactions

Agent	Condition induced
	Hepatotoxicity
Paracetamol metabolites, methotrexate, sodium valproate	Direct (predictable) hepatocellular damage
Methotrexate	Fibrosis
Clofibrate	Cholelithiasis
Oral contraceptives	Hepatic tumours
Chlorpromazine, erythromycin	Cholestatic jaundice (unpredictable)
INH, rifampicin, pyrazinamide, halothane, ethionamide	Hepatitis-like reaction (unpredictable)
	Renal Toxicity
NASIDs	Interstitial nephritis (allergic type)
Penicillins ACE inhibitors	Nephrotic syndrome
Sulfonamides	Glomerular nephritis
Aminoglycoside	Tubular necrosis
	Haematological toxicity
Primaquine, probenecid sulphomanides, chloramphenicol, sulphones, quinine, salicylates	Haemolytic anaemia in G-6PD deficiency.
Sulphonamides, sulphones, phenytoin, methotrexate	Megaloblastic anaemia
Nitrites and nitrates, sulphones,	Methemoglobinemia
Cytotoxic drugs	Aplastic anaemia
Chloramphenicol, gold salts, penicillamine, indomethacin, sulphonamides, sulphones, phenylbutazone	Agranulocytosis
Quinidine, quinine, α-methyldopa, aspirin, thiazide derivatives, heparin, valproic acid, rifampicin, gold preparation	Thrombocytopenia

Agent	Condition induced
	Endocrinal
Probenecid, aspirin, thiazide diuretics, loop susceptible diuretics, ethambutol, pyrazinamide, 6-mercaptopurine	Hyperuricacmia (with perception of gout in individuals)
	Hyperglycaemia
Corticosteroids, oral contraceptives, thiazide and loop diuretics	
	Teratogenicity (foetal abnormalities)
Thalidomide, penicillamine, warfarin, phenytoin, sod. valproate, trimethadione, folate antagonists (methotrexate), antithyroid drugs, androgens, progestogens, vitamin A	
	Neurotoxicity
Haloperidol, and other antipsychotic phenothiazines (except thioridazine)	Parkinsonism and other extrapyramidal disorders
Analeptics, xylocaine, INH, theophylline, amphetamine, cyclosporin, vincristine, lithium carbonate	Convulsions
INH	Peripheral neuritis
Iodochlorohydroxy quinoline (amoebicidal drug)	Subacute myelo-optic neuropathy (SMON)
Indomethacin, nitroglycerin, hydralazine	Headache
	Dermatological toxicity
Long acting sulphonomides, sulphones, barbiturates, phenytoin	Stevens-Johnson Syndrome
Heparin, cyclophosphamide and other cytotoxic drugs, oral contraceptives withdrawal	Alopecia
Tetracycline phenothiazines	Phototoxic
Sulphonamides, thiazides, griseofulvin	Photoallergic
	Disorders of GIT
Aspirin, indomethacin, glucocorticoids	Peptic ulceration or gastric haemorrhage

(Contd.)   *(Contd.)*

Agent	Condition induced
Opioids, ganglion blockers, aluminium hydroxide, ferrous sulphate, phenothiazines, tricyclic antidepressants	Constipation
	Psychiatric disorders
Reserpine, methyldopa, propranolol, cyclosporin corticosteroids, levodopa (rarely)	Depression
Amphetamine, ephedrine, l-dopa, amantadine	Insomnia
Amphetamine, l-dopa MAO inhibitors, corticosteroids	Schizophrenia-like state
l-dopa, amantadine, bromocriptine, pentazocine, propranolol	Hallucinatory states
	Cardiovascular disorders
Emetine, daunorubicin, doxorubicin, lithium carbonate	Cardimyopathy
Sympathomimetics, thyroid hormones, emetine	Cardiac arrhythmias
Corticosteroids clonidine withdrawal	Hypertension
	Disorders of the ear
Aminoglycoside antibiotics, salicylates (high doses), quinine, chloroquine, furosemide, ethacrynic acid (diuretic)	Ototoxicity
	Ocular toxicity
Glucocorticoides chloroquine, cardiac glycosides Quinine, ethambutol	Cataract Retinotoxic Optic neuritis
	Dental toxicity
Phenytoin	Gingival hyperplasia
Tetracycline	Dental toxicity
	Pulmonary toxicity
Busulfan, bleomycin	Pulmonary toxicity
	Miscellaneous
Rifampicin	Influenza - like syndrome
Metronidazole, captopril	Metallic taste in mouth

(Contd.)

Agent	Condition induced
Asparaginase (anticancer drug)	Pancreatitis
Hydralazine, procainamide	Lupus erythematosus
Loop diuretics	Gout
Tetracycline	Staining of teeth and bone deformities

Photosensitizing effects can be produced by substances (chemicals) used as medicines or as cosmetics. Photosensitivity includes phototoxic reactions which may be oxygen dependent i.e. photodynamic; or oxygen independent i.e. non-photodynamic. Acute phototoxicity reactions are more common and are manifested by erythema, oedema and blister followed by hyperpigmentation and desquamation. These reactions are confined to sun exposed skin.

Sunburn is induced by ultraviolet B (290 to 320 nm) radiation; chronic reaction in the form of wrinkling, atrophy, hypo- or hyperpigmentation is produced by UVA rays 320-400 nm radiations. Photosensitivity also includes photoallergic reactions which may appear promptly (characterized by immediate wheal and flare) being antibody-mediated (characterized by papular to eczematous process) or delayed being cell-mediated responses. The photoallergic reactions are rather uncommon.

The following are some examples of drug photosensitizers:

Agents	Clinical manifestations	Action spectrum nm
Nalidixic acid	Bullae, fragility	320-360
Phenothiazines	Delayed erythema, eczematous reaction, grey pigmentation	320-400
Quinidine	Delayed erythema	320-400
Sulphonylurea	Delayed erythema	315-400
Tetracyclines	Delayed erythema	350-420
Thiazides	Delayed erythema, delayed eczematous reaction	300-400

The basic law is that nonionizing radiation must be absorbed to produce photochemical and subsequently photobiological reaction.

The therapy is similar for both phototoxic and photoallergic reactions. It includes cool wet dressing, soothing lotions, topical corticosteroids and systemic antipruritic agents.

ADVERSE EFFECTS ON HUMAN FOETAL DEVELOPMENT

Foetal development passes through 3 main stages:
1. Blastocyst formation (gestation period to 16 days) where cell division continues until the primitive streak is formed. Cytotoxic drugs can inhibit cell division and result in death.
   Alcohol may also affect development at this very early stage.
2. Organogenesis (17 to 60 days, first trimester of pregnancy) can be affected by teratogens which can cause gross malformation of structural organs.
3. Histogenesis and functional maturation (60 days—term) can be affected by alcohol, nicotine, antithyroid drugs and steroids.

The following drugs can produce adverse effects on human foetal development.

Agent	Effects
Cytotoxic drugs, especially folate antagonists	Hydrocephalus, cleft palate, rib and limb defects
Heavy metals, especially mercury	Impaired brain development
Anticonvulsant drugs:	
Phenytoin	Cleft lip/palate, mental retardation
Trimethadione	High arched palate, delayed growth, facial abnormalities
Steroid hormones (oestrogens, androgen and progestogens)	Masculanization of female, testicular atrophy, reduced sperm count in male
Ethanol	Cardiac defects, mental retardation, facial abnormalities
Tetracyclines	Staining of teeth, thin tooth enamel, impaired bone growth
Antithyroid drugs	Goitre, hypothyroidism
Coumarin anticoagulants	Retarded growth, defects of limbs, eyes and CNS

The above drugs produce definite adverse effects on foetal development. But the following agents can also possibly produce adverse effects on the foetal development:

General anaesthetics especially halothane, antiemetics such as cyclizine, meclizine and antidepressants like imipramine.

Predisposing factors that influence ADRs

- Drug related factors
  - Drug itself: there are drugs with wide margin of safety and there are drugs with very narrow margin of safety.
  - Formulation: particle size, tablet disintegration and dissolution rate, presence of excipients in dosage form and degree of purity influence drug absorption, thus the potential for adverse effects.
  - Physicochemical properties such as pH, degree of ionization, lipid solubility, protein binding and extent of first-pass metabolism can alter bioavailability of a drug.
  - Dose: Ingestion of excessive amount of a drug will cause a more intense action.
  - Rate and route of administration: there is increased cardiotoxicity with a single I.V. bolus injection of doxorubicin; increased nephrotoxicity with faster infusion rates of cisplatin as compared to slower rates.
- Patient related factors
  - Age: at extremes of age ADR is more frequent. The adverse drug effects are more common in neonates and premature babies. They are more sensitive due to the following factors:
    - Hepatic microsomal drug metabolizing enzyme activity is low resulting in decreased metabolism.
    - There is reduced renal elimination
    - Blood brain barrier is not well developed.
  - In elderly: due to reduced hepatic and renal functions as well as reduced bodymass the adverse effects are more common.
- Sex: higher incidence in women as compared to men.
- Pregnancy: Special care should be taken to avoid any harm to the foetus.
- Disease: Hepatic dysfunction and renal

dysfunction increase severity and frequency of ADR.

• Extrinsic factors : Anticholinergic drugs, antipsychotics, and tricyclic antidepressants may precipitate heat strokes in persons exposed to hot temperature and high humidity environment.

• Multiple drug therapy: It increases the incidence of ADRs.

No drug is "safe" if it fails to cure a serious disease for which a cure is available.

No drug is dangerous to use if it will cure a fatal disease for which no other cure is available.

"Extreme remedies are appropriate for extreme diseases."   – Hippocrates

What was true 24 centuries ago is true today.

STUDY QUESTIONS

1. Define side effects, toxic effects, drug allergy and idiosyncrasy. Give examples.
2. Define teratogenicity and oncogenicity. Give examples.
3. List some important adverse effects manifested in CNS and GIT by certain drugs.
4. How do you measure therapeutic index?
5. Which drugs may produce the following adverse effects:
   (a) Extrapyramidal syndrome
   (b) Ototoxicity
   (c) Cardiotoxicity
   (d) Pulmonary toxicity
   (e) Nephrotoxicity
   (f) Optic neuritis/retinotoxicity
   (g) Hepatotoxicity
6. Name drugs and the effects produced by certain drugs on human foetal development.

GUIDE TO FURTHER READING

Adverse drug reactions (Editorial). Br Med J, 1981; 282:1819.

Chappell, WR. and Mordenti, J. Extrapolation of toxicological and pharmacological data from animals to humans, Adv Drug Res 1991;20:1.

Hurwitz, N. Predisposing factors in adverse reactions to drugs. Br Med J, 1969; 1:56.

Kalter, H., et al. Congenital malformations. N Engl J Med, 1983;308:424,491.

McKhann, G.M. The trials of clinical trials. Arch Neurol, 1989; 46:611.

Parker, C.W. Drug allergy. N Engl J Med, 1975; 292:511.

Rawlins, M.D. Clinical pharmacology: Adverse reactions to drugs. Br Med J, 1981; 282:974.

Rawlins, M.D. Postmarketing surveillance of adverse reactions to drugs. Br Med J, 1984; 288:879.

Riegelman, R.K. Studying a Study & Testing a Test. How to Read the Medical Literature. Little Brown, 1981.

Weller, P.C. Measuring the frequency of adverse drug reactions. Br J Clin Pharmacol, 1992; 33:249.

Zbinden, G and Flury-Reversi, M. Significance of LD_{50}-test for the toxicological evaluation of chemical substances. Arch Toxicol, 1981; 47:77.

MECHANISM OF DRUG ACTION

GENERAL PRINCIPLES

Drugs don't create new function, drugs modify the existing function or replace.

Stimulation : Selective increase in activity in specialized tissues, e.g. adrenaline produces increase in heart rate and force of contraction, caffeine stimulate cerebral cortex.

Depression : Selective decrease in activity in specialized tissues, e.g. barbiturates depress the central nervous system.

Dual action : Some drugs produce both stimulation and depression by acting at different sites, e.g. morphine stimulates vomiting centre and depresses respiratory centre.

Irritation : Produced on nonspecialized tissues, mild irritation produces stimulation and strong irritation produces inflammation and even necrosis.

Replacement : Iron in anaemia, vitamin D in rickets, insulin in diabetes mellitus.

Anti-infective action : Antibacterial drugs e.g. sulphonamides, antibiotics.

SITES OF DRUG ACTION

Drugs may act on (1) cell membrane, (2) intracellular constituents, (3) outside the cell, and (4) possess antimicrobial action.

On cell membrane

• Receptors as agonist or antagonist

- Enzymes and pump e.g. Na^+-K^+-ATPase, noradrenaline uptake pump
- Ion channels e.g. calcium channels
- Physicochemical action with lipid, protein or water constituent of nerve cell membrane e.g. general anaesthetics

---

Box 1.3. Terms associated with mechanism of drug action

- Affinity is ability of a drug to combine with a specific receptor.
- Intrinsic activity is the measure of drug's ability to produce an effect.
- Agonist has both affinity and intrinsic activity.
- Antagonist has affinity but lacks intrinsic activity.
- Partial agonist/partial antagonist has affinity but little intrinsic activity.
- Drug efficacy is its ability to produce a maximum drug effect.
- Drug potency is the relative concentration of two or more drugs that produce the same effect.

On intracellular constituents

- Nuclear receptors
- Enzymes e.g. monoamine oxidase, cholinesterase, xanthine oxidase
- DNA/RNA e.g. with anticancer agents
- Transport carrier molecules e.g. probenecid on renal tubules

Outside the cell

- Chemical interaction e.g. antacids, chelating agents, alkalizing and acidifying agents
- Physical mechanism e.g. osmotic diuretics, osmotic purgatives
- Antimicrobial agent such as penicillin interferes with bacterial cell wall formation

DIFFERENT WAYS OF MECHANISM OF DRUG ACTION (HOW DO DRUGS ACT?)

The following are the main modes of action:

Physical

Based on physical properties of drugs, e.g. bulk purgatives, tannins.

Chemical

Based on chemical properties of drugs, e.g. antacids neutralize gastric HCl.

$$NaHCO_3 + HCl = NaCl + H_2O + CO_2$$

Through enzymes

Enzymes are substances which speed up a wide variety of chemical processes within the body. Certain drugs have the property of inhibiting the action of enzymes and thus interfering with chemical processes.

- Nonspecific enzyme inhibition, e.g. acids, alkalies, heavy metals
- Specific enzyme inhibition
  - Competitive, e.g. PABA and sulphonamides
  - Noncompetitive, e.g. carbonic anhydrase inhibitor, diamox

Receptor concept

Receptors are reactive functionally important tissue components, chemical groups situated on cell surface, or within the cell. These are specialized structures which are either enzymes or part of enzymes, proteins, nucleic acid and are highly sensitive, specific and selective with distinct entity.

The receptor for a drug may be considered to be any functional macro-molecular component present in the organism. The drug is capable of altering (increasing or decreasing) the rate of any bodily function, but by interaction with such receptors it cannot initiate any function not already characteristic of a tissue acted upon.

If the drug interacts with receptors involved in functions common to most cells then its effects will be extensive throughout the body. This will not be so if the interaction of the drug is with more specialized receptors concerned with tissues involved solely with specific bodily functions. Therefore, these sites of action may be localized e.g. affecting a restricted area or particular organ or generalized, affecting most of the cells throughout the body.

The term receptor tends to be used loosely. Some use it to mean any target molecule with which a drug molecule has to combine in order to elicit its specific effect which can include any of the following four types of targets:

- receptors
- ion channels

- enzymes
- carrier molecules

Other types of protein targets include certain structural proteins, such as tubulin (target for colchicine), immunophilins (intracellular proteins) are target for immunosuppressive drugs such as cyclosporin. Targets for chemotherapeutic agents include DNA, cell wall constituents and other proteins.

Some examples are given in Table 1.11.

Table 1.11. Receptors.

Type of target	Agonists	Antagonists
Histamine (H$_1$ receptor)	Histamine	Mepyramine
Histamine (H$_2$ receptor)	Impromidine	Ranitadine
Oestrogen receptor	Ethinyloestradiol	Tamoxifen
Progesterone receptor	Norethisterone	Danazol
Insulin receptor	Insulin	Not known
Opiate (μ-receptor)	Morphine	Naloxone
Beta-adrenoceptor	Noradrenaline	Propranolol
Dopamine (D$_2$ receptor)	Dopamine	Chlorpromazine
Ion Channels		*Blockers*
Voltage - gated Na$^+$ Channels		Local Anaesthetics
Renal tubule Na$^+$ Channels		Amiloride
Enzymes		*Inhibitors*
Acetylcholinesterase		Neostigmine
Cyclo-oxygenase		Aspirin
Xanthine oxidase		Allopurinol
Carbonic anhydrase		Acetazolamide
HMG-Co A reductase		Simvastatin
Angiotensin - converting enzyme		Captopril
Dihydrofolate reductase		Trimethoprim
Carriers		*Inhibitors*
Na+ / K$^+$/ 2Cl Co-transporter (loop of Henle)		Loop diuretics
Na+ / K$^+$ pump		Cardiac glycosides
Proton pump (gastric mucosa)		Omeprazole
Others		*Inhibitors*
Immunophilins		Cyclosporin
		Tacrolimus
Tubuline		Colchicine
		Taxol

Receptor families

In terms of both molecular structure and the nature of transduction mechanism receptors can be distinguished into four types:

Type-I   : Channel-linked receptors (also called ionotropic receptors) e.g. nicotinic acetylcholine receptor or GABA receptor.

Type-II   : G-protein-coupled receptors (also called metabotropic receptors) e.g. muscarinic acetylcholine receptors and adrenergic receptors.

Type-III : Kinase-linked receptors, e.g. receptors for insulin and various cytokines and growth factors.

Type-IV   : receptors that regulate gene transcription (also known as nuclear receptors) e.g., receptors for steroid hormones and thyroid hormones.

Classification of Receptors

Receptors are usually classified on the basis of the effect of selective agonists and antagonists e.g. muscarinic and nicotinic receptors of ACh. However, as the diversity and selectivity have increased it has become clear that multiple subtypes exist which are of interest to researchers and of utility to the clinician. Expression of such subtypes allows a single agonist to produce unique response in specific cells or tissues, e.g. α_1 - and α_2 adrenergic receptors and the M$_1$ - and M$_2$ - muscarinic cholinergic receptors. All the four subtypes regulate G protein. The α_1 - adrenergic and M$_1$ - and of (M$_3$-) receptors initiate Ca^{2+} signaling via Gq whereas α_2 - adrenergic and the - M$_2$ - (and M$_4$-) muscarinic receptors regulate other signaling pathways via Gi.

The view that drugs interact with receptors still remains the cornerstone for theories on drug action, and it bears a close relationship to theories of enzyme action. Another modification of the receptor theory is the concept of spare receptors (receptor reserve)—this proposes that maximal effect may be obtained by an agonist without occupancy of the full available receptors. Spare receptors allow agonist with low affinity for receptors to produce maximal response even in low concentration.

Spare receptors are not hidden or unavailable and when occupied they can be coupled to respond.

When an agonist binds to a receptor and does not produce response, such receptor is termed a "silent receptor". On chronic use of a drug normal receptors of a neurotransmitter can be blocked on a target organ, then these silent receptors become active and tolerance to drug effects is manifested. On withdrawal of the drug, the silent receptors still remain active and with the normally active receptors (which become free of drug after withdrawal) result in the increased number of functional receptors. This results in "rebound hyperactivity" or withdrawal phenomenon in the neurotransmitter-effective system.

Drugs capable of forming a drug-receptor complex which initiates physiological activity have both affinity and efficacy and are called agonists. The ability of a drug to get bound to a receptor is known as affinity while the capacity of a drug to elicit response (action) after its interaction with receptor is termed as efficacy or intrinsic activity. A drug can bind with receptors without initiating a physiological response and may antagonise an agonist, because an antagonist possesses affinity and not efficacy (or intrinsic activity). The antagonism may be reversible (competitive or surmountable) if the inhibition can be reversed by increasing the concentration of the agonist; or irreversible (insurmountable) antagonism in case of irreversible inactivation of a receptor site.

Inverse agonists (negative antagonists) have full affinity but efficacy ranges between 0 to -1 and therefore they will produce an effect opposite to that of an agonist. For example Beta-carbolines act as inverse agonists at benzodiazepine receptor and produce the effects like anxiety, awakening and seizures which are just the opposite to the effects of benzodiazepines (anti anxiety, sedation and anticonvulsant) by binding with the same receptors. Inverse agonists have affinity with negative intrinsic activity. '

Some drug produces actions that are paradoxical in nature and are specifically opposite to those of the agonists.

Receptor desensitisation

Receptor mediated response to drugs often "desensitise" with time i.e. after reaching the initial high level, the response gradually decreases in the continuing presence of the agonist, e.g., at the neuromuscular junction.

Up and down regulation of receptors (change in number of receptors)

Prolonged exposure of high concentration of agonist causes a reduction in the number of receptors available for activation. This is known as down regulation of receptors. Down regulation of receptors may produce less effect in severe asthmatics who no longer respond to adrenoceptor agonist such as salbutamol.

Prolonged occupation of receptors by a blocker i.e. antagonist leads to an increase in the number of receptors, it is known as up regulation.

The phenomenon of down- and up- regulation of receptors may prove dangerous after sudden withdrawal of certain drugs. In such cases gradual tapering off should be done. For example, in endogenous depression there is down regulation of α-adrenoceptors with concomitant up regulation of β-adrenoceptors and prolonged use of tricyclic antidepressants results in down regulation of β-receptors with relatively up regulation of α-receptors.

An antihypertensive drug clonidine lowers BP due to α_2 adrenoceptor agonist action but after sudden withdrawal produces hypertensive crisis. It is so because the drug during the process down regulates the α_2 receptors which on sudden withdrawal respond vigorously to the sudden release of catecholamines.

PARTIAL AGONISTS

Some drugs, in addition to blocking access of the natural agonist to the receptor, are capable of a degree of activation, i.e. they have both antagonist and agonist action. Their effects can vary with circumstances, e.g. nalorphine in moderate doses antagonises opioid-induced respiratory depression, but in large doses increases it, whereas naloxone is a pure antagonist. The beta-adrenoceptor antagonists pindolol and oxprenolol have partial antagonist activity, in their case it is also called intrinsic sympathomimetic activity (ISA)], while propranolol is a pure antagonist.

Fig. 1.10 illustrates the drug-receptor interaction showing agonist and antagonist.

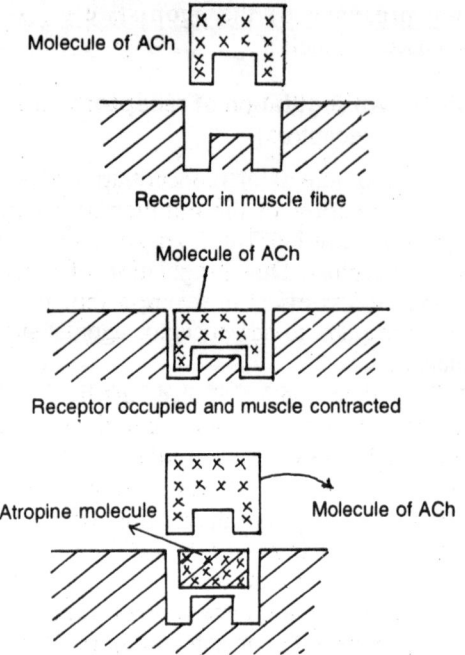

Fig. 1.10. Stimulation of muscle by acetylcholine (ACh) showing occupation of the receptor by the drug. After atropine the receptor site is blocked and no stimulation (contraction) occurs.

Drug-receptor interactions

It is schematically represented by the following equation:

$$D + R \underset{k_2}{\overset{k_1}{\rightleftharpoons}} DR \xrightarrow{k_3} E$$

where D = drug, R = receptor, DR = drug-receptor complex, E = biologic effect, and k_1, k_2 and k_3 = rate constants for adsorption, desorption from receptor, and production of effect, respectively.

The two step sequence involves an initial equilibrium between the drug and receptor followed by the observed effect as a result of the drug and receptor combination. Both the steps are strongly influenced by drug-receptor bonding and by stereochemical fit of the drug on the receptor. These two aspects of drug-receptor interactions are highly interdependent.

There are four kinds of bonds
1. Covalent,
2. Hydrogen bond,
3. Ionic bond, and
4. van der Waals' forces

Covalent bonds. Many drugs interact with biologic receptors through covalent bond formation. It has great bond strengths ranging from 40 to 110 kcal/mol. The mutual sharing of electron pairs between atoms in a covalent bond produces great bond strength. Spontaneous rupture of such a bond is unlikely at body pH and temperature; as a result these drugs exhibit prolonged pharmacologic effects and are thought of as acting irreversibly and exhibit long duration of action. However, eventually the drug effect is terminated through catalytic cleavage of the drug-receptor linkage or a metabolic turnover of the receptor molecule. The examples of covalent bonds are alkylation, acylation, and phosphorylation reactions.

If the forces that bind drug to receptor are weak e.g. hydrogen bonds, van der Waals' bonds, electrostatic bonds, the binding will be reversible; if the forces that bind are strong e.g. covalent bonds, then binding is irreversible.

An antagonist that binds reversibly to a receptor can be displaced from the receptor if the concentration of the agonist increases sufficiently, according to the law of Mass Action (rate of a chemical reaction is proportional to the concentration i.e. mass of reacting substances). This is competitive antagonism.

Drugs that bind irreversibly to receptors include phenoxybenzamine. This drug cannot be displaced from the receptor by increasing the concentration of agonist. Some toxins, including those present in snake venoms, bind irreversibly to the acetylcholine receptor. This is noncompetitive antagonism. Response after irreversible binding can be restored after elimination of the drug from the body and synthesis of new receptors and for this reason the effect may persist long after administration has ceased (hit and run drug).

Non-covalent bonds produce short-lived, reversible interactions between drugs and biologic receptors. As bond strength increases, a greater fraction of drug is bound to the receptor. These bond types are relatively weak.

The following are important noncovalent bonds:

	Bond strength (kcal/mol)	Illustration
Ionic	5	Na$^+$- - - - - Cl$^-$
Hydrogen	1-7	–C = O—H–N
van der Waals'	0.5-1	>C - - - - - C<

Fig. 1.11 shows different bonds in relation to ACh-receptor interaction.

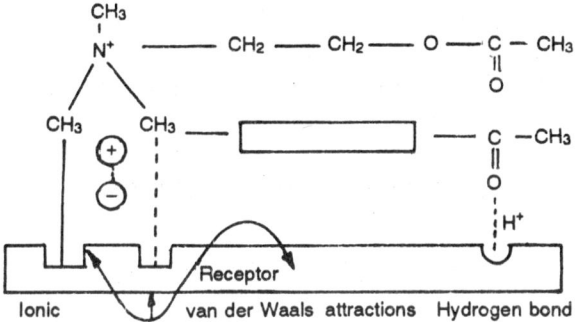

Fig. 1.11. Different bonds in relation to ACh-receptor interaction.

STUDY QUESTIONS

1. Define stimulation, depression, irritation. Give examples.
2. Give examples of certain drugs which act through physical and chemical processes.
3. Give examples of certain drugs which produce their action by (a) nonspecific enzyme inhibition and (b) specific enzyme inhibition.
4. Define enzymes. What are their important roles?
5. Explain receptor and binding of drugs to receptors.
6. Define agonist. Define 'affinity' and 'efficacy' in relation to agonist and antagonist.
7. Explain competitive or reversible antagonism and irreversible antagonism which are dependent upon the type of drug-receptor binding. Give examples. How are both terminated?
8. Draw diagrams to illustrate drug-receptor interaction: affinity and efficacy (intrinsic activity) resulting in drug effect and antagonism.
9. What are the types of bonds in case of drug-receptor complex?

GUIDE TO FURTHER READING

Ariens, E.J. Affinity and intrinsic activity in the theory of competitive inhibition. 1. Problems and theory. Arch Int. Pharmacodyn, 1994; 99:32.

Changeux, J.P. The acetylcholine receptor. Its molecular biology and biotechnological aspects. Bioessays, 1898; 10:48.

Dean, P.M. Molecular foundations of drug-receptor interaction. Cambridge University Press. Cambridge, 1987.

Goldstein, A., Aronow, L. and Kalman, S.M. Principles of Drug Action. The Basis of Pharmacology, 2nd ed. Wiley, 1974.

Kenakin, T.P., Bond, R.A., and Bonner, T.I. Definition of pharmacological receptors. Pharmacol Rev, 1992; 44:351.

Kenakin, T.P. Pharmacological Analysis of Drug-Receptor Interaction. Raven Press, New York, 1987.

Limbird, L.E. Cell Surface Receptors: A Short Course on Theory and Method, 2nd ed, M. Nijhoff, Boston, 1995.

Taussig, R. and Gilman, A.G. Mammalin membrane-bound adenylyl cyclases; J. Biol. Chem., 1995; 270:1.

Wong, S.K. and Garbers, D.L. Receptor guanylyl cyclases. J Clin Invest, 1992; 90:299.

DEVELOPMENT OF NEW DRUGS

Drug development is an extremely arduous, highly technical, time-consuming and very expensive process. It is only about 1% of compounds which are tested eventually become licensed medicines and carry the cost of 99% failures. Therefore for the successful developments, motivation and incentives of the organizations and the individuals working within them are important.

The principal approaches to drug discovery

- Idea is conceived from folklore or screening of natural products.
- Synthesis of analogues or antagonists of known hormone, autacoid, etc. or of molecules that modify understood biochemical processes, e.g. calcium channel blockers.
- Modification of the chemical configuration of a known drug. This is likely to yield derivatives

with similar properties or only minor differences. These can be called 'me-too' or 'me-again' drugs. However, now it is possible to utilize very sophisticated molecular design that it is possible to eliminate some actions and enhance other actions from the molecule. This may produce novel results. For example, sulphonamides, sulphonylureas, thiazides, acetazolamide are all derived from the earlier sulphonamides, synthesized in 1930s but possess different useful properties.

- Discovery of new properties of old drugs, e.g. aspirin for antithrombotic effect.

Usefulness and limitations of preclinical testing (animal studies)

Whatever be the source of the candidate molecule, it has to be tested experimentally (drug screening). It involves a variety of biologic assays at the molecular, cellular, organ, and whole animal levels. This indicates the activity and selectivity of the drug. The pharmacotherapeutic goal determines the type and number of initial screening tests.

In addition to in vitro studies, most of the biologic actions of the new drug must be tested in experimental animals before clinical trials can be started in humans. There are three conventional phases of clinical trial. A fourth phase follows after approval for general use. Table 1.12 shows the testing processes which are involved in the development of new drugs.

Preclinical testing (animal studies) is done in laboratory animals (dogs, cats, monkeys, rabbits, guinea pigs, rats and mice etc.).

The pharmacologic screening tests give information about the effect of a new substance on biological system and activity as well as on the experimentally induced disease models.

These studies also indicate mechanism of action, pharmacokinetics, dose ranges.

DIFFERENT TYPES OF TOXICOLOGICAL STUDIES

If the new compound shows promising results, the toxicity studies carried out in animals are listed below.

Table 1.12. Phases of drug development

Animal testing		Clinical testing	Marketing
Short-term ↓ Efficacy selectivity mechanism	Long-term ↓ Chronic toxicity Reproduction Teratogenicity Carcinogenicity	**Phase 1** WHO? Normal volunteers, special populations (renal and hepatic impairment) WHY? Safety, biological effects, metabolism, kinetics By WHOM? Clinical pharmacologist **Phase 2** WHO? Selected patients WHY? Therapeutic efficacy, dosage range, metbaolism, kinetics By WHOM? Clinical pharmacologist and clinical investigators **Phase 3** (Does it work, double blind?) WHO? Large samples of selected patients WHY? Safety and efficacy By WHOM? Clinical investigators	**Phase 4** (Post-marketing surveillance) WHO? Patients given drug for therapy WHY? Adverse reactions By WHOM? All physicians

Toxicity studies

Acute toxicity (single dose studies)	LD$_{50}$ (lethal dose in 50% animals). Maximum tolerated dose is determined. Single dose is given in 2 species of animals by two routes of administration.
Subacute toxicity (repeated dose studies)	Three doses and 2 species are used up to 6 months. The longer the clinical use, the longer the subacute test.
Chronic toxicity (long-term toxicology)	Studies carried out for 1-2 years.

Regarding the duration of repeated dose studies, the schedule depends on the intended duration of use in man as shown below:

Intended duration of use in man	Duration of study in animals
Single dose or several doses in one day	14 days
Up to 10 days	28 days
Up to 30 days	90 days
Beyond 30 days	180 days

Special toxicology

Carcinogenicity tests are not required prior to the early studies in man unless there is reason for suspicion of the drug. This test will be required if the drug is to be given to man for above 1 year. For this test 3 dose levels in 2 animal species are employed (which are known to have low incidence of spontaneous tumours) for 24 months in rats, 18 months in mouse i.e. most of animal's life and at the end of the test tissues are examined histologically.

For reproduction studies, two animal species are used for embryotoxicity and one species for fertility and perinatal studies. Three dose levels are employed.

Mutagenicity tests involving animals e.g. intraperitoneal injection of bacteria are required.

Use of animals in drug development

Many tests in drug development are done on anaesthetized animals and many on isolated organs of animals killed 'humanely'. The results obtained in whole animal may provide useful information because of the intact physiological systems who are capable of forming metabolites. In some respects animals are similar to man and in many respects they are not. The toxicity studies indeed cause a lot of suffering to the animals.

In order to decide if a chemical is a medicine or only a chemical, either animal experimentation is done or unknown substances are given to man. The first choice is preferred otherwise drug therapy will not advance. However, in future, when in vitro biochemical preparations and tissue cultures are so developed that basic mechanisms are well understood then it is possible that animal experimentations may not be necessary. It is likely to take a long time for cells in tissue culture develop characteristics e.g. new receptors. Researches designed to reduce the need to employ animals are welcome.

VALIDITY OF ANIMAL DATA

The therapeutic conclusions cannot be extrapolated directly to use in humans e.g. rabbit does not have a Bowman's membrane so studies carried out concerning corneal surface injury will give different results in monkeys and rabbits. Many strains of rabbits possess atropine esterase, which inactivates belladonna derivatives more rapidly than in humans.

Although the preclinical testing is essential but it has certain limitations.

It is important to recognize the limitations of preclinical testing. These include:

Large numbers of animals are used to obtain preclinical data. Attempts are being made to reduce the numbers required. Cell and tissue culture in vitro methods have been developed and are being used in some laboratories, however, their predictive value is very much limited at present. Some think that animal testing is unnecessary but it is really not so.

Extrapolation of toxicity data from animals to humans is not completely reliable. However, by using different species and different routes of administration and properly conducting the toxicity studies, the data do have predictive value for toxicity of any given compound in humans. Of course there are limitations on the amount of information obtained by toxicological testing in animals.

Rare adverse effects are unlikely to be detected.

CLINICAL TRIALS

When studies in animals predict that a new chemical may be effective and safe medicine, then it is tested in man. Prediction from animal studies about effectiveness and safety provide a useful guidance in most cases about the probable usefulness in humans.

The initial dose to be tried in humans is usually taken as 1/100-1/10 of the 'no-effect' dose in animals. The 'no-effect' dose is the maximum dose at which the specific toxic effect is not obtained.

The guidelines for studies in man usually include:

- Studies of bioavailability.
- Clinical trials which clearly indicate efficacy and safety of the drug.
- If the drug is meant for use in elderly, studies should be done in the elderly people.
- Interaction studies.
- If it is a fixed dose combination product, it should be justified that there is enhanced (potentiated) therapeutic effect, less toxicity for each component and adding of one ingredient is to counter the adverse effect of another ingredient.

Ethics of clinical trials

Physicians should withdraw the therapeutic trial if at any time they are convinced that it is not in the interest of patients to continue the trial.

Ethical objections that have been raised to the randomized controlled trial are :

- Double blind technique is an unethical deception.
- Use of dummy or placebo controls is an unethical deception.
- Patients in one group will get inferior treatment.
- Random allocation is unethical.
- The interest of the patient is always subordinated to the interest of society, ethics supersede 'individual' ethics, and this is unethical.

The above unethical considerations are looked after by taking informed consent from the volunteers or patients. Consent is central to the whole conduct of clinical research.

Need for statistics

Statistics may be defined as 'a body of methods making wise decisions in the face of uncertainty'.

Clinical impression is quite different from statistical therapeutic study. Unfortunately when general impressions are of long standing they become fixed rules of life.

By applying statistical tests the value of beliefs is ascertained.

No doubt, it is true that physicians deal with individuals and statistical therapeutic trial does not tell what will happen to any one individual. However, the knowledge gained that x% patients recover, y% improve and z% are unaffected, along with details of adverse effects, if any, provides more scientific basis for the choice of therapy than different clinical impressions of physicians.

Trials should be devised to have adequate power e.g. at least 80% chance of detecting the defined useful target effect within narrow confidence limits, at 5% statistical significance ($p = 0.05$). It is not worth starting a trial that has less than 50% chance of achieving the set objective, because the power (confidence interval) of trials is too low.

Role of placebo

Placebo or dummy medication as a control device in therapeutic trials:

The *double-blind technique* should be used if possible to exclude the psychological factors. Single-blind technique has little use as it may involve observer's bias.

The placebo (inert substance which patient believes it as an active substance) is useful to distinguish the pharmacodynamic effects of a drug from the psychological effects of the act of medication and certain circumstances e.g. enthusiasm of the investigator. The placebo administration also distinguishes drug effects from fluctuations in disease that occur with time e.g. rheumatoid arthritis. It also avoids false negative results, e.g. if only new drug and placebo are used which give identical results, it means that either the method used is insensitive or the new drug has only placebo effect. The therapeutic trial of a new analgesic should consist of a new drug, a placebo and a proved active analgesic. If all these three give identical results, it indicates that the methods employed cannot distinguish between the active and inactive drug.

The placebo or dummy medication as a control device should not deprive seriously ill patients for effective therapy, e.g. in epilepsy or tuberculosis, the control groups receive the best available therapy.

The aim is to determine the efficacy of the new drug in large population. After this the drug is released for general use.

The phases of clinical testing are summarized in Table 1.13.

Table 1.13. Phases of clinical trials

Phase 1	Clinical (20-50 subjects) Non-blind or open study healthy volunteers (or patients) Pharmacokinetics (ADME) Pharmacodynamics The aim is to observe activity, safety, tolerated dose range, efficacy and pharmacokinetics.
Phase 2	Clinical investigation (50-300 patients) Pharmacokinetics, pharmacodynamics, dose-range, efficacy and safety The limited aim is to find usefulness in disease and determine final dosage.
Phase 3	Formal therapeutic trials (250-1000 patients) to establish efficacy, safety, comparison with other drugs.
Phase 4	Post-licensing (marketing) studies (2000-10,000 + patients) It is surveillance during general use for safety and efficacy.

However, therapeutic trials are unlikely to reveal:

- Adverse effects that are uncommon or occur only after prolonged use e.g. oral contraceptives and vascular disease; renal damage due to analgesics.
- Effects in special population groups e.g. pregnancy, presence of renal and hepatic disease.
- Drug interactions.

STUDY QUESTIONS

1. Are animal studies essential for the development of a new drug? What are their limitations?
2. What different types of toxicological studies are carried out to ensure safety of a new drug?
3. Describe the phase 1, phase 2, phase 3 of testing in humans before marketing of a drug. What informations are obtained in each of these phases? What is phase 4 after marketing the drug?
4. What do you mean by placebo? What is its importance in clinical trials of a new drug?
5. What do you understand by double blind controlled study?
6. What are the different approaches in the process of development of a new drug?

GUIDE TO FURTHER READING

Alper, J. Drug discovery on the assembly line. Science, 1994; 264:1399.

Beecher, H.K. The powerful placebo. JAMA, 1955; 159:1602.

Brodie, B.B. Difficulties in extrapolating data on metabolism of drugs from animal to man. Clin Pharmacol Ther, 1972; 3:374.

Brody, H. The lie that heals: The ethics of giving placebos. Ann. Intern Med, 1982; 97:112.

Dimasi, J.A., Seibring, M.A., and Lasagna, L. New drug development in the United States from 1963 to 1992. Clin Pharmacol Ther, 1994; 55:609-622.

Gross, F. The present dilemma of drug research. Clin Pharmacol Ther, 1976; 19:1.

Gross, F. Drug research: Dead end or new horizon? Br Med J, 1982; 285:1444.

Guyatt. G., Sackett, D., Taylor, D.W., et al. Determining optimal therapy—randomized trials in individual patients. N Engl J Med 1986, 314:889-892.

If nothing goes wrong, is every thing alright? JAMA, 1983; 249:1743.

Kaitin, K.I., Manocchia, M., et al. The new drug approvals of 1990, 1991, and 1992: Trends in drug development. J Clin Pharmacol, 1994, 34:120-127.

Kuntz, I.D. Structure-based strategies for drug design and discovery. Science, 1992, 257:1078-1082.

Lasagna, L. Will all new drugs become orphans? Clin Pharmacol Ther, 1982; 31:285.

Mainland, D. Statistical ritual in clinical journals: Is there a cure? Br Med J, 1984; 288:841, 920.

McDevitt, D.G., and MacDonald., T.M. Post-marketing drug surveillance—How far have we got? Q J Med, 1991, 78:1-3.

Modell, W., et al. Factors influencing clinical evaluation of drugs with special reference to the double-blind technique. JAMA, 1958; 167:2190.

Nowak, R. Problems in clinical trials go far beyond misconduct. Science, 1994; 264:1538.

Passamani, E. Clinical trials—Are they ethical. N Engl J Med, 1991; 324:1589.

Sacks, H.S., et al. Meta-analyses of randomized controlled trials (pooling). N Engl J Med, 1987; 316:450.

Shaw, J. Medication errors a great hidden problem. Am Med News, Jan 1982; 8:18

Sheiner, L.B. The intellectual health of clinical drug evaluation. Clin Pharmacol Ther, 1991; 50:4

Strom, B.L., et al. Postmarketing studies of drug efficacy: When must they be randomized? Clin Pharmacol Ther, 1983; 34:1.

Drugs Acting on
Autonomic Nervous System (ANS)

GENERAL ASPECTS OF ANS

Nervous system comprises of central nervous system (CNS) and peripheral nervous system. The peripheral nervous system is further divided into autonomic nervous system (ANS) and somatic nervous system. The autonomic nervous system has two main divisions viz. sympathetic and parasympathetic nervous systems.

An organ is innervated by both sympathetic (adrenergic) and parasympathetic (cholinergic) nervous system and depending on the physiological need, one or the other system may dominate at any one time. However, spleen, sweat glands, most of the blood vessels and hair follicles have only sympathetic innervation; while ciliary muscles and exocrine glands of stomach and pancreas have only parasympathetic innervation.

The autonomic nervous system (ANS) is that part of the nervous system which controls all vital functions and supplies the viscera as distinct from the skeletal muscles. It is largely autonomous in that its activities are not under direct conscious control (autos = self; nomos = governing). The ANS is concerned primarily with visceral functions. The viscera include the gastrointestinal tract, the respiratory and urogenital systems, the heart and blood vessels, the intrinsic muscles of the eye and various secretory glands. The ANS maintains the constancy of the internal environment (homeostasis). Adrenergic system prepares body for active exertion whereas cholinergic system tends to conserve energy. The two divisions of the autonomic nervous system, i.e., sympathetic and parasympathetic, differ in their anatomical arrangement, their effects and mechanism of action.

On anatomical grounds, the sympathetic (thoracolumbar) and the parasympathetic (craniosacral) divisions both originate in nuclei within the central nervous system (CNS) and give rise to preganglionic efferent fibres. The sympathetic preganglionic fibres leave the CNS through the 12 thoracic segments and first 2 or 3 lumbar segments of the spinal cord hence called thoracolumbar system. The parasympathetic preganglionic fibres leave the CNS through the cranial nerves, especially the 3rd, 7th, 9th, and 10th in the brain stem and the 2nd, 3rd and 4th sacral segments of the spinal cord, hence this system is also called the craniosacral division. The autonomic system also carries a large number of sensory nerves which supply the various organs. These nerves enter the spinal cord where they may form a spinal reflex arc with the autonomic nerves leaving the cord or they may ascend to the brain where more complex reflexes are built up which may be influenced by impulses arising from highest levels of the brain. This is how some visceral sensations may enter consciousness and that events in consciousness may stimulate various visceral effects, for example, the rapid beating of the heart after a fright.

The autonomic nerves affect the organs which they supply by liberating a neurotransmitter at the nerve endings, which acts on a receptor in the organ concerned. This is known as the chemical transmission of nerve impulses. Neurotransmitters are chemical mediators that transmit nerve impulses across junctions such as synapses. This physiological understanding has made it much easier to understand how various drugs may modify the autonomic system.

Table 2.1 shows comparison between sympathetic and parasympathetic systems.

Table 2.1. Comparison between sympathetic and parasympathetic systems

	Sympathetic (adrenergic)	Parasympathetic (cholinergic)
Anatomical ground	Thoraco-lumbar (T1 to L2 or L3)	Cranio-sacral (3rd, 7th, 9th & 10th cranial; sacral 2nd, 3rd and 4th)
Distribution	Wide	Head, neck and trunk
Place of ganglia	Away from organs	On or near to organs
Postganglionic fibres	Long	Short
Neurotransmitter and its stability	NE, stable	ACh, rapidly destroyed
Role	Prepares body for active exertion, tackle stress and emergency	Conserves energy

Table 2.2 shows the main differences between the somatic and autonomic nervous system

Table 2.2. Comparison between somatic and autonomic nervous system

	Autonomic	Somatic
Organ supplied	All organs other than skeletal	Skeletal muscle
Nerve fibres	Preganglionic fibres are myelinated; postganglionic fibres are non-myelinated	Myelinated
Neurotransmitter	Acetylcholine, noradrenaline	Acetylcholine
Peripheral plexus formation	Present	Absent
Distal synapse	In central nervous system	Outside the central nervous system
Nerve section	Activity continues	Paralysis

The following organs receive only sympathetic innervation:

Blood vessels, ventricles, pilomotor muscles, kidney and liver.

The following organs receive only parasympathetic innervation:

Ciliary muscle of the eye, lacrimal glands, gastric secretions, bronchial glands.

The following organs receive both sympathetic and parasympathetic innervation:

Sinoatrial (SA) and atrioventricular (AV) nodes, iris, gastrointestinal smooth muscle.

Neurotransmitters

The following criteria should be fulfilled for a substance to be qualified as a postjunctionally acting neurotransmitter:

- It should be present in the presynaptic neuron along with enzymes which synthesize it.
- It should be released on stimulation of the nerve.
- When applied it should produce actions similar to those produced by the stimulation of the nerve.
- Its response should be terminated by a substance which will also antagonize the effect of nerve stimulation.
- If a substance potentiates the action of nerve stimulation it should also potentiate the response of the neurotransmitter.

Autonomic nervous system fibres release neurotransmitters at synapses as well as at points of contact with visceral effectors called neuroeffector junctions. On the basis of the neurotransmitter released, autonomic fibres are classified as either cholinergic or adrenergic.

Cholinergic fibres release acetylcholine (ACh) at following sites:

1. All parasympathetic and sympathetic pre-ganglionic axons.
2. All parasympathetic postganglionic axons.
3. Few sympathetic postganglionic axons such as those which supply to sweat glands, adrenals, and blood vessels in skeletal muscles.

Sympathetic or adrenergic fibres release nor-epinephrine (NE) at the postganglionic synapse. But the sympathetic transmitter at sweat glands and at some blood vessels, it is ACh.

Fig. 2.1 shows neurotransmitters associated with the autonomic nervous system.

Fig. 2.2 shows the sites of action of neuro-transmitters.

- Site 1 is stimulated by nicotine and blocked by ganglion blockers.
- Site 2 is stimulated by choline esters, anticholinesterases and pilocarpine.
- Site 3 is stimulated by sympathomimetics and blocked by adrenoceptor blocking agents.
- Site 4 is blocked by adrenergic neuron blockers.
- Site 5 is stimulated by choline esters and anticholinesterases and blocked by neuro-muscular blocking agents.

Synthesis, release and termination of ACh

Acetylcholine is synthesized by the interaction of acetyl CoA and choline in the presence of an enzyme choline acetylase. Acetyl CoA is formed by acetic acid Co-A-SH in the presence of ATP and enzyme acetyl thiokinase.

Acetylcholine is continuously hydrolyzed and resynthesized.

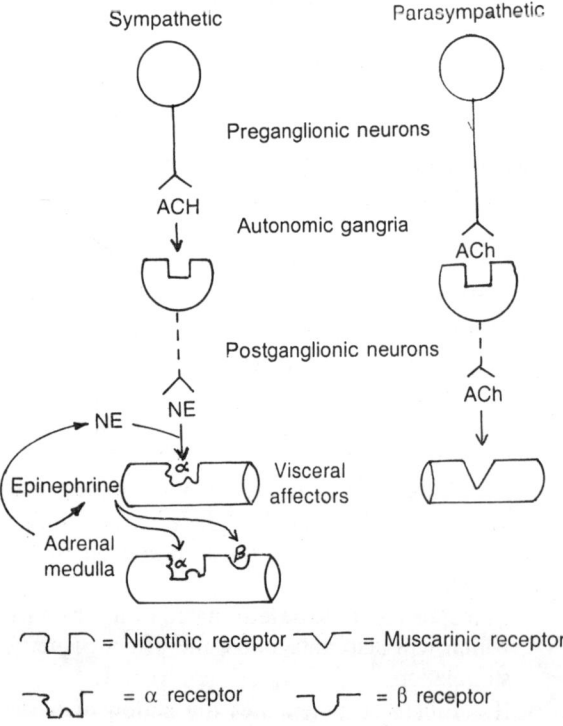

= Nicotinic receptor   = Muscarinic receptor

= α receptor   = β receptor

Fig. 2.1. Neurotransmitters and receptors associated with the autonomic nervous system.

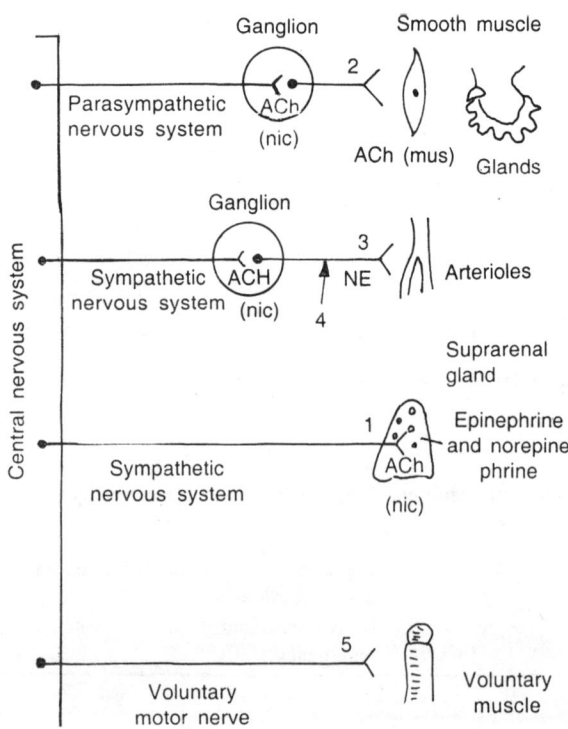

Fig. 2.2. Sites of action of neurotransmitters.

Following the release, ACh diffuses into the synaptic cleft to combine with receptors on the postsynaptic cell and the released ACh is hydrolyzed to choline and acetic acid within one millisecond so that it acts very briefly. The transmitter action is very rapid and very short.

Norepinephrine synthesis, storage and release

The metabolic precursor for norepinephrine is L-tyrosine, an amino acid present in the body fluids which is taken up (by specific transport system) by adrenergic neurons.

Tyrosine hydroxylase converts tyrosine to dihydroxyphenylalanine (DOPA). This first hydroxylation step is the main controlling point for norepinephrine synthesis. The next step is conversion of DOPA to dopamine by DOPA decarboxylase. It is a nonspecific enzyme and it is not rate-limiting and does not regulate norepinephrine synthesis. Dopamine β-hydroxylase (DBH) converts dopamine to norepinephrine. This enzyme is also nonspecific. This enzyme is located within the neurosecretory vesicle (NSV). Following depolarization of the neuron, NSV fuses with the neuronal membrane and by exocytosis discharges NE. Released NE may act on adrenoceptors, 'spill' into the blood stream, or be metabolized extraneuronally via COMT. NE pump transports NE back into the neuron and intraneuronal biotransformation occurs via MAO. Phenylethanolamine N-methyl transferase (PNMT) catalyses the N-methylation of norepinephrine to epinephrine.

The various steps of the biosynthesis, storage, release and termination of norepinephrine are shown in Figs. 2.3 and 2.4.

- Depolarization of the neuron leads to release of NE and by exocytosis discharges its soluble contents including NE.
- NE pump transports NE back into the neuron against a concentration gradient.
- Released NE may act on adrenoceptor, within 'spill' into the blood stream or be metabolized extraneuronally.

Norepinephrine storage :Under normal circumstances most of the norepinephrine is contained in

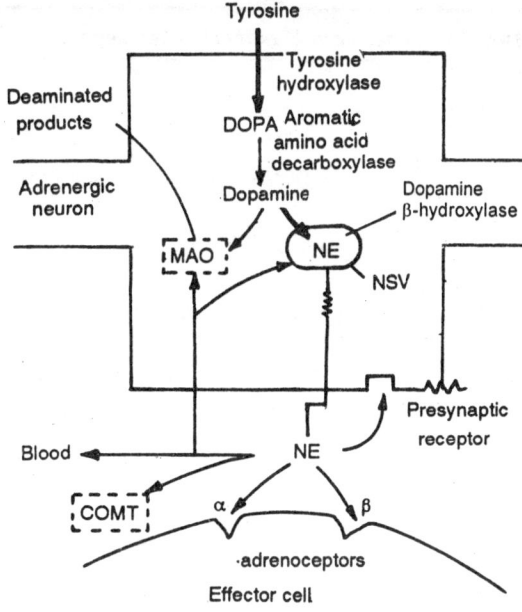

Fig. 2.3. Tyrosine is transported into the adrenergic neuron. The rate-limiting enzyme is tyrosine hydroxylase and the final enzyme dopamine beta-oxidase is located within the neurosecretory vesicle (NSV). Intraneuronal biotransformation occurs via MAO and extraneuronally via COMT.

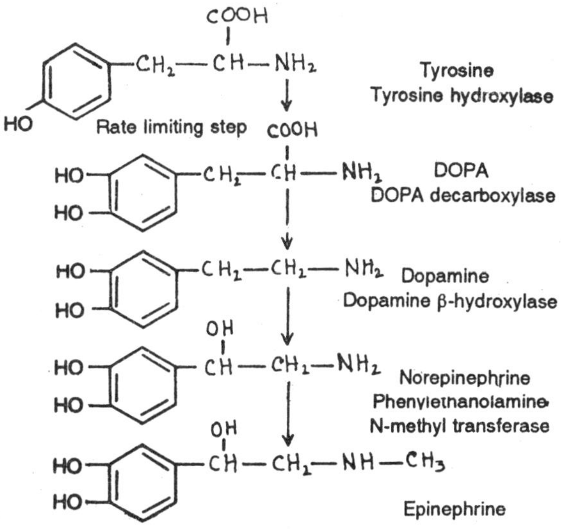

Fig. 2.4. Biosynthesis of norepinephrine and epinephrine.

Box 2.1. Metabolism of adrenaline (epinephrine)

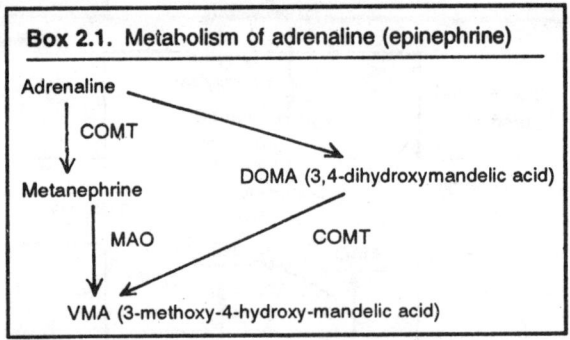

Box 2.2. Metabolism of noradrenaline (norepinephrine)

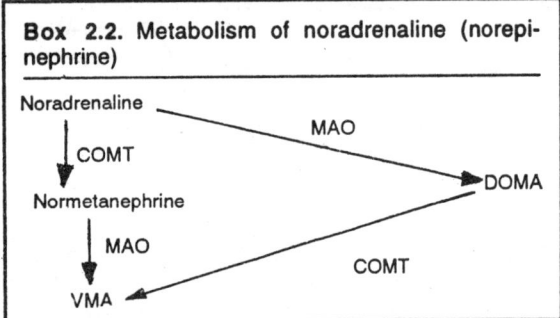

Box 2.3. Metabolism of dopamine

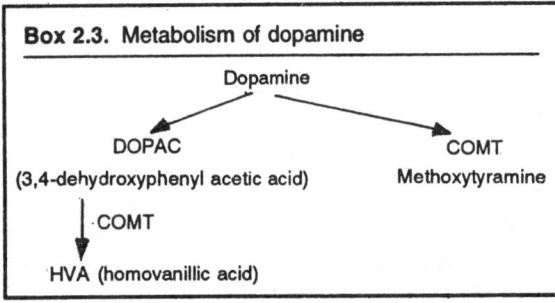

the vesicles at nerve terminals, only a little free form is present in the cytoplasm. As the concentration in the vesicles is very high, a special active carrier system is required to transport norepinephrine across the vesicle membrane. Some drugs such as reserpine interfere with this active process and cause nerve terminals to become depleted of their norepinephrine stores.

Release of norepinephrine : It is now recognized that norepinephrine by acting on presynaptic receptors can regulate its own release (auto-inhibitory feedback mechanism). This mechanism operates through α_2-receptors.

Uptake and degradation of catecholamines

Following release at the synapse, reuptake of norepinephrine by adrenergic nerve terminals is the main mechanism by which the released transmitter is inactivated.

The main effects of stimulating the autonomic nervous system are given in Table 2.3.

STUDY QUESTIONS

1. What are the functions of autonomic nervous system?
2. How is acetylcholine synthesized and terminated at the nerve terminals? At what sites acetylcholine is released?
3. Describe the synthesis, storage, release and termination of norepinephrine at the postganglionic sympathetic nerve terminals.
4. What do you understand by uptake (reuptake) of norepinephrine? What is its significance?

GUIDE TO FURTHER READING

Amara, S.G. and Kuhar, M.J. Neurotransmitter transporters: recent progress. Annu, Rev. Neurosci, 1993; 16:73.

Brownstein, M.J. and Hoffman, B.J. Neurotransmitters transporters: Recent Prog. Horm. Res., 1994; 49:27.

Burnstock, G. The changing face of autonomic neurotransmission. Acta Physiol. Scand., 1986; 126:67.

Hall, Z.W. and Sanes, J.P. Synaptic structure and development; the neuromuscular junction. Cell, 1993; 72 Suppl:99.

Parsons, S.M., Prior, C. and Marshall, I.G. Acetylcholine transport, storage, and release. Int. Rev. Neurobiol., 1993; 35:279.

Starke, K, Gothert, M. and Kilbinger, H. Modulation of neurotransmitter release by presynaptic autoreceptors. Physiol Rev, 1989; 69:864.

Taussig, R. and Gilman, A.G. Mammalian membrane-bound adenylyl cyclase. J. Biol. Chem., 1995; 270:1.

Taylor, G.S. and Bywater R.A.R. Novel autonomic neurotransmitters and intestinal function. Pharmacol Ther, 1989; 40:401.

Valtorta, F. et al. Neurotransmitter release and synaptic vesicle recycling. Neuroscience, 1990; 35:477.

Table 2.3. Response of effector organs to sympathetic and parasympathetic nervous system stimulation

Organ	Receptor	Sympathetic	Parasympathetic
Heart			
Atria	β_1, β_2	Contractility and conduction velocity increased ++	Force decreased
SA node	β_1, β_2	Increase in heart rate ++	Rate decreased
AV node	β_1, β_2	Automaticity and conduction increased ++	Conduction decreased; AV block +++
His-Purkinje system	β_1, β_2	Increase in automaticity and conduction velocity +++	—
Ventricles	β_1, β_2	Increase in contractility, conduction velocity and automaticity	—
Overall effect		Tachycardia and increase in cardiac output	Bradycardia, decrease in cardiac output
Arterioles			
Coronary	$\alpha_1, \alpha_2; \beta_2$	Constriction +; Dilatation ++	Dilatation
	β_2	Dilatation ++	—
Abdominal viscera	α_1, β_2	Constriction +++; Dilatation +	—
	β_2	Dilatation +	—
Salivary glands	α_1, α_2	Constriction +++	Dilatation ++
Renal	α_1, α_2	Constriction +++	—
	β_1, β_2	Dilatation +	—
Skeletal muscle	α	Constriction ++	Dilatation +
	β_2	Dilatation ++	—
Skin and mucosa	α_1, α_2	Constriction +++	Dilatation
Cerebral	α_1	Constriction (slight)	Dilatation
Pulmonary	α_1	Constriction +	Dilatation
	β_2	Dilatation	—
Veins	α_1, α_2	Constriction ++	—
	β_2	Dilatation ++	—
Lungs			
Tracheal and bronchial muscle	β_2	Relaxation +	Contraction ++
Bronchial glands	α_1	Decreased secretion	Stimulation +++
	β_2	Increased secretion	—
Stomach			
Motility and tone	$\alpha_1, \alpha_2, \beta_2$	Decrease +	Increase +++
Sphincters	α_1	Contraction +	Relaxation +
Secretion	α_1	Inhibition (?)	Stimulation ++
Intestine			
Motility and tone	$\alpha_1, \alpha_2, \beta_1, \beta_2$	Decrease +	Increase +++
Sphincters	α_1	Contraction +	Relaxation +
Secretion	α_2	Inhibition	Stimulation ++
Urinary bladder			
Detrusor	β_2	Relaxation +	Contraction +++
Trigone and sphincter	α_1	Contraction ++	Relaxation ++
Ureter			
Motility and tone	α_1	Increase	Increase (?)

(Contd.)

Organ	Receptor	Sympathetic	Parasympathetic
Eye			
Dilator pupillae (radial muscle of iris)	α_1 (mainly); very few β	Contraction (mydriasis) ++	—
Sphincter muscle of iris	α and β in equal amounts	—	Contraction (miosis) +++
Ciliary muscle	β_2 (mainly); α (very few)	Relaxation for far vision +	Contraction for near vision (accommodation) +++
Kidney			
Renal secretion	α_1	Decrease +	—
	β_1	Increase ++	—
Liver	α_1, β_2	Glycogenolysis and gluconeogenesis +++	—
Gall bladder and ducts	β_2	Relaxation +	Contraction +
Uterus			
Pregnant	α_1	Contraction	Variable
	β_2	Relaxation	—
Nonpregnant	β_2	Relaxation	Variable
Sex organs			
Male	α_1	Ejaculation ++	Erection +++
Skin			
Pilomotor muscle	α_1	Contraction ++	—
Sweat glands	α_1	Localized secretion +	Generalised secretion +++
Skeletal muscle	β_2	Increased contractility, glycogenolysis, K^+ uptake	
Spleen capsule	α_1	Contraction +++	—
	β_2	Relaxation +	—
Pancreas			
Acini	α	Decreased secretion +	Secretion ++
Islets (β cells)	α_2	Decreased secretion +++	—
	β_2	Increased secretion +	—
Pineal gland	β	Melatonin synthesis	—
Lacrimal glands	α	Secretion +	Secretion +++
Salivary glands	α_1	K^+ and water secretion +	K^+ and water secretion +++
	β	Amylase secretion +	—
Nasopharyngeal glands	—	—	Secretion ++
Posterior pituitary	β_1	Antidiuretic hormone secretion	—
Adrenal medulla	—	—	Secretion of epinephrine and norepinephrine (primarily nicotinic and secondarily muscarinic)
Adipose tissue	$\alpha_1, \beta_1, \beta_2$	Lipolysis	—

CHOLINERGIC DRUGS (PARASYMPATHETIC AGONISTS)

Cholinoceptors

Sir Henry Dale found that the alkaloid muscarine mimicked the actions of parasympathetic nerve discharge (parasympathomimetic action). The effects were mediated by receptor at the effector cells. But nicotine was found to stimulate autonomic ganglia and skeletal neuromuscular junctions. Later on, it was found that ACh acts at both the muscarinic and nicotinic receptors. Both are subtypes of cholinoceptors.

Classification of cholinergic (cholinomimetic) drugs

Drugs which mimic the effects of parasympathetic

Table 2.4. Types and locations of cholinergic receptors

Receptor type	Location	Responses	Agonist	Antagonist
Muscarinic receptors				
M_1	Autonomic ganglia	Depolarization Histamine release	ACh Carbachol	Atropine *Pirenzepine
	Gastric glands CNS	gastric secretion undefined		*Telenzepine
M_2	Heart SA node	Decreased rate of impulse generation	ACh Carbachol Methacholine	Atropine Gallamine
	Atrium	Shortening of duration of action potential, decreased contractile force		**AF-DX 116 methoctramine
	AV-node	Decreased velocity of conduction		
	Ventricle	Slight decrease in contractility		
M_3	Smooth muscle	Contraction	ACh Carbachol	Atropine
	Secretory glands	Increased secretion		***Hexahydro- siladifenidiol
Nicotinic receptors				
Muscle (N_M)	Neuromuscular Junction	End-plate-depolarization, skeletal muscle contraction	ACh Nicotine	d-tubocurarine
Nicotinic Neuronal (N_N)	Autonomic ganglia	Depolarization and firing of postganglionic neuron	ACh, Nicotine	Hexamethonium Trimethaphan
	Adrenal medulla	Liberation of catechola- mines		
	CNS	Excitation/Inhibition (site specific)		

M_4, M_5, Muscarinic receptors (location CNS): Genes have been cloned but functional receptors have not been incontrovertibly identified.

  * Selective antagonists to M_1
 ** Selective antagonists to M_2
*** Selective antagonists to M_3

stimulation are called parasympathomimetics or cholinergic agonists. These can be grouped in following categories:

Cholinergic receptors

Table 2.4 shows the types and locations of cholinergic receptors.

1. Direct acting cholinoceptor stimulants: These directly bind to and activate muscarinic or nicotinic receptors.

(a) Esters of choline
  Acetylcholine chloride
  Methacholine chloride
  Carbachol chloride
  Bethanechol chloride

(b) Cholinomimetic alkaloids
  Pilocarpine
  Muscarine (no therapeutic value)
  Arecoline (no therapeutic value)

2. Indirect acting cholinoceptor stimulants are drugs that inhibit cholinesterase (anticholinesterases) and thus increase the concentration of endogenous ACh. These are:
   (a) Short acting: Edrophonium
   (b) Medium duration anticholinesterases: Neostigmine, Physostigmine (eserine)
   (c) Long lasting: Organophosphorus compounds

   Table 2.5 shows the receptors and target organs of directly acting and indirectly acting cholinomimetics.

Table 2.5. Cholinomimetic drugs, receptors and target organs

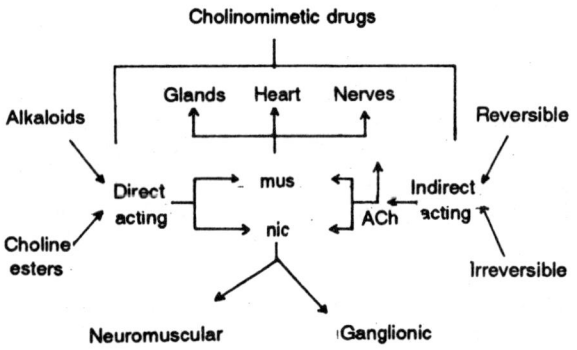

mus = muscarinic receptors; nic = nicotinic receptors

Table 2.6 shows comparison of some properties of choline esters.

Pharmacological actions of parasympathomimetics (cholinomimetics)

i. *Cardiovascular system* :
   Blood vessel : they do not receive parasympathetic innervation but the circulating, or exogenously administered cholinergic drugs cause vasodilatation.
   Heart : Atria – decrease in force of contraction, sino-atrial node–decrease in heart rate; atrioventricular node–decrease in conduction.

ii. *Gastrointestinal system* : increase in tone, amplitude, peristaltic and secretory activity.

iii. *Urinary tract* : contraction of detrussor muscle and relaxation of trigone and sphincter, leading to urination.

iv. *Eye* : miosis (contraction of circular muscle fibres of iris), spasm of accommodation (contraction of ciliary muscle), decrease in intraocular pressure through action on sphincter pupillae and ciliary muscle (enhances drainage of aqueous humour through the canal of Schlemm) and increase in lacrimal secretion.

v. *Bronchi* : bronchoconstriction, increase in bronchial secretion.

vi. *Salivary and sweat glands* : increase in secretion.

Table 2.6. Comparison of some properties of choline esters

	ACh	Methacholine	Carbachol	Bethanechol
Source	Physiological neurotransmitter	Synthetic	Synthetic	Synthetic
Susceptibility to ACh esterase	Rapidly destroyed	+	—	—
Stability	—	+	+++	+++
Actions (muscarinic)				
CVS	+	+++	+	±
GIT	+	+	+++	+++
Urinary bladder	+	+	+++	+++
Eye (topical)	+	+	+	+
Selectivity	Nonselective	CVS	GIT, urinary bladder	GIT, urinary bladder
Antagonism by atropine	+++	+++	+	+++
Actions (nicotinic)	+	+	+++	—

INDIVIDUAL CHOLINERGIC AGENTS

1. Directly acting cholinergic drugs

(a) Esters of choline

Acetylcholine

Acetylcholine produces a huge variety of actions and so rapidly destroyed that it is unlikely to be useful as a drug. Now a variety of drugs are available with longer action and varying degrees of selectivity.

Acetylcholine produces negative inotropic effect, negative chronotropic effect and vasodilatation. It increases GI motility and secretory activity. It contracts smooth muscle of uterus, ureters, bladder and bronchioles and constrictor muscle of iris. It stimulates salivary, sweat and lacrimal glands.

Methacholine

It acts selectively on muscarine receptors. It is rapidly hydrolyzed. It has more action on the cardiovascular system.

Carbachol

Carbachol is not destroyed by cholinesterase, its actions are most pronounced on the bladder and bowels. It is stable in the alimentary tract (oral dose 1-4 mg). It is dangerous if given intravenously but may be given subcutaneously (0.2-0.5 mg).

Bethanechol

Bethanechol (5, 10 mg) is not destroyed by cholinesterase. It acts chiefly on the bowel and bladder and may be more effective than carbachol. It can be given orally (5-30 mg) or 2-5 mg by subcutaneous injection.

(b) Alkaloids with cholinergic effects

Pilocarpine

Pilocarpine is an alkaloid from a plant Pilocarpus. It acts directly on end-organs innervated by postganglionic parasympathetic nerves. It also stimulates and then depresses the CNS. Its actions on autonomic ganglia and neuromuscular junction are very little.

Muscarine

It is obtained from amanita muscaria (oily agaric mushroom) and also present in some other mushroom species; pharmacological actions resemble those of pilocarpine. It has toxic neurologic effects. It has no therapeutic value.

Arecoline

It is obtained from areca nuts having parasympathomimetic actions similar to pilocarpine. It does not have any therapeutic use.

Therapeutic uses of directly acting cholinomimetics

Uses of pilocarpine :
1. Oral : 5-10 mg for xerostomia
2. Topical :
   - Wide angle glaucoma: 0.5% - 4% solution
   - Accommodative esotropia (convergent squint) in young children
   - Alternated with mydriatics to break adhesions between iris and lens
   - To overcome the mydriasis produced by atropine.

Acetylcholine chloride is only occasionally used in ophthalmic surgery. It is not used commonly since it is hydrolysed immediately by acetylcholinesterase (true AChE) and butyryl ChE (pseudo ChE) and it has diffuse actions. However, it is occasionally used in ophthalmic surgery. The topical ocular instillation of ACh produces no response as it is rapidly destroyed by cholinesterase before it can penetrate the cornea. But instillation of 1:100 solution directly on iris produces prompt and brief miosis at the time of surgery which may be preferred to the use of pilocarpine or physostigmine as the latter drugs cause prolonged miosis and postoperative pain.

Bethanechol is used in postoperative abdominal distension (postoperative atony), oesophageal reflux and urinary retention. *Carbachol* is used as 3% ophthalmic solution to produce miosis and in glaucoma resistant to pilocarpine or physostigmine.

Bethanechol or *methacholine* may be used as an alternative to pilocarpine to treat xerostomia (dryness of mouth due to diminished salivary secretion).

Adverse effects of directly acting cholinomimetic agents

The direct acting muscarinic agents (choline esters and pilocarpine) may produce nausea, vomiting, diarrhoea, salivation, sweating and bronchial constriction. These effects can be blocked by atropine and its congeners.

Contraindications of cholinergic agonists

- Bronchial asthma as they may aggravate bronchospasm.
- Peptic ulcer as they may increase secretion of gastric acid.
- Myocardial infarction.
- Hyperthyroidism, as it predisposes to atrial fibrillation.

Cholinesterases

These are of two types:

- Acetylcholinesterase (AChE) or true or specific cholinesterase, found in cholinergic neurons, cholinergic synapses and neuromuscular junctions. It hydrolyzes ACh at a greater velocity, it also hydrolyzes methacholine. Both nerves and muscles have the capacity to synthesize AChE.
- Butyrylcholinesterase (BuChE) or pseudocholinesterases are present in glial cells, plasma and liver. It is present in presynaptic and postsynaptic membranes and also basal lamina on neuromuscular junction. It hydrolyzes butyrylcholine at a greater velocity. It also hydrolyzes ACh but not methacholine, it is also more sensitive to inhibition by organophosphates. Liver and other tissues have the capacity to synthesize BuChE.

Table 2.7 shows comparison between true and pseudo cholinesterases.

Table 2.7. Comparison between AChE (true) and BuChE (pseudocholinesterase).

	True ChE (Acetylcholinesterase AChE)	Pseudo ChE (Butyryl cholinesterase) BuChE
Distribution	Cholinergic sites, RBC, gray matter	Plasma, intestine, liver, white matter
Hydrolysis		
ACh	Very fast (millisec)	Slow
Methacholine	Slower than ACh	Not hydrolyzed
Benzoylcholine	Not hydrolyzed	Hydrolyzed
Butyrylcholine	Not hydrolyzed	Hydrolyzed
Role	ACh action terminated	Hydrolysis of ingested esters
Inhibition	More sensitive to eserine	More sensitive to organophosphates

2. Indirectly acting cholinergic drugs

Anticholinesterase Agents (anti-ChE)

Classification

i. Naturally occurring: Physostigmine (a tertiary amine).
ii. Synthetic
   (a) Quaternary ammonium compounds
       (i) Short acting: Edrophonium
       (ii) Medium acting: Neostigmine, Pyridoxamine, Demecarium
   b) Long acting (irreversible)
       (i) Therapeutic agents: Diisopropyl fluorophosphate (DFP)
           Tetraethyl pyrophosphate (TEPP)
       (ii) Insecticides: Parathion, malathion
       (iii) Nerve gases: Tabun, sarin, soman

Table 2.8 shows reversible and irreversible anti-ChEs along with their uses and duration.

Table 2.8. Reversible and irreversible anti ChEs along with their uses and duration.

	Uses	Duration
Reversible		
Edrophonium	Myasthenia gravis, arrhythmias	2-10 minutes
Neostigmine	Myasthenia gravis, paralytic ileus	½-2 hours
Pyridostigmine	Myasthenia gravis	3-6 hours
Physostigmine	Glaucoma	½-2 hours
Ambenonium	Myasthenia gravis	4-8 hours
Demecarium	Glaucoma	4-6 hours
Irreversible		
Ecothiopate	Glaucoma	100 hours
Dyflos (DFP)	Insecticide	
Parathion	Insecticide	
Malathion	Insecticide	

Table 2.9 shows comparison between physostigmine and neostigmine.

Mechanism of action of anti - ChE agents

The reversible anti-ChEs resemble the structure of ACh. They combine with anionic and esteratic sites of ChE. this complex is less readily hydrolyzed than ACh esteratic site complex formed with ACh. This

Table 2.9. Differences between physostigmine (eserine) and neostigmine (prostigmine)

	Physostigmine	*Neostigmine*
Source	Calabar bean	Synthetic
Nature	Tertiary amine alkaloid	Quaternary ammonium compound
Stability	Less stable	More stable
Absorption	Good from GIT, conjunctiva	Absorption incomplete orally, good absorption after I.M. injection
Blood-brain barrier	Crosses	No
ChE inhibition	reversible inhibition	Reversible inhibition
Action on - cholinergic receptors	Acts on both muscarinic and nicotinic receptors	Acts on both receptors and also direct action
Antagonist	Atropine antagonizes completely	Incomplete antagonism
Toxicity	More toxic	Less toxic
Uses	Miotic, atropine poisoning	Myasthenia gravis, curare poisoning paralytic ileus, retention of urine

produces temporary inhibition of the enzyme. Edrophonium forms complex only at anionic site, so has a shorter duration of action (about 10 minutes).

The irreversible anti-ChEs organophosphorus compounds combine only with esteratic site and phosphorylate it. The hydrolysis of phosphorylated site is extremely slow and that is why they have long duration of action.

Therapeutic uses of anti-ChEs

- Wide angle glaucoma: Physostigmine, DFP, ecothiopate, demecarium.
- Paralytic ileus and atony of urinary bladder: Neostigmine
- Myasthenia gravis:
  (a) Diagnosis: Edrophonium is given intravenously to distinguish between myasthenic crisis and cholinergic crisis. Cholinergic crisis is due to excessive anti-ChE agent, myasthanic weakness is due to insufficient anti-ChE agent. When edrophonium is given cholinergic crisis is worsened but myas-

thenic weakness shows improvement. It is too short-acting (2-10 min.) for therapeutic use.
  (b) Treatment: Neostigmine, pyridostigmine
  (c) Prophylaxis of ChE inhibitors poisoning: Pyridostigmine.
- Atropine poisoning, overdosage of phenothiazines, antihistamines, tricyclic antidepressants.
- d-tubocurarine overdosage – neostigmine with atropine. Neostigmine may aggravate hypotension or bronchospasm caused by d-tubocurarine. Therefore atropine is given with neostigmine to counteract the muscarinic actions of neostigmine.
- Paroxysmal ventricular tachycardia: edrophonium (not commonly used these days), beta-blockers, calcium channel blockers or adenosine are preferred.
- Alzheimer's disease: physostigmine, tacrine, metrifonate.

MYASTHENIA GRAVIS

Myasthenia gravis is an auto-immune disease, with weakness and fatigability of skeletal muscle. It is a disease affecting skeletal muscle neuromuscular junctions. In myasthenia gravis, there is decreased number of functional nicotinic receptors on the postjunctional end - plates. There is weakness of skeletal muscles, particularly the small muscles of head, neck and extremities. Patient suffers from ptosis, diplopia, difficulty in swallowing and speaking. In severe cases all the muscles are affected including those required for respiration.

Drugs which aggravate myasthenia symptoms

Aminoglycosides, polymyxins, erythromycin, ciprofloxacin, norfloxacin, quinidine, procainamide, chlorpromazine, propranolol, lithium, phenytoin, d-tubocurarine.

Drugs which are given for the treatment of myasthenia gravis

Neostigmine 7.5 mg - 15 mg, six hourly; or pyridostigmine is given.

When anti-ChE agents do not promote near normal motor activity, corticosteroids are given.

In more advanced cases, immunosuppressants such as azathioprine or cyclosporin is beneficial.

Organophosphorus Poisoning

The toxicological aspects of the anti-ChE agents are of practical importance to the physician. The organophosphorus agents (pesticide-related) induce poisoning and it is a widespread global problem.

Acute intoxication due to anti-ChE agents

The effects of acute poisoning are manifested by muscarinic and nicotinic signs and symptoms.

Ocular effects include marked miosis, ocular pain and diminished vision.

Respiratory effects consist of tightness in the chest and wheezing respiration (due to combination of bronchoconstriction and increased bronchial secretion).

Gastrointestinal disturbances including vomiting, diarrhoea and abdominal cramps.

Additional muscarinic effects include extreme salivation, involuntary defaection, urination, sweating, lacrimation, bradycardia and hypotension.

Nicotinic actions at the neuromuscular junctions of skeletal muscle consist of generalized weakness, involuntary twitchings and eventually paralysis.

The most serious is the paralysis of the respiratory muscles.

CNS actions: Ataxia, slurred speech, excitation, convulsions.

Treatment

1. The effective antidotes are:
   (i) Atropine I.V. injection, 2-4 mg, followed by 2 mg every 5-10 minutes until muscarinic symptoms disappear or signs of atropinization (mydriasis, dryness of mouth, tachycardia) appear. Large doses are required to cross the blood-brain barrier; More than 200 mg may be needed on the first day.

   However, atropine is virtually without effect against the peripheral neuromuscular activation and subsequent paralysis. This action of anti-ChE agents as well as all other peripheral effects can be reversed by ChE reactivators.

   (ii) Cholinesterase reactivators:
   (a) Pralidoxime (PAM) 1-2 gram given over 15-30 min. by I.V. infusion.
   (b) Diacetyl monoxime (DAM)

When ChE is phosphorylated by organophosphate, pralidoxime exerts a nucleophilic attack on the phosphorus; the oxime - phosphate intermediate is split off leaving the regenerated enzyme (AChE) free to act normally to hydrolyze ACh. Oximes act on neuromuscular junction, action on ganglia and CNS are not significant.

Oximes are effective only if given at the earliest (upto 24 hours) because the phosphorylated enzyme undergoes a process of aging and becomes resistant to reactivation by the oximes, within a few hours. However, recent opinion is to give oximes even if the patient comes late.

PAM does not enter the CNS and is ineffective in reversing the central effects of organophosphate poisoning. PAM is most effective in regenerating the cholinesterase associated with skeletal muscle neuromuscular junctions.

DAM does cross the blood-brain barrier and can regenerate some of the central nervous system cholinesterase.

2. General supportive measures:
   • Termination of exposure i.e. removal of contaminated clothing etc.
   • Maintenance of patent airways - suction of respiratory secretion.
   • Administration of oxygen, artificial respiration, if required.
   • Control of convulsions with diazepam 5-10mg I.V. or sodium thiopental 2.5% I.V.
   • Treatment of shock.

STUDY QUESTIONS

1. What are the different types of cholinoceptors and their location?
2. What are muscarinic and nicotinic actions of acetylcholine?
3. Classify cholinomimetic drugs.
4. Compare choline esters regarding receptor specificity and hydrolysis by acetylcholinesterases.

5. Which alkaloids have cholinergic effects? What are the uses and adverse effects of carbachol and pilocarpine?
6. Describe the effects of cholinergic drugs on different organ systems.
7. List the drugs which inhibit cholinesterases. What are their uses and adverse effects? How are these adverse effects treated?

GUIDE TO FURTHER READING

Burnstock, G. and Hoyle, C.H.V. Autonomic Neuroeffector Mechanisms. Harwood Academic Publishers, 1992.

Brunning, T.A. et al. In vivo characterization of vasodilating muscarinic receptor subtypes in humans. Cir. Res, 1994; 74:912.

Caulfield, M.P. Muscarinic receptors-Characterization, coupling and function. Pharmacol Ther, 1993; 58:319.

Deighton, N.M. et al. Muscarinic cholinoceptors in the human heart: Demonstration, subclassification and distribution. Naunyn Schmiedebergs. Arch Pharmacol, 1990; 34:14.

dekort W.L.A.M., Kiestra, S.H. and Sangster, B. The use of atropine and oximes in organophosphate intoxications. A modified approach. Clin Toxicol, 1988; 26:199.

DeSilva, H.J., Wijewickrema, R. and Senanayake, N. Does pralidoxine affect outcome of management in acute organophosphorus poisoning? Lancet, 1992; 339:113.

Dettbarn, W.D. Pesticide induced muscle necrosis: Mechanisms and prevention. Fundam Appl. Toxicol, 1984; 4:518.

Drachman, D.B. Myasthenia gravis. N Engl J Med, 1994; 330:1797.

Eglen, R.M. and Whiting, R.L. Heterogeneity of vascular muscarinic receptors. J Auton Pharmacol, 1990; 19:233.

Engel, A.G. Congenital myasthenia gravis. Neurol. Clin, 1994; 12:401.

Epstein, J.B. et al. A clinical trial of bethanechol in patients with xerostomia after radiation therapy. A pilot study. Oral Surg, Oral Med, Oral Pathol, 1994; 77:610.

Farrar, H.C., Wells, T.G. and Kearns, G.L. Use of continuous infusion of pralidoxime for treatment of organophosphate poisoning in children. J Pediatr, 1990; 116:658.

Freedman, S.B., Beer, M.S. and Harley, E.A. Muscarinic M1, M2 receptor binding: Relationship with functional efficacy. Europ J Pharmacol, 1988; 156:133.

Goyal, R.K. Muscarinic receptor subtypes. Physiology and clinical complications. N Engl J Med, 1989; 321:1022.

Keeler, J.R., Hurst, C.G. and Dunn, M.A. Pyridostigmine used as a nerve agent treatment under wartime conditions. JAMA, 1991; 266:693.

Levy, M.N., Schwartz, P.J. (editors). Vagal Control of the heart. Futura, 1993.

Symposium (various authors). Subtypes of muscarinic receptors V. (Levine R.R. and Birdsall N.J.M. eds). Life Sci, 1993; 52:405.

Symposium (various authors). Subtypes of muscarinic receptors VI. (Levine R.R. and Birdsall N.J.M. ed). Life Sci, 1995; 56:801.

Wess, J. Molecular basis of muscarinic acetylcholine receptor function. Trends Pharmacol Sci, 1993; 14:308.

Arner, P. The beta 3-adrenergic receptor—a cause and cure of obesity? N Engl J Med., 1995; 333:382.

Brown, C.G. et al. A comparison of standard dose and high dose epinephrine in cardiac arrest outside the hospital. N Engl J Med, 1992; 327:1051.

Caron, M.G., Lefkowitz, R.J. Catecholamine receptors: structure, function, and regulation. Recent Prog Horm Res, 1993; 48:277.

Faure, C. et al. Identification of alpha 1-adrenoceptor subtypes in the human prostate. Life Sci, 1994; 54:1595.

Gingrich, J.A., Caron, M.G. Recent advances in the molecular biology of dopamine receptors. Annu Rev Neurosci, 1993; 16:299.

Hurvitz, L.M. et al. New developments in the drug treatment of glaucoma. Drugs, 1991; 41:514.

MacDonald, A. et al. Contributions of alpha 1-adrenoceptors, alpha 2-adrenoceptors, and P2d purinoceptors to neurotransmission in several rabbit isolated blood vessels: Role of neuronal uptake and autofeedback. Br J Pharmacol, 1992; 105:347.

McGrath, J.C., Brown, C.M. and Wilson, V.G. Alpha-adrenoceptors. A critical review. Med Res Rev, 1989; 9:407.

Ruffolo, R.R. Jr. et al. Pharmacologic and therapeutic applications of alpha 2-adrenoceptor subtypes. Annu Rev Pharmacol Toxicol, 1993; 32:243.

Ruffolo, R.R. Jr. et al. Structure and function of alpha-adrenoceptors. Pharmacol Rev, 1991; 43:475.

Seeman, P., Grigoriades, D. Dopamine receptors in brain and periphery. Neurochem Int, 1987; 10:1.

Spitzer, W.O. et al. The use of beta-agonists and risk of death and near death from asthma. N Engl J Med, 1992; 326:501.

Valtorta, F. et al. Neurotransmitter release and synaptic vesicle recycling. Neuroscience, 1990; 35:477.

Vincent, J., et al. Pharmacological tolerance to alpha 1-adrenergic antagonism mediated by terazosin in humans. J. Clin. Invest., 1992; 90:1763.

Zorgniotti, A.W. Experience with buccal phentolamine mesylate for impotence. Int. J. Impotence Res., 1994; 6:37.

ANTICHOLINERGIC DRUGS (PARASYMPATHETIC ANTAGONISTS)

The class of drugs referred to here as muscarinic receptor antagonists include atropine and a number of other agents having qualitatively similar effects.

Atropine

Atropine alkaloid is obtained from atropa belladonna (deadly night shade). Belladonna means a beautiful lady due to dilated pupils caused by atropine.

The other belladonna alkaloid scopolamine (hyoscine) is obtained from hyoscyamus niger.

Pharmacological properties

- *Secretions* : Atropine reduces salivary, lacrimal, bronchial and sweat secretions. This produces dryness in mouth and skin. The gastric secretion is only slightly reduced.
- *Cardiovascular system* : Although the dominant response is tachycardia, the heart rate often decreases transiently with average clinical doses (0.4-0.6 mg). This paradoxical effect was thought to be due to central vagal stimulation. Recent studies indicate that decrease in heart rate may result from blockade of M_1 receptors. The blood pressure is unaffected, since most resistance blood vessels do not have cholinergic innervation.

  Atropine counteracts the peripheral vasodilatation and fall in blood pressure caused by choline esters. However, when given alone atropine has no significant effect on blood pressure. It is so

because most vascular beds probably lack significant cholinergic innervation.

- *Eye* : The muscarinic receptor antagonists block the responses of the sphincter muscle of the iris and the ciliary muscle to cholinergic stimulation. Thus, they produce dilatation of the pupil (mydriasis) and cycloplegia (paralysis of accommodation). The rise in intraocular pressure (IOP) occurs when the anterior chamber is narrow. It will further raise intraocular pressure in glaucoma or in susceptible persons.
- *Gastrointestinal tract* : Motility is inhibited particularly in conditions in which there is increased gastrointestinal motility.
- *Other smooth muscles* e.g. bronchial, biliary and urinary tract are relaxed.
- *Uterine smooth muscle* is innervated by parasympathetic fibres but the effect of cholinergic impulses on uterine contractility is variable. Hence, atropine and scopolamine have negligible effect.
- *Central nervous system* : Atropine produces excitatory effects, in low doses mild restlessness, higher doses produce agitation and disorientation and in still larger doses, stimulation is followed by depression leading to circulatory collapse and respiratory failure after a period of paralysis and coma.
- *Respiratory tract* : The parasympathetic nervous system regulate bronchomotor tone, hence anticholinergic agents were used as bronchodilators which have been supplanted by adrenergic agents. However, owing to the introduction of ipratropium bromide anticholinergic therapy of respiratory disease has been revived.

Hyoscine

Hyoscine causes marked sedation in low doses unlike atropine. In high dosage, the effects of atropine and hyoscine are similar on the central nervous system. Hyoscine has a useful antiemetic effect.

Table 2.10 shows the differences between atropine and scopolamine (hyoscine).

Pharmacokinetics

The belladonna alkaloids are absorbed rapidly from

Table 2.10. Differences between atropine and scopolamine (hyoscine)

	Atropine	*Scopolamine*
CNS: Thereapeutic dose	No effect	Depression (sedation)
Toxic dose	Excitation	Excitation
Potency	More potent on heart, intestine and bronchial muscle	More potent on iris, ciliary body and secretory glands
Duration of action	More prologned action	Short duration of action
Motion sickness	Not used	Used. Effective in motion sickness. It has a useful antiemetic effect.

the GIT and can also reach circulation when applied topically. However, absorption from intact skin is limited. The half-life of atropine is about 4 hours. About half of the dose is metabolized in the liver and the remainder is excreted unchanged in the urine. Traces appear in various secretions including breast milk.

Synthetic and semisynthetic substitutes for belladonna alkaloids

Quaternary ammonium muscarinic receptor antagonists

Ipratropium bromide is formed by the introduction of an isopropyl group to the N atom of atropine. Oxitropium bromide is a derivative of scopolamine, formed by the introduction of an ethyl group. The most recently developed and bronchoselective drug is tiotropium bromide which has a longer duration of action.

Ipratropium bromide produces similar effects as atropine when administered parenterally, although somewhat more potent. However, it lacks appreciable effects on the CNS and has greater inhibitory effect on ganglionic transmission.

When solutions are inhaled, the effect is largely confined to respiratory tract. The absorption from lungs and GIT is inefficient.

Methscopolamine bromide is a quaternary ammonium derivative of scopolamine and so lacks the central actions of scopolamine; it is less potent than atropine and poorly absorbed but its action is prolonged. Its use is limited to gastrointestinal diseases. The usual oral dose is 2.5 mg acting for 6-8 hours.

Homatropine methylbromide is a quaternary derivative of homatropine, less potent than atropine but 4 times more potent as a ganglionic blocking

agent, indicated for relief of gastrointestinal spasm.

Methantheline bromide (banthine). It differs from atropine in having high ratio of ganglionic blocking activity to antimuscarinic activity. The usual dose is 50-100 mg lasting 6 hours. High doses produce impotence. Toxic doses paralyze respiration by neuromuscular block.

Propantheline bromide (pro-banthine). It is 2-5 times more potent than banthine. The dose is 15 mg which acts for about 6 hours.

Other drugs in this category include anisotropine methylbromide, clidinium bromide, glycopyrrolate, etc.

Tertiary-amine muscarinic receptor antagonists

Included in this group are homatropine hydrobromide (semisynthetic derivative of atropine), cyclopentolate hydrochloride and tropicamide. These agents are preferred to atropine and scopolamine because of their shorter duration of action.

Tertiary-amine muscarinic receptor antagonists gain access to CNS and so used to treat parkinsonism and extrapyramidal side effects of antipsychotic agents e.g. benztropine mesylate, artane and others.

Tertiary-amine used for antispasmodic properties includes dicyclomine hydrochloride (bentyl, others).

Selective muscarinic receptor antagonists

Pirenzepine is a tricyclic drug, has selectivity for M_1-, relative to M_2-, and M_3-muscarinic receptors.

Telenzepine is an analogue of pirenzepine, more potent having similar selectivity for M_1-muscarinic receptors. They are used for the treatment of peptic ulcer.

AF-DX116 is an analogue of pirenzepine, has greatest affinity for cardiac (M_2) muscarinic receptors, is being investigated for the treatment of bradyarrhythmias.

Methoctramine is more potent than AF-DX116 for cardiac M_2 receptors and is highly selective M_2 relative to M_3 receptors. A derivative tripitamine also discriminates between M_2- and M_3-muscarinic receptors.

Hexahydrosiladifenidol and 4-DAMP have greatest selectivity for M_3 receptors.

Himbacine is most useful for defining the M_4-muscarinic receptor subtypes.

The drugs listed above including pirenzepine do not discriminate M_4 receptors from the subtype for which they are otherwise selective.

Therapeutic uses of antimuscarinic drugs

1. *GIT disorders* :
   - Pirenzepine acts synergistically with H_2 receptor antagonists in the treatment of peptic ulcer.
   - To reduce salivary secretion in heavy metal poisoning and parkinsonism.
   - Diarrhoea due to adrenergic neuron blockers (lomotil, a combination of diphenoxylate and atropine).
   - Increased tone and motility of GIT.

2. *Ophthalmological uses* :
   - Topical use of mydriatic for funduscopic examination
   - Topical use of cycloplegic for iritis, iridocyclitis
   - Alternative, with miotic to prevent or break the adhesions between iris and lens

   Comparison of certain anticholinergic drugs employed in ophthalmic practice is given in Tables 2.11 and 2.12.

3. *Respiratory tract disorders* : Ipratropium (a synthetic analogue of atropine) inhalation in bronchial asthma and chronic obstructive pulmonary disease (COPD).

4. *CVS disorders* :
   - In the presence of sufficient depression of SA, AV node function which impairs cardiac output antimuscarinic drug is appropriate therapy.
   - To counteract reflex cardiac slowing
   - In AV block due to digitalis toxicity.

5. *CNS disorders* :
   - Benztropine for treating extrapyramidal disorder due to antipsychotic drugs.
   - Parkinson's disease, e.g., benztropine.
   - Scopolamine (oral, transdermal), for prevention and treatment of motion sickness.

6. *Genitourinary tract* :
   - Atropine with an opioid to treat renal colic
   - To relieve ureteral spasm and irritability of bladder (urinary urgency) after urologic surgery.

7. As *preanaesthetic* medicaments to inhibit excessive salivation and secretion of respiratory tract and prevent reflex vagal stimulation of the heart.

8. *Use in cholinergic poisoning* :
   - Antidote for organophosphate poisoning.
   - To antagonise muscarinic effects of neostigmine in myasthenia gravis and to reverse neuromuscular block in anaesthesia.

Box 2.4. Receptor-end-organ response		
Organ	*Receptor*	*Effect*
Heart	β_1	Increased inotropic and chronotropic
	M_2	Decreased inotropic and chronotropic
Coronary and pulmonary arterioles, blood vessels to skeletal muscle	β_2 (mainly)	Dilation
	α	Constriction
	M_2	Dilation
Other arterioles	α	Constriction
	β	Dilation
	M_2	Dilation
Veins	α	Constriction
	β_2	Dilation
Bronchi	β_2	Relaxation
	M_2	Constriction

Box 2.5. Autonomic pharmacology of the eye				
Tissue	*Adrenergic receptors*	*Response*	*Cholinergic receptors*	*Response*
Corneal epithelium	β_2	Unknown	Undefined	Unknown
Corneal endothelium	β_2	Unknown	Undefined	Unknown
Iris radial muscle	α_1	Mydriasis		
Iris sphincter muscle			M_3, m_3	Miosis
Trabecular meshwork	β_2	Unknown		
Ciliary epithelium	α_2/β_2	Aqueous production		
Ciliary muscle	β_2	Relaxation	M3	Accommodation
Lacrimal gland	α_1	Secretion	M_2, M_3, m_3	Secretion
Retinal pigment epithelium	α_1/β_2	H_2O transport/unknown		

Table 2.11. Anticholinergic drugs employed as mydriatics

Drug	% w/v	Onset in min	Duration	Reversed by	Mode of action
Atropine sulphate	1.0	40	7 days	Echothiophate	Antimuscarinic
Homatropine hydrobromide	1.0	40	2 days	Physostigmine	Antimuscarinic
Cyclopentolate hydrobromide	0.5-1.0	30	1 day	Physostigmine	Antimuscarinic
Tropicamide	0.5	15	8 hours	Physostigmine	Antimuscarinic
Eucatropine	5.0-10.0	20-30	6 hours	Physostigmine	Antimuscarinic

Table 2.12. Anticholinergic drugs employed before examination as cycloplegics

Drug	Cycloplegic strength	Cycloplegia onset	Duration
Atropine sulphate ointment	1%	36 hours	Up to 7 days
Hyoscine	1	90 min	24 hours
Homatropine	0.5%	60 min	24 hours
Cyclopentolate	1.0	45 min	12 hours
Tropicamide	1%	30 min	6 hours

Mode of action

Muscarinic receptor antagonists prevent the effect of ACh by blocking its binding to muscarinic cholinergic receptors at neuroeffector sites on smooth muscle, cardiac muscle, and gland cells; in peripheral ganglia; and in the central nervous system. In general, they cause little blockade of the effects of ACh at nicotinic receptors sites. Thus, at the neuromuscular junction where the receptors are nicotinic, extremely high doses are required to produce any degree of blockade.

Box 2.6. Terms associated with eye

Accommodation: A change in the curvature of the eye lens to be adjusted for vision at various distances, focussing.

Amblyopia: Loss of vision in an otherwise normal eye that, because of muscle imbalance, cannot focus in sync with the other eye.

Astigmatism: An irregularity of the lens or cornea causing the image to be out of focus producing faulty vision.

Blepharitis (blepharo = eyelid; itis = inflammation): An inflammation of the eyelid.

Keratitis (kerato = cornea): An inflammation of the cornea.

Miosis: Constricted pupil.

Mydriasis: Dilated pupil.

Nystagmus (nystazein = to nod): An involuntary movement of the eyeballs.

Photophobia (photo = light; phobia = fear): Abnormal visual intolerance to light.

Scotoma: An area of depressed or lost vision within the visual field.

Strabismus: An imbalance of extrinsic eye muscles that produces a squint.

Stroma: The tissue that forms the ground substance, foundation, or frame work of an organ, as opposed to its functional parts.

Atropine substitutes categorized according to their uses:

1. *As mydriatic agents* : Tertiary amine muscarinic receptor antagonists:

   Homatropine hydrobromide (semisynthetic derivative of atropine)

   Eucatropine

   Cyclopentolate hydrochloride

   Tropicamide

   These are short acting and less cycloplegic (advantages over atropine). Tropicamide is preferred because it has the quickest (20-40 min.) and briefest (less than 6 hours) action.

2. *As gastrointestinal antispasmodic agents* : Quaternary ammonium muscarinic receptor antagonists:

   Propantheline bromide (pro-Banthine)

   Oxyphenonium

   Tertiary amine muscarinic receptor antagonists:

   Dicyclomine hydrochloride

   Oxybutynin chloride

3. *As antiparkinsonian agents* : Tertiary amine muscarinic receptor antagonists gain access to CNS, so used to treat parkinsonism and extrapyramidal side effects of antipsychotic agents :

   Benztropine mesylate

   Procyclidine

   Ethopropazine

4. *Substitutes used specifically for urinary tract spasm* : Oxybutynin to relieve bladder spasm after urologic surgery, also to relieve ureteral spasm due to urolithiasis, and also for treating urinary urgency caused by minor inflammatory bladder disorders.

Adverse effects

- *Peripheral effects* : Tachycardia, dry mouth, mydriasis, hot and flushed skin, body temperature raised (hyperpyrexia).
- Central effects: atropine delirium, seizures, respiratory and cardiovascular failure, after a period of paralysis and coma, death.

  The traditional maxim (adage) may be like this: dry as a bone (due to inhibition of sweat glands), blind as a bat (due to cycloplegic effect), red as a beet root (as skin vessels dilate to compensate dryness) and 'mad as a hatter' (due to ataxia, confusion, hallucination and difficulty in speaking).

Contraindications to atropine use :

- Narrow angle (angle closure) glaucoma.
- Patients with shallow anterior chamber as angle-closure and acute glaucoma may precipitate in them.
- Enlarged prostate.
- Congestive heart failure with tachycardia.
- Pyloric stenosis.
- Chronic lung diseases as this reduces and dries up the respiratory tract secretions.

STUDY QUESTIONS

1. What are muscarinic antagonists? List these drugs.
2. What are the main effects of atropine? Describe atropine toxicity.
3. Compare the effects of atropine and other atropine substitutes as mydriatic and cycloplegic drugs.
4. Write notes on hyoscine, pirenzepine and pralidoxime.
5. Which anticholinergic drugs are used in the treatment of parkinsonism and how are they beneficial in this disorder?
6. How are antimuscarinic drugs useful as pre-anaesthetic medicaments?

GUIDE TO FURTHER READING

Ali-Melkkila, Kanto, J. and Iisalo, E. Pharmacokinetics and related pharmacodynamics of anticholinergic drugs. Acta Anaesthesiol Scand, 1993; 37:633.

Holtmann, G., Kuppers, U., Singer, M.V. Telenzepine, a new M1-receptor antagonist is a more potent inhibitor of pentagastrin-stimulated gastric acid output than pirenzepine in dogs. Scand, J. Gastroenterol, 1990; 25:293.

Rusted, J.M., Warburton, D.M. The effects of scopolamine on working memory in healthy young volunteers. Psychopharmacology, 1988; 96:145.

Vybiral, T. et al. Effects of transdermal scopolamine on heart rate variability in normal subjects. Am J Cardiol, 1990; 65:604.

Wellstein, A., Pitschner, H.F. Complex dose-response curves of atropine in man explained by different functions of M_1- and M_2-cholinoceptors. Naunyn Schmiedebergs. Arch Pharmacol, 1988; 338:19.

ADRENERGIC OR SYMPATHETIC ACTIVATING DRUGS (SYMPATHOMIMETICS)

The sympathetic nervous system regulates the activity of heart and other organs, particularly in response to stress. The effects are mediated by release of the neurotransmitter norepinephrine (noradrenaline) from the nerve ending which activate the adrenoceptor receptors on postsynaptic sites. The adrenal medulla, under condition of stress, also releases epinephrine (adrenaline).

Adrenoceptors

Ahlquist, in 1948, observed that catecholamines act on two receptors, alpha and beta. Soon after this, subtypes of these receptors were found.

α_1 and α_2 groups have been shown to have multiple subtypes existing within the groups. These are shown in Table 2.13.

Table 2.13. Receptor types

Receptors	Location
Adrenoceptors	
α_1	Postsynaptic effector cells, especially found on blood vessels, on radial muscle of eye, in GIT and on the splenic capsule
α_2	Presynaptic α_2 receptors are found at adrenergic and cholinergic nerve terminals
β_1	Postsynaptic effector cells especially heart and intestine
β_2	Postsynaptic effector cells, mainly on bronchial and avascular smooth muscle
β_3	Postsynaptic effector cells especially lipocytes
Dopamine receptors	
	Dopamine is an important neurotransmitter in the CNS. It acts on beta$_1$ receptors and releases NE from nerve terminals resulting in passive inotropic effect on the myocardium
D_1 (D_{A1})	Brain, renal vascular bed; the central D_1 receptor site is excitatory
D_2	Brain, renal vascular bed; D_2 receptor site is inhibitory in some brain tissues
D_3	Brain (limbic system); it is associated with emotional and cognitive behaviour
D_4	Brain, CVS

Table 2.14. Main adrenoceptor functions

α-adrenoceptor effects	β-adrenoceptor effects
Eye: mydriasis	↑ Heart (β_1) rate (SA node)
Arterioles: constriction (slight effect on coronaries and cerebral vessels)	↑ automaticity (AV node and muscle) ↑ conduction velocity
Skin: sweat, pilomotor	↑ myocardial contractility
Metabolic effect: hyperkalaemia	↓ refractory period Arterioles: dilation (β_2)
Bladder sphincter: contraction	Bronchi: relaxation (β_2) Uterus: relaxation of pregnant uterus (β_2) Skeletal muscle: tremor (β_2) Mast cells: release of autacoids inhibited (histamine, leukotrienes) Bladder detrusor: relaxation Metabolic effects: hypokalaemia (β_2); hepatic glycogenolysis (β_2); lipolysis (β_1).
Intestinal smooth muscle relaxation by both alpha and beta adrenoceptors	

Table 2.14 shows main adrenoceptor functions.

Classification by selectivity for receptors :

Agonists

- $\alpha + \beta$ effects—unselective: Epinephrine used as vasoconstrictor with local anaesthetic, as a mydriatic, in anaphylactic shock.
- α-effects: Norepinephrine has slight β_1 effect on heart. It has been superseded by dopamine.
- α-effects in CNS: Clonidine.
- β-effects—unselective: $\beta_1 + \beta_2$: Isoprenaline—it has been superseded by selective drugs.
- β_1-effects with some α-effects: Dopamine is used in vascular shock.
- β_1-effects: Dobutamine is used for cardiac inotropic effect.
- β_2-adrenoceptor agonists: Salbutamol, terbutaline, rimiterol, orciprenaline (partially selective) for treatment of asthma, and to relax the uterus.

Receptor specificity of adrenoceptor agonists

The specificity of different agonists is given in Table 2.15.

Table 2.15. Specificity of different agonists

Agonists	α_1	β_1	β_2
Norepinephrine	+++	+	+
Epinephrine	+	+++	+++
Isoprenaline	—	+++	+++
Phenylephrine	+	—	—
Salbutamol	—	+	+++
Dobutamine	—	+++	+
Terbutaline	—	+	+++

- α_1 type: α_{1A}, α_{1B}, α_{1C}, and α_{1D}. The spleen and liver contain mainly α_{1B}.
- α_2 type: α_{2A}, α_{2B}, α_{2C}.
- β type: β_1, β_2, β_3. β_1 receptors have equal affinity for epinephrine and norepinephrine, whereas β_2 receptors have a higher affinity for epinephrine than for norepinephrine. Molecular cloning has further shown that β_3 also exists.

Dopamine receptors

The endogenous catecholamine dopamine interacts with specific dopamine receptors which are particularly important in the brain and in the splanchnic and renal vasculature. The subtypes are termed D_1, D_2, D_4 and D_5 or D_{1A}, D_{2A}, D_{2C}, D_{1B}.

Relative selectivity of adrenoceptor agonists is shown in Table 2.16.

Table 2.16. Relative selectivity of adrenoceptor agonists

Relative receptor	Affinities
Alpha agonists	
Phenylephrine, methoxamine	$\alpha_1 > \alpha_2 >>>>> \beta$
Clonidine, methylnorepinephrine	$\alpha_2 > \alpha_1 >>>>> \beta$
Mixed alpha and beta agonists	
Norepinephrine	$\alpha_1 = \alpha_2; \beta_1 >> \beta_2$
Epinephrine	$\alpha_1 = \alpha_2; \beta_1 = \beta_2$
Beta agonists	
Dobutamine	$\beta_1 > \beta_2 >>>> \alpha$
Isoproterenol	$\beta_1 = \beta_2 >>>> \alpha$
Terbutaline	$\beta_2 >> \beta_1 >>>> \alpha$
Dopamine agonist	
Dopamine	$D_1 = D_2 >>\beta >> \alpha$

Classification of sympathomimetics based on site of action

- Directly acting on the adrenoceptors: Epinephrine, norepinephrine, isoprenaline, methoxamine, metaraminol, dopamine, phenylephrine.
- Indirectly acting by releasing norepinephrine from stores at nerve endings: Amphetamines, tyramine, ephedrine.
- By both mechanisms (directly as well as indirectly): Dopamine, ephedrine, other synthetic agents.

Pharmacological actions of sympathomimetic drugs

Sympathomimetic drugs mimic the actions of stimulation of sympathetic nervous system.

Cardiovascular system

Heart: Beta receptor activity largely determines the effects on the heart. The beta receptor activation produces increased influx of calcium into the cardiac cells resulting in increased contractility and conduction velocity.

Blood pressure: Phenylephrine which is almost pure alpha agonist increases peripheral arterial resistance and decreases venous capacitance. The blood pressure is enhanced and due to the marked rise in blood pressure vagal tone is increased (baroreceptor-mediated) resulting in bradycardia. However, cardiac output is not diminished due to the slowing of the heart rate because increased venous return increases the stroke volume.

Stimulation of beta receptors in the heart increases cardiac output. Isoprenaline which is almost pure beta agonist also decreases peripheral resistance by dilating certain vascular beds. Isoprenaline does not affect or slightly decreases the systolic pressure whereas it produces marked fall in diastolic pressure.

Blood vessels: Alpha receptors increase arterial resistance, whereas β_2 receptors produce smooth muscle relaxation. The overall effects of sympathomimetics on blood vessels depend on the relative action at α and β receptors and the sites of the vessels affected because their predominance differs at different sites, for example, the skin vessels have more alpha receptors.

Eye

The radial pupillary dilator muscle of the iris contains α receptors so drugs such as phenylephrine causes mydriasis. The α agonists enhance the outflow facility of aqueous humour while β agonists increase the production of aqueous humour. β agonists relax the ciliary muscle of the eye to a minor degree causing an insignificant decrease in accommodation. β-blockers reduce the secretory activity and reduce intraocular pressure.

Respiratory tract

Bronchial smooth muscles contain β_2 receptors that cause relaxation resulting in bronchodilation. The blood vessels of the upper respiratory tract contain α_1 receptors. The α agonists produce decongestant action.

Gastrointestinal tract

Both α and β stimulants relax the smooth muscle of gastrointestinal tract. β receptors are located directly on the smooth muscle cells. α stimulants (particularly α_2-selective) decrease muscle activity indirectly by presynaptically reducing the release of acetylcholine within the enteric nervous system.

Effects on endocrine and other functions

Stimulation of β receptors promotes insulin secretion which is inhibited by α_2 receptors. Renin secretion is stimulated by β_1 and inhibited by α_2 receptors.

Metabolic effects

Stimulation of beta receptors in fat cells leads to increased lipolysis.

Sympathomimetics enhance glycogenolysis in the liver mediated mainly by β receptors.

Central nervous system

The effects vary depending on the property of crossing blood-brain barrier. The catecholamines do not cross this barrier. It is only at the highest rates of infusion that subjective symptoms appear which may be only nervousness but in some cases feeling of impending disaster. However, the noncatecholamines such as ephedrine and amphetamine easily enter the CNS and produce CNS effects ranging from mild alerting, mood elevation, euphoria, anorexia and insomnia to psychotic behaviour. These effects are due to increase of dopamine-mediated processes in the CNS, rather than alpha or beta mediated effects.

SYMPATHOMIMETICS

Catecholamines

Epinephrine

Epinephrine (adrenaline in U.K.) causes positive chronotropic and positive inotropic actions on the heart (mainly β_1 receptors) and vasoconstriction in many blood vessels (α receptors). In some vessels, especially those supplying skeletal muscles which contain β_2 receptors, epinephrine produces their dilatation. The total peripheral resistance may thus decrease resulting in fall in diastolic blood pressure.

Epinephrine

Epinephrine interacts with both β- and α-receptors. At low concentrations, β effects predominate and at high concentrations, α effects predominate.

Routes of administration of epinephrine

- SC 0.3-0.5 mg of 1 : 1000 aqueous solution of epinephrine hydrochloride
- Intracardiac injection only in cardiac arrest
- Inhalation 1: 100 of a 1% aqueous solution
- Ophthalmic solution - epinephrine bitartrate, epinephrine hydrochloride
- Spray in ENT surgery

Therapeutic uses of epinephrine

- Acute hypersensitivity reactions
- Bronchial asthma (bronchodilation β_2) and decongestion of mucosa (alpha action)
- Along with local anaesthetics to prolong their action

- As a local haemostatic on bleeding surfaces - epistaxis
- As mydriatic
- For restoring cardiac rhythm in patients with cardiac arrest due to various causes.

Norepinephrine (noradrenaline in UK)

It has little effect on β_2 receptors and therefore the peripheral resistance is increased resulting in elevation of both systolic and diastolic blood pressure. Bradycardia is produced due to compensatory vagal reflexes.

Norepinephrine

Isoprenaline

Isoprenaline (isoproterenol) is almost a pure beta-receptor agonist and so a potent vasodilator. It has positive chronotropic and inotropic actions. Thus isoprenaline increases cardiac output as well as fall in diastolic pressure, and a lesser decrease or slight rise in systolic pressure.

Dopamine

Dopamine acts on D_1 receptors in vascular beds leading to vasodilation. Dopamine also activates β_1 receptors in the heart.

Uses of dopamine

- Shock associated with oliguria
- Cardiogenic and septic shock
- Chronic refractory CHF
  Caution : Hypovolaemia should be corrected before starting dopamine infusion
  Adverse effects of dopamine
  Nausea, vomiting, tachycardia, anginal pain, increased BP, arrhythmia, headache. Extravasation may produce ischaemic necrosis.

Dobutamine

Dobutamine is β_1 selective synthetic catecholamine.

It also activates α_1 receptors. It is not absorbed when given orally. It does not act on dopaminergic receptors although it resembles dopamine chemically. It has greater inotropic effect than chronotropic. Dobutamine is used to improve myocardial function in CHF, as oxygen demands are less than with other sympathetic agonists because it produces slight change in heart rate and systolic pressure.

Table 2.17 shows main differences between dopamine and dobutamine.

Table 2.17. Differences between dopamine and dobutamine.

Dopamine	*Dobutamine*
- Endogenous catecholamine	Synthetic agent
- Selectively stimulates dopamine receptor and causes selective dilation of renal and mesenteric blood vessels. Improves renal blood flow and urine output.	Selective stimulant at β_1 in heart
- Moderate doses exert positive inotropic effect (β_1 action)	Direct inotropic stimulation
- At high doses alpha stimulation produces vasoconstriction	Even at high doses has minimal effect on β_2 and alpha receptors.

Other sympathomimetics

Phenylephrine

Phenylephrine is almost a pure alpha agonist. It is not a catechol derivative so it is not inactivated by COMT and has more prolonged duration of action than catecholamines. It is an effective mydriatic and decongestant. It is also used to provide local vasoconstriction as 10% ophthalmic solution.

Adverse effects are similar to those of other catecholamines. It should be carefully employed in atrial fibrillation as it increases atrioventricular conduction.

Methoxamine

Methoxamine acts like phenylephrine. It can raise blood pressure for a long period due to vasoconstriction. It produces little CNS stimulation. It is used therapeutically in hypotensive states.

Ephedrine

Ephedrine acts primarily through the release of stored catecholamines. It also acts directly on adrenoceptors. It enters CNS so causes CNS stimulation. It can be given orally. It is used as a pressor agent in spinal anaesthesia, as a mydriatic and in the treatment of bronchial asthma and as a nasal decongestant.

Its action is prolonged as it is resistant to COMT and MAO.

Amphetamine

It enters CNS more readily and its CNS stimulant action is more marked than ephedrine. It also depresses appetite.

Adverse effects

Tolerance, psychic and physical dependence, toxic psychosis from large doses, prolonged use produces mental depression, fatigue, restlessness, insomnia, tachycardia, dry mouth, mydriasis.

Contraindications

Anorexia, insomnia

Methamphetamine

Methamphetamine has higher ratio of central to peripheral actions. The other variants of amphetamine are phenmetrazine, methylphenidate and pemoline. The pharmacologic actions and abuse potential are same as those of amphetamine.

RECEPTOR-SELECTIVE SYMPATHOMIMETICS

- α_1-selective drugs do not offer any advantage.
- α_2-selective agonists such as clonidine, methyldopa reduce blood pressure by acting in the CNS.
- β_1-selective drugs like dobutamine increases cardiac output, without increasing the heart rate.
- β_2-selective agents like terbutaline and ritodrine have important role in the treatment of asthma and as uterine relaxant in premature labor.

SPECIAL SYMPATHOMIMETICS

Cocaine inhibits reuptake of norepinephrine at noradrenergic synapses. It readily enters CNS and produces more intense amphetamine like action though of shorter duration.

Tyramine is a byproduct of tyrosine metabolism in the body. It is also found in fermented foods such as cheese.

Therapeutic uses of sympathomimetics

- **Hypotension.** Sympathomimetic drugs may be used in a hypotensive emergency to preserve cerebral and coronary blood flow, for example, in situations such as severe haemorrhage, spinal cord injury or overdoses of blood pressure lowering drugs or CNS depressant drugs. In these situations if vasoconstriction is desired, phenylephrine or methoxamine, norepinephrine may be utilized.
- **Shock.** The efficacy of sympathomimetics is unclear. A decision has to be taken whether to use vasoconstrictors or vasodilators.
- **Cardiogenic shock.** Dopamine or dobutamine may have a role. In small to moderate doses they increase cardiac output with little peripheral vasoconstriction.
- **To reduce blood flow.** Haemostasis is often necessary for facial, oral and nasopharyngeal surgery. Epinephrine in nasal packs (for epistaxis). α-agonists are combined with local anaesthetics to prolong the duration of local anaesthetic action. Epinephrine 1: 200,000 is usually employed.
- **Bronchial asthma.** β_2-selective drugs are as effective as and safer than the less selective agents.
- **Ophthalmic uses.** Epinephrine has mydriatic effect. Topical application of 1-2% epinephrine also lowers intraocular pressure by increasing outflow of aqueous humour. Dipivefrin is a prodrug of epinephrine which has greater ability to penetrate into the anterior chamber of the eye where it is converted to epinephrine by enzymatic hydrolysis.
- **Uterus.** β_2-selective agents relax the pregnant uterus, for this purpose ritodrine, terbutaline are used.
- **Central nervous system.** The amphetamines have alerting and sleep deferring action and may be used in the treatment of narcolepsy.
- **Hypertension.** α_2-agonist clonidine is useful in the treatment of hypertension by acting in the central nervous system. Clonidine also reduces

the craving for narcotics and alcohol during their withdrawal. It may also help in cessation of cigarette smoking. Clonidine can also diminish menopausal hot flushes.

The special uses of adrenergic drugs are given below:

Bronchodilators	Epinephrine, isoprenaline, orciprenaline, salbutamol, terbutaline, salmeterol
Pressor agents	Norepinephrine, ephedrine, dopamine, phenylephrine, mephentermine
Cardiac stimulants	Epinephrine, isoprenaline, ephedrine, dobutamine
CNS stimulants	Ephedrine, amphetamine, dexamphetamine, methamphetamine
Uterine relaxants	Salbutamol, terbutaline
Appetite suppressants	Fenfluramine, dexfenfluramine, mazindol
Nasal decongestants	Ephedrine, pseudoephedrine, phenylephrine, naphazoline, oxymetazoline, xylometazoline, isoxsuprine

Adverse effects of sympathomimetics

The pressor agents produce marked elevation of blood pressure which may be dangerous as it may lead to cerebral haemorrhage or pulmonary oedema. Due to increased cardiac work, angina or myocardial infarction may precipitate.

The beta-stimulant drugs may cause sinus tachycardia and damage myocardium.

Central nervous system toxicity may include restlessness, tremor, anxiety and insomnia.

Comparison of norepinephrine, epinephrine and isoprenaline is shown in Table 2.18.

Table 2.19 shows comparison among phenylephrine, epinephrine and isoproterenol in cardiovascular actions.

STUDY QUESTIONS

1. What are the different adrenoceptors and their subtypes?
2. Describe the relative selectivity of adrenoceptor agonists.

Table 2.18. Effects of norepinephrine, epinephrine and isoprenaline

Effect	Norepinephrine	Epinephrine	Isoprenaline
Heart			
Rate	Bradycardia (reflexly due to rise in B.P.)	Increased (direct action)	Increased (direct action)
Contractility	Little effect	Increased (direct action)	Increased (direct action)
Cardiac output	No change, decrease	Much increased	Much increased
Excitability	Insignificant or reduced	Increased	Increased
Conductivity	Increased	Much increased	Much increased
Blood pressure			
Systolic	Rises	Rises	Little change or may fall
Diastolic	Rises	Falls	Falls
Vascular beds in muscle	Constricted	Dilated	Dilated
Skin and viscera	Constricted	Constricted	Dilated
Total peripheral resistance	Increased	Decreased	Decreased
Metabolism			
Oxygen consumption	Insignificant	Increased	Insignificant
Glycogenolysis	Insignificant	Increased	Insignificant
CNS	Insignificant	Stimulated	Stimulated
Smooth muscle			
Bronchi	Little affected	Relaxed	Relaxed
Intestine and bladder	Relaxed	Relaxed	Relaxed
Sphincters	Constricted	Constricted	Constricted
Uterus (pregnant)	Stimulated	Inhibited	Inhibited
Capillary permeability	Little effect	Reduced	?

Table 2.19. Comparison among Phenylephrine, Epinephrine and Isoproterenol

Tissue	Phenylephrine	Epinephrine	Isoproterenol
Vascular resistance			
Cutaneous mucous membrane (alpha)	++	++	0
Skeletal muscle (β_2, alpha)	+	+/–	–
Renal (α_1, D_1)	+	+	–
Splanchnic (β)	++	–/+	–
Total peripheral resistance	+++	–/+	–
Venous tone	+	+	–
Cardiac			
Contractility (β_1)	0/+	++	+++
Rate (β_1)	vagal reflex	+/–	+++
Stroke volume	0, +, –	+	+
COP	–	+	++
Blood pressure			
Mean	++	+	–
Diastolic	++	–/+	–
Systolic	++	++	0 or –
Pulse pressure	0	++	++

+++ = Marked effect; ++ = Moderate effect; + = Slight effect; O = No effect; – = Decrease.

3. Classify adrenergic agonists according to selectivity for receptors.

4. Describe the distribution of adrenoceptor receptors in different tissues and their functions.

5. List sympathomimetics, classify them according to their site of action.

6. Tabulate the differences between epinephrine, norepinephrine and isoprenaline.

7. What are the clinical applications of epinephrine?

8. What are the main differences between ephedrine and adrenaline?

9. What are the uses and drawbacks of amphetamine?

10. Describe the pharmacological actions of sympathomimetics on cardiovascular system, gastrointestinal tract, eye and respiratory tract.

11. Describe the cardiovascular and ophthalmic applications of sympathomimetic drugs.

12. What are the possible adverse effects of sympathomimetics?

GUIDE TO FURTHER READING

Arner, P. The beta3-adrenergic receptor—a cause and cure of obesity? N Engl J Med., 1995; 333:382.

Brown, C.G. et al. A comparison of standard dose and high dose epinephrine in cardiac arrest outside the hospital. N Engl J Med, 1992; 327:1051.

Caron, M.G., Lefkowitz, R.J. Catecholamine receptors: structure, function, and regulation. Recent Prog Horm Res, 1993; 48:277.

Faure, C. et al. Identification of alpha1-adrenoceptor subtypes in the human prostate. Life Sci, 1994; 54:1595.

Gingrich, J.A., Caron, M.G. Recent advances in the molecular biology of dopamine receptors. Annu Rev Neurosci, 1993; 16:299.

Hurvitz, L.M. et al. New developments in the drug treatment of glaucoma. Drugs, 1991; 41:514.

MacDonald, A. et al. Contributions of alpha1-adrenoceptors, alpha2-adrenoceptors, and P2d purinoceptors to neurotransmission in several rabbit isolated blood vessels: Role of neuronal uptake and autofeedback. Br J Pharmacol, 1992; 105:347.

McGrath, J.C., Brown, C.M. and Wilson, V.G. Alpha-adrenoceptors: A critical review. Med Res Rev, 1989; 9:407.

Ruffolo, R.R. Jr. et al. Pharmacologic and therapeutic applications of alpha2-adrenoceptor subtypes. Annu Rev Pharmacol Toxicol, 1993; 32:243.

Ruffolo, R.R. Jr. et al. Structure and function of alpha-adrenoceptors. Pharmacol Rev, 1991; 43:475.

Seeman, P., Grigoriades, D. Dopamine receptors in brain and periphery. Neurochem Int, 1987; 10:1.

Spitzer, W.O. et al. The use of Beta-agonists and risk of death and near death from asthma. N Engl J Med, 1992; 326:501.

Valtorta, F. et al. Neurotransmitter release and synaptic vesicle recycling. Neuroscience, 1990; 35:477.

Vincent, J. et al. Pharmacological tolerance to alpha1-adrenergic antagonism mediated by terazosin in humans. J Clin Invest, 1992; 90:1763.

Zorgniotti, A.W. Experience with buccal phentolamine mesylate for impotence. Int J Impotence Res, 1994; 6:37.

ADRENERGIC (SYMPATHETIC) BLOCKING DRUGS (SYMPATHETIC ANTAGONISTS; ANTIADRENERGIC AGENTS, SYMPATHOLYTICS)

α-RECEPTOR BLOCKING DRUGS

Classification of alpha adrenergic blockers

Nonselective (α_1 and α_2)

- Non-competitive (irreversible) : Phenoxybenzamine.
- Competitive (reversible): Phentolamine, tolazoline, ergot alkaloids e.g. ergotamine, dihydroergotanine (Ergonovine is not a alpha blocker).

Selective blockers

- α_1 blockers: Prazosin, terazosin, doxazosin, trimazosin and indoramin.
- α_2 blockers: Yohimbine.

Table 2.20 shows receptor specificity of α receptors blocking agents

Table 2.20. Receptors specificity of alpha blockers

Drugs	α_1	α_2
Phentolamine	+++	+++
Phenoxybenzamine	+++	+++
Prazosin	+++	+
Indoramin	+++	+
Ergotamine	++PA	++
Dihydroergotamine	+	+
Yohimbine	+	+++

Selective α_1 blockers

Selective α_1 blockers have advantages over non-selective α blockers. As they have no effect on α_2 receptors neurotransmitter feedback inhibition is maintained, hence they do not produce tachycardia.

Mechanism of actions

Non-competitive (irreversible) : Phenoxybenzamine binds cova-lently to alpha receptors. The action is prolonged. The function is restored on synthesis of new receptors (may take several days).

Competitive : Phentolamine, tolazoline, ergotamine, dihydroergotamine act by reversible alpha adrenergic receptor blockade.

The half-life of reversible antagonist determines the duration of action, whereas the effect of irreversible antagonist lasts till new receptors are synthesised (may take several days).

Pharmacological effects

Cardiovascular system

The α receptors present on vascular smooth muscle determine the arteriolar and venous tone to a large extent and hence the alpha receptor blockers lower peripheral vascular resistance and blood pressure. These drugs may cause postural hypotension, palpitation and reflex tachycardia.

Other effects

Miosis is due to unopposed contraction of circular muscle due to loss of tone of radial muscle of iris; ejaculation is controlled by α-adrenoceptors so α-blockers may produce failure of ejaculation. Due to relaxation of sphincter of urethra and relaxation of the base of bladder, there may be incontinence of urine.

Miosis, nasal stuffiness and decreased adrenergic sweating also indicate blockade of α receptors.

INDIVIDUAL α-BLOCKERS

Phentolamine is almost equally potent in blocking the α_1 and α_2 receptors. It is also anti-5HT. Phentolamine is an agonist at muscarinic and H_1 and H_2 histamine receptors. It is poorly absorbed from GIT. Its actions are similar to those of phenoxybenzamine but of short duration.

The adverse effects include tachycardia, arrhythmia and angina. Diarrhoea and increased gastric hydrochloric acid may be produced due to agonist action at muscarinic, H_1 and H_2 histamine receptors.

Tolazoline is less potent but better absorbed from GIT and also rapidly excreted in urine. It is rarely used.

Ergot derivatives e.g. ergotamine causes reversible alpha-receptor blockade.

Phenoxybenzamine (dibenzyline) is an irreversible non-selective α-receptor blocker of long duration (16-48 hours). It also blocks H_1 histamine, acetylcholine and serotonin receptors. Phenoxybenzamine is absorbed satisfactorily after oral administration. However, its bioavailability is low. The adrenergic blocking activity is 6 to 10 times more than that of dibenamine.

The adverse effects of phenoxybenzamine include postural hypotension and tachycardia, nasal stuffiness and inhibition of ejaculation.

Prazosin is a very potent reversible alpha-receptor antagonist. It is highly selective for α_1 receptors with only slight affinity for α_2 receptors. Prazosin is effective as an antihypertensive drug. It is given orally and is well tolerated. The half-life is 3-4 hours. The reflex tachycardia is less than non-selective alpha-blockers such as phentolamine and phenoxybenzamine.

The dose of prazosin is 1 mg 2-3 times a day and gradually increased. Adverse reactions include first dose phenomenon (fainting after the first dose may be observed), headache, lassitude, constipation. It may produce retention of salt and fluid which can be corrected by diuretics.

Terazosin is another reversible α_1-receptor blocking agent. Its bioavailability is good. The half-life is about 9-10 hours. The dose is 5-20 mg once daily.

Doxazosin is α_1-selective antagonist with moderate bioavailability and its half-life is about 20 hours.

Indoramin is α_1-selective antagonist having efficacy as an antihypertensive. Urapidil is a new α_1-antagonist (with weak α_2-agonist and 5-HT_1 agonist actions and weak antagonist action at β_1 receptor.

Labetalol has both α_1-selective and β-blocking property.

Yohimbine (an alkaloid from a west African tree) is α_2-selective agent. It has no clinical usefulness.

Therapeutic uses of α-receptor blockers

- Pheochromocytoma is a tumour in adrenal medulla that releases a mixture of adrenaline and noradrenaline (norepinephrine) resulting in excess of catecholamines leading to hypertension, tachycardia and arrhythmias.

  As diagnostic test: Infusion of phentolamine can be given as a diagnostic test of pheochromocytoma. There will be greater than average drop in blood pressure in response to α blocking agents.

  In preoperative management: α-receptor antagonists are very useful in the preoperative management of patients with pheochromocytoma. Administration of phenoxybenzamine prevents acute hypertensive episodes. Oral doses of 10-20 mg daily are advised until hypertension is controlled. It may take 1 to 3 weeks after which surgery is undertaken.

- Essential hypertension: Mild to moderate hypertension may respond well with α_1-selective antagonists such as prazosin.

  Prazosin is well tolerated. However, postural hypotension is the major adverse effect.

- Hypertensive emergencies: The α-receptor blocking agents have limited value in the treatment of hypertensive emergencies.

- Haemorrhagic and endotoxic shock: Correction of fluid loss by i.v. infusion, and phenoxybenzamine 1 mg/kg by i.v. infusion helps in restoring perfusion of the tissues in haemorrhagic and endotoxic shock.

- Peripheral vascular disease: The α-receptor antagonists such as phentolamine, tolazoline, or phenoxybenzamine may benefit some patients with Raynaud's disease and such other conditions which involve reversible vasospasm in peripheral circulation. However, calcium channel blocking drugs are preferable.

- Local ischaemic tissue: If intense local vasoconstriction occurs due to inadvertent injection of α agonists such as norepinephrine during i.v. administration, the α antagonist such as phentolamine is useful if infiltrated into the ischaemic area.

- Urinary obstruction: In selected patients with urinary obstruction due to prostatic hypertrophy and who are poor surgical risks, phenoxybenzamine may be useful as the α-receptor antagonists produce partial reversal of smooth muscle contraction in the enlarged prostate or in the bladder base. Terazosin is preferred by many physicians for this purpose.
- Male sexual dysfunction: Phentolamine with a nonspecific vasodilator papaverine when injected into the penis may cause erection in men but its efficacy is not established. The drawbacks include fibrotic reactions locally, and systemic absorption may cause postural hypotension.

β-RECEPTOR BLOCKING DRUGS (BETA BLOCKERS)

These drugs antagonize the effects of catecholamines and other β agonists at β adrenoceptors. Most of these drugs are pure antagonists (there is no activation of receptor) while a few are partial agonists (cause partial activation of the receptor which is less than the full agonists). The other differences among the beta blockers are their relative affinities for β_1 and β_2 receptors, in their pharmacokinetic and membrane stabilizing effects.

The β-receptor blocking drugs can be classified as:

1. Non-selective β blockers lacking ISA (β_1, β_2): Sotalol, timolol.
2. β-blockers with membrane stabilizing activity and intrinsic sympathomimetic activity (ISA) e.g. oxprenolol, alprenolol and pindolol.
3. β-blockers with membrane stabilizing property e.g. propranolol.
4. β-blockers with cardioselective property e.g. atenolol and metoprolol. Acebutolol also has ISA.
5. β-blockers with α-blocking property e.g. labetalol.

Table 2.21 shows differences among β_1, β_2 and β_3 adrenoceptors.

Pharmacokinetics

The beta-receptor antagonists are well absorbed from GIT. The bioavailability of propranolol is low due to the extensive hepatic (first-pass metabolism). The beta-blockers are rapidly distributed. Most of them have half-lives in the range of 2-5 hours. There are certain exceptions, for example, the half-life of esmolol is only 10 minutes and nadolol has the longest half-life among all the beta blockers (about 24 hours).

Propranolol and metoprolol are extensively metabolized in the liver and only small amount of these drugs is excreted unaltered in the urine. Atenolol, celiprolol and pindolol are less completely

Table 2.21. Differences among β_1, β_2 and β_3 adrenoceptors

	β_1	β_2	β_3
Location	Heart, juxtaglomerular cells in kidney	Bronchi, blood vessels, uterus, GIT, urinary tract, eye	Adipose tissue
Agonist	Dobutamine	Salbutamol, terbutaline	BRL 37344
Antagonist	Metoprolol, Atenolol	Butoxamine alpha-methyl propranolol	CGP 20712A (also β_1) ICI 118551 (also β_2)

β_1 - receptor responds equally to E and NE and mediates cardiac stimulation and lipolysis.

β_2 - receptor is more responsive to E than to NE and mediates responses such as vasodilation and bronchodilation.

β_3 - adrenergic receptor has a much greater affinity for NE than E and unlike the β_1 and β_2 receptors, does not undergo desensitization. Systemic agonists for the β_3 - receptor, currently under development have a potential role in the treatment of obesity by increasing metabolic rate. β_3 subtype receptors mediate the metabolic responses in adipocytes and certain other tissues with atypical pharmacological characteristics.

Isoproterenol stimulates and propranolol blocks both β_1 and β_2 receptors.

metabolized. Nadolol is excreted unchanged in the urine.

Pharmacological Action of Beta Blockers

Cardiovascular system

- *Heart* : Negative inotropic and negative chronotropic effect.
  There is decrease in oxygen demand, so antianginal effect. Decrease in conduction through AV node, so antidysrhythmic effect.
- *B.P.* : Blood pressure is lower in hypertension (no effect on normal B.P.). Fall is due to:

decrease in heart rate

decrease in cardiac output

decrease in renin release

CNS effects

decreased release of NE from adrenergic neurons.

Respiratory tract : B_2 blockade may increase airway resistance in asthmatic patients

Eye : Aqueous humour secretion is decreased, so intraocular pressure decreases.

Metabolic and endocrine effects : Inhibition of lipolysis, inhibition of glycogenolysis, impairment of recovery from hypoglycaemia. If used for long term, serum VLDL increases and HDL decreases, LDL is not affected. HDL: LDL ratio is decreased so increased risk of coronary artery disease (CAD). These changes occur both with selective and non selective beta blockers, changes in lipids are less with drugs having intrinsic sympathomimetic activity i.e. which are partial agonists.

Effects unrelated to β-blockade

The membrane-stabilizing action (local anaesthetic action) is an important property of all β-blocking agents. It is due to blockade of sodium channels. However, after systemic administration as the concentration is very low for anaesthetic action, hence this effect is not likely to play any significant role. Satolol is a nonselective beta blocker which lacks membrane-stabilizing action but has marked antiarrhythmic effects that indicates potassium channel blockade.

Table 2.22 shows certain properties of β-blockers.

Pindolol, acebutolol are partial agonists i.e. β-blockers with intrinsic sympathomimetic activity.

Labetalol is nonselective beta- and selective α_1-blocker.

Table 2.23 shows the selectivity of some β-adrenergic blocking agents.

Table 2.22. Properties of some beta-receptor blocking drugs

β-blockers	Partial agonist activity	Local anaesthetic action	Lipid solubility	Elimination half-life	Approximate bioavailability (%)	Selectivity
Acebutolol	Yes	Yes	Low	3-4 hours	50	β_1
Atenolol	No	No	Low	6-9 hours	40	β_1
Betaxolol	No	Slight	Low	14-22 hours	90	β_1
Carteolol	Yes	No	Low	6 hours	85	β_1, β_2
Esmolol	No	No	Low	10 minutes	—	β_1
Labetalol	Yes	Yes	Moderate	5 hours	30	α, β
Metoprolol	No	Yes	Moderate	3-4 hours	50	β_1
Nadolol	No	No	Low	14-24 hours	33	β_1, β_2
Pindolol	Yes	Yes	Moderate	3-4 hours	90	β_1, β_2
Propranolol	No	Yes	High	3-6 hours	30	β_1, β_2
Sotalol	No	No	Low	12 hours	90	β_1, β_2
Timolol	No	No	Moderate	4-5 hours	50	β_1, β_2

Table 2.23. Selectivity

	α_1	α_2	β_1	β_2
Propranolol	—	—	+++	+++
Oxprenolol	—	—	+++ PA	+++
Practolol	—	—	+++	+
Atenolol	—	—	+++	+
Butoxamine	—	—	+	+++
Labetalol	+++	+	+	+

PA = Partial agonist; — = No effect; + = Mild effect; ++ = Moderate effect; +++ = Marked effect.

INDIVIDUAL DRUGS

Propranolol is a nonselective β-receptor antagonist (blocker). Its bioavailability is low due to extensive first-pass effect in the liver. It is not a partial agonist at β-receptors. It also blocks the central serotonin receptors moderately.

Metoprolol, atenolol

These are β_1-selective drugs. They are safer in patients who experience bronchoconstriction due to propranolol. However, it is better to avoid their use or employ them with great care in patients who give history of bronchospasm.

β_1-selective antagonists are preferred in case of diabetics or patients suffering from peripheral vascular disease when beta blockers are indicated.

Nadolol

Nadolol has long duration of action; its actions are the same as that of timolol. It is non-selective β-blocker. It is not metabolised and excreted unchanged in urine. Its effects and adverse reactions are similar to those of propranolol.

Pindolol, acebutolol, carteolol, ceteprolol and penbutolol

These possess partial β-agonist activity. Due to the intrinsic sympathomimetic activity these drugs cause less bradycardia and less adverse effects in plasma lipid profile than the pure beta antagonists. However, to what extent the partial agonist activity is clinically important is not clear.

Labetalol
$\beta_1 = \beta_2 \geq \alpha_1 > \alpha_2$

It is both α and β blocker. Its affinity for α-receptors is less than that of phentolamine but it is α_1-selective. Its β-blocking affinity is less than that of propranolol. The antihypertensive effect of labetalol is accompanied by less tachycardia than with other α-blockers.

Esmolol

It is β_1-selective with half-life of only 10 minutes (ultra-short-acting).

Butoxamine

It is β_2-selective but without any clinical application. $\beta_2 >>> \beta_1$.

Doses of some β-blockers

	Dose (mg)	Schedule
Propranolol	120-240	6-12 hourly
Metoprolol	150-300	12 hourly
Atenolol	50-100	Daily
Timolol	15-45	12 hourly
Pindolol	10-40	6 hourly

Therapeutic uses of beta-receptor blocking drugs

- Essential hypertension: The fall in blood pressure is gradual in onset, without postural hypotension. Propranolol 40 mg orally is given twice a day; this dose is gradually increased up to 120-240 mg/24 hours.
- Atenolol 50 mg is given once daily for 1-2 weeks and then increased up to 100 mg/24 hours.
- Ischaemic heart disease: In the prophylaxis of angina pectoris, propranolol has been found useful. It causes bradycardia, decreased myocardial contractility and fall in B.P. which decreases the work load of heart and decreases myocardial oxygen requirement even at rest. It also reduces cardiac response to sympatho-adrenal activity evoked by emotional changes and exercise. However, propranolol is not effective in variant or unstable angina, where vasospasm is the causative factor. β-blockers decrease the incidence and recurrence of myocardial infarction in patients of myocardial

ischaemia. Besides beta blockade, beneficial effects of propranolol to prevent platelet aggregation and promotion of fibrinolysis may also contribute to its usefulness.

- Cardiac arrhythmias: Propranolol is effective in all supraventricular tachycardia. It increases refractory period of A-V node and has membrane stabilizing effect. Dose is 10-30 mg orally 3-4 times a day.

- Glaucoma: The intraocular pressure is reduced due to reduced production of aqueous humour by the ciliary body.

  Timolol (0.25-0.5%) as eye drops is favoured because it lacks local anaesthetic action and is a pure antagonist. Its efficacy is same as that of epinephrine or pilocarpine in open-angle glaucoma. It has been observed that sufficient timolol may be absorbed from the eye (after topical use) to cause adverse effects on the heart and airways in susceptible persons.

  Betaxolol, carteolol, levobunolol, and metipranolol are also available for the treatment of glaucoma.

  Betaxolol is β_1-selective. Whether this advantage reduces systemic adverse effects remains to be determined.

- Hyperthyroidism : Beta receptor blockade prevents peripheral conversion of thyroxine to triiodothyronine. It is particularly effective in thyroid storm.

  Propranolol reduces tachycardia, tremor, sweating and nervousness in thyrotoxicosis. Dose is 10 mg thrice a day, increased by 10 mg weekly, maximum dose 80-240 mg/24 hours.

- As prophylactic in migraine (mechanism not known): Propranolol reduces frequency and severity of migraine.

- Pheochromocytoma: Propranolol in combination with alpha-adrenoceptor blockers is used during removal of tumour to prevent excessive cardiac stimulation by catecholamines released from the tumour.

- Propranolol is also helpful during withdrawal of alcohol.

- Beta-blockers also diminish portal vein pressure in patients with cirrhosis. Propranolol and nadolol have decreased the mortality rate associated with bleeding in cirrhosis.

Adverse effects of beta adrenergic blockade:

CNS: Muscle cramps, fatigue, lethargy, insomnia, depression, hallucinations, tremor, anxiety, restlessness.

CVS: Peripheral vascular diseases or Raynaud's disease may become worse; may produce cold extremities due to decrease in blood flow.

Beta-receptor blockade depresses myocardial contractility and excitability. Excessive bradycardia and hypotension may be produced.

Pulmonary: In asthmatics, there may be life threatening increase in airway resistance. The β_2-blokade may worsen asthma and other condition of airway obstruction.

Allergy: Allergic reactions such as rash, fever.

Metabolism: Hypoglycaemic action of insulin and oral antidiabetic agents may be potentiated by beta blockers. Delay in recovery from insulin induced hypoglycaemia.

Others: Constipation, diarrhoea, indigestion, sexual dysfunction.

Note : Abrupt withdrawal causes rebound phenomenon resulting in severe angina or M.I. and sudden death in patients of IHD.

Contraindications

- Heart block.
- Bronchial asthma; selective β_1-blockers may be tried.
- Mental depression.

STUDY QUESTIONS

1. Classify alpha-receptor blocking drugs, giving suitable examples. What are their clinical applications and reasons for limited use?

2. Compare phentolamine, phenoxybenzamine, prazosin and labetalol as alpha antagonists.

3. What are the pharmacological effects of alpha-receptor blocking drugs?

4. Classify beta-receptor blocking drugs. List these drugs showing relative affinities for β_1 and β_2 receptors, as well as differences among them in pharmacokinetic and membrane stabilizing

properties.

5. Describe the pharmacodynamics of beta-receptor antagonists.

6. Describe in detail the actions, mode of action, therapeutic uses, contraindications and adverse effects of propranolol.

GUIDE TO FURTHER READING

Babamoto, K. and Hirokawa, W.T. Doxazosin: A new alpha adrenergic antagonist. Clin Pharm, 1992; 11:415.

Benfield, P. and Sorkin, E.M. Esmolol: A preliminary review of its pharmacodynamic and pharmacokinetic properties, and therapeutic efficacy. Drugs, 1987; 33:392.

Benfield, P., Clissold, S.P. and Brogden, R.N. Metoprolol. Drugs, 1986; 31:376.

Brooks, A.M. and Gillies, W.E. Ocular beta blockers in glaucoma management. Clinical pharmacological aspects. Drugs Aging, 1992; 2:208.

Clark, J.A., Zimmerman, H.J. and Tanner, L.A. Labetalol hepatotoxicity. Ann. Intern. Med., 1990; 113:210.

Feely, J. and Peden, N. Use of beta adrenoceptor-blocking drugs in hyperthyroidism. Drugs, 1984; 27:425.

Fitzgerald, J.D. Do partial agonist beta-blockers have improved clinical utility? Cardiovasc Drugs Ther, 1993; 7:303.

Frishman, W.H. and Charlap, S. Alpha adrenergic blockers. Med Clin North Am, 1988; 72:427.

Frishman, W.H. Beta-adrenergic blockers as cardioprotective agents. Am J Cardiol, 1992; 70:21.

Harder, S. and Thurmann, P. Concentration/effect relationship of bunazosin, a selective alpha1-adrenoceptor antagonist in hypertensive patients after single and multiple oral doses. Int. J. Clin. Pharmacol Ther, 1994; 32:38.

Kyncl, J.J. Pharmacology of terazosin: an alpha1-selective blocker. J. Clin. Pharmacol., 1993; 33:878.

Shanks, R.G. Clinical pharmacology of vasodilatory beta-blocking drugs. Am. Heart J., 1991; 121:1006.

Lesar, T.S. Comparison of ophthalmic beta-blocking agents, Clin Pharm, 1987; 6:451.

Milne, R.J. and Buckley, M.M. Celiprolol. Drugs, 1991; 41:941.

Singh, B.N., Thoden, W.R. and Ward, A. Acebutolol: A review of its pharmacological properties and therapeutic efficacy in hypertension, angina pectoris and arrhythmia. Drugs, 1985; 29:531.

Taylor, S.H. Intrinsic sympathomimetic activity: Clinical fact or fiction? Am J Cardiol, 1983; 52:16D.

GANGLIONIC STIMULANTS AND BLOCKERS

The autonomic ganglia play an important physiological role in maintaining the constancy of internal environment.

Ganglion stimulating agents

Drugs such as dimethylphenylpiperazinium iodide (DMPP), tetramethylammonium (TMA), lobeline and nicotine (small doses) have no therapeutic utility.

Nicotine interacts ACh with receptor on the postsynaptic membrane of autonomic ganglia, causes initial stimulation of ganglia and releases catecholamines from the adrenal medulla. Large doses produce prolonged ganglionic blockade following initial stimulation. Larger doses prevent release of catecholamines from the adrenal medulla.

Nicotine is rapidly absorbed from skin, respiratory tract and buccal membranes. It is metabolised in liver, kidney, and lung. It is excreted via kidney. It is also excreted in the breast milk of lactating women who are heavy smokers.

Nicotine is a CNS stimulant via motor cortex excitation. It stimulates release of antidiuretic hormone (ADH). Small doses stimulate respiration but toxic doses depress it.

Due to stimulation of sympathetic ganglia and adrenal medulla there is increased total peripheral resistance, increased B.P., and tachycardia.

Due to stimulation of parasympathetic ganglia there is increased bowel motility.

Salivary and bronchial secretions are first stimulated and then blocked.

There is no therapeutic use of nicotine.

Ganglion blocking drugs

These drugs block the actions of acetylcholine and similar agonists of both sympathetic and parasympathetic autonomic ganglia. They have rarely a minor role in the short-term management of high blood pressure only because they are (i) nonselective and (ii) produce large number of adverse effects and (iii) tolerance develops rapidly. Hence these drugs are obsolete for therapeutic purposes.

Classification

A. Competitive blocking drugs

- Quaternary compounds: Hexamethonium, pentolinium, TEA.
- Sulphonium compounds: Trimetaphan.
- Amines: Mecamylamine, pempidine.

B. Persistent depolarizing agents

- Nicotine in large doses, cholinesterase (ChE) inhibitors in large doses.
- The quaternary and sulphonium compounds are poorly absorbed from gastrointestinal tract (GIT) and do not cross blood-brain barrier. They have to be given intravenously. The amines are absorbed from GIT but produce undesirable central effects such as tremors and psychosis.

Individual ganglion blocking drugs

Hexamethonium has a bridge of 6 methyl group between two quaternary nitrogen atoms. The addition of more intervening carbon groups decreases the activity at the ganglionic receptors and increases activity at the skeletal muscle receptors. Ten carbons as in decamethonium produce maximal activity at the skeletal muscle receptors.

Hexamethonium produces competitive ganglionic blockage by occupying ganglionic cholinergic receptors.

Hexamethonium reduces systemic vascular resistance, venous return, and cardiac output; gastric secretions are reduced in volume and acidity and gastric motility is reduced; salivary secretions are reduced, glomerular filtration rate is decreased, urinary bladder contractions are reduced so urinary excretion is impaired. It produces partial mydriasis and cycloplegia. Dryness of skin and flushing occur. Due to so many adverse effects, hexamethonium is not used therapeutically.

Tetraethylammonium (TEA) has very short duration of action, so hexamethonium (C6) was developed. The C10 analogue of hexamethonium called decamethonium was found to be an effective neuromuscular depolarizing blocking agent.

Mecamylamine, a secondary ammonium compound was introduced. It is better absorbed than the quaternary ammonium ganglion-blocking drugs.

Trimethaphan is given by i.v. infusion as it is inactived by oral administration.

Effects of ganglion-blockers

These are numerous and complex since both divisions of autonomic nervous system are blocked indiscriminately.

Central nervous system : The quaternary ammonium compounds do not cross the blood-brain barrier and hence are devoid of central nervous system effects. The secondary ammonium compound, mecamylamine, readily crosses the blood-brain barrier and therefore this drug can produce sedation, tremor and choreiform movements and mental aberrations.

Eye : These drugs cause predictable loss of accommodation (cycloplegia) because ciliary muscle is innervated by parasympathetic nervous system. The effect on pupil is not predictable because iris is innervated by sympathetic nervous system, however, in iris the parasympathetic tone is more marked; the ganglion-blockers usually produce moderate mydriasis.

Cardiovascular system : The innervation of blood vessels is mainly from sympathetic nervous system (vasoconstrictor fibres) so the ganglion-blockers diminish the arteriolar and venomotor tone, resulting in precipitous fall in blood pressure. As the postural reflexes which prevent venous pooling are blocked, orthostatic or postural hypotension becomes marked in the upright position.

The ganglion blockers diminish cardiac contractility. They produce tachycardia because the SA node is usually dominated by the parasympathetic nervous system.

Gastrointestinal tract : Motility and secretions are decreased leading to constipation.

Other systems : The genitourinary smooth muscles are affected resulting in hesitancy in urination and may precipitate urinary retention. Sexual functions may be impaired in that both erection and ejaculation may be prevented. These drugs also block thermoregulatory sweating. In very warm climate hyperthermia induced by these agents may be a problem otherwise normal body temperature is maintained by cutaneous vasodilatation.

Effects of autonomic drugs

As the effector cell receptors are not blocked, the autonomic drugs acting on the effector cells produce effects in patients who are receiving autonomic ganglion-blockers. The responses may even become greater because the homeostatic reflexes which moderate the autonomic responses are not present.

Clinical applications

The usefulness is limited in the treatment of hypertensive emergencies. Trimethaphan has been used. It is also used to reduce pulmonary vascular pressure in the treatment of acute pulmonary oedema.

Adverse effects

A large number of adverse effects can be produced as both sympathetic and parasympathetic ganglia are blocked.

Due to parasympathetic ganglionic blockade	Due to sympathetic ganglionic blockade
Palpitation,	Postural hypotension
Dilated pupils	Syncope,
Loss of accommodation	Inhibition of sweating
Constipation	Inhibition of ejaculation
Difficulty in micturition	
Dryness of mouth	
Dysfunction of penile erection	

STUDY QUESTIONS

1. Classify ganglion blocking agents. What are their main actions in central nervous system, GIT, eye and cardiovascular system?
2. Is there any therapeutic use of the ganglion blocking drugs? If yes, then for what purpose?
3. Why the use of ganglion blocking drugs has been abandoned for the treatment of many diseases?
4. Describe the disadvantages and adverse effects of ganglion blockers.
5. Name ganglion stimulating agents. Do they have any therapeutic utility?
6. Describe the pharmacology of nicotine.

GUIDE TO FURTHER READING

Benowitz, N.L. and Henningfield, J.E. Establishing a nicotine threshold for addiction. The implications for tobacco regulation. New Engl J Med, 1994; 331:123.

Mason, D.F.J. Ganglion-blocking drugs. In, Physiological Pharmacology: A Comprehensive Treatise. Vol 3. Root, W.S. and Hoffman, F.G. (editors). Academic Press, 1967.

Salem, M.R. Therapeutic uses of ganglionic blocking drugs. Int Anaesthesiol Clin, 1978; 16:171.

Unwin, N. Nicotinic acetylcholine receptor 9 A. resolution. J. Mol Biol, 1993; 229:1101.

Sargent, P.B. The diversity of neuronal-nicotinic acetylcholine receptors. Annu Rev Neurosci, 1993; 16:403.

Drugs Acting on Central Nervous System

ETHANOL

Aliphatic alcohols are hydroxy (OH) derivatives of aliphatic hydrocarbons. Depending on the number of OH groups these are designated as

- Monohydroxy e.g. ethyl, methyl, propyl.
- Dihydroxy e.g. ethylene glycol.
- Trihydroxy e.g. glycerol or glycerin.
- Polyhydroxy e.g. mannitol.

Ethanol (ethyl alcohol) is also simply referred as alcohol. It is a colourless liquid possessing an inflammable water soluble molecule.

Pharmacological properties

Local actions

- Rubefacient (40%) and counterirritant when rubbed on skin.
- Astringent due to dehydration and precipitation of surface proteins.
- Irritant to mucous membrane.

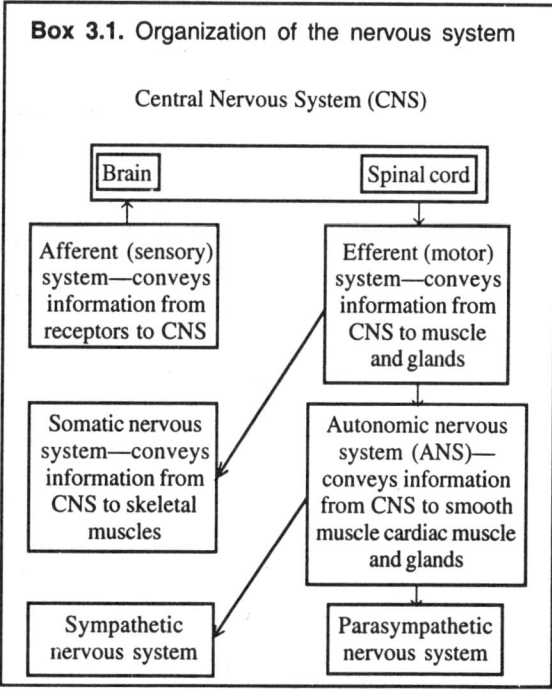

Box 3.1. Organization of the nervous system

Central Nervous System (CNS)

Brain — Spinal cord

Afferent (sensory) system—conveys information from receptors to CNS

Efferent (motor) system—conveys information from CNS to muscle and glands

Somatic nervous system—conveys information from CNS to skeletal muscles

Autonomic nervous system (ANS)—conveys information from CNS to smooth muscle cardiac muscle and glands

Sympathetic nervous system

Parasympathetic nervous system

- Cooling effect on skin due to rapid evaporation.
- Antiseptic due to precipitation of bacterial proteins. It is antiseptic against vegetative forms, spores are resistant.
- Irritant and painful on subcutaneous injection.
- Permanent damage when injected near the nerves.

Systemic actions

CNS: The most important action of ethanol is on central nervous system which it depresses. The apparent hyperactivity is due to depression of inhibitory control mechanisms.

The first mental processes to be affected are those that depend on training; memory, concentration, and insight are dulled and then lost.

The effects on the CNS are proportional to the concentration of ethanol in the blood as following:

Less than 50 mg/100 ml	No significant change.
50 to 100 mg/ 100 ml	Mild intoxication, euphoria, talkativeness, ataxia, exaltation, confidence abounds, personality becomes vivacious and uncontrolled mood swings and emotional outburst may be evident. Self criticism, restraint, hesitation and caution are lost.
150 mg/100 ml	Danger in driving, accident due to prolonged reaction time, bad judgement, over confidence.
200 mg/100 ml	Loss of self confidence.
300 mg/100 ml	Stupor, vomiting.
400 mg/100 ml	Deep anaesthesia. However, there is little margin between the full surgical anaesthetic dose and that which is dangerous to respiration.
500 mg to 700 mg/100 ml	Respiratory and circulatory failure, death.

Respiration: Due to buccal mucosal irritation, moderate amounts of ethanol reflexly stimulates respiration in conditions of collapse but it has direct depressant action on respiratory centre. Large amounts (blood concentration 400 mg/dl or more) produce dangerous or lethal depression of respiration.

Sleep: The acute use of ethanol in normal persons at bedtime reduces initial latency to sleep and REM-sleep and increases deep non-REM sleep. In chronic alcoholics, marked fragmentation of sleep occurs, with sleep interrupted by frequent awakenings.

Liver: Ethanol impairs gluconeogenesis, synthesis of lipoproteins is increased resulting in enhanced serum triglycerides.

Ethanol consumed on a regular basis in more than moderate amounts leads to deleterious effects in the liver principally from its metabolic process. A portion of the ingested ethanol is metabolised by microsomal mixed-function oxidases that are subject to induction by ethanol. The product of these reactions, acetaldehyde, is a toxic substance which leads to inhibition of a wide variety of enzymes.

The accumulation of acetaldehyde is in part owing to reduced activity of acetaldehyde dehydrogenase which causes a host of harmful effects including enhanced lipid peroxidation, damage to cellular membranes, depletion of glutathione, depletion of vitamins specially B_6, A and trace metals such as zinc and selenium and decreased transport and secretion of proteins due to inhibition of tubulin polymerisation. Thus hepatocytes are engorged with fat, protein, and water that progresses to cirrhosis of liver, as well as various metabolic disturbances produced in alcoholic individuals.

No doubt malnutrition can intensify hepatic damage but even excellent nutritional status does not prevent the development of alcoholic hepatitis or its progression to cirrhosis.

Chronic ingestion of ethanol can increase incidence of cancer and enhance toxicity of certain drugs such as acetaminophen because ethanol produces induction of microsomal oxidases coupled with depletion of glutathione which lead to accumulation of activated carcinogens or toxic metabolites.

Plasma lipoproteins: There is a negative correlation between chronic ingestion of small amounts of ethanol and the incidences of coronary heart disease. This protective effect seems to occur because ethanol increases HDL and decreases LDL in plasma.

Box 3.2. Terms associated with CNS

- Analgesia (an = without; algia = painful condition): Pain relief.
- Anaesthesia (esthesia = feeling): Loss of feeling.
- Dementia (de = away from; mens = mind): An organic mental disorder that results in permanent or progressive loss of intellectual abilities such as impairment of memory, judgement and changes in personality.
- Delusions: Firmly held but false beliefs are expressed that have absolutely no basis in fact.
- Delirium: A condition of extreme, mental, and usually motor excitement marked by defective perception, impaired memory, confused and unconnected ideas often with illusions and hallucinations.
- Hallucination (alucinari = to wander in mind): The apparent, often strong, subjective sense of perception of site, sound, smell, taste or touch without basis in external stimuli. Any sense may be affected.
- Hallucinogen: A substance eliciting hallucinations, depersonalization, perceptual disturbances, and disturbances of thought processes.
- Hallucinogenic: Relating to a hallucinogen.
- Illusion: A false perception; the mistaking of something for what it is not.
- Mania: An emotional disorder characterized by great psychomotor activity, excitement, and unstable attention.
- Neurosis (pl. neuroses): A functional nervous disease; disorder in which anxiety is primary characteristic. The patient knows that there is something wrong with him.
- Paranoid: Delusions of grandeur or persecution.
- Psychosis (pl. psychoses): A mental disorder causing gross distortion of a persons' mental capacity, and capacity to recognize reality, communicate and cope with ordinary demands of everyday life.
- Schizophrenia: The most common type of psychosis characterized by delusions and hallucinations and extensive withdrawal of the individual's interest from other people.
- Stupor: Unresponsiveness from which a patient can be aroused only briefly and by vigorous and repeated stimulation.

Kidney: Diuresis is produced after ethanol intake. The output of urine is increased due to ingestion of water (large amount of fluid is usually ingested with alcoholic beverages) and also due to inhibition of release of antidiuretic hormone (ADH) from posterior pituitary and resultant decrease in renal tubular reabsorption of water. However, ethanol in repeated doses, may have an antidiuretic effect.

GIT: The gastric secretion is increased in moderate doses (30-50 ml of 7-10%) due to release of histamine and gastrin in stomach. But above 15% concentration it inhibits motility and secretion. The activity of gastric and intestinal juices is inhibited above 20% concentration. Strong alcoholic drinks of 40% concentration and over are quite irritating to the mucosa and cause hyperaemia and inflammation and loss of plasma protein into gastrointestinal lumen. High concentrations of ethanol produce erosive gastritis. The gastric damage produced by aspirin is much enhanced by ethanol.

Ethanol produces lesions of oesophagus and duodenum and also produce acute and chronic pancreatitis because it increases secretion and also an obstruction of the pancreatic duct.

Body temperature: Ethanol enhances cutaneous blood flow. Heat is therefore lost more rapidly and the temperature falls. It produces feeling of warmth and sweating. With large amounts central temperature regulating mechanism is depressed and the fall in body temperature is pronounced.

Skeletal muscle: Small doses may lessen the appreciation of fatigue and increase muscular work, but large doses decrease muscular work due to CNS depression. It can also cause reversible damage to muscle signified by a marked increase in the activity of creatine phosphokinase in plasma. In chronic alcoholism skeletal myopathy may occur similar to alcoholic cardiomyopathy.

Ethanol as food: One gram of ethanol supplies seven calories, compared to nine calories from fat and four calories from carbohydrate and protein. However, ethanol is not an advisable food.

Cardiovascular system: Moderate doses produce cutaneous vasodilation, and produce warm, flushed skin. The vasodilation results partly from central vasomotor depression and partly from a direct vasodilation effect of ethanol on blood vessels. It has no significant effect on blood pressure, cardiac output and myocardial contractility. There is no beneficial increase in coronary blood flow in human beings.

Large doses depress cardiovascular system due to central vasomotor factors in acute poisoning. In chronic users of large amounts of ethanol, cardiomyopathy may be produced. There may be disturbances of conduction and rhythm.

Blood: Ethanol interferes with several aspects of folate metabolism and transport as well as its normal pattern of storage and release from the liver. These are reversible with the onset of abstinence. However, thrombocytopenia and vacuolization of precursors of red and white cells result due to direct depressant action of ethanol on the bone marrow.

The poor resistance of alcoholics to infection is due to depression of leukocyte migration into inflamed areas.

Biogenic amines: Ethanol elevates the concentrations of catecholamines in blood which may be partly responsible for the transient hyperglycaemia, pupillary dilation and slight rise in blood pressure.

Sexual functions: The popular notion is that ethanol is an aphrodisiac. The aggressive sexual behaviour after ethanol ingestion is due to loss of inhibition and restraint. The objective measurements indicate decrease in sexual responsiveness in both men and women. It has been reported that chronic ingestion of ethanol in men may lead to impotence, sterility, testicular atrophy and gynaecomastia. This feminisation in alcoholic man is due to (i) ethanol-induced hepatic injury leading to hyperoestrogenization and a reduced rate of production of testosterone, and (ii) ethanol markedly increasing the rate of metabolic inactivation of testosterone by increasing the activity of enzymes of the hepatic endoplasmic reticulum.

Teratogenic effects: The detailed characteristics of FAS are discussed under adverse effects.

Mechanism of action

Ethanol affects the functions of both excitatory (glutamate) and inhibitory (GABA) amino acid-activated ion channels.

Recently it has been found that ethanol potentiates the effect of 5-HT on the newly discovered 5-HT$_3$ receptor, thus it potentiates inhibitory drive through interneurons. The 5-HT$_3$ receptors are located primarily at inhibitory interneurons.

A relatively novel mode of action involves inhibition of the transport of adenosine.

Action of ethanol on other receptors and ion channels that may be relevant to its CNS effects include spatial inhibition of voltage-gate Ca^{2+} channels of the L-type. Such effects may be important in ethanol-induced inhibition of the release of ADH.

Pharmacokinetics

Absorption is very fast on empty stomach. It is absorbed unaltered from stomach and small intestines. It is distributed in total body water. It crosses placenta. The peak effect appears in 1-2 hours. Liver plays an important role in the metabolism, about 90% is metabolized by non-microsomal enzymes, the end products are carbon dioxide and water. Ethanol is metabolised (oxidised) by enzyme systems in the liver, into acetaldehyde and then to acetate, which is metabolised to carbon dioxide and water. Metabolites are responsible for organ damage in chronic over consumption, acetaldehyde in liver and fatty ethyl esters in other organs. About 10% of the total volume ingested escape metabolism and removed in perspiration, excreted in urine and exhaled through lungs (concentration in exhaled air is about 0.05% of blood concentration).

$$\text{Ethanol} \xrightarrow[\text{dehydrogenase}]{\text{Alcohol}} \text{Acetaldehyde} \xrightarrow[\text{dehydrogenase}]{\text{Aldehyde}}$$

$$\text{Acetate} \longrightarrow O_2 + H_2O$$

Metabolites are responsible for damage to organs in chronic over intake of ethanol, due to acetaldehyde in liver and fatty ethyl esters in other organs.

Therapeutic uses

The importance of ethanol in therapeutics is small. It is used in the treatment of methyl alcohol poisoning. Ethanol has been widely used and abused as a sedative. However, it has no medically approved use for this purpose.

Externally, ethanol has a number of medical uses. Based on its local action, ethanol can be used as a counterirritant when rubbed on the skin and for cooling effect on the skin (25% concentration) . It can be used to harden the skin in bed ridden patients. Its local application (50%) also reduces sweating and allays itching.

As a skin antiseptic, 70% by weight (76% by volume) is most effective; stronger solutions are less effective. Ethanol scrubs are common but the effect is transient, as it evaporates quickly and does not leave germicidal effect.

High concentrations of ethanol are often injected into nerves and ganglia for the relief of pain, accomplishing this by causing nerve degeneration e.g. trigeminal neuralgia and carcinoma involving nerves.

Ethanol retrobulbar injection: The retrobulbar injection of absolute or 95% ethanol has been advocated for the treatment of painful blind eyes, particularly on the old and severely ill patients.

Contraindications : Ethanol is contraindicated in peptic ulcer, hyperacidity, liver disease, epilepsy and pregnancy.

Drug interactions : Effects of ethanol are enhanced by other CNS depressants such as sedatives, hypnotics, anticonvulsants, antianxiety drugs and opioids.

Ethanol reduces clearance of phenytoin because both drugs compete for the same hepatic microsomal oxidase system.

The hepatic toxicity of acetaminophen is increased in individuals who consume ethanol regularly due to depletion of hepatic glutathione.

Unpleasant symptoms appear in patients treated with metronidazole, cephalosporins, or oral hypoglycaemic agents presumably due to inhibition of acetaldehyde dehydrogenase. These symptoms are similar to those experienced by patients who ingest ethanol with disulfiram.

Adverse effects

Acute intoxication with pure ethyl alcohol causes euphoria and occasionally causes temporary convergent strabismus with diplopia. The pupils may become dilated which continue to react to light except in severe stage of intoxication.

The side effects of moderate drinking include nausea, vomiting, hangover, traffic accidents. Acute ethanol intoxication produces fall in blood pressure, gastritis, hypoglycaemia, respiratory depression, coma, death.

Although no significant effects are produced on the sensory aspects of vision, but vision could be affected by nystagmus, poorly controlled eye movements, and diplopia. This may have considerable influence on the function of the eye in relation to automobile driving.

Management of acute alcohol poisoning

- Gastric lavage
- Supportive measures:
  Maintenance of fluid and electrolytes
  Artificial respiration, if needed (Analeptics should NOT be used as they may precipitate convulsions).

In case of **chronic alcoholism** there is psychic dependence, physical dependence associated with heavy drinking. Withdrawal symptoms include sweating, tremor, hallucinations, and convulsions. There may be ocular muscle palsies which appear rapidly as a result of haemorrhages in the nuclei of ocular motor nerves. Chronic alcoholism may cause disturbances ranging from nystagmus to complete ophthalmoplegia, in conjunction with ataxia and polyneuritis. Miosis and sluggish pupillary reaction to light have also been reported. Amblyopia which is partially or completely reversible has also been associated with chronic alcoholism. The toxic amblyopia of ethanol may be in reality a vitamin deficiency disease.

Correction of deficiencies of B vitamins if commenced early can produce complete recovery of vision and relief of peripheral neuritis. Apart from ethanol amblyopia with reduced visual acuity, an abnormally high incidence of defective colour vision has been reported in chronic alcoholism which gradually returns back during successful treatment of chronic alcoholism.

Visual hallucinations have been reported in both acute and chronic alcoholism.

Tobacco-ethanol amblyopia: In smokers and who drink ethanol and have poor nutrition, this combination has a synergistic effect on the optic nerve as the toxic effect of one alone with normal nutrition is much less. Treatment of tobacco-ethanol amblyopia with hydroxocobalamin I.M. 2 times weekly for 1 month and then weekly for several months is beneficial.

Chronic ethanol abuse is associated with a variety of cardiovascular disorders such as hypertension, cardiomyopathy, congestive heart failure, arrhythmias and sudden cardiac death.

Ethanol adversely affects the left ventricular function. Loss of potassium, altered calcium movement in the cell and altered lipid transport in the myocardium are the metabolic changes held responsible for the myocardial effects of ethanol. In addition to ethanol, its first metabolite acetaldehyde can depress left ventricular function. Due to the direct myocardial damaging effect of ethanol, typical MI with normal coronary arteries is well documented in patients of chronic alcoholism.

Ethanol consumption of more than 60 ml daily results in raising both systolic and diastolic blood pressure at all ages.

It is believed that consumption of ethanol in small amount has protective effect on the prevalence of coronary artery disease. But there is also a large body of data which suggests that there is no protective effect. Certainly the protective effect, if any, is lost if more than 60 ml of ethanol is used daily.

Cerebrovascular accidents, both subarachnoid haemorrhages and thrombotic strokes occur more in heavy ethanol users. There is a positive association between heavy drinking and mortality.

The non-cardiac ill effects of ethanol are liver cirrhosis, mental disorders such as alcoholic dementia, gastritis, pancreatitis and deaths due to accidents as a result of mental imbalance and violence.

Foetal alcohol syndrome (FAS): Chronic ethanol use by pregnant women results in malformation in offspring. There is a triad of symptoms consisting of growth retardation, CNS dysfunction, and congenital anomalies.

Foetal alcohol syndrome includes growth deficiency of prenatal origin (both height and weight), small eyeballs, mid face hypoplasia, smooth and long philtrum and thin upper lip, CNS manifestation are microcephaly, attention deficits, learning disabilities, intellectual deficits and seizures. FAS may lead to mental retardation.

Foetal alcohol syndrome can also involve eye and is manifested by short horizontal palpebral fissures and ptosis (seen more marked at 1 year of age). It is less apparent as the child grows. The other distur-

bances include reduced vision, higher incidence of myopia. Esotropia in 50-65% of all children is observed. Corneal opacities, anterior chamber angle abnormality, iris defects, optic nerve hypoplasia, pallor and tortuosity of retinal arteries have been reported.

Ethanol creates major problems

The overall health, social and economic problems related to ethanol outweigh its beneficial effects. Alcoholism is a major scourge of the human race and the most dangerous property of ethanol is the readiness with which it produces dependence. The abuse of ethanol creates a number of major problems. It has multiple destructive effects on brain tissue, the peripheral nervous system, liver, pancreas, GIT, CVS, endocrine organs and foetal development.

Management of chronic alcoholism

The main pharmacological approaches to alcohol dependence are the following : To alleviate the acute abstinence syndrome during "drying out", **benzodiazepines** are effective; clonidine and propranolol are also useful. Clonidine (Alpha 2 adrenoceptor agonist) inhibits the exaggerated transmitter release that occurs during withdrawal. Propranolol (Beta-adrenoceptor antagonist) blocks the effects of excessive sympathetic activity.

Disulfiram (tetraethylthiuram disulfide, Antabuse): It is relatively nontoxic when given by itself. But when ethanol is given to an individual, disulfiram increases blood acetaldehyde concentration 5-10 times above the level achieved without disulfiram.

The acetaldehyde syndrome includes nausea, vomiting, sweating, thirst, chest pain, blurred vision and hypotension. The face becomes hot and flushed, and there is intense throbbing in head and neck (due to marked vasodilation). The patient feels uneasiness, weakness, vertigo, panic and distress. The symptoms are extremely unpleasant.

The only use of disulfiram is in the management of chronic alcoholism. It is given 12 hours after stopping ingestion of ethanol. The dose is 500 mg daily for 1-2 weeks, then the maintenance dose is 125-500 mg daily.

Disulfiram is not a curative. It helps to abandon

the habit of taking ethanol. It can be used as aversion therapy to discourage people from taking alcohol.

Disulfiram

Calcium carbimide has actions and uses similar to those of disulfiram. The citrated form has been used as an adjunct in the treatment of chronic alcoholism in doses of 50 mg once or twice a day by mouth. It produces less intense interaction with alcohol than disulfiram. But, appreciable potentially dangerous cardiovascular changes have been observed during the carbimide-alcohol reaction. Peripheral neuropathy has also been observed.

Calcium carbimide is similar in action to disulfiram but is less effective and therefore safer, if the patient does drink.

Naltrexone, an orally effective opioid antagonist, has also been found to reduce the incidence of relapse in patients undergoing treatment for alcoholism, by reducing the euphorigenic or other positive reinforcing effects of alcohol ingestion.

Nalmefene

- Nalmefene an opiate antagonist is similar to naloxone and naltrexone but with longer elimination half-life; 50-80 mg/d can be helpful in chronic alcoholism.

Management of alcohol withdrawal syndrome

Objectives : prevent seizures, delirium and arrhythmias
- Restore electrolytes
- I.V. phenytoin for convulsions
- Give thiamine
- *Specific therapy* : substitute a long acting sedative-hypnotic drug, for alcohol and gradually taper the dose of the long acting drugs. Oxazepam is preferred in patients with liver disease. Phenothiazines are not used.

- Psychological and other supportive measures are needed so that there are no relapses.

METHYL ALCOHOL (METHANOL)

Methanol is used as an industrial solvent and is also used to adulterate industrial ethanol to make it unfit to drink. Methanol is sometimes consumed as a substitute for ethanol. Its acute toxicity is slightly less than ethanol i.e. it makes the subject less drunk. It is metabolised at only one fifth the rate of ethanol and it is the toxic metabolites produced over a long period that make methanol intoxication so serious. As little as 30 g may be fatal.

Methanol is metabolised in the same way as ethanol but produces formaldehyde instead of acetaldehyde from the first oxidation step. Formaldehyde is further oxidized to another toxic metabolite formic acid which produces intense acidosis. Formaldehyde is more reactive than acetaldehyde and reacts rapidly with proteins, causing the inactivation of enzymes involved in the tricarboxylic acid cycle. Conversion of alcohols to aldehydes occurs in the liver as well as in retina where the dehydrogenase responsible for the retinol/retinal conversion oxidizes exogenous ethanol. Formation of formaldehyde in the retina accounts for one of the main toxic effects viz. blindness which can occur after ingestion of as little as 10 g. The other main toxic effect is damage to peripheral nerves (neuropathy).

The effects of chronic methanol consumption are irreversible but acute poisoning may be treated by administration of large doses of ethanol which acts to retard methanol metabolism by competition for ethanol dehydrogenase. Methanol poisoning is manifested by severe malaise, vomiting, abdominal pain and tachypnoea (due to acidosis). Muscle cramps, coma and circulatory collapse may follow.

A prominent symptom is visual disturbances with scotomata and total blindness, which may occur early or late. It is due to formate accumulation. Although partial or complete recovery may occur but permanent blindness with optic atrophy is common. Very small doses can cause blindness and large doses may sometimes fail to do so, hence eye changes may be due to an idiosyncrasy.

There are 3 components of methanol poisoning

viz. (i) narcotic action 10 g/kg; (ii) uncompensated metabolic acidosis (latent period) caused indirectly by toxic metabolic products of methanol due to tissue damage by formaldehyde; and (iii) ocular and CNS necrosis including death of retinal ganglion cells and the basal ganglia. This component occurs only if the patient survives for 30 hours or more.

Treatment of methanol poisoning

- Gastric lavage with sodium bicarbonate
- Supportive measures to maintain respiration and circulation
- Acidosis to be treated by I.V. sodium bicarbonate in order to prevent retinal damage and other symptoms due to acidosis.
- Potassium is given to correct hypokalaemia
- Fluids and electrolytes
- Haemodialysis and peritoneal dialysis may remove both alcohols.
- Folate therapy (leucovorin) reduces blood formate levels by enhancing its metabolism.
- 4-methypyrazole inhibits alcohol dehydrogenase and thus retards its metabolism, 100 mg. I.V. slow infusion is effective. But somehow it is not commonly used.

Ethanol in methanol poisoning

Ethanol retards methanol metabolism by competing for alcohol dehydrogenase enzyme. Ethanol is markedly selective hence advocated in the treatment of methanol poisoning. Ethanol (100 mg/dl in blood) will saturate alcohol dehydrogenase sufficient to delay the metabolism of methanol. To achieve this, ethanol (10% in water) is given through a nasogastirc tube. The initial dose is 0.7 ml/kg followed by 0.15 ml/kg / hr drip, may have to be continued for several days. It is interesting, more theoretical than practical.

STUDY QUESTIONS

1. Describe the effects of ethanol on the central nervous system according to the different concentrations in the blood.
2. What are the local actions of ethanol?
3. Describe the effects of ethyl alcohol on GIT. Is it a suitable food?
4. What are the therapeutic uses of ethanol?
5. What are the contraindications, and drug-interactions of ethanol?
6. Describe acute and chronic alcoholism and their treatment.
7. What are the non-cardiac ill effects of ethanol?
8. Describe foetal alcohol syndrome (FAS).
9. Why ethanol is considered a major scourge of the human race?
10. In what way methyl alcohol (methanol) differs from ethyl alcohol?
11. What are the prominent toxic effects of methanol?
12. Can ethanol be useful in the treatment of methanol poisoning? If so, how?

GUIDE TO FURTHER READING

Abel, E.L. (ed). Fetal Alcohol & Syndrome. CRC Press, 1981.

Ballard, H.S. Hematological complications and alcoholism. Alcoholism. Clin. Exp. Res., 1989; 13:706.

Becker, C.E. Alcohol and drug use. Is there a "safe" amount? West J Med, 1984; 141:884.

Becker, C.E. Methanol poisoning. J Emerg Med, 1983; 2:47.

Chick, J. et al. Disulfiram treatment of alcoholism. Br J Psychiatry, 1992; 161:84.

Friedman, J.D., Klatsky, A.R. Is alcohol good for your health? N Engl J Med, 1993; 329:1882.

Iber, F.L., Lea, K. et al. Liver toxicity encountered in the Veterans Administration trial of disulfiram in alcoholics. Alcoholism Clin. Exp. Res., 1987; 11:301.

Olsen, J. Effects of moderate alcohol consumption during pregnancy on child development at 18 and 42 months. Alcohol Clin. Exp. Res., 1994; 18:1109.

Regan, T.J. Regional circulatory responses to alcohol and its congeners. Fed. Proc., 1982; 41:2438.

Roehrs, T. et al. Effects of alcohol, diphenhydramine, and triazolam after a nap. Neuropsychopharmacology, 1993; 9:239.

Rubin, E. and Urbano-Marquez, A. Alcoholic cardiomyopathy. Alcohol Clin. Res., 1994; 18:111.

Steinberg, W., Tenner, S. Acute pancreatitis. N Engl I Med, 1994; 330:1198.

Swift, R. M., Whelihan, W. et al. Naltrexone-induced alterations in human ethanol intoxication. Am. J. Psychiatry, 1994; 151:1463.

Wilson, G.T. Alcohol and human sexual behaviour. Behav. Res. Ther., 1977; 15:239.

Windham, G.C., Fenster, L., Swan, S.H. Moderate maternal and paternal alcohol consumption and the risk of spontaneous abortion. Epidemiology, 1992; 3:364.

Volpicelli, J.R. et al. Naltrexone in the treatment of alcohol dependence. Arch. Gen. Psychiatry, 1992; 49:876.

SEDATIVES AND HYPNOTICS

Sedatives are drugs which reduce excitement and produce quietness. Hypnotics are drugs which produce sleep. Sedatives act as hypnotics and vice versa, the main difference is quantitative. About one third dose of a hypnotic will act as sedative.

Normal sleep

Normal sleep is of two types, viz. :

- NREM (nonrapid eye movement) sleep: The eyeballs are motionless. Persons awakened at this phase of sleep say that they were "thinking".
- REM (rapid eye movement) sleep: The eyeballs show rapid movements. Persons awakened during this phase say that they were "dreaming".

A normal sleep begins with-NREM sleep (about 90 minutes) and is then interspersed with short periods of REM sleep (about 20 minutes) alternating with NREM sleep. Both NERM and REM sleep are essential for normal health.

Classification of sedatives-hypnotics

A. Barbiturates

- Long acting (8-12 hours): Phenobarbitone, mephobarbitone. They are used as antiepileptic and anticonvulsant.
- Intermediate acting (4-8 hours): Amytal is used in insomnia to maintain sleep.
- Short acting (2-4 hours): Pentobarbitone, secobarbitone. They are used to induce sleep in insomnia.
- Ultra short acting (1/2-1 hour): Thiopentone, methohexitone. They are used as intravenous general anaesthetic agents.

B. Non-barbiturates

- Benzodiazepines: Diazepam, nitrazepam.
- Newer nonbenzodiazepine hypnotics: Zopiclone, zolpidem.

- Chloral derivatives: Chloral hydrate.
- Aldehydes: Paraldehyde.
- Inorganic ions: Bromide.
- Miscellaneous: Meprobamate, antihistaminics, scopolamine, methaqualone.

BARBITURATES

Barbituric acid is malonylurea obtained by condensation of urea and malonic acid. Barbituric acid is not sedative-hypnotic but the derivatives of barbituric acid produce pharmacological actions.

Sequence of effects with barbiturates

Sedation → Hypnosis → Anaesthesia → Coma → Death

Pharmacological action

CNS: Barbiturates depress CNS, ranging from mild sedation to general anaesthesia. The anaesthetic dose is close to lethal dose, hence sedative-hypnotic barbiturates are not used to produce general anaesthesia.

Barbiturates were commonly used previously as sedative-hypnotics but now benzodiazepines are preferred.

All barbiturates are anticonvulsants but they are all not antiepileptics.

The ultra short acting barbiturates produce general anaesthesia on i.v. injection.

Barbiturates are not analgesics but enhance the analgesic effect of morphine etc.

The pain perception and reaction are relatively unimportant until unconsciousness, and in small doses barbiturates increase the reaction to painful stimuli. In the presence of pain, barbiturates produce overt excitement instead of sedation and this may be due to depression of inhibitory centres.

Effects on stages of sleep: Sleep latency, number of awakenings and duration of REM is decreased. However, tolerance develops to these effects if barbiturates are taken regularly. The effect on total sleep may be reduced by as much as 50% after two weeks of repetitive use. Drug dependence occurs with barbiturates.

Effect on peripheral nervous system: Barbiturates selectively depress transmission in autonomic ganglia and reduce nicotinic excitation by choline esters.

At skeletal neuromuscular junctions, the blocking effects of tubocurarine and decamethonium are enhanced. These actions are produced because barbiturates in hypnotic or anaesthetic doses inhibit the passage of current through nicotinic cholinergic receptors.

Respiration: Barbiturates in sedative-hypnotic doses do not affect respiration. High doses depress respiration.

CVS: When given orally in sedative and hypnotic doses there is no significant effect on cardiovascular system except for a slight decrease in blood pressure and heart rate such as occurs in normal sleep. However, direct depression of cardiac contractility occurs only when doses several times those required to cause anaesthesia are administered.

GIT: Hypnotic dose has no significant effect.

Kidney: The normal dose does not affect kidneys. However, larger doses decrease urinary output due to decrease in glomerular filtration and release of antidiuretic hormone. The oliguria or anuria in acute barbiturate poisoning occurs due to marked decrease in blood pressure.

Liver: Liver is unaffected at normal dose. However, large doses may produce hepatic dysfunction.

Acutely, barbiturates combine with several species of cytochrome P450 and competitively interfere with the biotransformations of a number of drugs such as steroids.

Chronic administration of barbiturates increases the protein and lipid content of the hepatic smooth endoplasmic reticulum as well as in the activities of glucuronyl transferase and the oxidases containing cytochrome P450. The inducing effect on these enzymes enhances the metabolism of a number of drugs including steroid hormones, cholesterol, bile salts, vitamin K and vitamin D.

An increase in the rate of barbiturate metabolism also occurs which accounts a part for the tolerance to barbiturates.

Mode of action

The mode of action of barbiturates is not very clear. They increase the inhibitory activity of GABA, primarily at synapses where neurotransmission is mediated by GABA acting at $GABA_a$ receptors. The mechanism of action of barbiturates on $GABA_a$ receptors appears to be distinct from those of either GABA or the benzodiazepines because although barbiturates enhance the binding of GABA to $GABA_A$ receptors, they promote (rather than displace) the binding of benzodiazepines.

Pharmacokinetics

Barbiturates are rapidly absorbed after oral as well as parenteral administration. They are widely distributed in the body. Liver plays main role in metabolizing barbiturates by

- oxidation at C 5 position,
- removal of N-alkyl radicals,
- cleavage of the ring, and
- thiobarbiturates are converted to oxygen analogues.

Phenobarbitone is metabolized slowly so 30% is excreted unchanged in urine as well as glucuronic acid conjugate. The sedative dose is 15-30 mg and hypnotic dose is 100 mg.

Therapeutic uses

- As sedative.
- Hypnotic.
- Barbiturates can be used as anticonvulsant.
- Preanaesthetic medicament.
- Potentiation of analgesics.
- Certain barbiturates such as phenobarbitone, mephobarbital and metharbital are used as antiepileptics.
- I.V. anaesthesia can be produced with ultra short acting barbiturates.

Barbiturates if used as sedative-hypnotic should be employed only when needed, in low doses and for shortest period. They may have value in insomnia of recent origin but not in chronic insomnia. If insomnia is due to pain, analgesics should be given to relieve pain. Barbiturates are not analgesic.

As sedative-hypnotic drugs barbiturates are not commonly used now as they lack specificity of effect in the CNS, have lower therapeutic index than benzodiazepines, tolerance occurs more frequently, liability of abuse is greater and number of drug interactions is considerable.

Adverse effects

- Tolerance.
- Drug dependence.
- Abstinence or withdrawal syndrome.
- Drug automatism.
- Enzyme induction is also responsible for many drug interactions.

Acute poisoning may be due to accidental or with suicidal intention. The overdose effects are hypotension, respiratory depression, oliguria and coma. If not treated properly, death results due to respiratory arrest.

The treatment of acute poisoning includes:

- Early gastric aspiration,
- Maintain respiration and circulation, and
- Alkalinization of urine increases urinary excretion of phenobarbitone but it is not so effective in case of short acting barbiturates.

Chronic poisoning (drug dependence)

The drug is withdrawn gradually as abrupt withdrawal may result in excitement, anxiety, tremors and even convulsions.

Deaths have also been reported due to abrupt withdrawal of barbiturates.

Contraindications

- Severe pulmonary insufficiency.
- Hepatic disease.
- Renal damage.

NON-BARBITURATES

Benzodiazepines

This group of drugs are more safe and also possess better sedative-hypnotic-antianxiety activity.

Benzodiazepines may be categorized on the basis of their pharmacokinetics :

1. Slow elimination of the drug or its active metabolite: Flurazepam produces an active metabolite having long half-life. If ingested daily, cumulative effect occurs. Flurazepam is useful in patients who awaken frequently in the night and in those who may accept sedative effect during the day.

2. Relatively slow elimination, but having marked redistribution: Diazepam produces active metabolites viz. desmethyldiazepam and oxazepam. If it is used regularly it has cumulative effect.

   Nitrazepam is useful for patients who complain of frequent awakenings during the night and who may accept some sedation during day time.

   Flunitrazepam is more potent having marked redistribution.

3. Rapid elimination with marked redistribution: Temazepam does not generate active metabolites. If it is taken daily, cumulative effect is obtained.

4. *Ultrarapid elimination* : Triazolam is very potent. Sleep is induced early and poorly maintained. It may produce withdrawal phenomenon and rebound insomnia. High doses may produce psychiatric disturbances. It is banned in UK, It is not marketed in India. Midazolam is very promptly absorbed, maximal effect reaches in 20 minutes. It is also employed as I.V. anaesthetic.

Pharmacological properties

CNS: The most prominent effects are sedation, hypnosis, decreased anxiety, muscle relaxation and anticonvulsant activity.

Effect on peripheral tissues: Only the coronary vasodilation observed after I.V. use and neuromuscular blockage with high doses are the effects which result from actions on peripheral tissues.

Respiration: Hypnotic doses of benzodiazepines do not affect respiration in normal persons. At higher doses used for preanaesthetic medication they slightly depress alveolar ventilation. This effect is exaggerated in patients suffering from chronic obstructive pulmonary disease (COPD).

CVS: Benzodiazepines produce minor effects in normal persons. In preanaesthetic doses they lower blood pressure and increase heart rate.

GIT: Benzodiazepines may be useful in anxiety-related gastrointestinal disorders. There is a paucity of evidence for direct action.

Absorption, fate and excretion

All the benzodiazepines are completely absorbed except chlorazepate which is rapidly decarboxylated in gastric juice to N-desmethyldiazepam (norda-zepam) which subsequently is absorbed completely.

Some drugs of this group e.g. prazepam and flurazepam reach systemic circulation only in the form of active metabolites.

On the basis of the elimination half-lives, benzo-diazepines can be categorized as :

- Short-acting agents ($t_{1/2}$ less than 6 hours) e.g. triazolam
- Intermediate-acting agents ($t_{1/2}$ 6-24 hours) e.g. estazolam and temazepam, and
- Long-acting agents ($t_{1/2}$ more than 24 hours) e.g. flurazepam

The volumes of distribution of benzodiazepines are large and increased in elderly patients. They cross placental barrier and are secreted into breast milk.

The benzodiazepines and their active metabolites bind to plasma proteins. The binding correlates with lipid solubility and occurs from about 70% for alprazolam to about 99% for diazepam. The concentration in cerebrospinal fluid is about the same as the concentration of free drug in plasma.

The several microsomal enzyme systems in the liver are responsible for the metabolism of benzo-diazepines.

Mechanism and site of action of benzodiazepines

They bind to benzodiazepine GABA$_A$ receptor which lead to increase in chloride conductance. They do not open chloride channels by themselves but they act allosterically to increase the affinity of the receptors for GABA.

Site : receptors are located in cerebral cortex, midbrain, ascending reticular formation, limbic system, cerebellum and spinal cord. They potentiate the neural inhibition mediated by GABA at all levels of neuraxis.

Therapeutic uses

Benzodiazepines are used as sedative-antianxiety (anxiolytic)-hypnotic drugs. These are very safe and effective hypnotics.

REM sleep remains relatively intact, hepatic microsomal enzymes are not affected, have low drug dependence potential, high therapeutic index. Fatal poisoning is very rare. They have almost replaced barbiturates as sedative-hypnotics.

All the benzodiazepines have very similar phar-macological profiles. However, they differ in selec-tivity and the clinical usefulness as shown below:

Benzodiazepines are used for the following con-ditions:

Hypnotic	Antianxiety	Anticonvulsant
Diazepam	Diazepam	Diazepam
Nitrazepam	Oxazepam	Clonazepam
Flurazepam	Lorazepam	Clobazam
Flunitrazepam	Chlordiazepoxide	
Temazepam	Alprazolam	
Triazolam		
Midazolam		

Some characteristics of benzodiazepines em-ployed as hypnotics are given in Table 3.1.

Drug	Duration	GI absorption rate	Active metabolite	Elimination half-life
Diazepam	Long	Rapid	Yes	2-4 days
Clonazepam	Long	Intermediate	Yes	2-3 days
Oxazepam	Intermediate	Slow	No	10 hours
Lorazepam	Intermediate	Intermediate	No	15 hours
Chlordiazepoxide	Long	Intermediate	Yes	2-4 days
Alprazolam	Intermediate	Intermediate	No	14 hours
Midazolam	Short	Intermediate	No	2.5 hours
Triazolam	Short	Intermediate	No	3 hours
Flurazepam	Long	Intermediate	Yes	2-3 days
Halazepam	Long	Slow	Yes	2-4 days
Prazepam	Long	Slow	Yes	2-4 days

Box 3.3. Pharmacokinetics of benzodiazepines

Table 3.1. Some characteristics of benzodiazepines employed as hypnotic

Benzodiazepine	half-life in hours	Dose (mg)	Uses
Long-acting			
Flurazepam	50-100	15-30	Chronic insomnia (short term frequent awakening in night)
Diazepam	30-60	5 - 10	
Nitrazepam	30	5-10	
Flunitrazepam	15-25	1-2	
Short-acting			
Temazepam	8-12	16-20	Sleep onset problem
Triazolam	2-3	0.125-0.25	
Midazolam	2	7.5	

Choice

The choice between different agents is dictated by the speed of action, its intensity and duration.

Substances with a short half-life that are not converted to active metabolite can be used for induction or maintenance of sleep. Substances with a long half-life are preferable for longer term anxiolytic treatment because they permit maintenance of steady plasma levels with single daily dosage. Midazolam enjoys use by the I.V. route in preanaesthetic medication and anaesthetic combination regimens.

Preference in certain situations

- In renal failure: chloral hydrate, nitrazepam
- In hepatic failure: Nitrazepam
- In respiratory disease: Temazepam
- In elderly: Chloral hydrate, lorazepam
- Prior to minor surgery: Diazepam or midazolam
- Elderly have more problems with benzodiazepines because both the metabolism and the renal functions are impaired, hence they accumulate. However, glucuronide conjugation is less affected than oxidative reaction, hence lorazepam which is metabolized by glucuronidation is preferred.

Nitrazepam is a useful drug for patients who complain frequent awakenings in the night. But it is likely to produce some day time sedation. Dose is 5 mg tablet 5, 10 mg capsule. It is relatively slowly eliminated but markedly distributed like diazepam and flunitrazepam.

Flunitrazepam is more potent and rapidly absorbed drug.

Temazepam dose not produce active metabolites. It is free of residual effects. It is suitable to treat patients who complain of sleep onset difficulty. This drug is relatively rapidly eliminated and markedly redistributed.

The important differences between benzodiazepines and barbiturates are given in Table 3.2.

Table 3.2. Important differences between benzodiazepines and barbiturates

Benzodiazepines	Barbiturates
1. Higher therapeutic index, wide margin of safety	Have narrow margin of safety
2. Tolerance mild	Marked tolerance
3. Physical dependence mild	More physical dependence
4. Withdrawal symptoms minor	Marked abstinence syndrome
5. Enzyme induction minimal	Marked inducer of hepatic microsomal enzymes
6. REM sleep less disturbed	Marked depression on REM sleep
7. Sleep resembles normal sleep with little hangover	Hangover is common.

Adverse effects

Benzodiazepines are relatively safe drugs. However, they may produce:

- Lightheadedness, lassitude, confusion, headache, impair driving.
- Hangover, dreaming with nightmares
- Weakness, blurred vision, impaired sexual function
- Allergic reactions, photosensitization, vertigo, menstrual irregularities

- Withdrawal syndrome includes insomnia, agitation, depression, anxiety, unpleasant dreams (but these are minor compared to barbiturates) anorexia, tremors.
- Administration to mother before delivery sometimes causes apnoeic spells, reluctance to feed, hypotonia and hypothermia in the new born (floppy baby syndrome).

Caution

- Care should be taken in respiratory diseases, renal and hepatic impairment, development of dependence.
- While using benzodiazepines for minor surgical procedures, the subject should not drive till the next day and avoid alcohol and to other CNS depressants.
- Midazolam can produce cardiac arrest and respiratory depression especially in elderly.
- Benzodiazepines can cause drug dependence when used on a regularly basis for prolonged periods. Doses should be tapered off gradually when therapy is to be discontinued.

The routes of administration, $t_{1/2}$ and therapeutic uses of commonly used benzodiazepines are given in Table 3.3.

Drug interactions

Ethanol increases rate of absorption of benzodiazepines and the associated CNS depression.

Valproate and benzodiazepines in combination may cause psychotic episodes.

Benzodiazepine antagonist

Flumazenil is a benzodiazepine analogue. It competes with benzodiazepine agonists as well as inverse agonists for benzodiazepine receptor, resulting in reversing their actions. It is a competitive antagonist at benzodiazepines site. Flumazenil is absorbed orally and undergoes high hepatic first-pass effect. The drug is well tolerated. It is used to reverse the effect of benzodiazepine anaesthesia. For this purpose, I.V. injection of 0.3-1 mg is indicated. The action begins within few seconds and the effect lasts for 1-2 hours. Its elimination half-life is 1 hour.

A dose of 0.2 mg/min/I.V. (maximum 5mg) is administered till the patient regains consciousness. Patients intoxicated due to the overdose of benzodiazepine respond within 5 minutes.

Flumazenil has been tried in cases of hepatic coma and acute alcohol poisoning with equivocal results.

Table 3.3. Routes of administration, $t_{1/2}$ and therapeutic uses of commonly used benzodiazepines

Drug, dosage	Route	Half-life (hours)	Condition
Alprazolam 0.25-0.5 mg b.i.d.	Oral	14 ± 2	Anxiety disorders, agoraphobia
Chlordiazepoxide (Librium, others) 15-40 mg/d in divided doses	Oral, I.M., I.V.	10 ± 3.4	Anxiety disorders, preanaesthetic medication, alcohol withdrawal
Clonazepam 1.5-10 mg/d in divided doses	Oral	2.3 ± 0.5	Seizures
Chlorazepate 3.75-20 mg b.i.d., q.i.d.	Oral	2.0 ± 0.9	Anxiety
Diazepam (Valium, others) 5-10 mg t.i.d., q.i.d. 50-100 mg q.i.d.	Oral, I.M., I.V.	14 ± 13	Anxiety, status epilepticus
Estazolam 1-2 mg	Oral	10-24	Insomnia
Flurazepam 15-30 mg	Oral	74 ± 24	Insomnia
Lorazepam 2-4 mg	Oral, I.M., I.V.	14 ± 5	Anxiety disorders, preanaesthetic medication
Oxazepam 15-30 mg t.i.d., q.i.d.	Oral	8 ± 2.4	Anxiety disorders
Temazepam 7.5-30 mg	Oral	11 ± 6	Insomnia
Triazolam 0.125-0.25 mg	Oral	2.9 ± 1.0	Insomnia

Adverse effects of flumazenil include agitation, anxiety, discomfort and feeling of cold.

Newer nonbenzodiazepine hypnotics

- Zopiclone
- Zolpidem

Zopiclone

Its half-life is 5-6 hours. It is a cyclopyrrolone hypnotic. Its actions resemble benzodiazepine effects on sleep. It potentiates GABA binding to a different site than benzodiazepines.

Dose : 7.5 mg.

It is used for short term treatment of insomnia. The side effects include impaired alertness and judgement, metallic taste in mouth and psychological disturbances.

Zolpidem

It is a recent imidazopyridine hypnotic. Its half-life is ½–2 hours. Dose 5–10 mg.

It reduces sleep latency and increases duration of sleep in patients suffering from insomnia.

OTHER SEDATIVE-HYPNOTICS

Chloral hydrate

It can produce refreshing sleep with 500 mg to 1 g/ oral dose for 4-8 hours. Its metabolite (trichloroethanol) is equally hypnotic. There is no enzyme induction and only mild addictive potential, but jaundice and proteinuria may occur.

The use of chloral hydrate is limited due to:
- gastric irritation,
- unpalatable taste,
- hepatic and renal toxicity, and
- overdose may affect cardiac muscle.

Triclofos is a stable ester of trichloroethanol which produces lesser side effects. Dose is 1-2 g orally.

Dichlorphenazone is a derivative of chloral and phenazone available in tablets. It is less irritant to GIT. The oral dose is 650 mg.

Paraldehyde

It is a cyclic ether, 4 to 8 ml orally is an effective hypnotic. Its action starts in 15 minutes and duration lasts for 4 to 8 hours. It can also be given by I.M. injection or per rectum. It is never given by I.V. inj. Although paraldehyde has wide margin of safety (no enzyme induction, mild addictive potential) but it is not commonly used as a hypnotic as it has several disadvantages including bad taste, offensive odour (10 to 30% is excreted through lungs) which lasts for about 24 hours. It is contraindicated in patients with liver diseases.

Meprobamate (Equanil, Miltown)

It is not superior to barbiturates as sedative-hypnotic and much less effective than benzodiazepines. Drug dependence develops.

Methaqualone

It possesses hypnotic, antitussive, spasmolytic and central muscle relaxant properties. It has similar actions as barbiturates and may be useful in patients who show idiosyncratic reactions to barbiturates. Dose is 150-300 mg orally at bed time. Its use is limited due to liability to develop severe drug dependence and marked hepatotoxicity. Mandrax is methaqualone plus diphenhydramine. It is a much abused drug.

Inorganic hypnotics: Bromides of sodium, potassium and ammonium can produce sedative-hypnotic effect as bromide ion produces non-specific depression of CNS. They are no more used since better drugs are available. Bromides are weak hypnotics and are required to be given for a few days to obtain full effect. They may also produce brominism characterized by gastric distress, dermatitis and neurological disturbances.

Treatment of Insomnia

Causes of insomnia include emotional stress (anxiety), physical complaints (cough, pain), and ingestion of substances possessing a centrally stimulating action (caffeinated beverages, sympathomimetics, theophylline, or antidepressants). Pharmacological intervention is not indicated unless causal therapy fails. Depending on the type of insomnia, sleep remedies with a short (oxazepam, t½–4-6 h) or an intermediate (nitrazepam) duration of action may be considered.

Use of a hypnotic drug should not be extended beyond 4 weeks, because tolerance may develop. The risk of a rebound decrease in sleep propensity after drug withdrawal is said to be avoidable by tapering off the dose over 2 to 3 weeks.

With any hypnotic, the risk of suicidal overdoses cannot be ignored. Compared with benzodiazepines, poisoning by barbiturates occurs more readily and is harder to treat. Thus, benzodiazepines have replaced barbiturates as hypnotics.

Hypnotics may exert "paradoxical" effects (restlessness, more excitement) and mental confusion, particularly in elderly individuals.

STUDY QUESTIONS

1. Define: narcotic, sedative, hypnotic, anxiolytic, tranquilizer, analgesic, anticonvulsant agent.
2. Explain how hypnotics produce adverse effect on normal sleep.
3. When are hypnotics needed?
4. What factors determine the choice of a hypnotic?
5. Why have benzodiazepines replaced the other hypnotics?
6. Classify barbiturates giving examples. Describe the pharmacokinetics and pharmacodynamics of barbiturates. What are their uses, contra-indications and drug interactions?
7. What are the different preparations, doses, and uses of benzodiazepines?
8. What are the advantages and disadvantages of chloral hydrate and paraldehyde as hypnotics?
9. Explain why bromides are no more used as hypnotics.

GUIDE TO FURTHER READING

Ballenger, J.C. Pharmacology of the pain disorders. J. Clin Psychiatry, 1986; 47 (Suppl): 27.

Balter, M.B. and Uhlenhuth, E.H. New epidemiologic findings about insomnia and its treatment. J. Clin. Psychiatry, 1992; 53 Suppl. 12:34.

Fleming, J.A.E. The difficult to treat insomniac patient. J. Psychosom Res, 1993; 37 Suppl. 1:45.

Lader, M. and File, S. The biological basis of benzodiazepine dependence. Psychol. Med., 1987; 17:539.

Mendelson, W.B. Pharmacologic alteration of the perception of being awake or asleep. Sleep, 1993; 16:641.

Pancrazio, J.J., Frazer, M.J. and Lynch, C. III. Barbiturate anesthetics depress the resting K$^+$ conductance of myocardium. J. Pharmacol. Expt. Ther., 1993; 265:358.

Prinz, P.N. et al. Geriatrics. Sleep disorders and aging. N. Engl J Med, 1990; 323:520.

Sloan, J.W., Wale, E. Effect of the chronic dose of diazepam on the intensity and characteristics of the precipitated abstinence syndrome in the dog. J Pharmacological Exp Therap, 1993; 265:1152.

Smith, M.C. and Riskin, B.J. The clinical use of barbiturates in neurological disorders. Drugs, 1991; 42:365.

Vogel, G. Clinical uses and advantages of low doses of benzodiazepine hypnotics. J. Clin. Psychiatry, 1992; 53 Suppli. 6:19.

Woods, J.H. et al. Abuse liability of benzodiazepines. Pharmacol Rev, 1987; 39:251.

OPIOID ANALGESICS AND ANTAGONISTS

There are endogenous opioid receptors, namely mu, kappa, delta, and sigma. The drugs which act on these receptors are shown below (agonists as well as antagonists). The mu and kappa receptors mediate actions of narcotic analgesic and sigma receptors are responsible for psychotomimetic effects. There are also fourth delta receptors which inhibit neurotransmission in the brain and periphery. Delta agonist have same actions as mu receptor agonists.

Tables 3.4, 3.5 and 3.6 show opiate receptors, functional effects of opioid receptors and selectivity of opioid drugs and peptides for receptor subtypes respectively.

ANALGESICS

These are drugs which selectively relieve pain by acting on the CNS and without altering consciousness.

Box 3.4. Opiate receptors	
Receptor	Action
Mu (μ)	Analgesia in supraspinal region, respiratory depression, euphoria, physical dependence
μ_1	Analgesia
μ_2	Respiratory depression
Kappa (κ)	Spinal analgesia, miosis, sedation
Sigma (σ)	Dysphoria, hallucinations, respiratory and vasomotor stimulation

Table 3.4. Opiate receptors—types and actions

Receptor	Agonist	Effect	Antagonist
Mu (μ) (supraspinal level)	Morphine	Euphoria, analgesia, respiratory depression, physical dependence	Nalorphine, pentazocine, naloxone
Kappa (κ) (spinal level)	Nalorphine (strong agonist) (morphine inactive)	Analgesia, sedation, miosis	Naloxone
Sigma (σ)	Pentazocine (strong agonist)	Dysphoria, hallucinogenic	Naloxone

Table 3.5. Functional effects associated with the main types of opioid receptor

Effect	μ	κ	σ
Analgesia			
Supraspinal	+++	−	−
Spinal	++	++	+
Peripheral	++	−	++
Respiratory depression	+++	++	−
Pupil constriction	++	−	+
Reduced GI motility	++	++	+
Euphoria	+++	−	−
Dysphoria	−	−	+++
Sedation	++	−	++
Physical dependence	+++	−	+

Table 3.6. Selectivity of opioid drugs and peptides for receptor subtype

Drug	μ	δ	κ
Endogenous peptides			
β-endorphin	+++	+++`	+++
Leu-enkephalin	+	+++	-*
Met-enkephalin	++	+++.	-*
Dynorphin	++	+	+++
Opiate drugs			
Pure agonists			
Morphine, codeine, oxymorphone, dextropropoxyphene	+++	+	+
Methadone	+++	-*	-*
Pethidine	++	+	+
Etorphine, bremazocine	+++	+++	+++
Fentanyl, sufentanil	+++	+	-*
Partial/mixed agonists			
Pentazocine, ketocyclazocine	+*	+	++
Nalbuphine	+*	+	(++)
Nalorphine	++*	-*	(++)
Buprenorphine	(+++)	-*	++*
Antagonists			
Naloxone	+++*	+*	++*
Naltrexone, diprenorphine	+++*	+*	+++*

Note : + symbols represent agonist activity; partial agonists in brackets; +* symbols denote antagonist activity; -* symbols represent weak or no activity.

Box 3.5. Narcotic analgesics

Agonists

Morphine-like
- Hydromorphone
- Oxymorphone
- Heroin

Codeine-like
- Dihydrocodeine
- Hydrocodeine
- Oxycodone

Mixed agonist/antagonist
- Pentazocine
- Butophanol
- Nalbuphine

Full antagonists
- Naloxone
- Naltrexone

Terminology

Opiates are drugs derived from opium and include morphine, codeine and semisynthetic congeners derived from them and from thebaine (another alkaloid from opium).

The term opioid is more inclusive. It applies to all agonists and antagonists with morphine-like activity, as well as to naturally occurring and synthetic opioid peptides.

Endorphin

It is a generic term that includes three families of endogenous opioid peptides viz. the enkephalins, the dynorphins and beta-endorphins.

Enkephalins : There are two most important enkephalins : methionine enkephalin and leuenkephalin.

They act on both mu and delta receptors. Enkephalins are present in pain areas in spinal cord, trigeminal nucleus, in limbic system and cortex. They are present peripherally at adrenal medulla, gastric and intestinal glands.

Dynorphins : Dynorphin A and B. They are more effective on kappa receptors but also effective on mu and delta receptors. Dynorphins have a distribution pattern similar to that of enkephalins. The enkephalins and dynorphins have short half-life which suggests neuromodulator or neurotransmitter

function. It seems that they regulate pain responsiveness (at spinal and supraspinal levels).

Beta-endorphins : They possess more potent analgesic activity compared to morphine. It is mainly localised in the hypothalamus and pituitary. It has long half-life. It has been suggested that it has a neurohormone function. It decreases FSH, LH, and enhances the release of growth hormone and prolactin.

The term narcotic means stupor (sleep producing) and it is associated with the strong opiate analogues. Now this term is used increasingly in a legal context to refer to abused substances.

Classification

- Narcotic analgesics/opiates/morphine-like.
- Non-narcotic/non-opioid/antipyretic, anti-inflammatory analgesics/aspirin-like.

OPIOID ANALGESICS

A. *Natural*

   Opium alkaloids
   - Phenanthrene derivatives: morphine (10%), thebaine (0.2%) and codeine (0.5%).
   - Benzylisoquinoline derivatives: papaverine (1%), noscapine (6%).

B. *Semisynthetic (opiates)*
   - Morphine analogues: oxymorphone, ethylmorphine, diacetylmorphine.
   - Codeine analogues: dextromethorphan, dihydrocodeine, dihydromorphinone, methyldihydromorphinone.

C. *Synthetic (opioids)*
   - Pethidine (Meperidine)
   - Pethidine analogues: alphaprodine, fentanyl, diphenoxylate.
   - Methadone and Methadone analogues: dextropropoxyphene.
   - Opioids with mixed action: Pentazocine, Buprenophine, Nalbuphine, Butorphanol.

MORPHINE AND RELATED OPIOID AGONISTS

Morphine

It is the main alkaloid present (10%) in opium. Opium is air dried dark brown resinous material (exudate)

Drug	Chemical radical and positions				Other changes	Receptor action
	3	6	17	14		
Morphine	–OH	–OH	–CH$_3$	–H		Agonist
Codeine	–OCH$_3$	–OH	–CH$_3$	–H		Agonist
Heroin	–OCOCH$_3$	–OCOCH$_3$	–CH$_3$	–H		Agonist
Levorphanol	–OH	–H	–CH$_3$	–OH	Lacks –O– at C4-C5 single bond between C7-C8	Agonist
Nalorphine	–OH	–OH	–CH$_2$CH=CH$_2$	–H		Partial agonist
Naloxone	–OH	=O	–CH$_2$CH=CH$_2$	–OH	Single bond instead of double bond between C7-C8	Antagonist
Naltrexone	–OH	=O	–CH$_2$–◁	–OH	Single bond instead of double bond between C7-C8	

obtained by incising the unripe poppy capsule of the plant papaver somniferum.

Chemical aspects

Morphine is a phenanthrene derivative, with two planar rings (A & B) and two aliphatic ring structures (C & D) which occupy a plane roughly at right angles to the planar rings.

Structure of morphine

The substitution at one or both of the hydroxyl groups (the phenolic OH at positions 3 and the alcoholic OH at position 6), and by substitution at the nitrogen atom at position 17, variants of the morphine molecule have been produced.

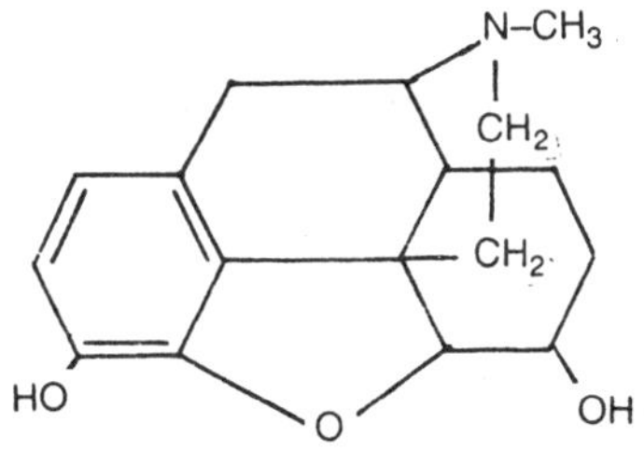

Codeine is methylmorphine, the methyl substitution being on the phenolic hydroxy group.

In thebaine both hydroxyl groups are methylated. This drug has little analgesic activity.

Heroin or diacetylmorphine is made by acetylation (OCOCH$_3$) at 3 and 6 positions of morphine.

Some examples are shown above which indicate the influence of chemical radical and positions on the receptor action.

Pharmacological effects

CNS: Analgesia is produced by

- Increasing the threshold to pain perception (effect on thalamus).
- Altering the emotional or psychological reaction to pain (cortical effect).
- Sleep is due to cortical depression. Sleep increases threshold to pain perception.

Morphine and related opioids produce there major effects on the CNS and bowel through mu receptors. Morphine is relatively selective for mu receptors, however, in higher doses it can interact with others.

When therapeutic doses are given to patients suffering with pain, the morphine-like drugs produce analgesia, drowsiness, changes in mood and mental clouding, and some patients experience euphoria. But if the same doses are administered to normal pain-free persons, nausea, vomiting, drowsiness, apathy and lessened physical activity may be produced.

The mechanism for these effect is not very clear.

Effects on medullary centres: some are stimulated and some depressed.

Stimulated	Depressed
Chemoreceptor trigger zone (CTZ)	Respiratory eentre
Vomiting centre	Vasomotor centre
Vagal centre	Cough centre
Oculomotor centre	Temperature regulating centre

Effect on pupillary size : Miosis is produced due to excitatory action on the oculomotor centre. High doses produced pin-point pupils. However, mydriasis occurs when asphyxia intervenes.

Therapeutic doses of morphine increase accommodative power and lower intraocular pressure in normal as well as in patients suffering with glaucoma.

Respiration : It is depressed even with doses too small to affect consciousness, and increases progressively when the dose is increased. Death occurs due to respiratory arrest.

Cough: It is suppressed in part by a direct effect on cough centre in the medulla. There is no relationship between depression on respiration and depression of coughing. Some drugs that suppress cough do not depress respiration.

Nauseant and emetic effect: Opioids produce these effects due to their direct stimulating effect on the CTZ. The vestibular component is also operative because nausea and vomiting occur more frequently in ambulatory patients and it is uncommon in recumbent patients.

Effects on the hypothalamus: The hypothalamus-heat-regulatory mechanisms are affected such that body temperature falls slightly with opioids. However, high doses taken for long period may increase body temperature.

Effect on neuroendocrine function: Morphine releases ADH (antidiuretic hormone).

Morphine decreases circulating concentrations of luteinizing hormone (LH) and follicle-stimulating hormone (FSH) and beta-endorphin.

Due to decreased concentrations of pituitary trophic hormones, the levels of testosterone and cortisol in plasma is reduced.

Tolerance and physical dependence: Tolerance develops after about a weak if 10-15 mg is injected twice by s.c. or i.m. injection. Tolerance develops to analgesia and respiratory depression, but not to GI effects and miosis. Psychic and physical dependence develops and abstinence syndrome is marked.

Gastrointestinal tract: Morphine produces spasmogenic effect, decreases biliary, pancreatic, and intestinal secretions, interferes with peristaltic movements. Due to non-propulsive spasm, morphine has constipative effect. This is due to peripheral action.

On other smooth muscles: The smooth muscles of ureter, bladder, biliary tract and bronchial muscle are contracted.

Cardiovascular system: Therapeutic doses of morphine-like opioids have no significant effect on blood pressure, heart rate and rhythm, but such doses produce peripheral vasodilation, partly due to central action and partly due to histamine release and dilatation of cutaneous blood vessels. Therefore, when supine patients assume the head up position orthostatic hypotension and fainting may occur.

Pharmacokinetics

Absorption of morphine from GIT is erratic and unsatisfactory, hence it is not given orally. The drug is readily absorbed after s.c./i.m. injection, onset of action is after 10-20 minutes and duration of action is about 4 hours. After absorption it is distributed in the body, can also cross placenta. Morphine is about 90% conjugated with glucuronic acid in the liver. Morphine-6-glucuronide is a major metabolite of morphine which has similar action as those of morphine. It is excreted in conjugated form and some in free form in urine. About 10% is excreted in faeces.

Preparations

Morphine sulphate, morphine hydrochloride inj.
Dose: 10-20 mg
Route: S.C. or I.M. inj., even I.V.

Uses

- To relieve severe life threatening excruciating visceral pain.
- Dyspnoea in left ventricular failure.
- Preanaesthetic medicament.

Contraindications

- Head injury
- Bronchial asthma
- Undiagnosed abdominal pain
- Presence of respiratory, hepatic or renal failure

- Patients with compromised respiratory function, such as those with emphysema.

In patients with chronic cor pulmonale, death has occurred even with therapeutic doses of morphine.

In head injury cases, the possibility of exaggerated depression of respiration and increased intracranial pressure must be considered. Opioids also produce miosis, vomiting, and mental clouding. These important signs for indicating the prognosis in head injury cases will be interfered. Hence, it is not advisable to use opioids in head injury cases.

Opioids can precipitate attacks of asthma in anaesthetized patients. During asthmatic attack, morphine and related drugs should be avoided, since they depress cough reflex and respiration and dry secretion.

Some opioids release histamine which will produce additional bronchoconstriction.

Patients with reduced blood volume are more susceptible to the hypotensive effects of morphine and related drugs.

In patients with hypotension (from any cause) the use of opioids should be avoided.

Patients with biliary colic may experience exacerbation rather than relief of pain, since the sphincter of Oddi constricts and the pressure in the common bile duct may rise more than tenfold.

Morphine poisoning

In acute poisoning there is pinpoint pupil and respiration is very slow (sometimes only 2 to 4 breaths per minute). The triad of coma, pinpoint pupil and depressed respiration strongly suggests opioid poisoning. The treatment includes gastric lavage with 1: 1000 KMnO$_4$ and 5% CO$_2$ inhalation.

Naloxone is a selective competitive antagonist. Naloxone hydrochloride 0.4 mg/ml is given by I.V. injection and the dose is repeated, if needed. It can produce dramatic reversal of the severe respiratory depression.

Chronic poisoning. Tolerance and drug dependence develops.

Withdrawal leads to abstinence syndrome (described elsewhere in this Chapter).

Codeine

It is methyl morphine. It is less effective than morphine as analgesic (1/4-1/6); less depressant (1/10) to respiratory centre. It seldom produces nausea and vomiting and drug dependence develops rarely.

Codeine phosphate 10-60 mg orally is given for the treatment of dry unproductive cough. It is also used as antidiarrhoeal agent.

Noscapine (Narcotine)

It is present in opium (about 6%). Its antitussive activity is similar to codeine. It dose not possess analgesic, sedative, constipative and respiratory depressant action. It does not have abuse liability.

Papaverine

It is present in opium (1%). It does not have any action on CNS. It is a good smooth muscle relaxant and vasodilator in animal studies but its action in humans is not satisfactory.

Apomorphine

It is a semisynthetic preparation. It has strong emetic action in dose of 0.1 mg/kg s.c. or i.m. injection. Oral route is not dependable. It produces emesis by acting on the chemoreceptor trigger zone. Its action can be antagonized by naloxone. It is not analgesic, drug dependence is rare as euphoria produced by it is much less.

Levorphanol (Levo-Dromoran)

It is opioid agonist of the morphinan series. The d-isomer is relatively devoid of analgesic action. The nonanalgesic isomer dextrophan has good antitussive activity.

The adult dose (2 mg) subcutaneously produces analgesia which lasts longer (6 hours) than morphine due to lipid solubility and cumulation of drug in body fat. It may produce marked sedation. It causes less nausea and vomiting than morphine.

Levorphanol acts mainly on the mu-receptor, it also has κ_3 action at higher doses, hence there is lack of complete cross-tolerance between morphine and this drug.

Oxymorphone

One mg is equianalgesic with 10 mg of s.c. morphine. It is not available as oral preparation. It produces at least equal or even more side effects.

Hydromorphone (Dilaudid)

1.5 mg i.m. injection is equivalent to 10 mg i.m. morphine. It is somewhat shorter acting and less constipating than morphine. It has better oral absorption but produces more respiratory depression.

Heroin

It is diacetylmorphine. It is rapidly hydrolyzed to 6-monoacetylmorphine 6-MAM, which in turn is hydrolyzed to morphine. Both heroin and 6-MAM being more lipid soluble than morphine enter the brain more readily. It is less sedative and also produces less nausea, vomiting and constipation. It is potent analgesic. But it produces marked euphoria, has high abuse potential. It is a banned drug.

Selection of an analgesic

Morphine is given subcutaneously or intramuscularly, at a dose of 10 mg/70 kg body weight. It relieves pain in 70% of patients. Morphine is available orally in standard tablets and controlled release preparations. However, due to first-pass effect, it is 2 to 6-fold less potent orally than parenterally.

Orally, codeine at 30 mg is equianalgesic to 325 to 600 mg of aspirin.

In pain due to biliary spasm, meperidine may be more effective than an equianalgesic dose of morphine.

For the management of pains of terminal illness and cancer pains opioid analgesics are recommended although tolerance and physical dependence may develop.

Adverse effects and precautions

Morphine and other opioids can produce several side effects including nausea, vomiting, dizziness, respiratory depression, pruritus, dysphoria, constipation, urinary retention and hypotension. Increased sensitivity to pain after the analgesic effect wears off, may occur in some patients.

Allergic phenomena also occur with opioid analgesics although not common.

Drug interaction

Opioids exaggerate the depressant effects of certain drugs such as phenothiazines, MAOIs, and tricyclic antidepressant.

Pethidine (meperidine, demerol)

It was discovered accidentally when new atropine-like drugs were being sought. It is a synthetic narcotic analgesic. Dose is 75-100 mg i.m. or s.c. injection. It differs from morphine in a number of ways:

- 1/10 as potent as morphine but more effective than codeine as analgesic.
- Equianalgesic doses depress respiration to a similar extent.
- Shorter duration of action (2-4 hours).
- Less constipating.
- Pupils are usually constricted, sometime produces mydriasis.
- Atropine like effect but undependable.
- Lacks antitussive action.
- Less euphoria but drug dependence develops.

In general, 75-100 mg of meperidine hydrochloride given parenterally is equianalgesic to 10 mg of morphine. In equianalgesic doses, it produces as much sedation, respiratory depression, and euphoria as does morphine.

It is less than one-half as effective orally as when given parenterally. It causes miosis like other opioids, increases the sensitivity of the labyrinthine apparatus and effects on secretion of pituitary hormones are similar to those of morphine.

The effects on cardiovascular system generally resemble those of morphine.

The effects of meperidine on smooth muscles are qualitatively similar to those observed with other opioids but less intense relative to its analgesic action. But it is less constipating than morphine.

Pharmacokinetics

Meperidine is absorbed by all routes of administration, however, site of absorption may be erratic after IM injection.

About 50% of orally administered dose escapes first-pass effect.

About 60% of the drug is protein bound.

It is hydrolyzed to meperidinic acid. It is also N-demethylated to normeperidine. Only a small amount is excreted unchanged in urine.

Adverse effects

The pattern of adverse effects is similar to that of morphine, except that constipation and urinary retention are less common.

In patients who are tolerant to meperidine, large doses repeated at short interval produce mydriasis, tremors, muscle twitches, and convulsions. These excitatory symptoms are due to accumulation of normeperidine which has a half-life of about 20 hours (half-life of meperidine is 3 hours). In this respect it differs from morphine.

Abrupt withdrawal differs from that of morphine, autonomic effects are fewer, symptoms develop more rapidly and are of shorter duration.

MEPERIDINE CONGENERS

Diphenoxylate

It is used in diarrhoea (dose 20 mg in divided doses). It is available only in combination with atropine sulphate (Lamotil, others). At high doses (40-60 mg) it shows opioid activity including morphine-like physical dependence after repeated administration.

Loperamide

For the treatment of chronic diarrhoea, it is as effective as diphenoxylate. The doses is 4 to 8 mg/ per day. The daily dose should not exceed 16 mg.

Fentanyl

It is a synthetic opioid which is about 80 times as potent as morphine as an analgesic. Its respiratory-depressant effect is of shorter duration than meperidine. The analgesic and euphoric effects are intensified and prolonged by droperidol (neuroleptic agent). Fentanyl is combined with droperidol for use as an i.v. anaesthetic. It is not favoured for the treatment of pain but used as an adjunct to anaesthesia.

Transdermal patches are now available. The congeners of fentanyl such as sufentanil citrate and alfentanil hydrochloride are also available.

Alphaprodine

It is a piperidine derivative, resembles meperidine. Its action is prompt but duration is short.

Anileridine

It is slightly more potent than meperidine. It is related to pethidine with comparable duration of effect i.e. 2-4 hours. Orally it has a more prolonged action.

Methadone

The pharmacological properties are qualitatively similar to those of morphine. It is a synthetic narcotic analgesic having actions almost similar to those of morphine. However, it differs from morphine in a number of ways.

- Longer half-life.
- Longer duration of action.
- Cumulation on repeated administration.
- Same or little more potent and effective orally.
- Less emetic and less constipating.
- Respiratory depression is more.
- Tolerance and drug dependence occurs, abstinence syndrome is less severe but more prolonged.

METHADONE CONGENER

Propoxyphene

d-propoxyphene produces analgesic action. It is recommended for mild to moderate pain at 65 mg of hydrochloride or 100 mg of the napsylate. Levopropoxyphene has some antitussive effect (less than codeine).

Dextropropoxyphene produces effects on the CNS that are similar to those with morphine-like opioids.

Propoxyphene is half to two-thirds as potent as codeine given orally; 90-120 mg propoxyphene hydrochloride given orally produces analgesic effects similar to that of 60 mg of codeine and as much analgesia as 600 mg of aspirin.

It is N-demethylated resulting in norpropoxyphene (half-life 30 hours).

Adverse effects

- It is one-third as potent as orally administered codeine in depressing respiration.
- Larger doses may produce convulsions in addition to respiratory depression. Cardiotoxicity, pulmonary oedema, confusion, delusion and hallucination have been reported. Its addiction liability is not marked.

Phenazocine hydrobromide

It is a synthetic analgesic with similar actions as morphine. However, its action is more rapid and of longer duration than morphine. It can be administered orally (5 mg tablets) sublingually, and also by i.m. and i.v. routes. It produces less respiratory depression than equianalgesic doses of morphine. It can produce slight hypertension and tachycardia rather than hypotension and bradycardia observed after morphine. It can be given during labor to provide relief from pain without adverse effects.

The main problems of use of phenazocine are:

- Due to sedative effect, the ambulatory patients should not drive or operate machines.
- Unpleasant and disturbing hallucinations.
- It should not be given in the presence of hepatic and renal impairment.

OPIOIDS WITH MIXED ACTIONS (MIXED AGONIST/ANTAGONIST AND PARTIAL AGONIST)

Pentazocine

It has both agonistic actions and weak opioid antagonistic actions. The pattern of effects on the CNS including analgesia, sedation, and respiratory depression are similar to that of morphine-like opioid. Higher doses (60-90 mg) produce dysphoric and psychotomimetic activity similar to those of nalorphine.

The analgesic activity is shown by l-isomer, the d isomer little activity for opioid receptors.

Low doses such as 20 mg administered parenterally depress respiration as much as 10 mg of morphine.

Pentazocine is well absorbed from the GIT and from s.c. and i.m. sites. It undergoes first-pass effect extensively (about 80%).

It passes through the placental barrier but to a lesser extent than does meperidine.

The adverse effects include lightheadedness, sweating, sedation, dizziness, anxiety, nightmares, hallucinations occur with parenteral doses above 60 mg. Higher doses produce marked respiratory depression associated with increased blood pressure and tachycardia.

Pentazocine produces drug dependence. However, the risk of drug dependence is lower than that associated with the use of morphine-like drugs.

The abuse pattern is less likely to develop with oral administration; thus this route should be employed whenever possible.

Nalbuphine

It is an agonist/antagonist opioid, and its effects qualitatively resemble those of pentazocine. However, it is more potent antagonist and therefore less likely to produce dysphoric side effects unlike pentazocine.

A dose of 10 mg (i.m.) nalbuphine is equianalgesic to 10 mg of morphine. Its respiratory depressant effect is also similar to morphine; however, it exhibits a ceiling effect as increased doses beyond 30 mg do not produce further respiratory depression.

Butorphanol

A parenteral dose of 2 to 3 mg has similar effect as analgesic and respiratory depressant equal to that produced by 10 mg of morphine.

Its major side effects include nausea, weakness, drowsiness and sweating. Psychotomimetic effects may occur but incidence is less than with pentazocine. This drug is more beneficial in the relief of acute rather than chronic pain. The usual dose is 1 mg and 4 mg of the tartrate given intramuscularly or 0.5 to 2 mg i.v. A nasal formulation is also available.

Buprenorphine

It is a derivative from thebaine, 25 to 50 times more potent and longer acting than morphine. The usual dose is 0.3 mg i.m. or i.v. for analgesia, sublingual dose is 0.4 to 0.8 mg.

Tramadol

It does not depress respiration or produce other side

effects seen with other opioid analgesics in therapeutic dose of 1 mg/kg. It also has antitussive action.

It is indicated in severe acute and chronic pain.

Tramadol does not produce tolerance or drug dependence. However, nausea, vomiting, stupor, or sweating have been reported as side effects.

OPIOID ANTAGONISTS

Nalorphine

In low doses it is a competitive antagonist, in higher doses it is analgesic. This reflects an antagonist action on mu receptors, along with a partial agonist action on k (kappa) and δ opioid receptors.

Nalorphine causes dysphoria, physical dependence can be produced by it and it can also precipitate a withdrawal syndrome in morphine addicts.

Nalorphine was the first morphine antagonist to be introduced as an effective antidote in acute morphine poisoning. Now it has been superseded by other drug such as naloxone because nalorphine in large doses itself depresses respiration.

Main uses of nalorphine:
- Along with morphine in an addict - withdrawal of mixture produces milder withdrawal syndrome.
- Diagnosis of drug dependence to morphine
- Acute intoxication of morphine or related drugs (naloxone is better).

Nalorphine is not used as an analgesic.

Naloxone

It is a true competitive antagonist at the opioid receptors. Its action is highest at mu receptors and to a great extent equally effective on other receptor subtypes.

The half-life is one hour. The duration of action is 1-4 hours.

Although it is readily absorbed from GIT but undergoes almost complete first-pass hepatic metabolism. Hence, it is parenterally administered.

Naloxone is used in the treatment of acute morphine poisoning as well as to precipitate withdrawal symptoms in dependent individuals who may be in coma and past history is not available.

For treating poisoning with opioids the dose is 0.4 to 0.8 mg i.v. repeated every 2-3 minutes for 2-3 doses, if needed.

For diagnosing opioid overdosage, the usual dose is 0.2-0.4 mg i.v.

Naltrexone

It is relatively a pure antagonist effective on oral administration (50 mg tablet). The half-life is 3 hours.

Therapeutic uses of opioid antagonists

- In opioid induced toxicity
- To diagnose physical dependence on opioids (but not to precipitate severe withdrawal syndrome)
- In the treatment of compulsive opioid users
- To decrease neonatal respiratory depression secondary to maternal opioid administration
- Naloxone is used in septic shock where opioid peptides are released by stress and may produces hypotension.

NON-OPIOID ANALGESICS (FOR OPIOID ADDICTS)

Benzoxazocine derivative

Nefopam: It is a nonopioid pain reliever. It does not inhibit synthesis of prostaglandins. It is an analgesic but poor antiinflammatory.

Nefopam has been found useful in the treatment of traumatic and postoperative pain and musculoskeletal pain. It is effective for relief of moderate pain, particularly useful in the treatment of pain in opioid addicts.

Its action is prompt and efficacy is similar to morphine.

Adverse effects include dryness in mouth, blurred vision and urinary retention due to its anticholinergic action. It produces nervousness, tachycardia as side effects due to sympathomimetic action. There are no adverse effects of opioids such as respiratory depression, dependence liability and constipation.

Dose: 30-60 mg orally three times a day or 20 mg I.M. 6 hourly/day.

STUDY QUESTIONS

1. Classify analgesics.
2. What are the main differences between narcotic and non-narcotic analgesics?
3. Describe the pharmacological effects, mode of action, preparations, doses, uses, contra-indications of morphine.
4. What are the differences between morphine and pethidine?
5. How is acute morphine poisoning treated?
6. Describe the characteristics of dependence on morphine and the withdrawal syndrome.
7. Describe the differences between morphine and codeine.
8. Name opioid antagonists. How do they act?
9. Describe the major classes of opioids receptors.
10. What are the various effects produced by opioid-receptor activation?
11. Discuss naloxone, nalorphine and naltrexone as narcotic antagonists.
12. Write notes on "brain's own opioids".

GUIDE TO FURTHER READING

Edwards, D.J. et al. Clinical pharmacokinetics of pethidine: 1982. Clin. Pharmacokinet., 1982; 7:421.

Frances, B et al. Further evidence that morphine-6D-glucuronide is a more potent opioid agonist than morphine. J Pharmacol Exp Therap, 1992; 262:25.

Kaiko, R.F. Age and morphine analgesia in cancer patients with postoperative pain. Clin. Pharmacol. Ther., 1980; 28:823.

Knapp, R.J. et al. Identification of a human delta opioid receptor: Cloning and expression. Life Sci., 1994; 54:463.

Martin, W.R. Pharmacology of opioids. Pharmacol Rev., 1983; 35:283.

Millan, M.J. k-opioid receptors and analgesia. Trends Pharmacol Sci 1990; 11:70.

Owen, J.A. et al. Age-related morphine kinetics. Pharmacol Ther., 1983; 34:364.

Pick, C.G. and Roques, B. et al. Supraspinal mu receptors mediate spinal/supraspinal morphine synergy. Eur. J. Pharmacol., 1992a; 220:275.

Pick, C.G. and Paul, D. et al. Potentiation of opioid analgesia by the antidepressant nefazodone. Eur. J. Pharmacol., 1992b; 211:375.

Portenoy, R.K. Chronic opioid therapy in nonmalignant pain. J. Pain Symptom Managements, 1990; 5:546.

Portenoy, R.K. et al. Transdermal fentanyl for cancer pain. Anesthesiology, 1993; 78:36.

Rossi, G., Pasternak, G.W. and Bodnar, R.J. Synergistic brain stem interactions for morphine analgesia. Brain Res., 1993; 624:171.

Weinberg, D.S. et al. Sublingual absorption of selected opioid analgesics. Clin. Pharmacol Ther., 1988; 44:335.

NON-NARCOTIC ANALGESICS

Non-narcotic analgesics (analgesic-antipyretics)

These drugs produce relief of pain and lower elevated body temperature. As these drugs also produce anti-inflammatory effect, so they are known as non-steroidal anti-inflammatory drugs (NSAIDs).

Properties of NSAIDs

Mildly analgesic, antipyretic and anti-inflammatory; act on subcortical sites such as thalamus and hypothalamus; they do not have affinity for morphine receptors; tolerance and drug dependence do not develop to these drugs.

Differences between narcotic and non-narcotic analgesics are given in Table 3.7.

Table 3.7. Differences between narcotic and non-narcotic analgesics

Narcotic analgesics	Non-narcotic analgesics
• Produce drug dependence	Do not produce drug dependence
• Produce CNS depression	No CNS depression
• Relieve deep seated pain	Relieve pain from integument
• No antipyretic or anti-inflammatory action	Have antipyretic and anti-inflammatory action
• No uricosuric action	Uricosuric action is present
• Central mechanism of action	Inhibit prostaglandins synthesis
• Used mainly as analgesic	Used as analgesic and in other inflammatory conditions

Classification

• Salicylic acid derivatives: Acetylsalicylic acid (aspirin), sodium salicylate, methyl salicylate.

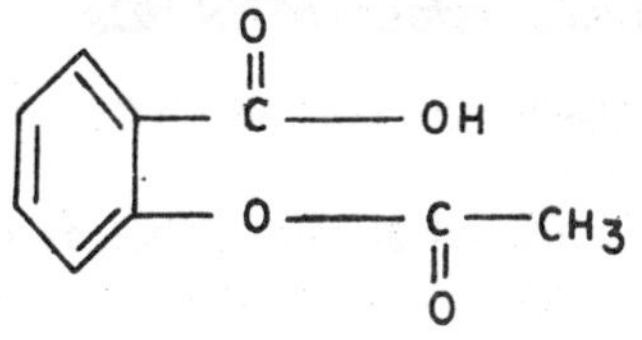

Structure of aspirin

- Para-aminophenol: Paracetamol.

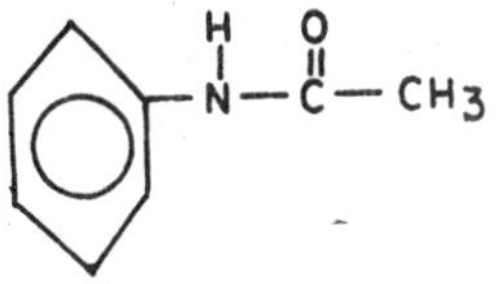

Structure of paracetamol

- Pyrazolone derivatives: Phenylbutazone, oxyphenbutazone.
- Indole derivatives: Indomethacin, sulindac.
- Propionic acid derivatives: Ibuprofen, fenoprofen, ketoprofen, naproxen, flurbiprofen.

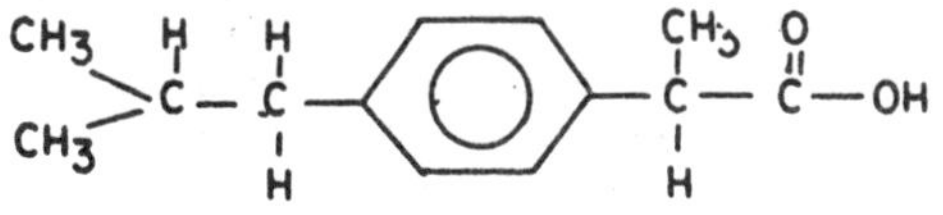

Structure of ibuprofen

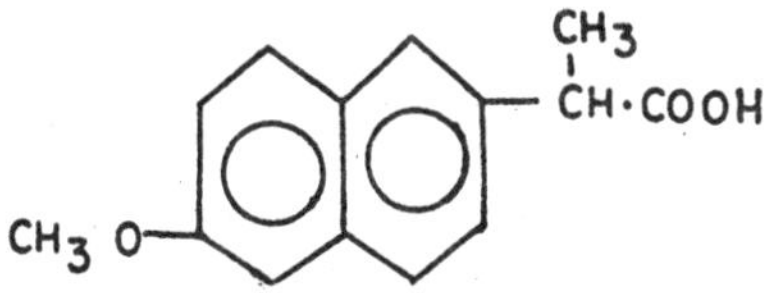

Structure of naproxen

- Fenamates (anthranilic acid derivatives): Mefenamic acid
- Arylacetic acid derivatives: Diclofenac, fenclofenac, tolmetin
- Oxicams: Piroxicam, Tenoxicam, Meloxicam
- Pyrrolo-pyrrole derivative: Ketorolac
- Alkanone: Nabumetone
- Sulfphonanilide derivative: Nimesulide

The nonsteroidal anti-inflammatory drugs (NSAIDs) can be classified according to their efficacy as antiinflammatory and analgesic drugs:

- Potent antiinflammatory and good analgesic:
  Salicylates: Aspirin, sodium salicylate, diflunisal
- Potent antiinflammatory and poor analgesic
  Pyrazolone: Oxyphenbutazone
  Indole derivatives: Indomethacin, sulindac, etodolac
- Moderate antiinflammatory and moderate analgesic:
  Propionic acid derivatives: Ibuprofen, fenoprofen, ketoprofen, fenbufen, flurbiprofen, naproxen
  Anthranilic acid derivatives: Mefenamic acid, flufenemic acid
  Arylacetic acid derivatives: Diclofenac, tolmetin, nabumetone
  Oxicam derivatives: Piroxicam, tenoxicam, meloxicam
  Pyrrolo-pyrrole derivative: Ketorolac
- Poor antiinflammatory and good analgesic:
  Para-aminophenol derivative: Paracetamol
  Pyrazolone derivative: Metamizole
  Benzoxazocine derivative: Nefopam

NSAIDs can also be classified according to their half-life:
Piroxicam: > 50 hours
Naproxen 14 $\pm$ 1 hours
Diflunisal 11 $\pm$ 2 hours
Sulindac: 10-30 hours
Aspirin, diclofenac, indomethacin, flurbiprofen: < 5 hours

Mechanism of action of NSAIDs

They inhibit the biosynthesis and release of prostaglandins, via the inhibition of cyclooxygenase pathways:
A. (i) • Irreversible inactivation, e.g., acetylation by aspirin competitive inhibition e.g., propionic acid NSAIDs (ibuprofen etc.) and piroxicam.
  • Reversible, no-competitive inhibition, e.g., paracetamol.
  (ii) Indomethacin inhibition phosphodiesterase thus increases c-AMP concentration which stabilize lysosomal membrane in polymorphs and prevents release of enzymes important in inflammatory response.
  (iii) Inhibition of activation of T lymphocytes which release lymphokines. Aspirin inhibits

the release of both prostaglandins and lymphokines.

(iv) Diclofenac and indomethacin inhibit lipoxygenase pathway which generates leukotrienes from leukocytes and synovial cells.

B. NSAIDs have oxygen radical scavenging effects (decrease production of free radicals and superoxides)

C. Some NSAIDs may interfere with the binding of mediators (such as chemotactic peptides derived from bacteria) to their receptors on inflammatory cells.

Pharmacological actions of NSAIDs

1. Antiinflammatory action: Decrease in vasodilator prostaglandins PGE_2, PGI_2 means less vasodilation and thus less oedema (antiinflammatory activity). Not all NSAIDs have the same degree of antiinflammatory activity; aspirin and indomethacin have strong antiinflammatory action; naproxen is moderately antiinflammatory while paracetamol is weak antiinflammatory

2. Analgesic effect: Decreased prostaglandins synthesis means less sensitization of nociceptive nerve endings to inflammatory mediators - bradykinin and 5-HT.

3. Antipyretic effect: Decrease in the mediator PGE_2 (generated in response to inflammatory interleukin-1)

4. Other actions: Aspirin inhibits aggregation of platelets. Sulindac inhibits aldose reductase and reduces conversion of glucose to sorbitol, used for cataract and peripheral neuropathy in diabetes.

Therapeutic uses

These drugs relieve pain within minutes of administration and lasts for a few hours. They are usually safe, do not lead to tolerance or drug dependence. They are commonly used for musculoskeletal pain, headache, toothache and other minor pains. On giving them regularly they have additional effect as anti-inflammatory and thus they not only act as analgesic but also reduce swelling, tenderness and stiffness.

General Adverse effects of NSAIDs

*   GIT: Nausea, vomiting, dyspepsia. Indigestion is very common.
*   Blood: Increased bleeding time by preventing thromboxane A formation, reduction in prothrombin level.
*   Haematemesis may occur with indomethacin.
*   Renal: Precipitation of acute renal failure in cirrhosis.
*   Nephropathy with analgesic mixture.
*   Allergy: Skin rashes, asthma, thrombocytopenia, particularly with fenclofenac.
*   Haemolysis in patients with G-6PD deficiency.
*   Salicylism (due to prolonged administration of salicylates)
*   Gastric damage in chronic users, with risk of haemorrhage, due to abrogation of the protective effect of PGE_2 on gastric mucosa e.g. with aspirin.
*   Reversible renal insufficiency due to lack of compensatory PGE_2 mediated vasodilatation.
*   Less commonly liver disorders, bone marrow depression. Aplastic anaemia has been reported due to phenylbutazone and oxyphenbutazone.

SALICYLATES

Salicylic acid (local application) is irritant to skin and mucous membranes, has keratolytic effect and some antifungal action.

Methyl salicylate is counterirritant as liniment; when applied to painful joints it produces comfort, warmth and relieves pain.

Aspirin (acetyl salicylic acid) is one of the oldest drugs still commonly used as analgesic, antipyretic, anti-rheumatic, uricosuric and anti-inflammatory. It is preferred to sodium salicylate.

Aspirin acts in following ways:
*   Reduces prostaglandin production.
*   Antibradykinin action.
*   Pain threshold is increased (site thalamus).
*   Antipyretic (site hypothalamus) through peripheral vasodilation.
*   Reduces platelet aggregation in low doses by preferentially blocking TXA_2 generation.
*   Uricosuric effect by inhibition of tubular secretion and reabsorption of uric acid.

Pharmacokinetics

Aspirin is rapidly absorbed from stomach and upper small intestine as such and is hydrolyzed to acetic acid and salicylate by esterases in tissues and blood. The peak plasma level reaches within 1-2 hours. The distribution is wide in the body. Liver plays an important role in the biotransformation. It is conjugated with glucuronic acid and with glycine, small portion is oxidized to gentisic acid. Salicylates are excreted in conjugated form, as gentisic acid and as free salicylates. The water-soluble conjugates are rapidly cleared by kidneys.

Aspirin soluble tablets (300 mg aspirin with citric acid and calcium carbonate) form calcium acetyl salicylate in water.

Aspirin should be avoided in patients using anticoagulants as it can cause hypoprothrombopenia.

Aspirin has been tested for the prevention of cystoid macular oedema following cataract extraction. Due to aspirin's long history of use, easy availability, low cost, and long history of safety, it remains the initial drug of choice for treating the majority of articular and musculoskeletal disorders, unless some contraindication exists or another NSAID offers advantage.

Therapeutic uses

Aspirin is widely used for its analgesic and anti-inflammatory effects. The other indications are for antipyresis, inhibition of platelet aggregation hence used as prophylactic agent to decrease the incidence of transient ischaemic attacks and unstable angina and may also be effective in reducing the incidence of thrombosis in coronary artery bypass grafts.

As analgesic (600 mg 4-6 hourly, if needed), antipyretic (600 mg non-specific, no effect on normal body temperature); anti-rheumatic (high doses 5-8 g/d in acute rheumatic fever), rheumatoid arthritis (600 mg 4 hourly), chronic gout (uricosuric effect, 2g or less/d increases serum uric acid level, dose more than 4g/d decreases urate levels).

Prevention of myocardial infarction (by preventing platelet aggregation) in small doses of aspirin.

Certain studies suggest that aspirin may reduce cataract formation but some other studies contradict it. Some epidemiologic studies suggest that low dosage of aspirin on long-term use is associated with a lower incidence of colon cancer.

Contraindications: Peptic ulcer, gastritis, hepatic and renal impairment, history of allergy to salicylates.

Adverse effects

Salicylism characterized by headache, nausea, vomiting, confusion, dizziness, tinnitus, deafness. Acid-base balance is disturbed. High plasma salicylate levels induce respiratory alkalosis due to increased ventilation, later acidosis due to accumulation of salicylic acid derivatives and depression of respiratory centre.

- GI upsets, gastric haemorrhage.
- Allergic manifestations.

Side effects due to NSAIDs include gastro-intestinal ulceration, blockade of platelet aggregation (inhibition of thromboxane synthesis), inhibition of uterine motility (prolongation of gestation), inhibition of prostaglandin-mediated renal function and hypersensitivity reactions.

Effects of plasma salicylate levels

The approximate relationships of plasma sali-cylate levels and the effects produced are as following:

- Upto 10 mg/ml produces analgesic, antipyretic and antiplatelet effects. The complications may include gastric intolerance, bleeding and hypersensitivity reactions.
- 10 to 50 mg/ml produce anti-inflammatory and uricosuric effects. Some patients may get tinnitus.
- 50 to 80 mg/ml, 80 to 110 mg/ml, 110 to 180 mg/ml produce mild, moderate and severe intoxication respectively.

The complication in mild intoxication is central hyperventilation, in case of moderate intoxication patient may have fever, dehydration and metabolic acidosis. The complications in severe intoxication are vasomotor collapse, coma and hypoprothrombinemia.

The blood level more than 160 mg/ml can prove lethal due to renal and respiratory failure.

Drug interactions

Aspirin displaces a number of drugs from protein

binding sites in the blood. These include tolbutamide, chlorpropamide, phenytoin, methotrexate and probenecid.

Drugs that increase salicylate intoxication include acetazolamide and ammonium chloride.

Corticosteroids may decrease salicylate concentration.

Treatment of toxic effects

- Gastric lavage with activated charcoal
- IV fluids to correct dehydration
- External cooling (cold sponge)
- Vitamin K and blood transfusion to treat haemorrhagic complications
- IV potassium to correct hypokalaemia and dextrose to treat ketosis
- IV sodium bicarbonate to correct acidosis
- Forced alkaline diuresis to promote excretion of salicylate (normal saline with 2% dextrose and 2% sodium bicarbonate 2 litres / hour with frequent determinations of blood pH and plasma CO_2).
- Peritoneal dialysis with a solution of albumin or haemodialysis or in small children exchange transfusion

PARA-AMINOPHENOLS

Paracetamol (acetaminophen)

It is a major metabolite of phenacetin. It has potent analgesic and antipyretic effect but weak anti-inflammatory activity. It does not have uricosuric action. It has replaced phenacetin as it does not produce renal damage unlike phenacetin. It also does not cause GI ulceration.

Paracetamol is rapidly absorbed when taken orally. It has wide distribution. It is largely conjugated in liver particularly with glucuronic acid. The conjugates and small amount of free drug are excreted in urine.

Paracetamol has analgesic-antipyretic effects without uricosuric and anti-inflammatory effects of aspirin.

Adverse effects are few in therapeutic doses (0.5-1 g, 3-4 times a day). Over-dosages produce deple-

tion of glutathione and the metabolite causes acute hepatic necrosis after ingestion of 10 gm.

It has potent analgesic and antipyretic effect but weak antiinflammatory activity. It does not have uricosuric property. It does not cause renal damage or GI ulceration.

Differences between aspirin and paracetamol are given in Table 3.8.

Table 3.8. Differences between aspirin and paracetamol.

Aspirin	Paracetamol
Has antiinflmmatory action	No antiinflmmatory action
Causes sever gastric irritation	Gastric irritation is less
Alters platelet function	Does not alter platelet function
Uricosuric in large doses	Not uricosuric
Affects CV system	Has no effect on CV system
Affects acid base balance	Does not affect acid base balance
Stimulates respiration	Does not stimulate respiration
Increases cellular metabolism, uncouples oxidative phosphorylation in large doses	Does not increase cellular metabolism Liver toxicity on continuous use for long time

Acute Paracetamol toxicity

Doses above 150mg/kg in children, more than 10g in adult can produce serious toxicity. In chronic alcoholics as low as 5 g/day taken for a few days can cause hepatoxicity. Dose more than 250 mg/kg may be fatal.

When large doses of paracetamol are taken glucuronidation capacity is saturated, hepatic glutathione is depleted and N-acetyl-benzoquinoneimine which is a metabolite of paracetamol (highly reactive metabolite) binds covalently to proteins in liver cells and renal tubules resulting in necrosis.

Acute paracetamol poisoning is more likely to occur in small children because they have low hepatic glucuronide conjugating capacity. Premature infants weighing less than 2 kg should not be given paracetamol for fear of hepatotoxicity.

Acute paracetamol poisoning is manifested initially as gastrointestinal disturbances. After about 10 to 15 hours centrilobular hepatic necrosis, renal tubular necrosis, hypoglycaemia leading to coma may occur. After 2 days jaundice appears. If plasma levels are above 200 microgram / ml at 4 hours and 30 microgram / ml at 15 hours hepatic failure and death occurs. In case these levels are lower recovery may take place with proper and adequate treatment. However, in most cases the treatment is ineffective if started 15 hours or more after ingestion of paracetamol.

Treatment of acute paracetamol overdosage

- Gastric lavage should be done or vomiting induced if the patient has been brought early.
- Supportive measures
- Specific therapy is provided: N-acetylcysteine 150 mg/kg I.V. infusion for 15 minutes, same dose IV. for next 20 hours, or 75 mg/kg orally every 4 hours for 2-3 days. This will replenish glutathione stores in liver

PYRAZOLONES

Phenylbutazone and oxyphenbutazone

Phenylbutazone is a pyrazolone derivative possessing potent anti-inflammatory properties. The daily dose is 300-400 mg in divided doses. However, aspirin and newer NSAIDs are superior.

Oxyphenbutazone is an active metabolite of phenylbutazone with similar properties. However, it may produce lesser GI irritation. It is white crystalline powder insoluble in water. It is a derivative of phenylbutazone, and with similar anti-inflammatory, analgesic and antipyretic properties. Oxyphenbutazone may be employed in a 10% concentration in an eye ointment base for nonpurulent inflammatory anterior segment eye conditions. Its use is free from the changes associated with topical steroid therapy.

Adverse effects of pyrazolone derivatives

These are frequent and serious including GIT disturbances, blurring of vision, euphoria, insomnia, agranulocytosis and aplastic anaemia (bone marrow depression) haemolytic anaemia retinal haemorrhages, optic neuritis, haematuria, convulsions,

nephrotic syndrome, gastric ulcers, deafness, sodium and water retention (oedema) and hepatic and renal tubular necrosis. Due to these toxic effects their use is limited although they are potent anti-inflammatory agents.

INDOLE DERIVATIVES

Indomethacin

It is well absorbed orally and 90% bound to plasma proteins. It is comparable to phenylbutazone in effectiveness in rheumatoid arthritis, osteoarthritis and gout. It should not be used as a simple analgesic. It is a better analgesic-antipyretic than phenylbutazone. It should not be used as a routine analgesic-antipyretic due to high incidence of serious side effects.

Systemic indomethacin can cause gastric irritation. Corneal deposits and pigmentary macular changes have been reported. It can cause sodium retention and transient elevation of blood urea and creatinine. It can aggravate psychiatric disturbances, epilepsy and parkinsonism. Hepatic, renal and haematological disturbances have also been described.

The usual dose is 50 mg tablets thrice a day orally. Indomethacin is not recommended for general use as an analgesic. It is beneficial in special situations such as acute gouty arthritis, osteoarthritis of the hip, pericarditis and pleurisy. A special application is in ductus arteriosus in premature infants.

1% eye drops is used as prophylactic against postoperative cystoid macular oedema instilled 4-6 times a day, prior to surgery.

Adverse reactions are dose-related and frequent. These include GI upsets, pancreatitis, severe headache, dizziness, confusion and depression. Psychosis has been reported though rarely. Serious haematologic reactions may occur including thrombocytopenia and aplastic anaemia. Hyperkalaemia may occur due to inhibition of the synthesis of prostaglandins in the kidney. Coronary vasoconstriction has been reported. Hepatic abnormalities may also occur but rarely. Indomethacin is less toxic than phenylbutazone.

Indomethacin is *contraindicated* in pregnancy, epilepsy, parkinsonism and renal disease, and should be employed carefully or may even be avoided in the presence of psychiatric disorders and peptic ulcer.

Drug interactions with indomethacin
- Frusemide - diuretic action is blunted
- Thiazide, frusemide, beta blockers, and ACEIs antihypertensive action is antagonized.
- Warfarin - displacement of warfarin
- Triameterene - increase in incidence of renal failure

Sulindac

It is prodrug, which is related to indomethacin. Its duration of action is longer than indomethacin and the incidence of side effects is less.

Sulindac is converted in the body to sulindac sulfide which is 500 times more potent than the parent drug.

The uses and adverse effects are similar to those of the other NSAIDs.

Serious adverse effects include Stevens - Johnson epidermal necrolysis syndrome, agranulocytosis, thrombocytopenia and nephrotic syndrome.

PROPIONIC ACID DERIVATIVES

These include ibuprofen, fenoprofen, flurbiprofen, ketoprofen and naproxen. These are well tolerated and possess anti-inflammatory actions similar to aspirin. Compared to indomethacin these drugs have comparable analgesic activity, slightly less anti-inflammatory activity and very much less tendency to cause side effects. They are better tolerated than aspirin.

The doses are as following:

Ibuprofen	0.2-0.6 gm thrice a day
Fenoprofen	0.3-0.6 gm thrice a day
Ketoprofen	0.5 gm twice or thrice a day
Flurbiprofen	0.5 gm twice or thrice a day
Naproxen	0.25 gm twice a day

Ibuprofen

In lower doses it is analgesic but inferior as an anti-inflammatory agent. It is extensively metabolized in the liver and only a little is excreted unaltered. Gastrointestinal irritation and bleeding may occur, but less frequently than with aspirin. The gastrointestinal symptoms can be modified by ingestion with meals. The other adverse effects include tinnitus, headache, dizziness, rash and fluid retention.

Serious haematologic effects include agranulocytosis and aplastic anaemia. All NSAIDs may affect kidney and the adverse effects include acute renal failure, interstitial nephritis, and nephrotic syndrome.

Naproxen and fenoprofen

Like ibuprofen, naproxen competes with aspirin for plasma protein binding sites. It also prolongs prothrombin time. Naproxen has a long half-life. Antacids delay its absorption. It is excreted as an inactive glucuronide metabolite in the urine.

Fenoprofen has a short half-life so multiple dosing is required.

Adverse effects of naproxen and fenoprofen are similar to those of ibuprofen (nephrotoxicity, jaundice, oedema, rash, CNS and cardiovascular effects, and tinnitus).

Flurbiprofen is readily absorbed and achieves high concentration in the synovial fluid. It is also available in a topical ophthalmic formulation for inhibition of intraoperative miosis.

The adverse effects are similar to other NSAIDs.

Ketoprofen

It has ability to inhibit both cyclooxygenase and lipoxygenase. However, in spite of dual effect it is not superior to other NSAIDs. It is metabolized completely in the liver. Its major adverse effects are on the CNS and GIT.

Oxaprozin

It is a new propionic acid derivative. Its distinguishing feature is a very long half-life. It is given once a day. It has the same benefits and risks as with other NSAIDs.

FENAMATES (ANTHRANALIC ACID DERIVATIVES)

Mefenamic acid

It is a useful analgesic in chronic and dull aching pain. It is less effective as antiinflammatory and more toxic than aspirin.

Its oral absorption is slow but complete.

The plasma half-life is 2-4 hours.

Mefenamic acid is mainly indicated in muscle, joint and soft tissue pain (where strong antiinflammaotry effect is not needed).

Dose: 250-500 mg thrice a day.

It should not be used for longer than one week and never in children.

Adverse effects include diarrhoea (most common), skin rashes and dizziness. Some cases of haemolytic anaemia have been reported which is no doubt rare but when it occurs it is serious.

PHENYLACETIC ACID DERIVATIVES (ARYLACETIC ACID DERIVATIVES)

Diclofenac is a potent cyclooxygenase inhibitor with anti-inflammatory, analgesic and antipyretic properties. It is rapidly absorbed and has a short half-life. Like flurbiprofen it accumulates in the synovial fluid. An ophthalmic preparation is available for prevention of postoperative ophthalmic inflammation.

Adverse effects include GI disturbances, CNS disturbances, skin rashes, allergic reactions. Renal function may be impaired though rarely.

Tolmetin

Its antiinflammatory action is more marked than ibuprofen but less marked than phenylbutazone. Its efficacy is similar to than of aspirin.

Dose: 400-600 mg twice a day.

Adverse effects are frequent and include GI disturbances (including ulceration), CNS adverse effects are similar to that of indomethacin though less severe. Tinnitus and vertigo have been reported but less severe than with aspirin.

Sulindac

It is a sulfoxide. It is a prodrug. Its active metabolite is, like diclofenac, an acetic acid derivative. This prodrug becomes active after being converted to a sulfide by liver. The uses and adverse effects are similar to those of other NSAIDs. Serious adverse reactions include Stevens-Johnson epidermal necrolysis syndrome, thrombocytopenia, agranulocytosis and nephrotic syndrome.

OXICAMS

Oxicam derivatives

Oxicams (piroxicam, tenoxicam, meloxicam) have certain advantages:

- They are less gastric irritant
- Have long duration of action
- They are administered once or twice daily
- They decrease production of IgM rheumatoid factor and lower its plasma levels in patients with rheumatoid arthritis.
- They also inhibit chemotaxis of leukocytes and decrease the ratio of T helper suppressor lymphocytes

Piroxicam possesses anti-inflammatory, analgesic and antipyretic properties. The main advantage is its long half-life which allows single daily dose.

Dose is 20 mg once a day. Its analgesic action is greater than aspirin, its anti-inflammatory potency is similar to indomethacin. It is rapidly and completely absorbed from GIT, 99% bound to plasma proteins. It is metabolized in the liver and excreted in urine.

Piroxicam is well tolerated. However, gastrointestinal disturbances and allergic reactions have been reported.

Tenoxicam

It is a congener of piroxicam having similar properties and indications.

Dose: 20mg once a day.

Meloxicam

It is a recently introduced piroxicam congener which has greater inhibitory effect against COX-2, which is implicated in the inflammatory response, than against COX-1, inhibition of which is associated with gastric renal and other adverse effects.

COX-2: COX-1 selectivity ratio of 11-14 times has been measured.

It should be borne in mind that the newer NSAIDs have been responsible for many instances of acute renal failure and nephrotic syndrome which develop insidiously. It is neither dose dependent nor related to duration of drug use. The condition may remain undetected until advanced. Because about 15% of patients develop adverse effects from aspirin, newer NSAIDs are indicated for such patients. Although less gastrointestinal irritation has been reported for most of them but some of them are proving more toxic in other ways.

PYRROLO-PYRROLE DERIVATIVE

Ketorolac

It is potent analgesic and moderate antiinflammatory agent. It is rapidly absorbed after oral and parenteral administration. Plasma half-life is 5-7 hours. It is mainly metabolized through glucuronidation. About 60% is excreted unaltered in urine.

Ketorolac has efficacy similar to morphine in relieving postoperative pain. It has no action on opioid receptors and is free from certain side effects of morphine such as respiratory depression, constipation, blood pressure lowering effect and liability to produce dependence.

Ketorolac can also inhibit platelet aggregation for short duration.

Ketorolac is used in postoperative, acute musculoskeletal pain, renal colic, migraine.

Dose: 10-20mg orally four times a day for maximum 5 days for the treatment of moderate pain.

15-30 mg IM (maximum 20 mg/day) 4-6 hourly is used to treat postoperative and acute musculoskeletal pain.

Ketorolac is not used as an obstetric analgesic.

Adverse effects include GIT upsets, headache, nervousness, fluid retention and dizziness.

Contraindications: Ketorolac should not be given in the presence of cardiac, renal and liver diseases, and in patients on anticoagulants. Its margin of safety in children, during pregnancy and in old age is not yet known.

SULFONALIDE

Nimesulide

Nimesulide (4-nitro-2-phenoxy methane sulphonanilide) is different from conventional NSAIDs. The serum concentration of 1.98 to 9.85 mg/L is achieved within 1.2 to 3.17 hours, bound 99% to plasma protein, and extensively metabolised to several metabolites and excreted mainly in the urine. 1-3% is excreted unchanged in the urine.

Nimesulide has potency similar to or greater than that of indomethacin, diclofenac, piroxicam and ibuprofen.

There are claim that nimesulide is better tolerated than other NSAIDs. But there are certain data that indicate that the GI tolerability of this drugs is the same as that of other NSAIDs and it exhibits the usual adverse effects (gastrointestinal, dermatological and haematological)

It has also been claimed that nimesulide can be safe in patients with bronchial asthma. However, further data is needed to confirm that it has any protective effect against allergen induced asthma. Some reports indicate that nimesulide may precipitate adverse reactions in asthmatic patients.

Dose: 100 mg twice a day orally in adults.

Mechanism of action

- It has selective prostaglandin synthetase inhibition. It also acts in ways other than prostaglandin synthesis inhibition.
- Reduction in superoxide anion production by activated neurotrophils by inhibition of phosphodiasterase and protein kinase.
- Inhibition of bradykinin and cytokine induced hyperalgesia.
- Inhibition of tumour necrosis factor (TNF-alpha) release.
- Direct scavenging hypochlorus acid (HOCl).
- Suppression of proteases like collagenase and elastase.
- Inhibition of histamine release from basophils and mast cells.
- Reduction in platelet activation factor (PAF) synthesis.

Uses

- Nimesulide is well tolerated with fewer side effects.
- Analgesic, antipyretic and anti-inflammatory.
- It is very effective agent to control pain and inflammation in patients with osteoarthritis and has the potential to limit cartilage damage and further disability. In inhibits metalloprotease synthesis and proteoglican degradation.
- It has also been found useful for the treatment

of tendinitis, bursitis, in ENT, dental and pelvic inflammatory conditions as well as in post-surgical pain disorders.

Adverse effects

These are similar to diclofenac but fewer.
- GI disturbance (stomatitis).
- Dermatological (rash, urticaria pruritus)
- CNS (dizziness, somnolence, headache, reduced visual acuity).

Contraindications

- Active peptic ulcer disease.
- Moderate and severe hepatic impairment.

Precautionary advice

As many cases of nimesulide induced hepatotoxicity have been reported some of which have been fatal it seems that both immunological and metabolic idiosyncratic reactions can be involved as the pathogenetic mechanism of nimesulide induced liver disease. The use of this drug in children appears unjustified when other safer alternatives are available.

Neonatal renal failure following the use of this drug has been reported.

Comparison of some commonly used NSAIDs is shown in Table 3.9.

Topical NSAIDs for musculoskeletal conditions:

A successful topical NSAID requires not only efficacy at the target site but the ability to reach that site, which may involve delivery via the systemic circulation and direct penetration. An important question in determining the potential advantages of topical NSAIDs is whether any clinical effect is

Table 3.9. Comparison of commonly used NSAIDs.

Drugs	Action			Dose (mg) and intervals
	Analgesic	Antipyretic	Anti-inflammatory	
Aspirin	+	+	+	300-600 4 hourly
Naproxen	+	+	+	250-500 12 hourly
Ibuprofen	+	+	+	400-800 6-8 hourly
Flurbiprofen	+	+	+	50-75 6-12 hourly
Fenbufen	+	+	–	300-600 6-8 hourly
Ketoprofen	+	+	+	50-100 6-8 hourly
Indomethacin	+	+	++	25-50 6-8 hourly
Sulindac	+	+	+	200 12 hourly
Meclofenamic acid	+	+	+	200-400 4-6 hourly
Mefenamic acid	+	+	±	250-500 4-6 hourly
Piroxicam	+	+	++	10-20 24 hourly
Tenoxicam	+	+	++	20, 24 hourly
Meloxicam	+	+	++	7.5 one daily
Phenylbutazone	+	+	++	400 daily in divided doses
Azapropazone	+	+	+	1200 daily in divided doses
Metamizol	+	+	–	500-1500
Propiphenazone	+	+	–	300-600, 8 hourly
Diclofenac	+	+	+	50, 6-12 hourly
Tolmetin	+	+	+	200-400, 4-6 hourly
Ketorolac	++	+	+	10-20, 6 hourly
				15-30 IM, 4-6 hourly
Nimesulide	+	+	+	100, 12 hourly
Nabumetone	+	+	++	100, 24 hourly
Paracetamol	+	+	–	500-1000, 4-6 hourly
Nefopam	+	+	–	30-60, 8 hourly
				20 IM, 6 hourly

achieved by direct transport to the tissue or by systemic absorption and redistribution.

The skin layers through which any drug must be transported are the stratum corneum (being the upper most layer of dead epidermal cells), viable epidermis (devoid of blood vessels), the basement membrane and the dermis (containing blood vessels). Absorption into the systemic circulation or penetration into deeper tissues occurs from this point. The stratum corneum is largely lipophilic and is best traversed by unionized drug, while the viable epidermal layer is predominantly aqueous. Thus, for optimal penetration through both layers, the drug requires both hydrophilic and hydrophobic qualities.

In recent years a growing number of topical nonsteroidal anti-inflammatory drugs (NSAIDs) have become available. This has been prompted in large part by the high incidence of serious GI adverse effects associated with the use of systemic NSAIDs, and the premise that minimization of plasma concentrations of active drug may result in fewer systemic adverse effects. Evidence in humans and animals with topical NSAIDs demonstrates lower plasma concentrations than with systemically administered drugs, while those in soft tissues are still of a magnitude considered consistent with exerting an anti-inflammatory effect. In joints, however, the evidence is less strong, and there is still dispute whether in this case the drug reaches the joint predominently via the transcutaneous or systemic route.

There has been a sufficient number of studies of soft tissue conditions to suggest equivalent efficacy in comparison with some oral NSAIDs. For anthropathies the literature is more sparse. The initial costs of topical agents tend to be higher than those of oral agents but a cost-effectiveness analysis suggests an overall benefit; this issue requires further clarification.

Choice based on activity

Good analgesic and potent anti-inflammatory	Aspirin
Good analgesic and poor anti-inflammatory	Paracetamol
Moderate analgesic and moderate anti-inflammatory	Ibuprofen, Piroxicam

---

Box 3.6. General untoward effects of NSAIDs

Unwanted effects are common, particularly in the elderly, and include :

- Dyspepsia
- Nausea
- Vomiting
- Gastric damage in chronic users; with risk of haemorrhage, due to abrogation of the protective effect of PGE_2 on gastric mucosa
- Skin reactions
- Reversible renal insufficiency due to lack of compensatory PGE_2-mediated vasodilation.
- Analgesic-associated neuropathy
- Less commonly liver disorders, bone marrow depression

Poor analgesic and potent anti-inflammatory	Phenylbutazone, Oxyphenbutazone, Indomethacin, Sulindac

Choice based on frequency of administration

Once-a-day-drugs	Piroxicam 20 mg/d
Twice-a-day-drugs	Naproxen 500 mg
3 or 4 times-a-day-drugs	Ibuprofen 400 mg Indomethacin 25 mg Diclofenac 50 mg

Choice based on suitability

Usually suitable for delicate stomach	Ibuprofen, Naproxen NOT-Aspirin, Indomethacin
Usually free from drug interactions with anticoagulants	Indomethacin, Naproxen, Ibuprofen, Piroxicam NOT-Aspirin, Phenylbutazone
Suitable for children	Aspirin, Ibuprofen, Naproxen

Choice based on relative suitability for COX-1 and COX-2 inhibition.

Cyclooxygenase (COX), the essential enzyme catalyzing the biosynthesis of prostaglandins was purified in 1976 and cloned in 1988. A second COX gene was discovered in 1991. It is now known that the two different genes express two similar but distinct isoform of the enzyme **COX-1** and **COX-2.** The two isoforms have similar primary protein structure (60% homology) and catalyze essentially the same reaction. The genes for COX-1 and COX-2 are located on separate chromosomes. There are clear differences in DNA mRNA structure and function between COX-1 and COX-2. But there is less difference between the protein structure and function of these enzymes. COX-1 also termed as "the good COX" which is constitutively present in virtually all tissues under basal conditions, whereas COX-2 termed as "the bad COX" is constitutively expressed under basal conditions in many areas of central nervous system and is also responsible for the production of prostanoid mediators of inflammation.

Most NSAIDs are inhibitors of both COX-1 and COX-2, though varying in the degree of inhibition. It has become clear now that the anti-inflammatory action of NSAIDs is mainly due to the inhibition of COX-2. Moreover, it is probable that, when used as anti-inflammatory agents, their unwanted effects are due largely to their inhibition of COX-1. Inhibition of COX-1 in stomach leads to gastric irritation while inhibition of COX-1 in platelets leads to prolonged bleeding.

New generation of NSAIDs (celecoxib and rofecoxib) has been developed that selectively targets the inducible isoform of cyclo-oxygenase, cyclo-oxygenase-2 (COX-2). This isoform was expressed at sites of inflammation, which has led to the speculation that its inhibition could provide all the benefits of current NSAIDs, but without their major side effects on GIT (which are due to the inhibition of COX-1). A third isoform, COX-3, a proposal that will have implications for the prescription of both existing and new generation NSAIDs, might represent a new therapeutic target.

It has been shown, in early clinical trials that several new selective COX-2 inhibitors are anti-inflammatory and analgesic but have no adverse gastric action.

A classification has been made of NSAIDs based on their relative selectivity for the two isoenzymes COX-1 and COX-2. NSAIDs relatively selective for COX-1 include Aspirin, Indomethacin, Sulindac, Piroxicam, Paracetamol and more selective inhibition for COX-2 includes Nimesulide. Non-selective inhibition is beneficial when, these drugs are prescribed to impart normal platelet function, to prevent

cardiovascular events. However, such inhibition may be harmful when normal gastrointestinal mucosal function is impaired, and unwanted mucosal damage occurs. Table 3.10 shows relative COX-1 and COX-2 inhibitors.

Table 3.10. Relative COX-1 and COX-2 inhibitors

Relatively selective COX-1 inhibitors	Equipotent COX-1 and COX-2 inhibitors	Relatively more selective COX-2 inhibitors
Aspirin	Diclofenac	Meloxicam
Indomethacin	Naproxen	Nimesulide
Sulindac	Ibuprofen	Newer compounds
Piroxicam	Flurbiprofen	
Tolmetin	Nabumetone	

SELECTIVE INHIBITORS OF COX-2

Celecoxib

It is a nonsteroidal anti-inflammatory drug, which selectively inhibits the enzyme, cyclo-oxygenase-2 (COX-2).

Dose: The recommended dose for osteoarthritis is 200 mg daily which may be given as a single dose or divided and given as 100 mg twice daily. The recommended dose for rheumatoid arthritis is 100 mg or 200 mg twice daily. The recommended dose for familial adenomatous polyposis is 400 mg twice daily. The recommended dose for acute pain and primary dysmenorrhoea is 400 mg initially with an additional dose of 200 mg as needed on day 1, then 200 mg twice daily as needed on subsequent days.

Pharmacokinetics

Celecoxib is 97% bound to plasma protein. Celecoxib is extensively metabolized in the liver via cytochrome P450 2C9 to 3 inactive metabolites; elimination is via the kidney (27%) and faeces (57%). Less than 3% is eliminated as unchanged drug. The half-life is 11 hours.

Cautions : Common adverse effects include dyspepsia, diarrhoea, and abdominal pain. Although the risk for ulcers and other serious gastrointestinal adverse effects is lower than for other NSAIDs, product labeling still includes warnings about the risk of ulceration, bleeding and perforation.

Clinical Applications

Celecoxib is indicated for the treatment of osteo-arthritis, rheumatoid arthritis, acute pain including primary dysmenorrhoea, and is also indicated for reducing the number of colon and rectal polyps in familial adenomatous polyposis (FAP). This treatment has NOT been shown to reduce the risk of gastrointestinal cancer or the need for FAP-associated surgeries and routine endoscopic surveillance.

Etoricoxib

It is a nonsteroidal antiinflammatory agent [selective inhibitor of cyclooxygenase-2 (COX-2)].

Dose : Oral doses of 30 or 60 milligrams once daily have shown efficacy in osteoarthritis of the knee or hip. In acute dental surgery pain, single doses of 120 milligrams have been effective.

Pharmacokinetics

Etoricoxib appears well-absorbed after oral doses, with peak plasma concentrations occurring after 1 to 1.5 hours. The drug is extensively metabolized in the liver; metabolites are excreted in urine and faeces. The elimination half-life of etoricoxib after single doses is approximately 22 hours.

Cautions

Gastrointestinal side effects have been reported. An increase in thrombotic events relative to naproxen was reported in one unpublished trial.

Clinical applications

Oral etoricoxib has been effective in treating signs and symptoms of osteoarthritis and rheumatoid arthritis; it has also been useful in acute dental pain. Whether this agent offers any advantage over other COX-2 inhibitors (e.g., celecoxib or rofecoxib) has not been determined; the prothrombotic potential of this agent requires further investigation.

Lumiracoxib

It is a second-generation selective cyclooxygenase-2 (COX-2) inhibitor.

Dose: In osteoarthritis, 200 to 400 milligrams daily has been effective. No dose adjustment is required in mild or moderate hepatic dysfunction.

Pharmacokinetics

Peak plasma levels occur 2 to 3 hours after oral doses. Lumiracoxib is metabolized in the liver and has a plasma elimination half-life of 3 to 6 hours.

Cautions

Gastroduodenal ulceration has been reported in 3 to 4% of osteoarthritis or rheumatoid arthritis patients receiving lumiracoxib, similar to that of celecoxib. The incidence of moderate-to-severe oedema has been reported about 1%.

Clinical Applications

Lumiracoxib has been effective in treating osteoarthritis and postoperative dental pain. It probably offers no clinical advantage over first-generation COX-2 selective inhibitors.

Parecoxib

It is a prodrug of the nonsteroidal antiinflammatory agent valdecoxib (a selective inhibitor of cyclooxygenase-2 (COX-2)).

Dose: Parecoxib is given by injection only. For postdental surgery pain, 20 or 40mg intramuscularly or 20 to 100 mg intravenously has been given. An intravenous dose of 40 mg has been effective in treating acute pain following gynaecological or orthopedic surgery. Data regarding multiple-dose schedules have not been published.

Pharmacokinetics

Data are limited. Parecoxib is rapidly hydrolyzed in the liver to valdecoxib, which accounts for all analgesic/antiinflammatory activity. Peak valdecoxib plasma concentrations are seen about 2 hours after intramuscular doses of 20 or 40 mg, and within one hour of intravenous administration of 20 to 100 mg. The elimination half-life of valdecoxib is approximately 8 hours.

Cautions

Complete adverse-effect data (including incidences) have not been published. When given for postsurgical pain, nausea, vomiting, abdominal pain, headache, dizziness, fever, pharyngitis, injection-site pain (intramuscular), and pruritus have been reported. Parecoxib has not significantly affected platelet function in healthy subjects (including those over 65 years); it has been associated with significantly fewer gastroduodenal ulcers/lesions than parenteral ketorolac involving healthy elderly subjects. Parecoxib has not altered the pharmacokinetics of midazolam or propofol.

Clinical Applications

Single doses of parecoxib have provided effective pain relief following dental surgery (intramuscular or intravenous) and orthopaedic/gynaecological surgery (intravenous). It appears particularly useful in postsurgical patients unable to tolerate oral therapy. This drug may replace parenteral ketorolac for postoperative pain management if subsequent multiple-dose studies confirm comparative efficacy and safety, and if cost is competitive.

Rofecoxib

It is a selective inhibitor of cyclooxygenase-2 (COX-2). It is now **banned** due to the increased incidences of adverse - effect data, concerning myocardial infarction and cerebral stroke.

Valdecoxib

It is a nonsteroidal antiinflammatory agent (selective inhibitor of cyclooxygenase-2 (COX-2)).

Dose: In rheumatoid arthritis and osteoarthritis, 10 mg orally once daily is effective. An oral dose of 20 mg twice daily is effective in dysmenorrhoea.

Pharmacokinetics

Peak plasma concentrations of valdecoxib occur within 3 hours of an oral dose; bioavailability is approximately 80%, and the extent of absorption is unaffected by food or aluminium-/magnesium-containing antacids. Valdecoxib is extensively metabolized in the liver; an active metabolite has been identified but does not appear to contribute significantly to clinical effects. Urinary excretion of unchanged drug is minimal (less than 5% of an oral dose). The plasma elimination half-life of valdecoxib is 8 to 11 hours.

Cautions

Adverse effects are similar to those observed with other nonsteroidal antiinflammatory agents (selective or nonselective), and include nausea, abdominal pain, dyspepsia, diarrhoea, and peripheral oedema. Gastrointestinal lesions/ulcers appear less frequent with valdecoxib compared to nonselective agents (e.g., naproxen), and valdecoxib does not significantly affect platelet aggregation. Anaphylaxis and severe skin reactions have occurred in some patients, possibly related to a history of sulfonamide allergy.

Clinical Applications

Oral valdecoxib has been effective in treating signs and symptoms of rheumatoid arthritis and osteoarthritis; it has also been useful in primary dysmenorrhoea and as a postoperative analgesic. Whether this agent offers any advantage over other COX-2 inhibitors has not been determined.

Present status of COX-2 inhibitors

Selective inhibitors of COX-2 were developed for the relief of inflammatory pain but without one of their side effects, gastronitestinal bleeding. However, the actual proof of enhanced safety turned out to be more elusive. Two large studies were published in year 2000. In the celecoxib studies the apparent gastrointestinal protective effect noted at the 6-month analysis had evaporated at the 12-month analysis.

COX-2 inhibitors reduced the production of antithrombotic product, prostacyclin, without changing the production of prothrombotic product, thromboxane.

In Sept. 2004, Merck withdrew rofecoxib because its trial showed increased cardiovascular toxicity.

Taken together, three large, randomized, control trials on celecoxib, rofecoxib, valdeocoxib, (and its i.v. prodrug parecoxib) confirmed the CV toxicity that had been suggested 5 years earlier.

It appears that this is a class effect. It is reasonable to ask whether the use of these drugs can now be justified.

After millons of patients have used COX-2 inhibitors, which were intended to avert gastrointestinal complications common to other NSIADs, serious

CV events have now been reported for three members of this class. Physicians are disarrayed, pharmaceutical companies are embarrased and financially threatened, and patients are injured.

COX-2 inhibitors not only lack the antiplatelet effects of aspirin; by inhibiting the production of prostacyclin, they also disable one of the primary defences of the endothelium against platelet aggregation, hypertension and atherosclerosis. COX-2 inhibitors also promote an imbalance in favour of vasoconstriction. These biologic actions, known since 1998; suggest that COX-2 inhibitors may increase the risk of cardivascular events, including mycocardial infarction, stroke, hypertension, and heart failure.

STUDY QUESTIONS

1. Classify non-steroidal anti-inflammatory drugs (NSAIDs). How do they act as anti-inflammatory and analgesic drugs?
2. Describe the pharmacology of salicylates.
3. Describe the main features of the different non-narcotic/analgesic-antipyretic/NSAIDs.
4. Name the various propionic acid derivatives and their formulations and usual antiinflammatory doses.
5. What are the adverse effects of phenylbutazone?
6. Write notes on Diclofenac, Mefanamic acid, and Piroxicam? What are their advantages and disadvantages?
7. Compare Aspirin and Paracetamol.
8. What are the uses and adverse effect of Indomethacin?
9. Discuss the choice of NSAIDs on the basis of activity, frequency of administration and suitability.

GUIDE TO FURTHER READING

Battistini, B. et al. COX-1 and COX-2: toward the development of more selective NSAIDs. Drug News Perspect., 1994; 8:501-512.

Borda, I.T. et al. NSAIDs: A Profile of Adverse Effects. Hanley and Belfus, Inc., Philadelphia, 1992.

Bresalier RS, Sandler RS, Quan H, et al. Cardiovascular events associated with rofecoxib in a colorectal adenoma chemoprevention trial. N Engl J Med 2005; 352: 1092-102.

Brooks, P.M. et al. Nonsteroidal antiinflammatory drugs—differences and similarities. N. Engl. J. Med., 1991; 324:1716-1725.

Clissold, S.P. et al. Paracetamol and phenacetin. Drugs, 1986, 32 Suppl. 4:46-59.

Clive, D.M. et al. Renal syndromes associated with nonsteroidal antiinflammatory drugs. N. Engl. J. Med., 1984; 310:563-572.

Derek A Willoughby, Adrian R Moore, Paul R Colville-Nash. COX-1, COX-2 and COX-3 and the future of treatment of chronic inflammatory disease. The Lancet Vol. 355. February 19, 2000.

Gabriel, S.E. et al. Risk for serious gastrointestinal complications related use of nonsteroidal anti-inflammatory drugs. A meta-analysis. Ann. Intern. Med., 1991; 115:787-796.

Giardiello, F.M. et al. Treatment of colonic and rectal adenomas with sulindac in familial adenomatous polyposis. N. Engl. J. Med., 1993; 328:1313-1316.

Gilroy DW, Tomlinson A, Willoughby DA. Differential effects of inhibitors of cyclooxygenase (cyclooxygenase 1 and cyclooxygenase 2) in acute inflammation. Eur J. Pharmacol 1998; 355: 211-17.

Graham, D.Y. et al. Duodenal and gastric ulcer prevention with misoprostol in arthritis patients taking NSAIDs. Misoprostol Study Group. Ann. Intern. Med., 1993; 119:257-262.

Imperiale, T.F. et al. A meta-analysis of low dose aspirin for the prevention of pregnancy-induced hypertensive disease. JAMA, 1991; 266:260-264.

Kantor, T.G. et al. Ibuprofen. Ann. Intern. Med., 1979; 91:877-882.

Kincaid-Smith, P. et al. Effects of non-narcotic analgesics on the kidney. Drugs, 1986; 32 Suppl. 4:109-128.

Lewis, A.J. et al. Nonsteroidal Anti-Inflammatory Drugs. Mechanisms and Clinical Use. Marcel Dekker, New York, 1987.

Leonards, J.R. et al. Gastrointestinal blood loss during prolonged aspirin administration. N. Engl. J. Med., 1973; 289:1020-1022.

Lubbe, W.F. et al. Low-dose aspirin in prevention of toxemia of pregnancy. Does it have a place? Drugs, 1987; 34:515-518.

Masferrer, J.L. et al. Selective inhibition of inducible cyclooxygenase-2 in vivo is anti-inflammatory and nonulcerogenic. Proc. Natl. Acad. Sci. USA., 1994; 91:3228-3232.

Meade, E.A. et al. Differential inhibition of prostaglandin endoperoxide synthase (cyclooxygenase) isozymes by aspirin and other non-steroidal anti-inflammatory drugs. J. Biol. Chem., 1993; 268:6610-6614.

Ment, L.R. et al. Low-dose indomethacin and prevention of intraventricular hemorrhage: a multi-center randomized trial. Pediatrics, 1994; 93:543-550.

Mitchell, J.A. et al. Selectivity of nonsteroidal anti-inflammatory drugs as inhibitors of constitutive and inducible cyclooxygenase. Proc. Natl. Acad. Sci. USA., 1993; 90:11693-11697.

Mukherjee D, Nissen SE, Topol EJ. Risk of cardiovascular events associated with selective COX-2 inhibitors. JAMA 2001; 286: 954-9.

Nussmeier NA, Whelton AA, Brown MT, et al. Complications of the COX-2 inhibitors parecoxib and valdecoxib after cardiac surgery. N Engl J Med 2005; 352: 1081-91.

Patrono, C. Aspirin as an antiplatelet drug. N. Engl. J. Med., 1994; 330:1287-1294.

Sandler, D.P. et al. Analgesic use and chronic renal disease. N. Engl. J. Med., 1989; 320:1238-1243.

Sibai, B.M. et al. The National Institute of Child Health and Human Development Network of Maternal-Fetal Medicine Units. Prevention of preeclampsia with low-dose aspirin in healthy nulliparous pregnant women. N. Engl. J. Med., 1993; 329:1213-1218.

Simmons DL, Botting RM, Robertson PM, Madsen ML, Vane JR. Induction of an acetaminophen-sensitive cyclooxygenase with reduced sensitivity to nonsteroid anti-inflammatory drugs. Proc Natl Acad Sci USA 1999; 96: 3275-80.

Smikstein, M.J. et al. Efficacy of oral N-acetylcysteine in the treatment of acetaminophen overdose. Analysis of the National Multicenter Study (1976 to 1985). N. Engl. J. Med., 1988; 319:1557-1562.

Solomon SD, McMurray JJV, Pfeffer MA, et al. Cardiovascular risk associated with celecoxib in a clinical trial for colorectal adenoma prevention. N Engl J. Med 2005; 352: 1071-80.

Vane, J. et al. Inflammation and the mechanism of action of antiinflammatory drugs. FASEB J., 1987; 1:89-96.

Vane, J. et al. Towards a better aspirin. Nature, 1994; 367:215-216.

Warner TD, Giuliano F, Vojnovic I, Bukasa JA, Mitchell JA, Vane JR. Nonsteroid drug selectivities for cyclo-oxygenase-1 rather than cyclo-oxygenase-2 are associated with human gastrointestinal toxicity: a full in vitro analysis. Proc Natl Acad Sci USA 1999; 96: 7563-68.

Willis D, Moore AR, Frederick R, Willoughby DA. Heme oxygenase: a novel target for the modulation of the inflammatory response. Nat Med 1996; 2: 87-90.

DRUGS USED IN MIGRAINE

Migraine is a specific neurological syndrome that has many manifestations. Migraine without aura is termed as 'common migraine'. Migraine with aura is termed 'classic migraine'. Migraine without aura has throbbing headache manifestation (usually unilateral) with associated nausea.

Migraine with aura (classic migraine)

In this condition headache is associated with characteristic premonitory sensory, motor or visual symptoms, the most common premonitory symptoms reported by migraineurs are visual, arising from dysfunction of occipital lobe neurons.

In classic migraine serotonin (5-HT) release from platelets causes vasoconstriction of intracerebral vessels which induces aura. The 5-HT is soon degraded by MAO and a state of 5-HT depletion occurs leading to vasodilation of intracerebral and extra cerebral vessels producing severe throbbing headache starting unilaterally often with photophobia, nausea, vomiting and prostration, which lasts for several hours.

Common migraine

In this condition, no focal neurologic disturbance precedes the recurrent headaches. Migraine without aura is the most frequent type of vascular headache. The International Headache Society criteria for migraine include moderate to severe head pain, pulsating quality, unilateral location, aggravation by walking stairs or similar routine activity, attendant nausea and/or vomiting.

5-HT in migraine

Molecular cloning studies have demonstrated that at least 14 specific 5-HT receptors exist in humans. The triptans (e.g., naratriptan, rizatriptan, sumatriptan and zolmitriptan) are potent agonists of 5-HT_{1B}, 5-HT_{1D} and 5-HT_{1F} receptors and are less potent at 5-HT_{1A} and 5-HT_{1E} receptors. Data indicates that antimigraine efficacy of the triptans relates to their ability to stimulate 5-HT_{1B} receptors, which are located both on blood vessels and nerve terminals. Selective 5-HT_{1D} receptor agonists fail to demonstrate clinical efficacy in migraine. Triptans that are weak $5\text{-}HT_{1F}$ agonists are also effective in migraine. However, only $5\text{-}HT_{1B}$ is currently thought to be essential for antimigraine efficacy.

Dopamine in migraine

Data support a role for dopamine in the pathophysiology of certain subtypes of migraine. Most migraine symptoms can be induced by dopaminergic stimulation. Moreover, there is dopamine receptor hypersensitivity in migraineurs. Conversely, dopamine receptor antagonists are effective therapeutic agents in migraine.

Management of migraine

Any known precipitating factors should be avoided. Migraine is triggered by a variety of factors including stress, anxiety, exertion, excitement, fatigue, anger and by food containing vasoactive amines (chocolate, cheese). These precipitating factors are associated with release of epinephrine, norepinephrine and also of arachidonic acid (precursor of prostaglandins) including thromboxane. These substances increase blood platelet aggregation and adhesion to vessel wall.

These trigger factors should be identified and avoided.

Antimigraine Therapies

Nonsteroidal anti-inflammatory drugs (NSAIDs)

Aspirin 650 mg	Every 4-6 hours
Paracetamol 650 mg	Every 4-6 hours
Ibuprofen 400-800 mg	Three times a day
Indomethacin 50 mg	Three times a day
Naproxen 550 mg followed by	275 mg three times day
Aspirin 300 mg + Caffeine 50 mg + Paracetamol 250 mg	Four times a day

These drugs are most effective when taken early in the migraine attack. The combination of paracetamol, aspirin and ceffeine is commonly used for the treatment of mild to moderate migraine.

Ergotamine, dihydroergotamine and triptans

Ergotamine and dihydroergotamine are non-selective $5\text{-}HT_1$ receptors agonists while triptans are selective $5\text{-}HT_1$ receptors agonists.

Ergotamine preparations offer a nonselective means of stimulating $5\text{-}HT_1$ receptors. Oral formulations of ergotamine also contain 100 mg caffeine (theoretically to enhance ergotamine absorption and possibly to add additional vasoconstrictor activity). The average oral ergotamine dose for a migraine attack is 2 mg. The sublingual formulation of ergotamine does not contain caffeine.

In general, ergotamine appears to have a much higher incidence of nausea than triptans but less headache recurrence.

Nasal

These include nasal formulation of dihydroergotamine or sumatriptan. The nasal sprays result in sustained blood levels within 30 to 60 minutes. However, the disadvantages include inconsistent dosing, poor taste and variable efficacy,.

Parenteral

Drugs such as dihyderogerotamine and sumatriptan are injected for rapid relief of a migraine attack.

Peak plasma levels of dihyderoergotamine are achieved 3 minutes after I.V. dosing, 30 minutes after I.M. dosing and 45 minutes after SC dosing. If an attack has not already peaked, SC or IM injection of 1 mg dihydroergotamine suffices for about 80 to 90% of patients. Sumatriptan, 6 mg SC is effective in about 70 to 80% of patients.

Dopamine antagonists

Metoclopramide, 10 mg is considered to enhance gastric absorption and also decrease nausea / vomiting and restore gastric motility. Dopamine antagonists should be considered as adjunctive therapy in migraine. Drug absorption is impaired during migrainous attacks because of reduced GI motility.

Parenteral

Drugs such as chlorpromazine, prochlorperazine and metoclopramide can also provide significant acute relief of migraine. They can be used in combination with parenteral 5-HT$_1$ agonists.

Triptans

Triptans are selective 5-HT$_1$, receptor agonists, the series of drugs known as triptans such as naratriptan, rizatriptan, sumatriptan, zolmitriptan are now available for the treatment of migraine. Among these triptans, rizatriptan appears to be the fastest acting and most efficacious. Sumatriptan and zolmitriptan have similar rates of efficacy as well as time to onset, whereas naratriptan is the slowest acting and the least efficacious. Triptans are not effective in migraine with aura unless given after the aura is completed and the headache initiated. Table 3.11 shows comparative pharmacology of oral triptans.

Table 3.11. Comparative pharmacology of oral triptans.

Drug	Dose (oral) mg	Oral bio-availability %	Clinical efficacy %
Rizatriptan	5-10 (max. 30/24hr)	45	71
Zolmitriptan	2.5-5 (max. 10/24hr)	44	65
Sumatriptan	25-100 (max. 100/24hr)	14	61
Naratriptan	1, 2, 5 (max. 5/24hr)	68	45

Sumatriptan

It is 5-HT$_{1D}$ agonist given orally or by subcutaneous injection. It is highly effective but short acting (half-life is about 2 hours)

Side effects include dizziness, tiredness.

It is contraindicated in IHD because of tendency to cause chest pain owing to coronary artery spasm.

Triptans are derived from serotonin molecule and act on the 5-HT$_{1B/1D}$ receptors. The receptors are on the blood vessels, trigeminal neurons and trigeminal nucleus caudalis. Activation of these receptors causes constriction of the extracerebral intracranial vessels, abolition of the dural extravasation and neurogenic inflammation and inhibition of trigeminal neuronal discharge. It is likely that 5-HT$_{1B/1D}$ agonist activity is the primary mechanism of the therapeutic effect of these drugs.

Almotriptan

It is a new antimigraine agent with nanomolar affinity for human 5HT$_{1B/1D}$ and 5-HT$_{1F}$ receptors. Almotriptan was effective in animal models predictive of antimigraine activity in humans and is safe in animals studies. It is well absorbed orally in humans. Its peak plasma levels are reached at 1-3 hours after its administration; its elimination t$_{1/2}$ is 3-4 h. No dose adjustment is required for gender or age except only in the case of severe renal impairment. The dose should not exceed 12.5mg over 24 h period.

Rizatriptan

This is a selective 5HT$_{1B/1D}$ receptor agonist for the acute treatment of migraine. It is available in a unique wafer formulations that dissolves rapidly in the mouth and can be taken without liquids, thereby offering patients a very convenient way to take treatment. Its t$_{1/2}$ is 2.4 h. Rizatriptan (5 and 10 mg) is effective in treating acute migraine with a dose related increase in efficacy.

Naratriptan

This is least potent among the triptans regarding the primary end points in the relief from acute migraine attack i.e. sustained freedom from pain or consistency (efficacy in at least two out of three treated attacks) of effect At 2.5mg dose it has better pharmacokinetic profile than 100 mg of sumatriptan. It is better tolerated.

Eletriptan

It is potent serotonin agonist at 5-HT$_{1B/1D}$ receptor and is indicated for the acute treatment of migraine headaches. It is administered orally and is rapidly absorbed, relatively high lipophilicity of eletriptan explains its fast oral absorption and shorter time for onset of action. It is more efficacious at 40 and 80mg dose as compared to 100mg of sumatriptan though modest increase in adverse events may be seen with 80 mg of eletriptan.

Zolmitriptan

It is a new antimigraine triptan having similar efficacy and tolerability at 2.5 and 5 mg as compared to 100mg of sumatriptan. Fast melt formulation of zolmitriptan represents real competition with other triptans in the usual tablet formulations. It is especially suitable for acute migraine patients for rapid relief.

Frovatriptan

It is a new 5-$HT_{1B/1D}$ agonist antimigraine triptan undergoing clinical trials. Preclinical data suggest that the pharmacokinetic and pharmacological profile of frovatriptan may differ from that of currently available triptans. It is longest acting triptan with $T_{1/2}$ 25 hours.

Newer drugs currently under development for acute attacks of migraine includes kainate antagonist LY 293558 and GR 79236, a selective adenosine A_1-receptor agonist. Various other approaches are blockade of calcitonin gene related peptide, neurokinin-1 antagonist and blockade of nitric oxide synthesis.

Although the triptans represent an important advance they are ineffective in some patients because of their coronary vasoconstrictive side effects LY334370, a selective 5-HT_{1F} agonist having exclusive neural action through trigeminovascular neuronal inhibition does not show any vasoconstrictive adverse effects. Exploring the mechanisms involved in onset of migraine will lead to development of more specific, more efficacious and better tolerated drugs.

The following drugs are effective in the treatment of severe migraine:

Ergotamine	1 mg, plus caffeine, 100 mg (tablet), at the onset 1-2 tablets then 1 tablet every half-hour (max. 6 tablets, 10 per week)
Ergotamine	2 mg, plus caffeine, 100 mg (suppository) at the onset 1 suppository then 1 after 1 hour (max. 2 per attack, 5 per week)
Dihydroergotamine	1 mg, i.m./i.v. at onset and every 1 hour (max. 2 mg i.v. or 3 mg i.m. per day, 6 mg per week)

Fig. 3.1 shows role of serotonin and mode of action of certain drugs used in migraine.

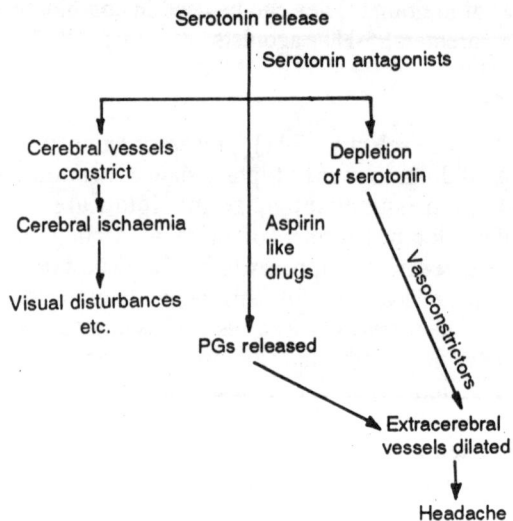

Fig. 3.1. Role of serotonin and mode of action of certain drugs used in migraine.

Drugs used for prophylactic treatment of severe migraine

- Tricyclic antidepressants may be effective even though patient is not depressed.

Amitriptyline	10-50 mg at bed times
Nortriptyline	25-75 mg at bed time

The antimigraine effect is independent of the antidepressant action.

- Beta-adrenergic receptor blockers (antagonists)

Propranolol	80-240 mg	qid
Atenolol	50-100 mg	daily
Metoprolol	50-200 mg	daily
Nadolol	40-80 mg	daily
Timolol	10-30 mg	daily

The effect is not due to beta-adrenergic blocking property because d-isomer of propranolol which lacks beta blocking effect is also effective in migraine.

Certain beta-adrenergic receptor antagonists such as acebutolol, oxprenolol, alprenolol are ineffective in the treatment of migraine.

- Calcium channel blockers such as diltiazem, verapamil, nifedipine, nimodipine are effective prophylactic drugs in migraine in usual therapeutic doses.
- Serotonin antagonist :

Methysergide maleate 4-8 mg qid is used only for prophylaxis of migraine and not for its treatment. One or two tablets (each tablet 1mg methysergide base, sublingual 2 mg tablet and for inhalation dispensing 0.36 mg in each inhalation are indicated. It is not generally used because although it is effective but has dangerous adverse effects.

Side effects include GI irritation, loss of appetite, lightheadeness, euphoria, hallucinations. Inflammatory fibrosis on prolonged use (retroperitoneal fibrosis, pleuropulmonary fibrosis, coronary and endocardial fibrosis).

- Clonidine (α_2 adrenoceptor agonist), 50-100 mg/day has been used as prophylactic agent. However, its efficacy is doubtful.
- Cyproheptadine (5-HT$_2$ receptor antagonist), 4-8 mg/day (max. 32 mg/d) has antihistaminic and calcium antagonist action. It is sometimes used in refractory cases.

It may produce drowsiness as side effect.

- Pizotifen (antihistaminic and 5-HT$_2$ antagonist), 1.5-3 mg orally in divided doses has similar prophylactic effect as cyproheptadine.

Adverse effects include weight gain, antimuscarinic effects.

Box 3.7 : Antimigraine drugs

For acute attack

- Simple analgesics, such as aspirin or paracetamol; metoclopramide may be given to speed up absorption.
- Ergotamine (5-HT$_{1D}$ receptor partial agonist)
- Sumatriptan (5-HT$_{1D}$ receptor agonist) is highly effective but short acting, newer compounds e.g. zolmitriptan is claimed to be faster-acting by mouth, and not to cause chest pain unlike sumatriptan.

For prophylaxis

- Pizotifen
- Propranolol, metoprolol
- Tricyclic antidepressants eg. amitriptyline,
- Methysergide (5-HT$_2$-receptor antagonist)
- Clonidine (Alpha2-adrenoceptor agonist)
- Calcium antagonists e.g. verapamil
- Cyproheptadine (5-HT$_2$-receptor antagonist)

- Anticonvulsant: Sodium valproate 250mg bid (max. 1000 mg/d). has also been used for prophylaxis of migraine.
- Monoamine oxidase inhibitors (MAOIs) such as : Phenelzine 15 mg tid and isocarboxazid 10 mg qid are not usually recommended as they may produce a large number of unwanted effects including postural hypotension.

STUDY QUESTIONS

1. What are the characteristics of migraine?
2. How is the acute attack managed?
3. What is the role of simple analgesics as well as ergot alkaloids?
4. Which drugs are useful for the prophylactic treatment of migraine?
5. What is the role of methysergide, its mode of action, uses and adverse effects?
6. Do propranolol and clonidine have any role in migraine?

GUIDE TO FURTHER READING

Ala-Hurula, V. Correlation between pharmacokinetics and clinical effects of ergotamine in patients suffering from migraine. Eur. J. Clin. Pharmacol, 1982; 21:397.

Albers, G.W., Simon, L.T. et al: Nifedipine versus propranolol for the initial prophylaxis of migraine. Headache, 1989; 29:215.

Allan, W.: Inheritance of migraine. Arch. Intern. Med., 1928; 42:590.

Bredberg, U et al: Pharmacokinetics of methysergide and its metabolite methylergometrine in man. Eur J Clin Pharmacol, 1986; 30:75.

Dalessio, D.J.: On migraine headache: serotonin and serotonin antagonism. JAMA, 1962; 181:318.

Ferrari, M.D. et al: Serotonin metabolism in migraine. Neurology, 1989; 39:1239.

Humphrey, P.P. et al: Serotonin and migraine. Ann NY Acad Sci, 1990; 600:587.

Moskowitz, M.A. et al: Pain mechanisms underlying vascular headaches. Rev Neurol, 1989; 145:181.

Moskowitz, M.A., Macfarlane, R: Neurovascular and molecular mechanisms in migraine headaches. Cerebrovasc Brain Metab Rev, 1993; 5:159.

Olesen, J et al: The common migraine attack may not be initiated by cerebral ischaemia. Lancet, 1981; 2:438.

Olesen, J., Tfelt-Hansen, P. and Welch, KMA. eds.: The Headaches. Raven Press, New York, 1993.

Sternbach, H: The serotonin syndrome. Am J Psychiatry, 1991; 148:705.

ANTIGOUT DRUGS

Gout is a genetically determined metabolic disorder in which there is overproduction of purines. It is characterized by intermittent attacks of acute arthritis. Acute gout is due to precipitation of sodium urate crystals (product of purine metabolism) in the synovial fluid and which evoke an inflammatory response, involving activation of kinin, complement and plasmin systems, generation of lipoxygenase products such as LTB_4 and migration of neutrophil granulocytes. These engulf the crystals by phagocytosis and release a glycoprotein which increases inflammation by (i) increasing lactic acid production from inflammatory cells → local pH is reduced → more urate crystals are precipitated in the affected joint and (ii) by releasing lysosomal enzymes which cause joint destruction.

Gout is characterised by hyperurecaemia. Primary gout is either due to overproduction or defective renal excretion of uric acid. Secondary gout is caused by certain agents such as thiazides, ethacrynic acid, pyrazinamide, levodopa, ethambutol, and clofibrate. In gout there is pain and swelling in joints and uric acid level in blood is raised.

Usually metatarsophalangeal of great toe is involved. Other joints may also be involved.

The therapeutic aims in gout are :

- To terminate the acute attack promptly and as gently as possible.
- To prevent recurrences of the disease from deposition of monosodium urate crystals in joints, kidneys and other sites.
- To prevent or reverse associated features such as obesity, hypertriglyceridaemia or hypertension.
- To prevent formation of uric acid kidney stones.

Drugs used in the treatment of gout

1. For acute attack:
   - NSAIDs: Indomethacin (drug of choice), naproxen, piroxicam, diclofenac.
   - Colchicine
   - Glucocorticoids
2. For chronic gout (prophylactic therapy against recurrent attacks):
   - Uricosuric agents: Sulfinpyrazone, probenecid, benzbromarone
   - Uric acid synthesis inhibitor: Allopurinol

The antigout drugs may act in the following ways:

- By general antiinflammatory and analgesic effect - NSAIDs
- By inhibiting leukocyte migration into the joint - Colchicine
- By increasing uric acid excretion (uricosuric agents) - Probenecid, sulfinpyrazone
- By inhibiting uric acid synthesis - Allopurinol

Colchicine

Colchicine (an alkaloid of Colchicum autumnale) is very effective, although it is not uricosuric but rapidly relieves pain and inflammation in gout.

It is a unique antiinflammatory agent in that it is effective only against gouty arthritis. It produces dramatic relief in acute attacks of gout, as well as an effective prophylactic agent against such attacks.

Colchicine is only occasionally beneficial in other types of arthritis; it is not an analgesic and does not produce relief of other types of pain.

Mode of action

Colchicine is neither analgesic nor anti-inflammatory. It neither inhibits synthesis nor promotes excretion of uric acid, hence there is no effect on blood uric acid levels. But colchicine specifically suppresses gouty inflammation.

Colchicine has no effect on phagocytosis of urate crystals but inhibits release of the glycoprotein, also inhibits granulocyte migration into the inflamed joint. Thus it interrupts the vicious cycle.

The inhibition of migration of granulocytes into the inflamed area and a decreased metabolic and phagocytic activity of granulocytes result in reduction of lactic acid and proinflammatory enzymes that occurs during phagocytosis. Thus, colchicine breaks the cycle that leads to the inflammatory response.

Colchicine is employed initially at 1 mg dose

orally followed by 0.5 mg every three hours till pain disappears or diarrhoea (adverse effect) occurs.

A total dose of 4 mg should not be exceeded and it should not be repeated within 7 days. In case colchicine is given within few hours of an attack about 90% of patients get relief within 12 hours and the symptoms of inflammation are completely gone in 48-72 hours.

Colchicine can also be administered intravenously, a single dose of 2 mg, diluted in 10-20 ml of 0.9% sodium chloride solution is usually adequate.

Colchicine can be used as a prophylactic agent for patients with chronic gout, for this purpose 0.5 mg 2-4 times a week may suffice.

Colchicine has also been used for the prevention and treatment of amyloidosis in patients suffering with familial paroxysmal polyserositis.

Colchicine has also been used in skin disorders such as psoriasis.

Adverse effects

Colchicine is not commonly used now because of severe adverse effects which include GI upsets such as nausea, vomiting, diarrhoea and abdominal pain. These side effects are most common and earliest adverse effects of colchicine overdoses. If the drug is used for a long period it may damage kidneys and suppress bone marrow (risk of agranulocytosis, aplastic anaemia); peripheral neuropathy and myopathy have also been produced by colchicine. Alopecia and azoospermia have also been described.

Role of NSAIDs is acute attack of gout:

Strong antiinflammatory agents like indomethacin, naproxen, piroxicam, diclofenac are given in high and repeated doses. They may take 12-24 hours to terminate an attack (slower than colchicine) but are better tolerated than colchicine. They are not used for prolonged period. Aspirin is avoided because of uric acid retention.

NSAIDs are now more commonly used as compared to colchicine.

The pharmacology of these drugs is described elsewhere in this chapter.

Glucocorticoids

Glucocorticoids such as prednisolone 40 mg orally in divided doses are given, if needed. The pharmacology of these drugs is described elsewhere in this chapter.

Systemically, they are rarely used in cases not responding or tolerating NSAIDs. Intraarticular injection of a soluble steroid suppresses symptoms effectively. However, it needs precautions.

DRUGS FOR CHRONIC GOUT

Uricosuric Agents

Uricosuric agents inhibit active reabsorption of uric acid by renal tubules and thereby increase the excretion of uric acid in urine.

Probenecid

Probenecid has been found useful in chronic gout in doses of 250-500 mg orally administered twice a day. Salicylates inhibit the uricosuric effect of probenecid so these two drugs should not be given simultaneously.

Probenecid inhibits the renal secretion of the glucuronides of NSAIDs such as naproxen, ketoprofen and indomethacin and thus may increase plasma concentration of such compounds.

The renal action of probenecid reduces the concentration of certain drug in urine and raises them in plasma e.g. in case of penicillin.

Probenecid is available for oral administration in the treatment of chronic gout at the dose of 250 mg twice a day for 1 week, followed by 500 mg twice daily.

Fluid intake should be liberal because probenecid has tendency to produce uric acid stones.

Uses of probenecid

- Chronic gout - given with plenty of water and urine is alkalinized to prevent crystallization of excess urate. NSAIDs are given in the beginning.
- Secondary hyperuricaemia due to drugs or disease but allopurinol is preferred.

  Note :

  - Therapy with probencid is not started in acute attack.
  - It is not useful in renal damage.

Adverse effects

Probenecid is well tolerated by most patients. However, in some patients adverse effects may appear including gastrointestinal upsets. Patients who are deficient in glucose-6-PD, it may precipitate haemolytic anaemia. Huge overdosage results in stimulation of CNS, convulsions, and death due to respiratory arrest.

Hypersensitivity reactions may also occur.

Interactions occurring with probenecid

- Probenecid inhibits tubular secretion of penicillin and cephalosporins, methotrexate, indomethacin.
- Inhibits biliary secretion of rifampin.
- Inhibits tubular secretion of nitrofurantoin.
- Salicylates block its uricosuric effect.

Sulfinpyrazone

Phenylbutazone and oxyphenbutazone possess uricosuric property. However, their long term use in chronic gout is not recommended because of frequent and severe adverse effects. For this reason several congeners were evaluated, one of these in which a phenylthioethyl configuration replaces the butyl side chain of the parent compound was found promising. It was found that the side chain oxidation in vivo of the metabolites of this new congener led to the formation of the sulphoxide, sulfinpyrazone, a potent uricosuric drug. It is a potent inhibitor of the renal tubular reabsorption of uric acid. However, it lacks the antiinflammatory and analgesic property of phenylbutazone.

Sulphinpyrazone has probenecid like uricosuric effect. It is used in chronic gout. It is contraindicated in peptic ulcer because the adverse effects on GIT may be severe.

Dose : 100-200 mg twice a day orally for the treatment of chronic gout, after first week the dose is gradually increased, if required up to 200-800 mg per day, divided in 2-4 doses.

Adverse effects

Adverse effects include gastric distress. The severe blood dyscrasias, and salt and water retention (hazards of phenylbutazone) have not been observed.

Hypersensitivity may occur but less frequently than with probenecid.

Benzbromarone

It is a potent and reversible inhibitor of the urate-anion exchanger in the proximal tubule. Its uricosuric action is inhibited by aspirin or sulfinpyrazone. It reduces the concentration of urate in plasma by inhibiting its tubular reabsorption.

Benzbromarone as the micronized powder in a single daily dose of 40 to 80 mg is more potent than other urocosuric agents. It is also useful in patients who are hypersensitive or refractory to other drugs used in gout or in patients with renal dysfunction.

Adverse effects of uricosuric agents:

- Gastric distress
- Skin rashes
- Aggravation of peptic ulcer
- Allergic reactions have been reported but less frequently, than with probenecid
- In the beginning of treatment with uricosuric agents acute attack may be precipitated due to mobilization of uric acid deposits

Contraindications of uricosuric agents

- Peptic ulcer
- History of renal stones
- Uric acid nephropathy
- Reduced GFR. Ineffective when GFR < 60ml / minute
- Age beyond 60 years
- Elevated uric acid excretion

The hypouricaemic therapy is not advocated for an acute attack of gout because the acute attacks of gout increase in frequency or severity during the early months of therapy when urate is being mobilized from affected joints.

Caution: Not effective in impaired renal function.

Uric acid synthesis inhibitors

These inhibit xanthine oxidase enzyme and thus synthesis of uric acid from hypoxanthine and xanthine is inhibited.

Allopurinol

It is not uricosuric, analgesic or antiinflammatory.

However, it can be given with uricosuric drugs. Allopurinol is an analogue of hypoxanthine.

Uric acid is formed primarily by the xanthine oxidase-catalyzed oxidation of hypoxanthine and xanthine. At low concentration allopurinol is a competitive inhibitor of the enzyme; at high concentrations it is a noncompetitive inhibitor. Alloxanthine is a metabolite of allopurinol formed by the action of xanthine oxidase which is a noncompetitive inhibitor of the enzyme. The actions of allopurinol are mainly due to this compound.

The urinary content of purines is solely uric acid in the absence of allopurinol. When it is administered the urinary purines are divided among hypoxanthine, xanthine, and uric acid. Each of these has its independent solubility, the concentration of uric acid in plasma is reduced without exposing the urinary tract to excessive load of uric acid. Allopurinol by lowering the uric acid concentration in plasma below its level of solubility, it facilitates the dissolution of tophi and prevent the development or progression of chronic gouty arthritis.

Due to the rapid renal clearance of the oxypurines during allopurinol therapy, the plasma concentration of xanthine and hypoxanthine are only little increased (not exceeding their solubility), hence their tissue deposition usually does not occur.

Inhibition of the enzyme xanthine oxidase by both allopurinol and its primary metabolite, alloxanthine (oxypurinol) accounts for the pharmacological effects of allopurinol.

The half-life of allopurinol is 2-3 hours, whereas the half-life of alloxanthine is 18-30 hours.

Allopurinol is effective for the treatment of both the primary hyperuricaemia of gout and that secondary to haematological disorders or antineoplastic therapy.

Allopurinol 100 mg, 300 mg tablets are available, dose is 100 mg/day increased to 300 mg daily, in some cases up to 600 mg/day may be given. The aim is to reduce plasma uric acid concentration below 6 mg/dl. It is not indicated during acute attack of gout. It is valuable in preventing acute attacks of gout. Allopurinol is specially used in patients with renal damage where uricosuric drugs are contraindicated.

Uses of Allopurinol

- Chronic gout. It is not effective in acute gout
- When uricosuric agents can not be used because of allergic or other adverse reactions
- For recurrent uric acid stones
- In patients with renal function impairment
- In secondary hyperuricaemia following the use of cytotoxic drugs

Uses of allopurinol in conditions other than chronic gout

- Myeloid leukaemia
- In visceral leishmaniasis (Kalazar)

Adverse reactions of allopurinol

- Acute attack of gouty arthritis may occur in the beginning by mobilizing uric acid deposits in tissues. Hence, concurrent prophylactic therapy with colchicine or NSAIDs are recommended.
- Hypersensitivity reactions
- GI upsets
- Liver damage
- Peripheral neuritis
- Depression of bone marrow
- Cataract formation

The uric acid metabolism and mode of action of antigout drugs are shown in Fig. 3.2.

STUDY QUESTIONS

1. What is primary and secondary gout?
2. What is the chief abnormality in gout?
3. Is colchicine uricosuric?
4. Describe drugs which are indicated in acute attack of gout.
5. Describe drugs used in chronic gout.
6. Describe the role and mode of action of uric acid synthesis inhibitors.
7. Explain why aspirin and probenecid should not be given simultaneously?

GUIDE TO FURTHER READING

Dan, T. et al: Uricosurics inhibit urate transporter in rat renal brush border membrane vesicles. Eur. J. Pharmacol., 1990; 187:303-312

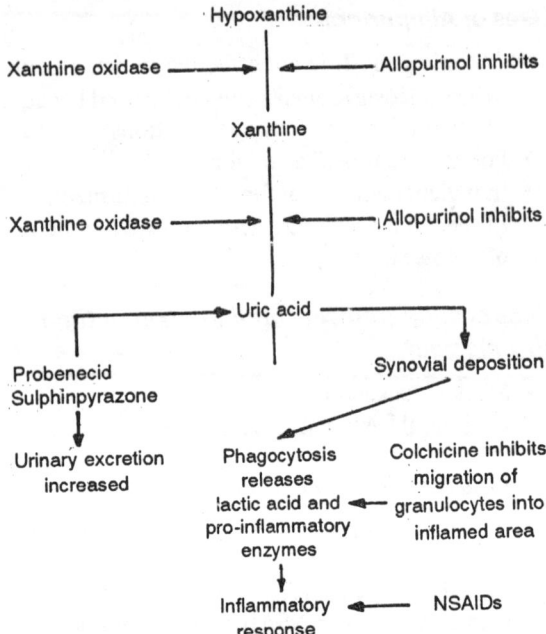

Fig. 3.2. Uric acid metabolism and mode of action of antigout drugs.

Emmerson, B.T. et al: Abnormal urate excretion associated with renal and systemic disorders, drugs, and toxins. In, Uric Acid. Handbook of Experimental Pharmacology, Vol, 51. Springer-Verlag, Berlin, 1978; pp. 287-324

Famey, J.P.: Colchicine in therapy. State of the art and new perspectives for an old drug. Clin Exp Rheum, 1988; 6:305.

Fanelli, G.M. et al: Urate excretion: drug interactions. J. Pharmacol. Exp. Ther., 1979; 210:186-195

Hande, K.R. et al: Severe allopurinol toxicity. Description and guidelines for prevention in patients with renal insufficiency. Am. J. Med., 1984; 76:47-56

Lerman, S., Megaw, J.M., Gardner, K.: Allopurinol therapy and cataract progenesis in humans. Am J Ophthalmol, 1982; 94:141.

Pascual, E., Castellano, J.A.: Treatment with colchicine decreases white cell counts in synovial fluid of asymptomatic knees that contain monosodium urate-crystals. J. Rheumatol, 1992; 19:600.

Star, V.L., Hochberg, M.C.: Prevention and management of gout. Drugs, 1993; 45:212.

Terkeltaub, R.A.: Gout and mechanisms of crystal-induced inflammation. Curr Opinion Rheumatol, 1993; 5:510.

Wallace, S.L. et al: Colchicine: Inflammation and the mechanism of action of antiinflammatory drugs. FASEB J., 1987; 1:89-96

Wallace, S.L. et al: Review: systemic toxicity associated with intravenous administration of colchicine-guidelines for use. J. Rheumatol., 1988; 15:495-499

Warnes, T.W. et al: Colchicine in primary biliary cirrhosis. Aliment. Pharmacol. Ther., 1991; 5:321-379

Yu, T.F. et al: Mutual suppression of the uricosuric effects of sulfinpyrazone and salicylate: a study in interactions between drugs. J. Clin. Invest., 1983; 42:1330-1339

Zemer, D. et al: Long-term colchicine treatment in children with familial mediterranean fever. Arthritis Rheum., 1991; 34:973-977

DRUG THERAPY OF RHEUMATOID ARTHRITIS

Rheumatoid arthritis (RA)

It is a chronic symmetrical inflammatory poly-arthritis of the synovial joints of the body. The brunt of the disease falls on the wrists (more in Indians and other Asians), the metacarpophalangeal joints and the proximal interphalangeal joints. However, all synovial joints in the body are at risk.

This chronic progressive inflammatory joint disease has a high prevalence in the Indian population (around 0.75%) with a female: male ratio of 3: 1. If the disease is left untreated it may lead to deformity, disability and eventual loss of movement.

Besides the joints, RA is a systemic disease. The most common ocular manifestation is keratoconjunctivitis sicca. In the lungs interstitial fibrosis, rheumatoid nodules and pleural effusion are common, inflammation of the pericardium may cause pericarditis. Rheumatoid nodules on the heart valves may lead to murmurs and the nodules in the heart muscle can cause electrical conduction disturbances.

Rheumatoid arthritis is a systemic immuno-inflammatory disease with natural remissions and relapses.

The activity of TNF-α and other cytokines are found to be responsible or many of the features of R.A. including tissue inflammation, cartilage and bone damage and systemic manifestations. Tissue necrosis factor (TNF) is a naturally occurring immune system protein (cytokine) with wide range of biological effects like important role in inflammatory process, activation of T cells and multiplication of both T and B cells. It also triggers the release of enzymes that damage cartilage and promotes bone destruction. The tissue damaging metalloproteinase enzymes eat away the cartilage.

All current treatments of RA are palliative

- NSAIDs are often given early in the course of disease to reduce pain and inflammation, These drugs do not stop the progression of RA. In addition at higher dose they produce unpleasant and serious GI events.
- When more aggressive therapy is required, disease modifying anti-rheumatic drugs (DMARDs) are used. Most common DMARDs used in rheumatology practices are methotrexate (MTX), hydroxychloroquine, sulfasalazine, gold, azathioprine etc. These drugs have the potential to interfere with the disease process by reducing or preventing joint damage. However, they do not reverse or completely arrest the damage. Onset of action of DMARDs is quite long. The potent side effects also limit their use in RA.
- Glucocorticoids which have beneficial anti-inflammatory effects, are commonly used in RA treatment along with NSAIDs and DMARDs. The adverse effects of systemic glucocorticoid administration, especially when given at sustained high dose, limit its use. It can give symptomatic relief.

Management of RA

The present-day treatment is aimed at:
1. Symptomatic control mainly of pain and stiffness
2. Physical measures to prevent deformities and disabilities and to preserve joint function. It is emphasized that physical therapy and rehabilitation are a must, are complimentary and do not replace medical therapy. Physicians add years to life, whereas physiotherapists add life to years
3. Control/suppression of immuno-inflammation for arresting progressive joint damage
4. Prevention of complications
5. Surgical intervention for correcting the joint deformities

NSAIDs in RA

It is a group of chemically diverse compounds that block the enzyme cyclooxygenase (COX), the key enzyme involved in prostaglandin synthesis, thereby exerting antiinflammatory and analgesic effects. These are used as first line agents in rheumatoid arthritis (RA). These are effective in controlling pain, swelling and morning stiffness, without any effect on progression of disease.

Controlled studies have failed to show any particular NSAID to be more effective than any other NSAID. Frequently a long acting NSAID is employed at bed time to provide relief in morning stiffness.

Gastrointestinal (GI) effects are the commonest NSAID associated side effects that include nausea, dyspepsia and abdominal pain. These are seldom serious. Serious side effects like GI perforation, ulceration and bleeding are not uncommon. Risk Factors for NSAID gastropathy include age > 65 years, smoking, concomitant steroid therapy and cardiovascular disease. In patients with impaired renal function, administration of even a single dose of conventional NSAID can lead to precipitous fall in glomerular filtration rate. If they are given for long time, they may produce fluid and sodium retention, hypertension, analgesic nephropathy, blunting of diuretic effects, hyperkalaemia and irreversible renal damage.

Studies have shown that COX enzyme exists as at least two distinct isomers that are structurally and functionally distinct labeled COX-1 and COX-2. COX-1 ixoenzyme is expressed at all sites of body function, the COX-2 is expressed on mobile pro-inflammatory cells.

This discovery has led to the hypothesis that selective inhibitors of COX-2 would block inflammation without blocking of COX-1 dependent normal physiological house keeping prostaglandins. Meloxicam, nabumetone, etodolac and nimesulide are preferential COX-2 inhibitors and celecoxib and rofecoxib are highly selective inhibitors of COX-2.

The pharmacology of NSAIDs (simple analgesic such as aspirin and paracetamol, other NSAIDs such as ibuprofen, indomethacin and piroxicam etc. is described elsewhere in this chapter.

COX-2 - selective drugs claim to improve therapies (as anti-inflammatory) while protecting the GI tract. Rofecoxib is banned.

Meloxicam in the dose of 7.5 and 15mg daily is as effective as piroxicam and naproxen in the treatment of RA. Similarly, celecoxib at 200mg twice daily has been shown to be equally effective as naproxen and diclofenac in RA.

However, the renal side effect profile of COX-2 inhibitors is expected to be similar to conventional NSAIDs.

Although newer and safer NSAIDs (COX-2 inhibitors) are now available but they alone only control the symptoms of the disease. Therefore treatment with disease modifying anti-rheumatoid drugs (DMARDs) along with NSAIDs has shown significant benefit as compared to those treated with NSAIDs alone.

Disease modifying anti-rheumatoid drugs (DMARDs)

They are classed such to point out the comparison with the NSAIDs which reduce the symptoms of RA but do not retard the progress of the disease, some indeed may make it worse.

DMARDs improve symptoms and reduce disease severity in RA. Whether they halt the long-term progress of the disease is controversial, so the term disease modifying is more appropriate.

The main uses of DMARDs are (i) to slow the progression of rheumatoid arthritis, (ii) juvenile idiopathic arthritis, and (iii) psoriatic arthritis. The choice depends on personal preference. Efficacy wise almost all DMARDs are equal. It is only in the toxic effects and contraindications in which they differ.

It is thought that most DMARDs inhibit the release or activity of cytokines involved in maintaining the inflammatory process, although other actions may also contribute. Any therapeutic effect may not be apparent for 4-6 months.

Indications of DMARDs

• Persistent signs and symptoms despite appropriate use of NSAID
• Evidence of progressive radiological damage
• Troublesome extraarticular symptoms

The salient features of DMARDs are (i) they should be used early i.e. within 6 months of disease activity, (ii) steroids and DMARDs together are used with the former as a bridge, (iii) the choice of DMARD chiefly depends on their toxic effects, (iv) these are used in conjunction with an NSAID regimen to treat rheumatoid arthritis.

Gold compounds in RA

Gold compounds produce subjective and objective improvement especially in early and aggressive disease, and often arrest at least temporarily, the progression of disease. However, their usefulness is limited in mild as well as in advanced disease.

The efficacy of gold compound in RA is comparable to other DMARDs. However, patients on gold are more likely to withdraw therapy due to adverse effects.

The exact mechanism of the antiarthritis effect is unknown, the best hypothesis is the capacity of gold compound to inhibit the maturation and function of mononuclear phagocytes and T cells.

The clinically used gold preparations are -
• Sodium aurothiomalate (I.M.) : 10 mg in first week, 25mg in second and third week.
• Auranofin (oral) : 6 mg daily.

Aurothioglucose and aurothiomalate sodium are rapidly absorbed after I.M. injection, but absorption is erratic on oral administration. They are given i.m. injection 100mg. as a test dose in first weak, 25mg in second and third weeks and than 25-50mg of aurothiomalate sodium or 50mg of aurothioglucose weekly till a cumulation dose of 1g is given.

Auronofin is more hydrophobic and is absorbed rapidly after oral administration (upto 25%).

The dose is 3-6mg/day in one or two doses.

Toxicity and poor long-term efficacy have led to debate over its place in antirheumatoid therapy. Oral gold preparation is less toxic but also much less effective.

Gold preparation should not be used if the disease is mild and it is also of little use if the disease is advanced.

Adverse effects

In about 15% of the patients, the common toxic effects involve skin (simple erythema to severe exfoliative dermatitis) and mucous membranes, particularly of the mouth (stomatitis, pharyngitis, tracheitis, gastritis, colitis, vaginitis, glossitis).

In areas of skin and mucous membranes, especially exposed to light, a gray-to-blue pigmentation (chrysiasis) may occur.

In about 5% of patients kidney functions may be affected. Transient and mild proteinuria occurs in about 50% of patients, and in 1 to 3% of cases, high albuminuria and microscopic haematuria have also been reported. In some cases gold induced nephrosis may occur.

Gold can also produce blood dyscrasias. Thrombocytopenia (due to accelerated degradation of platelets and/or effects upon bone marrow), leukopenia, agranulocytosis, and aplastic anaemia (rare but often fatal) may also occur.

Auranofin (Ridaura) is better tolerated than injectable preparations and the side effects are less. Proteinuria and incidence of nephrotoxicity may be less than with parenteral preparations.

The other toxic actions of gold preparation may also occur including encephalitis, peripheral neuritis, hepatitis and vasomotor crisis. However, these adverse effects are infrequent.

Contraindications

Renal disease, hepatic dysfunctions, history of infectious hepatitis or haematological disorders, pregnancy and breast feeding.

Concomitant use of antimalarial, phenylbutazone, oxyphenbutazone and immunosuppressants is contraindicated.

Gold is poorly tolerated by elderly patients.

Chloroquine and Hydroxychloroquine in RA

These are slightly less effective than other DMARDs, but as they are generally less toxic and better tolerated, they may be preferred in patients with milder forms of disease. Although chloroquine is more efficacious than hydroxychloroquine, yet hydroxychloroquine is preferred as its toxicity is more easily reversed on stopping treatment.

The mechanism of action is not known. They have been found to reduce monocytes IL-1 thus inhibiting B-lymphocytes.

These drugs should be used cautiously or not at all in the presence of hepatic disease or severe gastrointestinal, neurological or blood disorders.

Prolonged use of these drugs causes side effects such as blurring of vision, headache, diplopia, skin eruptions, bleaching of hair, widening of QRS interval and T wave abnormalities.

The major toxicity is ocular toxicity. They are deposited in cornea and the pigment epithelium of the retina. Mild maculopathy is reversible but severe retinopathy may advance even after stopping of drug and leads to permanent loss of vision. The general recommendation is that ophthalmological examination should be done every 6 months.

400 mg/d of hydroxychloroquine and 310 mg base per day of chloroquine are given for 3 months then 200 mg/day of hydroxychloroquine and 155 mg/day of chloroquine are given. In about half the patients, clinical benefits can be noted in 6-12 weeks, these drugs should be withdrawn if there is no effect.

Hydroxychloroquine is less efficacious than gold but is preferred in milder nonerosive cases.

Dose: 200-400mg/daily

Side effects include retinopathy, corneal deposits, rashes, graying of hair, myopathy and neuropathy. However, there is less risk of ocular toxicity than with chloroquine.

Penicillamine

It is a chelating agent. Its mechanism of action in RA is not understood. But it is useful, orally effective alternative to gold. It is indicated in mild, early and nonerosive disease. It is less effective than gold.

Enthusiasm for penicillamine has been curtailed by a high incidence of adverse effects, although better tolerability than gold or antimalarials has been reported if the dose is limited to 500mg daily or less.

Dose: 125-200 mg/d

Adverse effects

It includes nausea, anorexia, loss of taste sensation, proteinuria. It is more likely to produce serious toxicity including skin rashes and bone marrow depression.

Sulphasalazine in RA

It is commonly a first choice DMARD specially in the milder forms of rheumatoid arthritis. Its mode of action in RA is not yet clear. It is reported that it can scavenge toxic oxygen metabolites produced by neutrophils.

Sulphasalazine is a combination of sulphapyridine with a salicylate which is split into its component parts by bacteria in the colon.

Efficacy of sulphasalazine in RA has been shown in terms of clinical parameters (pain, morning stiffness and synovitis) and biological parameters i.e. cytokine levels (decrease TNFa). Radiographic progression is less with sulphasalazine as compared to hydroxychloroquine.

Dose: 1-3g/d in 2-3 portions.

Adverse effects

Nausea, vomiting, dyspepsia and abdominal pain, headache, irritability, depression, and dizziness. Other adverse effects reported are haemolytic anaemia, megaloblastic anaemia, aplastic anaemia and agranulocytosis (rare).

Other side effects may include systemic lupus erythomatosus (SLE) like illness and male sterility. These are usually reversible.

Immunosuppressants in rheumatoid arthritis

These are reserved for those cases who are refractory to the conventional treatment (rest, physiotherapy and NSAIDs).

Methotrexate in RA

Many rheumatologists consider methotrexate to be a first choice DMARD, although the risk of hepatotoxicity remains a concern.

It is a pro-drug and is metabolized intracellularly to long-lived active methotrexate polyglutamate. A spectrum of enzymatic inhibition occurs and there is an increase and release of adenosine which mediates anti-inflammatory effects via action on adenosine receptors.

Methotrexate-therapy takes several weeks to produce therapeutic effect in RA. Maximum effect reaches after several months. Withdrawal leads to RA flares, seen 3-4 weeks after drug discontinuation.

Methotrexate is generally given orally or SC/IM once weekly. Starting at 5 to 7.5 mg per week it is increased by 2.5 to 5 mg over 1-2 months until disease is controlled or limiting side effects occur. The maximum dose is 30 mg/week.

Methotrexate can improve disease activity when given once weekly in doses too small to produce systemic immunosuppression and in these doses adverse effects are usually mild.

Recent data suggest that treatment with a combination of DMARDs is more effective than monotherapy. Leflunomide, etanercept, infliximab, cyclosporin, and sulphasalazine use in combination with methotrexate, are more effective than methotrexate alone.

Adverse effects

Ulcerative stomatitis (10%) which may persist for days to weeks. Glossitis, gingivitis, minor oral ulcers, nausea, vomiting, diarrhoea, anaemia and intestinal perforation are dose dependent and usually appear soon.

Folic acid or folinic acid can reduce the toxicity, of methotrexate without reducing efficacy.

Drug interactions

Steroids should be given 12 hours apart from methotrexate as they may decrease uptake of methotrexate. NSAIDs/salicylates should be avoided as they may increase toxicity of methotrexate. Cyclosporin may increase renal toxicity. Sulphonamides and trimethoprim may increase haematologic toxicity. Tetracycline can decrease absorption of methotrexate. Hepatotoxic and nephrotoxic drugs should be avoided.

Contraindications

- Hypersensitivity to methotrexate
- Preexisting bone marrow depression
- Alcoholic liver disease
- Concurrent alcohol intake
- Severe renal or hepatic impairment
- Preexisting severe pulmonary impairment

Azathioprine

It has steroid sparing and disease modifying effects.

It has a slow onset of action, peak effect reaches around 4-6 months but the effect lasts for longer period of time.

It is used in some patients with severe disease who have failed to respond to other drugs.

Dose: 2-2.5mg/kg/day.

The main side effect of azathioprine are bone marrow depression, GI intolerance and infections.

Cyclosporin

It (2.5-5mg/kg/d) is effective in rheumatoid arthritis. However, it may damage kidney particularly in patients who are taking NSAIDs concurrently. It is reserved for refractory disease.

Cyclophosphamide

It is as effective as azathioprine and may be superior to IM gold and may retard the bone destruction as well. But the efficacy/toxicity ratio is a serious concern in the use of this agent in the long term treatment of non malignant disease like RA.

Recently, the immunosuppressant leflunomide and the cytokine modulators adalimumab, infliximab, etanercept and anakinra have been introduced for the treatment of rheumatoid arthritis.

Leflunomide, a pyrimidine pathway inhibitor has shown promising results in RA. It is a immuno-modulatory pro-drug. It converts into its active metabolite A77 1726 (teriflunomide) which is responsible for the majority of the in vivo activity. It has immunosuppressant and antiproliferative properties used as DMARD in the treatment of active RA and also used in the treatment of active psoriatic arthritis. The active metabolite inhibits dihydro-orotate dehydrogenase and protein tyrosine kinase C activity and thereby inhibit the rapidly proliferating lymphocytes.

Leflunomide is equally efficacious to sulpha-salazine and methotrexate in RA. However, it exerts an early onset of action as compared to sulpha-salazine and methotrexate and the effects last for a prolonged period of time. It has also been observed that this drug reduces functional disability to a greater extent as compared to sulphasalazine and metho-trexate. It appears to be a suitable alternative to methotrexate or sulphasalazine in RA.

The absence of major haematolgical, renal and liver toxicity with leflunomide monotherapy suggests that it may assume the position of second-line therapy after methotrexate.

Dose: Adult (usual):

Loading dose 100mg orally daily for 3 days, maintenance dose is 10-20mg orally daily in RA and 20mg once daily in psoriatic arthritis, may reduce dose to 10mg daily if higher dose not tolerated. It can be administered with or without food. Safety and effectiveness is not established in paediatric patients.

Contraindications

- Hypersensitivity to leflunomide.
- Pregnancy or women who may become pregnant (as teratogenic in animals).

Precautions

- Severe liver injury
- Use not recommended for patients with pre-existing liver impairment or evidence of hepatic infection.
- Use not recommended for patients with severe immunodeficiency, bone marrow dysplasia or severe uncontrolled infection.
- Renal insufficiency; free fraction of primary metabolite increased.

Adverse effects

Common

Alopecia, diarrhoea, increased liver enzymes, rash, GI disturbances, headache, weight loss, dry skin, dizziness, joint disorders.

Serious

Bronchitis, respiratory infection, hepatotoxicity, hepatic failure (rare), hypertension, leucopenia, pancreatitis, and severe infection including fatal sepsis have been reported. Few cases of Stevens - Johnson syndrome have been reported.

Caution

Use of leflunomide with other hepatotoxic and haematotoixc drugs should be avoided.

Change in approach

Until recently, the routine course of therapy was to treat patients with NSAIDs and to begin treatment with DMARDs when they showed radiological signs of joint damage. A major change in approach has taken place. Rheumatologists have started treatment with DMARDs early, when possible, before joint damage and loss of function can occur. It has been recommended that DMARD therapy be initiated not later than 3 months after diagnosis if the patient has on going joint pain, morning stiffness, fatigue, synovitis or persistent elevation of erythrocyte sedimentation rate (ESR) and C-reactive protein levels. Recent study has shown that early, consistent DMARD use can improve long-term functional outcome in rheumatoid arthritis. Early introduction of DMARDs in the course of the disease has been shown to have a better long term out come as compared to the delayed commencement of DMARDs (as little as 8 months delay).

It is now clear that irreversible joint damage commonly occurs early in the disease and rheumatologists generally add a DMARD shortly after RA has been diagnosed. U.S. guidelines recommend that DMARD is started within 3 months of diagnosis for patients not controlled by NSAIDs, although immediate treatment is recommended for those who present with persistent synovitis and joint damage.

Cytokine modulators (Biological response modifying drugs) in RA

Among the biological agents that have been evaluated in clinical trials, inhibitors of tumour necrosis factor alpha (TNF-Alpha) have shown perhaps the greatest promise as potential therapeutic agents for RA.

However, these agents are not appropriate with active disease who have insufficient response to methotrexate which is considered the standard for RA treatment. Patients with RA who have serious infection or malignancy, the use of anti-TNF therapies is not advised.

Understanding in the basic pathogenesis in RA have increased, the key players have identified as activated macrophages and T-cells and more importantly their released products, cytokines which are the main mediators responsible for the inflammation of the synovial membrane and cartilage and underlying bone damage.

Hence, targeted biological therapies which will neutralize the disease process have become possible.

Studies carried out on rheumatoid synovial tissue culture showed that TNF alpha is the pivotal cytokine amongst the many cytokines expressed in the synovial membrane and fluid and blocking TNF by its monoclonal antibody administration in collagen induced arthritis caused not only down regulation of all the pro-inflammatory cytokines, such as IL-1, IL-6 and TNF-Alpha but also amelioration of joint inflammation in collagen induced arthritis. This is the basis of anti TNF blockage using biological agents in patients with RA.

ADALIMUMAB

Adalimumab is a monoclonal tumour necrosis factor antibody used or along with methotrexate or other disease-modifying antirheumatoid drugs in the treatment of rheumatoid arthritis unresponsive to the latter alone.

It is given by subcutaneous injection in a dose of 4mg every other week; some patients not receiving methotrexate may benefit from increasing the dose to 40 mg every week.

Adverse effects, interactions and precautions are similar to infliximab.

INFLIXIMAB

It is one of the novel therapeutic agents that stops the progression of RA. It is chimeric IgG monoclonal antibody to tumour necrosis factor (TNF), a proinflammatory mediator. It is 75% human and 25% mouse protein, the mouse protein contains the binding site for TNF-a, whereas the human portion is responsible for effector function.

It is indicated in rheumatoid arthritis (in combination with methotrexate). It is a biologic response modifying agent for RA.

Dose: 3 mg/kg I.V. over 2 hours given at weeks 0, 2, 6 then every 8 weeks, thereafter, in combination with methotrexate. It is withdrawn if there is no response with 3 months of starting treatment. If signs and symptoms of RA recur, it may be given if within 16 weeks of the last infusion.

Safety and effectiveness in paediatric patients have not been established.

Contraindications

- Hypersensitivity to infliximab or murine products.
- Patients with moderate to severe congestive heart failure.

Adverse effects

Infliximab may cause **acute infusion reactions** during or within 1-2 hours: fever, chills, pruritus, urticaria, dyspnoea chest pain hypertension or hypotension.

Common adverse effects

Abdominal pain, nausea, vomiting, diarrhoea, fatigue, dizziness, headache and back pain.

Infections are common in patient treated with infliximab or other drugs that inhibit TNF, most often affect the upper respiratory tract and the urinary tract.

Delayed reactions

These have occurred 3 to 12 days after infusion: myalgia, arthralgia, fever and rash.

Serious

- Delayed hypersensitivity reaction
- Worsening of congestive heart failure
- Invasive fungal infections, opportunistic infections, tuberculosis
- Lupus - like syndrome has occurred rarely, treatment should be dicontinued if it develops.

ETANERCEPT

It is a recombinant version of soluble human tumour necrosis factor (TNF) receptor that binds specifically to TNF and blocks its interaction with endogenous cell-surface, TNF receptors.

It is a tumour necrosis factor binder.

Indications

- Ankylosing spondylitis, reduce signs and symptoms.
- Plaque psoriasis
- Active and progressive psoriatic arthritis

- Rheumatoid arthritis, may be used in combination with methotrexate.
- Polyarticular juvenile idiopathic arthritis.

Dose in rheumatoid arthritis (RA): 50 mg SC weekly, given as two 25 mg injections in one day or separated by 72 to 96 hours. If there is no response after 3 months, treatment is discontinued.

Juvenile (JRA) (4-17 years): 0.8mg/kg/week (max. 50mg/week) SC given as one or two injections (maximum 25mg per injection) in one day or twice weekly given 72 to 96 hours apart.

Contraindications

- Hypersensitivity to etanercept or components
- Active infections including chronic or localized infections including sepsis.

Precaution

- Discontinue if serious infection/sepsis occurs with treatment
- Poorly controlled or advanced diabetes (risk of infection)
- Concurrent, active, chronic or localized infection
- Concurrent immunosuppressive therapy
- May increase risk of malignancy

Adverse effects

Injection site reactions: erythema, itching, pain or swelling.

Common

Abdominal pain, nausea, vomiting, headache, dizziness, dyspepsia asthma

Serious

- Allergic reactions (< 2%)
- Infections including sepsis
- Anaemia, leukopenia
- Aplastic anaemia
- Tuberculosis
- Optic neuritis (rare)

It has been recommended to prescribe the anti TNF antibody at a dose of 3 mg/kg I.V. along with methotrexate, It should be given at interval of 2 months. If there is no response after 3 infusions, it is best not to repeat the agent.

The result of etanercept in patients with RA is similar to that of infliximab in a dose of 25mg subcutaneously twice a week, methotrexate is able to maximize the effect of etanercept.

Recombinant IL-1, receptor and monoclonal antibody to IL-6 have been tried (but only in small number of patients) with encouraging results.

ANAKINRA

Anakinra is a recombinant receptor antagonist of interleukin-I, an inflammatory mediator found in the plasma and synovial fluid of patients with rheumatoid arthritis.

The usual dose is 100mg once daily by subcutaneous injection.

Anakinra is used for the treatment of the signs and symptoms of moderate to severely active rheumatoid arthritis in patients who have had an inadequate response to methotrexate or another DMARD alone. In the U.K. it should only be given with methotrexate, however, in USA it may be given either alone or with another DMARD although not one which inhibits tumour necrosis factor.

Adverse effects and precautions

Mild to moderate injection site reactions with symptoms of erythema, bruising, swelling and pain are common. Other reactions include headache, nausea diarrhoea and abdominal pain. Rashes have been reported rarely. Upper respiratory tract infections have been reported. Serious infections have also occurred in patients with asthma. Blood dyscrasias, especially neutropenia have been reported rarely.

Interactions

Live vaccines should not be given with anakinra as its effect on vaccine efficacy or the risk of infections transmission is unknown.

The risk of serious infection and neutropenia is increased when anakinra and etanercept (or other TNF antagonists) are used together.

Besides anticytokine inhibitor, another approach is to use monoclonal antibody against CD4 molecule on the surface of T-cells. The activated T-cells are crucial in the pathogenesis of rheumatoid synovitis.

Its administration leads to lymphopenia but reduced inflammatory parameter in a limited trial.

The biological agents are available but they are very expensive. Long term safety of anti-TNF agents is yet not known.

The doses schedule needs to be optimised. Despite these considerations anti-TNF agents constitute a major therapeutic advance.

Choice of DMARDs

The choice depends on the severity of diseases. For mild disease, hydroxychloroquine, sulphasalazine and auranofin may be used as monotherapy.

For a moderately severe disease the choice would be low dose methotrexate, leflunomide and low dose cyclosporin as monotherapy. Systemic steroids may be used as "bridge therapy". Sodium aurothiomalate and d-penicillamine are also occasionally used for this category.

For severe disease, combination of DMARDs is recommended. In addition, some recommend administration of low-dose of prednisolone (7.5 mg/d) to the treatment regimen for severe RA.

Strategies for combining DMARDs include –

1. Step-up: start with single agent and then add others as and when needed.
2. Step-down: Start with 4 DMARDs achieve remission and then withdraw one drug at a time, leaving one DMARD at the end for maintenance of remission.
3. Parallel: Combine multiple agents from the start and continue on long-term basis.

Adjuvant Drugs

Corticosteroids

Steroids: These are very potent and useful drugs in rheumatoid arthritis, but their role is riddled with controversy. The role of steroids in rheumatoid arthritis can be described as –

(a) As an antiinflammatory agent: Low dose steroids with prednisolone (5mg/day in females and 7.5 mg/day in males) should be added if patients do not respond despite maximum tolerated dose of NSAIDs.

(b) Steroids act as antiinflammatory agent till the disease modifying antirheumatoid drugs

(DMARDs) start effects. As bridge therapy oral prednisolone should be started at 15 mg/day for one month and rapidly tapered to 10mg or less after 1 month. Steroids may or may not be continued after this bridge phase.

(c) Special indication: Steroids are the drugs of choice and first line agents in :

   (i) pregnant women with rheumatoid arthritis

   (ii) rheumatoid vasculitis (high dose 1mg/day), steroids with cyclophosphamide is indicated

   (iii) ocular disease and (iv) in elderly patients and in patients with mild to moderate renal insufficiency, low dose steroids are safe.

The most serious side effects of steroids is osteoporosis and a decrease in bone mass. The other side effects are gastritis, cataracts, hypertension.

Glucocorticoids provide quick and dramatic relief of symptoms. But they should be used judiciously and intermittently only for the periodic or acute inflammation. If they are used for chronic inflammation over prolonged periods they can have devastating ill-effects involving almost all the organ-system in the body.

Glucocorticoids do not arrest progress of rheumatoid arthritis. They are used only as adjuvants to other therapeutic agents.

They are indicated in few cases who do not respond to NSAIDs or the disease modifying drugs.

Dexamethasone or betamethasone 1.5 mg daily is sufficient.

In few cases if there is severe pain, swelling and immobility, single intra-articular injection of glucocorticoid may be given. It gives relief for a few weeks. Not more than 2-3 injections per year are recommended.

Adverse effects include (i) endocrine disturbances (moon face, truncal obesity, hirsutism, impotence, menstrual irregularities); (ii) GI (peptic ulcer); ocular (glaucoma, posterior subcapsular cataract); neurological side effect (psychosis); CVS (hypertension).

Future Developments

• New potential immunosuppressants are being investigated which include brequinar sodium, mizoribine and monoclonal antibodies.

• 5-lipoxygenase inhibitors that prevent conversion of arachidonate to 5-HPETE and hence inhibit synthesis of all leucotrienes, e.g. zileuton is under clinical trial. They reduce the generation of LTC_4, LTD_4 and LDE_4. Combined with suitable cyclo-oxygenase inhibitors, they may manifest many of the anti-inflammatory effects of glucocorticoids without the adverse effects of steroids.

• Cytokine targeted therapies and new biological response modifiers are being tried and coming on line. Cells involved in inflammatory response are mainly T-cells and macrophages secreting leucotrienes and TNF Alpha. Anticytokines and T-cell depleting agents therefore hold key to the treatment of rheumatoid arthritis in future.

• Many PDE_4 (Phosphodiesterase) inhibitors are under test as anti-inflammatory drugs.

• Stem cell transplants and gene therapies as treatment modalities are in experimental stage.

Matrix metalloproteinases

Matrix metalloproteinases (MMPs) are zinc dependent endopeptidases, which are capable of collectively degrading all kinds of extracellular matrix proteins.

MMPs can be divided into three general groups. Group one consists of collagenases, among which MMP-1 is particularly important in RA. Group-2 consists of gelatinases, and group 3 of stromelysin-I or metalloproteinase-3 (MMP-3).

MMPs are induced by numerous inflammatory stimuli, including IL-1Alpha and - Beta, platelet derived growth factor, endothelial growth factor (EGF), tumour necrosis factor alpha (TNF-alpha), urea crystals and even generalized phagocytosis.

Stromelysin-I or metalloproteinase-3 (MMP-3) is an enzyme capable of degrading many components of the extracellular matrix and has recently emerged as being of potential interest for the diagnosis and management of rheumatoid arthritis (RA). High levels of MMP-3 have been found in the synovial fluid and in the serum of RA patients, although concentrations are at least 250-fold lower in the latter. Serum MMP-3 levels in RA are correlated with disease activity, some radiological indices, erythrocyte sedimentation rate (ESR) and C-reactive protein levels; supporting the hypothesis that MMP-3 is a sensitive marker of the cytokine-driven local inflammation in this disease. However, elevated serum levels of MMP-3 are not specific for RA or for erosive joint diseases, as they have also been found in reactive arthritis (ReA) and in gout. Data show that MMP-3 levels in synovial fluid are elevated in all inflammatory arthropathies, whether acute or chronic and whether erosive or not, and correlate with all of the inflammatory variables. MMP-3 in synovial fluid is therefore a potential candidate for the assessment of the joint inflammatory process.

Matrix metalloproteinase inhibitors (MMPIs)

MMPIs may inhibit metalloproteinases by inhibiting enzyme activity, enzyme synthesis and enzyme release.

Some MMPIs are effective in RA. Their toxicities include GI toxicity, sun sensitivity and rare systemic lupus erythematosus like syndrome.

Although MMPIs development has been ongoing for a number of years, problems with immunogenicity, bioavailability, high clearance rates and distribution into cartilage have all prevented their rapid development. Recently some of these difficulties seem to have been overcome, as active development of MMPIs continues.

Presently available MMPIs: anthracycline antibiotics such as tetracycline, minocycline and doxycycline.

These antibiotics inhibit MMP-1 (interstitial collagenase) MMP-2 (gelatinase A) and MMP-3. They may work by chelating metal ions on the MMP molecule. This mechanism of action is independent of their mechanism of action as antibiotics.

Doxycycline, at subantimicrobial doses inhibits MMP activity, and has been used in various experimental systems for this purpose.

Minocycline can produce modest beneficial effects in patients with advanced RA, but the clinical significance of these improvements has been questioned.

Continued treatment with minocycline may reduce the need for DMARDs.

Despite the advances in the introduction of newer and safer NSAIDs (COX-2 inhibitors) as well as the changed approaches to the use of DMARDs, the therapy in rheumatoid arthritis is far from optimum.

Therefore search for newer modalities continues. The newer drugs include leflunomide, mycophenolate mofetil, iminocyclines and biological response modifiers like TNF-Alpha antagonist mainly etanercept and infliximab.

STUDY QUESTIONS

1. What is the aim of therapy in rheumatoid arthritis?
2. Which drugs are useful in arthritic conditions?
3. What is the role of simple analgesics, NSAIDs and corticosteroids?
4. Discuss the status of gold preparation in rheumatoid arthritis.

GUIDE TO FURTHER READING

Bomalaski, J.S. et al: Phospholipase A2 and arthritis. Arthritis Rheum., 1993; 36:190-198

Bomalaski, J.S. et al: Phospholipase A2 and arthritis. Arthritis Rheum., 1993; 36:190-198.

Brooks, P.M. et al: Tenidap-a new antiarthritic agent. Agents Actions Suppl., 1993; 44:161-163.

Cash, J.M., Klippel, J.H.: Second-line drug therapy for rheumatoid arthritis. N Engl J Med, 1994; 330:1368.

Edmonds, J.P. et al: Antirheumatic drugs: a proposed new classification. Arthritis Rheum., 1993; 36:336-339.

Faulds, D. et al: A review of its pharmacodynamic and pharmacokinetic properties and therapeutic use in immunoregulatory disorders. Drugs, 1993; 45:953-1040.

Friedel, H.A. et al: Nabumetone: a reappraisal of its pharmacology and therapeutic use in rheumatic diseases. Drugs, 1993; 45:131-156.

Fries, J. F et al: the relative toxicity of disease modifying antirheumatic drugs. Arthritis Rheum, 1993; 36:297.

Harris, E.D., Jr: Rheumatoid arthritis. Pathophysiology and implications for therapy N Engl J Med, 1990; 322:1277.

Hellman, D.B.: Arthritis and musculoskeletal disorders. In, Current Medical Diagnosis & Treatment, 1994.

Kavanaugh, A.F. et al: Treatment of refractory rheumatoid arthritis with a monoclonal antibody to intercellular adhesion molecule 1. Arthritis Rheum., 1994; 37:992-999

Kelley, W.N. et al: Textbook of Rheumatology, 4th ed., W.B. Saunders, Philadelphia, 1993.

Kidd, B.L. et al: Neurogenic influences in arthritis. Ann Rheum Dis, 1990; 49:649.

Konttinen, Y.T. et al: Peripheral and spinal neural mechanisms in arthritis with particular reference to treatment of inflammation and pain. Arthritis Rheum., 1994; 37:965-982.

Rainsford, K.O. et al: Inflammation Mechanisms and Actions of Traditional Drugs. Vol. I, Anti-Inflammatory and Anti-Rheumatic Drugs. CRC Press, Boca Raton, FL, 1985a.

Starkebaum, G.: Review of rheumatoid arthritis. Recent developments Immunol Allergy Clin North Am, 1993; 13:273.

Symposium. (Various authors). Arthrotec Investigators Meeting. Drugs, 1993a, 45 Suppl. 1:1-37.

Symposium. (Various authors). Anti-Rheumatic Drugs. Praeger Publishers, New York, 1983a.

Symposium. (Various authors). Sulfasalazine in rheumatic diseases. J. Rheumatol., 1988b, 15 Suppl. 16:1-42.

Todd, P.A. et al: Naproxen. A reappraisal of its pharmacology and therapeutic use in rheumatic diseases and pain states. Drugs, 1990; 40:91-137.

Todd, P.A. et al: Tenoxicam. An update of its pharmacology and therapeutic efficacy in rheumatic diseases. Drugs, 1991; 41:625- 646.

Williams, K.M., Day, R.O., and Briet, S.N.: Biochemical actions and clinical pharmacology of anti-inflammatory drugs. Adv Drug Res, 1993; 24:121.

PREANAESTHETIC MEDICAMENTS

These are given prior to induction of anaesthesia with the following important objectives:

- To decrease anxiety without producing excessive drowsiness
- To provide amnesia for the perioperative period while maintaining cooperation prior to loss of consciousness
- To relieve preoperative pain, if it is present
- To reduce the requirement of an inhalational anaesthetic agents
- To minimize the undesirable side effects associated with some of the general anaesthetic agents (salivation, bradycardia, coughing and postanaesthetic vomiting)

Drugs

- **Sedatives-hypnotics:** Short acting barbiturates e.g. pentobarbital and secobarbital produce sedation. These drugs do not have analgesic, cardiovagolytic, antiemetic and antisecretory properties. However, barbiturates can cause disorientation rather than sedation when the patient is in pain.

- **Antianxiety drugs:** Benzodiazepines are extensively used for preanaesthetic medication.

  Diazepam is used in doses of 5 to 10 mg orally. Its absorption is erratic and unreliable after parenteral administration due to poor solubility in water.

  Lorazepam produces prolonged sedation. The dose is 0.05 mg/kg (maximum 4 mg) intramuscularly. It can also be given orally.

  Midazolam is soluble in water, produces rapid action and has short duration of action. It produces fever side effects. Due to these reason this drug has become popular.

  The dose for preanaesthetic medication is 0.07 mg/kg body weight.

  Benzodiazepines produce sedative-antianxiety effects without any action on circulation and respiration. They do not produce analgesic, cardiovagolytic, antisecretory and antiemetic effects.

- **Analgesics:** Morphine (10-15 mg i.m.) will produce strong analgesic effects. However, it has certain undesirable side effects e.g. constipation and urinary retention. Nausea and vomiting are also not uncommon. Bradycardia and hypotension may occur. Morphine does not produce cardiovagolytic and antisecretory effects and may be even emetic.

  Pethidine (50-100 mg i.m.) is also given as preanaesthetic medication. Pethidine has cardiovagolytic and antisecretory actions. However, it shares all the other disadvantages of morphine.

  Fentanyl 0.05 to 0.10 mg i.m. may be used in some cases because of its short duration of action (1-2 hours).

- **Anticholinergic agents:** Atropine (0.6 mg i.m.) and hyoscine. These drugs possess cardiovagolytic and anti secretory effects, thus prevent bronchial secretions.

  Hyoscine 0.4 to 0.6 mg i.m. is superior to atropine as antisialagogue but less effective in preventing reflex bradycardia and possesses sedative action.

  Glycopyrrolate produces less sedation than

hyoscine and is a more effective antisialagogue and produces less tachycardia than atropine.

The dose is 0.1 mg i.v. which can be repeated at intervals of 2-3 minutes.

- **Antiemetics:** Droperidol and hydroxyzine sometimes are useful for their antiemetic effects.
- Promethazine 50 mg i.m. is antihistaminic with sedative, antiemetic and anticholinergic properties.
- Ranitidine 150 mg or famotidine 20 mg selectively block H_2-receptor for histamine, decreasing gastric acid secretion. The proton pump inhibitor omeprazole is an alternative.

  H_3-blocker ondensetron 4.8 mg i.v. is highly effective in reducing postanaesthetic nausea and vomiting.

  Metoclopramide 10-20 mg i.m. reduces postoperative vomiting.

No single drug can achieve all the above objectives, Hence combination of 2 or 3 drugs is recommended.

The effects of preanaesthetic agents are shown in Table 3.12.

Table 3.12. Effects of preanaesthetic agents

Drugs	Effects
H_2-receptor blockers	
Ranitidine	Antisecretory
Famotidine	
Anticholinergics	
Hyoscine	Antisecretory effect, reduction of vagal
Atropine	bradycardia, cardiac arrest and hypotension, prevention of laryngospasm. Hyoscine has antiemetic and amnesic action
Narcotic analgesics	
Morphine	For pre- and postoperative analgesia,
Pethidine	sedation reduces anaesthetic dose
Anxiolytics	
Diazepam	Anxiety relieved, postoperative amnesia
Lorazepam	
Sedatives	
Promethazine (phenargan)	Relieve anxiety and apprehension, also antiemetic and anticholinergic actions
Paraldehyde	Given rectally in children
Barbiturates	Sedative-hypnotic
Benzodiazepines	Preferred as sedative-hypnotic-anxiolytic

STUDY QUESTIONS

1. What is meant by preanaesthetic medication?
2. What is the objective of administering preanaesthetic medicaments?
3. Which drugs are used for this purpose?
4. Why combination of these drugs is required to be employed?
5. Explain the merits and limitations of the various preanaesthetic medicaments.

GUIDE TO FURTHER READING

Fragen, R.L. et al: Midazolam versus hydroxyzine as intramuscular premedicant. Can. Anaesth. Soc. J., 1983; 30:136-141

Moyers, J.R.: Preoperative medication. In, Clinical Anesthesia. J.B. Lippincott Co., Philadelphia, 1989; pp485-503

Meyers, E.F. et al: Glycopyrrolate compared with atropine in prevention of the oculocardiac reflex during eye-muscle surgery. Anesthesiology, 1979; 51:350-352

Newman, M et al: Midazolam is the sedative of choice to supplement narcotic anesthesia. J. Cardiothorac. Vas. Anesth., 1993; 7:615-619

Oduro, K.A. et al: Glycopyrrolate metholbromide. Comparison with atropine sulfate in anaesthesia. Can. Anaesth. Soc. J., 1975; 22:466-473

Reves, J.G. et al: Midazolam: pharmacology and uses. Anesthesiology, 1985; 62:310-324.

Walsh, J. et al: Premedication abolishes the increase in plasma beta-endorphin observed in the immediate preoperative period. Anesthesiology, 1987; 66:402-405

GENERAL ANAESTHETICS

General anaesthetics produce reversible loss of all sensations and consciousness. The main features are loss of reflexes and sensations and they produce unconsciousness and skeletal muscle relaxation.

The criteria for a desirable general anaesthetic agent are the following:

Induction should be pleasant and fast and recovery should be smooth and rapid.

Should produce good analgesia and adequate skeletal muscle relaxation.

Should have wide margin of safety. There should be no side effects.

These agents should be nonflammable.

Should be non-irritant to respiratory airways.

The general anaesthetics produce an irregular descending depression of CNS. There are four stages which can be observed with the use of ether. These are less likely to be demarcated with newer agents.

Stages of general anaesthesia

Stage 1   Stage of analgesia: The higher cortical functions are depressed but all reflexes are present.

Stage 2   Stage of delirium: The patient is in state of excitement, pupils are dilated but react to light, respiration is rapid and irregular and the muscle tone may be somewhat increased.

Stages 1 & 2 together form the induction phase of anaesthesia.

Stage 3   Stage of surgical anaesthesia: It is divided into four planes.

Plane i   The pupils are constricted and eyeballs are roving.

Plane ii   The eyeballs are fixed centrally. The pupils begin dilating, there is loss of corneal and largyngeal reflexes and skeletal muscles relax.

Plane iii   Pupils are dilated and light reflex is lost. There is marked muscle relaxation.

Plane iv   The pupils are widely dilated, there is shallow abdominal respiration. The anaesthetist never likes to reach this plane.

Stage 4   Stage of medullary paralysis: Patient is at shock level and there is respiratory and circulatory failure. Death results due to respiratory arrest.

General Anaesthetic Agents

Classification

1. Inhalational:
   Gases: Nitrous oxide
   Volatile liquids: Halothane, enflurane, isoflurane, desflurane, sevoflurane

Ether (used when modern facilities are not available)

2. I.V. anaesthetics:
   - Inducing agents: Thiopentone, etomidate, propofol
   - Slowing acting drugs, benzodiazepines (diazepam, lorazepam, midazolam)
   - Neurolept analgesia: Droperidol plus fentanyl
   - Dissociative anaesthesia: Ketamine

Pharmacokinetic aspects of inhalational general anaesthetics

Anaesthetics are small, lipid soluble molecules which cross the alveolar membrane with great ease. The pharmacokinetics of different anaesthetics vary due to their relative solubilities in blood and in fat.

The solubility in different media is expressed as partition coefficients. It is defined as the ratio of concentration of agent in 2 phases of equilibrium.

The speed of induction and recovery depends on following factors:

- Properties of the anaesthetics
  - Blood: Gas partition coefficient i.e. solubility in blood.
  - Oil: Gas partition coefficient i.e. solubility in fat.
- Physiological factors
  - Alveolar ventilation rate.
  - Cardiac output.

The lower the blood: gas coefficient the faster the induction and recovery.

The oil: gas partition coefficient (measure of fat solubility) determines potency and kinetics of distribution in the body.

High lipid solubility tends to delay recovery.

Table 3.13 gives blood: gas and oil: gas partition coefficients of some inhalation anaesthetics and effect on induction and recovery.

GASES

Nitrous oxide

Advantages

- Nonflammable i.e. non-explosive but supports combustion (process of burning).
- Induction and recovery prompt.

Table 3.13. Partition coefficients of some inhalation anaesathetics.

Drug	Partition Coefficient		Induction/ recovery
	Blood: gas	Oil: gas	
Ether	12.0	65	Slow
Halothane	2.4	220	Medium
Nitrous oxide	0.5	1.4	Fast
Enflurane	1.9	98	Medium
Isoflurane	1.4	91	Medium
Desflurane	0.4	23	Fast
Sevoflurane	0.6	53	Fast

- Does not affect respiration, liver and kidneys.
- Does not sensitize myocardium to catecholamines.
- Good analgesic.

Disadvantages

- Weak anaesthetic (about 80% gas with oxygen).
- Inadequate muscular relaxation.
- Supports combustion.
- Risk of bone marrow depression due to inhibition of methionine synthesis with prolonged use.

Ether (diethyl ether)

Advantages

- Safe, potent (10-15% in inspired air).
- Good analgesia, profound skeletal muscle relaxation.
- Does not sensitize myocardium to catecholamines.
- It is not toxic to liver and kidneys.

Disadvantages

- Flammable.
- Slow induction and prolonged recovery.
- Irritating odour, bronchial and salivary secretions are increased.
- Nausea and vomiting during recovery is common.

Halothane (fluothane)

Advantages

- Potent (2-3% concentration).

- Non-irritant or slightly irritant.
- Nonflammable.
- Induction is prompt and recovery fast but slower than cyclopropane.
- Skeletal muscle relaxation is good (more than cyclopropane).
- Sensitization of myocardium to catecholamines but less than cyclopropane.

Disadvantages

- Poor analgesic.
- Renal and hepatic blood flow is reduced.
- Poor skeletal muscle relaxation (less than ether, enflurane and isoflurane).
- Post-operative jaundice can be produced due to liver damage. Hepatitis in 1: 10,000 cases after repeated administration.
- Repeated administration can produce nephrotoxicity as well as liver damage. Post-operative jaundice may occur even after 5-21 days.

Ethyl chloride

Its use as a spray is based on its local anaesthetic action (refrigerating effect). However, it is not commonly used as it may produce tissue necrosis. It is flammable.

Enflurane

Advantages

- Induction and recovery are rapid.
- It is a better analgesic and better skeletal muscle relaxant than halothane.
- It is less likely to sensitize myocardium to adrenaline. Arrhythmias are rare.
- Noninflammable.
- Nonirritant.

Disadvantages

- Respiration is depressed more than halothane.
- Some risk of epilepsy like seizures.

Isoflurane

Advantages

- Induction and recovery are more rapid than halothane. It is one and half times more potent than halothane.

- Noninflammable.
- There is no renal or hepatic toxicity .
- It is less likely to sensitize myocardium to adrenaline than halothane.
- It lacks epileptogenic property.

Disadvantages

- Respiratory depression is prominent.
- Expensive.
- It may precipitate myocardial ischaemia in patients with CAD.

Desflurane and sevoflurane

These are new inhalational anaesthetics :
- They have low lipid solubility in blood and fat
- Induction and recovery are faster (like nitrous oxide)
- They are not much metabolized to fluoride
- More potent than nitrous oxide

Desflurane is chemically similar to isoflurane. However, its lower solubility in blood and fat produces faster induction and recovery (comparable to nitrous oxide). It is not appreciably metabolized, 10% is used for induction.

Desflurane can cause some respiratory tract irritation resulting in coughing and bronchospasm. Sevoflurane resembles desflurane but is more potent and thus less likely to cause respiratory tract irritation. About 3% is metabolized and fluoride levels can be detected. But it is not sufficient to cause toxicity.

Some important features of inhalation anaesthetics are given in Table 3.14.

I.V. ANESTHETICS (NON-VOLATILE ANAESTHETICS)

I.V. anaesthetics act much more rapidly than the fastest acting inhalation anaesthetics. They produce effect in about 20 seconds, i.e. as soon as the drug reaches the brain.

- Commonly used rapidly acting I.V. induction agents:
  - Thiopentone
  - Etomidate
  - Propofol
- Other rather less rapidly acting I.V. induction agents:
  Benzodiazepines such as -
  - Diazepam
  - Midazolam
- Other I.V. agents producing anaesthesia - like effects:
  - Droperidol + fentanyl (neurolept analgesia)
  - Ketamine (dissociative anaesthesia)

Pentothal sodium

Advantages

- Highly lipid soluble, enters brain immediately and is redistributed to muscle and fat leading to recovery of consciousness in 10-15 minutes.
- Nonirritant.
- Produces smooth, pleasant and quick (10-15 seconds) induction.
- Does not sensitize myocardium to adrenaline.

Disadvantages

- Respiratory depression (main disadvantage).
- Metabolized slowly, liable to accumulate in body fat.
- Poor or no analgesic effect.
- Weak muscle relaxant.
- Narrow margin between anaesthetic dose and the dose producing depression of respiratory centre and vasomotor centre.

Table 3.14. Some important features of general anaesthetics

Anaesthetic	Potency	Induction	Muscle relaxation	Heart depression	Inflammable	Liver damage
Ether	Potent	Slow	Good	No	Yes	No
Nitrous oxide	Weak	Prompt	Weak	No	No	No
Halothane	Very potent	Medium	Weak	Marked	No, May occur	
Enflurane	Very potent	Medium	Good	No/slight	No	No

Contraindications

- Allergy to barbiturates
- Severe cardiovascular disease or hypotension
- Dyspnoea or obstructive respiratory disease
- Status asthmaticus
- Hepatic dysfunction

Etomidate is used as an induction anaesthetic

Advantages

- It is a more popular I.V. anaesthetic agent because it has larger margin of safety (preferred over thiopentone.
- More quickly metabolized.
- Less risk of producing CV depression.
- Onset is fast and recovery is also fairly fast.
- No prolonged hangover unlike thiopentone.

Disadvantages

- Poor analgesic.
- More likely to produce involuntary movements during induction, as well as more likely to cause postoperative nausea and vomiting.
- Possible risk of adrenocortical suppression on its prolonged use.

Propofol is an oily liquid, used as 1% emulsion

- More rapidly metabolized than thiopentone.
- Induction in 30 seconds like thiopentone.
- Rapid recovery in about 4 minutes and there is no hangover.
- Does not cause involuntary movements and does not suppress adrenal cortex unlike etomidate.
- This drug can be used as a continuous infusion to maintain surgical anaesthesia.

The other rather less rapidly acting I.V. induction agents are benzodiazepines such as diazepam and midazolam. These are slower in onset and offset than other agents. However, the advantage is that there is less tendency to cause CV and respiratory depression.

Other I.V. agents producing anaesthesia - like effect

Neurolept analgesia

Opioid analgesic, fentanyl (related to pethidine) citrate 0.05mg plus a neuroleptic (potent tranquillizer like haloperidol) droperidol 2.5 mg IV, produces neurolept analgesia. There is intense analgesia without producing unconsciousness. It is a state in which the patient in completely disinterested and detached from environment without loss of consciousness, he is drowsy but cooperative. This state lasts for about 30 minutes. Minor surgical procedures such as endoscopy can be undertaken.

Neurolept anaesthesia

Neurolept analgesia is converted to neurolept anaesthesia by concurrent administration of 65% nitrous oxide and 35% oxygen.

Dissociative anaesthesia

It is a state of sedation, immobility (paralysis of movement) amnesia, and marked analgesia without loss of consciousness, by giving a single drug - ketamine. The other drug is phencyclidine but it produces more euphoria and sensory distortion than ketamine.

Ketamine produces sleep with profound analgesia but without muscle relaxation. It acts in 30 seconds - 1 minute and the effect lasts for about 10 minutes. Dose is 100mg, 500mg / 10ml injection, 2mg/kg I.V. or 10mg/kg I.M. (reflexes are lost, but respiration is not depressed).

Advantages

- Produces effect in 2.5 minutes (slower than thiopentone).
- Effect persists for 15 minutes.
- Good analgesic.
- Less vomiting and hypotension.
- Pharyngeal, laryngeal reflexes slightly impaired so can be given in asthmatic patients (does not induce bronchospasm).
- It lacks overall depressant action.

Disadvantages

- No muscle relaxation.
- Raise of blood pressure, heart rate, intracranial and intraocular pressure.
- Hallucinations, delirium and irrational behaviour may occur during recovery in about 50% of patients.
- Involuntary movements may occur during or following recovery.

Contraindications

- In hypertensives, it may raise B.P. unduly
- Cerebrovascular disease
- Pregnancy (it has oxytocic property)
- Cardiac failure
- Acute or chronic alcoholic intoxication
- Psychiatric disorders
- Increase in IOP
- Barbiturates and diazepam are incompatible with ketamine (not to be used in the same syringe)

These drugs do not have the controllability of inhaled drugs.

Theories of mechanism of action of general anaesthetics

The basic mechanisms by which these agents produce a reversible depression of nervous activity are not clear.

There are a number of theories including the following:

- Lipid theory: Anaesthetics dissolve in the lipid of the cell membrane and affect its physical state resulting in the alteration of the function of the membrane. Anaesthesia occurs due to expansion of volume. The more lipid soluble the anaesthetic, the more potent it will be.
- Hydrate (water theory): Anaesthetic forms anaesthetic - hydrate complex close to the surface of cell membrane.
  This disturbs the function of membrane proteins and interfere with ionic movements.
- Protein theory: Interaction of anaesthetic molecules with hydrophobic domains of various protein molecules affect their function disrupting the normal mechanisms by which the ion permeability of the membrane is controlled.

STUDY QUESTIONS

1. Describe the criteria for a desirable general anaesthetic agent.
2. What are the main signs of different stages of general anaesthesia?
3. What are the advantages and disadvantages of nitrous oxide, ether, halothane, enflurane and isoflurane?
4. What is neurolept analgesia?
5. What is dissociative anaesthesia?
6. Why induction and recovery are slow in case of general anaesthetics who are more soluble in blood?
7. Name the agents which sensitize the myocardium to catecholamines.
8. Name flammable anaesthetic agents.
9. Explain I.V. anaesthesia.

GUIDE TO FURTHER READING

Barden, J.M., Rice, S.A.: Metabolism and toxicity of inhaled anesthetics. In: Anesthesia, 4th ed. Miller RD (editor). Churchill Livingstone, 1994.

Blonin, R.T. et al: Proprofol depresses the hypoxic ventilatory response during conscious sedation and isohypercapnia. Anesthesiology, 1993; 79:1177.

Bovill, J.G. et al: Some cardiovascular effects of ketamine in man. Br. J. Pharmacol, 1971; 41:411P.

Calverly, R.K. et al: Voluntary and cardiovascular effects of enflurane anesthesia during spontaneous ventilation in man. Anesth. Analg, 1978; 57:610.

Elliott, R.H. and Strunin, L.: Hepatotoxicity of volatile anesthetics. Br. J. Anesth., 1993; 70:339.

Harper, M.H. et al: The magnitude and duration of respiratory depression produced by fentanyl and fentanyl plus droperidol in man. J. Pharmacol Exp. Ther., 1976; 199:464.

Johns, R.A.: Endothelium, anesthetics, and vascular control. Anesthesiology, 1993: 79:1381.

Marshall, B.E., Hanson, C.W. and Marshall, C.: Clinical physiology and pathophysiology of the respiratory system in a practical of Anaesthesia London, pp119.

Rebey, P.G., and Smith, G.: Anesthetic factors contributing to postoperative nausea and vomiting. Br. J. Anaesth, 1992; 69:4.

Sakai, T. and Takaori, M. Biodegradation of halothane, enflurane and methoxyflurane. Br. J. Anaesth, 1978; 50:785.

Seyde, W.C., Ellis, J.E. and Longnecker, D.E.: The addition of nitrous oxide to halothane decreases renal and splanchic flow and increases cerebral blood flow in rats. Br. J. Anaesth., 1986; 58:63.

Sweeney, B et al: Toxicity of bone marrow in dentists exposed to nitrous oxide. Br. Med J, 1985; 291:567.

White, P.F.: Ketamine update its clinical uses in anesthesia. Semin Anesth, 1988; 7:113.

Zbinden, A.M., Petersen-Felix, S, and Thomson, D.A. Anesthetic depth defined using multiple noxious stimuli during isoflurane/oxygen anesthesia; II. Hemodynamic Responses Anesthesiology, 1994; 80:261.

LOCAL ANAESTHETICS

Local anaesthetics are chemical agents that reversibly block regeneration and conduction of nerve impulses along sensory nerves when applied to or near nerves in appropriate concentration. They produce a temporary loss of sensation in localized area without loss of consciousness. They will also block motor nerves but in higher concentration than are normally obtained by topical application. Pain, which is carried by smallest fibres, is lost first, followed by touch and temperature sensitivity, pressure which is carried by the largest nerve fibres, is lost last, if at all.

The criteria for an ideal local anaesthetic

- It should be potent. Potency is related to the lipophilic chemical nature of the molecule as it must penetrate the lipid layer of nerve membranes. The more lipophilic, the more potent. Potency also varies with the extent of vasodilatation, which causes the local anaesthetic to be removed before it actually penetrates the nerve.
- Speed of onset of action should be quick. The onset of action of local anaesthetics is related to their physicochemical properties, to the concentration of the local anaesthetic agent and to the pH of the solution. As the pH of the local anaesthetic solution is increased more molecules of local anaesthetic are present in base form.
- It should be effective for a reasonable duration of time. The duration of local anaesthetics depends on the duration they remain bound to the nerve which itself is related to their chemical characteristics, concentration and to the amount of blood flow in the area surrounding the nerve. The duration of action of all local anaesthetics is more related to hydrophobicity, than to lipophilicity and to the intrinsic chemical nature of the drug.
- Non-irritant.
- Should not interfere with the healing process.
- Should not produce an effect on pupillary size, accommodation or intraocular pressure.
- Should not affect other drugs e.g. mydriatics, miotics, cycloplegics, antimicrobials etc.
- Should be available in a sterile and stable solution.

The above qualities differ from one drug to another.

The majority of operations in ophthalmological practice can be undertaken with the help of the local anaesthetic agents. Minor operations of the cornea, conjunctiva, eyelids can be carried out with topical anaesthetic. For extensive ocular surgery local anaesthetics have to be injected, e.g. injection anaesthesia in the form of infiltration of a localized area, blockade of nerve for regional anaesthesia, retrobulbar or peribulbar injection for anaesthesia of the orbit and globe.

Topical or surface anaesthesia means placing or instillation of anaesthetic solution in the conjunctival area or on the cornea or on mucous membranes.

Infiltration anaesthesia is the injection of local anaesthetic in the subcutaneous tissue or between tissue planes to distend that plane and fill it with local anaesthetic to block all the nerves that traverse the plane.

Nerve block refers to making an injection along side or in the fascial plane of major nerves.

Chemistry

These are tertiary amines separated by a bridge of ester or amide linkage of 6 to 9 Angstroms. The linkage gives rise to two major groups, the ester group and the amide group. The tertiary amine has a positive charge in aqueous solution, this end of the molecule has hydrophilic character, the aromatic end is lipophilic. The chemical configuration of these two ends of this molecule influences the potency, onset of action, duration of action, and selectivity.

Local anaesthetics are weak bases made available as salts for reasons of solubility and stability.

The local anaesthetics belong either to:

Ester group e.g. procaine and tetracaine or

Amide group e.g. lidocaine, etidocaine, mepivacaine and bupivacaine.

Structures of some local anaesthetics are shown in Fig. 3.3.

Tetracaine, etidocaine and bupivacaine have additional side chains which change the chemical nature resulting in prolonged action and cardiovascular toxicity.

All local anaesthetics are insoluble in water and unstable in their amine form. But they form soluble

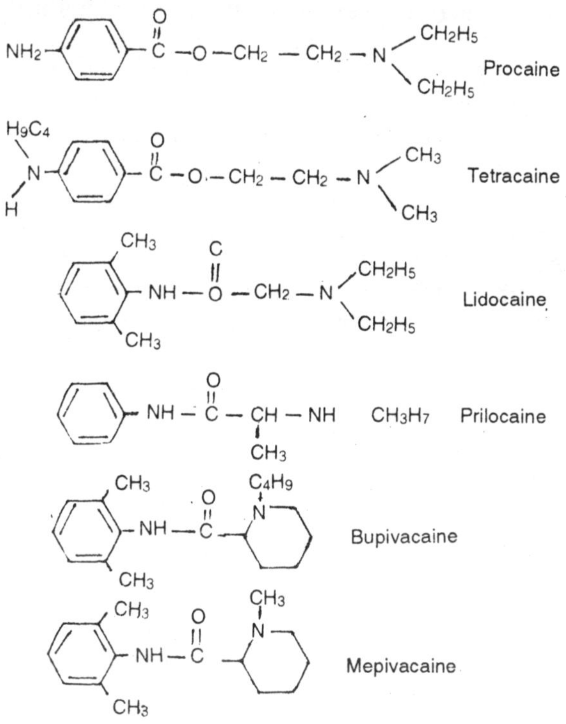

Fig. 3.3. Structural comparison of ester and amide local anaesthetics. If the connecting link between the intermediate group and the aromatic residue is an ester group the plasma pseudocholinesterase hydrolysis it. If the link is an amide bond, hydrolysis occurs in the liver.

salts with organic acids which are stable and can be autoclaved for sterilization.

Esters gradually lose effectiveness with repeated autoclaving, especially tetracaine. They become less stable as the pH is raised, for the same reason, they are bottled with a pH less than 6.5 for prolonged shelf life.

Amide drugs withstand repeated autoclaving. The potency is not decreased if the pH of the solution is kept between 3 and 6.5.

Alkalinization of the acid solution of these salts causes precipitation. Procaine and lidocaine form gradual precipitation, mepivacaine precipitates quickly at pH 7.2 and 2% concentration, bupivacaine and etidocaine form gummy mass rapidly below a pH of 6.9 and in strength above 0.25%.

When local anaesthetics are injected into tissues and tissue fluids, the effective concentration is decreased as agent partitions between cells and fluids. The higher the lipid solubility, the more likely the molecule will enter cells; the higher the water solubility the more will enter plasma and bind to proteins or lipoproteins.

The ester linkage breaks down rapidly by the plasma cholinesterase. The ester local anaesthetic is broken down to inactive products i.e. as the diffusion continues, the concentration is reduced more quickly than amide local anaesthetics which are not broken down during diffusion process. Certain persons may have low or absent plasma cholinesterase and in their case the use of ester local anaesthetics will be hazardous, even a lethal cardiac response. Thus, procaine like cocaine may cause unexpected death.

The ester group of local anaesthetics except propavacaine are hydrolyzed by esterases to paraminobenzoic acid which attaches as a ligand to many proteins and is thought to be highly allergenic. Because of these two demerits, ester local anaesthetics have little place in modern pharmacology except as topical anaesthetics in ophthalmology. The esters benoxinate and tetracaine should be used in the minimum soluble concentration if they are to be used. Proparacaine is not a PABA ester.

The amide group of local anaesthetic are not broken down in the tissues locally or in the blood stream with the exception of prilocaine. Prilocaine induces methaemoglobin formation in the blood stream so it is less than ideal drug. The amides are metabolized in the liver.

Mode of action

Differential sensitivity of nerve fibres

- Different types of nerve fibres differ significantly in their sensibility to local anaesthetic blockade on the basis of size and myelination, the smaller B and C fibres are blocked first, then small type A delta fibers are blocked next. The pain fibres are blocked first, other sensations disappear next and motor function is lost last.
- The smallest unmyelinated fibres which conduct impulses for pain, temperature, and autonomic activity conduct slowly are first to be blocked by local anaesthesia.
- Smaller nerve fibres have smaller critical length.

The critical length is the exposure time required by an anaesthetic to exert its action.

Local anaesthetics have also effect on other excitable membranes, besides nerve cell membranes. But local anaesthetics have weak neuromuscular blocking effect that are of little clinical significance. However, the effect on cardiac cell membranes are important. Some local anaesthetics are useful antiarrhythmic agents.

The nerve membrane is lipoidal and resists passage of cations except at pores known as transmembrane sodium channels. Local anaesthetics block these channels. The block occurs on the inner aspect of the channel, not on the outside of the membrane. The block is due to binding of cationic portion of local anaesthetic to the phospholipid membrane that surrounds the inner openings of the sodium channels resulting in occlusion of the channels which bars sodium entry and prevents axon depolarization. The local anaesthetics should exist alternately in ionized (water soluble) and unionized (lipid soluble) form. During lipid solubility the local anaesthetics traverse the nerve membrane to its interior and becoming ionized, the anaesthetic cation then binds to the inner end of the transmembrane sodium channel. There are million of sodium channel per square millimeter of axon surface. The local anaesthetics block the voltage gated sodium channels preventing opening of the channels and inhibiting their activation. The local anaesthetics diffuse into the axons and when the sodium channels are blocked, the nerve impulse is not propagated. It requires block of 3-7 mm of a myelinated nerve or 2-3 mm of a nonmyelinated nerve to prevent propagation of nerve impulse.

Thus, the local anaesthetics slow the propagation of nerve impulses by reducing the rate of rise of action potential and the rate of repolarisation.

- The conduction of impulse is completely blocked due to increased threshold for electrical excitability.
- Local anaesthetics specifically block nerve conduction by interfering with permeability of cell membrane to sodium, voltage dependent sodium channels. The interference with membrane permeability is explained either by (a) specific receptor theory according to which local anaesthetics displace calcium from a site near sodium channel and then block sodium channel

(b) membrane expansion theory postulates that because of the lipophilic properties of local anaesthetics, they incorporate into the cell membranes. This prevents the opening of the pores resulting in interference or passage of electrolytes.

The large number of Na^+ ions outside the membrane results in an external positive charge. Although there are more K^+ ions inside the cell membrane than outside, there are many more negative ions inside the membrane. This results in a net internal negative charge.

When a cell is at rest, there is considerable difference between the ion concentration outside and inside the plasma membrane. In a resting neuron (one that is not conducting an impulse) there is difference in electrical charges on either side of the membrane. This difference is partly the result of unequal distribution of potassium (K^+ ion concentration inside the cell is about 30 times greater than it is outside). The Na^+ ion concentration is about 14 times greater outside than inside. Another significant factor is the presence of large, nondiffusible negatively charged ions trapped in the cell. These include organic phosphate and protein anions (Fig. 3.4).

Even when a nerve cell is not conducting an impulse, it is actively transporting ions across its membrane. Na^+ ions are actively transported out and K^+ ions are actively transported in. The membrane system by which Na^+ and K^+ ions are actively transported simultaneously is called the sodium potassium pump. The operation of the pump requires the expenditure from ATP. The active transport of Na^+ and K^+ ions is unequal i.e. three Na^+ ions are actively transported out for every two K^+ ions actively transported in.

Nerves also contain a large number of negative ions, including organic phosphate and protein anions on the inside, that cannot diffuse outside or diffuse very slowly. Since sodium ions are positive and are actively transported outside the cells by the sodium potassium pump, a positive charge develops outside the membrane, even though K^+ ions are also positive and are actively transported to the inside of the cell by the sodium potassium pump, there are insufficient K^+ ions to equalize the even larger number of nondiffusible negative ions trapped in the cells. The

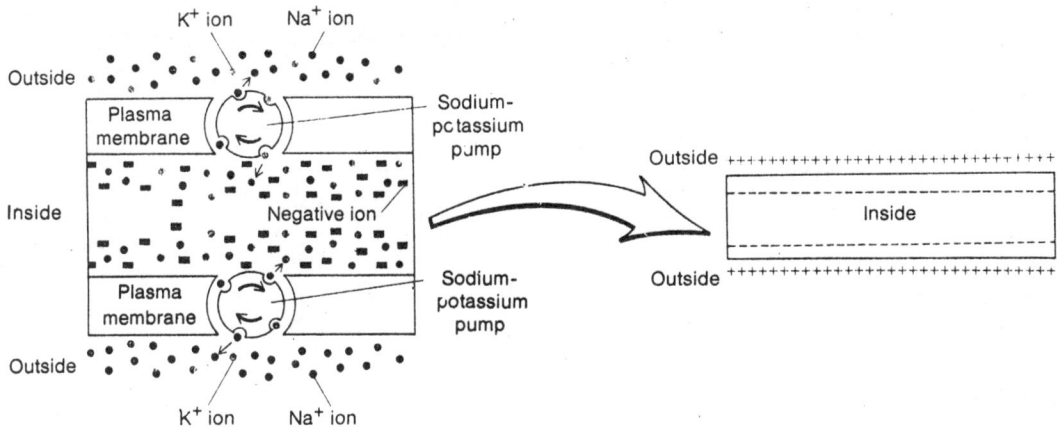

Fig. 3.4. Large number of Na$^+$ ions outside the membrane results in external positive charge. Although there are more K$^+$ ions inside the cell membrane than outside; there are many more negative ions inside the membrane. This results in a net internal negative charge.

sodium potassium pump, not only actively transports Na$^+$ and K$^+$ but also establishes concentration and electrical gradients for the ions. As a result, K$^+$ ions tend to diffuse (leak) into the cell.

Membrane permeability to K$^+$ ions is two times greater than that of Na$^+$ ions. If an excitatory stimulus is applied to a polarized membrane, the membrane permeability to Na$^+$ ions greatly increases at the point of stimulation. What happens is that voltage sensitive sodium channels open and permit the influx of Na$^+$ ions entering than leaving, the resting membrane potential begins to change. This process is called depolarization. Throughout depolarization, the Na$^+$ ions continue to move inside.

Voltage sensitive (gated) channels are ion channels. These channels contain one or more proteins that can undergo alterations in shape and thus function like gates by restricting or permitting the movement of ions. There are voltage sensitive sodium channels and voltage sensitive potassium channels.

Each voltage sensitive sodium channel has two separate gates, an activation gate near the exterior of the channel and an inactivation gate near the interior of the channel. In the resting membrane, the activation gate is closed and inactivation gate is also closed, resulting in inhibition of Na$^+$ ions to the interior of the cell. When a threshold stimulus is applied the voltage-sensitive sodium channels undergo a change from a resting to an activated state. In this state both the activation and inactivation gates

in the channels are open and Na$^+$ ions move inward in sufficient number.

In the resting state, the potassium channel gate is open to some degree, but K$^+$ ions are prevented from diffusing to the exterior (Fig. 3.5).

Systemic absorption of local anaesthetics from site of injection is influenced by:
- Drug tissue binding
- Presence of vasoconstrictor
- Physicochemical and pharmacological properties of the drug

Metabolism of ester group takes place by the plasma cholinesterase. As the hydrolysis is rapid they have short plasma half-lives. The amide type are hydrolysed by liver microsomal enzymes. The hydrolysis occurs in this sequences prilocaine (fastest) etidocaine lidocaine mapivacaine bupivacaine (shortest). The toxic effects of amide group of local anaesthetics are more likely to occur in patients with liver disease, e.g. average half-life of lidocaine may be increased from 1.8 hours in normal patients to over 6 hours in patients with liver disease.

The pharmacokinetic properties of some local anaesthetics are given in Table 3.15.

Individual agents

Cocaine (an alkaloid and ester): Even as a surface anaesthetic sufficient absorption may take place to cause serious adverse effects, although new era was ushered in ophthalmic surgery with the introduction

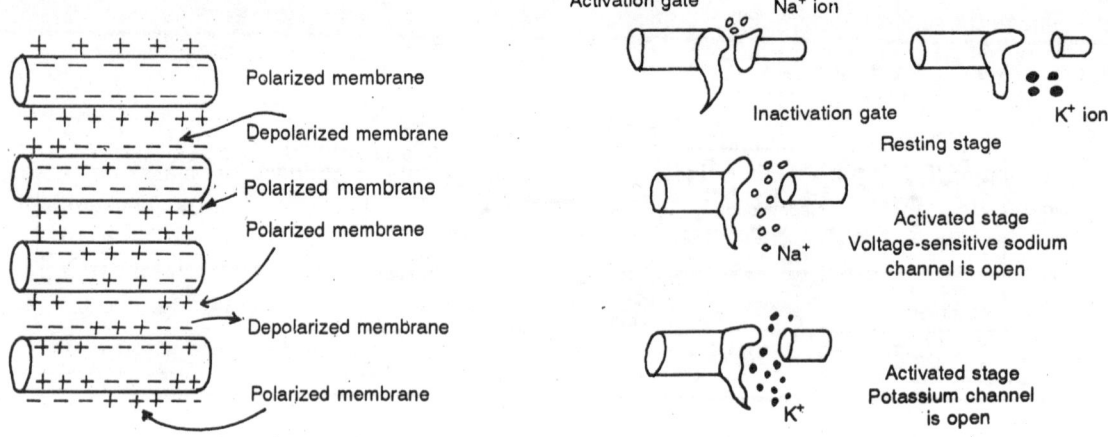

Fig. 3.5. Ion channels.

Table 3.15. Pharmacokinetic properties of some local anaesthetics

Drug	Rate of onset	Duration	Tissue penetration	Plasma half-life
Procaine	Moderate	Short	Slow	30 minutes
Lidocaine	Rapid	Moderate	Rapid	2 hours
Amethocaine	Slow	Long	Moderate	1 hour
Bupivacaine	Slow	Long	Moderate	3 hours
Prilocaine	Moderate	Moderate	Moderate	2 hours

of this first anaesthetic agent in the year 1804 by Koller but soon it was found that on topical application it did not diffuse deeply enough to abolish sensation from iris and did not eliminate pain when muscles were pulled or optic nerve was cut. It was found quite toxic to cornea. It was found very dangerous after giving injection as several deaths occurred. Hence cocaine has now no place as local anaesthetic agent.

Cocaine is so epitheliotoxic to the extent that it can be used to remove corneal epithelium when there is a severe epithelial oedema obstructing the view of the fundus.

Procaine (Novocaine, ester) replaced cocaine and became popular for injection. But it is useless as surface anaesthetic as it is not absorbed through mucous membrane. It has short duration of action after injection as it is rapidly hydrolysed in blood. It is injected in concentration varying from 0.5% to 4.0%.

Lidocaine (xylocaine, lignocaine, amide), is a successful drug for surface as well as for injection,

combining efficacy with comparative lack of toxicity. It has least toxicity on epithelium, produces adequate deep anaesthesia and has long duration of action. It appears an ideal topical ocular anaesthetic agent. It diffuses more readily through tissues so produces a wider area of anaesthesia. Its duration is longer than that of procaine (45 minutes to 1 hour). Most ophthalmic procedures rarely require more than 10-15 mg of solution hence there is a wide margin of safety. Lidocaine is more potent vasodilator than mepiva-caine which may be related to shorter duration of activity, but it has fastest onset of action, onset of corneal anaesthesia occurs within a minute. 1% lidocaine solution produces action for 30 to 60 minutes. It blocks ciliary ganglia when 2% solution is used. A 0.75% solution provides complete block of extraocular muscles in 5-10 minutes and the effect lasts for 45 minutes to 2 hours. A 4% solution provides complete akinesia in 5 minutes in 75% of patients and in 90% in 10 minutes.

Mepivacaine (amide-type) is chosen if there is history of allergy to other anaesthetic agents.

Mepivacaine of the same concentration as lidocaine has slower onset of action but in the orbit effect lasts one and half to two times as long as lidocaine when injected with the same amount of epinephrine. Mepivacaine has vasoconstrictor activity much greater than that of lidocaine or bupivacaine which led to its use in dentistry which will produce vasoconstriction and not require additional epinephrine.

In onset of action it is more rapid and duration about 20% longer than lidocaine. It does not have antiarrhythmic activity unlike lidocaine.

Tetracaine hydrochloride (Pontocaine, Amethocaine) is a derivative of para amino benzoic acid. It is about 10 times more toxic and more active than procaine after intravenous injection. For topical anaesthesia of the eye, a 0.5% solution or ointment is employed; for the mucous membranes of the nose and throat, a 2% solution; for spinal anaesthesia, a total dose of 5-20 mg is enough.

The effects are longer lasting than those of procaine. An ointment (0.5%) and cream (1%) for surface application to skin are available.

Proxymetacaine (proparacaine) is used in eye if it is important not to dilate the pupil e.g. for tonometry. It has greater potency than amethocaine but there is little clinical difference. Onset is 5-20 seconds similar to amethocaine. One drop is instilled every 5-10 minutes until 5-7 drops have been administered, deep anaesthesia is produced as required for cataract extraction. It causes much less stinging and squeezing of eye and is often painless.

Proparacaine 0.5% solution anaesthetizes the cornea and conjunctiva as well as or even better than 4% cocaine and with much less corneal damage.

Benoxinate hydrochloride is less irritating than tetracaine and causes less epithelial damage. One drop of 0.4% solution produces corneal anaesthesia within 60 seconds and the efficacy is similar to that of a 0.5% solution of proparacaine.

Etidocaine (amide) is similar to lidocaine but more potent and has longer duration of action.

Prilocaine (amide) is in general less toxic but it can cause methaemoglobinaemia (due to metabolite) at high doses. Its onset and duration of action are slightly more longer than lidocaine.

Bupivacaine (amide) is structurally similar to mepivacaine but more potent and has longer duration of action than mepivacaine. However, its onset of action is slower than mepivacaine. Its 0.5% concentration is comparable with 2% lidocaine. Its main advantage is prolonged duration of anaesthesia. The disadvantages include slow and unpredictable rate of onset of anesthesia. Bupivacaine's onset of activity is related to concentration, 0.25% is very sensitive to concentration and to the use of epinephrine.

Associated medication: Epinephrine

The concomitant use of a 1 : 200,000 solution of epinephrine with procaine or lidocaine enhances the duration of action. Epinephrine is vasoconstrictor. The anaesthesia is prolonged due to slow drug absorption from the site of injection. The chances of toxic reactions are also diminished because delayed systemic absorption allows more time for the detoxification and excretion. But in the presence of hypertension, cardiovascular diseases or thyrotoxicosis epinephrine should not be given.

Choice

The many agents available are proof that all have disadvantages and that no agent is unchallengeably the best for all occasions.

Choice is based on the duration of action required e.g. procaine and chloroprocaine are short acting. Lidocaine, mepivacaine and prilocaine have intermediate duration of action. Tetracaine, Bupivacaine, Etidocaine are long acting drugs.

The amide local anaesthetics currently employed permit the conjunctiva, the cornea or the whole orbit to be anaesthetized safely and without pain. Injections of local anaesthetic in the mid orbit can anaesthetize the entire globe and all the extraocular muscles if sufficient volume in administered there. The danger of injecting intravenous or intraarterially in the orbit in high concentrations or at high rate of injections has great risk of retrograde flow into the brain and risk of cardiac toxicity out of proportion to the amount of drug injected.

Combination of 2 or more local anaesthetics does not enhance activity beyond that which would be obtained to all equivalent concentration of the stronger drug. The therapeutic index is not improved except when the choice is to produce early onset and longer duration of action, in that case mixtures of injection anaesthetic of lidocaine and bupivacaine may be used.

Local anaesthetic vary most in producing initial stinging. In descending order of comfort they can be listed as following:

- Proxymetacaine (most comfortable)
- Benoxinate
- Lignocaine
- Amethocaine (least comfortable)

Tables 3.16, 3.17 and 3.18 show the percent used, onset, and duration of action of local anaesthetics employed as topical and infiltration anaesthetics respectively.

Table 3.16. Topical anaesthetics used in ophthalmology

Drug	Percent	Onset (min)	Duration (min)
Lidocaine (Xylocaine)	2-4	1	30
Proparacaine	0.5	1	15
Tetracaine	0.5, 1	1	20
Benoxinate (Oxybuprocaine)	0.4	1	15

Table 3.17. Local anaesthetics employed for infiltration

Drug	Percent	Onset (min)	Duration
Lidocaine	1, 2, 4	4-6	40-60 minutes
Lidocaine with epinephrine	1, 2	4-6	1 to 2 hours
Bupivacaine	0.25, 0.5 0.75	5-12	2 to 3 hours
Procaine (Novocaine)	1, 2	7-8	30-45 minutes

Indications for the use of local anaesthetics

Ophthalmological use

Local anaesthetics are instilled a single drop at a time. If required then successive drops are applied.

Foreign body removal: The blepharospasm which accompanies a foreign body makes examina-

Table 3.18. Preparations and uses of local anaesthetics

Local anaesthetic	Preparations	Uses
Cocaine	4-10%	Topical anaesthesia, use limited by abuse potential
Procaine	1-2%	Infiltration anaesthesia
	5-20%	Spinal anaesthesia
Tetracaine	10%	Spinal anaesthesia
	2%	Topical anaesthesia of mucous membranes
Lidocaine	1-2% solution, ointment, jelly or cream	Topical anaesthesia of mucous membranes
	0.5% solution	Infiltration anaesthesia
	< 5% solution	Spinal anaesthesia
Prilocaine	1-3%	Infiltration, regional, and spinal anaesthesia
Etidocaine	0.5-1.5%	Infiltration, regional, and epidermal anaesthesia
Mepivacaine	1-4%	Infiltration, regional nerve block
Bupivacaine	0.25-0.75%	Regional nerve block anaesthesia
Dibucaine	0.2%	Topical anaesthesia of mucous membranes

tion of the eye difficult. A drop of local anaesthetic will make location and removal of foreign body easy.

Tonometry: Topical anaesthesia is essential for the measurement of intraocular pressure.

Contact lens fitting: If initially a local anaesthetic is instilled, the fitting of contact lens can be easily done.

Certain diagnostic procedures can be carried out better if topical anaesthetic is used before hand e.g. Schirmer test of lacrimal function. Certain procedures are impossible without topical anaesthesia. Certainly procedures are made more comfortable for patients and are easier for ophthalmologists.

Local anaesthetics used to anaesthetize mucous membranes and skin: Certain local anaesthetics are irritating or ineffective for application to the eye, but they may be useful on the mucous membranes and skin. They are effective in the symptomatic relief of anal and genital pruritis.

Dibucaine as a cream or ointment for use on the skin is available.

Dyclonine hydrochloride is absorbed through skin and mucous membranes. It can be employed as 0.5% or 1.0% solution for topical anaesthesia during endoscopy and for anogenital procedures.

Pramoxime hydrochloride 1% is a surface anaesthetic agent and well tolerated.

Local anaesthetic used in wounds and ulcerated surfaces: Some local anaesthetics are poorly soluble in water and therefore too slowly absorbed. They remain localized for long time and produce a sustained anaesthetic action when applied directly to wounds and ulcerated surfaces. Benzocaine is one such local anaesthetic. It is incorporated into a number of topical preparations. Although it is too slowly absorbed to be toxic, however, it has been reported to cause methaemoglobinaemia in few cases.

Local anaesthetics used in some surgical procedures: Anaesthesia of mucous membranes of the nose, mouth, throat, tracheobronchial tree, oesophagus and genitourinary tract can be produced by direct application of aqueous solution of salts of many local anaesthetics or by suspension of the poorly soluble local anaesthetics.

Tetracaine 2%, Lidocaine 2% to 10%, and Cocaine 1% to 4% are used.

Local anaesthetics are injected directly into tissue which may include only skin or deeper structures (infiltration anaesthesia). For this purpose lidocaine, 0.5% to 1.0%, procaine, 0.5% to 1.0% and bupivacaine, 0.125% to 0.25% are used.

For nerve block anaesthesia e.g. brachial plexus blocks may be employed for procedures on the upper extremity and shoulder.

Intercostal nerve blocks are effective for anaesthesia of the anterior abdominal wall.

Cervical plexus block is appropriate for surgery of the neck.

Sciatic and femoral nerve blocks are useful for surgery distal to the knee.

For producing spinal anaesthesia, injection of local anaesthetics like lidocaine 1.5 to 5% or tetracaine 0.25-0.5% in 10% glucose (hyperbaric solution) into L2-L3 subarachnoid space is given. It is employed to perform surgical procedures on lower abdomen, pelvis and lower limbs.

Adverse effects of spinal anaesthesia include severe headache, hypotension, nausea, vomiting, rarely septic meningitis and respiratory arrest.

For producing spinal anaesthesia injection in subarachnoid space is given. The drugs most commonly used for this purpose are lidocaine, tetracaine, and bupivacaine. Procaine is used when a short duration of action is desired.

Adverse reactions to local anaesthetics

There is a possibility of both local and systemic adverse effects.

All local anaesthetics depress epithelial oxygen uptake to some extent. Repeated instillation may lead to desquamation of corneal epithelium and eventually loss of vision. Local anaesthetics may be used (rather abused) to remove temporarily the discomfort from the surface of the eye, e.g. the irritation persisting after the foreign body has been removed can lead some people to apply local anaesthetic repeatedly. This may result in exposure keratitis.

Disadvantages of topical anaesthesia include delay in healing processes, initial stinging by some topical anaesthetics and damage from superficial foreign bodies as the surface of the eye is insensitive.

Systemic effects can also be produced by local anaesthetics. In general, the CNS toxicity is stimulation followed by depression. Sometimes fainting or syncope may occur. The first symptom is circumoral or tongue numbness followed by lightheadedness or tinnitus and later on followed by visual disturbances, muscular twitching, convulsions and then unconsciousness. The respiratory arrest occurs at almost twice the concentration that produces unconsciousness. The convulsive activity of local anaesthetic is due to blockade of inhibitors in the brain stem and not by causing a hyperexcitable effect on the motor cortex. Recent studies indicate that barbiturates do not prevent central nervous system toxicity. The benzodiazepines seem to benefit in prevention and treatment of convulsions produced by local anaesthetics.

Myonecrosis may be produced by all local anaesthetics, lidocaine preferentially destroys white fibres and bupivacaine is more toxic to red fibres. At higher concentrations this specificity is lost and all striated muscle is damaged. Restoration of normal function occurs in 2 weeks to 3 months.

Bupivacaine is more cardiotoxic and produces adverse effect on conduction in the heart where its molecules actually enter cardiac cells and only slowly exit. Prilocaine converts haemoglobin to methaemoglobin, 3-5 mg in blood results in cyanosis.

Thus local anaesthetics have adverse effects on:

CNS: Convulsions, if they occur, are treated with i.v. diazepam, oxygenation and other supporting measures. Respiratory failure secondary to CNS depression is a late stage of toxicity.

Cardiovascular system: Hypotension is a late effect due to myocardial depression and peripheral arterial vasodilation.

Local anaesthetics block cardiac sodium channels leading to cardiovascular collapse. Cocaine differs from other agents in its cardiovascular effects. The blockade of norepinephrine reuptake results in vasoconstriction and may also precipitate cardiac arrhythmias.

Allergy to amide local anaesthetics is very rare. However, if ester group of local anaesthetics is used a test injection should be given in the skin to exclude allergy. It is worth mentioning that proparacaine does not break down into PABA, the high allergen.

Local anaesthetics are derivatives of para aminobenzoic acid (PABA) and sulphonamides compete with PABA and thus reduce the antibacterial effect of sulphonamides. It may be, but this antagonism is likely to have little significant effect because the level of sulphonamides is far more than the amount of PABA. Besides this, there will be a time delay in using local anaesthetic and applying the sulphonamide.

Prevention and management of the systemic toxicity is related to minimizing blood concentration which can be achieved by slow injection, avoiding intravascular injection of local anaesthetic.

Preoperative sedation has useful role. Sedatives have been a boon in the hands of some but not in all cases for ophthalmic procedures. Sedatives may make it difficult to determine whether the eye is totally anaesthetized. Sedatives also permit persons to lie in uncomfortable positions.

Thus sedatives do not have a primary place in ophthalmic local anaesthesia except in patients (rare) who are uncooperative for a block. These patients can be better handled with light general anaesthesia in operating room, rather than heavy sedation.

STUDY QUESTIONS

1. Define local anaesthetic agent. What are the qualifications for an ideal local anaesthetic agent?
2. Give examples of local anaesthetics which belong to (i) ester group and (ii) amide group. What are the main differences in characteristics of these two groups?
3. Describe the pharmacokinetics of local anaesthetics.
4. Explain why the use of xylocaine (lignocaine, lidocaine) is preferred to procaine.
5. Is there any advantage of combining 2 or more local anaesthetics? If yes, then how?
6. Compare in a tabulated form the commonly used topical anaesthetics regarding concentrations employed, onset and duration of action.
7. Compare in a tabulated form local anaesthetics employed for infiltration regarding % used, onset and duration of action.
8. Describe the mode of action of local anaesthetics.
9. Explain how the associated medication with epinephrine is useful with certain local anaesthetics. In which situations this combination is not used?
10. Discuss the indications for the use of local anaesthetics.
11. Write notes on (i) mepivacaine, (ii) tetracaine hydrochloride, and (iii) bupivacaine.

GUIDE TO FURTHER READING

Arora, R.B., and Vishweshwar N. Sharma, Local anaesthetic and pharmacological properties of 4n Butoxy B-(1-piperidyl) propiophenone HCl and B-diethyl amino ethyl p-n-Hexyloxy benzilate HCl. Jour. Pharm. & Exp. Therap., 1955; 115:413

Arora, R.B., Counsul, B.N., Sharma, V.N. and Kulshestra, O.P., Clinical trial of Dyclonine in intraocular ophthalmic surgery. The Eye, Ear, Nose and Throat Monthly, 1955; 34:593.

Arora, R.B., Sharma, V.N., Pharmacological investigations of Di- (B-O- methoxyphenylisopropyl) amine lactate, a new bronchodilator and local anaesthetic. Arch. Int. Pharmacodyn. 1956; 104:388.

Arora, R.B., Sharma, V.N., Pharmacology of Pyrollocaine and Bis (O investigations of (B-O- methoxyphenylisopropyl) amine lactate, Two new local anaesthetics. Ind. Jour. Med. Sci, 1956; 19:197.

Carpenter, R.L. and Mackey, D.C. Local anaesthetics. In, Clinical anaesthesia 2nd ed (Barash, P.G., Cullen, B.F., and Stoelting R.K., eds) JB Lippincott Philadelphia, 1992, pp 509-541

Catterall, W.A. Structure and function of voltage and sensitive ion channels. Science, 1988; 242: 50

Catterall, W.A. Cellular and molecular biology of voltage-gated sodium channels. Physiol. Rev. 1992;72:915

Counsins, M.J., and Bridenbaugh, P.O. (eds). Neural blockade in Clinical Anaesthesia and management of pain, 3rd ed. J.B. Lippincott Co., Philadelphia, 1995

Covino, B.G.: Pharmacology of local anaesthetic agents. Br. J. Anaesth, 1986; 58:701.

Drachman, D., Strichartz G. Potassium channel blockers potentiate impulse inhibition by local anesthetics Anesthesiology, 1991; 75:1051.

Fleming, J.A., Byck, R., Barash, P.G.: Pharmacology and therapeutic applications of cocaine, Anesthesiology, 1990; 73:518.

Ison L.L., De Jongh, K.S., and Catterall, W.A., Auxiliary subunits of voltage-gated ion channels. Neuron, 1994; 12: 1183.

Kendig, J.J., Courtney, K.R.: New modes of nerve block. Anesthesiology, 1991; 74:207.

Ragsdale, D.R. et al, Molecular determinants of state-dependent block of sodium channels by local anaesthetics. Science, 1994; 265:1724

Reiz, S. Nath S: Cardiotoxicity of proparavacaine compared to that of bupivacaine, Anesth Analg, 1989; 69:563.

Sharma, V.N., Bronchodilator activity of twelve recently synthesised local anaesthetics, Arch. Int. Pharmacodyn, 1960; 125:304.

Sharma, V.N., and Arora, R.B., The antiveratrinic action of some local anaesthetics, 1962; 14:515.

Sharma, V.N., Quinidine like activity of eight local anaesthetics, Ind. J. Physiol. & Pharmacol., 1962; 6:47.

Singh, K.P. and Sharma, V.N., Bronchodilator action of 5 recently synthesised local anaesthetics, Ind. Jour. Med. Sci., 1959; 13:507.

Stevens, R.A. et al: Back pain after epidural anaesthesia with chloroprocaine. Anaesthesiology, 1993; 78:492

Strichartz, G.R.: Pharmacology of local anaesthetics. In, Anesthesia, 4th ed. Miller R.D. (editor). Churchill Livingstone, 1994.

Tucker, G.T.: Pharmacokinetics of local anaesthetics Br. J Anaesth, 1986; 58:717.

SKELETAL MUSCLE RELAXANTS

Skeletal muscle relaxants can be grouped as:

1. Peripherally acting muscle relaxants which are
   - Neuromuscular blocking agents
   - Directly acting agents
2. Centrally acting muscle relaxants.

At the junction of a motor nerve and the skeletal muscle it supplies, there is a specialized portion of muscle membrane, called motor end-plate which contains the nicotinicreceptors of acetylcholine (ACh). When impulse reaches the nerve ending, ACh is released and permeability to ions of the motor end plate is modified which triggers action potential resulting in the contraction of the skeletal muscle.

1. Peripherally acting muscle relaxants
The neuromuscular blocking agents

Classification of neuromuscular blockers (muscle relaxants)

1. Depolarizing blocking agents: These are agonists at the nicotinic receptors:
   Succinylcholine, decamethonium
2. Non-depolarizing blocking agents (competitive). These act by blocking nicotinic receptors and some cases, also by blocking ion channels).
   - Isoquinoline derivatives:
     d-tubocurarine, metocurare, antracurium, doxacurium, mivacurium
   - Steroid derivatives:
     Rocuronium, pancuronium, vecuronium pipecuronium.

Neuromuscular blocking agents can also be classified according to their duration of action:
   - Long-acting (80-180 min): Pancuronium, pipecuronium, doxacurium, d-tubocurarine
   - Intermediate acting (30-40 min): Atracurium, rocuronium, vecuronium
   - Short-acting (12-18 min): Mivacurium
   - Ultra-short acting (5-10 min): Succinylcholine

Mechanism of action: Neuromuscular blockers act on cholinergic nicotinic receptors of the skeletal muscles at neuromuscular junction.

Pharmacokinetic characteristics of neuromuscular blockers

- They are not absorbed orally, given intravenously.
- They do not cross blood brain barrier, hence they do not produce CNS toxicity.
- They do not cross placental membrane, hence do not affect new born if they are used during caesarean section.
- d-tubocurarine, metocurine an gallamine are not metabolized.
- Steroidal drugs are metabolized in liver, 3-hydroxy metabolite is active.
- Long-acting drugs such as pancuronium, pipecuronium and doxacurium are excreted, mainly through kidney.
- Intermediate acting vacuronium and rocuronium are excreted through bile.
- Atracurium is inactivated by spontaneous breakdown. The breakdown products have no neuromuscular blocking action, but the metabolite can cross blood brain barrier and may produce seizures.
- Mivacurium is metabolized by BuChE, has short duration of action.
- Succinylcholine is metabolized by pseudo ChE.

Depolarizing agents (succinylcholine, decamethonium)

- Like acetylcholine (ACh) these react with nicotinic receptors at the muscle end-plate leading to depolarization of the excitable membrane. This phase I block is seen clinically as fasciculations.
- With prolonged exposure, a reduction in receptor sensitivity occurs leading to phase II block that is not competitive in nature.

Depolarizing blocking agents are also called persistent depolarizers. They cause prolonged depolarization of the motor end plate and prevent any response to ACh. In the presence of prolonged depolarization produced by these drugs there is no further generation of action potential after the initial twitch.

The depolarization agents prolong the normal depolarization process and thus become resistant to further stimulation, e.g. Suxamethonium and Decamethonium. Decamethonium is not used clinically as it is not metabolized and has a long lasting effect.

Anticholinesterases are not only ineffective as antidotes for such drugs but may also increase the paralysis.

Suxamethonium (Succinylcholine chloride) is a short acting (due to rapid metabolic degradation by pseudocholinesterase) neuromuscular blocking drug. The onset of action is 1 to 1.5 minutes and the duration of action is for 5 to 10 minutes.

Muscle fasciculations for several seconds precede relaxation. If plasma pseudocholinesterase is deficient, recovery from paralysis is prolonged.

Uses

Suxamethonium is used to produce muscle relaxation just after induction of anaesthesia to facilitate rapid tracheal intubation. It can also be used to protect against severe convulsions in electroconvulsive therapy.

Facilities for artificial respiration must be available as it is the only effective procedure for apnoea caused by succinylcholine.

Dose: 3-4 mg I.V. injection produces paralysis in 2-3 minutes and the effect lasts for 15-20 minutes.

Nondepolarizing (competitive) blocking agents (tubocurarine, gallamine, pancuronium, atracurium, vecuronium, mivacurium, pipecuronium, trocuronium, doxacurium)

- These combine with ACh receptors at the muscle end plate but do not activate them.
- By decreasing the number of available ACh receptors, these agents reduce the height of the end plate potential, the threshold for excitation is not reached.

Tubocurarine (d-tubocurarine)

It is a natural alkaloid (cyclic benzylisoquinoline) from roots of chondrodendron tomentosum. It is ineffective by mouth and so given by I.V. route. The onset of action is 4-6 minutes and the action lasts for about 80-120 minutes. It can also be given by I.M. injection.

Dose: 30 mg I.V.

The onset is not preceded by muscle fasciculations due to its some ganglionic blocking action.

The adverse effects include prolonged apnoea, hypotension, bronchospasm. The bronchospasm is due to histamine release.

The antidote for d-tubocurarine is anticholinesterase neostigmine. Artificial respiration may be needed.

Gallamine (Flaxedil)

It is a non-depolarizing muscle relaxant. It is less powerful with shorter duration of action compared to d-tubocurarine and unlike d-tubocurarine it does not release histamine (advantageous in asthmatic patients). But gallamine produces atropine like action on the cardiac branch of the vagus nerve so it can produce tachycardia.

Dose: 60-80 mg I.V., onset of action is 1-2 minutes.

Contraindications: Myasthenia gravis and renal failure.

Uses: same as d-tubocurarine.

Pancuronium dimethyl bromide

It is a steroidal bisquaternary ammonium compound, very effective neuromuscular blocker without producing any steroidal activity. It is a competitive nondepolarizing muscle relaxant like tubocurarine but has 5 to 8 times greater potency and lacks histamine releasing effect. The onset of action is 4-6 minutes and duration of action is 120-180 minutes.

Dose: 4-6 mg I.V. injection.

Uses: Same as d-tubocurarine.

Antidote: Anticholinesterases.

Atracurium

It is a competitive neuromuscular blocking agent, onset is very rapid (2-4 minutes) and duration is short(30-40 minutes). It seems that this drug produces actions on CNS less than other nondepolarizing muscle relaxants. This drug is also likely to be very useful in patients with renal failure. It is less histamine releaser than tubocurarine and metocurine.

Dose: 0.3-0.6 mg/kg body weight.

Antidote: Neostigmine.

Vecuronium

It is a monoquaternary analogue of pancuronium, onset of action is 2-4 minutes and duration of action is short (30-40 minutes). It produces fewer cardiovascular side effects than pancuronium. It does not release histamine so the risk of hypotension and bronchospasm is reduced.

Doxacurium is a benzylisoquinoline competitive neuromuscular blocker. Its onset of action is 4-6 minutes, and duration is 90-120 minutes.

Rocuronium is a competitive neuromuscular blocking agents, onset time is 1-2 minutes and duration of action is 30-40 minutes.

Mivacurium is a benzylisoquinoline. The onset of action of this competitive neuromuscular blocking agent is 2-4 minutes and the duration of action is 12-18 minutes.

Pipecuronium is a steroidal derivative. The onset of action of this competitive neuromuscular blocking agent is 2-4 minutes and duration of action is 80-100 minutes.

Table 3.19 shows comparison of d-tubocurarine, gallamine and succinylcholine.

Therapeutic indications of neuromuscular blocking agents

- The main clinical use is as an adjuvant to anaesthesia for promoting skeletal muscle relaxation and for facilitating endotracheal intubation.

Box 3.8. Comparison between depolarizing and nondepolarizing neuromuscular agents	
Depolarizing agents	*Nondepolarizing agents*
Persistent depolarization	Competitive block
Initial muscle fasciculations	Not preceded by fasciculation
Duration shorter	Duration longer
Synergistic to neostigmine	Antagonistic to neostigmine
Antagonistic to aminoglycosides, ether, halothane	Synergistic to aminoglycosides, ether, halothane
Synergistic to KCl	Antagonistic to KCl
Order of relaxation: limbs, head, neck, trunk	Order of relaxation: head, neck, limbs, trunk
No suitable antidote	Neostigmine

Table 3.19. Comparison of d-tubocurarine, gallamine and succinylcholine

	d-tubocurarine	Gallamine	Succinylcholine
Source	Natural	Synthetic	Synthetic
Mode of action	Nondepolarizing (competitive block)	Nondepolarizing (competitive block)	Depolarizing (persistent depolarization)
Elimination	Hepatic, renal	Renal	Plasma CHE
Initial fasciculation	Not preceded by fasciculations	Not preceded by fasciculations	Initial fasciculations present synergistic
Duration of action in normal person (in minutes)	80-120	15-20	5-10
In case of atypical pseudocholinesterase	30-40	15-20	Prolonged
Order of relaxation	Limbs, head, neck, trunk	Limbs, head, neck, trunk	Head, neck, limbs, trunk
Histamine release	Yes	No	No
Effect on heart	Rate increased	Rate increased	Rate decreased
Effect on B.P.	Fall	No effect	Slight fall
Effect on cardiac muscarinic receptors	None	Block	Agonist
Effect on autonomic ganglia	Block	No effect	Stimulation
Combination with non-depolarizing agents	Additive	Additive	Antagonist
Combination with depolarizing agents	Antagonistic	Antagonistic	Additive
Postoperative muscle pain	Absent	Absent	Present
Intraocular pressure	Not affected	Not affected	Elevated
Antidote for reversal of neuromuscular blockade	Cholinesterase inhibitors such as neostigmine, edrophonium, pyridostigmine	Cholinesterase inhibitors such as neostigmine, etc.	No antagonists exist. (i) Controlled ventilation is used till spontaneous recovery occurs. (ii) If anticholinesterase is given, phase I block will increase but it may reverse phase II block.

Adequate muscle relaxation can be obtained at lighter planes. The neuromuscular blocking agents of short duration often are used to facilitate intubation with an endotracheal tube. This facilitates laryngoscopy, bronchoscopy, and oesophagoscopy, in combination with a general anaesthetic.

- To prevent trauma associated with skeletal muscle contraction during electroconvulsive shock therapy. The seizures induced by electroconvulsive therapy of psychiatric disorders may cause dislocation or fractures.
- d-tubocurarine may be employed diagnostically for the detection of nerve-route compression masked by painful spasm of muscle involved in protective splinting. Tubocurarine can also assist in the diagnosis of myasthenia gravis.

Adverse effects of neuromuscular blockers

With depolarizing agents :

- Cardiac arrest and arrhythmic
- Malignant hyperthermia (a rare inherited condition determined by an autosomal recessive gene that gives rise to an abnormal type of plasma CHE

Neuromuscular blocker	Type	Onset	Duration	Histamine release	Cardiovascular effects
Tubocurarine	Nondepolarizing	Slow	Long	+3	Hypotension
Suxamethonium	Depolarizing	Rapid	Short	0	Bradycardia
Gallamine	Nondepolarizing	Slow	Long	0	Tachycardia
Pancuronium	Nondepolarizing	Slow	Long	0	Tachycardia (vagolytic)
Atracurium	Nondepolarizing	Intermediate		+2	0
Vecuronium	Nondepolarizing	Intermediate		0	0
Doxacurium	Nondepolarizing	Slow	Long	0	0
Pipecuronium	Nondepolarizing	Slow	Long	0	0
Mivacurium	Nondepolarizing	Rapid	Short	+1	0
Rocuronium	Nondepolarizing	Rapid	Short	0	0

Box 3.9. Neuromuscular blocking agents

0 = None; +1 = Slight; +2 = Mild; +3 = Moderate

- Hypokalaemia
- Temporary rise in intraocular pressure (IOP)
- Vomiting
- Muscle soreness

With non-depolarizing agents :
- Hypoxia
- Hypotension (due to both ganglionic blockade and histamine release)
- Decreased tone and motility of GIT due to ganglionic blockade
- Tachycardia and increased arterial pressure with gallamine (due to both vagolytic and tyramine like effects)
- Bronchospasm due to histamine release

Factors that modify the actions of neuromuscular blocking agents:

- In individuals, deficient in serum cholinesterase, the transient effects of succinylcholine are prolonged.
- In the presence of hepatic disease, the duration of action of succinylcholine is prolonged because serum cholinesterase is synthesised in the liver.
- Depolarizing neuromuscular blocking agents increase serum potassium.
- Aminoglycoside antibiotics exert a synergistic neuromuscular blockade when given with either depolarizing and competitive neuromuscular blocking agents. The mechanism is presynaptic.
- Inhalation general anaesthetic increase the effects of neuromuscular blocking agents.

- The duration of action of succinylcholine is also prolonged in case an irreversible anticholinesterases such as ecothiopate are used in the treatment of glaucoma.
- Patients suffering from myasthenia gravis are very sensitive to competitive neuromuscular blockers and phase II block will therefore occur sooner.

Directly acting muscle relaxants

Dantrolene is the only drug that comes under this category. It acts directly on the skeletal muscle. It has no effect on the CNS and neuromuscular junction.

Dantrolene interferes with excitation contraction coupling as it interferes with the release of Ca^{2+} from the sarcoplasmic reticulum.

It is absorbed from GIT, although the absorption is slow and incomplete. The main site of metabolism is liver and the metabolites are excreted in bile and urine.

Uses

- Neurological spastic disorders like multiple sclerosis, spinal injury.
- Malignant hyperthermia induced by halothane or succinylcholine.

Dose: 25 mg daily initially orally, may be increased to 100 mg 6 hourly; or 1 mg/kg/I.V. injection.

Adverse reactions are common and include

muscle weakness, drowsiness, dizziness, and hepato-toxicity.

Drugs such as aminoglycosides, polymyxins and local anaesthetics cause skeletal muscle relaxation as side effects. These are not used clinically for the purpose of relaxing skeletal muscles.

2. CENTRALLY ACTING MUSCLE RELAXANTS

- Mephenesin group: Mephenesin, Meprobamate, Carisoprodol, Chlorzoxazone, Methocarbamol
- Benzodiazepine: Diazepam
- GABA derivative: Baclofen

Skeletal muscle relaxation can also be brought about by centrally acting agents, e.g. Mephenesin, meprobamate, anti-anxiety agents including diazepam. These drugs act on internuncial spinal neurons to depress polysynaptic pathways. They also act on higher centres.

Mephenesin (Tolserol): It has selective action on spinal neurons but the action is rather weak. It has potent local anaesthetic and mild sedative action. It is available as 500 mg tablet or elixir 500 mg/5 ml.

Adverse effects include muscle incoordination, ataxia and diplopia. On i.v. administration it may cause thrombosis, haemolysis, haematuria.

Methocarbamol (Robaxin) is closely related to mephenesin, available as 500 mg and 750 mg tablet, for injection 100 mg/ml in 50% polyethylene glycol.

The indications and limitations are the same as mephenesin.

Chlorphenesin carbamate has similar action as mephenesin, available as 500 mg tablet.

Meprobamate (Equanil, Miltown) produces action similar to mephenesin, capsules containing 200 and 400 mg are available.

Carisoprodol is related to meprobamate, tablet contains 350 mg and capsule contains 250 mg.

Benzoxazole derivatives: Zoxazolamine (Flexin) is not used being hepatotoxic.

Chlorzoxazone (paraflex) has some usefulness in muscle spasms. However, some cases of jaundice have been reported.

Chlormezanone is used more as an antianxiety agent, without any specific effects on muscle rigidity.

Metaxalone (Skelaxin) is useful due to sedative effect.

Dose: 400 mg tablet.

Chlordiazepoxide (Librium) and Diazepam (Valium) are useful anti- anxiety drugs, beneficial in musculoskeletal disorders.

Cyclobenzaprine (Flexeril) is related to tricyclic antidepressants, employed for short term treatment of acute musculoskeletal painful conditions. It is not given for long term treatment otherwise numerous side effects occur like tricyclic antidepressants.

Baclofen: It is related to GABA (gamma-aminobutyric acid) acts similar to diazepam but less sedating. It is well absorbed orally and excreted unchanged in urine.

Dose: 5-20 mg twice or thrice a day.

The use of centrally acting muscle relaxants are limited.

They may be used in the following conditions:

Muscle spasm due to sprains, torticolis, arthritis, myositis, fibrositis, tetanus.

Adverse effects include drowsiness, ataxia, lethargy and allergic reactions.

Drug dependence is a problem with meprobamate and chlordiazepoxide (anti-anxiety) group of drugs.

Baclofen can produce fall in B.P., tachycardia, visual and auditory hallucinations (rarely).

Table 3.20 shows comparison of peripherally acting and centrally acting muscle relaxants.

Table 3.20. Comparison of peripherally acting and centrally acting muscle relaxants

Peripherally acting	Centrally acting
Produce loss of power of voluntary muscle movements.	Reduce muscular tone, but voluntary power of muscle movements is not lost
Neuromuscular transmission is blocked.	Polysynaptic reflexes in CNS are inhibited
Route of administration is i.v.	Generally given orally, also parenterally, if needed
CNS is not affected.	CNS depression occurs to some extent
Used as adjuvants to general anaesthesia.	Useful in acute muscle spasms, chronic spastic conditions such as torticolis, chronic backache, local injury or inflammation. Not effective in Parkinsonism

STUDY QUESTIONS

1. Classify skeletal muscle relaxants according to their mode of action, give suitable examples.
2. Tabulate the differences between d-tubocurarine and gallamine.
3. Compare depolarizing and non-depolarizing neuromuscular blocking agents.
4. Describe the pharmacology of succinylcholine.
5. Describe the therapeutic uses and adverse effects of neuromuscular blocking agents.
6. Describe directly acting muscle relaxant.
7. Name drugs that are centrally acting muscle relaxant. What are their therapeutic uses and adverse effects?
8. Comment on (i) mephenesin, and (ii) GABA derivative (baclofen) as muscle relaxant.
9. Compare peripherally acting and centrally muscle relaxant in a tabulated form.

GUIDE TO FURTHER READING

Agoston, S et at: Clinical pharmacokinetics of neuromuscular blocking drugs. Clin Pharmacokinet, 1992; 22:94.

Albright, A.L., Cervi, A., and Singletary, J.: Intrathecal baclofen for spasticity in cerebral palsy, JAMA, 1991;265:1418.

Basta, S.J., Modulation of histamine released by neuromuscular blocking drugs. Curr. Opin. Anaesthesiol. 1992; 5:512

Beran, D.R. et al: Reversal of neuromuscular blockade. Anesthesiology, 1992; 77:785.

Changeux, J.P. Chemical signalling in the brain. Sci. Am., 1993; 269:58.

Feldman, S.A. and Fauvel, N. Onset of neuromuscular block. In, Applied Neuromuscular Pharmacology, (Pollard B.J., ed) Oxford University Press, Oxford 1994, pp 69-84.

Hunter, J.M., Muscle relaxants in renal disease. Acta Anaesthesiol. Scand, 1994; 102 Suppl. ; 2-5.

Iaizzo, P.A., and Lehmann-Horn, F. Anesthetic complication in muscle disorders. Anesthesiology, 1995; 82:1093

Lazorthes, Y et al: Chronic intrathecal baclofen administration for control of severe spasticity. J Neurosurg, 1990; 72:393.

Lopez, J.R. et al: Effects of dantrolene on myoplasmic free [Ca^{2+}] measured in vivo in patients susceptible to malignant hyperthermia. Anesthesiology, 1992; 76:711.

Miller, R.D., Savarese, J.J.: Pharmacology of muscle relaxants and their antagonists. In, Anesthesia, 4th ed. Miller, R.D. (editor). Churchill Livingstone, 1994.

Strazes, K.P. and Fox,A.W. Malignant hyperthermia: A review of published cases. Anesth. Analg, 1993; 77:297

Stroud, R.M.: Acetylcholine receptor structure. Neurosci Comment, 1983; 1:124.

Watkins, J. Adverse reactions to neuromuscular blockers: frequency, investigations, and epidemiology. Acta Anaethesiol. Scand. 1994; 102:6.

Young, R.R., Delwaide, P.J.: Drug therapy; Spasticity. (Two parts) N Engl J Med, 1981; 28:96.

ANTIEPILEPTIC DRUGS

Antiepileptics are special class of anticonvulsant drugs which are clinically useful for the treatment of epilepsy. These are:

- Long acting barbiturates: All barbiturates have anti-convulsant properties, but only some of them such as phenobarbitone, mephobarbital and metharbital possess antiepileptic properties.
- Deoxybarbiturate: Primidone.
- Hydantoins: Phenytoin, mephenytoin.
- Oxazolidinediones: Tridione, paradine.
- Succinimides: Phensuximide (milontin), methsuximide (celontin), ethosuximide (zarontin).
- Acylureas: Phenacetamide (phenurone), pheneturide.
- Dibenzapine: Carbamazepine (tegretol).
- Benzodiazepines: Nitrazepam, clonazepam, diazepam.
- Dipropylacetate: Valproic acid (sodium valproate).
- Miscellaneous: Acetazolamide, dexamphetamine, progabide.

The term seizure refers to a transient change of behaviour due to the disordered, synchronous and rhythmic firing of population of brain neurons.

Seizure can be 'epileptic' when that occurs without provocation.

Seizure can be 'nonepileptic' when evoked in normal brain by electric or chemical convulsants.

The term epilepsy refers to a disorder of brain function manifested by the periodic and unpredictable occurrence of seizures. Table 3.21 shows types of seizures and drugs employed.

Table 3.21. Types of seizures and drugs employed

Types of epileptic seizures	Conventional drugs	Recent drugs
Partial seizures (begin focally in a cortical site)		
Simple partial (Manifestations determined by the area of cortex activated. Consciousness is preserved)	Carbamazepine, Phenytoin, Phenobarbital, Primidone, Valproate	Gabapentin, Lamotrigine
Complex partial (Consciousness is impaired from 30 sec to 2 minutes, with purposeless movements such as lip smacking or hand wringing)	Carbamazepine, Phenytoin, Phenobarbital, Primidone, Valproate	Gabapentin, Lamotrigine
Partial with secondarily generalized tonic-clonic seizure (Simple or complex partial seizure evolves into tonic-clonic seizures with loss of consciousness)	Carbamazepine, Phenytoin, Phenobarbital, Primidone, Valproate	Gabapentin, Lamotrigine
Generalized seizures (Involve both hemispheres from the onset)		
Absence seizure or petit mal (Abrupt onset of impaired consciousness associated with staring and cessation of ongoing activity, lasting less than 30 seconds)	Valproate, Ethosuximide, Clonazepam	Lamotrigine
Myoclonic epilepsy (A brief shock-like contraction of muscle, restricted to part of one extremity or may be generalize.)	Valproate	
Tonic-clonic seizure or grand mal (It is not preceded by a partial seizure.)	Carbamazepine, Phenytoin, Phenobarbital, Primidone, Valproate	
Status epilepticus	Diazepam I.V., Phenytoin I.V., Phenobarbitone I.V., Clonazepam, Lorazepam	

Spectrum of action of various antiepileptics

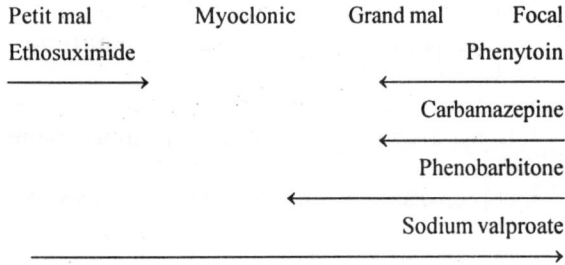

The ideal antiseizure drug should suppress all seizures without producing any adverse effects.

INDIVIDUAL AGENTS

Antiseizure Barbiturates

Phenobarbital (luminal): as an antiepileptic drug, it is employed when phenytoin, valproate or carbamazepine do not produce beneficial effects in grand mal type of epilepsy. It has only slight effect on petit mal. It is more suitable for grand mal type of epilepsy.

About 80% is slowly absorbed on oral administration, 45% is protein bound, 35% is excreted unchanged in urine and the rest is metabolized in the liver.

It is a cumulative drug. Tolerance develops. The usual dose is 100-300 mg/d.

Adverse effects include drowsiness, in severe cases there may be depression of respiratory and cardiovascular systems. It is a potent inducer of hepatic microsomal enzymes resulting in important drug interactions. The drug should be withdrawn gradually otherwise grand mal attack may precipitate.

Mephobarbital: Indications for its use are similar to phenobarbitone. Its effect is partly due to its conversion (demethylated) to phenobarbitone. Dose is 300-600 mg/d. It is more suitable for petit mal.

Metharbital: It is demethylated to barbital. Dose is 100 mg/d. It is more suitable for petit mal.

Deoxybarbiturates

Primidone (mysoline): It is not a pure barbituric acid

derivative, but its actions are similar to phenobarbital although less potent. It is indicated in all types of epilepsy except petit mal. It is favoured in grand mal and psychomotor seizures. Dose is 50 mg increased gradually to 250 mg thrice a day.

The adverse effects include folate deficiency anaemia, vitamin D deficiency, ataxia, visual disturbances, drowsiness. Agranulocytosis has been reported.

Hydantoins

Phenytoin (diphenylhydantoin, dilantin). It is one of the most widely used and powerful antiepileptic drug which does not cause general depression of the CNS.

It is indicated in all types of epilepsies, except absence seizures.

The drug is absorbed at rather slow rate from the small intestine. The absorption is slower after I.M. injection than after oral administration.

Dose 200-400 mg daily, if single dose is not tolerated then the drug is given in 2 or 3 divided doses.

I.M. injection is not recommended not only because its absorption is slower than after oral administration, but also because some drug precipitate occurs in muscle.

Phenytoin can be given by I.V. injection for status epilepticus as well as for its antiarrhythmic effect. The dose by I.V. injection is 1 to 3 mg/kg administered over 5 to 10 minutes.

Other uses of phenytoin include trigeminal and related neuralgias, but carbamazepine may be preferable.

Phenytoin is also used as an antiarrhythmic drug.

Adverse effects

- Hypertrophy of gums in 20% of cases due to disorder of fibroblastic activity.
- Hypocalcaemia as it interferes with vitamin D metabolism.
- Megaloblastic anaemia due to the interference with folate absorption.
- In some cases lupus erythematosus and pulmonary fibrosis have been reported.
- The idiosyncratic disturbances include blood dyscrasias.

Drug interactions

- Valproate displaces phenytoin from protein binding and inhibits its metabolism
- Carbamazepine and phenytoin (both enzyme inducers) enhance each other's metabolism
- Chloramphenicol, INH, dicumarol, warfarin inhibit phenytoin metabolism, phenytoin toxicity may occur
- A number of acidic drugs like salicylates etc. displace phenytoin from its binding sites
- Sucralfate decreases phenytoin absorption
- Phenobarbitone and ethanol competitively inhibit phenytoin metabolism, but on chronic administration by enzyme induction, they enhance each others metabolism

Other hydantoins

Mephenytoin (Mesantoin), unlike phenytoin is sedative and also rapidly absorbed after oral administration. Its antiepileptic spectrum is similar to that of phenytoin and it may exacerbate absence seizures.

Adverse effects : It causes less ataxia, gastric distress, gingival hyperplasia and hirsutism than does phenytoin and less sedation than does phenobarbital. However, serious toxicity is more common including rashes, fever, lymphadenopathy, aplastic anaemia, leukopenia, agranulocytosis, hepatotoxicity and lupus erythematosus. Therefore this drug is used only in those patients who do not respond or do not tolerate safer drug. The dose is 200-600 mg daily.

Ethotoin is relatively free of the typical adverse effects of phenytoin, but its efficacy is low. The dose is 2-3 g in 4-6 divided doses.

Oxazolidinediones

Tridione (Trimethadione) and Paradione (Paramethadione) : As antiepileptic drugs these are only indicated in the treatment of absence seizures who do not respond or tolerate other drugs. They may increase tonic-clonic seizures.

Dose is 0.9-1.8 g/d in divided doses.

Adverse effects include nausea, drowsiness, photophobia. The serious side effects though rare include blood disorders, aplastic anaemia and nephrotic syndrome.

Succinimides

Ethosuximide (zarontin): It is more effective than methsuximide and trimethadione and with lower side effects in absence seizures (petit mal). It is second choice to valproate. Dose is 250 mg twice a day, gradually increased to 1.75 g/d.

Methsuximide (celontin): dose is 150-300 mg capsules.

Phensuximide (milontin): dose is 500 mg capsules.

The mild adverse effects of succinimides include drowsiness, headache, dizziness, GIT upsets. Rare but serious side effects include leukopenia and aplastic anaemia.

Phenurone and Pheneturide: Indicated in psychomotor type of epilepsy, dose is 0.75-3.0 g/d. These may produce hepatic and renal toxicity, aplastic anaemia.

Iminostilbenes

Carbamazepine (Tegretol): It is one of the iminostilbenes. It is indicated in all types of epilepsy except absence seizures. It is also useful in trigeminal neuralgia.

Dose is 100-200 mg twice a day.

Adverse effects include dry mouth, drowsiness, nausea, vomiting, diarrhoea.

In idiosyncratic individuals it may produce generalized skin rashes, jaundice, and blood disorders.

It is a potent inducer of hepatic microsomal enzymes and so result in drug interactions, e.g. if given with phenytoin it reduces the plasma concentration of phenytoin.

Benzodiazepines

Benzodiazepines which are primarily sedative-antianxiety drugs, also possess antiepileptic properties but their usefulness is limited due to their pronounced sedative effect and development of tolerance.

Diazepam I.V., lorazepam I.V. are useful for status epilepticus; clonazepam related to nitrazepam is effective in all types of epilepsy. Nitrazepam and diazepam are now being replaced by clonazepam. Oral dose is 4-8 mg/d; 1-4 mg/I.V. is drug of choice for status epilepticus. Clonazepam is rapidly absor-

bed, peak plasma concentration reaches in 2-4 hours; 80% is protein bound. It is metabolized in liver to 3-hydroxyclozepam which is active and to 7-aminoclozepam and 7-acetaminoclozepam which are inactive metabolites.

Diazepam and the related drugs increase seizure threshold and act as anticonvulsant. They act on neurons containing GABA which is inhibitory in action and responsible for the anticonvulsant action.

Adverse effects include drowsiness, ataxia, visual disturbances, hypotension and respiratory depression.

Clobazam is 1,5-benzodiazepine and has slightly different chemical structure from that of diazepam and clonazepam which are 1,4-benzodiazepines. Due to this change in structure it is less sedative and results in less psychomotor retardation.

The peak serum levels reach after 1-4 hours after oral administration, its bioavailability is 87%, it is bound to plasma proteins 85%, its elimination half-life is 10-30 hours, its active metabolite is N-desmethyl clobazam.

Dose : Single bed time dose starting at 10 mg increasing to 60 mg (maximum upto 100 mg). It can also be given in two divided doses.

Uses

Clobazam is useful in the treatment of patients with refractory epilepsy. The most beneficial effects have been observed in patients with partial seizures, effective in absence seizures, also myoclonic and secondary generalised tonic-clonic and reflex epilepsies. It is useful in all age group.

Adverse effects

Sedation and dizziness are most common side effects. The other side effects include mood changes, occasional irritability, depression and fatigue.

Dipropylacetate

Valproic acid is a simple branched-chain carboxylic acid.

$$CH_3 - CH_2 - CH_2$$
$$CH_3 - CH_2 - CH_2 \Big\rangle CHCOOH$$

Sodium valproate

- It is a broad spectrum antiepileptic drug
- It is effective against all types of seizures (generalisd as well as partial)
- It is particularly very effective against absence seizures
- It is well absorbed from GIT, 90% is bound to plasma proteins and excreted as glucuronide in urine
- The plasma half-life is 15 hours

Dose: 200mg thrice a day orally, increased 200mg daily at 3 day interval until seizures are controlled

Mode of action

- Like phenytoin it blocks sodium channels
- It produces increase in GABA levels by inhibiting GABA-aminotransferase

Adverse effects

Anorexia, nausea, vomiting, drowsiness, headache, menstrual disturbances, weight gain, hair loss, thinning and curling of hair.

Serious adverse effects include hepatotoxicity, acute pancreatitis, leucopenia, prolongation of bleeding time and teratogenicity (spina bifida, cardiovascular orofacial and digital abnormalities).

Drug interactions

- It lowers plasma level of phenytoin by competition for protein binding.
- It increases 40% plasma phenobarbitone concentration, if used simultaneously.

Carbonic anhydrase inhibitor

Acetazolamide: It induces acidosis which reduces excitability of nerve cells. It may be used as adjuvant drug in grand mal and petit mal epilepsy, but seldom used now as an antiepileptic drug.

Tolerance developed with this drug.

Dose 250-1000 mg/d orally. The drug has usefulness as a diuretic, in glaucoma and premenstrual tension.

Mode of action of antiepileptics

General mechanisms of action of antiepileptic drugs:

- Reducing electrical excitability of cell membrane, possibly through block of sodium channels, e.g. carbamazepine, phenytoin and lamotrigine.
- Enhancing GABA mediated synaptic inhibition. This may be activated by an enhanced post-synaptic action of GABA i.e. GABA - mediated opening of chloride channels e.g. phenobarbitone and benzodiazepines; by inhibiting GABA - transaminase e.g. valproate, vigabatrin; or by drugs as $GABA_A$ and $GABA_B$ e.g. progabide.

Gabapentin has little or no action on GABA receptors but is an effective antiepileptic drug. Its mechanism of action remains uncertain.

Thus, antiepileptic drugs (i) prevent or reduce excessive discharge from pathologically altered neurons and/or (ii) reduce speed of epileptic electrical discharge from epileptic foci.

NEWER ANTIEPILEPTIC DRUGS

Felbamate

Felbamate is an analogue of meprobamate with less sedative action and having broader clinical spectrum than other earlier antiepileptic drugs. The mechanism of its action is not fully known. It has weak effect on sodium channels and a little effect on GABA.

The plasma half-life is 24 hours.

The use is limited to tonic-clonic and partial intractable epilepsy in children owing to severe allergic reactions.

The adverse effects include insomnia, irritability, nausea, occasionally severe reactions resulting in aplastic anaemia or hepatitis. It has been withdrawn from USA.

Topiramate

Topiramate is a newly introduced antiepileptic drug. The mechanism of action is complex and not fully understood. It appears to do a little of every thing i.e. blocking sodium channels, enhancing the action of GABA and weakly inhibiting carbonic anhydrase.

Topiramate has same spectrum of antiepileptic activity as that of phenytion with fewer adverse effects. It is a safe drug.

The main drawback is that it is not given to women of child bearing age because it is teratogenic in animals.

Tiagabine

Tiagabine is an analogue of GABA and acts by inhibiting GABA uptake. The mechanism of action is not yet fully understood. The clinical usefulness is also not yet fully assessed. It has short plasma half-life.

Adverse effects include drowsiness and confusion.

Vigabatrin

Vigabatrin is an analogue of GABA. It irreversibly inhibits GABA-transaminase and produces inhibitory effects, reduces hyper excitability. The half-life is short but produces a long lasting effect because the enzyme is blocked irreversibly so the drug is administered orally once daily. The dose is 2-4 g/d in adults and in children 40-100 mg/kg/daily. It is well absorbed orally and excreted unchanged in urine.

Its use is restricted to refractory cases of partial epilepsy with or without secondary generalized seizures.

This drug has been found useful in patients who are resistant to the established conventional drugs and hence it is an improvement in the therapy. It holds promise as monotherapy.

Its dose is decreased in elderly and in patients with renal dysfunction.

Side effects

Vigabatrin is relatively free from side effects. The main drawback is the occurrence of depression, and occasionally psychotic disturbances, drowsiness, behavioural and mood changes. Sedation, dizziness weight gain, agitation, confusion are other common side effects.

The sudden withdrawal of vigabatrin may precipitate seizures.

Contraindications : Mental illness

Gabapentin (Neurontin)

Gabapentin is a lipophilic GABA derivative. It enhances GABA release by an unknown mechanism. However, it does not act as an agonist at GABA receptor. The half-life is 6-8 hours. It is well absorbed orally and excreted unchanged in urine.

It has been found useful for partial seizures with and without secondary generalized seizures.

The dose is 800–900 mg daily in 3 divided doses.

It has been claimed that gabapentin is effective in patients who are resistant to conventional antiepileptic drugs but this claim remains to be established.

Adverse effects include mild sedation, ataxia and tiredness. However, it is relatively safe in case of overdosing because its absorption from the intestine depends on the amino acid carrier system and shows the property of saturability (saturable absorption).

Lamotrigine

Lamotrigine is a phenyltriazine derivative. It may be effective monotherapy for partial or generalized seizures. It can be effective against absence seizures. Its pharmacological effects are similar to that of phenytoin and carbamazepine although it is not chemically related. Addition of this drug to valproic acid produces a reduction of valproate concentration by 25% over a few weeks.

Lamotrigne acts by blocking sodium influx and thus inhibiting glutamate release in brain.

The plasma half-life is 24 hours.

It is well absorbed orally and completely metabolised in liver.

Dose: 50mg daily for 2 weeks, increased to 50 mg twice per day for 2 weeks then increased 100mg daily (maximum 300-500 mg/d divided in 2 doses).

Adverse effects include nausea, diarrhoea, dizziness, diplopia, sleepiness, ataxia and hypersensitivity reactions especially skin rashes.

Zonisamide

Zonisamide produces antiepileptic activity similar to phenytoin. It has been found useful in myoclonic seizures. The dose is 100-200 mg/daily, increased to 400-600mg/daily. The indications are the same as vigabatrin.

Adverse effects include ataxia, renal calculi.

Treatment of refractory epilepsy

About one-third patients with epilepsy do not respond to treatment with a single antiepileptic drug, and it becomes necessary to try a combination of drugs to control seizures. There are currently no clear guidelines for rational polypharmacy, but in most cases the initial combination therapy combines first-line drugs, i.e. carbamazepine, phenytoin, valproic acid and lamotrigine.

If these drugs are unsuccessful then the addition of a newer drug such as topiramate or gabapentin is indicated. Patients with myoclonic seizures resistant to valproic acid may benefit from the addition of clonazepam and those with absence seizures may respond to a combination of valproic acid and ethosuximide.

Antiepileptic drugs of choice are given in table 3.22.

Antiepileptic drug selection (grand mal)

- For generalized tonic-clonic seizures : The best initial choice is valproic acid and lamotrigine, followed by carbamazepine and phenytoin which are suitable alternatives (Note: Ethosuximide is NOT effective in grand mal)
- For absence seizures (petit mal)
  Valproic acid
  · Ethosuximide
- For myoclonic seizures
  Valproic acid
  Clonazepam
- When absence seizures coexist with tonic-clonic seizures, valproic acid is used since most drugs used in tonic-clonic seizures may worsen absence seizures
- For partial seizures : Carbamazepine is preferred because of low incidence of side effects

Other drugs used are :

Valproic acid, clonazepam, phenytoin
(Note: Ethosuximide is NOT effective in partial seizures)

- For status epilepticus (to be treated as a medical emergency)
  Diazepam i.v. 10mg, over 5 minutes, may be repeated twice more, at 15 minutes intervals (watch for hypotension and respiratory depression)
  As diazepam is short acting, it is followed by phenytoin 15-20mg/kg at not more than 50mg/minute

Clonazepam i.v. 1mg/ or upto 3mg by slow i.v. infusion may replace diazepam.

If seizures persist i.e. if above drugs fail, pentothal 25-100 mg is given slowly by i.v. injection. In very serious cases tubocurarine and artificial respiration may be required (though rarely).

The therapy must be individualized, as the

Table 3.22. Antiepileptic drugs of choice

	Primary Generalized Tonic-clonic	Partial	Absence Myoclonic Atonic	Atypical Absence
First-Line	Valproic acid Lamotrigine Valproic acid Lamotrigine	Carbamazepine Phenytoin	Ethosuximide Valproic acid	Valproic acid
Alternatives	Phenytoin Carbamazepine Topiramate Primidone Phenobarbitone Felbamate	Gabapentin Topiramate Tiagabine Primidone Phenobarbitone	Lamotrigine Clonazepam	Lamotrigine Topiramate Clonazepam Felbamate

effective dose of antiepileptic drug varies from patient to patient.

The choice of antiepileptic drug is based on seizure type and patient variables.

The advantages of monotherapy include :

- Equal or superior efficacy to many two drug or three drug regimens.
- Reduced frequency of adverse effects.
- Absence of interactions between antiepileptic drugs.
- Lower cost.
- Reduced risk of birth defects.
- Improved compliance (non-compliance is the most common cause of drug failure.
- Small number of patients requires two or rarely three antiepileptic drugs.

Therapeutic principles and general considerations

- One fit is fit for investigation but not for commencing antiepileptic treatment.
- The pharmacotherapy is selective, depends on the type of epilepsy.
- If one drug is not successful or adequate, second should be substituted or added.
- The treatment should be continued till there are no seizures for 2-3 years.
- The duration of antiepileptic therapy is for 2 years after the last seizure.
- The withdrawal of drug should be gradual, over a period of six months, otherwise there is danger of status epilepticus.
- Pregnancy should be avoided during antiepileptic therapy to avoid teratogenicity (more with sodium valproate and phenytoin). However, if pregnancy occurs, administration of these drugs should be continued to prevent seizures and status epilepticus (risk to both mother and unborn child).

Epileptic women on drugs run a 2-3 fold more chance of delivering deformed child. Foetal hydantoin syndrome consisting of cleft lip and palate, heart defects, digital and nail hypoplasia have been observed. Haemorrhagic disease of new born with phenytoin or phenobarbitone use has been observed.

STUDY QUESTIONS

1. What is the difference between convulsion and epilepsy; and between anticonvulsant and antiepileptic?
2. Are all barbiturates antiepileptics? Which among them possess antiepileptic property?
3. Classify antiepileptic drugs.
4. What are the main types of epilepsy and the choice of drugs indicated for each of them?
5. Describe the pharmacology of phenytoin.
6. What is the role of benzodiazepines in the treatment of epilepsy?
7. What is the mode of action of antiepileptic drugs?
8. Describe the pharmacology of sodium valproate. What is its spectrum of activity, mode of action and adverse effects?

GUIDE TO FURTHER READING

Akerman K.K. : Analysis of clobazam and its active metabolite norclobazam in plasma and serum HPLC/DAD. Scand J. Clin Lab Invest. 1996: 56: 609-614.

Ashton H. : Guidelines for the rational use of benzodiazepines. When and what to use. Drugs. 1994: 40: 25-40.

Bialer, M.: Comparative pharmacokinetics of the newer antiepileptic drugs. Clin Pharmacokinet, 1993; 24:441.

Brodie, M.J.: Drug interactions in epilepsy. Epilepsia, 1992; 33 (Suppl):513.

Brodie, M.J., Porter, R.J.: New and potential anticonvulsants. Lancet, 1990; 336:425.

Dalessio, D.J.: Current concepts: Seizure disorders and pregnancy. N. Engl. J. Med., 1985; 312:559.

Farwell, J.R. et al: Phenobarbital for febrile seizures-effects on intelligence and on seizure recurrence. N. Engl. J. Med., 1990; 322:364.

Freeman, J.M.: The best medicine for febrile seizures N. Engl. J. Med. 1992; 327:1161.

Goddard, G.V., McIntyre, D.C., and Leech, C.K.: A permanent change in brain function resulting from daily electrical stimulation. Exp. Neurol, 1969; 25:295.

McCutchen, C.B. et al: A comparison of carbamazepine, phenobarbital, phenytoin and primidone in partial and secondarily generalized tonic-clonic seizures. N. Engl. J. Med., 1985; 313:145.

McNamara, J.O. Cellular and molecular basis of epilepsy J. Neurosci, 1994; 14:3413.

Ramsay, R.E.: Treatment of status epilepticus. Epilepsia, 1993; 34 (Suppl):571.

Rogawski, M.A., Porter, R.J.: Antiepileptic drugs. Pharmacological mechanisms and clinical efficacy with consideration of promising developmental stage compounds. Pharmacol Rev, 1990; 42:223.

Shinnar, S et al: Discontinuing antiepileptic drugs in children with epilepsy: a prospective study. Ann. Neurol., 1994; 35:534.

Treiman, D.M.: The role of benzodiazepines in the management of status epilepticus. Neurology, 1990; 40 (Suppl 2):32.

Valproate: A new cause of birth defects Report from Italy and follow-up from France. MMWR Morb Mortal Wrly Rep, 1983; 32:438.

Working Group on Status Epilepticus, Recommended actions of the Epilepsy Foundation of American Working Group on Status Epilepticus. JAMA, 1993; 270:854.

Yerby, M.S.: Risks of pregnancy in women with epilepsy. Epilepsia, 1992; 33 (Suppl 1):523.

ANTIPARKINSONIAN DRUGS

Antiparkinsonian drugs are used for the treatment of parkinsonism. This disease is characterized by muscular rigidity, tremors, hypokinesia(slowness and poverty of movements), excessive salivation, mask like face, shuffling gait (impairment of postural balance) and pill rolling movements of fingers. These symptoms are due to a considerable decrease in the concentration of dopamine in the basal ganglia. There is an imbalance between acetylcholine and dopamine in the region of the basal ganglia.

The balance between acetylcholine and dopamine can be restored by:

- Anticholinergic drugs (cholinergic system is dominant in parkinsonism).
- Dopaminergic drugs (parkinsonism is a dopamine deficiency disease).

Antiparkinsonian drugs are listed below:

1. Drugs affecting brain cholinergic system:
   - Central anticholinergics:
     Benzhexol
     Benztropine
     Procyclidine
     Biperiden
   - Antihistamines:
     Orphenadrine
     Promethazine

     Diphenhydramine
     Ethopropazine
2. Drugs affecting brain dopaminergic system:
   - Dopamine precursor
     Levodopa
   - Dopamine agonists:
     Bromocriptine
     Pergolide
     Lisuride
     Pirbedil
   - Dopamine releaser :
     Amantadine
   - Peripheral decarboxylase inhibitors:
     Carbidopa
     Benserazide
   - MAO-B inhibitor :
     Selegiline

Anticholinergic drugs

These block acetylcholine in the CNS. Tremor and rigidity are reduced but do not affect hypokinesia. These are useful in drug induced parkinsonism, unlike levodopa and amantadine.

Several drugs with anticholinergic properties are currently used in the treatment of parkinsonism including:

Artane, 2-4 mg thrice a day.

Diphenhydramine hydrochloride, 25-50 mg, 3-4 times per day.

Benzhexol (Pacitane) 2 mg thrice a day orally is useful in decreasing rigidity and tremor.

Ethopropazine 100-500 mg/d is a phenothiazine with anticholinergic and antihistaminic properties. It diminishes tremor and rigidity.

Benztropine mesylate 1-4 mg 2 times per day or as a single dose is particularly useful against excessive salivation and muscular rigidity. It possesses both anticholinergic and antihistaminic effects.

Orphenadrine 50-300 mg/d produces general stimulating effect besides diminishing rigidity and tremor.

All have a modest antiparkinsonian action.

The adverse effects include sedation, confusion, constipation, urinary retention, and blurred vision (through cycloplegia).

Dopamine Receptor Agonists (dopaminergic drugs)

These reduce rigidity and hypokinesia substantially, as well as improve tremors. But they are not useful in drug induced parkinsonism.

Levodopa is a precursor of dopamine.

Amantadine (antiviral drug) enhances dopamine formation.

Bromocriptine stimulates dopaminergic receptors.

Levodopa (L-dopa)

Levodopa is a precursor of dopamine.

Dopamine is not well absorbed from GIT and does not penetrate CNS, hence, it is not effective.

Levodopa is well absorbed from GIT and freely passes through the blood-brain barrier and is decarboxylated to dopamine in the CNS and also in the periphery.

L-dopa is a very effective agent in the treatment of parkinsonism. However, it is itself largely inert, the effectiveness as well as the side effects are due to its conversion to dopamine by decarboxylation.

Dopamine reduces hypokinesia and rigidity and sometimes benefit tremor. However, it often loses efficacy after about 2 years.

The other limiting factors to levodopa therapy are psychoses and appearance of involuntary movements (dyskinesia - difficulty in performing voluntary movements).

Adverse effects of levodopa

At the beginning of therapy :

- Nausea, vomiting, postural hypotension cardiac arrhythmia, confusion, insomnia, night mares, anxiety disorientation, delirium, hallucinations.
- After prolonged therapy - Abnormal writhing movements (twist or roll oneself about) after two years of therapy involuntary choreiform movements (irregular involuntary jerky movements of muscles of face, neck, limbs, facial muscles).
- Fluctuations in motor performance (2-5 years of therapy), ON-OFF effect. This phenomenon consists of episodes in which patient's clinical state fluctuate rapidly between being 'OFF'

where the symptoms of parkinsonism suddenly become worse for a few minutes to a few hours, and being 'ON' (symptoms improve again). The 'OFF' period is so sudden that the patient stops walking or can not get up from the chair. This problem of 'ON-OFF' phenomenon is not seen in untreated parkinsonism patients or with other antiparkinsonian drugs.

Complications of treatment

Fluctuations in mobility has been reported in more than half of patients on levodopa after 5 years of therapy. They generally proceed through predictable 'end-of-dose' deterioration to the 'on-off' phenomenon with marked very sudden swings from mobility to immobility. The cause of the fluctuations is not know, but multiple factors including desensitisation of dopamine receptors, interference with the response to dopamine by other levodopa metabolites such as 3-O-methyldopa, fluctuating plasma concentrations, and the erratic transport of levodopa from blood to the brain have been suggested. Eventually the effect of various factors that produce even small changes in plasma concentrations of levodopa will progressively become more pronounced.

For the management of 'end-of-dose' fluctuations:
   More frequent but smaller doses, addition of selegiline or partial replacement of levodopa by a dopamine agonist with more prolonged action may also be tried.

To overcome the 'on-off' phenomenon:
- Continous I.V. infusion of levodopa reduces fluctuations in mobility but this is not practical for day-to-day management.
- Modified- release formulation of levodopa with a peripheral dopa- decarboxylase inhibitor may be useful. Taking levodopa on an empty stomach and delaying most of the day's protein consumption until the evening and addition of selegiline or a dopamine agonist is useful.

For dyskinesia:
   Dosage readjustment or partial replacement of levodopa with a dopamine agonist.

For severe pain and dystonia

Measures to increase 'on' periods will reduce or eliminate pain. If fluctuations remain a problem SC apomorphine is often effective.

Contraindications

Levodopa is contraindicated in psychotic patients

Box 3.10: Drugs used in parkinsonism (Parkinson's disease)

Drugs that replace dopamine:
  Levodopa usually with carbidopa or benserazide
Drugs that mimic action of dopamine:
  Bromocriptine, pergolide
MAO-B inhibitor:
  Selegiline
Drugs that release dopamine:
  Amantadine
Central anticholinergic drugs:
  Benztropine

The main drawback of levodopa is that only 5% of an oral dose reaches brain as it is extensively decarboxylated in the peripheral tissues. Dopa decarboxylase is an enzyme found in gut- wall and liver which breaks down levodopa to dopamine which does not cross the blood brain barrier. The inhibitor of this enzyme when combined with levodopa will enhance and prolong the effects of levodopa. As lesser dose of levodopa will be required there will be less incidence of side effects.

Carbidopa and Benserazide

These are dopa decarboxylase inhibitors which prevent the extracerebral breakdown of levodopa only and do not enter the CNS. Levodopa 250 mg plus 25 mg carbidopa or 100 mg levodopa plus 25 mg benserazide are recommended.

Dopa decarboxylase inhibitors :
  • Carbidopa
  • Benserazide

Advantages of levodopa - dopa decarboxylase inhibitor combination:
  • Plasma t½ of levodopa is prolonged , dose is reduced to 1/4 to 1/8
  • Effective levodopa dosage is attained quickly
  • Side effects are reduced

  • Pyridoxine reversal of levodopa effect does not occur (can give pyridoxine)
  • On-off effect is minimized as cerebral dopamine concentrations are more sustained

Vitamin B_6 (pyridoxine) increases the extracerebral metabolism of levodopa as it catalyzes peripheral decarboxylase activity resulting in decreased levodopa activity. But when decarboxylase inhibitor is combined with levodopa this problem is not there.

Contraindications

Levodopa is contraindicated in psychotic patients.

An alternative to levodopa is the use of drugs that are direct agonists of striatal dopamine receptors.

Bromocriptine and pergolide

Two dopamine agonists, **bromocriptine** and **pergolide** (both are ergot derivatives) are available. The duration of action of these drugs is longer than that of levodopa.

Bromocriptine is a strong agonist of D_2 class of dopamine receptors, while pergolide is an agonist at both D_1 and D_2 receptors subtypes.

Pergolide is more potent than bromocriptine.

Dose of pergolide is 0.75-3 mg daily (maximum 5 mg daily).

The dose of bromocriptine is 2.5-40 mg daily.

The actions and adverse effects are similar to those of levodopa.

Like levodopa they may cause orthostatic hypotension. They may induce hallucinations or confusion similar to that observed with levodopa. Besides these effects related to their actions at dopamine receptors, these drugs may induce pleuropulmonary and retroperitoneal fibrosis, and digital spasm (as they share properties with the parent family of ergot compounds).

The side effects of bromocriptine include nausea, vomiting and hypotension in the initial stages. The incidence of dyskinesias is similar or some what less than levodopa. But the psychiatric disturbances i.e. auditory and visual hallucinations are more frequent with bromocriptine as compared to levodopa. On long term treatment digital vasospasm, constipation, alcohol intolerance and psychiatric reactions have been reported. Unlike levodopa there is first dose phenomenon i.e. sudden cardiovascular collapse.

Amantadine Hydrochloride

It is an antiviral drug, capable of mobilizing dopamine. It produces slight improvement in all the symptoms of parkinsonism. It is less potent than levodopa but relief of symptoms appear more rapidly. It is less effective than levodopa but more useful than anticholinergics. However, the benefits are short lived and often disappointing.

Amantadine possibly potentiates dopaminergic function influencing synthesis, release or uptake of dopamine. Its dose is 100 mg daily, initially (once or twice a day), increase to 200-400 mg/d (100 mg twice a day) for 5-10 days.

As compared to levodopa and anticholinergic drugs amantadine produces less side effects. However, with excessive doses it can produce acute toxic psychosis, insomnia, ataxia, GI upsets, oedema and convulsions.

Amantadine is contraindicated in patients with history of seizures or congestive heart failure.

Selegiline (Deprenyl)

Monoamine oxidase-B inhibitor selegiline inhibits intracerebral metabolic degradation of dopamine. This results in the preservation of dopamine at the basal ganglia. Thus it enhances the therapeutic effect of levodopa and dose of levodopa can be reduced. But this effect is brief. This drug is not approved for general use.

Aporphines

Apomorphine is a potent emetic. It is a dopaminergic agonist, beneficial in parkinsonism. But its main disadvantage is renal damage. Its analogue N-propyl norapomorphine and similar substances are under trial.

Drugs which may cause parkinsonism like syndrome:

- Antipsychotics, e.g., phenothiazines such as chlorpromazine; butyrophenones such as haloperidol act by blocking the action of dopamine.
- Reserpine: Depletes dopamine stores.
- Alpha methyldopa: Decreases dopamine synthesis.

STUDY QUESTIONS

1. What are the characteristics of parkinsonism?
2. How can the balance between acetylcholine and dopamine be stored?
3. What is the basis of the use of anticholinergic and dopaminergic drugs in the treatment of parkinsonism?
4. Name anticholinergic agents employed in the treatment of parkinsonism.
5. Describe the pharmacology of levodopa. Why dopamine as such is not used?
6. What is the role of vitamin B_6 in relation to levodopa?
7. What is the use of dopa decarboxylase inhibitors?
8. Describe Amantadine.
9. Describe Bromocriptine.

GUIDE TO FURTHER READING

Agid, Y.: Parkinson's disease: Pathophysiology Lancet, 1991; 337:1321.

Calne, D.B.: Treatment of Parkinson's disease. New Engl. J. Med., 1993; 329:1029.

Chase, T.N., Engber, T.M., and Mouradian, M.M. Pathative and prophylactic benefits of continuously administered dopaminomimetics in Parkinson's disease. Neurol, 1994; 44 Suppl 6:515.

Cotzias, G.C., Papavasliou, P.S., and Gellene, R. Modification of parkinsonism-chronic treatment with L-DOPA. New Engl. J. Med., 1969; 280:337.

Factor, S.A., and Weiner, W.J.: Early combination therapy with bromocriptine and levodopa in Parkinson's disease. Mov. Dis., 1993; 8:257.

Fahn, S. and Cohen, G.: The oxidant stress hypothesis in Parkinson's disease: evidence supporting it. Ann. Neurol., 1992; 32:804.

Gibb, W.R.:Neuropathology of Parkinson's disease and related syndromes. Neural. Clin., 1992; 10:361.

Goetz, C.G.: Dopaminergic agonists in the treatment of Parkinson's disease. Neurol., 1990; 40 Suppl 3:50.

Golbe, L.I.: The genetics of Parkinson's disease: a reconsideration. Neurol., 1990; 40 Suppl 3:7.

Greene, P., Cote, L. and Fahn, S.: Treatment of drug-induced psychosis in Parkinson's disease with clozapine. Adv in Neurol., 1993; 60:703.

Hornykiewicz, O. Dopamine in the basal ganglia, Br. Med. Bull., 1973; 29:172.

Olanow, C.W., MAO-B inhibitors in Parkinson's disease. Adv. In Neurol., 1993; 60:666.

Ross, R.T.: Drug-induced parkinsonism and other movements disorders. Can J Neurol Sci., 1990; 22:155.

Standaert, D.G., and Stern, M.B. Update on the management of Parkinson's disease. Med. Clin. North Am., 1993; 77:169.

Drugs for Alzheimer's disease (AD)

Alzheimer's disease is a progressive neurodegenerative disorder. Atrophy of cortical and subcortical areas is associated with deposition of Beta-amyloid protein.

Alzheimer's disease refers to dementia that does not have an antecedent cause such as stroke, brain tumour and alcohol. Dementia is defined as an acquired syndrome of intellectual impairment produced by brain dysfunction.

Only advanced age and genetic predisposition have been known factors in the development of this disease. It is prevalent in about 2.3% in 65 to 75 years bracket, 3.9% in 70 to 80 age bracket and 22% in those beyond 80 years.

There is currently no treatment for Alzheimer's disease that will prevent or cure the process. Specific drugs that may check the cause of illness or regenerate the atrophic cells are not available. No doubt, restlessness and belligerence can be reduced by using antipsychotics or benzodiazepines. Emotional liability and paranoid tendencies may be helped by haloperidol. Alprazolam is useful when sleep is disturbed. These drugs may help in making the patient's life more comfortable.

It has been found that there is a relatively selective loss of cholinergic neurons in the basal forebrain nuclei (a region in which lesions produce cognitive and learning deficits). Choline acetyl transferase activity in the cortex and hippocampus is reduced (30-70%) in this disease but not in other disorders, acetylcholinesterase activity is also greatly reduced. Hence, it is presumed that approaches to restore cholinergic function may be useful in this condition.

Presently the most successful way is the inhibition of enzymatic degradation of acetylcholine for augmenting cholinergic transmission in Alzheimer's disease. On this basis, two compounds are available for trials.

Tacrine

It is a reversible cholinesterase inhibitor, initial dose is 10mg 6 hourly, dose increased at 6 weeks interval to a maximum of 40mg 6 hourly. It is orally bioavailable. It is metabolized in the liver.

Side effects include nausea, vomiting, diarrhoea, dizziness and rash. Hepatotoxicity may occur about 1 in 8000 cases.

Donepezil

It is a reversible cholinesterase inhibitor. The starting dose is 5 mg once a day at bed time, increased upto 10 mg a day.

Side effects include nausea, vomiting, diarrhoea dizziness, muscle cramps and insomnia.

As compared to tacrine, it has no significant hepatotoxicity.

Besides the above two compounds, selegiline (a MAO inhibitor) and vitamin E singly or a combination, may slow the progression of Alzheimer's disease in moderately affected persons.

Combination of tacrine and selegiline has been used with modest benefit in early cases of Alzheimer's disease.

Small uncontrolled trials have found that oestrogen may improve cognitive functions in female patients with Alzheimer's disease. Further studies are needed to test this idea.

There is a preliminary evidence that aspirin reduces the risk (and retards the onset of Alzheimer's disease).

Epidemiological studies show that life-long smokers have a reduced probability of developing Alzheimer's disease. However, too many adverse effects of nicotine preclude its use for this purpose.

Search for the main culprit involved in Alzheimer's disease has shown that the secret of this disease was closely held by an enzyme called 'γ secretase.' The secret behaviour of 'γ secretase' is modified by a pathological protein called 'presenilin'. It has been thought that a mutation in presenilin is instrumental in altering the behaviour of secretase resulting in an increased production of brain plaques, which is the cause of producing the dementia in these patients. Current research has suggested the dangerous protein 'presenilin' and γ secretase' enzyme are one and the same entity.

Based on this discovery, there appears a distinct possibility of bringing out specifically target drugs for treating Alzheimer's disease. New drugs may be developed to inhibit the formation of brain plaques, like it is possible today to prevent cholesterol deposition.

A characteristic feature of Alzheimer's disease is gray plaques, which are formed due to the accumulation of amyloid-beta peptide which is generated from its precursor and this requires the presence of a particular enzyme called 'γ secretase.'

STUDY QUESTIONS

1. What is Alzheimer's disease ?
2. Which drugs may make the patients of Alzheimer's more comfortable ?
3. What is the role of antioxidants such as selegiline and vitamin E in Alzheimer's disease.
4. Comment on (i) Tacrine, (ii) Donepezil.

GUIDE TO FURTHER READING

Aisen P.S., Davis K.L., 1977. The search for disease modifying treatment of Alzheimer's disease. Neurology 48 (suppl. 6): S35-41 (Good review article on current and prospective therapies).

Selkoe D.J. 1993, Physiological production of the β-amyloid protein and the mechanism of Alzheimer's disease. Trends Neurosci, 16:403-409 (Introductory review by one of the pioneers of the amyloid theory).

Selkoe D.J., Alzheimer's disease: genotypes, phenotype and treatments. Science 275: 630-631 (Short but informative summary of recent advances in Alzheimer genetics).

Yanker B.A., 1996, Mechanisms of neuronal degeneration in Alzheimer's disease. Neuron 16: 91-932 (Review focusing on reasons why neurons are damaged by amyloid deposition).

CNS STIMULANTS

A heterogeneous group of drugs can stimulate the central nervous system (CNS). These can be classified as under:

- Predominently cortical stimulants: Xanthine alkaloids, amphetamine, methylphenidate and pipradrol.
- Predominently medullary stimulants: Nikethamide, doxapram, amiphenazole
- Predominently spinal stimulants: Strychnine.

Xanthines (Methyl xanthines)

Caffeine, theophylline, theobromine are naturally occurring closely related alkaloids. They share in common several pharmacological actions of therapeutic interest. They relax smooth muscle, notably bronchial muscle, stimulate CNS, stimulate cardiac muscle, and act on the kidney as a diuretic.

Average cup of tea contains 50 mg caffeine and 1 mg theophylline; an average cup of coffee contains 75 mg caffeine and in an average cup of cocoa there is 200 mg theobromine and 4 mg caffeine.

Coffee seeds contain caffeine; tea leaves contain caffeine and theophylline; cocoa contains caffeine and theobromine.

Pharmacokinetics

Absorption after oral administration is generally satisfactory but may be erratic. They are metabolized by xanthine oxidase.

Actions

- CNS. The mental activity is stimulated (caffeine is more potent) when below normal. Fatigue is removed, and reaction time is decreased.
- CVS. Tachycardia and increased cardiac output.
- Smooth muscles. Relaxed (use of theophylline in asthma).
- Diuretic effect. It is due to (i) inhibition of renal tubular reabsorption of sodium, (ii) increasing renal blood flow by both cardiac and vascular actions. Better drugs are available for this purpose as xanthines are weak diuretics.
- Gastric secretion. Methylxanthines increase secretion of acid and pepsin in stomach.

Comparison of certain properties of caffeine, theophylline and theobromine is shown in Table 3.23.

Table 3.23. Main differences between caffeine, theobromine and theophylline

	Caffeine	Theophylline	Theobromine
CNS	+++	+++	+
CVS	+	+++	+
Smooth muscle of blood vessels	+	+++	+
Bronchial muscle	+	+++	+

+ mild, ++ moderate, +++ marked activity

Mode of action

- Uncoupling of intracellular calcium increases with muscle contractile elements.
  - Direct effect on intracellular calcium concentration.
  - Indirect effect on intracellular calcium concentrations via cell membrane hyperpolarization.
- Inhibition of phosphodiesterase, thereby increasing intracellular cyclic AMP.
- Antagonism of adenosine receptors. This is the most important factor responsible for most pharmacological effects of methylxanthines in therapeutic doses.

Uses

Theophylline (due to bronchodilator effect) is used in asthma. The preparation commonly used is aminophylline (100 mg) which is a combination of theophylline with ethylenediamine. It is administered by I.V. injection (250-500 mg in 20 ml of water) in about 10 minutes, it is dangerous to give it fast. Orally administered aminophylline is irritant so nonirritant preparation choline theophylline has been introduced which is given 100-400 mg orally 6 hourly.

Sustained release formulations are available. Suppositories and solutions for rectal administration are also available.

Uses of caffeine are (a) in analgesic mixture for removing tiredness. Caffeine is itself not an analgesic; (b) for the treatment of migraine combined with ergotamine. Caffeine directly constricts cranial vessels and also increases absorption of ergotamine from gastrointestinal tract.

Adverse effects of caffeine

Gastric irritation may occur as a side effect. The toxic effects include nervousness, insomnia and excitement. There may be tachycardia. The patients of peptic ulcer should not take caffeine.

Slight tolerance occurs to caffeine. In habitual heavy coffee drinkers (6 or more cups per day) abstinence syndrome includes headache and irritability.

Adverse effects of theophylline

Theophylline has a narrow margin of safety. With plasma levels above 15 microgram per ml, the side effects occur in following sequence:

- 15 µg/ml.: Dyspepsia, headache, insomnia
- 20 µg/ml.: Restlessness, palpitaion, vomiting
- 25 µg/ml.: Agitation, tachypnoea
- 30 µg/ml.: Increased muscle tone, extrasystole
- 40 µg/ml.: Arrhythmias, convulsion and coma

Amphetamines and related drugs

A group of drugs comprising its active dextro-isomer dextroamphetamine, with methamphetamine and methylphenidate have similar pharmacological properties. This group includes 'street drugs' such as methylenedioxymethamphetamine (MDMA or 'ecstasy'). Fenfluramine has chemical similarity but has different pharmacological actions.

The following actions are produced by amphetamine:

Fatigue is postponed
Locomotor stimulation
Excitement
Euphoria
Anorexia
Stereotyped behaviour (repeated actions)
Peripheral sympathomimetic actions (rise in BP and inhibition of GIT motility).

With large doses subjects develop tremors, confusion, dizziness.

Table 3.24 shows comparison of certain effects of amphetamines-like drugs.

Mechanism of action

Amphetamine acts by releasing noradrenaline stored in nerve endings in both the CNS and in periphery.

Table 3.24. Comparison of certain effects of amphetamines-like drugs

	Locomotor stimulation	Stereotyped behaviour	Anorexia	Euphoria
Amphetamine	+++	+++	++	++
MDMA	+++	+++	+	+++
Methylphenidate	+++	+++	+	+
Fenfluramine	–	–	+++	–

+++ = marked, ++ = moderate, + = slight, – = none
Note: Amphetamine - like drugs on continued intake lose anorexiant effect.

Dependence on amphetamine occurs, chiefly psychological but also physical dependence and on abrupt withdrawal there is withdrawal syndrome.

Pharmacokinetics

Amphetamine (t½ 12 hr) : It is readily absorbed by usual route, eliminated largely unchanged in urine.

Therapeutic uses

- Narcolepsy
- Appetite suppression. Alternatives are preferable
- Against fatigue: Seldom justified
- Use in sport is abuse.
- In some hyperactive children with attention deficit disorder, also methylphenidate (Ritalin).

The use of amphetamines and allied drugs is limited due to :

(i) dependence liability (drugs of abuse),
(ii) peripheral sympathomimetic activity (may cause rise in blood pressure and inhibition of GIT motility) and
(iii) risk of pulmonary hypertension.

Amphetamine is helpful but not completely effective for the treatment of narcolepsy (patient suddenly and unpredictably falls asleep at frequent intervals during the day).

For treating attention deficit and hyperactivity in children, phenylphenidate may be used (paradoxically). How it acts in this condition is not known.

Appetite suppression

Dexfenfluramine has replaced the racemic fenfluramine. It is structually related to amphetamine but it causes release of serotonin from nerve stores, rather than noradrenaline. It is sedative rather than stimulant to the CNS. It induces satiety i.e. the subject eats as frequently, but amount is less. In overdose amphetamine - like stimulation effects occur.

Uses

Choice for obesity (when a drug is needed). Weight loss begins is 2 weeks and lasts for 3 months.

Adverse drugs reactions

Sleepiness, depression, diarrhoea, impotence.

Heavy doses: CNS stimulation and cardiac arrhythmias.

Fluoxetine is an antidepressant that inhibits serotonin re-uptake into nerve endings. It has anorectic action.

Bulk preparations e.g., methylcellulose are given to provide feeling of satiety.

APPETITE STIMULATION

Cyprohepatadine

It blocks serotonin and histamine H_1-receptors. It increases appetite probably via an action on serotonin receptors in the hypothalamus.

Insulin increases appetite by reducing blood glucose concentration.

In general, little or nothing is gained by seeking to stimulate appetite by drugs.

Brain stem stimulants (Analeptics)

These stimulate medullary centres, and have the capacity to restore consciousness in patients in whom CNS is markedly depressed. They counteract respiratory depression caused by CNS depressants. However, their use has considerably declined as their margin of safety is very narrow and they can produce convulsions.

Bemegride (Megimide) : Its CNS stimulant action resembles pentylenetetrazol (leptazol) but it has wider margin of safety, produces effects more rapidly and of short duration. It was previously considered as a specific antagonist to barbiturates but it is not a specific antidote. It may be used by slow I.V. injection 50 mg every 5 minutes in acute respiratory failure as a general CNS stimulant.

Nikethamide (coramine) : After I.V. injection 0.5 to 2 g it produces effect promptly, but the duration of action is short. It is a weak analeptic. It can be repeated if required at intervals of 20-30 minutes to treat acute respiratory failure. Coramine 25% solution, 2.5 ml ampoules are available.

Doxapram : As a respiratory stimulant, its therapeutic index is higher as compared to other analeptics. The dose is 1-4 mg/minute I.V. injection; or 40-80 mg I.M. injection.

Ethamivan : It is related to nikethamide but more useful in acute respiratory insufficiency and barbiturate poisoning when administered I.V. 10 mg of 5% solution.

Prethcamide is a mixture of equal parts by weight of cropropamide and crotethamide. It has similar action and uses as doxapram. Dose is 100-250 mg orally, 250 mg/1.5 ml I.M. or I.V. injection.

Pentylenetetrazol (metrazol, cardiazol, tetrazol): It is a very potent CNS stimulant with very narrow margin of safety. As low doses produce excitation and high doses induce convulsions similar to picrotoxin, its therapeutic use is a thing of past. Now its use is limited as a convulsant for testing anticonvulsant drugs in experiment animals.

Picrotoxin : It is obtained from Anamirta cocculus. It produces respiratory and vasomotor stimulation as well as convulsions. It has no therapeutic value now.

Spinal convulsants

Strychnine : It is an alkaloid obtained from the seeds of strychnos nux vomica. It is a convulsant and acts as spinal stimulant.

It has now no therapeutic value.

STUDY QUESTIONS

1. Classify CNS stimulants according to their site of action.
2. Which drugs possess cerebral or psychomotor stimulant effect? What are the actions of caffeine on CNS and CVS?
3. What do you mean by the term analeptics? Name analeptic drugs. What are their uses and drawbacks?

GUIDE TO FURTHER READING

Aitken, M.L. et al: Life-threatening theophylline toxicity is not predictable by serum levels. Chest., 1987; 91:10-14.

Benowitz, N.L.: Clinical pharmacology of caffeine. Annu Rev Med, 1990; 41:277.

Benowitz, N.L.: Clinical pharmacology and toxicity of cocaine. Pharmacol Toxicol, 1993; 72:3.

Bertino, J.S. et al: Reassessment of theophylline toxicity. Serum concentrations, clinical course, and treatment. Arch. Intern. Med., 1987; 147:757-760.

Brackett, L.E. et al: Activities of caffeine, theophylline, and enprofylline analgos as tracheal relaxants. Biochem. Pharmacol., 1990; 39:1897-1904.

Bryant, D.H. et al: Effects of ipratropium bromide nebulizer solution with and without preservatives in the treatment of acute and stable asthma. Chest., 1992; 102:742-747.

Choi, O.H. et al: Caffeine and theophylline analogues: correlation of behavioral effects with activity as adenosine receptor antagonists and as phosphodiesterase inhibitors. Life Sci., 1988; 43:387-398.

Chou, J.M. et al Caffeine and Coffee: effects on health and cardiovascular disease. Comp. Biochem. Physiol., 1994; 109c:173- 189.

Curatolo, P.W. et al: The health consequences of caffeine. Ann. Intern. Med., 1983; 98:641-653.

D'Alonzo, D.E. et al: Salmeterol xinafoate as maintenance therapy compared with albuterol in patients with asthma. J. Am. Med. Assoc., 1994; 271:1412-1416.

Ernst, E. et al: Pentoxifylline for intermittent claudication. A critical review. Angiology, 1994; 45:339-345.

Fanta, C.H. et al: Treatment of acute asthma, Is combination therapy with sympathomimetics and methylxanthines indicated? Am. J. Med., 1986; 80:5-10.

Grabowski, J., Dworkin, S. I.: Cocaine: An overview of current issues. Int J Addict, 1985; 20:1065.

Graham, D.M. et al: Caffeine-its identity, dietary sources, intake and biological effects. Nutr. Rev., 1978; 36:97-102.

Graham, T.E. et al: Caffeine and exercise: metabolism and performance. Can. J. Appl. Physiol., 1994; 19:111-138.

Green, R.M. et al: The effects of pentoxifylline on patients with intermittent claudication. J. Vasc. Surg., 1988; 7:356-362.

McCubbin, M. et al: Does asthma or treatment with theophylline limit children's academic performance? N. Engl. J. Med., 1992; 327:926-930.

McFadden, E.R. et al: Methylxanthines in the treatment of asthma: the rise, the fall, and the possible rise again. Ann. Int. Med., 1991; 115:323-324.

Muttitt, S.C. et al: The dose response of theophylline in the treatment of apnea of prematurity. J. Pediatr., 1988; 112:115- 121.

Myers, M.G. et al: Effects of caffeine on blood pressure. Arch. Intern. Med., 1988a, 148:1189-1193.

Myers, M.G. et al: Caffeine and cardiac arrhythmias. Chest., 1988b, 94:4-5.

Nasser, S.S. et al: Theophylline. Current thoughts on the risks and benefits of its use in asthma. Drug Safety, 1993; 8:12-18.

Ogilvie, R.I. et al: Cardiovascular response to increasing theophylline concentrations. Eur. J. Clin. Pharmacol., 1977; 12:409-414.

Pomerleau, O.F.: Nicotine and the central nervous system. Biobehavioral effects of cigarette smoking . Am J Med, 1992; 93 (Suppl IA): IA.

Smith, D.E. et al (editors): Amphetamine use, Misuse and Abuse, GK Hall, 1979.

Stirt, J.A. et al: Aminophylline may act as a morphine antagonist. Anaesthesia, 1983; 38:275-278.

Stoloff, S.W. et al: The changing role of theophylline in pediatric asthma. Am. Fam. Physician, 1994; 49:839-844.

Tournaye, H. et al: Pentoxifylline in idiopathic male factor infertility: a review of its therapeutic efficacy after oral administration. Hum. Reprod., 1994; 9:996-1000.

PSYCHOPHARMACOLOGICAL AGENTS

Terminology associated with psychopharmacology

Illusions are misperceptions of external stimuli e.g., to mistake a rope for a snake at dark.

Hallucination is a percept experienced in the absence of an external stimulus to the sense organ e.g., flashes of light, bangs, whistles, hearing voices, seeing faces.

Delusion is a belief which is firmly held despite evidence to contrary. It could be persecutory delusion (paranoid delusion) or delusion of grandeur or delusion of guilt and worthlessness) nihilistic delusion is characteristic of extreme depressive state - is about to die or he has become bankrupt.

Hypochondriacal delusion is when the patient may believe that he is ill while all medical evidences show contrary.

Delusion of jealousy may lead to dangerous behaviour towards a person thought to be unfaithful.

Delusions of control is when the patient believes that his action, thoughts and impulses are controlled by an outside agency (characteristic of schizophrenia).

Acute dystonia: Spasm of muscles of tongue, face, neck, back.

Akathisia: Motor restlessness.

Parkinsonism: Rigidity, bradykinesia, mask facies, shuffling gait.

Tardive dyskinesia: Involuntary repetitive movements of lips, tongue, face, jaws and limbs.

The era of psychopharmacology commenced with the introduction of chlorpromazine by Laborit in 1952. The psychotropic drugs act on the psyche. These drugs may be grouped as:

1. Antipsychotics or neuroleptics (formerly called major tranquilizers). These produce calming effect without marked drowsiness.
2. Antianxiety (Anxiolytic-sedative, formerly called minor tranquilizers) drugs. These control tension and anxiety.
3. Drugs for affective disorders:
   (a) Antidepressants: These elevate mood
   (b) Antimanic drugs
4. Psychotherapeutic agents for cognitive disorders

1. Antipsychotic drugs or neuroleptics

These include substituted:
- Phenothiazines
- Butyrophenones
- Thioxanthenes
- Alkaloids of rauwolfia
- Dibenzodiazepines
- Few others such as pimozide

Substituted phenothiazines

- Aliphatic side chain
  - Chlorpromazine, triflupromazine (siquil)
- Piperidine side chain
  - Thioridazine (mellaril)
- Piperazine side chain
  - Trifluoperazine, fluphenazine, thioproperazine

Substituted butyrophenones

- Haloperidol, droperidol, trifluperidol

Substituted thioxanthenes

- Chlorprothixene, thiothixene

Rauwolfia alkaloids

- Reserpine (Serpasil)

Dibenzodiazepines

- Clozapine

Others

- Pimozide, molindone, loxapine

2. Antianxiety agents (anxiolytics, formerly called minor tranquilizers)

Benzodiazepines

- Diazepam (valium, calmpose), oxazepam, chlordiazepoxide (librium), flurazepam, nitrazepam, clonazepam, lorazepam

Carbamates

- Meprobamate (equanil, miltown)

Barbiturates

- Phenobarbitone (long acting tranquilo-sedative)

3. Drugs for affective disorders (drugs which relieve pathological changes in mood state)

Affective disorders are due to pathological changes in mood state.

These drugs are:
- Antidepressants
- Antimanic (mood stabilizer)

Depression

It is a mood of sadness or gloom. It occurs as a response to troubled circumstances. Most people can cope with it and are out of it in a matter of days. Such situational depression is often termed as grief etc. Distinction has to be drawn between depression as a response to troubled circumstances and depression as a symptom of manic depression disorders.

There are two extremes: "mania" and "depression". They occur in isolation or may accompany psychosis.

Types of depression

- Bipolar depression develops earlier in life and tends to be inherited. It may have features common with schizophrenia.
- Unipolar depression patients do not swing into bouts of mania and there is no genetic cause, occurs later in life. It is often associated with features of anxiety and aggression. Unipolar de-

pression may be "reactive" (distorted response to distressing circumstances) or 'endogenous' as a result of biochemical abnormality within the brain.

Symptoms of depression

- There is a general feeling of misery
- Indecisiveness
- Preoccupation with guilt and inadequacy
- Retardation of thoughts and action
- Loss of appetite
- Slowing of movements
- Sleep disturbances

Symptoms of mania

- Excessive exuberance
- Excessive physical activity
- Irritability
- Impatience
- Anger
- Mood generally inappropriate to the circumstances

Antidepressants

- Monoamine oxidase inhibitors (MAOIs)
  - (i) Hydrazines
    Phenelzine, nialemide
  - (ii) Nonhydrazine
    Isocarboxazid, tranylcypromine, pargyline
  - (iii) Isoenzyme selective
    Chlorgyline, deprenyl
- Monoamine reuptake inhibitors (thymoleptics)
  - Tricyclic antidepressants
    Imipramine, desipramine, amitriptyline, nortriptyline, doxepin
  - Bicyclic antidepressants
    Viloxazine
  - Monocyclic antidepressants
    Tofenacin
  - Tetracyclic antidepressants
    Minaserin, maprotiline
- Others
  - Flupenthixol (antipsychotic drug used in small doses in depression)

Anti-mania drugs

Lithium carbonate (mood stabilizer)

Types of mental diseases

Very broadly speaking, from the point of view of the clinical application of psychoactive drugs, the mental diseases are of two kinds: (1) Neuroses and (2) Psychoses.

Table 3.25 shows the differences between neurosis and psychosis.

Table 3.25. Differences between neurosis and psychosis.

Neurosis (pl : neuroses)	Psychosis (pl : psychoses)
Minor mental illness	Major mental illness
Patient's insight is intact	Lost
Hallucinations and delusions are not common	Common
Patient himself reports for treatment	Frequently brought by others
Adaptation to family and society good	Nuisance
Response to treatment good	Unpredictable, relapses common

Neuroses

The neurotic patients usually retain sufficient insight to realize that there is something wrong with them. It could be:

(a) Anxiety states out of proportion to the stress or fear which induces it. The abnormal fears or phobias could be to specific objects or even conditions viz. claustrophobia (fear of confined spaces), acrophobia (fear for heights) or agoraphobia (fear of crowded places).

(b) Hysteria mimicking symptoms of physical illness to escape from an unfavourable situation.

(c) Obsessional neuroses: obsessed and compulsive behaviour without any rationality, e.g. obsession with dirt.

(d) Depressive reactions: neurotic depression is usually reactive in nature, abnormally severe or prolonged reactions like sadness, self-criticism.

Psychoses

The psychotic patient lives in the world of his own, quite away from reality. He has no insight into his illness.

Schizophrenia

The most important and commonest type of psychosis is schizophrenia (split mind). It is a disorder of thinking, behaviour and expression appearing in clear consciousness. The patient is absorbed in his own thoughts, auditory hallucinations, social withdrawal, deterioration in personal care, purposeless stereotyped movements, crying or laughing inconsistent with environment or circumstances. There are delusions of paranoid thinking.

The psychotic patient lives in the world of his own, quite away from the reality. He has no insight into his illness. The four important symptoms of schizophrenia are: delusions, hallucinations, thought disorder and withdrawal from social contacts and blunting of emotions.

Drugs likely to cause psychoses - like condition:

Glucocorticoids	Indomethacin
Anticholinergics	L-dopa
Sympathomimetics	Amantadine
Carbamazepine	Lithium
Phenytoin	Digitalis
Disulfiram	

Affective psychoses : Endogenous depression (unipolar depression).

There is no obvious precipitating cause. It may be associated with anxiety, delusion or hallucinations. There is utter depression of mood (melancholia) and suicidal tendency.

Manic-depression psychoses (bipolar depression): There are swings of mood from elation and agitation (mania) to profound depression.

Clinical uses of chlorpromazine

Psychiatric indications

- Schizophrenia
- Schizoaffective disorders

- Nonmanic excited states
- Disturbed behaviour of senile dementia in Alzheimer's disease
- With antidepressants to control agitation or psychoses in depressed patients
- Relief of anxiety associated with emotional disorders
- Tourette syndrome (marked by tics, other involuntary movements), aggressive outbursts, grunts, and vocalizations that frequently are obscene

Nonspychiatric indications

- Antiemetic
- Antipruritic
- Preoperative sedative
- Anti hiccup
- Adjunct in tetanus (to produce muscle relaxation)

Neurochemical basis of mental diseases

Central neurotransmitters and neuroregulators seem to play role.

In schizophrenia (commonest psychosis), excessive dopaminergic activity is held responsible. Most drugs used in schizophrenia block dopamine receptors.

The other views in vogue are that the abnormal metabolites of endogenous NA, DA and 5-HT produce hallucinations.

Recently it has also been proposed that excessive endorphin, prostaglandin deficiency/excess, zinc deficiency, abnormal histamine metabolism, etc. may also be responsible for the abnormalities of schizophrenia.

Depression seems to be related to impairment of noradrenergic and/or serotonergic neurotransmission with uncompensated overactivity of cholinergic neurons in the CNS.

In mania, there may be hyperfunctioning of noradrenergic and/or serotonergic activity and dysfunction of cholinergic neurotransmission. Most of the drugs used in mania decrease availability of NA or DA as transmitter.

Antipsychotic agents

Chlorpromazine (CPZ)

It is the first neuroleptic introduced. It can be described as the prototype.

Pharmacological actions

CNS

- State of tranquillity, calming effect. Psychotic patients become less agitated, hallucinations decline.
- Hypothermic effect.
- Potentiate the narcotic and non-narcotic analgesia.
- Antiemetic effect (inhibits dopamine D_2 receptors in chemoreceptor trigger zone).
- Seizure threshold is lowered and may exacerbate epilepsy.
- Muscle relaxation.

Peripheral actions

- Local anaesthetic action.
- Quinidine like actions on heart.
- Weak anticholinergic, antihistaminic and 5-HT blocking activity.
- Alpha-adrenergic blocking action (hypotension, postural hypotension and failure of ejaculation).
- Neuroendocrine blocking activity on ACTH, gonadotrophins, growth hormone, ADH and insulin. Prolactin secretion is increased.
- Aggravates epilepsy and may antagonize antiepileptic drugs.

Metabolic actions

- Chlorpromazine depresses energy utilization by brain in therapeutic doses, larger doses interfere with energy production.

Adverse effects of chlorpromazine

1. Acute toxicity: 100 times the therapeutic dose is not lethal.
2. Side effects:
   Extension of pharmacological effects:
   (i) Anticholinergic effects - nasal stuffiness, dry mouth, blurred vision, urinary retention in elderly, constipation.

(ii) CV - Orthostatic hypotension, palpitation, faintness.

(iii) Neurological side effects:
- Seizures more with chlorpromazine, clopazine
- Acute reversible - acute dystonia akathisia, parkinsonism - like symptoms
- Late irreversible (after months or years of treatment) - tardive dyskinesia, perioral tremor (rabbit syndrome).

(iv) Endocrine disturbances –
Gynaecomastia (painful enlarged breasts, lactation)

3. Hypersensitivity reactions : Jaundice, opacities in cornea and lens with prolonged used, skin rashes.

In comparison with haloperidol, chlorpromazine is less potent, and produces less extrapyramidal effects. Haloperidol is more potent, less sedative, less hypotensive but exerts more extrapyramidal disorders.

There are two main receptor types: D_1 which increases adenylate cyclase activity, and D_2 which mediates the main presynaptic and postsynaptic inhibitory actions of dopamine.

D_3 and D_4 receptors belong to the same group as D_2.

The antipsychotic drugs owe their therapeutic effects mainly to blockade of D_2 - receptors. Antipsychotic effects require about 80% block of D_2 - receptors.

The main groups, phenothiazines, thioxanthenes and butyrophenones, show some preference for D_2- over D_1 - receptors; some of the newer agents, eg., sulpiride are highly selective for D_2-receptors, whereas clozapine is relatively nonselective between D_1 and D_2, but has high affinity for D_4.

- The antipsychotic effects is due to blockade of D_2 receptors in mesolimbic system.
- Blockade of dopamine receptors in nigrostriatal system produces motor effects.
- Blockade of dopamine receptors in tubero-infundibular region leads to hyperprolactinemia.
- Blockade of dopamine receptors at chemo-receptor trigger zone is responsible for their antiemetic effect.

The comparison of commonly used antipsychotic drugs is given in Table 3.26.

Mode of action of antipsychotic agents

Antipsychotic agents produce dopaminergic receptor blockade, as shown below.

Antianxiety is a subjective human phenomenon. It is unpleasant mood of tension and apprehension,

Table 3.26. Comparison of commonly used antipsychotic drugs (distinctive features of individual neuroleptics)

Drug	Antipsychotic dose (mg)		Sedation	Hypotension	Extra-pyramidal action
	Oral daily	Single i.m. dose			
Chlorpromazine hydrochloride	200-800	25-50	+++	++ oral, +++ i.m.	++
Trifluoperazine hydrochloride	5-20	1-2	+	+	+++
Thioridazine hydrochloride	150-600		+++	+++	+
Haloperidol and haloperidol decanoate	2-20	2-5 (haloperidol decanoate 25-250 every 2-4 weeks)	+	+	++++
Chlorprothixene	50-400	25-50	+++	++	++
Pimozide	2-6		+	+	+++
Molindone hydrochloride	50-225		++	+	++
Clozapine	150-450		+++	+++	0
Perfenazine	8-32	5-10	++	+	++

+++ marked effect, ++ moderate effect, + slight effect, — no effect

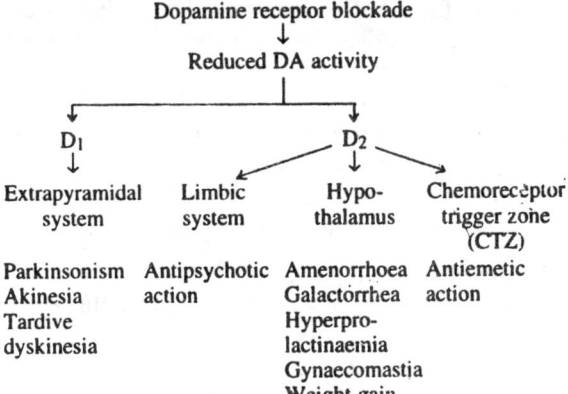

adrenals, heart and blood vessels. Reserpine combines with serotonin receptors and thus displaces this agent. The effects of depletion continue for some time after reserpine is no longer present (by contrast chlorpromazine does not deplete 5-HT or NA but does interfere with the action of serotonin). The antipsychotic effects of both the substituted phenothiazines and reserpine depend on adrenergic blocking effect, but these agents are antagonistic because the anti-adrenergic effects of reserpine are due to transmitter depletion while those of phenothiazines are due to prevention of the release of the transmitter.

usually imposed by distress or difficulties. Anxiety is an universal response of common people. However, it poses a problem where it is excessive. The manifestations of anxiety are - GIT: dry mouth, flatulence, epigastric discomfort, frequent lose stools; - CV: palpitation; Genitourinary: increased frequency and urgency of micturition, lack of libido; Musculoskeletal: headache, stiffness, tremor; Psychological: repetitive worrying thoughts, irritability, restlessness, uneasiness, sensitivity to noise; sleep: delayed, dreams, nightmares.

Reserpine

Reserpine is an alkaloid from Rauwolfia serpentina, a long time medicinal plant of Indian folklore. It has bradycardiac-hypotensive and tranquilizing effect. Reserpine reduces the concentration of serotonin in the brain and reduces concentration of NA in brain,

Butyrophenones

Haloperidol is pharmacologically but not chemically related to phenothiazines. It is a potent antipsychotic and potent antiemetic agent.

Thioxanthenes

Chlorprothixene and thiothixene are structural analogues of phenothiazines. The overall range of activity and adverse effects are similar.

Antianxiety drugs (Anxiolytic drugs)

Pharmacokinetics of Benzodiazepines

All benzodiazepines exert their actions at specific receptors. The choice between different agents is dictated by the speed of action, its intensity, and duration, These, in turn, reflect their physicochemical and pharmacokinetic properties. Individual benzodiazepines remain in the body for very different lengths of time and are chiefly eliminated through biotransformation. Inactivation may entail a single chemical reaction or several steps (e.g., diazepam) before an inactive metabolite suitable for renal elimination is formed. Since the intermediary products may, in part, be pharmacologically active and in part, be excreted much more slowly than the parent substance, metabolites will accumulate with continued regular dosing and contribute significantly to the final effect.

Biotransformation begins either at substituents on the diazepine ring (diazepam: N-dealkylation at position 1; midazolam: hydroxylation of the methyl group on the imidazole ring) or at the diazepine ring itself. Hydroxylated midazolam is quickly eliminated

Box 3.11. Common phenothiazine derivatives			
Drug	Main use	Adverse effects (frequency) Orthostatic hypotension	Extra-pyramidal symptoms
Chlor-promazine	Antipsychotic	Moderate	Moderate
Thioridazine	Antipsychotic	Moderate	Low
Triflu-promazine	Antipsychotic	Moderate	High
Prochlor-perazine	Antiemetic	Low	Moderate-low
Promethazine	Antihistaminic	Moderate	Low

following glucuronidation (t½-2 hr.) and N-Demethyldiazepam (nordiazepam, or nordazepam) is biologically active and undergoes hydroxylation at position 3 on the diazepine ring. The hydroxylated product (oxazepam) is pharmacologically active. By virtue of their long half-lives, diazepam (t½-32hr) and, still more so, its metabolite nordiazepam (t½-50-90 hr), are eliminated slowly and accumulate during repeated intake. Oxazepam undergoes conjugation to glucuronic acid via its hydroxyl group (t½-8hr) and renal excretion.

These were formerly called minor tranquilizers.

Benzodiazepines (Anxiolytics)

- Chlordiazepoxide (librium, equilibrium) 10 mg tablets, 20-100 mg dose. It has poor anticonvulsant effect. Active metabolites are slowly absorbed. It is administered orally or parenterally. The usual daily dose is 15-40 mg, 25-200 mg parenteral.
- Diazepam (valium, calmpose) 2.5 mg tablet, 10 mg/5ml syrup. The drug is quickly absorbed, metabolites formed are active. It is administered orally or parenterally.
- Oxazepam is slowly absorbed and duration is short as metabolites produced are not active. The dose is 30-60 mg in 2-3 divided doses. It is administered orally.
- Lorazepam has slower oral absorption than with diazepam, no active metabolites are produced, dose is 2-6 mg. It is an effective sedative when given by I.V. injection. It can be given orally or parenterally.
- Alprazolam has antidepressant action also. It is administered orally. The usual daily dose is 0.75-1.5 mg.
- Nitrozepam and Flurazepam are good sedative-hypnotic-antianxiety drugs.
- Clonazepam is preferred as antiepileptic. It is administered orally. The usual therapeutic dose is 1.5-10 mg.
- Flurazepam produces hypnotic effect in about 30 minutes after oral dose and duration is 6-8 hours. The major metabolite has long half-life which may cause daytime sedation and mental impairment.

The addiction potential is low and less suppression of REM sleep than other benzodiazepines. At higher dose, 30 mg it produces daytime residual sedation.

- Triazolam is very fast acting, duration is short which may not persist throughout the night. It may cause rebound insomnia.
- Temazepam may accumulate with repeated use. Its onset of action is intermediate-to-slow.

Some drugs likely to cause mania like condition

INH	Corticosteroids, Anticholinergics
Procarbazine	Sympathomimetics
L-dopa	Anticonvulsants
Disulfiram	Benzodiazepines

Pharmacological actions

Anxiolytics are useful as anticonvulsant, central muscle relaxant and also used in status epilepticus. But abrupt withdrawal may precipitate epileptiform seizures.

Benzodiazepines are not analgesic but potentiate analgesics, possess slight effect on ANS; do not induce hepatic microsomal enzymes; margin of safety is wide, and produce little respiratory depression even with over dosage. Tolerance and drug dependence develop but to lesser extent as compared to barbiturates.

The antianxiety drugs resemble sedative-hypnotics and markedly differ from antipsychotic drugs.

These do not affect thought disorders in schizophrenia.

These do not produce parkinsonism like condition.

They produce drug dependence and carry abuse liability unlike antipsychotic drugs.

Mode of action of benzodiazepines

Antianxiety effect may be due to stimulation of GABA and glycine (inhibitory transmitters) in limbic system, muscle relaxation is due to inhibition of polysynaptic reflexes in spinal cord.

Clinical uses

- For anxiety: diazepam, chlordiazepoxide
- As hypnotic: nitrazepam, flurazepam
- As antiepileptic: clonazepam

- For status epilepticus: I.V. diazepam
- As anticonvulsant: diazepam I.V., chlordiazepoxide
- I.M. or I.V. in tetanus, atropine poisoning, delirium tremens, strychnine poisoning.
- As premedicament: diazepam
- As muscle relaxant in chronic spastic disorders: diazepam
- For treating addiction with strong addiction producing drugs: diazepam.

Adverse effects

Sedation, confusion, lethargy, paradoxical aggression, drug dependence.

Non-benzodiazepine anxiolytics

Meprobamate (equanil,miltown) produces drug dependence similar to barbiturates. The withdrawal syndrome appears to be milder.

Dose 0.4-2.4 g; 0.2, 0.4 g tablets.

Hydroxyzine is H_1 antagonist with sedative, antiemetic and anticholinergic, antispasmodic and local anaesthetic properties.

Dose. 100-200 mg/d; 10-25 mg tablet; 10 mg/5 ml syrup; 6 mg/ml drops and 25 mg/2 ml injection.

Buspirone. It is an antianxiety drug that is not chemically or pharmacologically related to the benzodiazepines, barbiturates or other sedative - hypnotic drugs. It is rapidly and completely absorbed from GIT, this drug undergoes an extensive first-pass effect. One hydroxylated metabolite is active.

Buspirone is used for the short-term treatment of generalized anxiety. It may require 1-2 weeks for a therapeutic effect to take place.

Propranolol and other non selective beta blockers relieve symptoms of anxiety due to sympathetic overactivity.

Drugs for affective disorders

Affective disorders are due to pathological changes in mood state, viz. mania and depression. These drugs are:
- Antimanic (mood stabilizer)
- Antidepressants

Lithium carbonate is a very effective antimanic drug. As it takes about 8 days to achieve threshold level initially, so in initial or acute episodeofmania, the symptoms are required to be controlled by using antipsychotic drugs.

Lithium acts only in CNS if blood concentrations are kept within 2 mEq/litre. It is rapidly absorbed from intestine, is not protein bound and distributed both extracellularly and cellularly. It is excreted through kidneys.

Dose 600-900 mg on the first day, increased to 1200-1800 mg on the second day and then the dose is adjusted by monitoring plasma levels (optimum level 0.8-1.2 mEq/L).

Mode of action is not clear. It seems to act by modifying synthesis, release or action of 5-HT, dopamine and noradrenaline.

It inhibits adenylcyclase.

Adverse effects

Within therapeutic range adverse effects are mild: Thirst, polyurea, tremor, GI upsets.

Prolonged use leads to hypothyroidism.

Overdosage (> 2 mEq/litre conc. in blood):

Muscle twitches, ataxia, blurred vision, kidney damage (acute kidney failure), epileptiform convulsions, cardiac arrhythmias, coma, death.

Treatment of lithium overdosage: Alkaline diuresis with sodium bicarbonate and mannitol. Diuretics like furosemide are contraindicated as Li will replace Na in tissues and toxicity (particularly cardiac arrhythmias) will be enhanced.

Antidepressants

These fall into following categories :
1. Tricyclic antidepressants
2. Selective serotonin reuptake inhibitors (SSRIs)
3. Atypical antidepressants
4. Monoamine oxidase inhibitors (MAOIs)

1. Tricyclic antidepressants

Some clinically important tricyclic antidepressants are: Imipramine 75-300 mg is closely related to phenothiazines; Desipramine 75-300 mg, less sedative than imipramine; Amitriptyline 75-300 mg is better tolerated than imipramine; Nortriptyline 75-300 mg produces less sedation than its parent compound amitriptyline; Doxepin 75-300 mg is also effective in treating depression when anxiety is present; Protriptyline has a three-to-five day half-life and causes little sedation.

Imipramine

Mechanism of action of tricyclic antidepressants and related antidepressants

- Potentiate the action of biogenic amines, by blocking the inactivating reuptake of amines
- They possess antihistaminic (H_1-receptor blocking) and alpha-adrenergic properties.
- Possess antimuscarinic action and block reuptake of serotonin. Tertiary amines (imipramine, amitriptyline) are more effective at blocking serotonin uptake.

These drugs produce behavioral arousal and characteristic slowing of EEG, thymoleptic reactions. Higher doses produce depressant effect in the CNS.

Therapeutic uses of tricyclic antidepressants

- Treatment of depression
- Nocturnal enuresis
- Migraine
- Chronic pain
- Acute panic states
- Obscessive compulsive disorder
- Sleep apnoea
- Irritable bowel syndrome
- Doxepin is used in peptic ulcer
- Attention deficit disorder

Adverse effects of tricyclic antidepressants

- Antimuscarinic effect: Dry mouth, constipation, urinary retention, blurred vision, precipitation of glaucoma, impotence, hyperpyrexia, confusion, memory impairment. These are more with amitriptyline and doxepin, and less with desipramine.

- "Switch Process" - transition from depression to hypomania or manic excitement.
- CNS: headaches, drowsiness, confusion, disorientation, sedation, tremors, seizures. Amitriptyline causes more sedation, protriptyline causes less sedation.
- CVS: Postural hypotension, tachycardia, arrhythmias in overdosage.
- Allergic reactions: rashes, urticaria, photosensitivity.
- Jaundice, agranulocytosis.
- Increased appetite and weight gain.
- Sexual disturbances (impotence).

Interactions with tricyclic antidepressants

- Aspirin displaces tricyclic antidepressants from protein binding sites and cause toxicity.
- Tricyclic antidepressants potentiate CNS depressants e.g. alcohol.
- Barbiturates and cigarette smoking induce the metabolism of tricyclic antidepressants.
- Neuroleptics and steroids competitively reduce the metabolism of tricyclic antidepressants.
- Tricyclic antidepressants prevent the antihypertensive effects of guanethidine by interfering its transport into adrenergic neurons.

2. Selective serotonin (5-HT) reuptake inhibitors (SSRIs)

Used as antidepressants: Fluoxetine (most commonly used), Fluvoxamine, paroxetine, sertraline.

Advantages of SSRIs

- They lack anticholinergic and CVS side effects
- The do not cause weight gain
- They do not produce interaction with food containing tyramine
- Low acute toxicity

Adverse effects of SSRIs

- Nausea, vomiting, tremors, rashes
- In combination with MAOIs, they result in serotonin syndrome (tremor, muscle rigidity, hyperthermia, CV collapse)

- Fluoxetine produces increased aggression and violence. There is also increased suicide rate with this drug.

3. Atypical antidepressants

Nomifensine, trazodone, mianserin, maprotiline

Advantages of atypical antidepressants

- Less side effects than tricyclic antidepressants
- Most of these drugs are short acting except maprotiline

Mechanism of action

- Nomifensine is a selective dopamine uptake inhibitor
- Mianserine increases NE release.

Table 3.27 shows dose, side effects and certain characteristics of various groups of antidepressants.

Fluoxetine

It is a selective inhibitor of serotonin uptake in the CNS. It has little effect on central NE or dopamine function. It has less adverse effects because of minimal binding to cholinergic, histaminic, and alpha-adrenergic receptors.

It is well absorbed from GIT, undergoes extensive hepatic biotransformation to the active metabolite norfluoxetine. The inactive metabolites are excreted in the urine.

The onset of action is within 1-3 weeks after beginning treatment.

The elimination half-life for fluoxetine is 1-3 days and for norfluoxetine 7-15 days.

It is used for the treatment of mild to moderate endogenous depression.

Adverse effects include anorexia and unlike tricyclics does not cause weight gain. However, nausea, nervousness, headache, and insomnia occur more frequently than with tricyclics. It may precipitate mania or hypomania.

Sertraline and paroxetine

These are similar to fluoxetine. Sertraline is less likely than fluoxetine or paroxetine to interact adversely with other drugs.

Bupropion

It has no effect on amine uptake, increases NE release. Half life is about 12 hours.

It is rapidly absorbed from GIT and undergoes extensive first-class effect. It is used for the treatment of depression with anxiety. the improvement occurs within one week of treatment. This drug is sometimes effective in depressed patients who do not respond to tricyclic anti-depressants. It is also used to help stop smoking (alongwith nicotine patch).

It does not produce sedation, orthostatic hypotension, weight gain or sexual dysfunction associated with other antidepressants. However, it is contraindicated with eating disorders, seizures, or major head trauma because it may produce or exacerbate grand mal seizures.

Trazodone

It is a weak 5-HT uptake blocker, also blocks $5-HT_2$ and α_2-receptors. Half-life is 6-12 hours. It is safe in overdose, doesnot produce atropine-like effects.

Adverse effects include sedation, confusion, hypotension, cardiac dysfunction.

Maprotiline

It is a selective NE uptake blocker. Half-life is 40 hours (long acting drug). Adverse effects include atropine-like effects, sedation, seizures, allergic rashes, acute toxicity is similar to tricyclic antidepressants. This drug does not offer any major advantage.

Mianserin

It blocks α_2, $5-HT_2$, and H_1-receptors. It has no effect on monoamine uptake. Half-life is about 12 hours. It is safe in overdose. It has no atropine-like effects and no cardiovascular effects. However, unwanted effects such as sedation, seizures, hypersensitivity reactions including agranulocytosis have limited its use.

Venlafaxine

It is a weak 5-HT uptake inhibitor. It is a mixed NE/5-HT reuptake inhibitor. Half life is 6-12 hours. It is claimed to produce rapid effect (~ 1 week). Adverse effects include nausea, anxiety, sexual dysfunction. High doese cause a sustained diastolic hypertension.

Reboxetine

It is a type of antidepressant known as a selective norepinephrine reuptake inhibitor (NRI or NARI). It also has weak effect on serotonin reuptake. Dose in major depression in adults, is 4 mg twice daily.

Table 3.27. Antidepressants

Name	Usual Daily Dose, mg	Side effects	Comments
Tricyclic antidepressants			
Amitriptyline	150-300	Anticholinergic (dry mouth, tachycardia, consti-	Once daily dosing; nortri-
Nortriptyline	50-200	pation, urinary, retention, blurred vision; sweating,	ptyline best tolerated
Imipramine	150-300	tremor, postural hypotension, cardiac conduction	especially by elderly
Desipramine	150-300	delay, sedation weight gain)	
Doxepin	150-300		
Clomipramine	150-300		
Selective serotonin reuptake inhibitors (SSRIs)			
Fluoxetine	10-80	Headache, nausea and other GI effects, jitteri-	Once daily dosing,
Sertraline	50-200	ness, insomnia, sexual dysfunction	usually in A.M.;
Paroxetine	20-60		fluoxetine has very
Fluvoxamine	100-300		long half-life.
Citalopram	20-60		
Atypical antidepressant			bid-tid dosing
Venlafaxine	75-375	Nausea, dizziness, dry mouth, headache, increased B.P. anxiety and insomnia	
Mirtazapine	15-45	Somnolence, weight gain	Once daily dosing
Bupropion	250-450	Jitteriness, anorexia, tachycardia psychosis, flushing	tid dosing, fewer sexual side effects than SSRIs or TCAs
Trazodone	200-600	Sedation, dry mouth postural hypotension	Useful in low dose for slccp due to sedating effects with no anticho-linergic side effects.
Nefazodone	300-600	Sedation headache, dry mouth, nausea, consti-pation	Once daily dosing no effect on REM sleep un-like other antidepressants
MAOIs			
Phenelzine	45-90	Insomnia, hypotension weight gain, serious reactions with narcotics; hypertensive crisis; tyramine cheese reactions; lethal reactions with SSRIs	May be more effective in patients with atypical features or refractory depression

It is well-absorbed and not affected by food; peak plasma levels occur 1.5 to 2.5 hours after oral doses. Highly bound to plasma proteins. Extensive hepatic metabolism; no active metabolites; mostly excreted in urine as metabolites (9% unchanged). Elimination half-life: 12 to 14 hours.

It is effective in major depression.

4. Monoamine oxidase inhibitors (MAOIs)

The deficiency of the monoamine neurotransmitters, serotonin, dopamine and noradrenaline has been proposed as the cause of depression. MAO is the major metabolizing enzyme of these neurotrans-mitters. Thus the MAO inhibitors lead to increase intraneuronal concentration of monoamine trans-mitters and thereby act as antidepressants. How-ever, this enzyme inhibition is not specific as intesti-nal and hepatic oxidases are also inhibited.

The MAOIs can be classified as:
- Irreversible, not-selective between MAO-A and MAO-B subtypes :
- phenelzine, isocarboxazid, tranylcypromine
- Reversible, selective MAO-A :
  moclobemide, clorgyline (effective in depression)
  MAO-B specific :
  selegiline (not used as antidepressant, used in parkinsonism).

Pharmacological actions

- Enzyme inhibition starts early but the antidepressant action is evident after 1 to 3 weeks.
- Drugs whose effects are monoamine mediated viz. analgesics, hypnotics, antiepileptic are potentiated by MAOIs.
- Drugs whose effects are due to decrease in monoamine activity viz. neuroleptics including chlorpromazine and reserpine are antagonized by MAOIs.
- Pargyline produces hypotensive effect, may be due to sympathetic ganglion block. It is now no more used as an antihypertensive agent.
- Tranylcypromine (sympathomimetic action) potentiates action of indirectly acting sympathomimetics.

Clinical uses

Due to a large number of side effects and other severe interactions with food and many other drugs, MAOIs have few limited uses in clinical practice.

Adverse effects include hepatotoxicity, postural hypotension, insomnia, irritability, convulsions, impotency, leucopenia, skin rashes, etc.

Interactions with foods containing pressor amines like tyramine (cheese), broad beans (monoamine precursor dopa), and alcoholic beverages—beers, wines, yeast extracts (tyramine) will produce hypertensive crisis "cheese reaction".

Interaction with drugs

- Hypertensive crisis with indirectly acting sympathomimetic e.g. amphetamine, ephedrine, dopamine.
- Marked respiratory depression, hypertension and coma with narcotic analgesics.
- Toxicity of barbiturates, alcohol, anticonvulsants, sedative-hypnotics is increased as MAOIs potentiate the action of these drugs.
- Potentiate tricyclic antidepressants. When MAOIs are to be replaced by tricyclic antidepressants, at least 2 to 3 weeks gap should be given.
- With L-dopa: hypertension.
- Excessive hypoglycaemia with oral hypoglycaemic agents and insulin.
- Increased toxicity with antimalarials.

As frequently encountered severe adverse effects and interactions of MAO inhibitors had made these drugs almost obsolete, recently specific MAO inhibitors have been introduced. MAO exists in A and B form. MAO B inhibitors are not expected to produce hypertensive crisis because NA (and serotonin) are substances for MAO A but not MAO B form.

Deprenyl is MAO B inhibitor which has been successfully used in depression without producing "cheese reaction" Chlorgyline inhibits MAO A; Dopamine is a common substances for MAO A & B.

4. Psychotherapeutic agents for cognitive disorders (cerebroactive drugs)

The cognitive disorders are commonly associated with definable neuropathological, metabolic, or toxic (including drug induced) changes and are characterized by confusion, disorientation.

It has been claimed that certain drugs improve cerebral circulation. However, in many cases this claim has not been substantiated. The therapeutic benefits are uncertain.

Nootropic drugs are new psychotherapeutic agents which facilitate the acquisition of learning and increase retention of memory. They may act by improving cerebral circulation and cerebral metabolism.

The following nootropic drugs have diverse chemical nature:

- Acetylcarnitine
- Aniracetam
- Citicoline
- Fampridine
- Idebenone
- Piracetam
- Vincamine
- Vinpocetine
- Cyclandelate
- Nicergoline
- Oxiracetam

Uses of nootropic drugs

- Cognitive deficits. Cognition is the process of acquiring (registration), storing (retention of

memory) and utilizing (recall of memory) the knowledge of learning.
- Children with learning and attention deficits.
- Memory disorder in neurological and psychiatric conditions.
- Amnesia following seizures, alcoholism, cerebral trauma.
- Senile dementia (Alzheimer type).
- Cerebrovascular accidents - stroke.

INDIVIDUAL AGENTS

Acetylcarnitine

It is a naturally occurring substance related to acetylcholine.

Dose: Oral doses of 1500 to 3000 mg daily have been administered to patients with Alzheimer-type dementia. For children with hyperactivity, the dosage is 50 milligrams/kilogram orally twice daily. The drug has also been given in intravenous doses of 20 mg/kg/day.

The elimination half-life of acetylcarnitine is 1.7 hours following an intravenous dose.

Cautions

Acetylcarnitine has been well tolerated in studies to date; agitation, nausea, vomiting, and occasional psychiatric disturbances have been reported with oral therapy.

Clinical Applications

Acetylcarnitine has been reported to slow progression of cognitive and behavioral impairment in patients with Alzheimer's disease; further long-term studies and comparisons with other agents used in Alzheimer's disease are needed to evaluate its therapeutic status.

Aniracetam

It is a "nootropic" agent used in the treatment of Alzheimer's disease and other disorders associated with cognitive impairment.

Dose: Oral aniracetam 500 mg twice daily has been used in the treatment of Alzheimer's disease.

Pharmacokinetics

Pharmacokinetic data for aniracetam are limited; the drug is rapidly absorbed after oral doses, although plasma levels are low due to first-pass metabolism. The primary metabolite of aniracetam is N-anisoyl gamma-aminobutyric acid, which is pharmacologically active.

Cautions

Confusion has been the main adverse effect of aniracetam in studies to date; the drug has not significantly affected blood pressure and heart rate, and has not been associated with haematologic or hepatic toxicity.

Clinical Applications

Aniracetam has shown some acute efficacy for Alzheimer's disease, however, larger and longer trials are needed.

Citicoline

It is a pyrimidine 5'-nucleotide used for its cerebro-active/dopaminergic properties in a variety of neurological disorders.

Dose: Citicoline has been administered orally, intramuscularly, and intravenously; usual doses have ranged from 500 to 1000 milligrams daily.

Pharmacokinetics

Citicoline is well absorbed following oral or intramuscular administration; plasma choline levels are increased significantly by either route. The drug is metabolized in the gut wall and liver to cytidine diphosphate and choline, and only small amounts of a dose are recovered in urine and faeces (less than 3% each); approximately 12% of a dose is eliminated as respiratory carbon dioxide. A substantial portion of a dose appears to be stored in tissue or utilized by the body for phospholipid synthesis.

Cautions

Only a few adverse effects have been reported during citicoline therapy, the most frequent of which are gastrointestinal disturbances, dizziness, and fatigue; no significant organ toxicity has been reported.

Clinical Applications

Citicoline has improved some symptoms in patients with Parkinson's disease when added to Levodopa therapy; conclusive evidence of efficacy in other conditions is lacking (stroke, vascular dementia, Alzheimer's disease, head injury). Flaws in design are evident in most studies evaluating this agent, and further well-controlled trials are needed to establish its role in therapy.

Fampridine

It is a potassium channel blocking agent.

Dose: Oral Fampridine 10 to 50 mg daily has been used in patients with multiple sclerosis; higher oral doses have been used in disorders of neuro-muscular transmission (e.g., myasthenia gravis). Fampridine has also been given by intravenous bolus or continuous infusion in varying doses; dose adjust-ments should be considered in renal impairment.

Pharmacokinetics

Fampridine is well absorbed after oral administration of enteric-coated tablets, with peak serum levels occurring in approximately 3 hours; protein binding is negligible. The drug is not metabolized to an appreciable extent; 90% of a dose is excreted unchanged in the urine. An elimination half-life of approximately 3 hours has been reported.

Cautions

Adverse effects of Fampridine are primarily confined to the central nervous system and include paresthesias, dizziness, restlessness, anxiety, and gait instability; confusional episodes and seizures can occur with higher doses (greater than 1 to 1.5 mg/kg/day). Oral therapy has been associated with nausea, vomiting, abdominal pain, and diaphoresis; pain on injection is frequent with intravenous ad-ministration.

Clinical Applications

Fampridine has shown some degree of efficacy in multiple sclerosis, myasthenia gravis, congenital myasthenia, Eaton-Lambert syndrome, spinal cord injury, botulism, verapamil overdose, and as an antagonist to neuromuscular blockade; results in Alzheimer's disease are equivocal. The toxicity of fampridine, particularly seizures, has limited its use for all indications, and at present its use should be restricted to selected patients with multiple sclerosis and neuromuscular transmission disorders.

Idebenone

It is a nootropic agent.

Dose: The oral dose of Idebenone has ranged from 90 to 300 mg/day and up to 5 mg/kg/day.

Pharmacokinetics

The pharmacokinetics of idebenone have not been extensively studied. Therapeutic serum levels remain undefined, although dose-dependent changes in peak serum levels are documented over the range of 10 to 100 mg and are approximately 300 to 400 mcg/L following doses of 45 to 50 mg. serum levels were similar in healthy volunteers, patients with renal insufficiency, and patients with hepatic dysfunction; time to peak was delayed in patients with liver failure. Food enhances absorption, with doubling of peak serum concentrations. No evidence of drug accumulation with prolonged therapy has been noted. Therapeutic effects have been observed from 2 to 8 months after initiation of therapy.

Cautions

Side effects are usually mild and rarely cause withdrawal of therapy. Gastrointestinal complaints were recorded by 7%; headache, anxiety, drowsi-ness, and tachycardia may be noted. Although urinary retention and oedema have been reported with idebenone, a causal relationship has not been deter-mined.

Clinical Applications

Idebenone has shown modest therapeutic effects in a variety of neurologic disorders; however, clinical trials are needed to determine the safety, efficacy, and optimal dose of the drug, and its ultimate role in therapy.

Piracetam

It is a "nootropic" agent, which is believed to en-hance learning and memory.

Dose: Oral piracetam 2 to 4 grams three times daily, increasing to 18 to 24 grams daily, has been effective in various types of myoclonus when given in combination with other antimyoclonic agents; in children with dyslexia (incomplete alexia i.e. reduced reading ability) 1.65 g orally twice daily has been effective.

Pharmacokinetics

Peak serum levels of piracetam are observed within 30 to 45 minutes of oral administration; relatively high levels have been reported in brain tissue. Piracetam is primarily excreted unchanged in the urine; its elimination half-life is 5 to 6 hours.

Cautions

Very few adverse effects have been reported with piracetam in clinical studies to date; nervousness, irritability, headache, confusion, nausea, and abdominal pain have been reported occasionally. Piracetam has been reported to enhance the anticoagulant effects of warfarin.

Clinical Applications

Piracetam may have a role in the treatment of dyslexia in children. Potential efficacy of the drug has been reported in myoclonus, sickle cell anaemia and alcoholism, although further studies are needed. Consistent clinical benefits of piracetam in Alzheimer's disease have not been adequately demonstrated.

Vincamine

It is an alkaloid compound derived from the Vinca minor plant.

Dose: The recommended range for vincamine is 30 milligrams given orally one to three times a day. The dosing regimen should be determined individually and depends on the responsiveness to the therapy.

Pharmacokinetics

Vincamine is quickly absorbed enterally after oral administration, reaching the initial half-life after approximately 2 hours, followed by a slower elimination phase. The distribution of vincamine is extensive and it can also pass the blood-brain barrier. Vincamine is mainly metabolized in the liver and excreted by the kidneys.

Cautions

Vincamine should not be used if intracranial tumours are present (or any disease related to increased intracranial pressure), cerebrovascular accident (CVA in the acute phase), during pregnancy and lactation, or for convulsive disorders due to lack of data. Vincamine is also contraindicated in cardiac arrhythmias, acute myocardial infarction, or severe electrolyte imbalances (hypokalaemia or hypocalcaemia).

Clinical Applications

Vincamine has therapeutic value for patients with mild to moderate dementia, chronic cerebrovascular insufficiency, psychosis due to cerebral cell or tissue damage, and vertebro-basal ganglia insufficiency. Vincamine is also used for inner ear defects (dizziness, vascular circulatory disturbances and Meniere's syndrome), as well as for eye disorders (acute retinopathy and circulatory disturbances in the retina).

Vinpocetine

It is a synthetic vincamine derivative used for the treatment of cerebrovascular disorders.

Dose: Oral doses of 15 to 30 milligrams daily have been used in vascular or degenerative cerebral insufficiency.

Pharmacokinetics

Peak serum levels of vinpocetine occur within 1.5 hour of oral doses. The drug is metabolized in the liver, with only small amounts appearing unchanged in the urine. The elimination half-life of oral vinpocetine is 1 to 2 hours.

Cautions

Vinpocetine is generally well-tolerated. Adverse effects reported, following therapeutic use of vinpocetine include hypotension, dry mouth, weakness, tachycardia, stomach upset, rash or urticaria, and facial flushing.

Clinical Applications

Oral vinpocetine is claimed to increase cerebral blood flow and stimulate cerebral metabolism. It has shown some degree of efficacy in cerebrovascular disorders, although larger and better designed trials are needed to confirm benefits. The drug was ineffective in Alzheimer's disease in one study.

Cyclandelate

It is a mandelic acid derivative with vasodilating and antispasmodic properties. The drug also has in vitro antiplatelet aggregating effects.

Dose: Dosing with Cyclandelate is empiric; generally, 1600 mg/day is given orally in 4 equal doses. Doses can be reduced to a maintenance dose of 400 to 800 mg/day; beneficial effects may not appear until after 8 to 12 weeks of therapy.

Pharmacokinetics

Pharmacokinetic data with Cyclandelate is nonexistent. An assay for the compound and its metabolites has been developed, but has not been used to define pharmacokinetic data for the drug.

Cautions

Caution regarding a vascular "steal" syndrome should be recognized with cyclandelate use; blood vessels less affected by atherosclerosis, but more responsive to the drug, may vasodilate and shunt blood away from the more ischaemic areas. Patients with gastric disorders, bleeding, or platelet function abnormalities should exercise caution.

Clinical Applications

Cyclandelate should be used rarely, if at all. Little consistent, reproducible data supports its use in senility or dementia and other indications such as thrombophlebitis, nocturnal leg cramps, and Raynaud's phenomenon are not documented in the literature. Little pharmacological or pharmacokinetic data is available to assist in optimizing dosing regimens.

Nicergoline

It is a semisynthetic ergotamine derivative with alpha-adrenergic blocking activity.

Dose: For symptoms due to cerebrovascular insufficiency, oral doses of 5 to 15 mg 3 times daily, intramuscular doses of 2 to 4 mg/day or twice daily, or IV infusions of 4 to 8 mg/day have been used. Oral doses of 15 to 30 mg/day have been used in neurogenic bladder dysfunction, various ophthalmic disorders due to vascular insufficiency, and pruritus.

Pharmacokinetics

Peak serum levels are reached within 1 to 1.5 hours after oral dosing, 90 to 100% of an oral dose is absorbed, and the elimination half-life is 2.5 hours.

Ninety percent of a dose is metabolized, primarily by hydrolysis and demethylation; 70 to 80% of nicergoline and its metabolites are excreted renally.

Cautions

Nicergoline has been well tolerated in clinical trials; most side effects were mild and transient. It should be used with caution in acute haemorrhage; severe bradycardia; concurrent anticoagulant or platelet aggregation inhibitor therapy; concurrent anti-hypertensive therapy.

Clinical Applications

The clinical efficacy of nicergoline is unclear; however, it has been used in cerebrovascular insufficiency and peripheral vascular disease, vascular insufficiency in the eye and ear, as an adjunct in arterial hypertension and prophylaxis of venous thrombosis.

Oxiracetam

In a controlled trial, piracetam and oxiracetam (each 6 grams intravenously once daily) were compared in the treatment of 60 elderly patients with chronic cerebrovascular insufficiency. Treatment duration was 60 days. Both drugs produced favourable effects on psychosomatic and neurologic symptoms. Oxiracetam was better tolerated and was associated with a significant decrease in platelet aggregation. This trial was not randomized; further well-designed studies involving larger patient numbers are needed to more adequately assess the role of these drugs in chronic cerebrovascular disorders.

STUDY QUESTIONS

1. Define psychotropic drugs, and classify them.
2. What was the line of treatment of mental disorders before the introduction of chlorpromazine?
3. Define neuroleptics (antipsychotics) and classify them.
4. Describe the pharmacological actions, mode of action, doses, therapeutic uses, and adverse effects of chlorpromazine.
5. Which drugs are usually employed for the treatment of affective disorders (drugs which relieve pathological changes in mood state)?

6. Describe the pharmacology of tricyclic antidepressants.
7. What is the use of Lithium? What are its advantages and disadvantages?
8. Explain the neurochemical basis of mental diseases.
9. What are the main differences between neuroleptics (formerly called major tranquilizers) and anxiolytics (formerly called minor tranquilizers)?
10. How do antianxiety (anxiolytic) drugs act?
11. What are monoamine oxidase inhibitors? Why are they not commonly used in the treatment of depression? Describe their adverse effects and drug interactions.
12. What are psychostimulants? Describe their uses and limitations?
13. What are the uses and adverse effects of amphetamine?
14. Describe briefly serotonin reuptake inhibitors.
15. Define nootropic drugs. What are their uses ?
16. Comment on the mode of action of nootropic drugs.
17. Give a list of nootropic drugs
18. Write short-note on (i) Nicergoline; (ii) Cyclandelate; (iii) Piracetam.

GUIDE TO FURTHER READING

Alvir, J.M.J. et al: Clozapine-induced agranulocytosis: incidence and risk factors in the United States. N. Engl. J. Med., 1993; 329:162.

Amsterdam, J., Brunswick, D., and Mendels, J.: The clinical application of tricyclic antidepressant pharmacokinetics, and plasma levels. Am. J. Psychiatry, 1980; 137:653.

Baldessarini, R.J.: Current status of antidepressants; clinical pharmacology and therapy. J. Clin. Psychiatry in psychiatry Principles and practice 3rd ed. Harvard University Press, 1996 (in press).

Balderssarini, R.J., Cohen, B.M., and Teicher, M.H.: Significance of neuroleptic dose and plasma level in the pharmacologic treatment of psychoses. Arch. Gen. Psychiatry, 1988; 45:79.

Baldessarini, R.J.: Enhancing treatment with psychotropic medicines. Bull. Menninger Clin., 1994; 58:224.

Baumgartner, A., Bauer, M., and Hellweg, R.: Treatment of intractable non-rapid cycling bipolar affective disorder with high-dose thyroxine; an open clinical trial. Neuropsychopharmacology, 1994; 10:183.

Bellibas, S.E. et al: Lithium and anticholinergic combination of maintain a stable lithium plasma level. Hum. Psychopharmacol Clin. Exp., 1994; 9:33.

Biederman, J.: Sudden death in children treated with a tricyclic antidepressant. J. Am. Acad. Child Adolesc. Psychiatry, 1991; 30:495.

Biederman, J., and Jellinek, M.S.: Psychopharmacology in children. N. Engl. J. Med. 1984; 310:968.

Brown, W.A., and Khan, A.: Which depressed patients should receive antidepressants? CNS Drugs, 1994; 1:341.

Cade, J.F.J. Lithium salts in the treatment of psychotic excitement. Med. J. Aust., 1949; 2:349.

Calabrese, J.R. et al: Spectrum of efficacy of valproate in 78 rapid-cycling, bipolar patient, J. Clin. Psychopharmacology, 1992; 12:535.

Cassem, N.: Cardiovascular effects of antidepressants. J. Clin. Psychiatry, 1982; 43: 22.

Chandra, D., Sharma, V.N. and Mittal, R.L., Thin layer chromatography of some new phenothiazines. Chemist-Analyst, 1967; 56:100.

Coplan, J.D., Gorman, J.M., and Klein, D.F.: Serotin related functions in panic-anxiety: a critical review. Neuropsychopharmacology, 1992; 6:189.

Cusack, B., Nelson, A., and Richelson, E.: Binding of antidepressants to human brain receptors; focus on newer generation compounds. Psychopharmacology, 1994; 114:559.

Czeizel, A., and Lendvay, A.: Lack of teratogenic effects of benzodiazepines. Lancet, 1987; 1:628.

Dabiri, L.M., Pasta, D., Darby, J.K., and Mosbacher, D.: Effectiveness of Vitamin E for treatment of long-term tardive dyskinesia. Am. J. Psychiatry; 1994; 151:925.

Gerlach, J. New antipsychotics: Classification, efficacy and adverse effects. Schizophrenia Bull., 1991; 17:289.

Goff, D.C., and Baldessarini, R.J.: Drug interaction with antipsychotic agents. J. Clin. Psychopharmacol, 1993; 13:57.

Keck, P.E. et al: Valproate oral loading in the treatment of acute mania. J. Clin. Psychiatry, 1993; 54:305.

Kind, P., and Sorensen, J.: The costs of depression. Int. Clin. Psychopharmacol., 1993; 7:191.

Lader, M.:Benzodiazepines: A risk-benefit profile. CNS Drugs, 1994; 1:377.

Laegreid, L., Hagberg, G., and Lundberg, A.: The effect of benzodiazepines on the fetus and the newborn. Neuropediatrics, 1992; 23:18.

Leonard, B.E.: Biochemical strategies for the development of antidepressants. CNS Drugs, 1994; 1:285.

Sharma, H.L., Sharma, V.N. and Mittal, R.L., Studies on the synthesis of nitrophenothiazines by Smiles rearrangement. Tetrahedron Letters, 1967; 17:1657.

Sharma, H.L., Banergee, S.P., Sharma, V.N. and Mittal, R.L., Phenothiazines exhibiting lesser extrapyramidal manifestations. J. Med. Chem., 1968; 11:1244.

Sharma, H.L., Sharma, V.N. and Mittal, R.L., Studies on nitrophenothiazines; Part I. Their synthesis and an explanation for their peculiar behaviour of halonitrobenzenes with aminothiophenol. Aust. Jour. Chem., 1968; 21:3-81-3086.

Sharma, H.L., Sharma, V.N. and Mittal, R.L., Studies on nitrophenothiazines; Part II. IR and UV Spectral characteristics of some nitrophenothiazines and nitrodiphenylsulphides. Aust. Jour. Chem., 1968; 21:3087.

Sharma, V.N., Singh, K.P., and Rathod, D.S., Central nervous system actions of some phenothiazine derivatives. Ind. Jour. Med. Res., 1967; 55:897.

Singh, K.P., Sharma, V.N. and Rathod, D.S., Pharmacological actions of some recently synthesized phenothiazine derivatives. Ind. Jour. Med. Res., 1967; 55:889.

Zarate, C.A., Tohen, M., and Baldessarine, R.J.: Clozapine therapy in severe mood disorders. J. Clin. Psychiatry, 1995 (in press).

DRUG DEPENDENCE AND DRUG ABUSE

Since ancient civilization, man has been in search of substances that provide him with an escape from reality.

The term drug abuse denotes use of a drug for non-medical purposes and almost always for altering consciousness, to obtain chemical vacation and an escape from reality. The drug abuse is intermittent or continuous, invariably self administered, for escape from personal problems which may be real or imaginary, for fun, excitement or recreation or amusement.

The term drug misuse includes taking it for wrong indication, in wrong dosages, or for too short or too long a period.

Drug abuse and drug dependence should be distinguished. For example, drug abuse without drug dependence i.e. giving a harmful drug is abuse without dependence. Similarly drug dependence can be without abuse, i.e. a diabetic may be dependent on insulin without abuse. However, drug abuse and drug dependence can also co-exist.

Drug abuse

What constitutes abuse depends on the opinions of a particular society and cultural considerations, for example, temperate use of alcohol and tobacco is generally accepted in U.K., U.S.A. and many other countries, whereas in most Arabic countries tobacco is accepted but not the use of alcohol. Taking cannabis is considered a serious abuse in U.K. and U.S.A. but generally not so in India. Thus, non-medicinal drug use may be a term preferable to abuse.

The nonmedicinal use means either continuous or occasional use of drugs by the individual according to his own choice or due to some compulsive desire to achieve 'chemical vacation'.

Drugs used for nonmedicinal purposes may be divided into 2 groups, hard and soft. The hard group includes heroin, morphine and analogues. These produce severe emotional and physical dependence. Soft drugs include sedatives, anxiolytics, cannabis, alcohol and tobacco. There is little or no physical dependence except with large doses of depressants such as alcohol and barbiturates.

The above classification is unsatisfactory as it does not recognize individual variation in drug use. It is hard-use (life centers around the use) and soft-use (use is occasional) rather hard drugs and soft drugs.

Drug dependence

It is a state arising from repeated, periodic or continuous administration of a drug, that results in harm to the individual and sometimes to the society. The subject feels a desire, need or compulsion to continue using the drug and feels ill if he does not take it (abstinence or withdrawal syndrome).

Drug dependence is characterized by the following:

(i) Psychic dependence (emotional) is first to appear. It is manifested by compulsive drug-seeking behaviour. The subject uses it repetitively in spite of known risks to health, for example, heavy cigarette smoking. Psychic dependence precedes physical dependence but does not always lead to it. There is emotional stress, if the drug is withheld.

(ii) Physical dependence occurs if the withdrawal produces symptoms and signs which are usually opposite of those sought by the user. It develops with cerebral depressants to a substantial extent, but is minor or absent with stimulant drugs.

(iii) Tolerance signifies a decreased response to the effects of the drug. It becomes essential to employ ever larger doses to achieve the same effect. It is closely associated with the phenomenon of physical dependence but may also occur to certain drugs such as LSD that do not produce dependence.

The World Health Organization Expert Committee on Addiction producing Drugs has recommended the use of the term drug dependence in place of the previously used words 'habit' and addiction. In case of drug habit, the subject merely had a desire to take the drug and it was harmful to the individual. In addiction, the subject becomes both emotional and physically dependent and resulted in harm to both the individual and the society. But in many instances the distinction fails. Alcohol provides a good example. For some it is a 'habit' but it merges into 'addiction'. The use of the term drug dependence is welcome, because there was never a true difference between habit-forming and addicting drugs. The term addiction is too imprecise to be useful.

The Motives for nonmedicinal drug use

• To escape from harsh reality of personal problems and to relieve stress and depression.
• Fun, recreation and curiosity.
• Rebellion against the family or society, or orthodox social values.
• To get mystical or religious experience.

Mechanism of drug dependence

Emotional dependence may occur to any drug that alters consciousness. In case of mild dependence it is not necessary that the drug should have important psychic effects, the belief as to what it does is equally

important. Some people develop a strong emotional dependence on food and eat too much.

Physical dependence and development of tolerance imply that adaptive changes have taken place in the body, and when the drug is withheld these adaptive changes are left unopposed resulting in rebound activity.

Types of drug dependence according to WHO

Morphine-type	Emotional dependence severe; physical dependence severe; tolerance develops quickly and is marked; cross-tolerance with related drugs; naloxone induces abstinence syndrome
Barbiturate-type	Emotional dependence severe; physical dependence develops slowly but very severe; tolerance less marked than with morphine; cross-tolerance with alcohol, chloral hydrate, paraldehyde, meprobamate, diazepam, chlordiazepoxide
Amphetamine-type	Emotional dependence severe; physical dependence slight; tolerance occurs
Cannabis-type	Emotional dependence; physical dependence slight or absent so no withdrawal syndrome; tolerance slight.
Cocaine-type	Emotional dependence severe; physical dependence absent (or slight); tolerance absent
Alcohol-type	Emotional dependence severe; physical dependence with prolonged heavy use; cross-tolerance with other sedatives
Tobacco-type	Emotional dependence strong; physical dependence slight

DRUGS OF ABUSE

Opioids

The most commonly abused drugs in this group are heroin, morphine and meperidine (pethidine).

These drugs produce intense emotional dependence, marked tolerance and marked physical dependence develop. If these drugs are withdrawn, withdrawal or abstinence syndrome develops.

> ## Box 3.12. Opioid withdrawal syndrome
> - Craving for opioids
> - Irritability, restlessness
> - Nausea, cramps
> - Anxiety, insomnia
> - Mydriasis
> - Sweating
> - Piloerection ("gooseflesh")
> - Vomiting, diarrhoea
> - Tachycardia
> - Yawning
> - Fever

> ## Box 3.13. Benzodiazepine withdrawal syndrome
> - Agitation, Anxiety
> - Muscle cramps
> - Sleep disturbance
> - Increased sensitivity to light and sound
> - After high dose usage
> - Seizures
> - Delirium

> ## Box 3.14. Nicotine withdrawal syndrome
> - Anxiety
> - Irritability
> - Dysphoria
> - Depressed mood
> - Difficulty in concentration
> - Restlessness
> - Increased appetite or weight gain

The signs and symptoms of withdrawal begin 8-10 hours after the last dose, characterized by lacrimation, rhinorrhoea, yawning and sweating. It is followed by restless sleep, nausea and vomiting myalgia and involuntary movements ("kicking the habit"), hyperthermia and hypertension appear in later stages. The acute course of withdrawal may last 7-10 days.

Barbiturates and other sedatives

Emotional dependence, tolerance and physical dependence are produced. Benzodiazepines produce less drug dependence as compared to the barbiturates. The withdrawal syndrome appears late and is characterized by convulsions, tremors, delirium, hallucinations and other psychosis-like symptoms.

Tobacco

The tobacco smoke is complex (about 500 compounds).

The main pharmacologically active ingredients are nicotine (acute effects) and tars (chronic effects).

Nicotine is readily absorbed from oral, nasal and respiratory mucosa to reach the brain tissue within 7 seconds of inhalation Nicotine content of tobacco varies from 0.2 to 5% and that of each cigarette from 0.05 to 2 mg, fatal dose of nicotine is 60mg. 20 cigarettes a day gives 100 mg of nicotine a week which in single dose will kill him as rapidly as a bullet. If one smokes 25 cigarettes a day the average loss of life is about 5 years i.e. 5 minutes per cigarette smoked.

Tar contains polycyclic aromatic hydrocarbons some of which are documented carcinogens, among these are - non- volatile nitrosamine and aromatic amines causing bladder cancer; benzopyrene causing lung cancer.

The health hazards are also contributed by acrolein, hydrocyanic acid, nitric oxide, nitrogen dioxide, cresol and phenols.

Smoke of pipes and cigars is alkaline (pH 8.5) and nicotine is relatively un-ionized and lipid soluble so it is quickly absorbed in the mouth, so these smokers obtain nicotine without inhaling.

Smoke of cigarettes is acidic (pH 5.3) and nicotine is relatively ionized and insoluble in lipids. Desired amounts of nicotine are only absorbed if taken into the lungs. Cigarette smokers therefore inhale (they have high rate of death from lung cancer).

Characteristics of dependence of tobacco

Psychological dependence is extremely strong, and tolerance and some physical dependence occur. Transient withdrawal effects include sleep changes and impaired performance and disturbance of mood.

Effects of chronic tobacco smoking

Cancers

- Lung cancer, pipe and cigar smokers have less risk than cigarette smokers, because they inhale less.
- Cancer of the mouth and throat. It is as great for pipe and cigar smokers as it is for cigarette

smokers. The risk is 5-10 times more than that of non-smokers.

- Cancer of the pancreas, kidney and urinary tract are also more common in smokers.

There is no longer any doubt that tobacco use causes death and disease on a very large scale. Since the middle of the 20th century, tobacco products have killed more than 60 million people in developed countries alone. In another 30 years, unless the trend changes drastically, about 10 million would be killed each year by tobacco products with 70% of these deaths occurring in developing countries. At present, it is estimated that tobacco kills over 3 million people per year and if current trends continue, the death toll would rise to 10 million deaths per year by the 2020s or 2030s, with majority of deaths occurring in developing countries. Since 80s and 90s, India's consumption of tobacco has increased by 40% and it now ranks third in the world. In India alone, tobacco-related disease claims 2200 lives every day. Beedi and cigarette smokers have three-two-four times higher risk of suffering a heart attack when compared to non-smokers. Women who smoke may have irregular periods and reach menopause 2 years earlier than non-smokers. Smoking during pregnancy can result in a low birth weight baby, premature birth or intrauterine growth retardation.

In spite of such known hazards, it is estimated that about 20 crore men and 5 crore women above the age of 15 are slaves to the tobacco habit in India.

Chronic lung disease

- Chronic mucus hypersecretion which produces persistent cough with phlegm is caused by smoking (smoker's cough).

Box 3.15. Diseases caused by smoking.

- Cancers of the oral cavity, larynx, lung, oesophagus, bladder, pancreas, renal pelvis, stomach, and cervix.
- Smoking is also a cause of heart disease, peripheral disease, chronic obstructive lung diseases and low birth weight babies.
- Smoking is a probable cause of: peptic ulcer disease, unsuccessful pregnancies, increased infant mortality (including Sudden Infant Death Syndrome—SIDS).

(Source: WHO)

- Chronic obstructive lung disease may be produced by smoking. It causes difficulty in breathing due to narrowing of the air passages in the lungs.

Diseases of CVS

Smokers are about twice as likely to die of coronary heart disease as are non-smokers and the heavy smokers about three and half times as likely. Atherosclerotic narrowing of the coronary arteries is increased, platelet adherence is increased by smoking which increases the readiness with which thrombi form and the carboxyhaemoglobinaemia of habitual smokers causes polycythaemia, which increases blood viscosity.

Women and smoking

Infertility. Women who smoke are more likely to be infertile or take longer to conceive than non-smokers. Smoking adversely affects ovarian function (how is unclear). Smokers are more liable to have an earlier menopause.

Complications of pregnancy. There is a twofold risk of spontaneous abortion in women who smoke 20 or more cigarettes a day during pregnancy (although incidence of toxaemia of pregnancy is lowered but this minor advantage does not offset the large number of disadvantages).

The placenta is heavier in smokers. The enlarged placenta and placental abnormalities may represent adaptations to lack of oxygen due to smoking. This lack of oxygen is due to increased concentrations of circulating carboxyhaemoglobin.

Unborn child. There is usually low birth weight.

Contraception. The risk of myocardial infarction, stroke and other cardiovascular diseases (particularly over 45 years of age) is increased three-to four fold by either contraceptive use or by smoking. But when two are combined there is about 10-fold increase in overall risk.

Ethanol

Alcohol dependence syndrome (chronic alcoholism)

Alcoholism is a major scourge of the human race and the most dangerous property of alcohol is the readiness with which it produces dependence. The major factors determining physical dependence are dose, frequency of dosing, and duration of abuse.

Box 3.16. Alcohol withdrawal syndrome

- Alcohol craving
- Irritability, Tremor
- Nausea
- Sleep disturbance
- Sweating
- Seizures (12-48 hours after last drink)
- Delirium tremens
- Visual hallucinations
- Tachycardia
- Mydriasis

Sudden withdrawal of alcohol can precipitate an acute psychotic attack (delirium tremens) and convulsions, agitation, anxiety and increased sympathetic autonomic activity.

Foetal alcohol syndrome characterized by microcephaly, mental deficiency with irritability in infancy, low body weight and length, small eyeballs and short palpebral fissures, lack of nasal bridges, may be produced in children of about 10% of alcohol abusers.

Effects of chronic alcohol abuse on drug metabolism, toxicity and tolerance:

Increase drug metabolism	*Increase drug toxicity*
Phenobarbitone	Paracetamol
Meprobamate	Vitamin A
Sulfonylureas	INH
Phenytion	
Barbiturates	*Increase drug tolerance*
Benzodiazepines	Anaesthetics

Table 3.28 shows list of main drugs of abuse.

Hallucinogens (Psychodysleptics, psychotomimetics)

Hallucinogens are drugs which produce hallucinations. However, hallucinations may be uncommon or only a part of overall effects of hallucinogenic drugs. These are also called psychotomimetic drugs because their actions mimic the naturally occurring psychoses, but the effects do not closely resemble

Table 3.28. Main drugs of abuse

Type	Dependence liability
• Narcotic analgesics	Very strong
Morphine	
• CNS depressants	
Ethanol	Strong
Barbiturates	Strong
• Anxiolytic drugs	
Benzodiazepines	Moderate
• Psychomotor stimulants	
Amphetamine	Strong
Cocaine	Very strong
Caffeine	Weak
Nicotine	Very strong
• Psychotomimetic agents	
LSD	Weak or absent
Cannabis	Weak or absent
Mescaline	Weak or absent
Phencyclidine	Moderate

schizophrenia. The term psychedelic was used to denote a supposed "mind-releasing" aspect of such drug used. However, it is also not very accurate since many other disinhibiting drugs e.g. alcohol may achieve the same insights.

Long time back, the peyote cactus (containing mescaline) and mushrooms (containing psilocin) were used to induce psychedelic effects by the natives of Mexico and Southwestern United States.

Lysergic acid diethylamide (LSD)

LSD causes curious effects in animals, green sunfish become aggressive, siamese fighting fish float nose up, tail down, the elephant exhibits episodically a form of sexual or delinquent behaviour. LSD has remarkable potency (30 mcg is effective oral dose) psychological dependence occurs, physical dependence does not occur.

In humans, vision is blurred, objects appear distorted, auditory acuity increases, food appears coarse and gritty in the mouth. Time seems to stop or to pass slowly or gets faster. There are tremors, dilated pupils, ataxia. The walls of a room appear as if taking respiration. Music is heard which is not there, smell comes from colours.

> **Box 3.17.** Cannabis withdrawal syndrome
> - Irritability
> - Mild agitation
> - Sleeplessness
> - Nausea
> - Cramps
> - Restlessness

> **Box 3.18.** Cocaine withdrawal syndrome
> - Cocaine craving
> - Depression, Dysphoria
> - Fatigue, Sleepiness
> - Bradycardia

Mescaline

It is an alkaloid from mexican cactus (peyote) and psilocybin from fungus psilocybe (magic mushrooms) produce similar effects as LSD.

Cannabis

It is obtained from the annual plant *Cannabis sativa*, *C. indica* and *C. americana*. The term cannabis includes bhang (leaves), ganja (crushed leaves and flowers) and the resin scrapped off the plant is known as charas or hashish.

Marijuana is a mixture of ground-up flowers and small leaves of plant materials.

Cannabis is a hallucinogen. The oily cannabinoids including tetrahydrocannabinol (THC) is the chief cause of the psychic action. Besides cannabinoids, there are certain water-soluble substances (atropine like substance which may produce dryness of mouth) and some acetylcholine like substances that may produce irritant effect, if smoked.

Cannabis produces a variety of effects. Euphoria is common, with laughter which seems pointless and the subject can not control it. Size of objects and distance are distorted, sense of time disappears, the beginning of the sentence may be forgotten before it is finished.

Cannabis smoked or taken by mouth produces reddening of the eyeballs (vasodilatation), ataxia. Appetite is increased.

Stimulants

Cocaine

Cocaine is an alkaloid obtained from the leaves of Erythroxylon coca. It is used as snuff, swallowed, smoked or injected I.V. Emotional dependence is severe but physical dependence is slight or absent, as is tolerance. Cocaine is a stimulant of the central nervous system.

If cocaine is used in high doses it produces paranoid psychosis. The subject suffers from megalomania. He is very suspicious in nature and the paranoid behaviour (delusion of persecution) may be such that he may shoot first and then discuss.

Amphetamines

Amphetamine is phenylisopropylamine. Its pharmacokinetics are similar to those of ephedrine, but amphetamine enters the CNS more readily and has more marked stimulant effect on mood and alertness and depressant effect on appetite.

Methamphetamine is very similar to amphetamine.

Phenmetrazine is a variant with amphetamine like actions. It is also a drug of abuse.

Methylphenidate and pemoline are amphetamine variants with similar effects and abuse potential as those of amphetamine.

Amphetamines cause alertness, wakefulness, euphoria and less fatigue. They stimulate the CNS.

The emotional dependence is severe, tolerance occurs but the physical dependence is slight.

Large doses cause aggressiveness, irritability, toxic psychosis and the thinking process is generally impaired.

Treatment of drug dependence (general aspects)

- The person must have a strong will power to get himself treated. No amount of preaching helps.
- The reasons for the drug abuse must be identified and the factors leading to it must be eliminated.

- Supportive therapy. The symptoms of withdrawal should be treated according to the needs as they are varied in nature dependent on the type of drug used.
- Psychological treatment is important.
- Rehabilitation of the patient is usually required.
- The patient should be watched for any relapse.

STUDY QUESTIONS

1. Define drug abuse and how does it differ from misuse of drugs. Explain with examples.
2. Define drug dependence. What are the main characteristics of drug dependence? Why the word addiction is not proper in relation to drug abuse?
3. What are the usual and general motives of persons involved in drug abuse?
4. List the drugs which lead to drug dependence.
5. Describe the different types of drug abuse.
6. What is psychic dependence, physical dependence and withdrawal syndrome?
7. Explain drug tolerance and its relation to drug dependence.
8. What are the differences between barbiturate type, cannabis type, LSD type and cocaine type of drug dependence?
9. What are the effects of chronic tobacco smoking?
10. List hallucinogens.
11. Describe ethanol type drug dependence.
12. Explain foetal alcohol syndrome.
13. Briefly indicate the different measures which should be taken to manage a case of drug dependence.

GUIDE TO FURTHER READING

Bagiotti G & Cavallini G: Acetyl-L-carnitine vs tamoxifen in the oral therapy of Peyronie's disease: a preliminary report. BJU Internat 2001; 88(1):63-67.

Block, R.I., Ghoneim, M.M.: Effects of chronic marijuana use human cognition. Psychopharmacology, 1993; 110:219.

Clark WM, Wechsler LR, Sabounjian LA et al: A phase III randomized efficacy trial of 200 mg citicoline in acute ischemic stroke patients. Neurology 2001; 57:1595-1602.

Dewit, H., Pierri, J., and Johanson, C.E.: Assessing individual differences in alcohol preference using a cumulative dosing procedure. Psychopharmacology, 1989; 1:113.

Gorelick, D.A., Rose, J., and Jarvlk, M.E.: Effect of naloxone on cigarette smoking. J. Subst. Abuse, 1989; 1:153.

Hollister, L.E.: Health aspects of cannabics. Pharmacol Rev, 1986; 38:1.

Lobaugh NJ, Karaskov V, Rombaugh V et al: Piracetam therapy does not enhance cognitive functioning in children with Down Syndrome. Arch Pediatr Adolesc Med 2001; 155:442-448.

Mariotti C, Solari A, Torta D et al: Idebenone treatment in Friedreich patients: One-year-long randomized placebo-controlled trial. Neurology 2003; 60:1676-1679.

Marzuk, P.M. et al: Fatal injuries after cocaine inglia use as a leading cause of death among young adults in New York City, N. Engl. J. Med., 1995; 332:1753.

McLellan, A.T., Woody, G.E., and O'Brien, C.P.: Development of psychiatric illness in drug abusers. N. Engl. J. Med., 1979; 301:1310.

Montgomery SA, Thal LJ, & Amrein R: Meta-analysis of double blind randomized controlled clinical trials of acetyl-L-carnitine versus placebo in the treatment of mild cognitive impairment and mild Alzheimer's disease. Int Clin Psychopharmacol 2003; 18:61-71.

Nestler, E.J.: Molecular mechanisms of drug addiction. J. Neurosci, 1992; 12:2439.

Ray, O.A.: Drugs, Society and Human Behavior, 6th ed. Mosby, 1993.

Schuckit, M.A.: Low level of response to alcohol as a predictor of future alcoholism. Am. J. Psychiatry, 1994; 151:184.

Silverman, K et al: Withdrawal syndrome after the double-blind cessation of caffeine consumption. N. Engl. J. Med., 1992; 327:1109.

Smith, D.E. et al (editors): Amphetamine use, Misuse and Abuse, GK Hall, 1979.

Tang WK, Ungvari GS & Leung HCM: Effect of piracetam on ect-induced cognitive disturbances: a randomized, placebo-controlled, double-blind study. J ECT 2002; 18(3):130-137.

Thal LJ, Grundman M, Berg J et al: Idebenone treatment fails to slow cognitive decline in Alzheimer's disease. Neurology 2003; 61:1498-1502.

Tomaassini V, Pozzilli C, Onesti E et al: Comparison of the effects of acetyl L-carnitine and amantadine for the treatment of fatigue in multiple sclerosis: results of a pilot, randomised, double-blind, crossover trial. J Neurol Sci 2004; 218(1-2):103-108.

Vicari E & Calogero AE: Effects of treatment with carnitines in infertile patients with prostato-vesiculo-epididymitis. Hum Reprod 2001; 16(11):2338-2342.

Volpe, J.J.: Effect of cocaine use on the fetus. N. Engl. J. Med., 1992; 327:399.

Waegemans T, Wilsher CR, Danniau A et al: Clinical efficacy of piracetam in cognitive impairment: a meta-analysis. Dement Geriatr Cogn Disord 2002; 13:217-224.

Cardiovascular Agents

Terminology associated with heart

Palpitation : Abnormal rate or rhythm of heart : A fluttering of the heart.

Paroxysmal tachycardia : A period of rapid heart beats that begins and ends suddenly.

Stokes-Adams syndrome : Sudden attacks of unconsciousness sometimes with convulsions, that may accompany heart block.

Cardiomegaly : Heart enlargement.

Terminology associated with blood vessels :

Phlebitis : Inflammation of a vein, often in a leg.

Thrombophlebitis : Inflammation of a vein with clot formation.

Raynaud's disease : A vascular disorder characterized by bilateral attacks of ischaemia, usually of the fingers and toes, in which the skin becomes pale, and exhibits burning and pain.

ANTIANGINAL DRUGS

Heart supplies blood to all parts of the body, gets its own supply of blood through the coronary arteries. The coronary blood flow is only 4% of the cardiac-output and the O_2 extraction is 75%. Coronary blood flow occurs during diastole only.

In normal persons, the coronary blood flow increases to meet the increased myocardial oxygen demand. If need arises, there may be as much as five-fold increase in the coronary flow. But this capacity is reduced in patients suffering from angina pectoris. The characteristic anginal pain develops when coronary artery disease causes inadequate blood supply to the myocardium. The myocardial oxygen demand outstrips the supply of oxygen. There is retrosternal pain that radiates to chest, left shoulder, upper arm and neck.

The autoregulation of myocardial O_2 supply and demand is shown in Fig. 4.1.

Angina is due to imbalance between supply and demand (Table 4.1 and Fig. 4.2).

Types of angina

1. Stable or classical angina: The anginal attacks usually appear during physical or mental exertion. If the coronary vessels are narrowed as a result of atherosclerosis, there is hardly any scope to increase the coronary blood flow by employing coronary dilators. The beneficial effects can be obtained by using drugs which

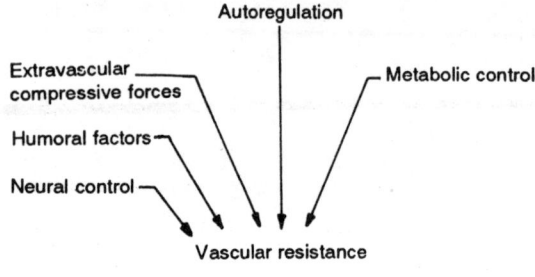

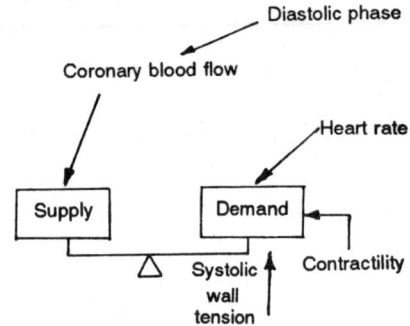

Fig. 4.1. Myocardial O_2 supply and demand.

Table 4.1. Factors which decrease oxygen supply/increase oxygen demand

O_2 supply decreases due to	O_2 demand increases due to
1. Coronary spasm	1. Physical exercise
2. Platelet emboli producing temporary block	2. Severe anaemia
3. Atherosclerosis	3. Anxiety, physical and mental stress and strain
	4. Thyrotoxicosis

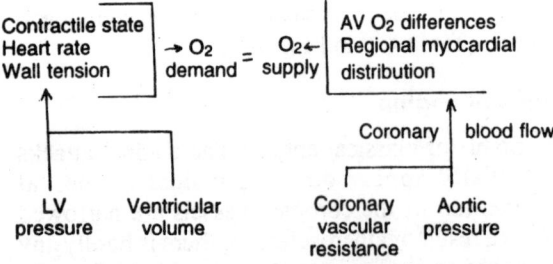

Fig. 4.2. Myocardial O_2 supply-demand relationship.

decrease the work load of the heart by reducing preload or after load or both.

2. Unstable angina (preinfarction angina): It is characterized by recurrent attacks with minimal exertion due to restriction in coronary flow.

3. Variant angina (Prinzmetal's angina): The attacks occur even during rest or during sleep. The pain is not associated with physical or mental exertion. It is due to recurrent coronary vasospasm and in some cases due to temporary blocking of a coronary artery by platelet embolism, i.e. caused by reduction in coronary flow and not due to increase in O_2 demand.

The main factors which influence the myocardial oxygen consumption are (i) stress on the ventricular wall during systole, (ii) cardiac rate and (iii) force of myocardial contractility.

The stress on ventricular wall is determined by preload and afterload.

Preload is the venous filling pressure. It depends on venous filling and distension of the myocardium during diastole (ventricular end-diastolic pressure and volume).

The reduction in preload results in pooling of blood in peripheral veins → decrease in venous return → decrease in left ventricular end-diastolic pressure, volume, ventricle size and wall tension → increased ventricular efficiency and decreased oxygen requirement.

Afterload is the ventricular wall tension or force developed during systole. It is dependent on peripheral resistance against which the heart is working. The reduction of the peripheral arterial resistance reduces afterload which results in decreasing the myocardial consumption of oxygen.

The main antianginal therapy is (i) to reduce the workload of the heart and/or (ii) to increase the coronary blood flow, and (iii) both.

If the coronary vessels are narrowed due to atherosclerosis, there is little scope to increase the coronary blood flow by coronary dilators. In such situations, the use of drugs which decrease the work load of the heart, preload or afterload or both, will be useful.

Drugs which reduce afterload

- Calcium channel blockers
- phentolamine, hydralazine

Drugs which reduce both preload and afterload

- Organic nitrates
- ACE inhibitors
- Sodium nitroprusside
- Prazosin

Antianginal drugs

These can be grouped in the following categories:

1. Nitrites-Nitrates
    - Rapid onset, short acting: Amyl nitrite and glyceryl trinitrate (nitroglycerin)
    - Slow onset, long acting: Erythrityl tetranitrate, pentaerythritol tetranitrate (peritrate) and mannitol hexanitrate, isosorbide dinitrate (sorbitrate), isosorbide mononitrate.
2. Beta-adrenergic blocking drugs: propranolol, atenolol and metoprolol.
3. Calcium channel blockers, e.g. nifedipine, verapamil and diltiazem.
4. Miscellaneous group (other antianginal drugs), e.g. perhexilene, dipyridamole, diazepam, and prenylamine; antihyperlipidaemic agents and oral anticoagulants.

Nitrite-nitrate group

Nitrites are esters of nitrous acid and nitrates are polyesters of nitric acid.

Pharmacokinetics

Absorption from GIT is variable after oral administration. Amyl nitrite (destroyed by gastric HCl and so not given orally) is inhaled and is rapidly absorbed from lungs. Glyceryl trinitrate is promptly absorbed from the mucous membrane of the mouth when given sublingually (not orally due to extensive first-pass effect). The orally administered nitrates are less effective than sublingual tablets as they are primarily degraded in the liver.

The nitrites and organic nitrates are quickly removed from the blood, two third is converted into ammonia and one third is excreted unaltered in the urine.

Pharmacological actions & Mechanism of action

1. Effects on heart

The nitrates relax all smooth muscles, including vascular smooth muscle. They relax smooth muscles by direct action. The proposed biochemical action involves the formation of free radical nitric oxide (NO), which stimulates guanylate cyclase, the resultant guanosine 3′,5′-monophosphate (cyclic GMP) activates a protein kinase, which mediates dephosphorylation of myosin. The formation of endothelial-derived relaxation factor (EDRF) is also a contributory action.

The venous dilatation (venous tone reduced) results in decreased cardiac filling pressure, decreased ventricular diastolic size and reduced systemic blood pressure and cardiac output.

Nitrates decrease peripheral arteriolar resistance. The arterial dilatation decreases the work load of the ventricles. However, the compensatory tachycardia due to hypotension is a disadvantage. But this can be countered by employing a beta-blocker.

Thus the organic nitrates reduce both the preload and afterload due to dilatation of venous capacitance and arteriolar resistance respectively. The major action is reduction in the myocardial oxygen requirement relative to myocardial oxygen delivery.

In addition, decrease in left ventricular end-diastolic pressure reduces tissue pressure around subendocardial vessels, favouring the redistribution of coronary blood flow to this area.

These drugs do not increase the total blood flow in patients suffering from angina (unlike normal person). However, these drugs possibly promote redistribution of coronary blood flow. The dilated arterioles of non-ischaemic myocardium may redistribute the blood flow towards ischaemic areas. Further studies have revealed that in normal persons, the ratio between endocardial and epicardial blood flow is even and in acute myocardial ischaemia, the endocardial blood flow is disproportionately decreased. It has been reported that nitroglycerin preferentially enhances the endocardial blood flow. This occurs both in normal and in acute myocardial ischaemia. However, the total coronary blood flow is not increased. They do not increase the total coronary blood flow in patients with atherosclerosis.

2. Extra-cardiac effects

Effect on other smooth muscles: These drugs relax the smooth muscles of bronchi, biliary tract, GIT, gall bladder, ureter and uterus.

The nitrates dilate vessels in the skin, resulting in flushing. The vasodilation of cerebral vessels results in intracerebral pressure and sometimes in headache.

To terminate an acute attack of angina, amyl nitrite and glyceryl trinitrate are effective agents.

Amyl nitrite: It is available in small glass pearls containing 0.2 ml volatile liquid. The glass pearl is crushed in a handkerchief (to avoid injury from glass particles) and vaporous are inhaled. Its chief advantage is that it acts very fast (10 seconds). The effect lasts for 5 to 10 minutes. This drug is no more popular due to certain disadvantages, viz.

- It is inconvenient to use.
- It has bad odour.
- It produces fall in B.P. and tachycardia.

Glyceryl trinitrate (Nitroglycerin): This drug is very popular. The onset of action is rapid (1 to 2 minutes) and the effect lasts for 15 to 30 minutes when it is administered sublingually. The sublingual route of administration has certain advantages. The drug can be spit out after the pain is relieved and hence the incidence of side effects is reduced. The other advantage is that the hepatic first-pass inactivation is avoided. The usual dose is 0.5 mg tablet, up to 2 tablets at a time may be administered sublingually. The maximum daily dose is 6 mg per day.

Nitroglycerin is also now available as an aerosol buccal spray, 0.4 mg in a metered dose.

The recently introduced drug delivery system for nitroglycerin is in the form of 2% ointment applied on the skin, attached as a transdermal patch, 4-hourly. The usual dose is 5 mg in 24 hours. The effect is more prolonged (3 to 4 hours) than the sublingual tablet. Nitroglycerin ointment can be usefully employed to prevent nocturnal angina.

Nitroglycerin terminates acute attack of angina pectoris. It is also effective prophylactically if taken before performing a task which precipitates angina.

Besides nitroglycerin (glyceryl trinitrate), isosorbide dinitrate (sorbitrate) 2.5 to 5 mg can be given sublingually. The effect begins within 2 to 5 minutes and lasts for 1 to 2 hours.

Erythrityl tetranitrate 5 mg by sublingual administration acts in 2-5 minutes and the effect lasts longer than with nitrogylcerin.

To prevent attacks of angina, the following long acting antianginal drugs have been employed :

Isosorbide dinitrate, 40 to 120 mg given orally in divided doses per day, acts within 15 to 30 minutes. The effect lasts for about 4 hours.

Pentaerythritol tetranitrate (peritrate) 20 to 40 mg, three or four times a day given by the oral route starts effect in about 30 minutes and lasts for 4 to 5 hours.

Erythrityl tetranitrate, 30 to 60 mg administered orally per day in divided doses will produce effect lasting for 2 to 4 hours.

The prophylactic value of the long acting nitrates in angina is controversial. Some studies claim that these drugs reduce severity and frequency of anginal attacks, while some other studies claim that their effects are not better than placebo.

The long acting nitrates produce venous dilatation and can be of some value with digitalis and diuretics in treating cardiac failure.

The formulation and dosages of commonly employed nitrite-nitrates are given in Table 4.2.

Clinical uses of nitrites-nitrates

- Angina pectoris (main use): The short acting drugs are used to terminate acute attacks; and the long acting drugs are used as prophylactic agents (but now are being replaced by other drugs).
- Acute pulmonary oedema: The short acting agents bring about relief of paroxysmal nocturnal dyspnoea.
- Severe CHF: The short acting agents reduce afterload.
- Acute myocardial infarction: I.V. nitroglycerin (very carefully monitored) decreases left ventricular filling pressure due to venodilatation.
- Biliary colic, GIT spasm and urethral spasm: Nitrates can be given to treat those cases who are refractory to the conventional treatment.
- Cyanide poisoning: Nitrites induce methaemoglobinaemia.

Table 4.2. Organic nitrates for clinical use

Amyl nitrite	Inhalation 0.18 or 0.3 ml
Nitroglycerin	Tablet for sublingual use 0.15 to 0.6 mg as needed
	Aerosol buccal spray 0.4 mg per spray as needed
	Sustained-release tablet or capsule 2.5 to 9 mg 2-4 times/day
	Buccal tablet 1 mg every 3 to 5 hours
	Ointment 1.25 to 5 cm (1/2 to 2″) topically to skin every 4-8 hours
	Transdermal disc 1 disc (2.5 to 15 mg every 24 hours)
	I.V. 5 mcg/min
Isosorbide dinitrate (Sorbitrate, others)	Tablet for sublingual use 2.5 to 10 mg every 2-3 hours
	Chewable tablet 5-10 mg every 2-3 hours
	Oral tablet or capsule 10-40 mg every 6 hours
	Sustained-release capsule or tablet 40-80 mg every 8-12 hours
Isosorbide-5-mononitrate	Tablet for sublingual use 10-40 mg twice a day
	Sustained-release capsule or tablet 60 mg/day
Erythrityl tetranitrate (Cardilate) (Imdur, others)	Tablet for sublingual use 5-10 mg as needed
	Oral tablet or capsule 10 mg 3 times/day

Methaemoglobin is a form of heamoglobin consisting of globin with an oxidized haem, containing ferric iron. This pigment is unable to transport oxygen.

- Trigeminal neuralgia: Nitrites may be given to reduce severity of pain.
- The long acting nitrates with digitalis and diuretics are sometimes useful in treating cardiac failure as they produce venous dilatation.

Adverse effects

- Tolerance and cross tolerance develops if nitrite - nitrate group of drugs are administered repeatedly. The tolerance develops fairly early, within 2-3 weeks. But it is also lost quickly within a few days after stopping the intake. The prolonged use of long acting nitrates can render the short acting drugs ineffective. However, tolerance is not a problem if these drugs are administered intermittently.

- Methaemoglobinaemia can result as nitrite oxidizes haemoglobin to methaemoglobin.
- Excessive hypotension with syncope.
- Due to sudden lowering of the systemic blood pressure due to generalized vasodilatation and compensatory reflex tachycardia, patients often complain of dizziness, fullness in head, skin flushing and throbbing headache (meningeal vessels dilated).
- The organic nitrates may aggravate ischaemia and precipitate an anginal attack in some cases. It is paradoxical because they are effective antianginal agents. The statement regarding this adverse effect seems self contradicting but it is true. These drugs in high doses may markedly reduce the diastolic pressure resulting in reflex tachycardia and increased myocardial contractility which will counteract the beneficial effect and may precipitate an anginal attack.

Contraindications

Glaucoma, severe anaemia, hypotensive state, increased intracranial pressure.

Beta-adrenergic blockers

Increased sympathetic activity results in increased cardiac work. The myocardial oxygen demand is increased.

The beta-adrenergic blocking agents reduce heart rate, velocity of myocardial contractility, decrease systemic blood pressure and increase diastolic pause. Although all the actions of beta blockers are not useful, as reduced heart rate and contractility increase the systolic ejection period and left ventricular end diastolic volume which tend to increase the oxygen consumption, but the net result is decreased cardiac work and so reduction in myocardial oxygen demand. They do not produce coronary dilatation.

The beta-blockers are useful prophylactic agents in stable and unstable types of angina. They are not beneficial in Prinzmetal's angina (variant or vasospastic angina), which is caused by coronary vasospasm and may even make this condition worse because the unopposed effects of catecholamines on alpha receptors may increase the coronary resistance.

Propranolol, a non-selective beta-blocker is popularly employed (not in variant type) as no other beta-blocker has been found superior to it. The usual dose is 20 mg three or four times a day administered orally. If required, the dose is gradually increased till angina is controlled.

Metoprolol and atenolol which are cardioselective beta1-blockers are not superior to propranolol as prophylactic antianginal drugs, but they should be preferred if the patient of angina pectoris is also suffering from bronchial asthma or diabetes mellitus.

Major adverse effects of beat-blockers

These include severe bradycardia, hypotension, bronchospasm and rarely heart failure, but these are uncommon, if patients are appropriately selected. More subtle side effect which may go unrecognised unless sought, include fatigue, lassitude, nightmares, and cold extremities.

Combination therapy : β-blockers plus nitrates have synergistic effect. β-blocker counteracts nitrate induced tachycardia.

Caution: β-blocker can precipitate congestive heart failure if cardiac reserve is poor. Such patients should be first treated with digitalis and diuretics.

Sudden cessation may trigger a withdrawal syndrome which can exacerbate anginal attacks.

Calcium channel blockers (Nifedipine, verapamil and diltiazem)

These inhibit inward movement of Ca^{++} into cardiac and smooth muscle cells, resulting in the following effects:

- Heart rate and contractility are reduced resulting in decreased oxygen demand.
- Peripheral arterial vessels are dilated as the peripheral resistance is reduced (afterload is reduced). They have only little effect on venous beds so do not affect cardiac preload.
- Coronaries are dilated which increase the oxygen supply. They increase the coronary blood flow more than the nitrates. The onset is slower but better maintained. Nifedipine has greater action on the blood vessels, whereas verapamil has more marked action on the heart.

In stable (classic- or exertional) angina the usefulness is mainly due to decreased myocardial oxygen demand, secondary to reduced B.P., heart rate and contractility. The beneficial effect is also due to coronary arterial dilatation. It has also been found effective in unstable and variant angina (Prinzmetal's angina). The limitation of nifedipine is its short duration of action.

After sublingual administration, nifedipine is promptly and completely absorbed. After oral administration its bioavailability is about 50%, peak effect reaches in 1 to 3 hours and the duration of action is for about 10 hours. It is about 98% bound to plasma proteins. It is excreted by kidneys as inactive metabolites.

Calcium channel blockers are used as third line antianginal agents.

Dosage : In acute anginal attack, 10 mg is administered sublingually.

For prophylaxis of angina, 10 to 20 mg thrice a day orally is advocated.

The relative cardiovascular effects of some Ca^{2+} channel blockers are given in Table 4.3.

Table 4.3. Relative cardiovascular effects of Ca^{2+} channel blockers

Drug	Vaso-dilation (coronary flow)	Suppre-ssion of cardiac contrac-tility	Suppres-sion auto-maticity (SA node)	Supp-ression of conduc-tion (AV node)
Nifedipine	5	1	1	0
Verapamil	4	4	5	5
Diltiazem	3	2	5	4
Nimodipine	5	1	1	0
Nicardipine	5	0	1	0

0 = No effect; 1-5 = Slight to most prominent effects

Pharmacokinetic characteristics of calcium channel blockers

	Bioavail-ability	Active metabolite	Elimination $t_{1/2}$ (hrs)
Verapamil	15-30%	yes	4-6
Diltiazem	40-60%	yes	5-6
Nifedipine	30-60%	minor	2-5
Felodipine	15-25%	none	12-18
Nicardipinie	20-40%	?	1-3
Amlodipine	60-65%	none	35-45

Uses of calcium channel blockers

Cardiovascular :

- Prinzmetal's variant angina
- Stable angina pectoris
- Unstable angina
- Silent myocardial ischaemia
- MI
- Atrial fibrillation and flutter
- Paroxysmal supraventricular tachycardia
- Systemic hypertension
- Anti-atherogenic properties (decreased calcium accumulation within arterial wall cells)

Non-cardiovascular :

- Neurological disorders (nimodipine and flunarizine have been tried, use limited)
- Migraine prophylaxis (well established)
- Epilepsy (flunarizine reduces seizures not responding to conventional therapy)
- Vertigo (beneficial effects of cinnarizine, a selective calcium channel blocker)

Second generation calcium channel blockers

Ultra-long acting :

- Amlodipine 5-10 mg OD for angina, hypertension
- Benidipine 4-8 mg OD for hypertension

Medium duration of action :

- Isradipine 2, 5 mg capsule BD for hypertension, angina
- Felodipine 5, 10 mg tab OD for hypertension, angina
- Nisoldipine 5, 20 mg tab OD for hypertension, angina

Short duration of action :

- Nicardipine 20, 30 mg capsule TDS for hypertension, angina
- Nimodipine 30 mg capsule for cerebral spasm, subarachanoid haemorrhage

Adverse effects

- Vasodilatation results in sodium retention, weight gain, oedema, vertigo, headache, flushing, reflex tachycardia, negative inotropic and conduction delay.

- Verapamil increases serum level of digitalis and thus can cause acute digitalis toxicity.
- Calcium channel blockers, perhaps especially when combined with beta-blocker can produce or aggravate the following:
  - Hypotension
  - A-V block
  - CHF
  - Asystole
- Nifedipine can increase anginal symptoms in about 10% of patients as peripheral vasodilatation may result in increased sympathetic tone. Verapamil or diltiazem produce less marked peripheral vasodilatation and reflex tachycardia and hence these two drugs are not likely to aggravate myocardial ischaemia.

Combination therapy

- Nifedipine can be combined with nitrates, particularly when beta-blocker is either ineffective or contraindicated.
- Simultaneous use of nifedipine and propranolol produce better results in stable angina as beta-blocker suppresses reflex tachycardia. Nifedipine unlike verapamil and diltiazem does not delay A-V conduction. Verapamil or diltiazem should not be combined with propranolol, otherwise increased A-V block, severe bradycardia and decreased left ventricular function will counteract any advantage offered by these drugs.
- Nifedipine (reduces afterload) and nitrates (reduce preload) can be usefully combined.

Miscellaneous group (other antianginal drugs)

Sedative-anxiolytic drugs such as diazepam are useful in stress-induced angina.

Prenylamine depletes catecholamines, it is a weak beta-blocker and inhibits calcium influx. If 15 to 30 mg doses are given thrice a day, central catecholamines are depleted which produce sedative effect.

Perhexiline maleate: It is an effective and promising drug being clinically tried in doses of 100 mg/ 3-4 times a day. It resembles verapamil in its actions. It is an effective antianginal drug which :

- Produces direct smooth muscle relaxation
- Decreases the left ventricular work and myocardial oxygen consumption and
- Produces transient depletion of catecholamines in myocardium.

Thus, it is effective due to both reduction in oxygen demand and increased oxygen supply. But it is not a first line antianginal drug as it may frequently produce severe side effects which include hepatotoxicity, neuropathy, loss of vision. The other side effects are GIT upsets, tremors, insomnia, hypoglycaemia, dizziness and rashes.

Dipyridamole (persantin): It is a coronary dilator but as it does not reduce venous return, the cardiac work is not decreased.

It acts on small vessels of coronary bed which are already dilated. It has very little action on vascular resistance in ischaemic areas. It also induces 'coronary steal' due to generalized vasodilatation. Therefore it is not effective as an antianginal agent, though some use it for prophylaxis in angina.

This drug inhibits aggregation of platelets and hence may have the ability to prevent future thrombosis in coronary and cerebral vessels. The recommended dose is 25 to 50 mg thrice a day orally.

Papaverine relaxes smooth muscles and cyclandelate is also papaverine like direct smooth muscle relaxant. However, they are practically of no value in angina pectoris.

Aminophylline increases coronary flow but also increases the cardiac work, hence it is no longer employed in angina.

Nicotinyl xanthinate combines xanthine and nicotinic acid, both are vasodilators, but value in angina is doubtful.

Molsidomine : It belongs to a newly discovered class of sydnonimines, which resemble nitroglycerin in their mode of action. It appears to act more slowly than nitrates, but its effect lasts longer.

Nicorandil : It is a potassium channel activator, also possesses nitrate-like activity. It relaxes vascular smooth muscle and does not appear to cause tolerance with chronic dosing.

It is basically not metabolic in action but shows haemodynamic control and cytoprotective activity by acting as potassium channel opener and nitric oxide donor. This results in :

- increased transmural blood flow (arteriolar dilation)
- spasmolytic action (epicardial vessel dilation)
- decrease in preload (venodilation)
- decrease in afterload (systemic arterial dilation)
- no cardiac depression (safe in CHF)
- cytoprotection

The above effects improve oxygen supply/demand balance.

It has beneficial effect on exercise-induced angina, it relieves coronary spasm. It exerts cardioprotective effect by decreasing energy expenditure in ischaemic zone, it increases regional myocardial flow (collaterals).

The dose is 5-10 mg twice a day.

An understanding of the metabolic process leading to myocardial ischaemia has led to the development of a new therapeutic approach that may complement or be an alternative to the conventional haemodynamic medical approach whilst offering potential additional benefits to interventional strategies.

The metabolic abnormalities that occur as a consequence of myocardial ischaemia are complex. In the absence of an adequate oxygen supply mitochondrial oxidative metabolism decreases and oxidation of carbohydrates and free fatty acids (FFAs) declines dramatically. Circulating FFAs increase and may further depress cardiac function, increase ischaemic damage and promote arrhythmias. Pyruvate dehydrogenase is inhibited and glucose and lactate oxidation is impaired with a subsequent increase in acidosis. In order to reverse this process, metabolic agents have been developed with the aim of stimulating glucose and lactate oxidation.

Metabolic agents act directly to increase pyruvate oxidation and help remove the lactate that has accumulated during the ischaemia and/or reduce the amount of fatty acids in the blood.

Evidence exists for clinical benefit in patients with stable angina of varying severity principally using the drug trimetazidine, and ranolazine, a similar agent, is currently commencing clinical trials in a large population study. The concept of using a metabolic agent to tackle a metabolic problem is attractive and the clinical trial data are encouraging with trimetazindine as monotherapy but in particular as combination therapy with conventional haemodynamic agents.

Trimetazidine : It is a piperazine derivative. It protects myocardium by preserving energy-producing metabolism at the cellular level.

- It limits intracellular acidosis.
- It avoids loss of potassium and intracellular accumulation of Na^+ and Ca^{2+}.
- Prevents free-radical induced damage.
- Improves oxygen availability.
- Slows down and delay anaerobic glycolysis.
- Reduces fatty acids oxidation.
- Reduces excessive accumulation of neutrophils at the site of ischaemia which may help to reduce the infarct size.
- Reduces platelet adhesiveness and aggregation prior to cyclooxygenase pathway.

Trimetazidine provides a synergistic effect when combined with other conventional anti-anginal drugs. It allows reduction of the dosages of other concomitant drugs.

It improves left ventricular function in severe ischaemic cardiomyopathy.

The dose is 20 mg thrice a day.

Levo-carnitine : It is a naturally occurring nontoxic substance essentially for fatty acid oxidation and energy production. More than 90% of its total body content is found in cardiac and skeletal muscle tissue.

It has been recently shown that both chronic and acute ischaemia provoke a relative or absolute deficiency of carnitine in the myocardium which leads to accumulation of toxic fatty acid groups (Acetyl CoA) which in turn leads to inhibition of adenine nucleotide transferase enzyme which is responsible for ATP transport from mitochondria to cytoplasm; decrease in oxidative utilisation of glucose results in the production of lactic acid which is highly toxic to the cells; the damage to myocardial cell membrane ultimately leads to reduced myocardial contractility and arrhythmias.

Sodium and calcium blocker

Bepridil : It has anti-anginal action. It has bioavailability 60%, protein binding 99%, half-life 25-40 hours and extensively metabolised. It is administered orally 200-400 mg once a day.

The role of oral anticoagulants and antihyperlipidaemic agents in patients of angina, is controversial. Some advocate their use in unstable and severe cases.

Choice of anti-anginal agent

Patients with very clear-cut effort-related angina should be offered a beta-blocker as should those with a prior myocardial infarction. Diltiazem and verapamil may also be given but should be avoided in the presence of significant left ventricular dysfunction. Nitrates are valuable where there is left ventricular dysfunction; beta blockers and some vascular selective long-acting dihydropyridines can also be given cautiously in such circumstances. Patients with asthma and peripheral vascular disease may be best treated with a long-acting nitrate or a calcium antagonist, although selective beta-blockers may be given with caution.

The other measures such as weight reduction in obese persons, stopping of smoking, removal of etiological factor if possible; correction of anaemia if that be the cause are beneficial in the management of angina pectoris.

STUDY QUESTIONS

1. What causes anginal pain?
2. Which conditions lead to decrease in O_2 supply, and increase in O_2 demand?
3. What are the main types of angina?
4. Explain preload and afterload.
5. Classify antianginal drugs.
6. What is the status regarding efficacy, mode of action and adverse effects of nitrite-nitrates as antianginal drugs?
7. Describe pharmacokinetics, route of administration, dosage and mode of action of nitroglycerin.
8. Which drugs are useful in treating acute attack of angina, and which drugs are used for prophylactic purpose?
9. How are beta-blockers useful in patients of angina?
10. What is the role of calcium channel blockers in

the treatment of angina? What may be their adverse effects?

11. List drugs which are coronary dilators.
12. Which drugs lower preload/afterload or both? What is the significance?
13. Write notes on the value of (i) perhexiline maleate (ii) dipyridamole and (iii) diazepam as antianginal agents.

GUIDE TO FURTHER READING

Anon: Optimizing antianginal therapy: consensus guidelines. Am. J. Cardiol., 1992; 70:72G-76G.

Bauters, C et al: Physiological assessment of augmented vascularity induced by VEGF in ischemic rabbit hindlimb. Am. J. Physiol., 1994; 267:H1263-H1271.

DeMots, H., and Glasser, S.P.: Intermittent transdermal nitroglycerin therapy in the treatment of chronic stable angina. J. Am. Coll. Cardiol., 1989; 13:786-795.

DeWood, M.A. et al: Randomized double-blind comparison of side effects of nicardipine and nifedipine in angina pectoris. The Nicardipine Investigators Group. Am. Heart J., 1990; 119:468-478.

Egstrup, K et al: Transient myocardial ischemia during nifedipine therapy in stable angina pectoris, and its relation to coronary collateral flow and comparison with metoprolol. Am. J. Cardiol., 1993; 71:177-183.

Fox, K.M. et al: Unstable and stable angina. Eur. Heart. J., 1993; 14 Suppl. F:15-17.

Furberg, C.D., Psaty, B.M. et al: Dose-related increase in mortality in patients with coronary heart disease. Circulation, 1995; 92:1326-1331.

Hanet, C et al: Effects of nicardipine on regional diastolic left ventricular function in patients with angina pectoris. Circulation, 1990; 81:III48-54.

Hansen, J.F. et al: Treatment with verapamil after an acute myocardial infarction. Review of the Danish studies on verapamil in myocardial infarction (DAVIT I and II). Drugs, 1991; 42 Suppl. 2:43-53.

Jugdutt, B.I.: Effects of nitrate therapy on ventricular remodeling and function. Am. J. Cardiol., 1993; 72:161G-168G.

Kloner, R.A. et al: Nifedipine in ischemic heart disease. Circulation, 1995; 92:1074-1078.

Lablanche, J.M. et al: Potassium channel activators in vasospastic angina. Eur. Heart J., 1993, 14 Suppl. B:22-24.

Lacoste, L.L. et al: Antithrombotic properties of transdermal nitroglycerin in stable angina pectoris. Am. J. Cardiol., 1994; 73:1058-1062.

Lehmann, G et al: Pharmacokinetics and additional anti-ischaemic effectiveness of amlodipine, a once-daily calcium antagonist during acute and long-term therapy of stable angina pectoris in patients pretreated with a beta-blocker. Eur. Heart J., 1993; 14:1531-1535.

Lowenstein, S et al: Nitric oxide: a physiologic messenger. Am. Intern. Med., 1994; 120:227-237.

Moncada, S et al: The L-arginine-nitric oxide pathway. N. Engl. J. Med., 1993; 329: 2002-2012.

Nabel, E.G. et al: Gene therapy for cardiovascular disease. Circulation, 1995; 91:541-548.

Ohno, T et al: Gene therapy for vascular smooth muscle proliferation after arterial injury. Science, 1994; 265:781-784.

Opie, L.H. and Messerli, F.H.: Nifedipine and mortality: grave defects in the dossier. Circulation, 1993; 92:1068-1073.

Parker, J.O.: Eccentric dosing with isosorbide-5-mononitrate in angina pectoris. Am. J. Cardiol., 1993; 72:871-876.

Pitt, B.: Blockade of the renin-angiotensin system. Effect on mortality in patients with left ventricular systolic dysfunction. Cardiol. Clin., 1994; 12:101-114.

Robertson, D., and Stevens, R.M. et al: Nitrates and glaucoma, JAMA., 1977; 237:117.

Rutherford, J. D et al: Pharmacologic management of angina and acute myocardial infarction. Am. J. Cardiol., 1993; 72:16C-20C.

Takeshita, S., Zheng, L.F. et al: Therapeutic angiogenesis: a single intraarterial bolus of vascular endothelial growth factor augments revascularization in a rabbit ischemic hindlimb model. J. Clin. Invest., 1994; 93:662-670.

Taylor, S.H. et al: Usefulness of amlodipine for angina pectoris. Am. J. Cardiol., 1994; 73:28A-33A.

Thadani, U et al: Role of nitrates in angina pectoris. Am. J. Cardiol., 1992; 70:43B-53B.

Vane, J.R. et al: The endothelium: maestro of the blood circulation. Philos. Trans. R. Soc. Lond. [Biol.], 1994; 343:225-246.

Van Zwieten, P.A. et al: Similarities and differences between calcium antagonists: pharmacological aspects. J. Hypertens., 1993; 11 Suppl. 1:S3-S11.

Vogt, M et al: ACE-inhibitors in coronary artery disease? Basic Res. in Cardiol., 1993; 88 Suppl. 1:43-64.

Why, H.J. et al: A potassium channel opener as monotherapy in chronic stable angina pectoris: comparison with placebo. Eur. Heart J., 1993; 14 Suppl. B25-29.

Yusuf, S. et al: Update of effects of calcium antagonists in myocardial infarction or angina in light of the second Danish Verapamil Infarction Trial (DAVIT-II) and other recent studies. Am. J. Cardiol., 1991, 67:1295-1297.

Yusuf, S et al: Calcium antagonists in coronary artery disease and hypertension. Time of revaluation? Circulation, 1995; 92:1079-1082.

TREATMENT OF HYPERTENSION AND OTHER VASCULAR PROBLEMS

The normal blood pressure (B.P.) depends on:
- Peripheral vascular resistance
- Cardiac output
- Volume of blood within circulation.

By decreasing one or more of these factors it is possible to lower the B.P.

Fig. 4.3 shows some factors involved in the control of B.P. that affect the basic equation: B.P. = CO × PR.

Blood Pressure = Cardiac Output × Peripheral Resistance

Hypertension (persistently raised B.P.) is a common disease. The higher the blood pressure more is the risk of cardiovascular diseases. Hypertension has damaging effect on brain, heart and kidneys. The incidence of coronary artery disease (CAD), cerebral haemorrhage and renal failure is increased. Hypertension is of two types, viz. (i) primary or essential where the cause of sustained raised blood pressure is not known and (ii) secondary hypertension where the cause is known and therefore the treatment is not difficult.

The level of systolic pressure is also important in assessing the incidence of arterial pressure on cardiovascular morbidity. Some data suggest that it may be more important than diastolic pressure. For example, males with normal diastolic pressure (<82 mmHg) but elevated systolic pressures (> 158 mmHg) have a cardiovascular mortality rate 2.5 times higher than individuals who have similar pressures but whose systolic pressures are normal (<130 mmHg). A reduction in mortality and morbidity with treatment, specially in the elderly, has been documented in these patients. Systolic and diastolic B.P. in normal persons and in hypertensive cases are shown in Table 4.4.

Table 4.4. Classification of B.P. for adults aged 18 years and older

Category	Systolic pressure mmHg	Diastolic pressure mmHg
Optimal	< 120	< 80
Normal	< 130	< 85
High normal	130-139	85-89
Hypertension		
Stage 1 (mild)	140-159	90-99
Stage 2 (moderate)	160-179	100-109
Stage 3 (severe)	180-209	110-119

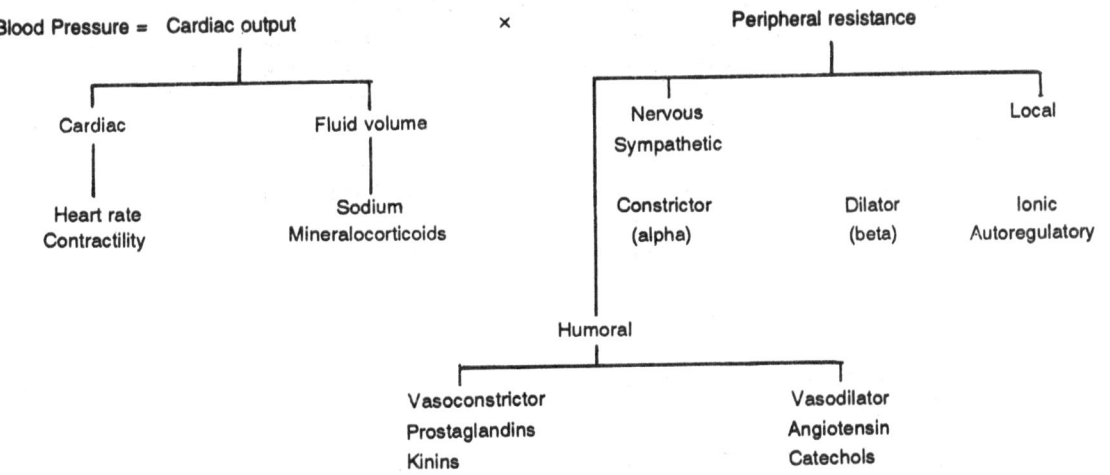

Fig. 4.3. Factors involved in the control of B.P.

The Seventh Report of the Joint National Committee on Prevention, Detection, Evaluation and Treatment of high blood pressure (JNC, USA) has introduced a new classification that includes the term "prehypertension" for those with BPs ranging from 120 to 139 mm Hg systolic and/ or 80 to 89 mm Hg diastolic blood pressure. Another change in classification is the combining of stage 2 and stage 3 hypertension into a stage 2 category.

Arterial pressure fluctuates in most persons, whether they are normotensive or hypertensive. Patients who are classified as having labile hypertension are those who sometimes, but not always, have arterial pressure in the hypertensive range. These patients are often considered to have borderline hypertension.

Sustained hypertension can become accelerate or enter a malignant phase, although that is unusual in treated cases. Accelerated hypertension is defined as a significant recent increase over previous hypertensive levels associated with evidence of vascular damage on funduscopic examination but without papilloedema. Malignant hypertension is defined by the presence of papilloedema, usually accompanied by retinal haemorrhages and exudates, rather than by the absolute pressure level, though a patient with malignant hypertension often has a blood pressure above 200/140.

A strong family history of hypertension, along with the reported finding of intermittent pressure elevation in the past favours the diagnosis of essential hypertension.

Secondary hypertension may be due to the use of steroids or oestrongens. A history of repeated urinary tract infections, renal or endocrine disease also indicate secondary hypertension.

Classification of antihypertensive agents based on sites and modes of action (Fig. 4.4)

1. Sympathetic inhibitors

- Adrenergic mechanisms in the CNS i.e. centrally acting at brain stem: Clonidine, Methyldopa, Reserpine
- Reflex stimulation of baroreceptors: Veratrum alkaloids
- Sympathetic ganglia: Mecamylamine, Pentolinium, Pempidine.

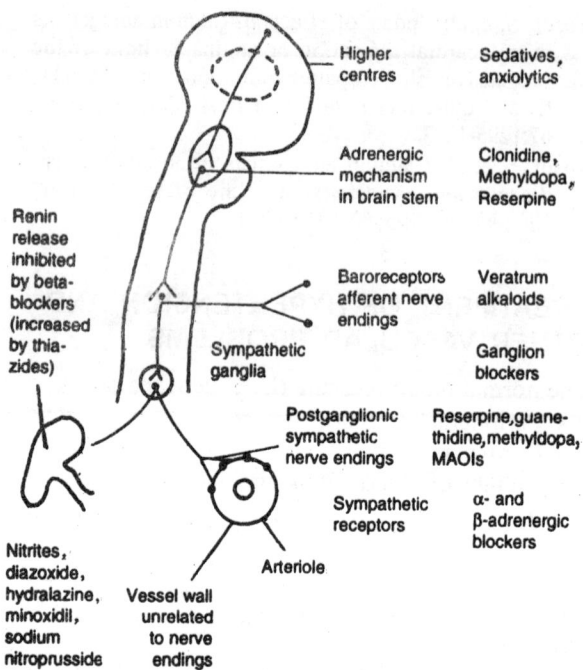

Fig. 4.4. Sites and modes of action of antihypertensive agents.

- Adrenergic neuron blockers:
  - Guanethidine, Bethanidine (inhibit release of NA).
  - Reserpine depletes axonal stores of NA.
  - Pargyline inhibits MAO
- Adrenergic receptors:
  - Alpha-blocker: Prazosin.
  - Beta-blocker: Propranolol, atenolol.
  - Alpha and beta-blocker: Labetalol.

2. Renin-angiotensin-aldosterone system

- Beta-blockers block renin release.
- Captopril, enalapril and lisinopril block conversion of angiotensin I to angiotensin II by inhibiting angiotensin-converting enzyme.
- Saralasin blocks competitively angiotensin II at vascular receptor site.
- Spironolactone counteracts action of aldosterone.

3. Vascular smooth muscle

- Ca^{++} channel blockers: Verapamil, Nifedipine, Diltiazem. These are arteriolar vasodilators.

Box 4.1 Summary of factors that affect arterial blood pressure
- Cardiac output
- Blood volume
- Peripheral resistance

Box 4.2. Classes of antihypertensive medications

Diuretics	
Thiazide	Hydrochlorothiazide
Loop	Frusemide
Potassium-sparing	Amiloride
	Triamterane
	Spironolactone
Beta blockers	
Nonselective	Propranolol
Cardioselective	Atenolol
	Metoprolol
Ca^{2+}-Channel blockers	Nifedipine
Vasodilators	
Arteriolar (direct)	Hydralazine
	Minoxidil
Nonselective	Nitroprusside
Alpha-blockers	Prazosin
Centrally acting	Clonidine
Peripherally acting	Reserpine
	Guanethidine
ACE inhibitors	Enalapril
	Lisinopril

- Diuretics: Thiazides, Loop diuretics, K-sparing diuretics (spironolactone, triamterone).
- Direct acting:
  - Arteriolar vasodilators: Diazoxide, Hydralazine, Minoxidil.
  - Arteriolar-venular vasodilators: Sodium nitroprusside.

Criteria for an ideal antihypertensive drug

- It should produce smooth, predictable and reliable blood pressure lowering effect in both systolic and diastolic pressures in supine as well as erect posture.
- Leave intact the normal B.P. responses to exercise and posture.
- Produce no immediate or remote side effects, nor affect cardiac output or reduce blood flow to vital organs such as brain, heart and kidneys.

- It should be available by all routes of administration and tolerance should not develop on long term use.

The ideal remains unattained. However, judicious use after proper selection of the drug alone or in appropriate combinations, it may be possible to satisfy most of these requirements.

ANTIHYPERTENSIVE AGENTS

DRUGS ACTING ON CNS

Clonidine

It is an imidazole derivative having moderately potent antihypertensive effect. It is well absorbed on oral administration, half-life is 12 hours. About 40% is excreted unchanged in urine and the rest is excreted by kidneys as metabolites.

Initial dose is 0.05 to 0.1 mg thrice a day orally. In emergencies it can be given by I.M. injection.

The main advantages of clonidine are that postural hypotension is less and there is no significant reduction in renal blood flow. However, it is not the first line drug for the treatment of hypertension due to frequent side effects and risk of withdrawal syndrome. The abrupt withdrawal is characterized by increased B.P., headache, tremor, and restlessness.

Clonidine also has some usefulness as a prophylactic agent in migraine. But it has not proved very effective for this purpose. Its mode of action in migraine is not clear.

Clonidine is a centrally acting alpha2-adrenergic agonist and thus diminishes sympathetic outflow from hypothalamus and medulla oblongata.

The adverse effects include fluid retention, sedation, constipation, dryness of mouth.

Drug interactions: Tricyclic antidepressants interfere with the antihypertensive effect of clonidine.

Methyldopa (Aldomet)

It reduces the total peripheral resistance without any significant change in cardiac output or heart rate.

It acts within CNS, stimulates the presynaptic alpha adrenergic receptors of vasomotor centers (as clonidine acts).

Previously it was thought that a false neuro-transmitter alpha- methyl noradrenaline was formed which was released on nerve stimulation. It is now known that methyldopa acts on central adrenergic mechanisms through its metabolite alpha-methyl noradrenaline.

Methyldopa is well absorbed from GIT following oral administration and largely excreted by the kidneys. One advantage of methyldopa is that it produces much less postural hypotension than guanethidine or ganglionic blocking agents or MAOIs. It is indicated in moderate to severe hypertension.

Dosage : 250 mg tablets twice or thrice a day initially, then increments of 250 mg every third day, maximum 2 g/d. In hypertensive crisis it is given by I.V. injection (250 mg/5 ml).

Adverse effects : Sedation, marked drowsiness, depression, GI upsets, nasal stuffiness, impotence and nightmares.

Contraindications : Active hepatic disease.

Reserpine

It is one of the alkaloids from rauwolfia serpentina plant. It depletes catecholamines and serotonin centrally as well as peripherally. The blood pressure lowering effect is due to peripheral depletion of noradrenaline. The central actions such as bradycardia, sedation and tranquilization also helps patients suffering from hypertension. Reserpine is useful in uncomplicated mild hypertension. It is a slowly acting drug, takes 2-3 weeks for full effect.

Dosage : 0.1, 0.25 and 1 mg tablets, solution for injection 2.5 mg/ml are available. The usual dose is 0.3-0.5 mg orally daily.

The *adverse effects* include nasal stuffiness, hyperacidity, diarrhoea, postural hypotension (more than methyldopa), parkinsonism like condition, marked depression (due to central serotonin depletion) which may be severe and induce suicidal tendencies.

REFLEX INHIBITORS OF SYMPATHETIC FUNCTIONS

Veratrum alkaloids

Veratrum alkaloids (protoveratrines A and B mixture less than 2 mg I.V. were previously used to control severe malignant hypertension). They reflexly stimulate the baroreceptors in left ventricle, lungs, aorta and carotid sinus. They lower B.P. by decreasing the peripheral resistance. As these drugs have very narrow margin of safety there is no justification for using them.

DRUGS ACTING ON AUTONOMIC GANGLIA

Mecamylamine, pentolinium and pempidine

These may be used for the emergency treatment of malignant hypertension. But these drugs are not commonly used as they do not act specifically at sympathetic ganglia but also on parasympathetic ganglia resulting in many undesirable effects.

The adverse effects include postural hypotension, constipation, paralytic ileus, dry mouth, blurred vision, retention of urine and GI upsets.

ADRENERGIC NEURON BLOCKERS

Guanethidine, bethanidine and debrisoquine

These are taken up into adrenergic neurons by active membrane amine-pump system. These block release of NA which takes place in response to sympathetic stimulation.

Guanethidine unlike other members of this group also produces depletion of NA from storage sites within the nerve terminals.

The hypotensive effect is mainly due to decrease in the cardiac output. It is indicated only in severe cases, now it is less frequently used as compared to vasodilators.

Guanethidine is absorbed about 50% from GIT on oral administration. The onset of action is slow and the desired effect is observed after 3 days. However, the effect lasts for about a week after the drug is stopped. It does not cross the blood brain barrier. About 50% is metabolized and the rest is excreted unchanged in the urine.

Dosage : Initial dose is 10 mg orally per day, if required the dose is increased by 10 mg after every week.

Ampoules containing 10 mg/ml are also available for parenteral use.

Adverse effects : Postural hypotension (more than reserpine), reduced sympathetic activity resulting in parasympathetic predominance which produce nasal congestion, diarrhoea, and bradycardia.

The other side effects include GI upsets, and parotid tenderness.

Drug interactions : Tricyclic antidepressants oppose the effects of guanethidine as they block its uptake into adrenergic neurons.

Bethanidine and Debrisoquine block sympathetic postganglionic neuron transmission without depleting the tissue stores of catecholamines. The duration of their action is shorter than guanethidine. The dose of bethanidine is 10 mg tablets thrice a day orally after meals; debrisoquine 10 mg is administered once or twice a day. These drugs are excreted unchanged in urine. Tricyclic antidepressants oppose their actions.

The adverse effects of these drugs include postural hypotension, and fluid retention.

Bretylium

It is a postganglionic adrenergic neuron blocker. Initially it induces release of noradrenaline followed by impairment of neurotransmission. It has been found unsuitable as antihypertensive drug due to frequent and severe side effects and quick development of tolerance.

MAO INHIBITORS

Pargyline

It is the only member of this group used as an antihypertensive drug. The dose is 10-15 mg tablets once a day orally.

But it is not commonly used due to too many side effects including postural hypotension and adverse interactions with a large number of drugs and also with foods containing tyramine.

ADRENOCEPTOR BLOCKERS

Alpha adrenergic blockers such as **phenoxybenzamine, phentolamine** and **tolazoline** can lower the blood pressure but these are not used for this purpose due to (i) marked reflex tachycardia and (ii) postural hypotension.

Prazosin hydrochloride: It is a selective or specific postsynaptic α_1-blocker.

It causes vasodilation of both the arteries and veins. It reduces peripheral vascular resistance and lowers arterial blood pressure in supine and erect patients. Unlike non-selective alpha- blockers, it does not produce reflex tachycardia. Unlike beta blockers prazosin does not affect blood lipids. It does not increase plasma renin activity. It produces minimal changes in cardiac output, renal blood flow and glomerular filtration rate.

The plasma half-life is 2-3 hours but can be prolonged by CHF. It is extensively metabolised, may undergo significant first-pass metabolism, has a bioavailability of about 60%, and is probably excreted in bile and faeces.

It is indicated in mild to moderate hypertension.

Dose: 0.5 mg orally thrice a day.

Adverse effects include sodium and fluid retention. It may show 'first dose phenomenon' resulting in marked orthostatic hypotension and syncope one hour after the first dose.

Terazosin has a longer half-life (12 hours) and longer duration of action (24 hours) than prazosin but is otherwise similar to prazosin. Terazosin is used to treat benign prostatic hyperplasia (improves urine flow and decreases symptoms of obstruction) as well as hypertension.

Beta adrenoceptor blockers

These are useful for the treatment of hypertension, angina pectoris and cardiac arrhythmias.

Beta blockers can be regarded as belonging to one of six sub-groups.

- β_1 selective (cardioselective) without ISA (e.g. atenolol, metoprolol).
- β_1 selective (cardioselective) with ISA (e.g. acebutolol).
- β_1 selective (cardioselective) with ISA (e.g. celiprolol).
- Non-selective without ISA (e.g. propranolol).
- Non-selective with ISA (e.g. oxprenolol).
- Non-selective β-blocker with α blocking (e.g. labetalol).

Cardioselectivity : The advantage of cardioselective beta blockers over non-selective agents can be demonstrated in at least six areas :

- Relative blood pressure lowering effects
- In airways disease

- In insulin-dependent diabetic hypertension
- In smokers
- During exercise
- On serum lipids

Beta blockers cause little change in total serum cholesterol but may lower serum HDL cholesterol and raise serum LDL cholesterol and triglycerides. Cardioselective agents without ISA exert lesser effects on these parameters than non-cardioselective agents without ISA. Furthermore, at low doses, cardioselective agents can control blood pressure, in which case these changes are minimal.

Effect of ISA

Partial agonist effect (Intrinsic sympathomimetic activity, ISA)

Some beta blockers also have ISA which is the ability to cause weak stimulation of beta adrenergic receptors while simultaneously blocking the effect of endogenous catecholamines. Possession of ISA may result in fewer adverse effects related to unopposed beta blocked effects (bradycardia, heart block, bronchoconstriction, peripheral vascular constriction). Pindolol exhibits the most ISA of the beta blockers currently available. Carteolol and oxprenolol have moderate ISA. Acebutolol has mild to moderate ISA and the other members of the group have little if any such ISA activity.

Mechanism of action of beta adrenergic blockers

They lower blood pressure in hypertensive patients. They do not lower B.P. in normotensive persons. The fall of B.P. is due to following mechanisms :

- reduction of pulse rate, hence cardiac output
- decrease in plasma renin
- diminished venous tone
- reduction in norepinephrine release
- reduction in peripheral vascular resistance
- modulation of baroreceptor reflexes
- diminished sensitivity to catecholamines

Hypertensive patients in whom beta adrenergic blockers are suitable

- Patients with angina or post myocardial infarction.
- Coexisting anxiety or tachycardia
- Tense and young patients
- Non-obese, hypertensive
- Pregnancy

Hypertensive patients in whom beta adrenergic blockers should be avoided

- LVF
- CHF
- Patients with bradycardia and conduction defects
- Patients with asthma
- Diabetics or patients with borderline glucose tolerance
- Patients with abnormal lipid profile
- Elderly patients
- Peripheral vascular disease

β-adrenoceptor blocking drugs impair the sympathetic mediated (β$_2$-receptor) release of glucose from the liver in response to hypoglycaemia due to insulin and sulphonylureas, and also reduce the adrenergic-mediated symptoms of hypoglycaemia except sweating (sweat glands have α receptors). The hypoglycaemia is thus both profound and less noticeable.

A diabetic needing a β-blocker should be given β$_1$-cardioselective member e.g. atenolol. The nonselective beta blockers e.g. propranolol will enhance hypoglycaemia and produce hypertension with bradycardia due to the unopposed α vasoconstrictor activity.

These are useful drugs for the treatment of hypertension, angina pectoris and cardiac arrhythmias. The beta blockers are:

Propranolol

It is well absorbed from the intestines. There is 'first-pass' metabolism to a significant extent (40-70%) in the liver before it reaches the systemic circulation. The main metabolite is 4-hydroxypropranolol which is active but with shorter half-life.

Initial dose is 10-20 mg three or four times a day. It is used in mild to moderate hypertension.

Atenolol

It does not have partial agonist activity, lipid solubility is low, elimination half-life is 6-9 hours, bioavailability is about 40%, acts selectively on β_1 receptors.

Metoprolol

Its partial agonist activity is nil, lipid solubility moderate, elimination half life 3-4 hours, bioavailability about 50%. Its acts selectively on β_1-receptors.

Nadolol has no partial agonist activity, has low lipid solubility, elimination half-life is 14-24 hours, bioavailability about 33%. It acts on both β_1 and β_2-receptors.

Acebutolol

It has partial agonist activity, lipid solubility is low, elimination half-life is 3-4 hours, bioavailability is about 50%. It acts selectively on β_1-receptors.

Pindolol

It has partial agonist activity, moderate lipid solubility elimination half-life is 3-4 hours, bioavailability is 90%. It acts both on β_1 and β_2-receptors.

Adverse effects of beta blockers: Beta blockers can worsen asthma and heart failure, produce hypoglycaemia, CNS disturbances including poor concentration, lethargy and vivid nightmares.

Labetalol blocks both alpha and beta adrenoceptors. Its usefulness as an antihypertensive agent is due to:

- Blocking effect on alpha adrenergic receptors in peripheral arterioles resulting in reduction of peripheral resistance and thus fall in B.P.
- Blocking effect on beta adrenergic receptors results in prevention of compensatory reflex sympathetic activity induced by peripheral vasodilatation.

The antihypertensive effectiveness on oral administration is similar to that of methyldopa. However, postural hypotension is not a problem with Labetalol.

Dose: 100 mg thrice a day orally. It can also be given by I.V. injection for rapid control of severe hypertension.

Adverse effects : Epigastric pain, nasal stuffiness and vivid dreams.

Contraindications : Bronchial asthma.

The effect of beta and alpha adrenergic antagonists on serum lipids is shown in Table 4.5.

Table 4.5. Effects of beta and alpha antagonists on serum lipids

	LDL	HDL	TG	Lipoprotein lipase	LCAT
Beta blockers	↑	↓	↓↓	↓	↓
Alpha blockers	↓	↑↑	→	↑	↑

LCAT = lecithin:cholesterol acyltransferase; ↑ = increased; ↓ = decreased; → = no change

ANGIOTENSIN-CONVERTING ENZYME INHIBITORS (ACEIs)

These are specific competitive inhibitors of ACE which results in reducing the synthesis of angiotensin II and preserving the concentration of bradykinin. This lowers B.P. due to reduction of peripheral vascular resistance. The adrenergic activity is also reduced which contributes to the antihypertensive effect.

The heart rate and cardiac output are not affected. ACE inhibitors reduce both preload and afterload.

Advantages of ACEIs

- No postural hypotension, electrolyte disturbances, and CNS effects.
- Safe in asthmatics, diabetics and peripheral vascular disease.
- Renal blood flow is maintained.
- No hyperuricaemia, no deleterious effect on plasma lipid profile.
- No rebound hypertension on sudden withdrawal.
- Reversal of LVH seen in hypertensives.
- Prevention of secondary hyperaldosteronism and K^+ loss due to diuretics.

Angiotensin converting enzyme inhibitors are:

Specially beneficial for	*Not to be used in*
• Young patients	• Pregnancy
• Diabetic patients	• Bilateral renal artery
• Co-existing angina	stenosis or in single kidney

- Post MI cases
- CHF
- LV hypertrophy
- Gout
- Dyslipidaemic patients

Precaution in –
- High salt intake
- Presence of dry cough
- Patients receiving high dose diuretic therapy

Uses of ACE inhibitors

- Hypertension
- Cardiac failure
- Following MI
- Diabetic nephropathy
- Progressive renal insufficiency

These appear to confer a special advantage in the treatment of patients with diabetes, slowing the development of diabetic glomerulopathy, and also slow the progression of other forms of chronic renal disease such as glomerulosclerosis. Such drug is probably the preferred initial agent in the treatment of hypertensive patients with left ventricular hypertrophy.

The endocrine consequences of ACEIs are important in a number of facets of hypertension treatment. They blunt the normal aldosterone response to Na^+ loss, the normal role of aldosterone to oppose diuretic-induced natriuresis is diminished, thus they enhance the efficacy of diuretic drugs. It means that even very small dose of diuretics may substantially improve the antihypertensive efficacy of ACEIs. It also means that if high does of diuretics are given together with ACEIs it may lead to excessive reduction in BP and Na^+.

Captopril was the first such agents to be develop, since then enalapril, lisinopril, quinapril, ramipril, benazepril, moexipril and fosinopril have become available.

The three major effects of angiotensin II and the mechanism that mediate them are listed in Table 4.6.

Figs. 4.5 and 4.6 show the role of angiotensin in hypertension and renin angiotensin and kinin relationship in Fig. 4.7.

The actions of angiotensin II and kinin-angiotensin system are shown in Fig. 4.7.

Renin release is reduced by clonidine, methyldopa, reserpine, Beta-blockers and adrenergic neuron blockers.

Renin release is increased by thiazides, loop diuretics, spironolactone, hydralazine and diazoxide.

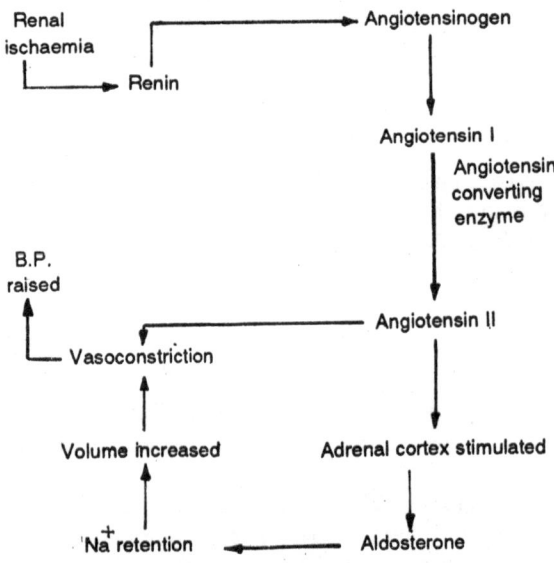

Fig. 4.5. Role of angiotensin in hypertension.

Table 4.6. Three major effects of angiotensin II and mechanisms

Altered peripheral resistance	Altered renal function	Altered cardiovascular structure
Direct vasoconstriction Increased NE release Decreased NE reuptake Increased sympathetic discharge in CNS Release of catecholamines from adrenal medulla Rapid pressure response	Direct action of increased Na^+ reabsorption in proximal tubule Release of aldosterone from adrenal cortex Direct renal vasoconstriction Increased renal sympathetic tone (CNS) Increased noradrenergic neurotransmission in kidney Slow pressure response	Increased production of growth factors Increased synthesis of extracellular matrix proteins Increased afterload (cardiac) Increased wall tension (vascular) Vascular and cardiac hypertrophy

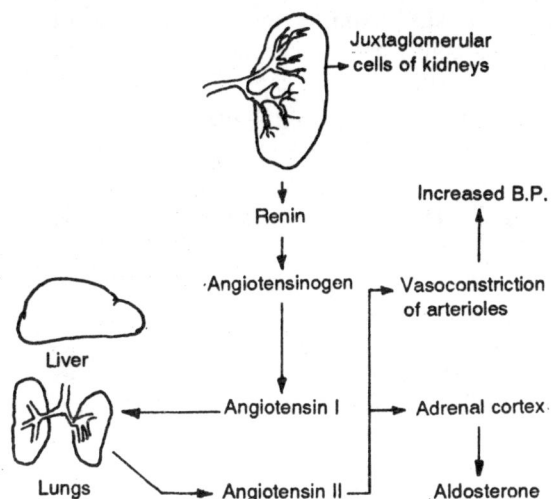

Fig. 4.6. Role of renin and involvement of liver and lungs.

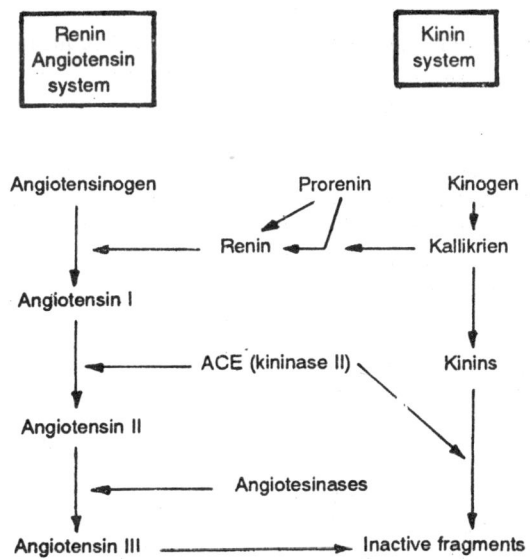

Fig. 4.7. Renin-angiotensin system.

Prazosin does not change renin secretion.

Captopril produces antihypertensive effect as it inhibits conversion of angiotensin I to angiotensin II, by competitive inhibition of angiotensin-converting enzyme. Angiotensin II produces direct pressor activity and stimulation of aldosterone secretion from adrenal cortex. These effects are inhibited by captopril.

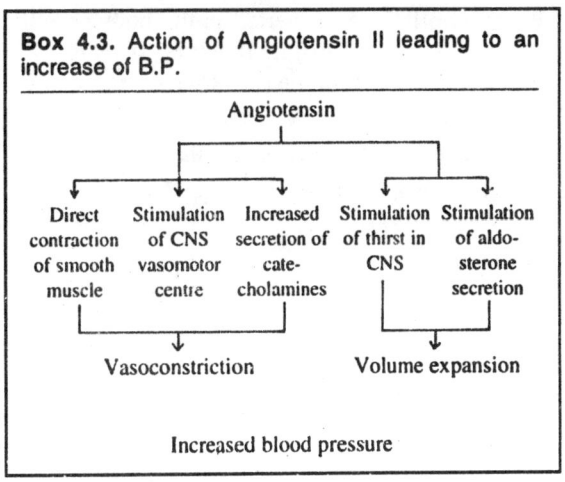

Box 4.3. Action of Angiotensin II leading to an increase of B.P.

Captopril is rapidly absorbed from GIT.

Dose: 25-75 mg twice or thrice a day, it is useful in severe resistant cases where standard therapy has failed. It is often combined with a diuretic.

It is safe in asthmatic and diabetic patients.

Renal blood flow is well maintained.

Enalapril (Invoril)

It is a prodrug converted in liver into active drug enalaprilat. It has certain advantages over captopril. It is more potent, dose is 10-20 mg once a day, has longer duration of action than captopril (half-life 11 hours). Its absorption is not affected by food. Side effects are less frequent, e.g. alteration in taste sensation is only in 1.5 % cases compared to 10% with captopril.

Lisinopril : It is a lysine derivative of enalaprilat. Its half life is 12 hours. It is absorbed more slowly than enalapril and has a slower onset of action.

Dose: 10-80 mg once daily.

Benazepril and **ramipril** are excreted in urine and may require dosage adjustment when renal function is impaired.

Fosinopril is excreted in bile and does not require dosage adjustment in presence of impaired renal function.

Quinapril is a prodrug that is rapidly converted to its active form in the small intestine and liver.

Perindopril is also a long acting ACE inhibitor

like lisinopril. It is converted in the body to active metabolite perindoprilat. It tends to restore the reduced elastic properties of arteries and heart in hypertensives.

Dosage : Initial 4 mg once a day.

Contraindications :
- Hypersensitivity
- Pregnancy

Adverse effects

- Common : cough, dizziness, hyperkalaemia, hypotension, nausea.
- Serious : angioedema, hepatic failure (rare)
- Hypotension has followed the first dose of ACE inhibitors in sodium depleted patients.
- Dry cough is common and bronchospasm may occur.
- Neutropenia can occur; and, in patients who have impaired renal function; or serious autoimmune disease (e.g., systemic lupus erythematosus), captopril should be used with caution. Neutropcnia is rare with enalapril or lisinopril.
- Proteinuria can occur, especially in patients with compromised renal function monitoring of urinary protein levels should be done.
- About 10% of patients treated with captopril develop reversible skin rashes, alteration in taste, proteinurea, and leukopenia. The incidence is lower (1.5%) with enalapril and lisinopril because they lack a sulphydryl group.
- Headache, dizziness, and fatigue are the most common side effects associated with enalapril.
- Hyperkalaemia has been reported. Rarely angioedema occurs.

Contraindications: Presence of renal dysfunction, in patients with bilateral renal artery stenosis because acute renal failure may ensue.

Saralasin : It is an angiotensin II analogue. It acts on angiotensin II receptors of vascular smooth muscle. It is a peptide angiotensin II receptor antagonist. It may be employed as a diagnostic agent to find renal cause of hypertension or for emergency treatment of angiotensin II-dependent hypertension. It may be given by I.V. infusion at a rate of 20 mcg/kg/min in these situations. However, the clinical value

of saralasin is limited because of lack of oral bioavailability and unacceptable partial agonist activity. Its half life is very short (4 minutes). Therefore attempts were to develop orally active, potent, and selective nonpeptide angiotensin II receptor antagonist, Losartan.

Losartan is a angiotensin to receptor antagonist. It is available as a single agent or in a fixed dose regimen containing 50 mg of losartan and 12.5 mg of hydrochlorothiazide.

Losartan 25 mg is administered twice a day which reduces blood pressure but the effect is not so great as that obtained with an ACEI. The effect is also obtained after 3-6 weeks with Losartan.

There are certain advantages of this drug. Cough and angioedema have not been observed unlike ACEIs because ACEIs not only prevent conversion of angiotensin I to II but also prevent ACE-mediated degradation of bradykinin and substance P.

The *adverse effects* like those of ACEIs will occur e.g. hypotension, hyperkalaemia and reduced renal function. i.e. those related to a diminished level of angiotensin II.

Adverse effects that are independent of reduced effects of angiotensin II are not yet known.

Contraindication : Pregnancy, breast-feeding.

DRUGS AFFECTING THE VASCULAR SMOOTH MUSCLE

Ca++ channel blockers

All Ca^{2+}-channel blockers are equally effective when used alone for the treatment of mild to moderate hypertension and are as effective in lowering BP as beta-adrenergic receptor antagonists or diuretics.

These drugs block entry of calcium and thus relax smooth muscle of blood vessels. They also have negative inotropic effect resulting in decreasing the cardiac output.

Verapamil, Nifedipine and Diltiazem belong to this group. All the three drugs are powerful dilators of coronary and peripheral arteries. The vasodilator effect makes these drugs useful in the treatment of hypertension. Nifedipine is more powerful than the other two drugs as vasodilator. Verapamil has more marked effect on heart.

Therapeutic uses of calcium channel blockers

- Hypertension – Nifedipine
- Bronchial asthma – nifedipine
- Angina (variant, exertional, unstable) - nifedipine, nimodipine, nicardipine
- Cardiac arrhythmias - verapamil, diltiazem
- In migraine - flunarizine
- Nocturnal leg cramps
- Reynaud's disease - nifedipine, diltiazem and felodipine
- To slow progression of renal failure and to protect transplanted kidney
- Hypertrophic cardiomyopathy

Advantages of calcium channel blockers as antihypertensives

- Rapid   onset and long duration of action, can be given once daily
- No cardiac depression
- Effective irrespective of renin status of the patient
- No adverse effect on foetus
- No impairment of renal perfusion
- Central perfusion is maintained with no sedation
- Can be used in patients with asthma, angina or COPD.
- No effect on male sexual function
- No effect on electrolytes, lipids and uric acid (unlike beta-blockers).

Calcium channel blockers are more suited for

- Elderly patients
- Isolated systolic hypertension
- Asthma/COPD patients
- Hypertensive patients with associated renal disease
- Patients with angina
- Pregnant women with hypertension

Caution observed in use of calcium channel blockers

- May aggravate diabetes. Nifedipine decreases insulin release

- Should not be used in patients with cardiac failure or conduction defects.

Adverse effects include flushing, sensation of heat, oedema around shins and ankles.

Ca^{2+}-channel blockers should not be used in patients with SA node or AV node abnormalities or in patients with overt CHF. However, they are safe in patients with asthma, and adrenal dysfunction. Unlike beta-blockers they do not affect plasma concentration of lipids, uric acid, and electrolytes.

Benzothiadiazines (Thiazides) and related diuretics

Saluretics

It has been suspected that certain hypertensive persons have abnormal salt metabolism and a relationship between salt intake and blood pressure has been established.

The rationale for use of saluretic drugs is almost self-evident in essential and expanded blood volume and high sodium burden. However, certain saluretic drugs have been found to lower blood pressure of persons with essential hypertension who have small extracellular fluid volumes. The smooth muscles in such persons have a high intracellular sodium content.

When thiazide saluretics are given, the fall in blood pressure in the first week or two correlates with saluresis and the decrease in extracellular fluid volume (hence, in venous return, stroke volume and systolic blood pressures). In this phase, heart rate is accelerated and peripheral resistance is increased. The antihypertensive action passes into a phase in which the extracellular volume and heart rate return toward normal and peripheral resistance falls.

Not all saluretics are alike in this effect, which suggests that something more than saluresis is involved. For example, high-ceiling saluretics never lower the vascular resistance, and blood pressure is lowered only because cardiac output is decreased. Spironolactone is a useful antihypertensive agent only when aldosterone or 18-hydroxycorticosterone levels are high.

At present, thiazide-like saluretics often are the first drugs to be used in the treatment of essential hypertension, used alone in mild essential hypertension, other drugs are added in moderate and severe essential hypertension.

Thiazides also correct the counter productive salt and water retention that occurs as a side effect to most other antihypertensive drugs.

Hypertensive patients in whom diuretics are suited

- Elderly patients
- Renal disease
- Obese patients with volume overload with Na+ retention
- Isolated systolic hypertension

Hypertensive patients in whom diuretics should be avoided

- Young active hypertensive patients
- Diabetics
- Hypertension with gout
- Patients with hyperlipidaemia

Chlorothiazide and **hydrochlorothiazide** reduce blood volume resulting in reduction of cardiac output. They also have direct relaxant effect which develops more slowly. The advantages of thiazides are that they are well tolerated and do not produce postural hypotension and no fluid retention. The disadvantages are that they are weak and side effects include hyperuricaemia, hypercalcaemia and hyperglycaemia as they decrease renal excretion of uric acid and calcium and inhibit insulin release.

These drugs initially decrease extracellular volume and cardiac output; long-term use decreases peripheral resistance.

Dose: 50-100 mg.

Nonthiazide diuretic agent, **Indapamide** exerts antihypertensive effect primarily by vasorelaxation. All in all, new data provide very strong evidence that indapamide is a unique diuretic agent, one that does not alter lipid levels, that does not regress left ventricular hypertrophy and that protects against progressive renal damage. The dangers of dyslipidaemia and the left ventricular hypertrophy and knowledge that proteinuria, too, is a major risk factor, the potential for greater protection from the cardiovascular sequelae of hypertension with indapamide compared to other diuretics seems almost certain.

Loop diuretics (high ceiling diuretics)

Frusemide (furosemide) and ethacrynic acid selectively inhibit NaCl reabsorption in the thick ascending limb of the loop of Henle.

They are given in hypertension in patients in whom other diuretics or antihypertensives do not produce satisfactory response.

Frusemide dose : 20-80mg is single or in 2 divided doses orally

Ethacrynic acid dose : 50-200 mg orally.

Indications for high ceiling diuretics in the treatment of hypertension

- Chronic renal failure
- Coexisting refractory CCF
- Resistance to combination regimens containing a thiazide
- Marked fluid retention due to use of potent vasodilators

Spironolactone is a K-sparing diuretic. It may produce K-retention. It is an aldosterone antagonist. It is sometimes given along with thiazides to prevent K-loss.

It produces arteriolar as well as venous dilatation.

Hydralazine decreases peripheral resistance thus lowers B.P. It is not commonly used alone as it produces frequent side effects including nasal stuffiness, tremors, reflex tachycardia, headache, dizziness and palpitation. It is usually given combined with propranolol or a diuretic.

It can worsen coronary artery disease because of the myocardial stimulation it produces.

Dose: 25 mg tablet thrice a day.

Diazoxide is a nondiuretic congener of thiazides which is not suitable for long term use as it produces sodium and water retention unlike thiazides and may precipitate diabetes and gout. It is used only in hypertensive emergencies by I.V. route. It produces arteriolar dilatation without any effect on venules. The usual dose is 75 mg I.V. then 150 mg at 5 minute intervals till B.P. is controlled. The oral absorption is erratic. The plasma half-life averages 28 hours, but the antihypertensive effect usually lasts only 4-12 hours.

Diazoxide inhibits insulin release from pancreas. It can be given orally to treat hypoglycaemia due to insulinoma.

Adverse effects include severe hypotension, oedema due to retention of salt and water. Its reflex sympathetic stimulation can cause angina and worsen myocardial ischaemia. It may produce hyperglycaemia as it inhibits release of insulin from the pancreas.

Sodium nitroprusside has rapid action but short lived (2-10 minutes). It is indicated in hypertensive emergencies. It produces arteriolar as well as venous dilatation. 50mg/5ml in amber coloured vials are available, used as I.V. infusion in hypertensive crisis.

It acts directly on arterial and venous smooth muscle but has little effect on other smooth muscles.

Adverse reactions include hypotension, diaphoresis, restlessness, palpitation, retrosternal pain, nausea, vomiting, headache, hypothyroidism (interferes with iodine transport). Methaemoglobinaemia has been reported.

Minoxidil is a potent drug, indicated in severe hypertension that does not respond adequately to more conventional antihypertensive therapy. It directly relaxes arteriolar smooth muscles. It is rapidly absorbed from GIT. About 85% is excreted as metabolites and the rest in unchanged form in the urine.

It is indicated only for severe hypertension. It is a vasodilator selective for arterioles, rather than for veins, similar to diazoxide and hydralazine.

Dose: 10-40 mg orally once a day or in divided doses.

Adverse effects : Sodium and fluid retention, oedema, hirsutism, tachycardia, pericardial effusion, increased hair growth of male type in females. Hirsutism occurs for unknown reasons; it is not associated with virilism or other endocrine abnormalities.

Table 4.7 shows certain comparative features of antihypertensive agents.

Regimen of treatment of essential hypertension

Mild hypertension: Sedatives such as diazepam may be useful, however, if it is unsuccessful then thiazides are advocated. In case these are unsuc-cessful then beta-blocker or reserpine are added to the regimen.

Moderate hypertension: Thiazide with reserpine or beta blocker or methyl dopa or hydralazine.

Severe hypertension: Oral diuretic plus beta blocker plus vasodilator or oral diuretic with guanethidine or clonidine.

Hypertensive crisis (emergencies): Sodium nitroprusside I.V. or Labetalol I.V. infusion or Hydralazine I.V. infusion or Diazoxide I.V.

Antihypertensives to be avoided in pregnancy (unsafe) are :

- Nonselective β-blockers : Propranolol may cause low birth weight, decreased placental size, neonatal bradycardia. However, proof is lacking.
- Sodium nitroprusside is contraindicated in eclampsia
- Reserpine : Suicidal depression in mother ; nasal stuffiness, deranged respiratory and temperature control in the new born.
- Labetalol may be hepatotoxic.
- ACE inhibitors, Losartan : growth retaradation and risk of foetal damage, oligohydramnios. Captopril produces foetal anuria.
- Diuretics should not be used as they deplete intravascular volume, increase utero-placental perfusion deficit, increase risk of placental infarcts and may cause neonatal thrombocytopenia, still birth, miscarriage.

Antihypertensives which are safer in pregnancy

- Prazosin/clonidine (provided postural hypotension can be avoided).
- Methyldopa is safe both for the mother and the baby.
- Cardioselective $β_1$-blocker such as atenolol and those with ISA such as pindolol and acebutolol.
- Dihydropyridine, calcium channel blockers (but discontinue before labour as they weaken uterine contractions).

Combination Therapy

It is rational to combine drugs with different

Table 4.7. Some comparative features of antihypertensive agents

Mode of action	Drugs	Postural hypotension	Sodium retention	Others	Special features
Inhibitors of sympathetic discharge	Clonidine	–	–	Dry mouth, drowsiness ++	Rebound
	Methyldopa	+	+	Drowsiness ++	hypertension
Ganglion blockers	Trimetaphan	+	–	Constipation	Not used
Sympathetic neuron blockers	Guanethidine,	+	+	Diarrhoea	
	Reserpine	+	+	Drowsiness, severe depression	Little used
Adrenoceptor blockers					
α	Prazosin	+	–	Tachycardia	
β	Propranolol,			Bronchoconstriction, cardiac	
	Atenolol	–	–	failure	
α and β	Labetalol	+	–	Drowsiness	
Vasodilators	Hydralazine	+	–	Tachycardia	
	Diazoxide	+	+		
	Nitroprusside	+	–		
	Thiazides	–	–	Hyperglycaemia, hyperuricaemia,	
	Ca-antagonists	+	–	Headache, reflex, tachycardia	
Block of renin-angiotensin system	Captopril	–	–		
	Saralasin	–	–		
	Enalapril	–	–	Rashes, fever, cough	
	Lisinopril	–	–	Cough	
Reduction of blood volume	Diuretics	–	–	K-loss, deafness	

mechanisms of action in certain hypertensives whose hypertension is not adequately controlled by single drug.

- ACE inhibitors are synergistic with diuretics. This combination is suitable for patients who have associated CHF and LV hypertrophy.
- All sympathetic blockers (except β-blockers) and vasodilators cause fluid retention. Combination with diuretic checks fluid retention and development of tolerance.
- Diuretics, vasodilators, calcium channel blockers, ACE inhibitors increase plasma renin activity. Those may be combined with β-blockers, clonidine, methyldopa which lower plasma renin activity.
- Other useful combinations include :
  ACE inhibitors + Calcium channel blockers or β-blocker or clonidine or methyl dopa

Combination to be avoided in

- Alpha or Beta adrenergic blocker with clonidine: antagonism of clonidine action has been observed.

- Nifedipine with diuretic : no additional antihypertensive action of diuretic seen.
- Hydralazine with prazosin : similar haemodynamic action.
- Reserpine with β-blockers : marked bradycardia.
- Verapamil/diltiazem with β-blockers : marked bradycardia, A-V block.
- Methyldopa with clonidine : same class.

Nonpharmacological approaches such as reduction of weight in obese persons, sodium salt restriction, avoidance of stress and strain as far as possible, and avoidance of smoking and tobacco chewing are helpful in the management of hypertension.

Obesity and hypertension are closely related, mechanism is unclear but increased secretion of insulin in obesity results in insulin-mediated enhancement of renal tubular reabsorption of Na^+ and an expansion of extracellular volume. Obesity is also associated with increased activity of sympathetic nervous system.

Heavy consumption of alcohol increases the risk of cerebrovascular accident but not CHD. It has been reported that small amount of alcohol protects CHD. However, alcohol increases B.P.

Other vascular problems

Chronic hypotension

It may be due to low cardiac output, malnutrition, primary adrenocortical insufficiency.

Patients of chronic hypotension complain of dizziness, faintness, lethargy, weakness and easy fatiguability.

There is no specific treatment for this condition. Administration of high salt diet (NaCl 10-20 g a day) or 9-alpha-fluorohydrocortisone 0.1-0.5 mg a day will produce expansion of extracellular fluid volume.

Orthostatic pooling of blood (causes faintness) can be prevented by applying tight full length elastic bandages on legs.

Regional vascular problems

In peripheral arterial occlusive diseases e.g. atheromatous occlusive conditions in limbs, Buerger's disease and Raynaud's disease, the aim of therapy is to improve blood flow or change the distribution of blood flow. For this purpose tolazoline is given by intraarterial route. It produces only temporary relief. The other better drug is pentoxyfylline (a derivative of methyl xanthine). The dose is 800-1600 mg orally in three divided doses daily for about 2 months.

Calcium channel blockers like nifedipine dilate the arteries.

Ketanserin (5-HT antagonist)

It has vasodilator and antiplatelet activity. It is effective in hypertension, however it does not offer any significant advantage over other antihypertensive agents.

After oral administration, peak effect reaches after 1-2 hours. Its bioavailability is low due to first-pass effect. About 50% is metabolized by the liver to ketanserinol an inactive metabolite, only small quantity, is excreted unchanged in the urine. The elimination half-life is 10-18 hours.

Dose : 40 mg twice a day orally, I.V. 5mg followed by infusion of 5-10mg / hour. It is a specific serotonin antagonist.

Adverse effects include postural hypotension (not frequent), palpitation (frequent). Headache, dizziness fatigue, sedation (most frequent).

Carnitine is claimed to enhance the metabolic efficacy of ischaemic muscle.

Ischaemic cerebro-vascular accidents

The aims of treatment are :

- Improvement of circulation and oxygenation (O_2 40% + CO_2 5%)
- To decrease oedema. 10% glycerol is given by I.V. infusion about 8-10 mg/min, total dose being 1-2 g/kg. Infusion of mannitol or low molecular weight dextran are also recommended. Dexamethasone 10 mg I.V. in divided doses for at least a week initially (and then reduced) are also helpful.
- To prevent further thrombosis aspirin 75 mg with 100 mg dipyridamole daily.
- Heparin 2500-5000 units I.V. every 3 hours till the patient is stabilized. The dose should be tailed off.
- Muscle spasticity should be reduced by dantrolene sodium 25-50 mg twice a day or diazepam or baclofen.

STUDY QUESTIONS

1. Why is it necessary to treat hypertension? Define primary (essential) and secondary hypertension; hypotensive and antihypertensive agents.
2. Classify antihypertensive drugs based on sites and mode of action.
3. What is the role of antianxiety drugs in the treatment of hypertension?
4. Which antihypertensive act centrally at brain stem? Describe their pharmacology.
5. Why veratrum alkaloids are not used now?
6. Describe the adverse effects of ganglion blocking drugs.
7. Name blockers of adrenergic receptors which may be used as antihypertensive drugs.
8. Explain renin-angiotensin-aldosterone system. How do angiotensin converting enzyme inhibitors act? Name these drugs and describe their status and adverse effects.
9. Write short notes on (i) hydralazine, (ii) sodium nitroprusside, (iii) minoxidil, (iv) diazoxide.
10. Describe the role of calcium channel blockers in the treatment of hypertension.

11. What is the importance of thiazides, loop diuretics and K-sparing diuretics as antihypertensive? What are the adverse effects of thiazide diuretics?

12. What are the adverse effects of the following: Clonidine, Reserpine, Guanethidine?

13. Describe propranolol regarding its use in the treatment of hypertension. How does it lower the blood pressure? What are its contraindications?

14. Explain the rational combination of certain antihypertensive drugs.

15. Which antihypertensive drugs are
    (i) more likely to produce postural hypotension
    (ii) sodium retention

16. Describe the management of
    (i) chronic hypotension
    (ii) peripheral arterial occlusive diseases and
    (iii) ischaemic cerebrovascular accidents

GUIDE TO FURTHER READING

AIRE Study Group. Effect of ramipril on mortality and morbidity of survivors of acute myocardial infarction with evidence of heart failure. Lancet, 1993; 342:821-828.

Ambrosioni, E et al: The effect of the angiotensin-converting- enzyme inhibitor zofenopril on mortality and morbidity after anterior myocardial infarction. N. Engl. J. Med., 1995; 332:80-85.

Bralet, J et al: Effects of alatriopril, a mixed inhibitor of atriopeptidase and angiotensin I-converting enzyme, on cardiac hypertrophy and hormonal responses in rats with myocardial infarction. Comparison with captopril., J. Pharmacol. Exp. Ther., 1994; 270:8-14.

Calhoun, D.A., Oparil, S.: Treatment of hypertensive crisis. N. Engl. J. Med., 1190; 323:1177.

Cambien, F et al: Deletion polymorphism in the gene for angiotensin-converting enzyme is a potent risk factor for myocardial infarction. Nature, 1992; 359:641-644.

Cody, R.J. et al: Comparing angiotensin-converting enzyme inhibitor trial results in patients with acute myocardial infarction., Arch. Intern. Med., 1994; 154:2029-2036.

Croog, S.H. et al: The effects of antihypertensive therapy on the quality of life. N. Engl. J. Med., 1986; 314:1657.

Daemen, M.J., Lombardi, D.M. et al: Angiotensin II induces smooth muscle cell proliferation in the normal and injured ral arterial wall, Circ. Res., 1991; 68:450-456.

Danser, A.H., van kats, J.P. et al: Cardiac renin and angiotensins. Uptake from plasma versus in situ synthesis. Hypertension, 1994; 24:37-48.

Davidoff, R.A.: antispasticity drugs. Mechanisms of action, Ann Neurol, 1985; 17:107.

Dzau, V.J.: Vascular renin-angiotensin system and vascular protection. J. Cardiovasc. Pharmacol., 1993; 22Suppl. 5:S1-S9.

DelliPizzi, A.M., Hilchey, S.D. et al: Natriuretic action of angiotensin (1-7). Br. J. Pharmacol., 1994, 111:1-3.

Dzau, V.J., Sasamura, H et al: Heterogeneity of angiotensin synthetic pathways and receptor subtypes: physiological and pharmacological implications. J. Hypertens., 1993; 11:S13-S18.

Fletcher, A.E., Bulpitt, C.J.: How far should blood pressure be lowered? N. Engl. J. Med., 1992; 326:251.

French, J.F., Flynn, G.A. et al: Characterization of a dual inhibitor of angiotensin I-converting enzyme and neutral endopeptidase. J. Pharmacol. Exp. Ther., 1994; 268:180-186.

Frishman, W.H., Fozailoff, A: Renin inhibition: a new approach to cardiovascular therapy. J. Clin. Pharmacol., 1994; 34:873-880.

Gifford, R.W. Jr: Management of hypertensive crisis. JAMA, 1991; 266:829.

Gruppo Italiano per lo Studio dell Sopravvivenza nell'Infarto Miocardico. GISSI-3: effects of lisinopril and transdermal glyceryl trinitrate singly and together on 6-week mortality and ventricular function after acute myocardial infarction., Lancet, 1994; 343:1115-1122.

Hanssens. M et al: Fetal and neonatal effects of treatment with angiotensin-converting-enzyme inhibitors in pregnancy. Obstet Gynecol, 1991; 78:128.

Hartford, M et al: Cardiovascular and renal effects of long term antihypertensive treatment. JAMA, 1988; 259:2553.

Hata, A et al: Angiotensinogen as a risk factor for essential hypertension in Japan. J. Clin. Invest., 1994; 93:1285-1287.

Hoelscher, D.D., Weir, M.R.: Hypertension in diabetic patients: an update of interventional studies to preserve renal function. J. Clin. Pharmacol., 1995; 35:73-80.

ISIS, Collaborative Group. ISIS-4: Randomised study of oral captopril in over 50,000 patients with suspected acute myocardial infarction. Circulation, 1993; 88:I394.

Iwai, N., Ohmichi, N et al Genotype of the angiotensin-converting enzyme gene is a risk factor for left ventricular hypertrophy, Circulation, 1994; 90:2622-2628.

Jeunemaitre, X., Soubrier, F et al: Molecular basis of human hypertension: role of angiotensinogen. Cell, 1992; 71:169-180.

Joint National Committee on Detection, Evaluation, and Treatment of High Blood Pressure: The fifth report of the Joint National Committee on Detection Evaluation, and Treatment of High Blood Pressure (JNCV). Arch Intern Med, 1993; 153:154.

Kambayshi, Y et al: Molecular structure and function of angiotensin type 2 receptor. Kidney Int., 1994; 46:1502-1504.

Kaplan, N.M.: Calcium entry blockers and future prospects. JAMA, 1989; 8:444.

Kaplan, N.M.: The appropriate goals of antihypertensive therapy ; Neither too much nor too little. Am Intern Med, 1192; 116:686.

Keilani, T et al: Selected aspects of ACE inhibitor therapy for patients with renal disease: impact on proteinuria lipids and potassium. J. Clin. Pharmacol., 1995; 35:87-97.

Lam, YWF, Shepher, M.M.: Drug interactions in hypertensive patients: Pharmacokinetic, Pharmacodynamic and genetic considerations. Clin Pharmacokinet, 1990; 18:295.

Law, M. R., Frost, C.D., Wald, N.J.: Analysis of data from trials of salt reduction. Br. Med. J, 1991; 302:819.

Lewis, E.J. et al: The effect of angiotensin-converting-enzyme inhibition on diabetic nephropathy. N. Engl. J. Med., 1993; 329:1456-1462.

Luke, R.G.: Essential hypertension; A renal disease? A review and update of the evidence. Hypertension, 1993; 21:380.

Maheswaran, R et al: High blood pressure due to alcohol: A rapidly reversible effect. Hypertension, 1991; 17:787.

Makino, N et al: Effect of angiotensin-converting enzyme inhibitor on regression in cardiac hypertrophy. Mol, Cell Beochem, 1993; 119:23.

Materson, B.J. et al: Single-drug therapy for hypertension in men: A comparison of mix antihypertensive agents with placebo. N. Engl. J. Med., 1993; 328:914.

Mattu, R.K., Needham, E.W. et al: DNA variant at the angiotensin-converting-enzyme gene locus associates with coronary artery disease in the Caerphilly Heart Study. Circulation, 1995; 91:270-274.

Pfeffer, M.A.: ACE inhibition in acute myocardial infarction. N. Engl. J. Med., 1995; 332:118-120.

Pfeffer, M.A., Braunwald, E et al: Effect of captopril on mortality and morbidity in patients with left ventricular dysfunction after myocardial infarction. N. Engl. J. Med., 1992; 327:669-677.

Saavedra, J.M.: Brain and pituitary angiotensin. Endocr. Rev., 1992; 13:329-380.

Setaro, J.F., Black, H. R.: Refractory hypertension. N. Engl. J. Med., 1992; 327:543.

SHEP Cooperative Research Group: Implications of the Systolic Hypertension in the Elderly Program. Hypertension, 1993; 21:335.

SOLVD, Investigators. Effect of enalapril on survival in patients with reduced left ventricular ejection fractions and congestive heart failure. N. Engl. J. Med., 1992; 329:1768.

SOLVD, Investigators. Effect of enalapril on mortality and the development of heart failure in asymptomatic patients with reduced left ventricular ejection fractions. N. Engl. J. Med., 1992; 329:1768.

Timmermans, P.B. et al: Angiotensin II receptors and angiotensin II receptor antagonists. Pharmacol. Rev., 1993; 45:205-251.

TRACE Study Group. The TRAndolapril Cardiac Evaluation (TRACE) study: rationale, design, and baseline characteristics of the screened population. Am. J. Cardiol., 1994; 73:44C-50C.

Villarreal, F.J., Kim, N.N. et al: Identification of functional angiotensin II receptors on rat cardiac fibroblasts. Circulation, 1993; 88:2849-2861.

Weber, M.A.: Hypertension: Step forward and Step backward - The Joint National Committee Fifth Report. Arch Intern Med., 1993; 153:149.

World Health Organization: The 1986 guidelines for the treatment of mild hypertension. Hypertension, 1986; 8:957.

Zusman, R.M.: Angiotensin-converting enzyme inhibitors: more different than alike? Focus on cardiac performance. Am. J. Cardiol., 1993; 72:25H-36H.

DRUGS USED IN THE TREATMENT OF CONGESTIVE HEART FAILURE

The normal heart weighs 250-300 gram. The heart relies on aerobic metabolism for its energy supply. At rest it extracts 60-65% of O_2 passing through it.

The blood volume in normal adult is 5 litres and of this 1.5 litres is in heart and lungs, of the 3.5 litres of blood in systemic circulation 60% is within the veins.

The prime function of the heart is to maintain circulation so that the tissues receive O_2 and nutrients and get rid of metabolic wastes.

CARDIOTONIC DRUGS

Cardiac glycosides

The term digitalis designates the entire group of cardiac glycosides. This term is given as the shape of the flower of the plant is digit like. These drugs are also known as cardiotonic glycosides. These differ from cardiac stimulants e.g. adrenaline, as their actions are prolonged, myocardial contractility is increased with only little increase in oxygen consumption, and usually accompanied by bradycardia.

Sources, composition, chemical nature and structure-activity relationship (SAR)

Plant source of cardiac glycosides	Active glycosides
Digitalis purpurea (leaves)	Digitoxin, gitoxin, gitalin
Digitalis lanata (leaves)	Digitoxin, gitoxin, digoxin
Strophanthus grates (seeds)	Ouabain (G-strophanthin)
Strophanthus kombe (seeds)	Strophanthin K
Thevetia nerifolia (fruit)	Thevetin

In the above plants, there are precursor glycosides which on enzymatic/alkaline hydrolysis yield cardiac glycosides and on acid hydrolysis aglycone or genin is produced, e.g. the leaves of digitalis purpurea has purpurea glycoside A as a precursor glycoside, it yields digitoxin and digitoxigenin on hydrolysis.

Chemically, digitalis has a steroidal structure with an unsaturated lactone ring attached to the C-17 position. The sugar moieties (1 to 4 molecules of sugar) are attached to the C-3 position. The structure without sugar is called aglycone or genin (Fig. 4.8).

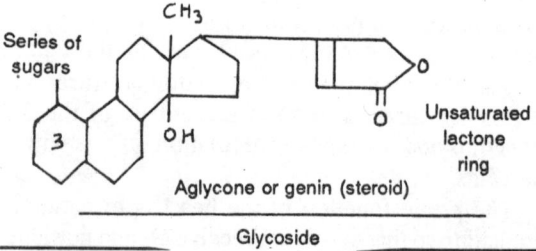

Fig. 4.8. Basic structure of digitalis glycoside.

Structure activity relationship

- The aglycone or genin structure i.e. steroid nucleus plus lactone ring is essential for pharmacological activity. The basic structure of aglycone is cyclopentanoperhydrophenanthrene nucleus and an unsaturated lactone ring at C-17 position.
- Saturation of lactone ring brings about 10-fold decrease in pharmacological actions; and if the ring is opened the activity is completely lost.
- The presence of sugars linked to C-3 position of the steroid nucleus enhances
  - water solubility
  - potency of the aglycone
  - absorption
  - cell penetration
  - half-life and
  - drug metabolism.

The removal of sugars from the glycoside produces shorter acting and weaker agents.

Mechanism of action of digitalis

Normally sodium ions are concentrated extracellularly and K^+ ions intracellularly. The passive diffusion of equalization of these ions is checked by the active transport of Na^+ and K^+ cations which actively moves Na^+ ions out of the cell and K^+ ions inside the cell. The intracellular concentration of Na^+ and K^+ are maintained by the activity of ATPase energized membrane pump system which actively moves sodium ions outside the cell and K^+ ions inside the cell.

All cardiac glycosides are potent and highly selective inhibitors of the active transport of Na^+ and K^+ across cell membranes, by binding to a specific site on the extracytoplasmic face of the alpha subunit of Na^+, K^+ ATPase, the enzymatic equivalent of the cellular Na^+ pump

The cardiac glycosides specifically bind to the membrane Na^+, K^+ ATPase enzyme associated with the sodium pump and inhibit its activity. The inhibition of Na^+, K^+ ATPase by cardiac glycosides results in reduction of energy available to the sodium pump. This impairs the active transport of Na^+ and K^+ cations. This permits large amounts of Na^+ to enter passively. When the intracellular Na^+ is increased ex-

Box 4.4. Effects of cardiac glycosides on the heart

Effects	Atrial	AV-node	Ventricles
Direct			
Contractility	↑	→	↑
ERP	↑	↑	↓
Conduction velocity	↓	↓	→
Automaticity	→	→	↑
Indirect			
ERP	↓	↑	→
Conduction velocity	↑	↓	→
Effect on ECG	P changes	PR prolonged	QT, T and ST depressed
Adverse effects	Extra-systole tachy-cardia	A-V depression or block	Fibrillation, extra-systole, tachycardia

Box 4.5. Factors affecting sensitivity to cardiac glycosides

- Hypokalaemia or hyperkalaemia
- Hypercalcaemia
- Hypomagnesemia
- Thyroid status
- Abnormal renal function
- Respiratory disease

Box 4.6. Toxic effect of cardiac glycosides

Cardiac	Proarrhythmic effects
Noncardiac	Visual: Disturbed colour vision, GI: Loss of appetite, nausea, vomiting, abdominal pain, Psychiatric: Confusion, dizziness, fatigue, abnormal dreams, delirium Respiratory: Increased ventilatory response to hypoxia

change of intracellular Ca^{++} is decreased. This is responsible for inotropic effect. Calcium and digitalis have synergistic effects. The administration of calcium in digitalized patients is dangerous.

The factors that influence cardiac output are shown in Fig. 4.9.

Pharmacological actions

The most important property of digitalis is the positive inotropic action. The increase in the force of myocardial contractility is the basis of usefulness of digitalis in the treatment of congestive heart failure (CHF). CHF is defined as the inability of the heart to meet the metabolic requirements of the peripheral systems. Digitalis increases the cardiac output, decreases the dilated cardiac size, venous pressure and blood volume. The improved haemodynamic state results in diuresis and relief of oedema.

Table 4.8 shows site and mode of action of cardiac glycosides. Table 4.9 shows pharmacokinetics and routes of administration of cardiac glycosides.

The second important action is its ability to slow the ventricular rate and that makes it a useful drug in atrial fibrillation/flutter.

Effects on heart

1. Direct stimulation effects of myocardium

Table 4.8. Summary of the effects of cardiac glycosides, site and mode of action

Effect	Site and mode of action
Vasoconstriction	
Direct	Vascular smooth muscle inhibition of Na^+, K^+-ATPase and increased Ca^{2+} entry by Na^+-Ca^{2+} exchange (transient effect with rapid administration)
Indirect	
CNS	Augmented sympathetic discharge in the area postrema, enhanced alpha-adrenergically mediated vasoconstrictor tone at higher or rapidly administered doses
Efferent neural	Release and/or reduced reuptake of Na^+ from nerve terminals at sympathetic adrenergic neuroeffector junction
Vasodilation Withdrawal of elevated sympathetic vasoconstrictor tone accompany CHF	Direct inotropic effect on cardiac muscle Enhanced baroreceptor sensitivity Reflex withdrawal of elevated sympathetic tone
Cholinergic modulation	Inhibition of NE release by ACh at the prejunctional adrenergic nerve terminal in vascular smooth muscle

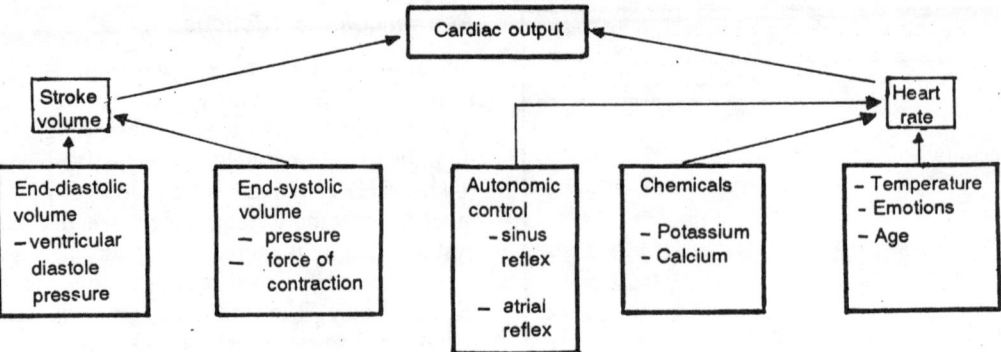

Fig. 4.9. Summary of factors that influence cardiac output.

Effects of digitalis on the myocardium

(i) In normal heart, the positive inotropic effect may be produced with slight or no effect on cardiac output. In some cases digitalis produces decrease in heart size and cardiac output which may decrease the efficiency of the heart as a pump.

(ii) In failing heart, the myocardial contractility is significantly increased. The cardiac output and stroke volume are increased. The size of the dilated heart is reduced and brought within the normal physiological range.

Effect on heart rate: In normal heart there is usually no effect.

In failing heart, the rate is decreased by two mechanisms :

(a) In low doses due to vagal effect, the A-V conduction is slowed. This bradycardia or negative chronotropic effect can be reversed by atropine.

(b) In high doses, the extravagal or direct cardiac effect produces bradycardia which is not antagonized or reversed by atropine.

2. Excitability and automaticity are increased under the influence of cardiac glycosides.

3. Conducting tissue: A-V conduction is slowed due to vagal as well as extravagal action. The conducting tissue is depressed with increase in refractory period which protects ventricles in atrial arrhythmias.

4. Effect on refractory period
   On atrium
   (a) RP shortens by vagal stimulation in small doses so flutter is converted to fibrillation.

Table 4.9. Pharmacokinetics and routes of administration of three cardiac glycosides

	Route of administration	GIT absorption	Plasma protein binding	Potency	Duration	Onset in min	Plasma $t_{1/2}$	Peak effect	Excretion
Digitoxin	Oral	95%	95%	Least	3 weeks	30-60	5-7 days	6-12 hrs	90% metabolised in liver, renal excretion is minimal
Digoxin	Oral/I.V.	75%	30%	Intermediate	6 days	15-30	36 hrs	2-6 hrs	80% renal excretion, mostly unchanged, some GI excretion
Ouabain	I.V.	Poor, unreliable	Negligible	Most potent	1-2 days	5-10	1/2-2 hours	20 hours	Renal, some GI excretion

(b) RP increases by direct action by large doses.

On A-V node and bundle of His

RP is increased by both vagal and extravagal effects.

On ventricles

RP is decreased by direct action.

5. Coronary flow: No direct effect, improvement in coronary circulation is due to increase in cardiac output and prolonged diastole.

6. ECG: Digitalis produces characteristic effects which indicate whether the patient is taking digitalis or not.
   (a) Early effects: P wave changes, ST. segment depressed and inverted.
   (b) Late effects: PR interval is prolonged (slowing of A-V conduction), QT interval shortened (shortening of systole).

Extracardiac effects

Blood vessels: The B.P. tends to be normalized as the circulation improves. The direct constricting effect of digitalis on peripheral blood vessels is not of much significance. It may constrict coronary arteries but this action is not prominent. The coronary circulation improves due to increased cardiac output.

Kidneys: The diuretic effect is chiefly due to improved renal circulation as a result of increased cardiac output. However, in large doses digitalis inhibits sodium reabsorption directly in the renal tubules.

CNS: Therapeutic doses of digitalis do not produce any effect on CNS. But in large doses it produces central sympathetic stimulation (confusion, visual disturbances, etc.) and activation of chemoreceptor trigger zone (nausea, vomiting).

The most commonly used cardiac glycosides are digoxin, digitoxin and ouabain.

All the cardiac glycosides are more concentrated in heart, liver and kidneys. They are all cumulative drugs.

Digitoxin: It is found in both digitalis purpurea and digitalis lanata. As it is highly lipid soluble it is completely absorbed from GIT. On oral administration it persists in the body for longer time. Digitoxin is safe in the presence of renal failure as very small amount of the drug is excreted in urine. It is metabolized slowly so toxicity may continue for long

time even after the drug is discontinued. It can be given orally as well as by I.M. injection or I.V. injection but there is no use giving it parenterally as it is absorbed 100% on oral administration and produces equally rapid action. It produces more cumulative action among cardiac glycosides.

Dosage: Digitoxin tablets 0.05, 0.1, 0.15 and 0.2 mg strength and elixir 0.5 mg/ml are available for oral administration. Solution for injection (rarely used) contains 0.2 mg/ml.

Digoxin: It is derived from digitalis lanata. It is the most commonly used preparation among the cardiac glycosides. It is less lipid soluble than digitoxin so its absorption from GIT is about 75%. It is excreted mostly unchanged in urine and about 10-20% in stool. It should not be given in the presence of renal failure.

Dosage: 0.125, 0.25, 0.5 mg tablets; 0.05, 0.1, 0.2 mg capsules, and elixir 0.05 mg/ml for oral administration and solution for parenteral administration containing 0.1 and 0.25 mg/ml.

Initial dose is 0.5-1 mg I.V. in serious cases, in less serious cases 0.5-1 mg I.M.; after parenteral administration, digoxin 0.25 mg three or four time a day is administered daily orally till desired effect is obtained. The maintenance dose is 0.25 to 0.5 mg orally per day.

Medigoxin is claimed to have better bioavailability.

Lanatocide C (cedilanid) is very poorly absorbed from GIT. It is injected intravenously.

Ouabain: It is obtained from strophanthus plant. Its absorption is erratic, poor and unreliable on oral administration. It is given only intravenously for quick effect.

Dose: The single full digitalizing dose is 0.12-0.25 mg by I.V. injection. It produces effect within 3-10 minutes.

Gitalin is a mixture of glycosides obtained from digitalis purpurea which does not offer any advantage over others.

Digitalization (full therapeutic effect) and maintenance

- Rapid oral digitalization (24-36 hours):
  - Digoxin 1 mg followed by 0.25 mg 6 hourly for 24 hours.

- Rapid I.V. digitalization:
  - Digoxin/Ouabain 0.25 mg I.V. hourly.
- Slow digitalization:
  - Digoxin 0.25 mg per day (5-7 days), if not then 0.5 mg per day.

If maintenance doses are given from the beginning, the digitalization is obtained after 4 half lives i.e. 6-7 days with digoxin and after 4 weeks with digitoxin.

The signs of full digitalization are clinical improvement, bradycardia (heart rate below 60/min). The loss of appetite and nausea appear first as adverse effects.

Once optimal benefit is achieved, the maintenance dose usually is adjusted to 10% of the digitalising dose.

Indications

- Congestive heart failure: The primary beneficial effect in low output (due to hypertension, valvular defects) is due to the positive inotropic action of digitalis. This increases the cardiac output (in spite of bradycardia). Digitalis improves the efficacy of the heart as a pump. Due to the improvement of haemodynamic state, renal circulation is improved and diuretic effect produced relieves oedema.

  The results are poor when digitalis is given in cases of high output failure (due to severe anaemia, thyrotoxicosis, cor pulmonale).

  The use of digitalis in heart failure is being re-evaluated. It should be given only if clearly indicated. The drug has low therapeutic index. It is no more an essential drug for all cases of heart failure, as diuretics and vasodilators have been found effective.
- Left ventricular failure: The initial drug administered is morphine, then furosemide and digitalis.
- Atrial fibrillation with or without CHF.
- Paroxysmal supraventricular tachycardia. The beneficial effect is due to its vagal effect on S-A node and on the conducting tissue.

Adverse effects of digitalis : The therapeutic index is low. The adverse effects occur more fre-

quently in elderly persons and in the presence of hypokalaemia.

Mild to moderate side effects include loss of appetite, nausea, vomiting and bradycardia.

Severe toxic effects include blurred vision, white borders are seen on dark objects (white vision), disorientation, S-A and A-V block, ventricular tachycardia and even ventricular failure. Almost any type of arrhythmias or disturbances of conduction may occur.

Allergy has been reported in very rare cases.

Treatment of digitalis toxicity

- The administration of digitalis preparation is stopped.
- Potassium chloride is given to correct hypokalaemia, 5-7 g/d in divided doses orally or by slow I.V. infusion (0.3-0.5 mol per minute in normal saline (glucose increases hypokalaemia).
- Phenytoin, lidocaine or procainamide are effective against digitalis induced ventricular arrhythmias. For supraventricular tachycardia, propranolol is effective.
- Atropine is indicated to counteract heart block as it reduces vagal tone.

Drug interactions

1. Drugs which increase serum levels of digitalis glycosides :
   - Quinidine
   - Verapamil
   - Methyldopa
   - Indomethacin
   - Diuretics (by producing hypokalaemia, precipitate digitalis toxicity).
   - Adrenergic drugs and methyldopa may induce arrhythmias in digitalized patients.
2. Drugs which reduce serum levels of digitalis glycosides :
   - Rifampin by induction of hepatic microsomal enzymes.
   - Antacids and neomycin reduce bioavailability of digitalis glycosides.
   - Metoclopramide, cholestyramine and sucralfate reduce absorption of digitalis glycosides.

Contraindications

- Hypokalaemia (enhances toxicity).
- Partial A-V block (converted to complete block).
- Constrictive pericarditis.
- Renal failure (digitoxin can be given).
- Ventricular tachycardia may progress to ventricular fibrillation.
- Acute myocarditis (digitalis may precipitate arrhythmias).

Digitalis improves myocardial contractility (positive inotropic effect) most effectively in the dilated failing heart. This property is responsible in patients of congestive heart failure (CHF) to increase cardiac output, decrease heart size, venous pressure and blood volume. The increased renal blood flow improves glomerular filtration leading to excretion of oedema fluid which further reduces ventricular preload and the danger of pulmonary oedema.

The improved haemodynamic state can reverse the signs and symptoms of CHF.

However, digitalis is not without serious faults (narrow margin of safety i.e. low therapeutic index, high incidence of adverse effects and drug interactions).

Later, dopamine and dobutamine were introduced for their positive inotropic actions in the management of acute, refractory congestive heart failure. Dopamine, initially, was focus of attention because its vasodilator action decreases the cardiac impedance (unload the left ventricle), which increases stroke output beyond that achieved by the positive inotropic action. But its pharmacokinetics (it is ineffective orally, given by I.V. infusion) and side effects restrict its use.

Angiotensin-converting enzyme inhibitors

Angiotensin-converting enzyme inhibitors e.g. enalapril, lisinipril produce beneficial haemodynamic effects resulting in increased cardiac output by reducing afterload and by decreasing total peripheral resistance, pulmonary resistance, and preload. Initially, ACE inhibitors were used in patients not responding adequately to digitalis and diuretics. Today, they are used as first-line agents for CHF therapy. Adding an ACE inhibitor to therapy with diuretics and digitalis has increased the survival rate among patients with mild to severe CHF.

Drugs that combine inotropic with vasodilator actions (Phosphodiesterase inhibitors)

These drugs have become known as inodilator drugs. They may displace digitalis.

These are bipyridine compounds. They increase myocardial contractility without inhibiting $Na^+ K^+$ AT Pase.

Amrinone (inamrinone)

The name of the drug amrinone has been changed to inamrinone in U.S.A.

It inhibits phosphodiesterase III and thus increases myocardial cAMP and transmembrane influx of Ca^{2+}. It has no action on $Na^+ K^+$ - ATPase.

Its main actions are positive inotropic and direct vasodilatation. It decreases systemic vascular resistance. Both these effects improve cardiac output in CHF. But the more important effect is in ventricular unloading consequent to arteriolar dilatation.

If administered intravenously to patients of CHF, its action starts within 5 minutes and lasts for 2-3 hours.

It is used intravenously in severe and refractory CHF as an additional drug to conventional therapy with digitalis, diuretics and vasodilators.

At present its use should be limited to patients found to be refractory to other drugs. Only short-term treatment is advised.

Adverse effects after I.V. use include nausea, vomiting, anorexia and abdominal pain. Hepatotoxicity, arrhythmia and in some cases thrombocytopenia have been reported.

Dose : 0.75 µg/kg bolus injection is followed by 2 to 20 µg/kg per min. infusion.

Milrinone lactate

It is related to amrinone having similar actions. But it is 20 to 30 times more potent than amrinone as a positive inotropic drug and some what more potent as an arteriolar and venous dilator. It does not affect renal function significantly.

It is superior to amrinone in that it is orally effective and also does not cause thrombocytopenia or fever but probably it is more arrhythmogenic.

However, the oral form is still not available. The drug may be used in the long term treatment of CHF. Its half life is 2.3 hours. It is excreted rapidly in urine.

Milrinone acts as a positive inotropic and vasodilator agent with little chronotropic activity.

Mechanism of action

The mechanism action of milrinone is similar to that of amrinone.

Milrinone does not interact with beta adrenergic receptors, nor does it inhibit sodium-potassium triphosphatase activity, as do the digitalis glycosides. Its ionotropic activity is well preserved in the presence of inotropic concentrations of dopamine or ouabain.

Pharmacodynamic properties

Both inotropic and vasodilator effects have been observed with milrinone plasma concentrations in the 100-300 ng/ml range.

In patients with depressed myocardial function loading doses of milrinone lactate produce prompt, significant improvements in cardiac output without significant increases in myocardial oxygen consumption. In addition to increasing myocardial contractility, milrinone improves diastolic function as evidenced by improvements in left ventricular diastolic relaxation.

Pharmacokinetics

Milrinone has been shown (by ultracentrifugation) to be in excess of 70% bound to human plasma proteins at plasma concentrations of 70-400 ng/ml.

The primary route of excretion is via the urine. The major urinary excretion products of orally administered milrinone in humans are unchanged milrinone (83%) and its O-glucuronide metabolite (12%). About 60% elimination occurs within the first two hours following the dosing and about 90% recovered within the first eight hours following dosing.

No information is available to indicate whether milrinone is excreted in breast milk.

Indications

Milrinone is indicated for the short term IV therapy of heart failure, including low output states following cardiac surgery.

Contraindications

Hypersensitivity to milrinone.

Warnings

- Even though milrinone has not increased myocardial oxygen consumption in patients with chronic heart failure, the use of milrinone lactate injection during the acute phase of myocardial infarction should be undertaken with caution as it may lead to an undesirable increase in myocardial oxygen consumption.
- In patients with severe obstructive aortic or pulmonary valvular disease or hypertrophic subaortic stenosis, milrinone should not be used.
- Safety and effectiveness in children have not been established.
- There have been no adequate and well controlled studies in pregnant women. It is used during pregnancy only if the potential benefit justifies.

Drug Interactions

- Milrinone should not be diluted in sodium bicarbonate IV infusion.
- Furosemide or bumetanide should not be administered in intravenous lines containing milrinone lactate (precipitate is formed).

Dosage and administration

Loading dose: I.V. 50 µg/kg given slowly over 10 minutes.

Maintenance dose : 0.25 to 0.75 µg/kg/min. intravenous.

The maximum daily dose should not exceed 1.13 mg/kg.

The duration of therapy should depend on patient responsiveness. Patients have been maintained on infusions of milrinone lactate for upto 5 days.

Overdosage

High doses may produce hypotension and cardiac arrhythmia.

No specific antidote for milrinone is known, general measures of circulatory support should be undertaken.

Adverse Effects

CVS : Supraventricular and ventricular arrhythmias, hypotension and angina/chest pain. In exceptional cases torsade de pointes (paroxysms of ventricular tachycardia) have been reported.

CNS : Headache

Skin : Rashes

Liver : Abnormality in liver function tests has been observed

Other events reported are : Hypokalaemia, tremor, bronchospasm and thrombocytopenia.

Enoximone

It is a congener of amrinone, equipotent but is better tolerated.

It is effective for short-term treatment of chronic CHF in patients refractory to conventional therapy.

Dosage : Oral 75-450mg, daily in 3 divided doses.

I.V. 0.25mg/kg every 6-8 hours.

Flosequinan

It is a fluoroquinolone derivative that produces both venous and arterial vasodilatation and increases heart rate and contractility. It is a nonselective inhibitor of phosphodiesterase. Its precise mechanism of action remains unknown, it appears to influence intracellular release of calcium by attenuating levels of inositol triphosphate or inhibiting protein kinase C. It increases cardiac output, stroke volume, heart rate and decreases preload and afterload. Its half-life is 1.7 hours.

It is absorbed rapidly after oral administration and undergoes slow conversion to an equally active sulfone metabolite. The half-life of the metabolite is 30 to 40 hours. The active and several inactive metabolites are excreted in the urine.

Dose : Oral : initial dose 50mg once a day in morning.

OTHER DRUGS

Carvedilol (nonselective beta-adrenergic blocking agent)

It is used as an adjunct in CHF along with digitalis, diuretics and ACE inhibitors for the treatment of mild to moderate CHF.

Carvedilol is rapidly and extensively absorbed. Food slows rate of absorption. It is 98% protein bound. The elimination half-life is 7-10 hours.

Its bioavailability is 25-35% due to significant first-pass metabolism.

Dosage : 3.125 mg twice a day for 2 weeks with food, gradually increased to 6.25mg twice a day, then every two weeks doubled.

The usual adult dose is 25mg twice a day.

Trandolapril (nonsulfhydryl ACE inhibitor)

It is absorbed 10% from GIT, food slows the rate of absorption but not the extent of absorption. Its onset of action is 2 hours, lasts for 24 hours. Its biotransformation occurs in liver. It is hydrolyzed to trandolaprilat which is an active metabolite.

The half-life of trandolapril is 6 hours, and that of the active metabolite 10 hours.

The drug is excreted about 33% in urine (15% of which as metabolite), 66% is excreted in faeces (38% as metabolite).

Nesiritide

It is a recently introduced drug, manufactured from E. coil using recombinant DNA technology.

It is indicated for acutely decompensated CHF patients who have dyspnoea at rest or with minimal activity.

Its elimination half-life is 18 minutes

Dosage : 2 mcg/kg as bolus given for 60 seconds initially , then continuous I.V. infusion at a dose of 0.01 mcg/kg/minute.

Side effects : More frequent side effect is hypotension, less frequent side effects include angina, apnoea (bluish lips or skin, difficulty in breathing, dizziness, lightheadedness.

STUDY QUESTIONS

1. How do cardiotonic glycosides differ in their actions compared to cardiac stimulants such as adrenaline (epinephrine)?
2. Describe the sources of cardiac glycosides.
3. Explain the stature-activity relationship (SAR) of cardiac glycosides.
4. In what respects digitoxin, digoxin and ouabain differ?

5. What are the cardiac effects of digitalis on (i) normal heart (ii) failing heart.

6. How and what effect digitalis produces on heart rate?

7. Describe the extra cardiac actions of digitalis.

8. Explain the beneficial effects of digitalis in congestive heart failure (with low cardiac output).

9. Explain the procedure for (i) rapid digitalization (ii) slow digitalization.

10. Describe the indications, contraindications, precaution, drug interactions and adverse effects of digitalis. How is digitalis toxicity treated?

11. How does digitalis act (mode of action)?

12. Discuss the role of thiazide diuretics with K-sparing diuretics, certain other inotropic drugs such as dopamine and its congener dobutamine in the treatment of heart failure.

13. Describe the role of calcium channel blockers like nifedipine in heart failure.

14. Write short notes on (i) prazosin, (ii) amrinone.

GUIDE TO FURTHER READING

Acute Infarction Ramipril Efficacy (AIRE) Study Investigators.: Effect of ramipril on mortality and morbidity of survivors of acute myocardial infarction with clinical evidence of heart failure. Lancet, 1993; 342:821-828.

Armstrong, P.W. et al: Medical advances in the treatment of congestive heart failure. Circulation., 1994; 88:2941-2952.

Bigger, J.T. et al: Diuretic therapy, hypertension, and cardiac arrest. N. Engl. J. Med., 1994; 330:1899-1900.

Blaustein, M.P. et al: Physiological effects of endogenous ouabain: control of intracellular Ca^{2+} stores and cell responsiveness. Am. J. Physiol., 1993; 264:C1367-C1387.

Bristow, M.R. et al: Dose-response of chronic B-blocker treatment in heart failure from either idiopathic dilated or ischemic cardiomyopathy. Circulation, 1994; 89:1632-1642.

Califf, R.M., Bengtson, J.R.: Cardiogenic shock. N. Engl. J. Med., 1994; 330:1724.

Carvero, P.G. et al: Flosequinan, a new vasodilator: Systemic and coronary hemodynamics and neuroendocrine effects in congestive heart failure. J. Am. Coll Cardiol, 1992; 20:1542.

Chatterjee, K: Digitalis, catecholamines, and other positive inotropic agents. In: Cardiology. Parmley, W.W., Chatterjee K. (editors). Lippincott, 1988.

Cohn, J.N. et al: A comparison of enalapril with hydralazine- isosorbide dinitrate in the treatment of chronic congestive heart failure. N Engl J Med, 1991; 325:303.

Cody, R.J. et al: Clinical trials of diuretic therapy in heart failure: research directions and clinical considerations. J. Am. Coll. Cardiol., 1993; 22:165A-171A.

Cohn, J.N. et al: Vasodilator therapy of cardiac failure. N. Engl. J. Med., 1977; 297:27-31, 254-258.

Cohn, J.N. et al: Treatment of infarct related heart failure: vasodilators other than ACE inhibitors. Cardiovasc. Drugs Ther., 1994; 8:119-122.

Conti, C.R. et al: Use of calcium antagonists to treat heart failure. Clin. Cardiol., 1994; 17:101-102.

Davies, D.L. et al: Do diuretics cause magnesium deficiency? Br. J. Clin. Pharmacol., 1993; 36:1-10.

Doughty, R.N. et al: Beta-blockers in heart failure: promising or proved? J. Am. Coll. Cardiol., 1994; 23:814-821.

Eisner, D.A. et al: The Na-K pump and its effectors in cardiac muscle. In, The Heart and Cardiovascular System, 2d ed. (Fozzard, H.A., Haber, E., Jennings, R.B., Katz, A.M., and Morgan, H.E., eds.) Raven Press, New York, 1991; pp. 863-902.

Elkayam, U et al: Calcium channel blockers in heart failure. J. Amer. Coll. Cardiol., 1993; 22:139A-144A.

Ferguson, D.W.: Digitalis and neurohormonal abnormalities in heart failure and implications for therapy. Am J Cardiol, 1992; 69:24G.

Fisher, M.L. et al: Beneficial effects of metoprolol in heart failure associated with coronary artery disease: a randomized trial. J. Am. Coll. Cardiol., 1994; 23:943-950.

Fowler, M.B. et al: In, Congestive Heart Failure. Springer-Verlag, New York, 1994; pp. 400-453.

Gamba, G et al: Primary structure and functional expression of a cDNA encoding the thiazide-sensitive, electroneutral sodium- chloride cotransporter. Proc. Natl. Acad. Sci. U.S.A., 1993; 90:2749-2753.

Goto, A., Yamada, K., Sugimoto, T.: Endogenous digitalis: Reality or myth? Life Sci, 1991; 48:2109.

Gruppo, Italiano per lo Studio della Sopravvivenza nell'Infarto Miocardico. GISSI-3 Investigators. Effects of lisinopril and transdermal glyceryl trinitrate singly and together on 6-week mortality and ventricular function after acute myocardial infarction. Lancet, 1994; 343:1115-1122.

Hall, D., Zeitler, H., Rudolph, W.: Counteraction of the

vasodilator effects of enalapril by aspirin in severe heart failure. J Am Coll Cardiol, 1992; 20:1549.

Harrison, D.G. et al: The nitrovasodilators. New ideas about old drugs. Circulation, 1993; 87:1461-1467.

Humes, H.D. et al: The kidney in congestive heart failure. In, Contemporary Issues in Nephrology, Vol.1. Churchill Livingstone, New York, 1978.

Kelly, R.A. et al: Recognition and management of digitalis toxicity. Am. J. Cardiol., 1992a; 69:108G-119G.

Kelly, R.A. et al: Use and misuse of digitalis blood levels. Heart Dis. Stroke, 1992b; 1:117-122.

Kelly, R.A. et al: Digoxin in heart failure:implications of recent trials. J. Am. Coll. Cardiol., 1993; 22:107A-112A.

Kelly, R.A. et al: Endogenous cardiac glycosides. Adv. Pharmacol., 1994; 25:263-288.

Kelly, R.A., and Smith, T.W. et al: Antibody therapies for drug overdose. In, Therapeutic Immunology. Blackwell Scientific, Cambridge, MA, 1996(In Press).

Lahav, M. et al: International administration of furosemide vs. continuous infusion preceded by a loading dose for congestive heart failure. Chest, 1992; 102:725-731.

Leier, C.V. et al: Clinical relevance and management of the major electrolyte abnormalities in congestive heart failure: Hyponatremia, hypokalemia, and hypomagnesemia. Am. Heart J., 1994, 128:564-574.

Lenfant, C et al: Report of the Task Force on Research in Heart Failure. Circulation, 1994; 90:1118-1123.

Lewis, R.P. et al: Digitalis. In Cardiotonic Drugs: A Clinical Survey. (Leier, C.V., ed.) Marcel Dekker, Inc., New York, 1987; pp 85-150.

Lingrel, J.B. et al: Structure-function studies of the Na, K- ATPase. Kidney Int., 1994; 44:S32-S39.

Mahdyoon, H et al: The evolving pattern of digoxin intoxication: observations at a large urban hospital from 1980 to 1988. Am. Heart J., 1990; 120:1189-1194.

McGarry, S.J. et al: Digoxin activates sarcoplasmic reticulum Ca^{2+} release channels: a possible role in cardiac inotropy. Br. J. Pharmacol., 1993; 108:1043-1050.

Mehra, A et al: Potentiation of isosorbide dinitrate effects with N-acetylcysteine in patients with chronic heart failure. Circulation., 1994; 89:2595-2600.

Packer, M et al: The development of positive inotropic agents for chronic heart failure: how have we gone astray? J. Am. Coll. Cardiol., 1993; 22:119A-126A.

Packer, M et al: Withdrawal of digoxin from patients with chronic heart failure treated with angiotensin-converting enzyme inhibitors. RADIANCE Study. N. Engl. J. Med., 1993; 329:1-7.

Smith, T.W.: Digitals: Mechanisms of action and clinical use. N. Engl. J. Med., 1988; 318:358.

Smith, T.W. Digoxin in heart failure. N. Engl. J. Med., 1993; 329:51-53.

St. John Sutton, M. et al: Quantitative two-dimensional echocardiographic measurements are major predictors of adverse cardiovascular events after acute myocardial infarction. The protective effects of captopril. Circulation, 1994; 89:68-75.

SOLVD Investigators.: Effect of enalapril on survival in patients with reduced left ventricular ejection fractions and congestive heart failure. N. Engl. J. Med., 1991; 325:293-302.

The SOLVD Investigators: Effect of enalapril on mortality and the development of heart failure in asymptomatic patients with reduced left ventricular ejection fraction. N Engl J Med, 1992; 327:685.

Sweadner, K.J.: Multiple digitalis receptors. A molecular perspective. Trends Cardiovasc Med, 1993; 3:2.

Swedberg, K: Initial experience with beta blockers in dilated cardiomyopathy. Am. J. Cardiol., 1993; 71:30C-38C.

Uretsky, B.F. et al: Randomized study assessing the effect of digoxin withdrawal in patients with mild to moderate chronic congestive heart failure: results of the PROVED trial. J. Am. Coll. Cardiol., 1993; 22:955-962.

Waagstein, F et al: Beneficial effects of metoprolol in idiopathic dilated cardiomyopathy. Lancet, 1993; 342:1441-1446.

ANTIARRHYTHMICS

Cardiac arrhythmias are defined as abnormalities in the site of origin of the impulse, its rate or regularity or a disturbance in conduction of the impulse.

Antiarrhythmics are the drugs which are employed to prevent or treat cardiac arrhythmias.

For the proper understanding of the basic mechanisms of arrhythmias as well as the actions of antiarrhythmics, it is necessary to consider the following cardiac electrophysiology:

1. Action potential phases
2. S-A and A-V nodes and Purkinje fibres have the capacity to discharge impulses automatically. The S-A node has the highest degree of automaticity and it is the normal pacemaker of the heart. If it is depressed or it

fails to function, the other specialized conducting tissues (A-V node, His-Purkinje system) contain latent pacemaker cells which can initiate impulse generation resulting in ectopic impulse formation. Most antiarrhythmic agents have more effect on latent pacemakers than on the S-A node pacemaker.

Arrhythmias may result from
• Faulty impulse initiation
• Faulty impulse conduction
• Combination of the above

In areas of injured myocardium, conduction may be slow, or refractoriness shortened, or both, resulting in the reentry of aberrant impulses and, hence, a cardiac arrhythmia. Thus it may be due to
• partial or complete conduction block or
• re-entry in case of imbalance of conductivity and refractoriness in branching conducting tissue.

As alterations in impulse generation, impulse conduction or both produce arrhythmias, therefore the basic actions of antiarrhythmic drugs are either to decrease the automatic discharge or to affect conduction in re-entry circuits.

ACTION POTENTIAL

There are 4 phases of the action potential (AP) (Fig. 4.10):
• Phase 0: Rapid depolarization. Sodium enters cell. The inward movement of Na$^+$ ion through fast channels is responsible for inward sodium current producing 0 phase of the action potential (AP). The cell membrane's electrical charge changes from negative to positive.
• Phase 1: Rapid repolarization. Potassium briefly leaves cell. Short initial rapid repolarization to the plateau level of AP is brought about by inactivation of sodium current and transient K$^+$ current. As fast Na$^+$ channels close and K$^+$ ions leave the cell, the cell rapidly repolarizes and returns to resting potential.
• Phase 2: Sustained depolarization (plateau). Calcium enters cell. Plateau or period of more gradual repolarization is associated with influx of Ca^{++} ions. Calcium ions enter cells through

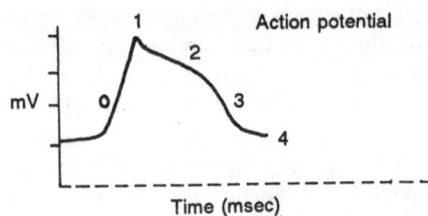

Fig. 4.10. Cardiac action potential.

slow channels while K$^+$ ions exit (represented by notch in the beginning of the phase).
• Phase 3: Rapid repolarization. Potassium leaves cell. Second final rapid period of repolarization to resting (diastolic) levels of transmembrane voltage is associated with flow of K$^+$ ions out of the cell.
• Phase 4: Slow depolarization (diastole). Gradual increase in sodium permeability. Slow depolarization phase is fully repolarized state when K$^+$ moves into and Na$^+$ moves out of the cell i.e. the cell returns to resting state. When the spontaneous phase 4 depolarization opens M gate in the channel the inward Na$^+$ current is very intense though very brief, it is terminated due to rapid closure of H gate in the sodium channel.

Beginning during phase 1 and ending at the start of phase 3, the cell is in absolute refractory state. During phase 3 cell responds to strong stimulus i.e. there is relative refractory period.

Classification of antiarrhythmic drugs on the basis of their electrophysiological effects
(Table 4.10)

Some of these drugs have more than one action, e.g. class I group A drugs also have class III effects; propranolol has predominantly class II effects but it also has class I effect.

Etiology

Arrhythmias may be due to heart disease, myocardial infarction, large doses of digitalis, increased sympathetic tone, decreased parasympathetic tone, vagal stimulation (e.g. straining at stool), increased O$_2$ demand (from stress, fever, exercise), metabolic disorders, hypertension, hyperkalaemia, thyroid disorders, chronic bronchitis.

Table 4.10. Classification of antiarrhythmic drugs on the basis of their electrophysiological effects

Class I: Sodium channel blockers	These decrease inflow of sodium during phase 0 of AP. The subgroups A, B, C differ in degree and onset of myocardial depression. I Group A: Quinidine, procainamide, disopyramide. Decrease in slope of phase 4. I Group B: Lidocaine, phenytoin, mexiletine, tocainamide. Minimal phase 0 depression. I Group C: Encainide, lorcainide, flecainide. Marked phase 0 depression.
Class II: Beta-adrenoceptor antagonists	Propranolol, sotalol, metoprolol. Depress phase 4 of Action potential (AP).
Class III: Potassium channel blockers	Bretylium, amiodarone. Prolong AP duration i.e. increase effective refractory period.
Class IV: Calcium channel blockers	Verapamil, nifedipine, diltiazem. Inhibit entry of calcium into the cardiac cell. Excitation is reduced in S-A and A-V nodes which depend on calcium current for depolarization.
Class V: Drug employed in arrhythmias but is not antiarrhythmic	Digitalis

PRINCIPLES IN THE CLINICAL USE OF ANTIARRHYTHMIC DRUGS

1. Precipitating factors should be identified and eliminated.
2. The goals of treatment should be established the therapy should be initiated only when a clear benefit to the patient can be identified.
3. The risks should be minimized by observing the following:
   - Antiarrhythmic drugs can cause arrhythmias.
   - The dose should be adjusted to maintain the plasma concentration within therapeutic range.
   - Patient-specific contraindications e.g. patient with history of CHF are prone to develop heart failure during disopyramide therapy.
   - History of MI: Flecainide should not be given.
   - Asthma: Beta adrenergic blockers will worsen the condition.
   - Constipation: Verapamil should be avoided.
   - Diarrhoea: Quinidine should not be given.
   - Lung disease: Amiodarone is to be avoided.

The drug-provoked arrhythmias must be recognized, since further treatment with antiarrhythmic agent will exacerbate the problem.

CLASS I: SODIUM CHANNEL BLOCKERS

Class I Group A

Quinidine

Wenckebach in 1914 reported the arrhythmia combating property of quinidine for the first time and since then it has been used as an antiarrhythmic drug. Although this cinchona alkaloid also possesses some antimalarial, antipyretic and oxytocic actions but these are of no clinical utility.

Actions on heart: Quinidine decreases automaticity, excitability, conduction velocity and contractility.

Quinidine depresses automaticity in the cardiac pace maker cells and also in ectopic foci, by increasing threshold to electrical stimuli. It reduces slope of phase 4 depolarization due to reduction of diastolic Na^+ influx. It also reduces the movement of Na^+ across cell membrane during phase 0 of action potential resulting in reduction of conduction velocity and prolongation of refractory period. The decrease in diastolic depolarization suppresses ectopic focal activity. The lengthened refractory period tends to stop re-entry.

Pharmacokinetics : Quinidine is well absorbed from GIT, peak plasma level in reached in 1 to 3 hours, half-life is about 3 hours and the duration of action is 6 to 8 hours. The therapeutic plasma levels are 3 to 6mcg/ml. Quinidine is bound (60 to 80%) to plasma albumin. About 30% is excreted uncharged in urine and the rest is metabolized (hydroxylated) in liver.

Preparations and dosage : Quinidine gluconate tablets 200, 300 mg for oral administration. Quinidine gluconate 300 mg tablets for oral as well as I.M. injection are available. Quinidine should not be given by I.V. route as it lowers B.P. and cardiac output and increases left ventricular diastolic pressure.

Indications : Quinidine depresses automaticity so it can be useful both in supraventricular as well as ventricular tachyrhythmias. But due to several frequently occurring adverse effects, it has now limited clinical applications:

- Prevention of paroxysmal ventricular tachycardia and ventricular extrasystoles.
- Prevention of atrial tachycardia, extrasystoles, atrial fibrillation and atrial flutter.
- To maintain sinus rhythm after DC shock.

DC shock has largely replaced the use of quinidine for correcting tachyrhythmias to normal sinus rhythm and its chief use is to maintain sinus rhythm after cardioversion.

Actions

Cardiac action is due to its (i) vagolytic activity and (ii) direct depressant activity.

- Automaticity : Quinidine depresses sodium entry thus depresses ectopic activity in all tissues except SA node, hence depress arrhythmias due to enhanced impulse formation.
- Excitability : Depressed
- Conduction velocity: Depressed
- Refractory period : By depressing K^+ efflux (direct action), it prolongs RP of all tissues but by its vagolytic action it increases RP of atria and shortens that of AV node. The overall effect is to increase RP of atria, decrease RP of AV node, increase RP of ventricle.
- AV conduction : Enhanced. In atrial flutter it may increase ventricular rate.
- Contractility : Negative inotropic action due to decreased calcium influx. Hyperkalaemia enhances this effect, hypokalaemia antagonizes this.
- ECG : Increase in QT interval, inversion of T wave and depression of ST segment.
- B.P. : Fall in B.P. due to alpha blocking action and direct relaxation on arterioles.
- Other actions : Like quinine - skeletal muscle depressant, antimalarial, antipyretic and oxytocic activity. These are of no clinical utility.

Adverse effects : GIT upsets such as nausea, vomiting and diarrhoea are common. Tinnitus, headache and blurred vision are manifestations of cinchonism.

Allergic manifestations are also not uncommon due to hypersensitivity and idiosyncratic reactions in many cases, hence it is recommended to give test dose initially.

Quinidine should be considered as a dangerous drug as in large doses it can cause serious cardiotoxicity, affecting cardiac dynamics.

It is a myocardial depressant drug, contractility of the heart is depressed and peripheral vasodilation produces hypotension.

Quinidine produces S-A or A-V conduction block, ventricular ectopic beats, even ventricular tachycardia or fibrillation.

Procainamide hydrochloride (Pronestyl)

It is produced by replacing the ester linkage by amide linkage in procaine molecule. This little change makes the compound more stable in the body with fewer side effects as compared to procaine.

Actions on heart : These are similar to those of quinidine. It decreases excitability, conduction velocity and prolongs refractory period more in the atria compared to the ventricle.

Pharmacokinetics : On oral administration, it is completely absorbed from GIT, peak plasma level reaches within 1-2 hours. The plasma half-life is 2-4 hours. The effective plasma levels are 0.4-0.8 mg/100 ml. It is bound only to about 15% to blood proteins. About half of the dose is excreted unaltered in the urine and the rest is metabolized by the liver. Its chief metabolite is N-acetyl procainamide which possesses antiarrhythmic property. The rate of acetylation of procainamide is genetically determined. There are slow and fast acetylators.

Dosage : 250/500 mg tablets are available for oral administration, every 3 to 4 hourly (as half life is short). Solution for injection containing 100 or 500 mg/ml is available for parenteral administration. 100 to 250 mg, 4 to 6 hourly by I.M. injection and in severe life threatening cases it can be injected by I.V. route at the rate of 25 to 50 mg/minute, total maximum dose is 1 g under ECG monitoring.

Therapeutic uses : These are similar to that of quinidine. Procainamide may be effective in cases who do not respond to quinidine. Favourable results are obtained in ventricular arrhythmias, except in digitalis induced cases.

Adverse effects : GIT upsets, depression, psychosis, hypotension, agranulocytosis. Allergic reactions such as urticaria, angioneurotic oedema, joint and muscle pains have been reported.

If procainamide is given orally for prolonged periods in doses exceeding 2g/day, there may appear a syndrome resembling systemic lupus erythematosus (LES) in about 30% cases. For this reason, procainamide is not preferred for prolonged oral use.

Contraindications : Complete A-V block.

Disopyramide phosphate

The electrophysiological actions are similar to those of quinidine.

It depresses automaticity, conduction velocity and increases refractory period.

It also has anticholinergic as well as direct effect on A-V conduction like quinidine.

Pharmacokinetics : It is well absorbed from GIT, peak plasma level reaches within 2 hours, half life is 4-5 hours. About 80% is excreted unaltered in the urine and the rest is metabolized (N-dealkylation) by the liver.

Therapeutic uses : Prevention of ventricular premature beats, ventricular extrasystoles and ventricular tachycardia. The drug is also useful in atrial tachycardia.

Dosage : 100, 150 mg capsules. Initially 300 mg orally 100-150 mg 6 hourly. It can also be given in dose of 2 mg/kg, up to 150 mg, by slow (5-10 min) I.V. injection.

Adverse effects : Dry mouth, urinary retention, tachycardia, blurred vision and constipation can be produced due to its anticholinergic activity.

Other side effects include GIT upsets, psychosis, hypoglycaemia, hepatic damage and skin rashes.

It can precipitate acute angle closure glaucoma, though rarely.

Caution : In glaucoma, prostate hypertrophy, renal failure.

Contraindications : Cardiogenic shock.

Class I Group B

Lidocaine hydrochloride (Xylocaine, lignocaine)

It is a local anaesthetic. Its mechanism of action as an antiarrhythmic drug differs from quinidine and procainamide.

It shortens the duration of action potential and reduces the effective refractory period. It has slight effect on contractility.

It does not have any vagolytic effect.

It depresses automaticity and diastolic depolarization.

Pharmacokinetics : It is not given by mouth as it is hydrolyzed in the gut and on first pass through liver, it is inactivated very rapidly.

The plasma half life after one injection is 15 minutes. It is bound to plasma proteins to a minor extent. The drug is rapidly metabolized in the liver. Hence it is necessary to give loading dose initially followed by I.V. infusion. The therapeutic plasma levels are 2 to 5 mcg/ml.

Lidocaine solution containing 20, 40, 200 mg/ml are available for I.V. injection (bolus injection in 2-5 minutes).

Dosage: 50 to 100 mg I.V. loading dose followed by constant I.V. infusion 500-750 mg/12 hours, at the rate of 2 mg/minute are generally employed.

Therapeutic uses : It is widely employed for prevention and treatment of ventricular ectopic activity following myocardial infarction. It is also effective in digitalis induced arrhythmias. It seems to be the drug of choice in acute ventricular arrhythmias. However, lidocaine does not have any significant role in the treatment of supraventricular tachyarrhythmias.

Adverse effects : Lidocaine is relatively quite a safe drug. Some patients complain of GIT symptoms, bradycardia, hypotension, difficulty in swallowing and talking. There may be neurological disturbances such as drowsiness, disorientation and convulsions. Very large does can depress A-V conduction and cause negative inotropic effect.

Contraindications : Hypersensitivity to amide type of local anaesthetics, bradycardia, A-V block and other conduction disorders, if there is pre-existing bundle branch block, administration of lidocaine will result in heart block and even cardiac stand still.

Phenytoin sodium (Dilantin)

It is an antiepileptic drug which has antiarrhythmic activity.

Actions : It resembles lidocaine in its cardiac actions. It acts on myocardial cell membrane and (i) enhances Na^+ influx during depolarization and potassium efflux during repolarization, (ii) depresses pace maker activity in Purkinje tissue.

Phenytoin neither depresses the excitability nor prolongs the refractory period of atrial or ventricular muscle. It may shorten the effective refractory period and the duration of action potential like lignocaine. It may often increase the A-V conduction and occasionally increase intraventricular conduction. It prevents local spread of ectopic focus with only little effect on conductive tissue.

Pharmacokinetics : The drug is slowly absorbed following oral administration, peak plasma levels reach after several hours.

Absorption from the I.M. injection site is erratic so not given by this route. For the treatment of arrhythmias it is usually given intravenously. The therapeutic serum levels are 10-18 mg/l.

Dosage : 100 mg capsules, and solution for injections 50 mg/ml are available. The infusion rate is 25-50 mg/ml, maximum dose being 0.5 to 1 g. In severe cases I.V. infusion 50-100 mg every 5 minutes, maximum 10-15 mg/kg of body weight can be given.

Indications :
- The real indication of this antiarrhythmic drug is in digitalis-induced tachyarrhythmias both atrial and ventricular, without adversely affecting intraventricular conduction.

  It depresses the ventricular automaticity produced by digitalis. It also reverses the prolongation of A-V conduction induced by digitalis.
- It may also be used as an alternative to lidocaine in ventricular arrhythmias.

The drug is not effective in atrial flutter, atrial fibrillation or in chronic ventricular arrhythmias.

Adverse effects : These are not common. With large I.V. doses, A-V block, bradycardia, impairment of cardiac contractility and even cardiac arrest may occur.

Mexiletine and Tocainide

These are analogues of lidocaine with structures that have been modified to reduce first pass-hepatic metabolism to make the oral therapy effective. Their electrophysiological actions are similar to those of lidocaine.

Both have been use for the treatment of ventricular arrhythmias.

Mexiletine is well absorbed from GIT, peak plasma level reaches in 2 to 4 hours and plasma half-life is about 10 hours.

The daily dosage is 600-750 mg orally; I.V. dose is 1 to 3 mg/kg followed by infusion of 20-45 mcg/kg/minute, followed by 0.6- 1.2 g orally in divided doses daily, given 8 hourly.

The drug is indicated in ventricular arrhythmias following myocardial infarction and in digitalis induced arrhythmias. It is as effective as procainamide with fewer side effects.

Adverse effects are similar to lidocaine. Nausea, vomiting, hypotension, ataxia, and sinus bradycardia may occur.

Tocainide : It is a lidocaine analogue, well absorbed from GIT, peak effect reaches in about 1 hour, and plasma half-life is about 15 hours. The therapeutic blood concentration is 18-45 mmol/l. Only about 15% is bound to plasma proteins. About 40% is excreted unchanged in the urine and the rest is metabolized in the liver.

Indications are similar to those of lidocaine, with two advantages i.e. it is effective orally and it has long half-life.

In severe conditions it can be injected I.V. 500-750 mg in 15 to 30 minutes, followed by 600-800 mg orally. The usual maintenance dose is 1.2 g orally in divided doses per day.

Adverse effects include nausea, hypotension and bradycardia and in few cases hepatotoxicity has been reported.

Class I Group C

Encainide, lorcainide and flecainide

These three are local anaesthetic antiarrhythmic drugs having rather selective effects on fast sodium channels.

These are quickly absorbed from GIT after oral administration. Flecainide is not subject to first pass hepatic extraction unlike the other two drugs of this group.

The investigations carried out so far, indicate that these drugs may be useful in the long term therapy of premature ventricular beats, particularly in those patients who do not respond satisfactorily to other antiarrhythmic agents.

Propafenone

It is a Na^+ channel blocker, like flecainide it also blocks K^+ channels. It is used for supraventricular tachycardias, including atrial fibrillation. It can also be used in ventricular arrhythmias but like other Na^+ channel blocker, it is only moderately effective.

It is well absorbed and eliminated by both hepatic and renal routes. It undergoes extensive first pass-effect (metabolized to 5-Hydroxypropaphenone).

Adverse effects include acceleration of ventricular response in patients with atrial flutter.

Moricizine

It is a phenothiazine analogue used in the chronic treatment of ventricular arrhythmias.

Its electrophysiological effect is to depress Na^+ current. Some reports indicate a recovery similar to that of flecainide; other reports indicate that like lidocaine, moricizine shortens AP and QT interval.

CLASS II: B-ADRENOCEPTOR BLOCKING DRUGS

Propranolol hydrochloride (Inderal)

It possesses membrane stabilizing property on the myocardium. It inhibits adrenergic stimulation of heart, reduces heart rate, prolongs A-V conduction and reduces contractility.

The direct effects are similar to those of quinidine and procainamide but unlike quinidine it does not have anticholinergic effect.

Propranolol decreases diastolic influx of Na^+ during 0 phase of the action potential and increases efflux of K^+ during repolarization. These two effects result in:
- reducing automaticity,
- reducing conduction velocity
- increasing refractory period.

Propranolol also has class I effects but usually in doses higher than the therapeutic range.

The drug is well absorbed from GIT, and mainly metabolized in the liver. The metabolites are excreted in the urine. One of the metabolites 4-hydroxypropranolol retains the beta blocking activity.

Dosage : 10 to 40 mg orally 2-3 times a day; 0.1 to 0.15 mg/kg of body weight in divided doses by I.V. injection.

Adverse effects : Withdrawal syndrome after abrupt withdrawal has been reported. These symptoms are indicative of adrenergic overactivity.

Therapeutic uses

- β-blockers are more beneficial than quinidine in the treatment of digitalis induced arrhythmias and in arrhythmias due to excess of catecholamines.
- These can abolish exercise/emotion induced tachycardia due to anxiety and hyperthyroidism.
- Effective in suppressing atrial tachycardia associated with Wolff-Parkinson-White syndrome.
- Particularly useful in converting paroxysmal atrial tachycardia to normal sinus rhythm.
- Employed to control ventricular rate in atrial flutter and atrial fibrillation, although these disorders are rarely abolished by β-blockers.

Sotalol

It is a non-selective beta-adrenergic receptor antagonist that prolongs action potential and is used for ventricular tachyarrhythmias. It is at least as effective as most Na^+ channel blockers. It is also effective in atrial arrhythmias including atrial fibrillation.

Sotalol prolongs AP and QT interval, decreases automaticity, slows AV nodal conduction and prolonged AV refractoriness both by K^+ channel block and block of beta-adrenergic receptors.

Sotalol is eliminated by renal excretion of unchanged form.

Sotalol can cause torsades de points especially when serum K^+ is low. This is the major toxicity with sotalol. The other adverse effects are those associated with beta-adrenergic receptor blockade.

CLASS III: POTASSIUM CHANNEL BLOCKERS

Bretylium tosylate

Initially introduced as an antihypertensive agent but

now it is not at all used for this purpose due to severe side effects and development of tolerance.

It prolongs the durations of action potential with prolongation of the effective refractory period. Automaticity and conduction velocity are not suppressed.

It is poorly absorbed from GIT. After I.V. injection it is excreted unaltered in the urine. Its plasma half-life is 7 hours and therapeutic plasma levels range between 0.5 to 1 mcg/ml.

Dosage : Solution containing 50 mg/ml is available for I.M./I.V. injection. The usual dose is 5 to 10 mg/kg I.V. or I.M.

Therapeutic uses : Its use is limited to severe refractory ventricular arrhythmias. Although it is very effective in ectopic ventricular rhythms but this drug is not very desirable.

Adverse effects : Hypotension due to adrenergic neuron blockade, bradycardia, diarrhoea and parotid pain.

Amiodarone

It was initially introduced as an antianginal drug.

It prolongs the duration of action potential and the effective refractory period. In higher doses it also shows β-blocking and quinidine like activity.

The drug is absorbed from GIT, strongly bound to plasma proteins and slowly excreted.

The usual dose in 300 to 600 mg orally daily. The initial dose is 200 mg thrice a day for one week followed by maintenance dose of 200 mg per day.

Indications : Resistant recurrent supraventricular and ventricular arrhythmias refractory to the usual therapy.

Adverse effects : GIT symptoms, photosensitivity and vertigo, peripheral neuropathy have been reported after long term use.

Interactions : Amiodarone can potentate anticoagulant therapy. It may increase plasma digoxin level.

Contraindications : Sinus bradycardia, A-V block, thyroid disease (as the drug contains iodine so it may impair thyroid function). It should not be given with verapamil or beta blockers.

CLASS IV: CALCIUM CHANNEL BLOCKERS OR CALCIUM ANTAGONISTS

The slow channel or calcium channel inhibitors or calcium entry blockers, represent a major development in cardiovascular pharmacology. Verapamil, nifedipine and diltiazem belong to this group. Verapamil is a benzene acetonitrile; nifedipine is a dihydropyridine and diltiazem is a benzothiazepine.

All the three drugs are powerful dilators of coronary and peripheral arteries and so useful as antianginal agents. Verapamil and diltiazem (not nifedipine) are useful as antiarrhythmics. The vasodilator effect makes them useful as antihypertensive. Nifedipine is more powerful in this respect than the other two drugs (Table 4.11).

Table 4.11. Comparison among the three calcium channel blockers

	Verapamil	Diltiazem	Nifedipine
S-A node automaticity	↓	↓	—
Ventricular automaticity	↓	—	—
Effective refractory period			
A-V nodal	↑↑	↑	↑↓
Ventricular	—	—	—
Vasodilation	±	+	+++
Dose	40-120 mg thrice a day	30-60 mg thrice a day	5-40 mg twice or thrice a day
Uses	Angina, arrhythmias	Angina, hypertension, arrhythmias	Angina, hypertension, CHF

It is more appropriate to designate them as slow channel blockers than calcium channel blockers as they permit entry of some Na^+ in addition to Ca^{++} and are activated much slower than the fast channels through which Na^+ enters and causes rapid phase of the action potential.

These drugs do not directly antagonize the effects of calcium, they act at the slow channels of cell membrane and inhibit the influx of Ca^{++} into cells.

They also seem to inhibit mobilization of calcium from intracellular stores.

Drugs such as nitroprusside, hydralazine, papaverine and diazoxide interfere with the availability of Ca^{++} ions but act at sites other than the calcium channels.

The slow channel blockers act as cardioprotectives as these:
- Prevent ischaemic myocardium from calcium injury
- Dilate coronary arteries and collateral vessels
- Decrease cardiac work
- Lower afterload (have little effect on venous beds so don't affect cardiac preload)
- Decrease myocardial oxygen consumption
- Prevent coronary spasms
- Prolong A-V conduction and refractory period (not nifedipine) resulting in prevention of re-entry or excitation (antiarrhythmic property)
- Decrease platelet adhesion
- Decrease blood viscosity

Verapamil hydrochloride (Isoptin)

It blocks the slow Ca^{++} dependent ionic channels. The inward movement of Ca^{++} into cardiac muscle cells, smooth muscle cells of the coronaries and systemic arteries and cells of the cardiac conduction system is inhibited. This leads to the following effects:
- In the heart, automaticity and conduction velocity are reduced and refractory period is increased.
  The calcium channel blockers have little effect on venous beds so do not affect cardiac preload. There is reduction of phase 4 depolarization due to inhibition of slow Ca^{++} dependent ionic channels in the sarcolemma.
- In the coronary and systemic arteries, the vascular resistance is decreased resulting in peripheral vasodilatation. It minimally affects the rapid sodium current.

Pharmacokinetics : Verapamil is well absorbed from GIT on oral administration, but not more than 20% reaches the systemic circulation as it is markedly metabolized in the gut and undergoes first-pass metabolism in the liver. About 90% is bound to plasma proteins. The plasma half life is 3 to 4 hours. A number of metabolites are active but less than the parent drug.

Dosage : 80 to 100 mg orally 3-4 times a day; 5-10 mg by slow I.V. injection, 1 mg/minute up to 10 mg, I.V. infusion 5-10 mg/hour, total daily dose 25-100 mg. The I.V. route is employed only to monitored patients.

Uses : Atrial tachyarrhythmias and angina pectoris. It is a drug of choice in atrial tachycardia. It is effective in slowing ventricular rate in atrial flutter or atrial fibrillation, the degree of block is increased and sinus rhythm may be restored.

The drug is very useful in supraventricular arrhythmias, particularly in re-entry supraventricular arrhythmias, but it has only slight effect or may be even ineffective in ventricular arrhythmias.

Contraindications : Low blood pressure states, cardiogenic shock, advanced heart failure, partial heart block and digitalis toxicity.

Interactions : Verapamil should not be given with beta-adrenergic blockers otherwise additive bradycardia will result. It increases plasma digoxin level, adverse effects can develop.

Adverse effects : Hypotension, sinus bradycardia, nausea, vomiting, headache, dizziness, constipation and myocardial depression. Flushing, headache and ankle oedema are less common. But nausea, vomiting and constipation are quite frequent with verapamil.

Nifedipine

The main action is arteriolar dilatation, total peripheral resistance is decreased, blood pressure falls. It does not depress S-A node or A-V conduction. Marked improvement of ventricular function occurs in CHF cases. Coronary flow is increased.

Nifedipine undergoes lesser first pass metabolism. As it is highly lipid soluble, absorption from sublingual route is rapid.

It is extensively bound to plasma proteins, metabolized in liver, inactive metabolites are excreted in urine.

Adverse effects include vasodilatory features i.e. sensation of heat, palpitation, flushing, dizziness, vertigo occur more with nifedipine. Shins and ankle oedema, hypotension, headache and nausea may also occur.

Diltiazem

It is a potent coronary dilator but less potent than nifedipine. It has modest direct negative chronotropic, inotropic and dromotropic action.

It is quickly absorbed from GIT on oral administration.

Dose is 30-60 mg thrice or four times a day orally.

Adverse effects are similar to that of verapamil though less frequent.

Tables 4.12 and 4.13 summarise the effects of antiarrhythmic drugs and their metabolism respectively. Table 4.14 lists the undesirable effects of antiarrhythmic drugs.

Tables 4.15 and 4.16 summarise the utility and uses of antiarrhythmic drugs respectively.

Class V : Drugs used in arrhythmias but not antiarrhythmic

Cardiac glycosides prolong refractory period of the AV node and thus control the rate and force in supraventricular arrhythmias/supraventricular tachycardia, atrial fibrillation and flutter.

Table 4.12. Effects of antiarrhythmic drugs

Drug	Automaticity		Refractory period		Membrane responsiveness (Purkinje fibres)
	SA node	Purkinje fibres	AV node	Purkinje fibres	
Quinidine, Procainamide, Amiodarone, Disopyramide	→	↓	↑ → ↓	↓	↓
Lidocaine, Tocainide, Mexiletine	→	↓	↑ → ↓	↓	↓
Propranolol	↓	↓	↑	↑	↓
Acebutolol	↓	↓	↑	↑	↓
Bretylium	↑↓	↑↓	↓ → ↑	↑	→
Verapamil	↓	→ ↓	↑	→	→

↑ = Increased; ↓ = Decreased; → = No change

Table 4.13. Metabolism of antiarrhythmic drugs

Drug	% metabolized	Major metabolite	Metabolites active
Quinidine	60-70	3-hydroxyquinidine	Yes
Procainamide	40-50	N-acetyl procainamide	Yes
Disopyramide	25-35	Mono-N-dealkylated disopyramide	Yes
Lidocaine	90	Monoethylglycine xylidide	No
Phenytoin	90	Para-hydroxyphenyl hydantoin	Yes

Table 4.14. Undesirable effects of antiarrhythmic drugs

	Effect on cardiac rhythm	Hypotension	CNS effects	Other effects
Quinidine	Sinus arrest, S-A block, A-V block, Asystole	+++	Cinchonism	GI distress, fever, thrombocytopenia
Procainamide	A-V block, asystole	+	Psychosis, giddiness, depression agranulocytosis	Lupus-like syndrome, fever, nausea, cramps,
Disopyramide	A-V block, asystole	+		Cardiac decompensation
Lidocaine	Sinus arrest	+	Paresthesias, disorientation, convulsions	
Pheytoin	Sinus arrest	+	Ataxia, nystagmus, lethargy, coma	Megaloblastic anaemia, rash
Propranolol	Sinus arrest, A-V block, asystole	+	Nightmares	Bronchospasm, fatigue, GI distress, marked hypoglycaemia
Bretylium	Sinus arrest, initial aggravation of arrhythmias	++++		Nausea, vomiting, increased sensitivity to catecholamines

Table 4.15. Utility of antiarrhythmic drugs in the treatment of specific arrhythmias

Arrhythmia	Quinidine	Procainamide	Disopyramide	Lidocaine	Phenytoin	Propranolol	Bretylium
Supraventricular atrial flutter	1	1	—	0	0	1	0
Paroxysmal supraventricular tachycardia	3	3	3	0	1	3	0
Ventricular tachycardia	2	4	3	4	2	1	3
Induced by digitalis ventricular arrhythmias	1	1	1	3	3	2	0

0 = none; 1 = poor; 2 = fair; 3 = good; 4 = excellent

Table 4.16. Uses of antiarrhythmic drugs

	Choice	Alternative
1. Supraventricular (atrial fibrillation or flutter) Paroxysmal atrial or nodal tachycardia	Digitalis to control ventricular rate Verapamil	Verapamol or beta-blocker Digoxine and beta-blocker
2. Ventricular Premature complexes Ventricular tachycardia	Beta-blocker Lidocaine	Procainamide Beta-blockers, mexiletine
3. Digitalis induced	Lidocaine	Phenytoin, beta-blocker, procainamide

Digitalis is contraindicated in ventricular arrhythmia.

In toxic doses, digitalis enhances automaticity of ventricles : ventricular fibrillation.

Choice of antiarrhythmics

Properties of an ideal antiarrhythmic drug: It should be an effective, long acting drug without any adverse effect and available by all routes of administration. It should not unduly depress myocardial contractility or slow conduction. It should be capable of preventing or eradicating local block. It should not have undue vagal stimulating action.

There is no single ideal antiarrhythmic drug.

Tachyarrhythmias: Sinus tachycardia: Treatment is rarely required.

Atrial premature systoles: If these are not due to cardiac disease (MI or thyrotoxicosis), anxiolytics are beneficial. If they are due to cardiac disease then digitalis, propranolol or quinidine are indicated.

Atrial tachycardia: Verapamil if A-V block is not present.

Atrial flutter: digitalis, digitalis followed by quinidine, verapamil or propranolol.

Atrial fibrillation: Digoxin, verapamil or disopyramide.

Ventricular ectopic beats: Propranolol, lidocaine or procainamide.

Ventricular tachycardia: Lidocaine or cardioversion followed by I.V. infusion of lidocaine or I.V. procainamide or I.V. phenytoin.

Ventricular fibrillation: It needs most urgent treatment. Electric cardioversion followed by lidocaine, or procainamide or phenytoin or propranolol.

Digitalis induced arrhythmias: Lidocaine, phenytoin or propranolol.

Bradyarrhythmias

Sinus bradycardia: If severe, atropine sulphate blocks ACh, so heart rate and A-V conduction velocity are increased; or isoprenaline hydrochloride (isuprel) by I.V. infusion. For sustained therapy isoprenaline is given orally or sublingually.

STUDY QUESTIONS

1. What are the main causes of arrhythmias? What are the basic mechanisms involved?
2. What is likely to happen if arrhythmias are not corrected?
3. Classify antiarrhythmics, giving suitable examples in each class of drugs.
4. How do the following classes of antiarrhythmics act?
   - Sodium channel blockers
   - B-adrenoceptor antagonists
   - Calcium channel blockers
5. Describe quinidine, procainamide and lidocaine regarding their pharmacokinetics, mode of action, efficacy as antiarrhythmics and adverse effects.
6. Describe propranolol regarding its mode of action and uses as an antiarrhythmic drug.
7. Discuss how calcium channel blocking agents act as cardioprotectives?
8. What are the main differences between verapamil, nifedipine and diltiazem.
9. Write notes on:
   (i) Combination therapy in the treatment of arrhythmias
   (ii) Choice of antiarrhythmics in supraventricular tachycardia, supraventricular fibrillation, flutter and ventricular arrhythmias.
10. How does digitalis help in supraventricular arrhythmias? Why is it contraindicated in ventricular arrhythmias? Which antiarrhythmic in particular is useful in digitalis induced arrhythmias?

GUIDE TO FURTHER READING

Arora, R.B., Sharma, V.N., and Madan, B.R., Antiarrhythmics Part I, Chloroquine in auricular fibrillation. IJMR, 1955; 43:659.

Arora, R.B., Sharma, V.N., and Madan, B.R., Ortho substituted benzoic acid esters of dialkyl amino alkanol in experimental cardiac arrhythmias. Jour. Pharm. and Pharmac. 1956; 8:323.

Arora, R.B., Sharma, V.N., and Madan, B.R., Antiarrhythmics Part V, Tridiuricane. A new local anaesthetic in experimentally induced atrial flutter, fibrillation and ventricular arrhythmia. IJMR, 1956; 44:271.

Dusman, R.E. Stanton, M.S et al: Clinical features of amiodarone-induced pulmonary toxicity. Circulation, 1990; 82:51-59.

Feely, J et al: Increased toxicity and reduced clearance of lidocaine by cimetidine. Ann. Intern. Med., 1982; 96:592-594.

Fozzard, H.A. et al: Cardiac electrophysiology. In, The Heart and Cardiovascular System: Scientific Foundations. (Fozzard, H.A., Haber, E. Jennings, R.B., Katz, A.M., and Morgan, H.E., eds.) Raven Press, New York, 1991; pp. 63-98.

Gupta, S.C., Sharma, V.N. and Sharma, H.L., Antiarrhythmic and anti-parkinsonian activity of two new phenothiazine salts. Ind. J. Exp. Biol., 1974; 12:504.

Krapivinsky, G et al: The G-protein-gated atrial K+ channel IKACh is a heteromultimer of two inwardly rectifying K+-channel proteins. Nature, 1995; 374:135-141.

Lelorier, J et al: Pharmacokinetics of lidocaine after prolonged intravenous infusions in uncomplicated myocardial infarction. Ann. Intern. Med., 1977; 87:700-706.

Levy, S et al: Stories about the origin of quinquina and quinidine. J. Cardiovasc. Electrophysiol., 1994; 5:635-636.

Lie, K.I. et al: Lidocaine in the prevention of primary ventricular fibrillation. N. Engl. J. Med., 1974; 291:1324-1326.

Madan, B.R., Sharma, V.N., Surpentine and Ajmaline in ventricular ectopic activity. Arch. Int. Pharmacodyn. 1959; 122:323.

Madan, B.R., Sharma, V.N., and Vyas, D.S., Study of the cardiovascular actions of some new antihistamine compounds. IJMR, 1967; 53:250.

Morady, F et al: Disopyramide. Ann. Intern. Med., 1982; 96:337-343.

Morike, K.E. et al: Quinidine-enhanced beta-blockade during treatment with propafenone in extensive metabolizer human subjects. Clin. Pharmacol. Ther., 1994; 55:28-34.

Nademanee, K. et al: Amiodarone and post-MI patients. Circulation, 1993; 88:764-774.

Richens, A. et al: Clinical pharmacokinetics of phenytoin. Clin. Pharmacokinet., 1979; 4:153-169.

Roden, D.M. et al: Current status of class III antiarrhythmic drug therapy. Am. J. Cardiol., 1993; 72:44B-49B.

Roden, D.M. et al: Clinical Pharmacology of antiarrhythmic agents. In, Sudden Cardiac Death. (Josephson, M.E., ed.) Blackwell Scientific, 1993; pp. 182-185.

Roden, D.M. et al: Risks and benefits of antiarrhythmic drug therapy. N. Engl. J. Med., 1994; 331:785-791.

Sanguinetti, M.C. et al: Two components of cardiac delayed rectifier K$^+$ current: differential sensitivity to block by class III antiarrhythmic agents. J. Gen. Physiol., 1990; 96:195-215.

Seller, R.H. et al: The role of magnesium in digitalis toxicity. Am. Heart J., 1971; 82:551-556.

Sharma, V.N., and Singh, K.P., Effect of some antihistaminic compounds in experimental cardiac arrhythmias. Arch. Int. Pharmacodyn. 1961; 131:24.

Sharma, V.N., Antiacetylcholine, antiaccelator and local anaesthetic activity of some quinidine like drugs. Arch. Int. Pharmacodyn. 1962; 137:410.

Sharma, V.N., and Arora, R.B., Antiarrhythmic activity of nine benzoic acid derivatives with special reference to their mode of action. IJMR, 1963; 51:327.

Singh, K.P., and Sharma, V.N., Suppression of acute ventricular tachycardia in dogs by three benzoic acid derivatives. Arch. Int. Pharmacodyn. 1964; 147:69.

Singh, K.P., and Sharma, V.N., Arrhythmia combating properties of some local anaesthetics. Arch. Int. Pharmacodyn. 1961; 121:1-2, 1-9.

Singh, K.P., and Sharma, V.N., 10-N-Substituted phenothiazine derivatives in auricular arrhythmias. Arch. Int. Pharmacodyn. 1969; 177:168.

Singh, K.P., and Sharma, V.N., Chemical constitution and drug action of N-Substituted phenothiazines in ventricular ectopic tachycardia, Jap. J. Pharmac., 1970; 20:173.

Singh, B.N. et al: Advantages of beta blockers versus antiarrhythmic agents and calcium antagonists in secondary prevention after myocardial infarction. Am. J. Cardiol., 1990, 66:9C-20C.

Singh, B.N. et al: Arrhythmia control by prolonging repolarization: the concept and its potential therapeutic impact. Eur. Heart J., 1993; 14 Suppl H:14-23.

Wang, Q et al: SCN5A mutations associated with an inherited cardiac arrhythmia, long QT syndrome. Cell, 1995; 80:805-811.

Vaughan Williams, E.M. et al: Classifying antiarrhythmic actions: by facts or speculation. J. Clin. Pharmacol., 1992; 32:964-977.

Weiss, J.N. et al: Ventricular arrhythmias in ischemic heart disease. Ann. Intern. Med., 1991; 114:784-797.

Wenckebach, K.F. et al: Cinchona derivatives in the treatment of heart disorders. JAMA, 1923; 81:472-474.

Wilde, A.A. et al: Electrophysiological effects of ATP sensitive potassium channel modulation: implications for arrhymogenesis. Cardiovasc. Res., 1994; 28:16-24.

Woods, K.L. et al: Long-term outcome after intravenous magnesium sulphate in suspected acute myocardial infarction: the second Leicester Intravenous Magnesium Intervention Trial (LIMIT-2). Lancet, 1994; 343:816-819.

DRUGS USED IN THE TREATMENT OF HYPERLIPIDAEMIA (HYPOLIPIDAEMIC AGENTS)

The lipoproteins are special proteins which carry lipids in plasma.

They contain a nonpolar core of triglycerides and cholesterol esters, surrounded by a polar coat of phospholipids, free cholesterol and apoproteins. The lipid in chylomicron and VLDL is mainly triglycerides, in LDL it is mostly cholesterol. LDL and VLDL are atherogenic whereas HDL has a protective effect.

The protein constituents of the lipoproteins are called apoproteins. The major apoproteins are called apo-E, apo C, and B. There are two forms of apo B, a low-molcular-weight form called apo B-48 which is characteristic of the exogenous system that transports ingested lipids, and a high-molecular-weight form called apo B-100 which is characteristic of the endogenous system.

Atherosclerosis is a multifactorial disease which requires multipronged approach

Cholesterol is an essential component of membranes and is intimately involved in many aspects of cellular structure and functions e.g. it affects the fluidity of cell membrane, membrane permeability, transmembrane exchange and other cell properties. It is the precursor of all steroids in the body such as corticosteroids, sex hormones, bile acid and vitamin D. Thus it plays a general, fundamental, and highly specific role in the economy of the body. However, elevated levels are harmful. The words 'good' and 'bad' cholesterol are used for the high density lipoprotein cholesterol and low density lipoprotein cholesterol respectively. Too much of 'bad' and too little of 'good' cholesterol are considered dangerous risk factors for coronary heart disease (CHD).

Evidence linking elevated serum cholesterol to CHD is overwhelming. The circulating LDL-cholesterol is the exclusive source of cholesterol deposited in the intimal cells of arterial wall, which may form bulky atherosclerotic plaques resulting in heart attacks or a stroke.

Thus high cholesterol level is harmful and lowering the elevated cholesterol is beneficial.

The drug treatment of hyperlipidaemia is lifelong and therefore should be prescribed only after excluding the secondary causes of the disorder and after dietary advice fails to produce the desired effects on the lipid profile. This will prevent the occurrence of hepatomegaly, splenomegaly, eruptive xanthomas and pancreatitis.

Hyperlipidaemia also called hyperlipoproteinaemia is rise in plasma lipids mainly cholesterol and triglycerides.

Hyperlipoproteinaemia is present when cholesterol levels exceed 240 mg/dl or triglyceride level exceeds 200 mg/dl. In this condition the cholesterol or triglyceride carrying plasma lipoproteins exceeds normal limits. It is a matter of concern because :

- increased lipoproteins can enhance process of the development of atherosclerosis, thrombosis and myocardial infarction;
- hypertriglyceridaemia can produce life threatening pancreatitis.

Hyperlipidaemia may be primary or secondary. The primary hyperlipidaemia is of 5 types viz.

Types	Cholesterol	TG	LDL	Risk of CHD	Treatment
I	+	+++			Dietary
IIa	+		+	High	Resin, niacin, statin
IIb	+	+	+	High	Niacin, fibrates
III	+	+		Moderate	Niacin, fibrates
IV	+	+		Moderate	Niacin, fibrates
V	+	+			Niacin, fibrates

The secondary hypercholesterolaemia may be due to hypothyroidism and nephrotic syndrome. Maturity onset diabetes is often associated with hypertriglyceridaemia.

The iatrogenic causes include thiazide diuretics, beta blockers. Ethanol is a common cause of hypertriglyceridaemia.

Box. 4.7. Common forms of secondary hyperlipidaemia

Condition	Lipid abnormalities
Diabetes mellitus	↑ TG ↓ HDL
Nephrotic syndrome	↑ Chol (± ↑ TG) ↑ LDL
Uraemia	↑ TG ↓ HDL
Hypothyroidism	↑ Chol (± ↑ TG) ↑ LDL
Alcoholism	↑ TG
Beta-adrenergic blocker	↑ TG ↓ HDL
Oral contraceptives	↑ TG ↓ HDL
Obstructive liver disease	↑ Chol

This cause should be treated first in these cases.

It has been shown that the atherosclerotic lesion can regress at all stages of lesion development.

Regression may be achieved by :
- dietary therapy
- hypolipidaemic drugs

Effect of diet

Prior to the use of hypolipidaemic drugs, dietary control trial is essential because high intakes of saturated fatty acids, cholesterol and excess calories leading to obesity are causally related to atherosclerotic cardiovascular disease.

LIPID LOWERING DRUGS

The drug treatment of hyperlipidaemia is life long and therefore prescribed only after excluding the secondary causes of the disorder and if dietary advice fails to produce the desired effects on the lipid profile. This will prevent the occurrence of hepatomegaly, splenomegaly, eruptive xanthomas and pancreatitis. This will also reduce the long term risk of atherosclerosis.

A plasma lipid lowering drug should possess the following properties:
- It should be efficacious on a long term basis
- Simplicity of application
- Lack of side effects and safe on long term use
- It should have a documented effect on the clinical end-point e.g. MI or atherosclerosis

- It should fulfill conditions for long term compliance

Classification of hypolipoproteinemic drugs :

- Interfere with intestinal absorption of cholesterol by :
  - Binding resins : Cholestyramine, colestipol
  - Plant sterol : Beta sitosterol
  - Ezetimibe by inhibiting absorption of cholesterol
- Fibric acid : Gomfibrozil, clofibrate, fenofibrate, bezafibrate.
- HMG-CoA - reductase inhibitors : Lovastatin, simvastatin pravastatin, mevastatin, atorvastatin.
- Inhibitor of VLDL production and lipolysis : Nicotinic acid
- Antioxidants : Probucol
- Others : Neomycin, gugulipid.

Lipid lowering drugs should be prescribed only after excluding the secondary causes of hyperlipidaemia and if dietary advice fails to produce the desired effects on the lipid profile.

Drugs which mainly reduce plasma cholesterol

Binding resins

Cholestyramine and **colestipol** are non-absorbable bile binding resins which bind bile acid in intestinal tract and bile acids are excreted in faeces. This depletes hepatic bile acids and liver shall need CH for the synthesis of bile acids. This will produce decrease in CH level in the body.

These drugs produce reduction in plasma cholesterol and LDL cholesterol. However, there may be increase in VLDL and TG levels. Hence, these drugs are useful in hypercholesterolaemia but not for hypertriglyceridaemia.

Dosage

Cholestyramine 8g twice a day, colestipol 10g twice a day, It is more acceptable than cholestyramine.

Adverse effects

As bile acid binding resins are not absorbed, systemic toxicity is low but GI disturbances are common.

- Unpalatable, nausea, flatulence, abdominal distension, constipation or diarrhoea.
- Interfere with the absorption of fat soluble vitamins, and of drugs such as chlorothiazide, digoxin, warfarin which should be taken at least 1 hour before or 4-6 hours after the resin.
- Bulky and unappetising

Drugs interactions

They bind and reduce absorption of digoxin, warfarin, thiazides, barbiturates, aspirin, iron salts, tetracyclines, thyroxine.

- Malabsorption of vitamin K may occur as bile salts are needed for absorption of vitamin K.
- Synergism occurs with HMG-CoA reductase inhibitors or nicotinic acid.

Plant sterols : Beta sitosterols interfere with absorption of dietary cholesterol from GIT.

Dose : 10-20g in divided doses daily.

Beta sitosterol is unpalatable due to bad taste. The dose is also too large.

Ezetimibe

It reduces blood cholesterol by inhibiting absorption of cholesterol by the small intestine. It localizes and appears to act at the brush border of the small intestine and inhibits the absorption of cholesterol, leading to a decrease in the delivery of intestinal cholesterol in the liver. This causes reductions in hepatic cholesterol stores and increase in the clearance of cholesterol from the blood, this distinct mechanism is complementary to that of the HMG-CoA reductase inhibitors.

Indications

Hypercholesterolaemia, primary; alone or in combination with statin.

Contraindications :

- Hypersensitivity to ezetimibe
- Active liver disease

Ezetimibe can the administered with or without food administration (high-fat or non-fat meals) have no effect on the extent of absorption. It is absorbed and extensively, conjugated to a pharmacologically active phenolic glucuronide. Ezetimibe and ezetimibe - glucuronide are bound to human plasma protein (very high > 790%).

Ezetimibe is rapidly metabolized to ezetimibe - glucuronide in the small intestine and liver.

Half life : Ezetimibe and ezetimibe-glucuronide 22 hours for both.

Dose : Adult usual dose : 10mg orally once daily.

Elimination : Renal : 9%; ezetimibe - glucuronide is the major component.

Faecal : 69%; ezetimibe is the major component.

Adverse effects

Abdominal pain, back ache, arthralgia, cough, diarrhoea, fatigue, headache, sinusitis.

Drug interaction

- cyclosporin
- fibric acid derivatives

Precaution

- Ezetimibe should be used during pregnancy only if the potential benefit justifies the risk to the foetus.
- It should not be used in nursing mothers unless the potential risk justifies the potential risk to the infant.
- Treatment with ezetimibe in children less then 10 years of age is not recommended.
- Greater sensitivity of some older individuals cannot be ruled out.

Drugs which mainly reduce plasma triglycerides : Fibric acid derivatives (fibrates) :

Gemfibrozil, clofibrate, fenofibrate, bezafibrate.

Fibrates

- Increase plasma HDL
- Decrease hepatic lipid synthesis
- Cause marked reduction in circulating VLDL and hence TGs
- Reduce release of plasma TG by liver and
- Decrease plasma LDL by stimulating hepatic uptake resulting in clearance of LDL

Clinical uses of fibrates

- Fibrates e.g., bezafibrate, gemfibrozil are well tolerated, taken at night or in divided doses during the day
- Marked effect in lowering TG (in patients in whom resins are contraindicated)
- Mixed dyslipidaemia (increased TG and increased cholesterol)
- In combination with other lipid-lowering drugs in patients with resistant dyslipidaemia

Adverse effects

- GI disturbances
- Myositis like syndrome (unusual but can be severe, more common in the presence of kidney disease)

Clofibrate is not preferred as it may produce gall stones. It may produce hair loss, GI disturbances, decrease in libido. It may induce myositis particularly when combined with lovastatin. Its t½ is 12 hours, dose 2g/d in 2-4 divided doses orally.

Gemfibrozil is preferred over clofibrate because it is more effective and better tolerated. It is commonly used drug.

Bezafibrate, ciprofibrate and **fenofibrate** are third generation fibrates. They are effective lipid lowering drugs but their long-term safety is yet to be demonstrated.

Fenofibrate has a uricosuric effect which is useful is patients in whom hyperuricaemia coexists with mixed dyslipidaemia.

Drug interactions

As they are highly protein bound so may displace sulphonylureas and warfarin (displacement drug interaction).

Contraindications

- Hepatic and renal dysfunction
- Pregnancy
- Lactating mothers

HMG-CoA reductase inhibitors

HMG-CoA reductase is the rate limiting enzyme in cholesterol synthesis. It catalyses the conversion of HMG-CoA to mevalonic acid (MVA).

Recently a new class of lipid lowering drugs, HMG CoA reductase inhibitors, have been introduced. These drugs act by decreasing liver cholesterol synthesis resulting in up regulation of LDL receptors, increased clearance of LDL from plasma, and diminution of plasma LDL levels.

INDIVIDUAL AGENTS

Lovastatin

It has excellent cholesterol lowering effect, well tolerated and fulfills conditions for long term compliance. It has low level of subjective side effects and given once daily at a dose of 20-80 mg. It is easy to administer and patients' acceptance is outstanding.

It lowers LDL by about 35-45% in subjects with familial hypercholesterolaemia (FH) and non familial hypercholesterolaemia (non FH).

Triglyceride levels are decreased by 15-20% and HDL cholesterol is increased by 2-15%. The LDL/HDL ratio is reduced by 40 percent.

Simvastatin

It is lovastatin, chemically modified by the synthetic addition of methyl group on its alkyl side chain which renders it most potent hypocholesterolaemic agent. Both lovastatin and simvastatin are administered as prodrugs in their lactone form which readily undergo first pass metabolism, hepatic sequestration and hydrolysis to active hydroxy acid forms in liver, the target organ.

Contraindications : Pregnancy lactation, liver disease and children.

Pravastatin

It is administered in its active form as a sodium salt. About 34 % is absorbed, undergoes extensive first-pass hepatic effect, and about 50% is bound to protein.

The liver is the chief route of excretion, and about 20-40% is excreted in urine.

Fluvastatin

It is administered in its active form. Its absorption is almost complete, hepatic extraction is extensive and about 90% is protein bound.

The peak plasma concentration occurs in 0.6 hour.

Liver is the chief route of elimination, less than 5% is excreted in urine and more than 90% in faeces.

Pharmacokinetics

HMG-CoA reductase inhibitors are given orally, last thing before going to bed at night.

They are well absorbed and extracted by the liver, their site of action and are subject to extensive presystemic metabolism.

Clinical uses

- Simvastatin and pravastatin reduce mortality as well as morbidity in appropriately selected patients.
- In patients who have symptomatic atherosclerotic diseases, or who are at increased risk of CHD due to elevated blood cholesterol.
- Useful in patients with heterozygous familial hypercholesterolaemia.

Adverse effects

These drugs are well tolerated; mild and infrequent adverse effects include GI disturbances, insomnia, rash. Serious adverse effects include severe myositis, hepatitis and angioedema. Serious adverse effects are rare.

Caution

- Statins should be given with caution or not at all in patients with liver diseases.
- Most statins are ineffective in patients with homozygous form of familial hypercholesterolaemia who can not make LDL receptors. Atorvastatin is an exception, having some useful effect on serum cholesterol in such patients.

Contraindications

- Pregnancy
- Itraconazole and cyclosporin increase the risk of myositis

Certain characteristics of statins are given in Table 4.17.

Table 4.17. Characteristics of statins

Characteristic	Lovastatin	Simvastatin	Atorvastatin	pravastatin	Cerivastatin
Maximal dose (mg/day)	80	80	80	40	0.3
Maximal LDL cholesterol decrease (%)	40	47	60	34	28
Average LDL cholesterol reduction (%)	34	34	50	34	28
Average triglyceride reduction (%)	16	18	29	24	13
Average HDL cholesterol increase (%)	8.6	12	6	12	10
Plasma half life (hr.)	2	1-2	14	1-2	2-3
Effect of food on absorption	Increased absorption	None	None	Decreased absorption	None
Optimal time of administration	with meals (morning and (evening)	Evening	Evening	Bedtime	Evening
Penetration of central nervous system	Yes	No	No	No	Yes
Renal excretion of absorbed dose (%)	10	13	2	20	33

Atorvastatin Calcium

It produces long-lasting inhibition of HMG-CoA reductase and lowers triglycerides as well as cholesterol.

Indications

- Dysbeta lipoproteinaemia
- Hypercholesterolaemia, primary
- Hypercholesterolaemia, familial (children 10-17 years)
- Hyperlipidaemia
- Hypertriglyceridaemia

Contraindications

- Hypersensitivity to atorvastatin
- Liver disease
- Pregnancy or lactation (breast feeding)
- Unexpected, persistent elevation of serum transaminases

Precautions

- Concomitant therapy with fibrates, niacin, cyclosporin, erythromycin or azo antifungals may increase the risk of myopathy
- Heavy alcohol use
- History of liver disease
- Reduce doses or discontinue therapy if serum transaminase levels 3 times the upper limit of normal persist
- Withhold temporarily or discontinue therapy in

any patient who develops a condition suggestive of or predisposing to myopathy or renal failure

Dosage, adult (usual): 10-80 mg orally once daily.

Dosage, pediatric (usual) : 10 mg orally daily, upto maximum 20 mg orally daily.

Administration

- May be administered with or without food.
- Patient should be maintained on a low cholesterol diet.
- Concomitant statin therapy with fibrates should generally be avoided (risk of rhabdomyolysis).

Adverse effects

Common : Abdominal pain, constipation, flatulence, nausea, headache, mild liver enzyme elevation.

Serious :
- hepatotoxicity (rare)
- rhabdomyolysis (rare)

Drugs which mainly reduce plasma triglycerides

Inhibitors of VLDL production

Nicotinic acid (niacin)

It is a water soluble vitamin but its hypolipidaemic activity is not related to its activity as vitamin. Nicotinamide is not hypolipidaemic.

Nicotinic acid (i) decreases hepatic secretion of

VLDL and thus lowers LDL; (ii) inhibits cholesterol synthesis in liver and (iii) increases clearance of VLDL by tissue resulting in lowering the plasma triglycerides; (iv) decreases catabolism of HDL resulting in elevation of HDL level; (v) decreases plasma fibrinogen leading to decreased tendency to thrombosis.

Dose : 0.5 to 2 g thrice a day orally.

The adverse effects are frequent and include sense of warmth (due to cutaneous vasodilation), flushing and dryness of skin, diarrhoea.

Carbohydrate intolerance, hyperuricaemia (gout is precipitated), and hepatic dysfunction may also occur.

Tolerance develops to niacin after a few days to the side effects such as flushing and itching.

Contraindications

Peptic ulcer, pregnancy, gout and small children.

Acipimox

It is an antihyperlipidaemic analog of niacin.

Pharmacokinetics

Acipimox is rapidly and completely absorbed; peak plasma levels occur approximately 2 hours after oral administration. It is poorly bound to plasma proteins. It is not metabolized, and is mainly excreted un-changed in the urine.

Clinical Applications

Preliminary data suggest that acipimox may be useful in the treatment of hyperlipoproteinemias, especially hypertriglyceri-daemia.

Cautions

Acipimox is generally well tolerated; flushing, gastric upset, and headache are the most commonly occurring adverse effects. Hyperglycaemia has not been reported with acipimox. Vomiting, hypotension, heartburn, loose stools, itching, rash, tingling of the extremities, and cutaneous blisters have also occurred.

Adult Dosage

Oral : The optimal dose of acipimox has not been determined. In the treatment of hyperlipidaemias, the usual dose employed has been 250 mg orally 2 to 3 times a day either alone or in conjunction with other drugs. Some investigators have reported similar results with doses of 500 mg once a day.

Dosages in Renal Failure

Acipimox is eliminated almost exclusively via the kidneys. Dosage reduction in patients with renal failure is recommended.

Dosage adjustment during dialysis

Acipimox is efficiently removed with haemodialysis. In uraemic patients, elimination of acipimox was negligible until initiation of remodialysis.

Antioxidant

Probucol

There is a growing interest in the possible role of free radicals in the development of atheroma. Oxidative modification of LDL particles in the arterial sub-endothelium results in structural changes, which are postulated to make them more atherogenic than native LDL.

Probucol has antioxidant action (desirable property) which prevents hydroperoxidation of lipoproteins. this inhibits formation of foam cells in the arterial intima. Thus it protects against atherogenesis.

It produces regression of tendon xanthomas which results due to deposition of lipids in tendons and skin. These are painful and disfiguring lesions.

Probucol decreases HDL (underisable property).

Dose : 250-500 mg twice a day.

The side effects include diarrhoea and other GIT upsets, fatigue, dizziness, headache, itching, insomnia, different odour of skin, palpitation and tremors.

Probucol should be avoided in patients with long Q-T interval on ECG.

Others

Neomycin sulphate is not absorbed from GIT. It reduces plasma LDL cholesterol. However, it is not recommended for this purpose. It produces ototoxicity and nephrotoxicity.

Oestrogens in large doses decrease cholesterol

but increase TG. These are not clinically employed for this purpose because of feminizing effects and increased incidence of thromboembolism.

d-Thyroxine increases the synthesis of LDL receptors which increases LDL cholesterol uptake. It is not used for this purpose due to adverse effects (such as tremors, nervousness, insomnia, sweating) and more effective, better tolerated and safer drugs are available.

Guggulipid is clinically used.

It is an oleo gum resin obtained from a medicinal plant commiphora mukul.

It reduces seurm cholesterol, LDL cholesterol and triglycerides. It increases HDL level.

It acts like fibrates and in addition reduces platelet aggregation (useful in atherosclerosis).

Precaution : In cases with hepatic disease.

The decision to prescribe cholesterol lowering drugs depends on the LDL level as well as on the associated CAD risk factors in an individual patient as following :

Without CAD and < 2 risk factors –
Drug therapy is considered at > 190 mg/dl LDL and the aim is to reduce it to < 160 mg/dl
Without CAD but > 2 risk factors –
Drug therapy is considered at > 160 mg/dl LDL and the goal is to reduce it to < 130 mg/dl
Without CAD or other atherosclerotic disease –
Drug therapy is considered at > 130 mg/dl

Box 4.8. Dosages of statins	
Lovastatin	10 or 20 mg/d with food (increments at 6-8 weeks interval), maximum 80 mg/d
Simvastatin	5-10 mg once daily at bedtime, maximum 40 mg/d
Pravastatin	10-20 mg/d once at bedtime, maximum 40 mg/d
Fluvastatin	20 mg/d once at bedtime, maximum 40 mg/d

Table 4.18 : choice of hypolipidaemic agents in hyperlipidaemia

Hyperlipidaemia	Drug for monotherapy	Drug combinations
↑ LDL and normal TG (<200 mg/dl)	HMG- CoA reductase inhibitor Bile acid sequestrant Nicotinic acid	HMG-CoA reductase inhibitor+Bile acid sequestrant Bile acid sequestrant + Nicotinic acid
↑ LDL and TG (200-400 mg/dl)	HMG-CoA reductase inhibitor Gemfibrozil Nicotinic acid	HMG-CoA reductase inhibitor + Gemfibrozil HMG-CoA reductase inhibitor + Nicotinic acid Bile acid sequestrant + Nicotinic acid Gemfibrozil + Nicotinic acid

Box 4.9 : Mode of action of hypolipidaemic drugs

Drugs		Mechanism
HMG-CoA (3-hydroxy-3-methyl glutaryl coenzyme A) Reductase inhibitors	Simvastatin, Lovastatin, etc.	Competitively inhibit conversion of HMG-CoA to mevalonate. ↓ cholesterol synthesis by inhibition of rate limiting HMG-CoA reductase to mevalonate
Bile acid sequestrants	Cholestyramine Colestipol	↓ Bile acid absorption, ↑ Hepatic conversion of cholesterol to bile acids ↑ LDL receptors on hepatocytes
Fibric acid derivatives	Gemfibrozil Bezafibrate, etc.	↑ Activity of lipoprotein lipase ↓ Release of fatty acids from adipose tissue
Nicotinic acid		↓ Production of VLDL ↓ Lipolysis in adipocytes

LDL and the goal is to reduce it to < 100 mg/dl

The guidelines regarding TG levels are as following :

Serum TG (mg/dl)	Recommendation
< 200 (normal)	Nil intervention. Some recommend to lower it to < 150 mg/dl by changing life style.
200–400	Life style to be modified. However, drugs considered if CAD is present or total blood cholesterol is > 240 mg/dl or HDL < 35 mg/dl or family history of premature CAD or multiple risk factors.
400–1000 (high) > 1000 (very high)	Drug therapy is required. Vigorous intervention needed as risk of acute pancreatitis is high; diabetes if present must be controlled, drug therapy should be instituted, and very low fat diet advised.

The following is the risk classification based on the Lipid levels.

LDL cholesterol :	Desirable	< 100
	Borderline	100-129
	High	130-159
	Very high	> 160
HDL Cholesterol :	Ideal	> 60
	Desirable	40-59
	Low	< 40
Triglycerides :	Ideal	< 100
	Above normal	100-149
	Borderline	150-199
	High	200-399
	Very high	> 400

Choice of hypolipidaemic agents is given in Table 4.18.

Table 4.19 shows **therapeutic status of certain hypolipidaemic agents**.

The following are **cut-off levels** as advised by the U.S. National Cholesterol Education Programme:

	Total cholesterol mg/dl	LDL-cholesterol mg/dl
Desirable	< 200	< 130
Borderline	200-239	130-159
High risk	> 240	> 160

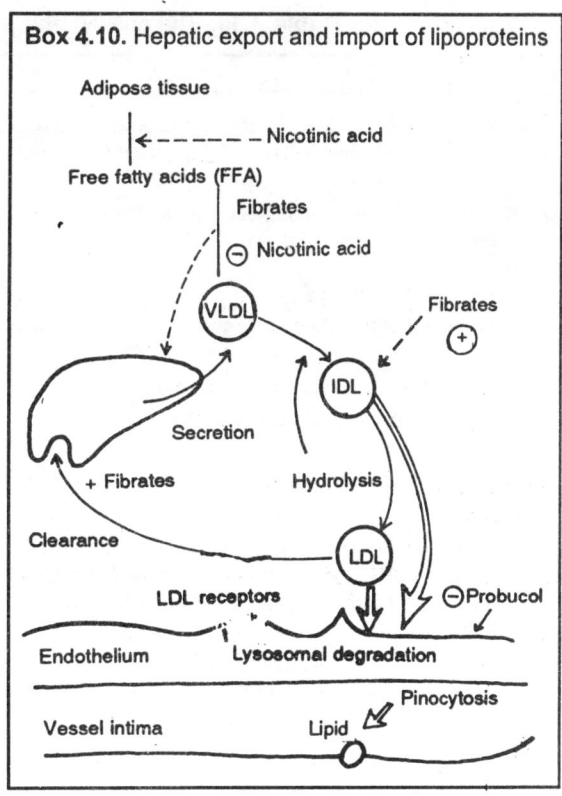

Box 4.10. Hepatic export and import of lipoproteins

Two cut off points which are uniform for both sexes and all ages can be used to classify patients into desirable, borderline and high blood cholesterol.

Patients with 200 mg/dl total blood cholesterol are given dietary advice.

If blood cholesterol is 200 mg/dl, the test should be repeated to confirm the level.

Patients with 200-239 mg/dl who are not otherwise at high risk are advised to adopt a fat controlled diet.

Patients with 240 mg/dl of total blood cholesterol should undergo a lipoprotein analysis as should those with levels 200-239 mg/dl who are at high risk for other reasons.

'High risk' patients are those who already had a heart attack. They are given intensive intervention at a lower cut off point.

LDL cholesterol is a better indicator of risk. Patients with LDL cholesterol of 160 mg/dl or more as well as with 130-159 mg/dl who are at high risk should be given intensive lipid lowering treatment.

Table 4.19. Therapeutic status of certain hypolipidaemic agents

Drug	Merit	Demerit
Clofibrate	Moderate efficacy, well tolerated, increases HDL-CH, lowers VLDL synthesis, lowers TG, increases catabolism of LDL-CH	Risk of cholelithiasis, several side effects, myocytic syndrome, long term safety in dispute
Bezafibrate, Ciprofibrate, Fenofibrate	Fairly good effect, easy to administer, increase HDL-CH, lower VLDL-CH & TG	Long term safety is not known
Nicotinic acid	Good efficacy, increases HDL-cholesterol, lowers VLDL-CH & LDL-CH, 5 yrs. safety established	Many side effects, gout precipitated, risk of stone formation
Probucol	Moderate efficacy, regression of tendon xanthoma, anti-oxidant, easy to administer, inhibits LDL oxidation	Variable or no effect, several side effects, diarrhoea common, long term safety not known
Cholestyramine, Cholestipol	Moderate efficacy, increase HDL-CH, long term safety known	Large dose, troublesome to take, plasma TG increased, GI side effects, do not fulfill conditions for good compliance
Gemfibrozil	Moderate efficacy, 5 years safety established, increases HDL-CH, decreases plasma TG level, inhibits VLDL production and enhances VLDL clearance	Less effect on LDL levels
Lovastatin, Simvastatin	Excellent effect, well tolerated, less side effects, given once daily, increase HDL-CH, lower CH synthesis and thus lower plasma LDL levels	Troublesome myopathy, teratogenic in animals, cataract in dogs, long term safety not known, headache, transient and inconsistent changes in bowel habits, nausea, insomnia, increase in alkaline phosphates, transaminases, creatinine, kinase

---

Box 4.11. Coronary arterial luminal obstruction

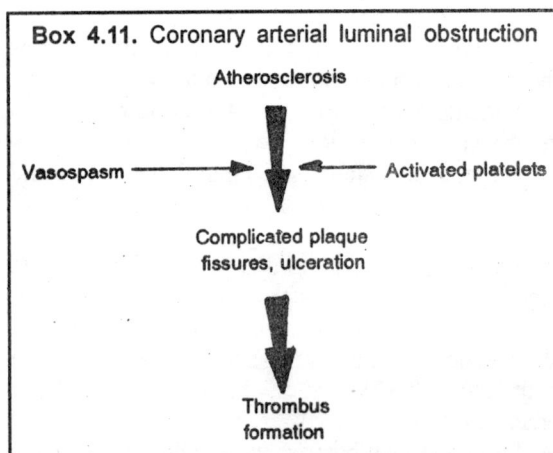

Box 4.12. Risk factors for ischaemic heart disease

- Hyperlipidaemia
- Excess serum cholesterol level especially LDL-cholesterol
- Increased ratio of LDL to HDL
- Excess triglycerides
- Hypertension
- Diabetes mellitus
- Cigarette smoking/tobacco chewing
- Obesity
- Lack of regular exercise
- Genetic predisposition (family history of ischaemic heart disease at an early age)
- Sedentary life style
- Fibrinogen level
- Left ventricular hypertrophy (enlarged left ventricle)
- Oral contraceptive use
- Chronic stress or type A personality (aggressive, competitive, chronically impatient, ambitious)
- Age and sex (incidence higher among men than among premenopaused women and increases in both sexes with age)

The therapeutic status of the commonly used hypolipidaemic agents is summarized in Table 4.19.

Drug combination

• Bile acid sequestrant cholestyramine or

cholestipol plus lovastatin or simvastatin will act at different levels and therefore this combination may be considered better.

- Bile acid sequestrant plus nicotinic acid combination is considered very good for lowering LDL cholesterol in familial hypercholesterolaemia (FH). Bile acid sequestrant increases LDL removal and nicotinic acid decreases LDL production. But many patients may not tolerate this combination as both these drugs produce gastrointestinal side effects.

- Bile acid sequestrant plus a fibrate: This is a useful combination as bile acid sequestrant lowers LDL cholesterol but often increases VLDL. By addition of a fibrate e.g., gemfibrozil the VLDL increases will be counteracted.

- If triple drug therapy is required, then bile acid sequestrant with lovastatin and nicotinic acid combination may be given. However, lovastatin with nicotinic acid combination should be given with extreme caution, because impaired hepatic excretion of lovastatin may result in severe myopathy.

- In case there is increased plasma triglycerides and low HDL cholesterol concentration, gemfibrozil and nicotinic acid are preferred.

In order to avoid or at least delay the development of atherosclerosis and its sequelae, besides dietary control and hypolipidaemic agents, the other steps should also be taken to correct modifiable risk factors such as cigarette smoking, diabetes mellitus, hypertension, obesity, hypertriglyceridaemia and sedentary life style.

STUDY QUESTIONS

1. What is the physiological role of cholesterol in the body?

2. How do elevated serum levels of cholesterol produce damaging effect? Is it a modifiable major risk factor for producing atherosclerosis? What are the cut-off levels for total cholesterol, desirable, borderline and high risk serum levels.

3. What are the major types of primary hyperlipidaemia? What may be the causes of secondary and iatrogenic hyperlipidaemia?

4. What is the role of dietary control in the man-

agement of atherosclerosis? What are the properties of desired hypolipidaemic drugs?

5. Describe the merits and demerits, mode of action and adverse effects of the following drugs as hypolipidaemic agents:
   (a) Nicotinic acid
   (b) Fibric acid derivatives
   (c) Anion exchange resins
   (d) Guggulipid
   (e) HMG CoA inhibitors

6. Write notes on
   (i) Probucol
   (ii) Sitosterols

7. Discuss combination therapy of hypolipidaemic agents.

8. Explain why the following are not considered suitable as hypolipidaemic agents although they reduce serum cholesterol level:
   (a) Neomycin
   (b) d-Thyroxine
   (c) Oestrogens

9. What are the other modifiable risk factors for producing atherosclerosis and CHD, besides hyperlipidaemia?

GUIDE TO FURTHER READING

Alberts, A.W. et al: Cardiol, Drug Rev., 1989; 7:89-109.

Alpana Ram, Lauria, P., Kumar, P. and Sharma, V.N., The lipid lowering drugs - updated. The Indian Journal of Hospital Pharmacy, 1993; Sep-Oct: 167

Alpana Ram, Effect of Plumbago Zeylanica in hyperlipidaemic rabbits and its modification by vitamin E, Ind. Jour. Pharmacol., 1996;28:161.

Alpana Ram, Lauria, P., Gupta, R. and Sharma, V.N., Hyperlipidaemic effect of Myristica fragrans fruit extract in rabbits. Jour. of Ethnopharmacology, 55; 49-53, 1996.

Alpana Ram, Lauria, P., Gupta, R., Kumar, P., Sharma, V.N.: Hypocholesterolaemic effects of Terminalia arjuna tree bark. Jour. of Ethnopharmacology, 55; 165-169, 1997.

Arsenian M.A.: Magnesium and Cardiovascular Disease. Progress in cardiovascular disease xxxv, 271-310, 1993.

Assmann M.D. and Schulte H.: Relation of high density lipoprotein cholesterol and triglycerides to incidence of atherosclerotic coronary artery disease (the

PROCAM experience) Am. J. Cardiol. 70: 733-737, 1992.

Austin M.A.: Plasma triglyceride and coronary heart disease. Atheroscler. Thromb. 11: 2, 1991.

Bainton D., Miller N.E., Bolton C.H. et al: Plasma triglyceride and high density lipoprotein cholesterol as predictors of ischemic heart disease in British men. Br Heart J. 68: 60-66, 1992.

Berglund, L.F. et al: Altered apolipoprotein B metabolism in very low density lipoprotein from lovastatin-treated guinea pigs. J. Lipid Res., 1994; 35-956-965.

Breslow, J. et al: Familial disorders of high-density lipoprotein metabolism. In, The Metabolic and Molecular Bases of Inherited Disease, 7th ed. McGraw-Hill, New York, 1995; pp. 2031-2052.

Brown, B.G. et al: Lipid lowering and plaque regression. New insights into prevention of plaque disruption and clinical events in coronary disease. Circulation, 1993; 87:1781-1791.

Brown M.S. and Goldstein J.L.: A receptor mediated pathway for cholesterol homeostasis. Science 232: 34-37, 1986.

Brunzell, J.D. et al: Familial lipoprotein lipase deficiency and other causes of the chylomicronemia syndrome. In, The Metabolic and Molecular Bases of Inherited Disease, 7th ed. McGraw-Hill, New York, 1995; pp. 1913-1932.

Chopra K. and Singh M.: Involvement of oxygen free radicals in cardioprotective effect of rutin - a naturally occurring flavonoid. Ind. J. Pharmacol. 26: 13 - 18, 1994.

Connor W.E.: Dietary fibre - nostrum or critical nutrient. N. Engl. J. Med. 322: 193 - 195, 1990.

Denke, M.A. et al: The cholesterol lowering diet. In, Lowering Cholesterol in High-Risk Individuals and Populations. Marcel Dekker, Inc., New York, 1995; pp. 183-208.

Durrington P.N.: Can any agreement be reached on cholesterol lowering (Conference Report). Br. Heart J. 71: 125 - 128, 1994.

Esterbauer H., Dieber-Rothenderr M., Striegl G. and Waeg G.: Role of vitamin E in preventing the oxidation of low density lipoprotein. Am. J. Clin. Nutr. 53(Suppl.): 3145- 3215, 1991.

Gail Vines: Diet, drugs and heart disease. New Scientist, 25, 44-48, 1989.

Ginsberg, H.N.: Lipoprotein physiology and its relationship to atherogenesis. Endocrinol. Metab. Clin. North Am., 1990; 19:211- 228.

Goldstein, J.L. et al: Familiat hypercholesterolemia. In, The Metabolic and Molecular Bases of Inherited

Disease, 7th ed. McGraw-Hill, New York, 1995; pp. 1981-2030.

Grundy, S.M.: HMG CoA reductase inhibitors: clinical applications and therapeutic potential. In, Drug Treatment of Hyperlipidemia. Marcel Dekker, Inc., New York, 1991; pp. 139-167.

Gupta K.D. and Gupta R., Dietary Treatment of Coronary Heart Disease, 1993, Centre for Heart Disease Production and Rehabilitation, Jaipur, pp 19-29.

Halliwell B.: Drug antioxidant effects-a basis for drug selection? Drugs 42 (4): 569-605, 1991.

Havel, R.J. et al: Introduction: structure and metabolism of plasma lipoproteins. In, The Metabolic and Molecular Bases of Inherited Disease, 7th ed. McGraw-Hill, New York, 1995; pp. 1841- 1851.

Hemila H.: Vitamin C and Plasma Cholesterol. Critical Reviews in Food, Science and Nutrition 32 (1): 33-57, 1992.

Hertog M.G.L., Feskens J.M., Hollman P.C.H. et al.: Dietary antioxidant flavonoids and risk of coronary heart disease The Zutphen Elderly Study. Lancet: 342: 1007 - 1011, 1993.

Illingworth, D.R. et al: Fibric acid derivatives. In, Drug Treatment of Hyperlipidemia. Marcel Dekker, Inc., New York, 1991; pp. 103-138.

Illingworth, D.R. et al: Treatment of heterozygous familial hypercholesterolemia with lipid-lowering drugs. Arteriosclerosis, 1989; (Suppl 1):I121-I124.

Illingworth, D.R. et al: A review of clinical trials comparing HMG-CoA reductase inhibitors. Clin. Ther., 1994; 16:366-385.

Illingworth D.R.: An overview of lipid lowering drugs. Drugs 36(Suppl.3): 63-71, 1988.

Kagan V.E., Serbinova E.A., Forte T., Scita G., and Packer L.: Recycling of vitamin E in human low density lipoproteins. J. Lipid Res. 33; 385-397, 1992.

Kane, J.P. et al: Disorders of the biogenesis and secretion of lipoproteins containing the B apolipoproteins. In, The Metabolic and Molecular Bases of Inherited Disease, 7th ed. McGraw-Hill, New York, 1995; pp. 1853-1885.

Karpe F., Bard J.M., Steiner G. et al: HDLs and elementary lipemia: studies in men with previous myocardial infarction at a young age. Arteriosclerosis Thrombosis 13: 11-22, 1993.

Larsen, M.L. et al: Drug treatment of dyslipoproteinemia. Med. Clin. North Am., 1994; 78:225-245.

Levine, G.N. et al: Cholesterol reduction in cardiovascular disease. Clinical benefits and possible mechanism. N. Engl. J. Med., 1995; 332:512-521.

Mahley, R.W. et al: Type III Hyperlipoproteinemia: the

role of apolipoprotein E in normal and abnormal lipoprotein metabolism. In, The Metabolic and Molecular Bases of Inherited Disease, 7th ed. McGraw-Hill, New York, 1995; pp.1953-1980.

Myerson R.M.: Magnesium - a neglected element? J. Pharm. Med. 2: 89-97, 1991.

National Cholesterol Education Program: Second report of the expert panel on detection, evaluation and treatment of high blood cholesterol in adults (Adult treatment panel II). Circulation 89: 1329-1445, 1994.

Nuglisch J. and Krieglstein J.: Pharmacological treatment of cerebral ischemia. Drugs of Today 28: 431-438, 1992.

Packer L.: Protective role of vitamin E in biological systems. Am. J. Clin. Nutr. 53(Suppl.): 10505-10555, 1991.

Oliver M.F.: Might treatment of hypercholesterolaemia increase non-cardiac mortality? Lancet 337: 1529-1531, 1991.

Paterson, R.W. et al: Impact of intensive lipid modulation on angiographically defined coronary disease: clinical implications. South, Med. J., 1994; 87:236-242.

Quinet, E.M. et al: Adipose tissue cholesteryl ester transfer protein mRNA in response to probucol treatment: cholesterol and species dependence. J. Lipid Res., 1993; 34:845-852.

Reddy K.S. Why is preventive cardiology essential in the Indian context? In Wasir H.S. (ed) Preventive cardiology. An introduction, 1991, Vikas Publishing House, New Delhi, pp 1- 14.

Rimm E.B., Stampfer M.J., Ascherio A., Giovannucci E.: Vitamin E consumption and risk of coronary heart disease in men. N. Engl. J. Med. 328: 1450 - 1456, 1993.

Richard, B.M. et al: Transport of HDL cholesterol esters to the liver is not diminished by probucol treatment in rats. Arterioscler. Thromb., 1992; 12:862-869.

Rossouw J.E., Lewis B. and Rifkind B.M. The value of lowering cholesterol after myocardial infarction. N. Engl. J. Med. 323: 1112 - 1119, 1990.

Sasahara, M. et al: Inhibition of hypercholesterolemia-induced atherosclerosis in the nonhuman primate by probucol. I. Is the extent of atherosclerosis related to resistance of LDL to oxidation? J. Clin. Invest., 1994; 94:155-164.

Scandinavian, J. et al: Randomised trial of cholesterol lowering in 4444 patients with coronary heart disease: the Scandinavian Simvastatin Survival Study (4S). Lancet, 1994; 344:1383-1389.

Schonfeld, G.: Inherited disorders of lipid transport.

Endocrinol. Metab. Clin. North Am., 1990; 19:229-257.

Second Report of the Expert Panel on Detection, Evaluation, and Treatment of High Blood cholesterol in Adults presenting the National Cholesterol Education Program's recommendation. Circulation 89: 1337-1445, 1994.

Sheu W.H.H., Shieh S.M., Shen D.D.C. et al: Effect of pravastatin treatment of glucose, insulin and lipoprotein metabolism in patients with hypercholesterolemia. Am. Heart J. 127; 331-336, 1994.

Silva J.M. and Silva P.S.,: Sexless HDL. Lancet 343: 129-130, 1994.

Smith D. and Pekkanen J.: For debate. Should there be a moratorium on the use of cholesterol lowering drugs? Br. med. J. 304: 431 - 443, 1992.

Steinberg, B. Lipoproteins and atherosclerosis. A look back and a look ahead. Atherosclerosis. 1983; 3:283.

Stampfer M.J., Charles H., Hennekens J., Ann E.M., Graham A.C., Bernard R. and Walter C.W.: Vitamin E consumption and the risk of coronary disease in women. N. Engl. J. med. 328: 1444- 1449, 1993.

Steinberg D.: Antioxidants and Atherosclerosis: A current assessment. Circulation 84: 1420-1425, 1991.

Steinberg D. (Editorial): Antioxidants, vitamins and coronary heart disease. N. Engl. J. Med. 328: 1487-1489, 1993.

Superko, H.R. et al: Coronary artery disease regression. Convincing evidence for the benefit of aggressive lipoprotein management. Circulation, 1994; 90:1056-1069.

Tan K., Betteridge D.J., Marmot M.G. et al: Hypertriglyceridaemia and vascular risk. Report of a meeting of physicians and scientists, University College London Medical School. Lancet 342: 781-787,1993.

Tobert J.A.: Cholesterol lowering and non-cardiac mortality (letter) Lancet 338: 126, 1991.

Tyroler, H.A. et al: Lowering plasma cholesterol levels decreases risk of coronary artery disease: An overview of clinical trials. In, Hypercholesterolemia and Atherosclerosis. Churchill Livingstone, New York, 1987; pp. 99-115.

Utermann, G.: Lipoprotein (a). In, The Metabolic and Molecular Bases of Inherited Disease, 7th ed. McGraw-Hill, New York, 1995; pp. 1887-1912.

Witztum, J.L. et al: Current approaches to drug therapy for the hypercholesterolemic patient. Circulation, 1989b, 80:1101-1114.

Witztum, J.L.: The oxidation hypothesis of athero-scle-rosis. Lancet, 1994; 344-793-795.

Witztum, J.L. et al: Disorders of lipoprotein metabolism. In, Cecil Textbook of Medicine, 20th edition. WB Saunders Co., Philadelphia, 1996; In press.

DRUG THERAPY OF VARIOUS TYPES OF SHOCK (Fig. 4.11)

Shock is a clinical state of acute circulatory failure. No matter what the cause of shock may be, the basic defect is a wide spread and serious reduction of perfusion of the vital organs. If it is not treated properly, it leads to generalized impairment of cellular function.

The hypoperfusion is precipitated by the decreased cardiac output. Besides decreased cardiac output, in majority of patients, low blood pressure is also a prominent accompaniment. However, shock may occur in the presence of normal or even raised blood pressure.

The real problem in shock is low blood flow (hypoperfusion) rather than low blood pressure.

The aims of drug treatment of shock is therefore (i) to restore tissue perfusion, (ii) to restore intravascular blood volume and (iii) early diagnosis of causative factors.

The management of shock is a kleidoscopic manoeuvring as there is no single approach that can be applied to all shock patients, e.g. hepatic shock is treated one way and cardiogenic shock another. The treatment depends on the pathogenesis of shock.

There is marked reduction in tissue perfusion. The anoxic tissues liberate vasodilators such as bradykinins, histamine and 5-HT. Due to anoxia and tissue acidosis the pressure within capillaries is increased (pre-capillary sphincter open widely, post-capillary sphincter is much less affected by anoxia), resulting in loss of plasma by exudation and circulating blood volume is further decreased. If the condition is not promptly and properly treated and ischaemic necrosis of small bowel mucous membrane occurs, shock becomes irreversible.

Cardiogenic shock may be myopathic (reduced systolic function):

- acute myocardial function, myocardial depression in septic shock;

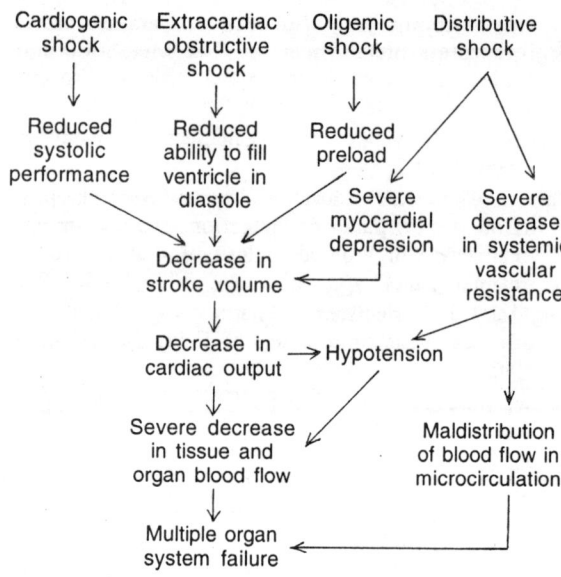

Fig. 4.11. Different types of shocks and their pathogenesis.

- may be mechanical due to mitral regurgitation, aortic stenosis etc.

Extracardiac obstructive shock may be due to constrictive pericarditis, pulmonary embolism, pulmonary hypertension.

Oligemic shock may be due to haemorrhage, fluid depletion secondary to vomiting, diarrhoea, burns.

Distributive shock includes septic shock, anaphylaxis, neurogenic shock, all of these usually cause a profound decrease in peripheral vascular resistance.

There are 5 main types of shock, viz.

1. Hypovolaemic
2. Cardiogenic (Acute myocardial infarction)
3. Septic
4. Anaphylactic shock
5. Neurogenic shock

1. Hypovolaemic shock

It is due to loss of fluids from vascular or extravascular compartment, after haemorrhage, burns, excessive vomiting or diarrhoea, and potent diuretics. If the loss of blood, plasma or water is not replaced, there is reduction in venous return and cardiac output.

The agent of choice is whole blood but if it is

not available, plasma or artificial plasma expanders should be used for fluid replacement. Any drug therapy in shock is secondary to the appropriate fluid replacement. The aim is to restore effective blood volume and correction of electrolyte imbalance.

Plasma Expanders

Plasma expanders are substances when infused intravenously retain fluid in the vascular compartment as they exert colloidal osmotic (oncotic) pressure.

The colloidal solutions are used as substitutes for plasma in conditions where plasma has been lost e.g., in burns, hypovolaemic and endotoxin shock; also used in cases of the whole blood loss till the same can be arranged. However, plasma expanders do not possess oxygen carrying capacity.

Contraindication

- Severe anaemia
- Cardiac failure
- Pulmonary oedema
- renal insufficiency

Human plasma would be ideal but it carries risk of transmitting serum hepatitis. The reconstituted human albumin is also best but it is expensive. Hence, synthetic high molecular weight substances are often employed.

Desirable plasma expanders should possess following properties

- Pharmacodynamically inert
- Stable, easily sterilizable and inexpensive
- Remain in circulation for adequate duration of time, not leak out in tissues
- Not rapidly disposed
- Osmotic pressure exerted comparable to that of plasma
- Should not have pyrogenic or antigenic/allergenic effect
- Without any adverse effect on any visceral function
- Should stand long periods of storage

Substances used as plasma expanders

- Human Albumin
- Dextran
- Degraded gelatin polymer
- Hydroxyethyl starch
- Polyvinylpyrrolidone (PVP)

Human Albumin

It is obtained from pooled human plasma; 100ml of 20% human albumin solution exerts osmotic pressure similar to that of 800ml of whole blood or 400 ml of fresh frozen plasma. Human Albumin is free of risk of transmitting serum hepatitis unlike whole blood or plasma. There is also no risk of sensitization. It is expensive.

20% solution is employed in burns, hypovolaemia, shock, acute hypoproteinemia and acute liver failure.

Dextran

Dextrans can be stored for several years. They are cheap and they are therefore most commonly employed.

Dextran (polysaccharide obtained from sugar beat) is available as (1) Dextran-70 (molecular weight 70,000), (2) Dextran-40 (molecular weight 40,000 low molecular weight dextran).

Dextran-70 expands plasma volume for about 24 hours. Six percent solution in dextrose or saline is used, whereas Dextran-40 10% solution is used in dextrose or saline.

Dextran-40 acts faster than dextran-70. It reduces blood viscosity, improves microcirculation, but rapidly filtered at the glomerulus and thus expands plasma volume for shorter time. It is a stable plasma expander but may produce platelet dysfunction bleeding tendency and acute renal failure.

Dextran fulfills the criteria of an ideal plasma expander except that :

- Dextran may interfere with blood grouping and cross matching.
- Dextran used clinically is not antigenic. But as its structure resembles to antigenic polysaccharides, therefore if some polysaccharide reacting antibodies are present in the patient (in sufficient quantity), they may react with dextran occasionally resulting in anaphylactic reaction (urticaria, fall in B.P. itching, bronchospasm). However, anaphylactic shock is rare.

• Dextran may interfere with coagulation and platelet function (prolong bleeding time).

Degraded Gelatin Polymer

The molecular weight is 30,000 that exerts colloidal (oncotic) similar to albumin. It is not antigenic, does not interfere with blood grouping and cross matching of blood. It remains stable for about 3 years.

It expands plasma volume for 12 hours. It is more expensive than dextran.

Hypersensitivity reactions (though rare) such as urticaria, rigor, fall in B.P., flushing may occur.

Hydroxyethyl starch

It is effective, cheap volume expander with fewer side effects. It is a complex mixture of ethoxylated amylopectin of various molecular sizes (range 10,000 to 1 million). Six percent of this substance has colloidal activity similar to that of human albumin.

Adverse effects include fever, chills, itching and swelling of salivary glands. Anaphylactic reactions (urticaria, bronchospasm) may also occur.

Polyvinylpyrrolidone (PVP)

It is a synthetic polymer of molecular weight 40,000. It is used as 3.5% solution in buffered normal saline. It is less used as plasma expander because it interferes with blood grouping and cross matching and is histamine releaser.

Vasopressors: After correction of volume deficit, infusion of adrenaline, noradrenaline, metaraminol or mephentermine is used.

Vasopressor drugs are most effective in hypovolaemic shock which is not associated with decrease in blood volume e.g. shock associated with spinal anesthesia and neurogenic shock. In other cases, the reflex vasoconstriction is already so intense that use of vasoconstrictors will further decreases the blood flow. In such cases use of vasopressors is not advocated.

Vasodilators: On the basis of the concept, that the blood flow to the vital organs determines the survival in shock, rather than blood pressure, alpha-adrenergic blockers have been advocated, their I.V. infusion diminish vasoconstriction and improve tissue perfusion.

They produce 3 important beneficial cardiovascular effects, viz.

1. Increase cardiac output and total circulating volume.
2. Induce local redistribution of blood flow so that larger amount passes through channels that exchange metabolites with tissue cells.
3. Reverse the vasoconstriction induced shift of fluid from vascular to interstitial compartment.

Alpha-blockers reduce the extreme vasoconstriction produced by the reflex overactivity of sympathetic nervous system and thus remove the harmful effects of vasoconstriction on microcirculation and permit rapid administration of I.V. fluid without increasing the central venous pressure.

Phenoxybenzamine, 1 mg/kg/slow I.V. infusion well diluted in 500 ml 5% dextrose solution may be administered for this purpose.

Phentolamine has shorter duration of action, and regitine effect lasts only for half an hour.

Caution: Alpha-adrenergic blocker should follow adequate replacement of fluid volume. There may be precipitous fall of blood pressure.

Corticosteroids: Some investigators do not find convincing evidence of their efficacy in shock, while others often advocate their use. The point for emphasis is that higher doses should be employed to produce pharmacological effect rather than physiological effect. In high doses glucocorticoids decrease peripheral resistance and produce positive inotropic effect resulting in improvement of tissue perfusion.

Glucocorticoids are likely to be beneficial as:
• They restore or enhance effects of vasopressors
• Inhibit histamine synthesis and correct the abnormal permeability of endothelium
• Stabilize lysosome membranes and
• Reduce platelet adhesiveness

Glucocorticoids are of proved volume in anaphylactic shock. In septic shock, they decrease the sensitivity to endotoxins but may increase susceptibility to infection.

2. Acute myocardial infarction (cardiogenic shock)

The commonest cause of cardiogenic shock is myocardial infarction.

Acute myocardial infarction (MI) is a serious medical emergency due to sudden coronary occlusion resulting in ischaemic necrosis of some area in the myocardium. The main impact is on the left ventricular function. The patient suffers from cardiogenic shock characterized by severe, persisting precordial pain, shock, hypotension and feeling of impending death. These symptoms unlike angina do not disappear after rest and if not properly treated cardiac arrhythmias may also develop.

The pharmacologic approaches for the treatment of MI are:

1. During initial stage

(a) Potent pain relievers such as morphine sulphate 4-8 mg injection repeated frequently or pethidine HCl 75-100 mg I.V. or pentazocine.
Sedative anxiolytics such as diazepam 2-5 mg given 2-3 times a day or nitrazepam.

(b) Oxygen inhalation for 2-3 days to counteract hypoxia and strict bed rest for 6-8 weeks after MI when infarct size is reduced.

(c) Blood pressure should be maintained enough to restore perfusion of vital organs. But the B.P. should not be raised so high that myocardial oxygen demand is increased.
To maintain blood pressure in severe hypotension, dopamine HCl 200 mg in 5% glucose solution by I.V. drip at a rate of 2.5 mcg/kg/min is given which increases myocardial contractility without affecting heart rate. It dilates renal and mesenteric vascular beds which helps to maintain blood volume, tissue perfusion and microcirculation. Dobutamine is also suitable as it has positive inotropic effect along with modest peripheral vasoconstriction. If beneficial effect is not produced then hydrocortisone hemisuccinate 200 mg I.V. is recommended. It protects tissues against damaging effects of hypoxia, in a nonspecific manner.

(d) In case of acidosis, sodium bicarbonate by I.V. drip or other alternative alkalizing agents are employed to correct metabolic acidosis.

2. Steps for treating left ventricular failure (low cardiac output failure or forward L.V. failure)

Drugs which reduce afterload are useful. These are prazosin or sodium nitroprusside, or hydralazine with dopamine or dobutamine.

3. For backward left ventricular failure with pulmonary congestion

Drugs which reduce cardiac preload are useful. Glyceryl trinitrate reduces preload. I.V. infusion of glyceryl trinitrate in patients with acute myocardial infarction with doses which maintain or improve stroke work of the heart relieves pulmonary congestion, by decreasing the left ventricular filling pressure and also by decreasing the myocardial oxygen demand. I.V. glyceryl trinitrate has also been reported to decrease the size of the affected zone in case of inferior infarcts but without such effect on patients with anterior infarcts.

These findings are based on few studies and convincing results of other similar studies will help to show the utility of organic nitrates in myocardial infarction.

4. Prevention and treatment of arrhythmias

- Tachyarrhythmias: I.V. lidocaine, procainamide or disopyramide.
- Ventricular fibrillation: Cardioversion
- Bradycardia and heart block: Atropine, artificial pacemaker if complete heart block is present.
- Supraventricular arrhythmias in the absence of LV failure: I.V. verapamil or I.V. propranolol.
- Supraventricular arrhythmias in the presence of LV failure: I.V. digoxin, followed by digoxin orally with verapamil.

5. Prevention of extension of thrombus

The incidence of thrombo-embolic complications may thus be reduced.

Heparin followed by oral anticoagulants have been employed. Low doses of heparin provides primary prophylaxis against thrombolism after myocardial infarction. Regarding the use of oral anticoagulants, there are controversial reports. There is lack of data to indicate their definite usefulness for this purpose. They are being used by several physicians in the hope that the risk of recurrent myocardial infarction will become less.

Drugs used in the treatment of coronary artery Thrombosis

Streptokinase, urokinase and tissue-type plasminogen activator (t-PA) are available for i.v. administration in the treatment of coronary artery thrombosis associated with myocardial infarction.

These facilitate conversion of plasminogen to plasmin. Plasmin is fibrinolytic.

As t-PA is more selective than kinases, it has high affinity for fibrin and induces the degradation of plasminogen to plasmin only in the presence of fibrin.

The plasma half-life of t-PA is five minutes, for urokinase 16 minutes and 23 minutes for streptokinase.

Uses

- t-PA and streptokinase have comparable efficacy in reducing mortality and improvement of left ventricular function.
- Streptokinase is most effective when given less than three hours after the onset of symptoms. It is given by intravenous or intracoronary infusion.
- Urokinase is infused into occluded coronary artery.
- t-PA is given by intravenous route only.

Adverse effects and contraindication:

- Serious bleeding may occur, most important, gastrointestinal and intracranial haemorrhages are possible.
- Streptokinase can cause anaphylaxis.
- With any throbolytic agent, cardiac arrhythmias can occur upon reperfusion of the occluded vessels.
- Contraindications include internal bleeding, cerebral vascular accidents, recent intracranial or intraspinal trauma, recent surgery, known bleeding diathesis or severe uncontrolled hypertension.

6. Limitation of infarct size and secondary prevention

To prevent reinfarction in patients who have had myocardial infarction i.e. future attacks; platelet antiaggregatory drugs such as aspirin 75 mg once a day or dipyridamole 50-100 mg thrice a day.

Aspirin in low doses has potent and long lasting effect on platelet function. Due to this effect aspirin can be useful for prophylaxis or treatment of diseases such as CAD, M.I. and postoperative deep-vein thrombosis, which are associated with platelet hyperaggregability. The emphasis is on low doses 75-100 mg per day. Aspirin in low doses selectively inhibits TXA_2 synthesis so the platelet aggregation is inhibited for long time, 1 to 2 weeks.

This long lasting effect is because platelets do not have nucleus and in the absence of DNA, new enzyme can not be synthesized and it takes time for new platelets to be derived from marrow megakaryocytes.

Aspirin in high doses, 900 mg/d inhibits cyclo-oxygenase and therefore TXA_2 and PGI_2 are both inhibited and the net effect is quite small. But in low doses selectively inhibits TXA_2 synthesis.

The low doses of aspirin with or without dipyridamole benefit transient cerebral ischaemic attacks but do not prevent thrombotic stroke.

There is also no clear indication that these drugs which have platelet antiaggregating action have any effectiveness in primary prevention or prophylactic role in ischaemic heart disease.

Dipyridamole 100 to 200 mg twice a day inhibits platelet aggregation. It is given alone or with aspirin.

Sulphinpyrazone, 200 mg four times a day reduces platelet adhesions and also has some antiarrhythmic action. However, it does not have selective inhibitory effect on TXA_2 synthesis.

Beta-adrenergic blockers such as propranolol, metoprolol, timolol or oxprenolol may reduce incidence of reinfarction and death after MI as they reduce cardiac work and myocardial oxygen demand. The infarct size is also reduced.

7. Antihyperlipidaemic agents

Their role has been a controversial issue. However, according to the studies conducted by the Lipid

Research Clinics Coronary Prevention Trial in 1984, the risk of CAD is decreased by lowering the plasma levels of low density lipoprotein-cholesterol.

3. Septic shock (septicaemic shock, endotoxic shock)

The endotoxins are liberated, venous return and cardiac output are decreased.

Treatment

- Appropriate antibiotic therapy is promptly instituted. Septic shock occurs usually when a person is suffering from Gram negative microorganisms and less commonly during the course of Gram positive bacterial infections.
- Adequate circulatory volume should be maintained.
- Correction of acid-base balance is important by sodium bicarbonate or molar lactate.
- Blood pressure should be raised and maintained at respectable level but not excessive, by administration of sympathomimetics. If noradrenaline is given then it should be only for a short time, isoprenaline can be given. Dopamine is generally employed.
- Adequate oxygenation is required.
- Corticosteroids in large doses are given to suppress systemic reactions to endotoxins.

4. Anaphylactic shock

It is severe, wide spread and life threatening hypersensitivity reaction. Tl.ere is marked vasodilatation resulting in precipitous fall in blood pressure and severe bronchospasm with increased capillary permeability.

It may be (i) immediate due to circulating antibodies or (ii) delayed due to cell bound antibodies.

Drugs to combat anaphylactic shock

- Adrenaline HCl 0.5 ml 1 : 1000 solution, I.M. or 0.1 ml 1 : 1000 diluted in 10 ml saline I.V. injection.
- Oxygen inhalation to antagonize hypoxia.
- In case of severe vasomotor collapse, dopamine HCl 200 mg in 5% glucose saline I.V. drip at the rate of 2.5 mcg/kg/min.
- Corticosteroids (hydrocortisone 200 mg I.V.).

5. Neurogenic shock

In this condition, there is paralysis of sympathetic vasoconstriction mechanism resulting in hypotension, e.g. in spinal anaesthesia, spinal cord injury, acute barbiturate poisoning, abdominal injury and perforation of hollow viscus.

The treatment is similar to that given for hypovolaemic shock, with dopamine.

STUDY QUESTIONS

1. What are the different types of shock? What may be the causes of shock? What is the main defect produced due to shock?
2. Describe the mechanism of shock.
3. What are the aims of treatment in general for the treatment of shock?
4. What may cause hypovolaemic shock? Describe the agent of choice and if that is not available, what are the merits and demerits of plasma expanders? Describe dextrans.
5. Discuss the role of vasopressors as well as vasodilators in the treatment of shock.
6. Discuss the role of dopamine and corticosteroids in shock.
7. How is septic shock treated?
8. What are the characteristics of anaphylactic shock? Which drug is notorious to produce this kind of shock? How is it treated?
9. What is the drug therapy of neurogenic shock?
10. What is the commonest cause of cardiogenic shock? What is the mechanism of this type of shock? Describe the pharmacologic approach during initial stage as well as steps for treating forward or backward left ventricular failure and prevention or treatment of arrhythmias.
11. Describe drugs which are given to limit the infarct size in MI and for the prevention of future attacks.
12. Explain why only low doses of aspirin are effective as platelet antiaggregatory agent. What are other drugs used for the same purpose?

GUIDE TO FURTHER READING

Barach, E.M. et al: Epinephrine for treatment of anaphylactic shock. JAMA 1984; 251:2118.

Ruffolo, R.R. Jr: Fundamentals of receptor theory: Basics for shock research. Circ Shock, 1992; 37:176.

Bone, R.C. et al: A Controlled clinical trial of high-dose methylprednisolone in the treatment of severe sepsis and septic shock. N. Engl. J. Med., 317; 653:1987.

Connors, A.F. et al: Evaluation of right-heart catheterization in the critically ill patient without acute myocardial infarction. N. Engl. J. Med., 308; 263:1983.

Ellrodt, A.G. et al: Left ventricular performance in septic shock: Reversible segmental and global abnormalities. Am. Heart J, 110:402, 1985.

Guyton, A.C. et al: Local control of blood flow by the tissues; and nervous and humoral regulation, in Human Physiology and Mechanisms of Disease, 3rd ed. Philadelphia, Saunders, 1982; pp. 161-169.

Guyton, A.C. et al: Cardiac output and circulatory shock, in Human Physiology and Mechanisms of Disease, 3rd ed. Philadelphia, Saunders, 1982; pp. 187-200.

Natanson, C. et al: Gram negative bacteremia produces both severe systolic and diastolic cardiac dysfunction in a canine model that stimulates human septic shock. J Clin Invest, 77:259; 1986.

Ognibene, F.P. et al: Neutrophil aggregation activity and septic shock in humans: Neutrophil aggregation by a C5a-like material occurs more frequently than complement component depletion and correlates with depression of systemic vascular resistance. J Crit Care 3:103, 1988.

Ognibene, F.P. et al: Depressed left ventricular performance in response to volume infusion in patients with sepsis and septic shock. Chest, 93:903, 1988.

Parker, M.M. et al: Septic shock in humans: Clinical evaluation, pathogenesis, and therapeutic approach, in Textbook of Critical Care, 2 d ed, W.C. Shoemaker et al (eds). Philadelphia, Saunders, 1989, pp 1006-1023.

Parrillo, J.E. et al: A circulating myocardial depressant substance in humans with septic shock: Septic shock patients with a reduced ejection fraction have a circulating factor that depresses in vitro myocardial cell performance. J. Clin. Invest., 76:1539, 1985.

Rock, P. et al: Efficacy and safety of naloxone in septic shock. Crit Care Med 13:28, 1985.

Scharer, G.L. et al: Norepinephrine alone versus norepinephrine plus low-dose dopamine: Enhanced renal blood flow with combination pressor therapy. Crit Care Med 13:492, 1985.

Ziegler, E.J. et al: Treatment of gram-negative bacteremia and shock with human antiserum to a mutant Escherichia coli. N Engl J Med 307:1225, 1982.

Drugs Acting on the Kidney

Terminology associated with Renal System

Dysuria	Painful urination
Enuresis (nocturia)	Bed-wetting; involuntary passage of urine, usually occuring at night or during sleep
Polyurea	Excessive urine formation
Uraemia	Toxic levels of urea in the blood resulting from severe malfuncting kidneys

FUNCTIONS OF KIDNEY

The functional unit of the kidney is the nephron.

Functions of different parts of nephron are as following:

- Proximal convoluted tubule
  - Reabsorption of water, Na^+, Cl^-, $NaHCO_3$, glucose, amino acids
  - Excretion of uric acid, acetates, phosphates, thiazides, furosemide, probenecid, indomethacin, penicillin, morphine, atropine, procainamide, creatinine
  - Plays role in regulatory mechanism of Na^+/K^+ ATPase

- Loop of Henle
  - Thin ascending limb concerned with reabsorption of water.
  - Thick ascending limb (medulla): reabsorption of Na^+, K^+, Cl^-, Mg^{2+}. This part plays regulatory role in Na^+, K^+, Cl^- co-transport system.
  - Cortical diluting segment: reabsorption of Na^+ Cl^- and plays role in regulatory mechanism of Na^+/K^+ ATPase, carbonic anhydrase.

- Distal convoluted tubule
  - Reabsorption of Na^+, Cl^-, HCO^-_3, Ca^{2+}
  - Excretion of K^+, H^+, NH_3, phosphate
  - Regulatory mechanism: Aldosterone, parathormone, angiotensin II

- Collecting tubule and duct
  - Reabsorption of Na^+, Cl^-, water
  - Excretion of K^+, H^+, NH_3
  - Regulatory mechanism: Aldosterone, Antidiuretic hormone

OEDEMA

There is an abnormal accumulation of fluid in the body. Oedema may result due to several causes, particularly due to kidney, heart and liver diseases. There is no general treatment which will suit every case. The particular cause, in each case, has to be removed.

The treatment of oedema consists of :

1. Correction of underlying cause i.e. malnutrition, hepatic, cardiac and renal diseases.
2. Salt restricted diet
3. Diuretic therapy

Diuretics are drugs that increase the rate of urine flow; however, clinically beneficial diuretics also increase the rate of excretion of Na^+ (natriuresis) and an accompanying anion, usually Cl^-. Diuretics not only alter the excretion of Na^+, but also may modify renal handling of other cations, e.g., K^+, H^+, Ca^{++}, Mg^{++}; and anions, e.g. Cl^-, HCO_3^-, $H_2PO_4^-$ and uric acid.

These act in two ways, viz.

1. By increasing the renal blood flow and glomerular filtration rate, e.g. cardiac glycosides, xanthines, plasma volume expanders and dopamine. These are not conventional diuretics.
2. By augmenting solute excretion in the glomerular filtrate and tubular fluid, e.g. osmotic diuretics and drugs which inhibit sodium reabsorption from the glomerular filtrate.

Diuretics can be classified based on mechanism of action as:

- Osmotic diuretics (agents that enhance water excretion): mannitol, urea, sucrose.

- Acidifying and alkalinizing salts: ammonium chloride, potassium citrate, potassium acetate.
- Mercurials: mersalyl
- Xanthines: theophylline
- Carbonic anhydrase inhibitors: acetazolamide
- Thiazides
- High ceiling diuretics: furosemide, ethacrynic acid
- Potassium sparing diuretics: spironolactone, amiloride

Sites of action	Diuretics
Proximal tubule	Carbonic anhydrase inhibitors, osmotic diuretics, xanthines
Ascending loop of Henle medullary portion	Loop diuretics (furosemide, ethacrynic acid), mercurials
Ascending limb of loop cortical part	Thiazides, mercurials
Distal tubule and collecting duct	Spironolactone

The anatomy and nomenclature of nephron are shown in Fig. 5.1.

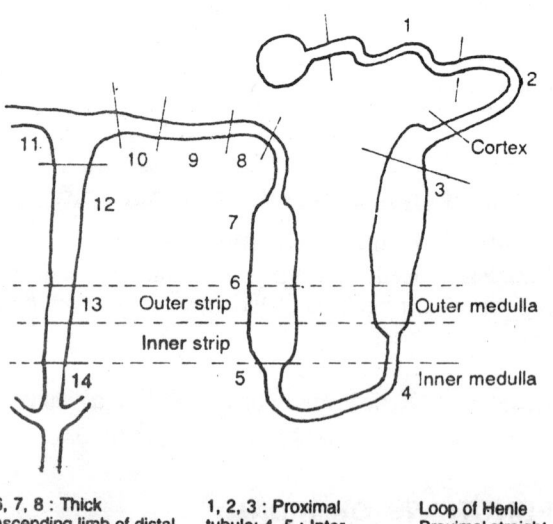

6, 7, 8 : Thick ascending limb of distal straight tubule; 8, 9 : Early distal tubule; 10, 11 : Late distal tubule; 12, 13, 14 : Collecting duct.

1, 2, 3 : Proximal tubule; 4, 5 : Intermediate tubule; 6, 7, 8, 9 : Distal tubule; 10, 11, 12, 13, 14 : Collecting system.

Loop of Henle Proximal straight tubule 3 to distal tubule 8 Distal convolution

Fig. 5.1. Anatomy and nomenclature of nephron.

Box 5.1. Mechanism of oedema formation

Increased blood hydrostatic pressure	Decreased plasma proteins	Increased capillary permeability	Increased extracellular fluid volume coupled with fluid retention

OEDEMA

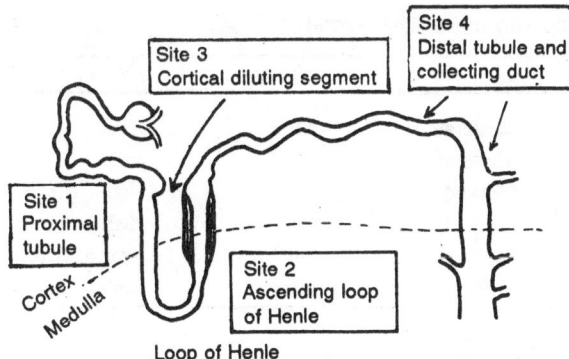

Fig. 5.2. Sites of action of different diuretics.

The sites of action of different diuretics are shown in Fig. 5.2.

Diuretics can also be grouped as following:

1. High efficacy diuretics e.g. furosemide which act at ascending loop of Henle (medullary portion).
2. Medium efficacy diuretics e.g. thiazides which act at ascending loop of Henle (cortical part).
3. Weak diuretics e.g. carbonic anhydrase inhibitors, potassium sparing diuretics, xanthines, osmotic diuretics, acidifying and alkalinizing diuretics which act at proximal tubule, distal tubule and collecting duct.

OSMOTIC DIURETICS

The commonly used osmotic diuretics are glycerin, isosorbide, mannitol, and urea. These agents are freely filtered at the glomerulus, their reabsorption by the renal tubule is limited and they are relatively inert pharmacologically. They increase significantly osmolality of plasma and tubular fluid.

Box 5.2. Some urinary alkalinizers and acidifiers	
Urinary alkalinizers	*Urinary acidifiers*
Potassium citrate	Ascorbic acid
Sodium citrate	Ammonium chloride
Sodium bicarbonate	Calcium chloride
Sodium acetate	Phenylbutazone
Acetazolamide	Sodium acid phosphate

Mechanism

Osmotic diuretics by extracting water from intracellular compartments expand extracellular fluid volume, decrease bold viscosity, and inhibit renin release.

Osmotic diuretics act both in the proximal tubule and the loop of Henle, the latter is the primary site of action.

Osmotic diuretics increase urinary excretion of nearly all electrolytes, Na^+, K^+, Ca^{++}, Mg^{++}, Cl^-, HCO_3 and PO_4^-.

Table 5.1 shows effect of some diuretics on electrolyte excretion.

Table 5.2 gives the oral availability, half-life and route of elimination of the four currently available osmotic diuretics.

Uses

- To control intraocular pressure (IOP) during acute attacks of glaucoma.
- For short-term reduction in IOP, preoperatively as well as postoperatively in patients who require ocular surgery.
- To reduce cerebral oedema of brain mass before and after neurosurgery.
- The osmotic diuretics are not used to mobilize oedema fluid as they produce minimal effect on the excretion of electrolytes. They are used to lower intracranial and intraocular pressure.
- Mannitol 15-20% solution, 50-100 ml is given intravenously (not absorbed orally). Urea orally or intravenously can be given. Orally urea has unpleasant taste and may produce nausea and vomiting. It can precipitate pulmonary oedema. Mannitol should not be administered intramuscularly or subcutaneously, or added to whole blood for transfusion (increased osmotic pressure will cause crenation and agglutination of red blood cells). Solutions of Mannitol should be infused using an in-line filter. Mannitol has a tendency to crystallize. If crystals are apparent, the solution should be warmed to 70 degrees centigrade and then cooled to room temperature before administration.
- Urea and sucrose are now no more preferred.

Table 5.1. Effect of different diuretics on electrolyte excretion

Diuretics	Na+	K+	Cl-	HCO3-	Efficacy
Osmotic diuretics	Moderate	Moderate	Moderate	Mild	Low
CAI (diamox)	Moderate	Moderate	Moderate	Mild	Mild
Furosemide	Marked	Marked	Marked	Nil	High
Ethacrynic acid	Marked	Marked	Marked	Nil	High
Thiazides	Moderate	Moderate	Moderate	Nil	Intermediate
K-sparing	Mild	Retains	Mild	Nil	Low

Table 5.2. Oral availability, half-life and route of elimination of osmotic diuretics

Drug	Oral absorption	Half-life (hours)	Route of elimination
Glycerin	Orally active	0.5-0.75	Metabolism
Isosorbide	Orally active	5-10	Renal excretion of intact drug
Mannitol	Very little	0.25-1.7*	Renal excretion of intact drug
Urea	Very little	Insufficient data	Renal excretion of intact drug

* In renal failure 6-36 hours

The usual dose of mannitol to reduce intraocular pressure is 1.5 to 2 grams/kilogram intravenously over 30 to 60 minutes as a 15% to 20% solution.

Mannitol infusion may be discontinued when adequate reduction of intraocular pressure is accomplished. Usually 1 gram/kilogram is sufficient, and effects will last for 6 to 8 hours.

Adverse effects

- As water is extracted from intracellular compartments, and the extracellular fluid volume gets expanded, this may cause pulmonary oedema in patients with heart failure or pulmonary congestion.
- Extraction of water also causes hyponatraemia resulting in headache, nausea and vomiting.
- Urea may cause thrombosis if extravasation occurs.

Contraindications

- Patients who are anuric.
- Glycerin is metabolised and can cause hyperglycaemia.
- Mannitol and urea are contraindicated in patients with active cranial bleeding.

- Urea is contraindicated in case of impaired renal function (risk of elevation of blood ammonia levels).

CARBONIC ANHYDRASE INHIBITORS

Acetazolamide (diamox)

The inhibition of carbonic anhydrase is associated with a rapid rise in urinary HCO_3^- excretion.

Carbonic anhydrase is present in a number of extrarenal tissues including the eye, gastric mucosa, pancreas, CNS and red blood cells.

Carbonic anhydrase in the ciliary processes of the eye mediates the formation of large amounts of HCO_3^- in aqueous humour. Due to inhibition of carbonic anhydrase, carbonic anhydrase inhibitors decrease the formation of aqueous humour and consequently reduce IOP.

The efficacy of acetazolamide in epilepsy is in part due to the production of metabolic acidosis. However, its direct actions in the CNS also contribute to its anticonvulsant action.

The oral bioavailability, plasma half-life and routes of elimination of certain carbonic anhydrase inhibitors are listed in Table 5.3.

Acetazolamide and ethoxzolamide act on proximal tubule and inhibit carbonic anhydrase enzyme.

Table 5.3. Inhibitors of carbonic anhydrase (primary site of action is proximal tubule)

Drug	Relative potency	Oral absorption	Half-life in hours	Route of elimination
Acetazolamide	1	Almost complete	6-9	Renal excretion of intact drug
Dichlorphenamide	30	Good	Insufficient data	
Methazolamide	> 1 < 10	Almost complete	14	25% renal excretion of intact drug, 75% metabolism

They produce excretion of HCO_3^-, Na^+ and K^+. They are weak diuretics.

Dose of diamox is 250 mg, orally once daily or every other day as a diuretic.

Carbonic anhydrase Inhibitors thus block sodium bicarbonate reabsorption causing sodium bicarbonate diuresis.

It is also used to lower the intraocular pressure as carbonic anhydrase is essential for the production of aqueous humour. For use in glaucoma, it is given orally 2-4 times a day.

Carbonic anhydrase inhibitors have some beneficial effect in petit mal epilepsy (how, is not clear).

These may be used to alkalinize the urine e.g. in the treatment of salicylate or barbiturate poisoning.

Adverse effects

Adverse effects are not common, some patients complain of headache, drowsiness, dizziness and fatigue. Diamox way depress bone marrow rarely but if it occurs it may produce leukopaenia, agranulocytosis, aplastic anaemia which is a serious matter.

Contraindications

Liver disease, hepatic coma may be precipitated.

Xanthines

Theophylline, aminophylline which act on proximal tubules, inhibit reabsorption of Na^+ and produce mild transient diuresis.

Dose: 250-500 mg I.V. slowly.

THIAZIDES AND THIAZIDE-LIKE DIURETICS

These inhibit Na^+-Cl^- symporter, perhaps by competing for the Cl^- binding site and thus there is increased Na^+ and Cl^- excretion.

They are moderately efficacious.

The relative potency, oral bioavailability, plasma half-life and route of elimination of thiazides and thiazide-like diuretics are listed in Table 5.4.

Chlorothiazide, hydrochlorothiazide, flumethiazide, hydroflumethiazide interfere with the reabsorption of salt and water. They increase excretion of Na^+ and K^+. They mainly inhibit Na^+ reabsorption.

Table 5.4. Thiazide and thiazide-like diuretics

Drug	Relative potency	Oral absorption	Half-life in hours	Route of elimination
Bendroflumethiazide	10	Almost complete	3-4	30% renal excretion of intact drug, 70% metabolism
Benzthiazide	1	Incomplete data	Incomplete data	Incomplete data
Chlorothiazide	0.1	10-20%	1.5	Renal excretion of intact drug
Hydrochlorothiazide	1	65-75%	2.5	Renal excretion of intact drug
Hydroflumethiazide	1	50%	12-27	40-80% renal excretion of intact drug, 20-60% metabolism
Polythiazide	25	Almost complete	25	25% renal excretion of intact drug; 75% unknown pathway of elimination
Chlorthalidone	1	60-70%	44	60% Renal excretion of intact drug, 10% excretion of intact drug into bile; 25% unknown pathway of elimination

They act at cortical portion of loop of Henle (at origin of distal tubule).

Uses

- Oedema associated with heart (CHF), liver (hepatic cirrhosis) and renal (nephrotic syndrome, chronic renal failure, acute glomerulonephritis) disease and for oedema caused by corticosteroid therapy.
- Hypertension either alone or in combination with other antihypertensive drugs.
- Nephrogenic diabetes insipidus reduces urine volume up to 50%).
- Management of bromide intoxication (as other halides are excreted by renal processes similar to those for Cl^-).
- Calcium nephrolithiasis (thiazide diuretics reduce urinary excretion of Ca^{++}).

Adverse effects

- Adverse effects include hypercalcaemia (due to Ca retention), hyperuricaemia (as urinary excretion of uric acid is decreased), hyperglycaemia (due to suppression of insulin), uric acid retention and excess loss of K^+.
- Thiazide diuretics rarely cause CNS (headache, vertigo), gastrointestinal (nausea, vomiting, diarrhoea, constipation), sexual (impotence and reduced libido), haematological and dermatological (skin rashes) disorders. However, serious adverse effects are related to abnormalities of fluid and electrolyte balance including extracellular volume depletion, hypotension, hyperkalaemia, hyponatraemia, metabolic alkalosis, hypermagnesemia, hypercalcaemia and hyperurecemia.
- Chlorthalidone (thiazide congener) is similar to thiazides with more prolonged effect.

Dose: 50-100 mg. It is twice as potent as chlorothiazide and duration of action is for 48 hours.

Mercurial diuretics

Calomel, mersalyl, thiomerin, mercumatilin, meralluride are organic mercurial diuretics which are no longer used due to their high toxicity and can be considered of historical interest. These have been replaced by better drugs. They primarily inhibit Cl^- reabsorption, mainly act on ascending limb of Henle. They are contraindicated in kidney diseases. The only use appears to be refractory cases of cardiac oedema.

In an acidic environment mercuric ion (Hg^{2+}) dissociates so reabsorption of Na^+ is reduced and excretion of Na^+ and Cl^- is increased. More Cl^- ion than Na^+ is lost.

In an alkaline environment, Hg^{2+} does not dissociate to take an active form so patients become refractory to the mercurials in about seven days. However, an acidifying agent, such as ammonium chloride can be combined with the mercurial diuretic which creates metabolic acidosis, counteracting the metabolic alkalosis which will combat refractoriness.

LOOP DIURETICS

Loop diuretics (high ceiling diuretics) with a 'ceiling' of diuresis much higher than that of the thiazides are frusemide or furosemide (lasix), and Ethacrynic acid. Loop diuretics selectively inhibit NaCl reabsorption in the thick ascending limb of the loop of Henle. The two prototypical drugs of this group are furosemide and ethacrynic acid.

Table 5.5 shows some characteristics of loop diuretics.

These have an ability to block Na^+-K^+-$2Cl^-$ symporter in the thick ascending limb of Henle (so referred as loop diuretics). The inhibitors of Na^+-K^+-$2Cl^-$ symport are very potent and for this reason they are often called high ceiling diuretics.

The loop diuretics are a chemically diverse group of drugs. These drugs attach to the Cl binding site of the symporter. They also inhibit Ca^{++} and Mg^{++} reabsorption in the thick ascending limb.

Loop diuretics cause a profound increase in the urinary excretion of Na^+ and Cl^-.

The relative potency, oral absorption, half-life and route of elimination of loop diuretics are listed in Table 5.5.

The dosage of certain loop diuretics are given below:

- Furosemide 20-80 mg daily as single dose or in 2 divided doses.
- Bumetanide: 0.5-2 mg once a day (40 times potent).

Table 5.5. Loop diuretics, high-ceiling diuretics (primary site of action is thick ascending limb)

Drug	Relative potency	Oral absorption	Half-life in hours	Route of elimination
Furosemide	1	10-90%	0.3-3.5	60% renal excretion of intact drug, 40% metabolism
Bumetanide	40	58-90%	0.3-1.5	65% renal excretion of intact drug, 35% metabolism
Ethacrynic acid	0.7	Almost complete	0.5-1	60% renal excretion of intact drug, 35% metabolism
Torsemide	3	78-90%	0.8-6.0	30% renal excretion of intact drug, 70% metabolism

- Ethacrynic acid: 50-200 mg orally.
- Torsamide: 2.5-20 mg

Clinical applications

- Acute pulmonary oedema
- CHF
- Hypertension (in patients in whom other diuretics or antihypertensives do not produce satisfactory response)
- Oedema of nephrotic syndrome
- Oedema of ascites of liver cirrhosis
- Hyponatraemia (combined with hypertonic saline)
- Oedema associated with chronic renal insufficiency (combined with isotonic saline)
- To treat hypercalcemia
- To prevent volume depletion
- They are good for acute emergency conditions as their action is prompt and potent.

Adverse effects

The adverse effects are common and include hypokalaemic metabolic alkalosis, hyperglycaemia, hyperuricaemia, ototoxicity, nephrotoxicity, hypotension, allergic reactions.

Box 5.3. Conditions which lead to hyperkalemia

Patients at increased risk of developing hyperkalaemia
- Patients with renal failure
- Patients taking ACEs
- Patients taking K^+ supplements
- Patients receiving other K^+-sparing diuretics

Even NSAIDs can increase the likelihood of hyperkalaemia in patients receiving Na^+ channel inhibitors

---

Contraindications

Hepatic cirrhosis, borderline renal failure, or congestive heart failure.

K^+-SPARING DIURETICS

Potassium sparing or retaining diuretics are spironolactone, triamterene and amiloride.

Spironolactone antagonizes the effects of aldosterone at the cortical collecting tubule and late distal tubule. Spironolactone acts through direct pharmacological antagonism of mineralocorticoid receptors; whereas amiloride, and triamterene inhibit Na^+ transport through ion channels in the luminal membrane. The action of amiloride and triamterene is independent of aldosterone.

Spironolactone is usually given four times a daily. Dose is 25-200 mg. Duration of action is 3-5 days.

Triamterene (100-200 mg) is administered orally twice a day (duration of action is 8 to 12 days) and amiloride (50-100 mg) is given once daily (duration of action is 4 to 5 days).

These drugs cause excretion of Na^+ and retention of K^+. The site of action is distal tubule. These are relatively ineffective if given alone. Their chief use is to give them along with other diuretics to counter loss of K^+ and enhance excretion of Na^+.

As the late distal tubule and collecting duct have a limited capacity to reabsorb solutes, blockade of Na^+ channels at this site of nephrone produces only a small increase in the excretion rate of Na^+ and Cl^- (about 2% of the filtered load).

At higher doses amiloride also blocks Na^+-H^+ and Na^+-Ca^{++} antiporters and inhibits Na^+ pump.

The relative potency, oral absorption, half-life and route of elimination of K^+ sparing diuretics are given in Table 5.6.

Table 5.6. Inhibitors of renal epithelial Na^+ channels (primary site of action is late distal tubule and collecting duct)

Drug	Relative potency	Oral absorption	Half-life in hours	Route of elimination
Amiloride	1	15-25%	20	Renal excretion of intact drug
Triamterene	0.1	30-70%	4.2	Metabolism (Triamterene is transformed into an active metabolite which is excreted in the urine)
Mineralocorticoid receptor antagonist (aldosterone antagonist; K^+-sparing diuretics)				
Spironolactone		60-70%	1.5	Metabolism in liver; canrenone is active metabolite

Table 5.7. Adverse effects of diuretics

	Hyperglycaemia	Hyperuricaemia	Hypokalaemia	Ototoxicity	Ca excretion
Thiazide	+	+	+	–	Decreased
Ethacrynic acid	+	+	+	+	Increased
Furosemide	+	+	+	+	Increased
Bumetanide	+	+	+	+	Increased
Torsemide	+	+	+	+	Increased
Acetazolamide	–	–	+	–	×
Indapamide	+	+	+	–	Decreased

+ = side effect; – = no side effect; ′ = no effect

Table 5.7 gives adverse effects of certain diuretics.

Uses

- Seldom used as sole agents in the treatment of oedema or hypertension (due to mild natriuresis).
- Major utility is in combination with other diuretics.

Adverse effects

These include hyperkalaemia, mental confusion, benign prostatic hypertrophy, drowsiness, hirsutism, GI upsets, lethargy, ataxia, gynaecomastia and other adverse effects such as menstrual disorders and deepening of the voice (due to androgenic effects). Acute renal failure with combination of triamterene with indomethacin, and kidney stones with triamterene (which is poorly soluble) may be produced

Triamterene is metabolised to an active 4-hydroxytriamterene sulphate and this metabolite is excreted in urine, its activity is comparable to the parent drug hence toxicity of this drug may be increased in both hepatic disease (decreased metabolism) and renal failure (decreased urinary excretion of active metabolite).

Triamterene is a weak folic acid antagonist so cirrhotic patients are prone to megaloblastosis. Triamterene may also reduce glucose tolerance and induce photosensitisation and has been associated with interstial nephritis and renal stones (1 in every 200-250 cases of renal stones).

Spironolactone competitively inhibits the binding of aldosterone and block the biological effects of aldosterone (hence also called aldosterone antagonist).

Spironolactone is diuretic of choice in patients with hepatic cirrhosis.

Uses

- Coadministered with thiazides or loop diuretics in the treatment of oedema or hypertension (adrenal adenomas).
- Treatment of refractory oedema associated with secondary aldosteronism (cardiac failure, hepatic cirrhosis, severe ascites).

Drug interactions

- Potentiation of antihypertensives by thiazides and loop diuretics.
- Enhanced toxicity of digitalis, competitive neuromuscular blocking agents because of their hypokalaemic action.
- Enhanced ototoxicity of aminoglycosides when given with loop diuretics.
- Enhanced nephrotoxicity of first generation cephalosporins and aminoglycosides with loop diuretics.
- Decreased action of loop diuretics with NSAIDs especially indomethacin.
- Increased lithium toxicity with diuretics (due to increased reabsorption of lithium in proximal tubule. However amiloride and frusemide are useful in lithium overdosages.

Clinical applications of diuretic agents and choice

Oedematous states

Diuretics are used to reduce peripheral or pulmonary oedema due to diseases of the heart, kidney, vasculature, or abnormalities in the blood osmotic pressure.

1. Congestive heart failure: Oedema associated with congestive heart failure can be generally managed by loop diuretics. Sometimes combination of loop diuretics and thiazides is necessary.

   Hypokalaemia induced by diuretics in cardiac patient can exacerbate underlying cardiac arrhythmias and enhance digitalis toxicity and therefore this aspect must be kept in mind while giving diuretics to cardiac patient.

2. Kidney disease: If a patient has kidney disease acetazolamide should be avoided because of its tendency to exacerbate acidosis, and K^+-sparing diuretics should also not be given as they will exacerbate hyperkalaemia.

   Loop diuretics are the best choice in treating oedema associated with kidney failure.

   It is emphasized that overzealous use of diuretics can cause renal function to decline in all patients, particularly in patients having underlying kidney disease.

3. Hepatic cirrhosis: Cirrhotic patients are usually resistant to loop diuretics, and highly responsive to spironolactone. Combination of loop diuretics and K^+-sparing agent may be effective. However, overzealous diuretic therapy causes marked reduction in intravascular volume, hypokalaemia and metabolic alkalosis. Hepatorenal syndrome and hepatic encephalopathy may be dangerous consequences in cirrhotic patients.

4. Idiopathic oedema: It should be controlled by mild salt restriction alone if possible rather than by diuretic agents.

Nonoedematous states

1. Hypertension

Diuretic and mild vasodilator actions of the thiazides are useful in the treatment of mild essential hypertension. Diuretics play an important role in patients who need multiple drugs to manage their blood pressure. Diuretics increase the efficacy of angiotensin-converting enzyme inhibitors. If powerful vasodilators such as hydralazine are used they usually require simultaneous use of diuretics to avoid volume retention and oedema.

2. Nephrolithiasis

Most of the renal stones contain calcium phosphate or calcium oxalate and may cause hypercalcuria due to a renal 'leak' of calcium. Calcium stones are also formed due to an increased intestinal absorption of calcium. In such cases also thiazides are effective as adjunctive therapy with other measures. It can be treated with thiazide diuretics which reduces urinary calcium concentration by increasing calcium reabsorption in the distant convoluted tubules.

3. Hypercalcaemia

Loop of Henle is the main site of absorption of calcium, loop diuretics and saline administration simultaneously will produce calcium diuresis.

4. Diabetes insipidus

Thiazide diuretics can reduce polyuria and polydipsia (appears paradoxical) in patients who do not respond to antidiuretic hormone; the effect is mediated through plasma volume reduction, enhanced proximal reabsorption of NaCl and water, and decreased delivery of fluid to the diluting segments. In this way the volume of dilute urine is reduced.

Diuretic Combinations

Loop diuretics and thiazides in combination will often produce diuresis which is more than an additive diuretic response. This combination can mobilize large amounts of fluid, even in patients who may have been refractory to single agent.

Potassium-sparing diuretics and loop diuretics or thiazides: The hypokalaemia induced by loop diuretics and thiazide diuretics can be prevented by the addition of a potassium-sparing diuretic. This combination is indicated if the hypokalaemia can not be managed with dietary salt restriction which will limit sodium delivery to the collecting tubule or with potassium chloride supplements. Combination of loop agent or thiazide diuretic with K-sparing diuretic is fairly safe. However, it should be avoided in the presence of renal insufficiency which may develop severe hyperkalaemia due to K-sparing diuretics.

Antidiuretics

These are agents that reduce urine volume which are primarily used in diabetes insipidus.

These drugs are:
- Antidiuretic hormone (ADH, Vasopressin);
- Thiazides and
- Other drugs such as chlorpropamide, clofibrate.

ADH (Antidiuretic hormone, vasopressin)

Vasopressin is a posterior pituitary peptide hormone. It is important mainly for its action on the kidney, but it is also a powerful vasoconstrictor. Its effects are initiated by two different types of receptors termed V_1 and V_2 - receptors.

Water retention (antidiuretic effect) is mediated through V_2 - receptor. It occurs at low plasma concentrations of vasopressin and involves activation of adenylate cyclase and increased production of cAMP in renal collecting ducts.

Vasoconstriction is mediated through V_1- receptors (2 types V_{1a} and V_{1b} are coupled to the phospholipid C/IP3 system), requires much higher concentrations of vasopressin and involves intracellular calcium mobilization. Vasopressin causes generalized vasoconstriction, including coeliac, mesenteric and coronary vessels. It also affects other smooth muscle e.g. gastrointestinal and uterine.

The contraction of smooth muscle by ADH, particularly in the CV system is by acting on V_{1a} - receptors. ADH promotes the release of corticotrophin from anterior pituitary by an action on V_{1b} - receptors. It tends to increase the concentration of factor VIII in the blood.

Preparations of ADH used and pharmacokinetic aspects

- Vasopressin (ADH) itself. It has short duration of action, weak selectivity for V_2 - receptors, usually given by SC or IM injection or by IV infusion. It is rapidly eliminated, plasma half-life is 10 minutes.
- Desmopressin. It has increased duration of action. It is V_2-selective and usually given as nasal spray. It has 12 times the diuretic action of ADH and 0.4% of its vasopressor activity. Its half-life is 75 minutes.
- Lypressin. It is similar in potency to vasopressin but is given as a nasal spray. It is rapidly eliminated. Its plasma, half-life is 10 minutes.
- Telipressin. It has increased duration of action, is V_1-selective and is given intravenously.
- Felypressin. It has short duration of action and is V_1-selective.

Therapeutic uses of vasopressin peptides

1. V_1-receptor mediated therapeutic applications :
   - Telipressin is used for GI contractions - postoperative ileus and abdominal distension - to expel gases before abdominal x-ray.
   - For oesophageal varices (emergency treatment) simultaneous administration of nitroglycerin and vasopressin to reverse cardiotoxic effects of vasopressin.
   - During surgery for portal hypertension.
   - Acute haemorrhagic gastritis

2. V_2-receptor mediated therapeutic applications :
   - Central diabetes insipidus - desmopressin (intranasal spray twice-a-day).
   - Bleeding disorders - Von Willibrand's disease, moderately severe haemophilia A, haemo-

static abnormality in uraemia.
- Primary nocturnal enuresis.
- Postlumbar puncture headache.

Adverse effects

If antidiuretic peptides are used intranasally in therapeutic doses, there are few adverse drug reactions. Nausea and abdominal cramps, and hypersensitivity reactions have been reported.

I.V. vasopressin may cause spasm of the coronary arteries and resultant angina and it frequently causes abdominal and uterine cramps.

Thiazides and other drugs

These decrease urine flow in diabetes insipidus (both renal and pituitary origin). They produce sustained electrolyte depletion.

Hydrochlorothiazide 25-50 mg thrice a day is more convenient though less effective than antidiuretic hormone.

Chlorpropamide may be given in diabetes insipidus of pituitary origin and not of renal origin like ADH. However, Hypoglycaemia limits its usefulness.

Clofibrate and carbamazepine reduce urine volume in diabetes insipidus of pituitary origin but their value in uncertain.

ADH antagonists

ADH antagonists are lithium salts and demeclocycline (tetracyline derivative). These inhibit the effects of antidiuretic hormone at the collecting tubule.

Serum levels of lithium must be monitored because concentrations more than 1 mmol/L are toxic. Demeclocycline 600-1200 mg/d is less toxic and more reliably effective.

Both lithium and demeclocycline can cause acute renal failure.

STUDY QUESTIONS

1. Classify diuretics and indicate their sites of action.
2. Describe the uses, mode of action and adverse effects of acetazolamide.
3. Describe pharmacology of thiazides.
4. Describe loop diuretics including uses, contraindications and adverse effects. Why are they

called 'high ceiling diuretics'?
5. Write notes on (i) Osmotic diuretics, (ii) Acidifying and alkalinizing salts and (iii) Xanthines as diuretics
6. Comment on (i) diuretic combinations and (ii) ADH antagonists, and (iii) Treatment of diabetes insipidus.
7. What is likely to happen due to overzealous use of diuretics?
8. Describe the effects of different diuretics on electrolyte excretion.

GUIDE TO FURTHER READING

Brater, D: Pharmacodynamic considerations in the use of diuretics. Annu. Rev. Pharmacol. Toxicol., 1983; 23:45-62.

Brater, D: Resistance to loop diuretics. Why it happens and what to do about it. Drugs, 1985; 30:427-443.

Brater, D: Clinical pharmacology of loop diuretics. Drugs, 1991; 41:14-22.

Burg, M et al Furosemide effect on isolated perfused tubules. Am. J. Physiol., 1973; 225:119-124.

Canessa, C et al: Amiloride-sensitive epithelial Na^+ channel is made of three homologous subunits. Nature, 1994; 367:463-467.

Guyton, A: Blood pressure control—special role of the kidneys and body fluids. Science, 1991; 252:1813-1816.

Levinsky, N.G. et al: Mannitol and loop diuretics in acute renal failure. In, Acute Renal Failure, 2nd ed. Churchill Livingstone, New York, 1988, pp. 841-856.

Oates, J.A. et al: The participation of prostaglandins in the control of renin release. Fed. Proc., 1979; 38:72-74.

Payne, J.A. et al: Alternatively spliced isoforms of the putative renal Na-K-Cl cotransporter are differentially distributed within the rabbit kidney. Proc. Natl. Acad. Sci. U.S.A., 1994; 91:4544-4548.

Tannen, R: Diuretic-induced hypokalaemia. Kidney Int., 1985; 28:988-1000.

Williamson, H.E. et al: Inhibition of ethacrynic acid induced increase in renal blood flow by indomethacin. Prostaglandins, 1974; 8:297-301.

Xu, J.C. et al: Molecular cloning and functional expression of the bumetanide-sensitive Na-K-Cl cotransporter. Proc. Natl. Acad. Sci. U.S.A., 1994; 91:2201-2205.

Zahykevich, A.: Amiloride for lung disease in cystic fibrosis. D.I.C.P., 1991; 25:1340-1341.

Drugs Acting on Respiratory System

Terminology associated with respiratory system

Asphyxia	Oxygen starvation
Dyspnoea	Painful or laboured breathing
Epistaxis	Loss of blood from the nose
Haemoptysis	Spitting of blood from the respiratory tract
Orthopnoea	Dyspnoea that occurs in the horizontal position
Rhinitis	Chronic or acute inflammation of the mucous membrane of the nose
Tachypnoea	Rapid breathing
Rales	Sounds sometime heard in the lungs that resemble bubbling or rattling. Rales are to the lungs what murmurs are to the heart.

BRONCHIAL ASTHMA

The development of asthma involves (i) genetic and (ii) environmental factors. The asthmatic attack consists of two main phases viz. (A) the immediate phase and (B) delayed phase.

(A) Immediate phase (initial phase) : In allergic asthma, in this phase allergen provocation occurs. It is due to spasm of the bronchial smooth muscle. Allergen interaction with mast cell-fixed IgE releases histamine, LTC_4, LTD_4, PDG_2 and neurokinin. Various chemotaxin such as LTB_4 and chemokines attract eosinophils and mononuclear cells in the area which set the stage for the delayed phase.

(B) Late phase (delayed response): It is a progressing inflammatory phase.

Asthma can be considered as a predominantly inflammatory illness. The asthmatic airway narrowing is due to inflammation. There is increase in the numbers of inflammatory cells, including eosinophils, macrophages and lymphocytes in bronchoalveolar lavage fluid from asthmatic patients. This is true for both allergic and nonallergic asthmatic patients.

In the classic immunologic model, asthma is a disease mediated by reaginic (IgE) antibodies bound to mast cells in the airway mucosa. On exposure to an antigen, antigen-antibody interaction takes place on the surface of the mast cells. This triggers the release of mediators stored in the granules of the cells as well as synthesis and release of an enormous variety of inflammatory mediators (Fig. 6.1). The substances released are histamine, tryptase and other neutral proteases, leukotrienes C_4 and D_4, prostaglandin D_2, eosinophil chemotactic factor (ECF), neutrophil chemotactic factor (NCF) and other compounds. The effects of various mediators are listed in Tables 6.1 and 6.2.

The effects of mast cell mediators are given in Table 6.2.

These mediators constrict bronchial smooth muscle, produce mucosal oedema, hyperaemia and produce viscid secretions resulting in airway obstruction (reversible).

It has been shown that there is a correlation between increasing IgE levels and prevalence of asthma and this indicates that majority of asthma cases have an allergic component which may not be readily identified by standard procedures.

Allergen-specific IgE is bound to the mast cell and activates it resulting in releases of inflammatory mediators, hence drugs that more broadly address asthmatic inflammation are of greater benefit than drugs that only address bronchoconstriction per se.

The exposure to antigen produces synthesis of IgE which binds to mast cells of the target organ. On reexposure to antigen, antigen-antibody interaction on mast cell surfaces triggers release of inflammatory mediators (Fig. 6.2).

Table 6.1. Effects of mast cell mediators of inflammatory processes

Preformed	
Histamine	Vasodilation, vasopermeability, cough, bronchoconstriction
TNF-alpha	Adhesion molecule regulation
Proteases	Vasodilation, vasopermeability, bronchoconstriction
Heparin	?
Lipid-derived	
LTC_4	Bronchoconstriction, vasodilation, vasopermeability
LTB_4	Leukocyte chemotaxis
PGD_2	Mucus secretion, vasodilation, vasopermeability, bronchoconstriction
Platelet activating factor (PAF)	Leukocyte chemotaxis, bronchoconstriction
Clytokine	
Tumor necrosis factor (TNF-α)	Adhesion molecule regulation
IL-1	Promotion of inflammation
IL-3	Mast cell division
IL-4	Mast cell division, B lymphocyte immunoglobulin class switching to produce IgE

There are 3 major components of reversible airways obstruction:

1. Bronchospasm i.e. narrowing of air pathways
2. Thick tenacious sputum
3. Mucosal oedema

The bronchial smooth muscle tone is controlled by:

- Humoral factors: histamine, bradykinin, serotonin, PGF_2 and LTC_4, LTD_4 and LTE_4

Table 6.2. Actions of mediators released from mast cells.

	Leukotrianes	*Histamine*	*PAF*	*PGs*
Bronchoconstriction	LTD_4, C_4, E_4	+++	++	PGD_2 PGF_{2a}
Mucosal oedema	LTC_4, D_4	+++	++	PGE_2
Mucus secretion	LTC_4, D_4	–	++	–
Chemotaxis and cellular activation	LTB_4	–	++++	–

These mediators constrict bronchial smooth muscle, produce mucosal oedema, hyperaemia and produce viscid secretions resulting in airway obstruction (reversible).

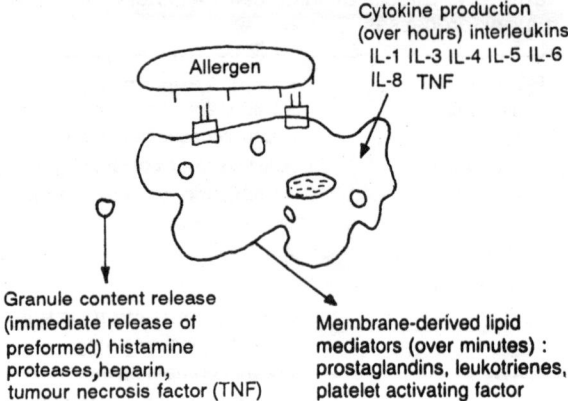

Fig. 6.1. Release of inflammatory mediators from activated mast cells.

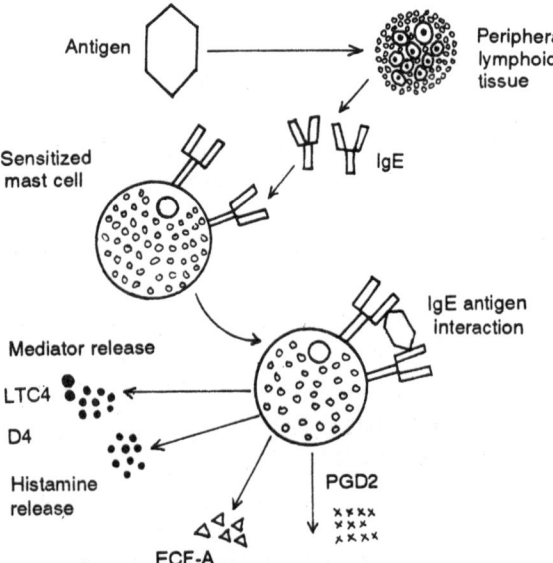

Fig. 6.2. IgE-antigen interaction and release of mediators. Exposure to antigen causes synthesis of IgE which binds to mast cells. On reexposure to antigen antigen-antibody interaction on mast cell surface triggers release of mediators.

leukotrienes together previously called slow-reacting substances of anaphylaxis (SRS). These cause bronchoconstriction.

• Autonomic nervous system: Parasympathetic stimulation causes bronchoconstriction mediated by acetylcholine.

Sympathetic stimulation through noradrenaline causes bronchodilatation.

Prevention

Asthma is often preventable if environmental and other triggering factors can be identified and eliminated. For example, measures to control house dust, mite antigen etc. should be employed. Discontinuance of cigarette smoking, avoidance of exposure to environmental tobacco smoke are essential aspects of preventive care.

Drug treatment of bronchial asthma

1. Relievers (bronchodilators), which give immediate relief of symptoms by causing relaxation of airway smooth muscle.
2. Preventers (controllers), which suppress the underlying inflammatory process and provide long-term control of symptoms.

Relievers and preventers of asthma are given in Table 6.3.

Table 6.3. Relievers and preventers of asthma

Relievers	Preventers
Short-acting beta-agonists Salbutamol, terbutaline	Corticosteroids Inhaled-beclomethasone dipropionate, Budesonide,
Short-acting theophylline Aminophylline	fluticosone propionate Oral-prednisolone Cromones
Anticholinergic agents Ipratropium bromide	Sodium cromoglycate, nedocromil sodium Long-acting bronchodilators
Epinephrine infection	Inhaled long-acting beta$_2$-agonists salmeterol, formoterol Oral sustained release beta2-agonists Sustained-release-theophylline Antileukotriene drugs Zileuton Zafirlukast, Montelukast, Pranlukast

ANTIASTHMATIC DRUGS

The drugs for asthma therapy include :
- Bronchodilators
- Leukotriene inhibitors
- Inhibitors of mediator release
- Corticosteroids

The formulations and initial dosages of some drugs used in treating asthma are given in Tables 6.4 and 6.5.

BRONCHODILATORS

These open air passages and facilitate breathing as well as diminish bronchospasm by relaxing the smooth muscle of bronchioles.

1. Sympatomimetics
   - α_1, β_1 and β_2 agonists: Adrenaline, ephedrine.
   - β_1 and β_2 agonist: Orciprenaline
   - β_2 agonists: Salbutanol, terbutaline
2. Methylxanthines: aminophylline
3. Anticholinergics: Ipratropium, tropitropium

Sympathomimetics

α_1, β_1, and α_2 agonists:

Adrenaline 0.2-0.5 ml of 1 in 1000 solution by deep SC/IM/aerosol is given to control acute attack. It produces prompt and potent action, but the duration is very brief. It is not given orally or by I.V. injection. It has no prophylactic use.

Ephedrine 30-60 mg orally 3-4 times a day produces slow and less potent bronchodilator effect, though the duration of action is longer. It is also orally effective. It is not useful to control acute attack, it can be used as a prophylactic. It produces CNS stimulation and tachyplylaxis.

β_1 and β_2 agonists:

Isoprenaline produces prompt and marked bronchodilation when given parenterally or by aerosol. It produces tachycardia (disadvantage). After oral or sublingual route its absorption is unreliable.

Dose: 0.5% from a nebulizer 5-15 inhalations. Metered-dose inhaler 1-2 inhalations.

Sublingual 10-20 mg/d.

Orciprenaline (isoprenaline derivative) has longer duration of action, can be given orally and produces less action on heart.

Table 6.4. Some drugs used in the treatment of asthma

Antiinflammatory drugs	
Corticosteroids	
Beclomethasone dipropionate	Metered-dose inhaler (42 µg/puff) 2-4 puffs 2-4 times a day for adults; 2 puffs 4 times a day or 4 puffs twice a day for children
Budesonide	Metered-dose inhaler (50, 200 µg/puff) 400-2400 µg divided 2-4 times a day for adults; 200-400 µg twice a day for children
Triamcinolone acetomide	Metered-dose inhaler (100 µg/puff) 2 puffs 3-4 times or 4 puffs twice a day for adults; 1-2 puffs 4 times or 4 puffs twice a day for children
Prednisone or prednisolone	For adults: Oral tablets (5, 10, 20 mg); Oral liquid—Acute: up to 50 mg/day for 5-14 days, Chronic: up to 40 mg every other day. For children: Acute: 10-40 mg twice a day for 5-14 days, Chronic: 20-40 mg every other day
Cromolyn	Spinhaler powder (20 mg/capsules) 1 capsule 4 times a day for adults and children. Metered-dose inhaler (800 µg/ puff) 2-4 puffs for both. Nebulized solution (10 mg/ml) 20 mg 4 times a day for both adults and children
Bronchodilators	
β_2-selective adrenergic drugs	
Albuterol	Metered-dose inhaler (90 µg/puff) 2 puffs every 4-6 hours as needed, same for both adults and children Powder inhaler (200 µg/capsules) 1-2 capsules 4-6 hours as needed, same for both adults and children Nebulized solution (5 mg/ml) 2.5 mg 3-4 times a day for adults; 0.1-0.15 mg/kg every 4-6 hours as needed in children Syrup or tablets 2-4 mg 3-4 times a day for adults; 0.1 mg/kg (max. 2 mg) every 6-8 hours as needed
Salmeterol	Metered-dose inhaler (21 µg/puff) 2 puffs twice a day for adults; 1-2 puffs twice a day for children
Terbutaline	Metered-dose inhaler (200 µg/puff) 2 puffs every 4-6 hours as needed and same for both adults and children
Theophylline	Extended release capsule or tablet 300-600 mg/daily. For children less than 1 year: 1 mg/kg/day = (0.2) (age in weeks) + 5; 1-9 years: 12-20 mg/kg/day; 10-16 years: 12-16 mg/kg/day

Table 6.5. Drugs for the treatment of chronic asthma in children

Mild	Brief, intermittent, infrequent (< 2 times/month)	Pretreat with 1-2 puffs of a beta-adrenergic agonist (as needed) and/or cromolyn before exposure to exercise, allergen or other stimuli
Moderate	Symptoms > 1 to 2 times/week requires occasional emergency care	Inhaled beta-adrenergic agonist (as needed), 3-4 times/day and cromolyn. If symptoms persist, inhaled steroids used
Severe	Continuous symptoms, frequent nocturnal symptoms, occasional hospitalization and emergency care	Inhaled beta-adrenergic agonist (as needed), 3-4 times/day and inhaled steroids with or without cromolyn. Oral steroids may also be considered

Dose: 20 mg 3-4 times a day orally.

0.65 mg per inhalation, 2-3 inhalations.

β_2 agonists: Salbutamol, terbutaline.

- These relax the bronchial muscle whatever the spasmogens involved.
- They also inhibit the release of mediators from the mast cells and release from monocytes of one of the primary mediators of inflammation - tumour necrosis factor (TNF-Alpha).
- They increase mucus clearance by an action on cilia.
- They do not produce cardiac stimulation.

Salbutamol 4 mg thrice a day orally has no action on β_1 receptors so does not produce cardiac stimulation. It is safer than isoprenaline. It can be given by oral/aerosol/SC/IM/slow I.V. injection. It is usually given by inhalation, maximum effect is within 30 minutes and effect lasts for 4-6 hours. It is used to control symptoms on 'as needed basis'.

Terbutaline 5 mg thrice a day orally has similar action as salbutamol. It can also be given as aerosol or by SC injection (0.25 mg). It is usually given by inhalation, maximum effect occurs within half an hour and effect lasts for 4-6 hours.

Rimiterol produces rapid and potent action on inhalation. It has similar activity as salbutamol and terbutaline. However, it is short acting.

Dose: Metered-dose inhaler (200 mcg/puff), 1-3 puffs daily

Salmeterol is longer-acting (duration 12 hours) agent given by inhalation. It is not used 'as needed' unlike salbutamol and terbutaline but given regularly twice daily.

Dose: metered-dose inhaler (21 mcg/puff) 2 puffs twice a day.

Tremor is the commonest side effect of β_2-adrenergic agonists in the context of their use in asthma.

Tolerance can also occur with beta agonists in asthmatic airways. Steroids can reduce development of tolerance as they inhibit beta receptor down regulation.

Certain β_2 adrenergic agonists which can be inhaled are listed in Table 6.6

Table 6.6. Inhaled β_2 adrenergic agonists

Drug	Comments
Albuterol	Rapid onset (<5 min), duration of 3 to 5 hours.
Bitolterol	Faster prodrug, similar to albuterol
Metaproterenol	Similar to albuterol
Pirbuterol	Similar to albuterol
Terbutaline	Similar to albuterol
Salmeterol	Slower onset (20 min), long duration (12 hours).
Fenoterol	Similar to salmeterol

Methylxanthines

Aminophylline (theophylline plus ethylenediamine) 50-100 mg by slow I.V. injection produces prompt relaxation of bronchial muscle. It acts directly on bronchial muscle (increase concentration of cyclic AMP leading to relaxation.

Methylxanthines are not important for asthma therapy because :
- Side effects are more than β_2 - receptor agonists
- CNS stimulation
- Hypotention
- Palpitation

The bronchodilator action of aminophylline depends upon its theophylline content.

Dose: 300-600 mg/d in 3-4 divided doses.

Anticholinergic agents

These are useful for reducing bronchospasm. The bronchial muscles are controlled by autonomic nervous system with parasympathetic fibres predominating in number and effect, stimulation of parasympathetic nervous system induces bronchospasm. Consequently, anticholinergic drug are useful for reducing bronchospasm. The anticholinergics are less effective than sympathomimetics. They thicken bronchial secretion (disadvantage).

Atropine sulphate is not recommended as its onset of action is slow, has low efficacy and may produce many side effects.

Atropine methyl nitrate is more potent and produces less side effects. It can be given orally, by I.M. injection and as an aerosol.

Ipratropium bromide is administered by inhalation and also used as a nasal spray. The half-life is 3-4 hours. It is more active with longer duration of action. It produces less anticholinergic side effects, does not affect bronchial secretion. It is poorly absorbed after oral use. It is given by inhalation. On inhalation its actions are confined exclusively to the airways.

Adverse effects from inhalation are cough, mouth dryness, nausea, headache, dizziness. Use as a nasal spray induces epistaxis, nasal dryness, drythroat, and nasal congestion in some patients.

LEUKOTRIENE INHIBITORS (ANTILEUKOTRIENES)

Leukotriene antagonists represent an important advance in non-steroidal antiinflammatory therapy in asthma. They exhibit both antiinflammatory and bronchodilator activity; along with a high therapeutic index.

Leukotriene-receptor antagonists are the first novel class of antiasthmatic drugs to become available over the past three decades. They have an unique profile in that they are a hybrid of an antiinflammatory and bronchodilator drugs and they can be taken as a tablet once or twice daily. The published data with leukotrine-receptor antagonists such as montelukast or zafirlukast show good antiasthmatic activity over a wide spectrum of asthma severity either as monotherapy or with inhaled steroids. Another potential spin-off of leukotrine-receptor antagonists is

that they also seem to be effective in treating allergic rhinitis, which commonly coexists in patients with asthma.

- Leukotriene synthesis inhibitor: Zileuton.
- Leukotriene receptor antagonists: Montelukast, pranlukast and zafirlukast.

Leukotriene synthesis inhibitor

Zileuton is a 5-lipoxygenase inhibitor. Such drugs prevent the production of not only the spasmogenic leukotrienes LTC_4 and LTD_4, but also LTB_4 (a chemotactic that recruits leukocytes into the bronchial mucosa and then activates them).

Zileuton is approved for oral prophylaxis and chronic treatment of asthma in patients ≥ 12 year of age. It is a specific inhibitor of 5-lipoxygenase which results in inhibition of LTB_4, LTC_4, LTD_4, and LTE_4.

Zileuton is a prototype compound, given orally, has low potency and hence administered 3-4 times daily. It blocks antigen - and exercise - induced bronchospasm and inhibit or reduce late phase inflammation.

Dosage, 12 years and older: 600 mg orally 4 times daily (may take with or without food). Safety and efficacy have not been established in children under 12 years of age.

Contraindications

- Active liver disease
- Hypersensitivity to zileuton

Precautions

- Alcohol intake
- History of liver diseases
- Not indicated for acute asthma attacks

Hepatic transaminases prior to therapy, once a month for 3 months then every 2-3 months while on therapy, should be monitored.

Adverse effects include nausea, dyspepsia, myalgia, abdominal pain, asthenia, hepatic function impairment.

Leukotriene receptor antagonists

Montelukast Sodium

It is approved for oral prophylaxis and chronic treatment of asthma.

It is a selective cysteinyl leukotriene ($CystLT_1$) receptor antagonist. Its mean bioavailability is about 60-70% which is not influenced by food. It is extensively metabolizd by CYP3A4 and CYP2C9 but does not inhibit these enzymes in therapeutic doses. Metabolism occurs (presumably hepatic); excretion is mainly via the bile.

Indications :
- Prophylaxis and chronic treatment of asthma
- Seasonal allergic rhinitis.
- Shows some efficacy in exercise-induced asthma but should not be used as monotherapy for this condition.

Dosage: The usual adult dose is 10 mg orally once a day. Paediatric patients: 5 mg once a day for children ages 6 to 14 years, and 4 mg once daily for children ages 1 to 5 years.

It is well-tolerated; adverse effects include GI disturbances, headache liver function abnormalities and eosinophilic conditions have been reported rarely.

Drug interaction: Phenobarbital can induce its metabolism.

Because of the incorporation of glutathione, LTC_4, LTD_4, LTE_4 are called cysteinyl leukotrienes (CysLTs)

LTC_4 and LTD_4 are extremely potent bronchoconstrictors, about 1000 times more potent than histamine. Their rapid onset of action is similar to that of histamine, but their duration of effect is longer.

In the affinity binding studies LTD_4 had the maximum affinity for $CysLT_1$ receptors, about 200 times greater than LTE_4.

$CysLT_2$ receptor has not yet been identified in human airways.

Comparison of lukotriene antagonists and long-acting β_2 agonists is given in Table 6.7.

Pranlukast

It is a selective LT-receptor antagonist, food enhances its absorption.

Indications:
- Chronic asthma patients.
- Pranlukast can blunt or eliminate bronchoconstrictor responses to numerous asthma challenges.

Dose : 450 mg orally twice daily after meals.

It is well - tolerated; adverse effects include headache, dyspepsia, nausea, flatulence.

Zafirlukast

It is a leukotriene receptor antagonist. It is rapidly absorbed following oral administration. Intake of zafirlukast with food decreases the bioavailability by about 40%, therefore, the drug should be taken at least 1 or 2 hours after eating. It is extensively metabolized in the liver, about 10% is excreted unchanged in urine.

Indications :
- As an alternative to inhaled steroids in patients with mild persistent asthma symptoms and as add-on therapy for moderate persistent symptoms.
- British but not US asthma guidelines support the use of leukotriene modifiers in more severe stages of asthma as well.
- Prophylaxis and treatment of asthma.
- May be effective for exercise-induced asthma and atopic dermatitis.

Dosage: 20 mg twice daily for adults and adolescents and 10mg twice daily for children 5 through 11 years of age.

Table 6.7. Comparison of leukotriene antagonists and long-acting β_2 agonists.

Drug	Route	Frequency	Antiinflamatory/ Tolerability	Symptoms control & action	onset of action	tachyphylaxis	Indication
Leukotrine antagonists	Oral	o.d/b.i.d	Yes	Good	Hours	No	Preventer, Controller
Long-acting β_2 agonists	inhaled	b.i.d	No	Good	Minutes	Yes	Controller

Zafirlukast should be taken on an empty stomach as food reduces the bioavailability of the drug.

Zafirlukast is well-tolerated; adverse effects include headache, nausea, gastritis, somnolence, elevation of liver enzymes, and asthma exacerbation. Churg-Strauss syndrome, a rare and sometimes fatal reaction has been reported with zafirlukeast, usually when patients are reducing their oral steroid dose.

MAST CELL STABILIZERS

Cromolyn sodium and **nedocromil sodium** inhibit the release of mediators of inflammation from mast cells. These mediators include histamine, leukotrienes, platelet activating factor (PAF), prostaglandins, proteases, interleukins, and numerous cytokines.

The inhibitors of mediator release, cromolyn and nedocromil are not used to treat acute bronchospams as they require administration for several days to weeks (2-4 weeks) before decrease of bronchospasm and congestive symptoms associated with the release of inflammatory mediators (from mast cells, eosinophils, neutrophils, basophils and alveolar macrophages that are involved in the inflammatory components of this disease).

They are ineffective in acute attack.

Sodium cromoglycate (cromolyn)

Sodium cromoglycate and the related drug nedocromil sodium are not bronchodilators, have no direct action on smooth muscle.

If given prophylactically, they reduce both the immediate and the late-phase responses in asthma and reduce bronchial hyper-reactivity in many but not all patients. Children respond better than adults.

They are effective in :
- Antigen - induced
- Exercise - induced
- Irritant - induced asthma

Mechanism of action

Cromoglycate is a mast cell stabilizer (prevent histamine release from mast cell). However, it is not the basis of its anti-asthmatic effect because several compounds have been synthesized which inhibit mast cell histamine release but they are devoid of anti-asthmatic effects.

The mechanism of action is not fully known. But there is evidence that cromoglycate (i) depresses the exaggerated neuronal reflexes that are triggered by stimulation of the "irritant receptors," (ii) may inhibit the release of preformed T cell cytokines.

Pharmacokinetics

Cromoglycate is very poorly absorbed from GIT, hence it is administered by inhalation and acts locally. When it is given by inhalation 10% is absorbed into the circulation.

It is rapidly excreted unaltered, 50% in the bile and 50% in the urine.

Its plasma half-life is 90 minutes.

Dose: Usual starting dose for adults is 2 metered sprays (800 mcg/spray) from the metered dose inhaler inhaled 4 times daily at regular intervals.

Adverse reactions with inhalation include dizziness, headache, cough, wheezing, nasal congestion, bad taste and rash.

Nedocromil Sodium

Nedocromil inhibits release of mediators including histamine, leukotriene C_4, and prostaglandin D_2. It inhibits the activation and mediator release from a variety of inflammatory cell types associated with asthma including eosinophils, neutrophils, macrophages, mast cells, monocytes and platelets.

It provides the basis for inhibition of the development of early and late bronchoconstrictor response to inhaled antigen and other causes of bronchoconstriction e.g., sulphur dioxide. The mean half-life is 3.3 hours.

It is administered by inhalation.

Dose: Metered - dose inhaler (1.75mg/puff, 2 puffs four times a day)

Adverse reactions

The drug is well tolerated with few adverse reactions such as unpleasant taste, upper respiratory tract infections, headache, nausea, and dyspepsia. Allergic reactions have been reported (rarely).

Ketotifen

It acts like cromoglycate, but it is orally active. It

inhibits release of histamine and other mediators from the mast cell. the dose is 1-2 mg twice a day orally.

The most common adverse effect is drowsiness.

CORTICOSTEROIDS

Glucocorticoids are not bronchodilators and are ineffective in the treatment of immediate response to the eliciting agent. However, they are efficient in the management of chronic asthma (where inflammatory component is predominant). They are also life-saving in status asthmaticus. They are indicated in severe chronic asthma not controlled by bronchodilators alone and in status asthmatics.

The basis of their anti-inflammatory action in asthma is that they decrease formation of cytokines that recruit and activate eosinophils and are responsible for promoting the production of IgE. They also inhibit generation of the vasodilators, PGE_2 and PGI_2.

Corticosteroids are not only effective anti-inflammatory agents but also potentiate the bronchodilator effect of adrenergic drugs.

They produce following effects:

- Anti-inflammatory effect
- Reduce oedema
- Can restore responsiveness in patients who have developed resistance to inhaled bronchodilators
- Improvement comes after 6 hours, so during first few hours bronchodilator therapy is instituted

Therapy with corticosteroids is the mainstay in patients who have failed to respond to bronchodilators. They restore patient's sensitivity to bronchodilators. Bronchodilator therapy with β_2 agonist is continued in full doses.

The dose of hydrocortisone is 3 mg/kg I.V. infusion 6 hourly, and 30-60 mg of prednisolone per day orally or I.V. dose of 1 mg/kg of methylprednisolone every 6 hours.

To correct acidosis sodium bicarbonate is administered. Once patient improves, prednisolone 50-60 mg is given as single dose orally. On improvement, dose is tapered slowly by 5 mg every 3-4 days.

Table 6.8. Inhaled corticosteroids.

Drug	Comments
Beclomethasone dipropionate	High topical activity, active metabolite formed in lung fluids, low systemic bioavailability.
Budesonide	High topical activity, used as powder, rapid hepatic metabolism, limited systemic bioavailability.
Flunisolide	Good topical activity, higher systemic bioavailability, short plasma half-life.
Fluticasone propionate	Very high topical activity, very low systemic bioavailability
Triamcinolone acetonide	Good topical activity, short plasma half-life, limited systemic bioavailability.

The corticosteroids which are given by inhalation are listed in Table 6.8.

Beclomethasone, triamcinolone are advocated. Two puffs 4 times daily or 4 puffs twice daily produce effect equivalent to 10-15 mg/d of prednisone with fewer systemic side effects.

Adverse effects

These are not common with inhaled steroids.

If corticosteroids are administered by aerosol, systemic adverse effects are less.

Betamethasone and beclomethasone are active topically (inhalational) and do not produce suppression of pituitary adrenal axis.

Thrush (oropharyngeal candidiasis) and dysphonia (voice problems) can occur (rarely). If part of an inhaled drug is ingested unwanted effects may be observed. But this is less likely with fluticasone as its absorption from GIT is very limited and undergoes almost complete first-pass metabolism.

The adverse effects of oral glucocorticoids is described in Chapter 10.

OTHER DRUGS

Nifedipine and verapamil given by inhalation significantly inhibit bronchoconstriction. However, in majority of cases relief provided is partial and there is considerable variation among subjects.

In elderly asthmatics, infection is commonly found to be a precipitating factor. Hence, wherever suspected appropriate antibiotics should be added during acute exacerbation.

Histamine H_1 - receptor antagonists have no place in the therapy of asthma. However, some newer, non-sedating antihistamines, such as loratidine are moderately effective in mild atopic asthma.

In young asthmatics with dominating manifestations of upper respiratory allergy, antihistaminics may be used. However, they are not beneficial in elderly asthmatics as they most often have non-allergic disease (intrinsic asthma).

Expectorants are not very useful unless associated with chronic bronchitis.

Various immunosuppressive agents like methotrexate, gold compounds and cyclosporin have been tried for controlling asthma in patients developing the adverse effects of systemic steroids, however, none has found a place in regular practice due to the significant side effects.

Management of asthmatic attack

In mild cases, inhalation of a beta-receptor agonists are as effective as subcutaneous injection of epinephrine. These are more effective than intravenous aminophylline. However, if the attack is severe, oxygen inhalation, bronchodilators and corticosteroids are to be employed. β_2-agonist is given by aerosol and subcutaneous injection; aminophylline by continuous intravenous infusion, and intravenous corticosteroids may all be necessary to be administered in severe cases.

The therapeutic interventions are shown in Fig. 6.3.

Among the xanthines, theophylline is the most effective bronchodilator. The two commonly used salts are aminophylline which contains 86% theophylline and oxtriphylline which contains 64% by weight.

The intracellular levels of cyclic AMP can be increased by beta-adrenergic receptor agonists which increase the rate of its synthesis by adenylyl cyclase or by phosphodiesterase inhibitors such as theophylline which slows the rate of its degradation or block it (Fig. 6.4).

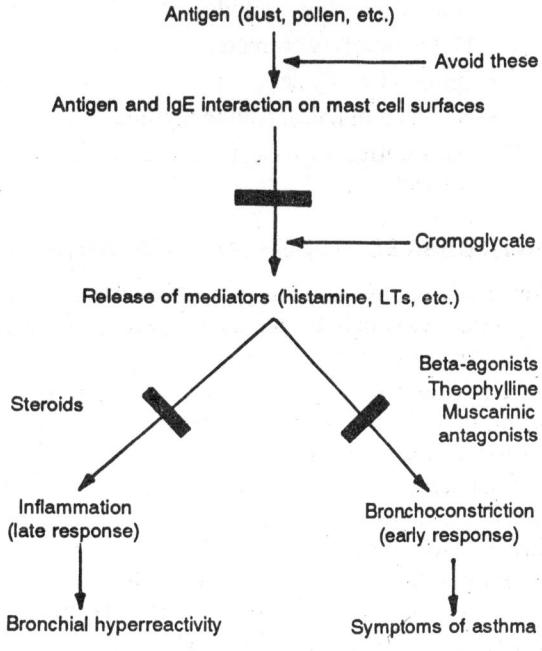

Fig. 6.3. Therapeutic interventions.

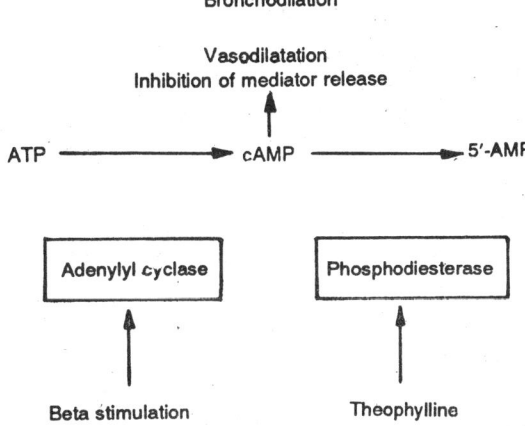

Fig. 6.4. Role of beta-agonists and theophylline.

Status asthmaticus

It is a medical emergency. The treatment includes:
- Oxygen is administration
- Salbutamol inhalation in oxygen given by nebulizer
- Hydrocortisone I.V. followed by a course of oral prednisolone

Additional measures include –

- Dehydration is corrected
- Ipratropium by nebulizer
- Salbutamol I.V. or Aminophylline
- Antibiotics in case bacterial infection is present

ANTITUSSIVES (COUGH SUPPRESSANTS)

Antitussives are valuable in suppressing dry and unproductive cough. It is necessary to find the cause of cough for proper treatment.

Codeine is a commonly used narcotic antitussive agent. It is highly effective having much less liability to produce drug dependence as compared to strong narcotics such as morphine and other opiate-like drugs. Dose of codeine phosphate is 8-15 mg thrice or four times a day orally.

Pholcodine is a non-analgesic opiate of the same chemical class as papaverine. Although, structurally related to opioids, if has no opioid like actions. It is at least as effective as codeine and longer acting and hence given once or twice a day.

Dose: 10-15 mg once or twice a day.

Carbetapentane has no dependence inducing liability. Besides antitussive action it has weak local anaesthetic and anticholinergic properties.

Oxeladin is devoid of opioid adverse effects.
Dose : 15-30 mg.

Chlophedianol is similar to oxeladin. However, acts slowly but has longer duration of action.

Dose : 20-40 mg.

Adverse effects include irritability, vertigo and dryness of mouth.

Pipazethate is a phenothiazine having antitussive action with little sedative and analgesic actions.

Dose : 40-80 mg.

Dextromethorphan is as potent as codeine as a cough suppressant. Dose is 10-20 mg orally 3-4 times daily. It is neither analgesic nor it produces drug dependence. It produces less constipation than codeine.

Levopropoxyphene, in contrast to its dextro form has antitussive action without being an analgesic. It is claimed to be as potent antitussive as codeine. It is devoid of opioid effects but sedation may be produced as a side effect.

Dose : 50-100 mg every 4 hours.

Noscapine is a naturally occurring opium alkaloid of benzylisoquinoline group. It has no significant actions on CNS in doses within the therapeutic range. It does not produce drug dependence. It has good antitussive property.

However, noscapine is a potent releaser of histamine and large does can cause bronchoconstriction and transient hypotension.

Dose : 15-30 mg orally thrice a day.

Adverse effects include headache, nausea. It can produce bronchoconstriction in asthmatics as it releases histamine.

Antihistamines such as chlorpheniramine (2-5 mg), diphenhydramine (15-25 mg) and promethazine (15-25 mg) are commonly used.

Due to their sedative and anticholinergic actions, cough is relieved.

EXPECTORANTS

Expectorants are drugs which are useful in loosening and liquefying mucus, in soothing irritated bronchial mucosa and making cough more productive.

They act by (i) decreasing the viscosity of the bronchial secretions and facilitating their elimination; (ii) by increasing the amount of respiratory tract fluid.

Examples : Acetylcysteine, ammonium chloride, ammonium carbonate, antimony potassium tartarate, terpin-hydrate, sodium citrate, glycerin, potassium iodide.

These increase bronchial secretion, facilitating its removal by coughing. The following drugs act as cough expectorants.

Sodium and potassium citrate or acetate (act by salt action); KI produces irritation being secreted by bronchial glands; ammonium salts produce gastric irritation thereby reflexly increase bronchial secretion. Guaiacol, terpin hydrate, vasaka syrup are also used as expectorants.

MUCOLYTICS

These drugs make sputum less viscous so more easily cleared. They produce fragmentation of mucopolysaccharide fibres in sputum and thus increase the volume of sputum, decrease the viscosity, and facilitate expectoration. These are indicated in patients who find it difficult to expectorate their viscous sputum.

Bromhexine is a synthetic derivative of vascine an alkaloid from plant adhatoda vasaca.

Dose : 8-16 mg thrice a day orally.

Acetylcysteine (mucomyst) depolymerizes mucopolysaccharides. Liquefaction after inhalation occurs within a minute, peak effect occurs in 5-10 minutes. The agent is marketed as a 10 or 20% sterile solution. A nebulized solution 1-10 ml of a 20% solution or 2-20 ml of a 10% solution is inhaled every 2-6 hourly.

Carbocisteine (mucolex) is a derivative of sulphur containing amino acid cysteine Its aerosol spray decreases viscosity and increases volume of sputum. It splits disulphide bonds linking strands of mucus.

Dose : 10-15 ml thrice a day as 5% w/v syrup. It produces more prompt and greater effect than bromhexine. It should be avoided in patients with history of peptic ulcer.

RESPIRATORY STIMULANTS

These are clinically disappointing as no drug is available which can specifically stimulate the respiratory drive.

Xanthines

Xanthines do improve medullary blood flow and hence regarded as respiratory stimulant but they have limitations.

ANALEPTICS (DRUGS WHICH RESTORE FAILING RESPIRATION)

Analeptic, a Greek word meaning restorative or strengthening drug. Some of them act directly on respiratory center in the medulla but not specifically on this area alone but stimulate all levels of cerebrospinal axis resulting in general arousal. They all induce convulsions in large doses.

Nikethamide

It is a pyridine derivative, water soluble and slightly viscous oil.

Dose: 2 ml of a 25% solution repeated every 4-6 hours, if needed.

Structure of nikethamide

It is suitable for short term use only, stimulates all levels of CNS, However, respiratory stimulation is produced in doses that cause little central excitation, due partly to stimulation of carotid and aortic chemoreceptors. It increases sensitivity of respiratory center to CO_2, acts more powerfully on a depressed respiratory center than on a normal one.

It is absorbed from all sites of administration but usually given intravenously.

It is converted to nicotinamide, excreted as N-methylnicotinamide. The effect is over in 2 minutes after I.V. injection.

Indications

- Acute respiratory failure cases who are drowsy and unable to cough properly.
- To counteract overdosage of respiratory depressant drugs such as morphine.

Adverse effects

Large doses produce clonic convulsions followed by depression of CNS including respiratory center. Other side effects are pruritus, anxiety and GI upsets.

Doxapram

It has a wider margin of safety than nikethamide. It is an analeptic, used intravenously as a respiratory stimulant, in post anaesthetic respiratory depression.

Dose : 0.5-1mg/kg as a single dose.

Adverse effects include hypertension tachycardia, arrhythmia, muscle twitchings, tremors, convulsions and vomiting.

Ethamivan

It is a derivative of vanillic acid having almost similar

actions, uses and toxicity as those of nikethamide. Its duration of action is 10 minutes after I.V. injection.

Dose: 150-400 mg I.V. injection; available in 2 ml ampoules containing 5% solution of ethamivan.

It is a nonspecific analeptic used to stimulate respiration.

It is claimed to have better safety margin than nikethamide.

Contraindications and drug interactions

- Hypertension, coronary artery disease, airways obstruction, thyrotoxicosis, status asthmaticus, history of past cerebral vascular accident.
- The effects are potentiated by MAOIs.

Adverse effects

Hypertension, tachycardia, dysrhythmias and vomiting have been reported.

STUDY QUESTIONS

1. What are the major components of reversible airways obstruction in a patient of asthma? And how these are tackled by drugs?
2. List the mediators which are released from mast cell surfaces and what effects are produced by them?
3. Describe bronchodilators and discuss their mode of action.
4. What are the advantages and disadvantages of corticosteroids in the treatment of bronchial asthma? How are they administration? How do they act?
5. Why H1 antihistaminics are not adequately effective in asthma?
6. Discuss the role of anticholinergic versus sympathomimetics in the treatment of asthma.
7. Describe beta2-agonists in the treatment of asthma.
8. Discuss the mast cell stabilizers in the treatment of asthma.
9. At what sites the therapeutic interventions can act in the treatment of asthma?
10. How is status asthmaticus managed?
11. Describe the commonly used antitussives.
12. Write notes on (i) expectorants (ii) mucolytics.

13. What do you mean by the term analeptics? What are their indications and limitations?
14. What is the mechanism of action and therapeutic status of antileukotrienes in the treatment of asthma ?
15. Write notes on (i) Montelukast, (ii) Zafirlukast, (iii) Zileuton.

GUIDE TO FURTHER READING

Allen, D.B. et al: A meta-analysis of the effect of oral and inhaled corticosteroids on growth. J. Allergy Clin. Immunol., 1994; 93:967-976.

Anonymous. Guidelines for the Diagnosis and Management of Asthma. NIH Publication No. 91-3042, 1992.

Bagenstose SE, Levin L & Bernstein JA: The addition of zafirlukast to cetirizine improves the treatment of chronic urticaria in patients with positive and autologous serum skin test results. J Allergy Clin. Immunol 2004; 113(1):134-140.

Barnes, P.J.: Inhaled glucocorticoids for asthma. N. Engl. J. Med., 1995; 332:868-875.

Barnes, P.J. et al: Efficacy and safety of inhaled corticosteroids in asthma. Am. Rev. Resp. Dis., 1993; 148:S1-S26.

Barnes PJ. Drugs for airway diseases. Medicini 1999; 27; 37-45.

Barnes PJ, Grunstein MM, Leff AR and Woolcock AJ (eds.) Asthma 1997; 1507-1568.

Blair Jarvis and Anthony Markano. Montelukast - A review of its therapeutic potential in persistent asthma. Drugs 2000 Apr; 59(4).

Brackett, L.M., Shamim, S et al: Activities of caffeine, theophylline, and enprofylline analogs as tracheal relaxants. Biochem. Pharmacol, 1990; 39:1897-1904.

Brian J Lipworth. Leukotrine - receptor antagonists. The lancet vol. 353: Jan. 2, 1999.

British Thoracic society et. al. 1997 The British guidelines on asthma management. Thorax 52 (suppl.); 51-521.

Brogden, R.N. et al: Nedocromil sodium. An updated review of its pharmacological properties and therapeutic efficacy in asthma. Drugs, 1993; 45:693-715.

Bryant, D.H. et al: Effects of ipratropium bromide nebulizer solution with and without preservatives in the treatment of acute and stable asthma. Chest, 1992; 102:742-747.

Bryant, D.H.: Nebulized ipratropium bromide in the treatment of acute asthma. Chest, 1986; 88:24-29.

Busse, W.W.: What role for inhaled steroids in chronic asthma? Chest, 1993; 104:1565-1571.

Campbell, R.K.: Clinical update on pentoxifylline therapy for diabetes induced peripheral vascular disease. Ann. Pharmacother., 1993; 27:1099-1105.

Chou, J.M. et al: Caffeine and Coffee: effects on health and cardiovascular disease. Comp. Biochem. Physiol., 1994; 109c:173-189.

Curatolo, P.W. et al: The health consequences of caffeine. Ann. Intern. Med., 1983; 98:641-653.

David Price. Tolerability of montelukast; drugs 2000; 59 suppl. 1:35-42.

D'Alonazo, G.E. et al: Salmeterol xinafoate as maintenance therapy compared with albuterol in patients with asthma. J. Am. Med. Assoc., 1994; 271:1412-1416.

Dompeling, E. et al: Slowing the deterioration of asthma and chronic obstructive pulmonary disease observed during bronchodilator therapy by adding inhaled corticosteroids. A 4- year prospective study. Ann. Intern. Med., 1993; 118:770-778.

Drazen JM and Israel E et.al.: Treatment of asthma with Drugs Modifying the leukoteriene pathway. N Eng. J. Med. 1999 Jan. 21; 340: 197-206.

Ernst, E.: Pentoxifylline for intermittent claudication. A critical review. Angiology, 1994; 45:339-345.

Fanta, C.H. et al: Treatment of acute asthma. Is combination therapy with sympathomimetics and methylxanthines indicated? Am. J. Med., 1986; 80:5-10.

Fredholm, B.B. et al: Nomenclature and classification of purinoceptors. Pharmacol. Rev., 1994; 46:143-156.

Funk, J.O. et al: Horizons in pharmacologic intervention in allergic contact dermatitis. J. Am. Acad. Dermatol., 1994; 31:999-1014.

Graham, T.E. et al: Caffeine and exercise: metabolism and performance. Can. J. Appl. Physiol., 1994; 19:111-138.

Greening, A.P. et al: Added salmeterol versus higher-dose corticosteroid in asthma patients with symptoms on existing inhaled corticosteroid. Lancet, 1994; 344:219-224.

Hall I.P. 1997 The future of asthma. Br. Med. J. 314: 45-49.

Harel Z, Riggs S, Vaz R et al.: The use of the leukotriene receptor antagonist singulair (montelukast) in the management of dysmenorrhea in adolescents (abstract). J Adolescent Health 2004; 34(2): 127.

Helenius I, Lumme A, Ounap J et al: No effect of montelukast on asthma-like symptoms in elite ice hockey players. Allergy 2004; 59(1): 39-44.

Hill, M. et al: Asthma pathogenesis and the implications for therapy in children. Pediatr. Clin. North Am., 1992; 39:1205- 1224.

Hoag, J.E. et al: Long-term effect of cromolyn sodium on nonspecific bronchial hyperresponsiveness: a review. Ann. Allergy, 1991; 66:53-63.

Holgate, S.T.: Antihistamines in the treatment of asthma. Clin. Rev. Allergy, 1994; 12:65-78.

Israel, E.: Moderating the inflammation of asthma: inhibiting the production or action of products of the 5-lipoxygenase pathway. Ann. Allergy, 1994; 72:279-284.

Israel, E. et al: Treating mild asthma-when are inhaled steroids indicated? N. Engl. J. Med., 1994; 331:737-739.

Kamada, A.K. et al: Salmeterol: its place in asthma management. Ann. Pharmacother., 1994; 28:1100-1102.

Kay, A.B. et al: Disodium cromoglycate inhibits activation of human inflammatory cells in vitro. J. Allergy Clin. Immunol., 1987; 80:1-8.

Kobayashi S, Ishizuka S, Tamura N et al.: Churg-Strauss syndrome (CSS) in a patient receiving pranlukast. Clin Rheumatol 2003; 22(6) 491-492.

Lindgren, S. et al: Does asthma or treatment with theophylline limit children's academic performance? N. Engl. J. Med., 1992; 327:926-930.

Lipworth, B.J.: Clinical pharmacology of corticosteroids in bronchial asthma. Pharmacol. Ther., 1993; 58:173-209.

McFadden, E.R. et al: Dosages of corticosteroids in asthma. Am. Rev. Resp. Dis., 1993; 147:1306-1310.

McFadden, E.R. et al: Exercise-induced asthma: N. Engl. J. Med., 1994; 330:1362-1367.

McGill K.A. Busse W.W. 1996 Zileutin, Lancet 348: 519-523.

Meltzer, E.O. et al: Long-term comparison of three combinations of albuterol, theophylline, and beclomethasone in children with chronic asthma. J. Allergy Clin. Immunol., 1992; 90:2-11.

Micheletoo C, Tognella S, Visconti M et al: Montelukast 10mg improves nasal function and nasal response to aspirin in ASA-sensitive asthmatics: a controlled study vs placebo. Allergy 2004; 59(3) 289-294.

Moffitt, J.E. et al: Management of asthma in children. Am. Fam. Physician, 1994; 50:1039-1050, 1053-1055.

Nasser, S.S. et al: Theophylline. Current thoughts on the risks and benefits of its use in asthma. Drug safety, 1993; 8:12-18.

Nelson, H.S.: Beta-adrenergic bronchodilators. N. Engl. J. Med., 1995; 333:499-506.

NIH. Management of asthma during pregnancy. NIH Publication No. 93-3279, NIH, Bethesda, Md., 1993.

Page, C.P.: Beta agonists and the asthma paradox. J. Asthma, 1993; 30:155-164.

Rachelefsky, G.S. et al: International consensus on the management of pediatric asthma: a summary statement. Pediatr. Pulmonol., 1993; 15:125-127.

Rosenwasser I.J. 1997 Interleukin-4 and the genetics of atopy. N. Engl. J. Med. 337: 1766-1767 (Editorial comment).

Sears, M.R. et al: The Beta2 agonist controversy. Observations, explanations and relationship to asthma epidemiology. Drug Safety, 1994; 11:259-283.

Stoloff, S.W.: The changing role of theophylline in pediatric asthma. Am. Fam. Physician, 1994; 49:839-844.

Taburet, A. et al: Pharmacokinetic optimisation of asthma treatment. Clin. Pharmacokinetic., 1994; 26:396-418.

Texeira N.M. et. al. 1997. Phosphodiesterase (PDE) 4 inhibitors: anti-inflammatory drugs of the future. Trends Pharmacol Sci. 18: 164-170.

Van Bever, H.P. et al: Pharmacotherapy of childhood asthma. An inflammatory disease. Drugs, 1992; 44:36-46.

Van Schayck, C.P. et al: Bronchodilator treatment in moderate asthma or chronic bronchitis: continuous or on demand? A randomised controlled study. Br. Med. J., 1991; 303:1426-1431.

Weinberger, M.: Pharmacologic management of asthma. J. Adolesc. Health Care, 1987; 8:74-83.

Weinberger M.E. Hendeles I. 1996 Theophylline in asthma. N. Engl J. Med. 334: 1380-1388.

Drugs Affecting Haematopoiesis and Haemostasis

HAEMATINICS

Haematinics are agents that are required for the formation of blood. These are mainly iron, folic acid, and vitamin B_{12}. Their deficiency results in anaemia.

Anaemia results when the quality or quantity of blood is decreased. It may be due to haemorrhage, malabsorption, deficient intake, hypoplasia or aplasia of bone marrow, pregnancy, lactation.

IRON

The body of a 70 kg man contains about 4 g of iron, 65% of which circulates in the blood as oxygen carrying molecule, haemoglobin. About one-half of the remainder is stored in the liver, spleen and bone marrow, chiefly as ferritin and haemosiderin. The iron in these molecules is available for fresh haemoglobin synthesis. The rest is present in myoglobin, cytochromes and various enzymes. This iron is not available for haemoglobin synthesis.

Total iron content is 3-5 g, 2/3 in RBCs as Hb, rest 1/3 in stores in marrow, spleen, liver, muscles. Table 7.1 shows body contents of iron.

Table 7.1. Body contents of iron

Essential iron	Male	Female
	mg/kg body weight	
Hb	31	28
Myoglobin and enzymes	6	5
Storage iron	13	4
Total	50	37

Iron rich food: liver, heart, egg yolk, dry beans, fruits.

Iron moderately rich food: meat, fish, green vegetables.

Iron content is low in milk and non-green vegetables.

Daily average diet supplies about 20 mg of iron out of which about 10% is absorbed, anaemic person absorbs about 30%. The absorption takes place in upper part of small intestine.

Iron requirement is 0.5-1.0 mg daily for adults; during pregnancy requirement is 2.5-3 mg per day.

The dietary iron or medicinal iron is in ferric or ferrous form but only ferrous iron is absorbed. The absorption is increased by acidic pH of gastric juice (< 5) due to reduction of ferric iron and delayed by alkaline pH, antacids. Ascorbic acid reduces ferric iron and forms absorbable complex.

The ferric state of iron (Fe^{3+}) in methaemoglobin is less able to carry oxygen than the ferrous form (Fe^{2+}) in haemoglobin.

Microcytic anaemia is due to iron deficiency.

The symptoms of anaemia include loss of appetite, weakness, palpitation, early fatigue and pallor of skin and mucous membranes. These are due to reduced O_2 carrying capacity of red blood cells.

Haemolytic anaemia is due to excess blood loss.

Macrocytic (megaloblastic) anaemia is due to B_{12} and folic acid deficiency. Deficiency of folic acid or vitamin B_{12} may result in maturation defect in pernicious anaemia and other megaloblastic anaemia. Pernicious anaemia is due to B_{12} deficiency.

Aplastic anaemia is due to aplasia of bone marrow.

Pharmacokinetics of iron preparations

Non-haem iron and inorganic iron salts are converted to ferrous iron and then absorbed by the intestinal mucosal cells. Vitamin C increases iron absorption. Haem iron from haemoglobin and myoglobin can be absorbed as haemin (ferric form of haem) without being converted to ferrous form.

The absorption of iron occurs in duodenum and proximal jejunum, and transported by active transport. In the mucosal cell the absorbed ferrous iron is converted to ferric iron and together with the ferric iron split from haemin is either stored in the mucosal cell as haematin or transported to the blood via transferrin (plasma transport protein). It is the serum iron carrier. The rate of absorption is controlled by the need of the body. Iron is bound in ferric form to plasma B_1-globulin. It is transported to the storage sites (liver, spleen) as ferritin, or its aggregate, haemosiderin.

Iron is stored in 2 forms—soluble ferritin and insoluble haemosiderin. The precursor of ferritin is apoferritin. Apoferritin takes up ferrous iron oxidizes it and deposits the ferric iron in its core. In this form, it constitutes ferritin which is the primary storage form of iron. Iron is most readily available from ferritin. The life-span of this iron-laden protein is only a few days. Haemosiderin is a degraded form of ferritin.

Small amounts of iron (1 mg daily) are lost due to exfoliation of intestinal mucosal cells into the faeces; traces are excreted in urine, bile and sweat. Fig. 7.1 shows transport of iron.

Iron preparations

Oral preparations :
- Ferrous sulphate (cheapest).
- Ferrous succinate
- Ferrous fumarate
- Ferrous gluconate
- Colloidal ferric hydroxide

Ferrous sulphate 200-600 mg daily, contains 20% elemental iron, ferrous fumarate 200-600 mg daily contains 33% elemental iron, ferrous gluconate 200 mg daily contains 12% elemental iron.

The effective dose of all these preparations is based on iron content.

Liquid preparations stain teeth.

Ascorbic acid enhances absorption of iron.

As ferrous salts are rapidly changed to ferric salts in the air so they are given as coated tablets.

Iron sulphate makes stool black.

Parenteral preparations :
- Iron-dextran injection (I.M. or I.V.)
- Iron sorbitol-citric acid complex (only I.M.)

Uses

- Prevention of iron deficiency
- Treatment of anaemias due to iron deficiency (microcytic hypochromic anaemia)

Orally administered ferrous sulphate, the least expensive of iron preparations, is the drug of choice for iron deficiency. Ferrous salts are absorbed about 3 times as well as ferric salts.

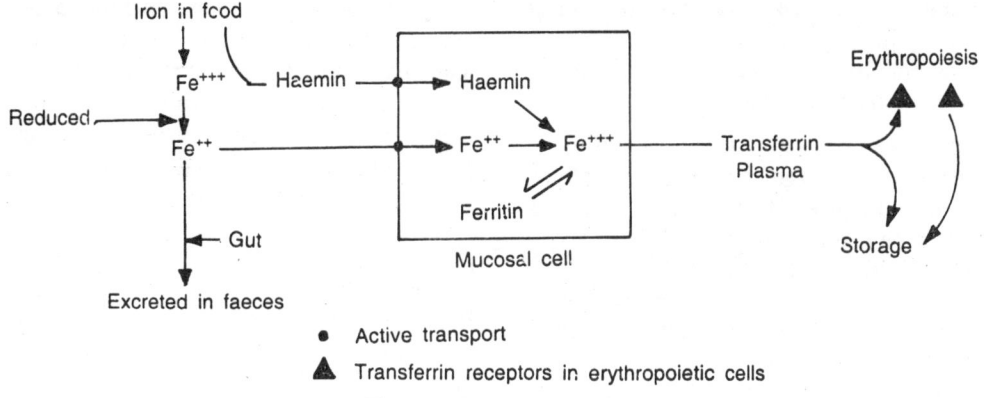

Fig. 7.1. Transport of iron.

Variations in particular ferrous salts have little effect on the bioavailability, and the sulphate, fumarate, succinate, gluconate are absorbed to about the same extent.

Ferrous sulphate or ferrous fumarate 200-600 mg are given orally with meals daily that should increase haemoglobin within 2-4 weeks and become normal within 1-3 months. This therapy should increase 1 g % haemoglobin per week. However, the therapy should be continued for 3-6 months for replenishment of iron stores in the body. For an adult of 70 kg body weight, 250 mg iron for Hb deficit of each g/dL is calculated as the required amount.

Iron can also be given parenterally but only under certain circumstance, for example, (i) if patient is not able to tolerate oral therapy, (ii) malabsorption and (iii) severe deficiency.

• Patients with a disease such as sprue, which prevents absorption of iron from the gastro-intestinal tract.

The parenteral preparations of iron are iron dextran and iron sorbitol.

Iron dextran is a complex of ferric hydroxide with 5000 to 7000 daltons in a viscous solution, containing 50 mg/ml of iron. dextran having 50 mg elemental iron per ml of solution.

100-250 mg iron (2-5 ml) is injected I.M. daily, total dose is given for about 15 days.

If it is given by I.V. route (infusion over 1-2 hours, diluted in saline), test should be done for any allergic reactions.

Iron sorbitol (iron-sorbitol-citric acid complex) complex with MW less than 5000 contains 50 mg elemental iron/ml.

Dose is 100 mg (2 ml) daily by I.M. injection.

I.M. injection is painful.

I.M. route is appropriate when I.V. route is inaccessible.

Differences between iron-dextran and iron sorbitol are given in Table 7.2.

Table 7.2. Differences between iron-dextran and iron sorbitol.

Iron Sorbitol	Iron-dextran
Low molecular weight	High molecular weight
Given only I.M.	Can be given I.M. or I.V.
30% excreted in urine	Not excreted
Absorbed directly into circulation	Given I.M., absorbed through lymphatics
May saturate transferrin	Not bound to transferrin
Directly available	Taken up by macrophages, and slowly made available to RBC.

Adverse reactions

• Oral therapy: Nausea, constipation or diarrhoea, heartburn, upper gastric discomfort. Iron tablets should be taken with meals or soon after meals to avoid GIT upsets.

If the liquid is given, iron solution may be placed on the back of the tongue with a dropper to prevent transient staining of teeth.

• Parenteral therapy: I.M. injections are painful. Headache, joint pains may occur. Allergic reactions, anaphylactoid reactions in case of I.V. therapy have been reported.

Iron toxicity can be acute as well as chronic.

Acute toxicity: If a large number of iron tablets are taken by mistake (even 10 tablets in case of children) there will be necrotizing gastroenteritis (vomiting, bloody diarrhoea and shock) that needs immediate treatment by gastric lavage with carbonate solution (to form insoluble salt) or with desferrioxamine 2g/L. In addition to gastric lavage, 10 g desferrioxamine is instilled in stomach, and also 1-2 g given by I.M. or I.V. route to neutralize (chelate) absorbed iron.

Chronic toxicity (haemosiderosis): Excess iron is deposited in liver, pancreas, heart and other organs resulting in organ failure.

Haemochromatosis or haemosiderosis may also be due to excess iron absorption or due to repeated blood transfusion (each transfusion gives about 250 mg iron).

An orally absorbable iron chelator, deferiprone 75 mg/kg/daily in divided doses may be given to treat iron overload. Deferoxamine 1-2 g I.M./I.V. chelates ferric iron and forms nontoxic ferrioxamine which is excreted in urine. The maximum dose is 6 g/24 hours.

Drug interactions: Iron chelates with tetracycline, ciprofloxacin, levodopa, penicillamine and methyldopa. These should not be given simultaneously.

COPPER

Copper deficiency is extremely rare in human beings. There is no evidence that copper ever needs to be added to a normal diet. However, anaemia due to copper deficiency has been noted in individuals who have undergone intestinal bypass surgery, in those who are getting parenteral nutrition, in malnourished infants and in patients ingesting excessive amounts of zinc.

Copper deficiency in experimental animals interferes with the absorption of iron and its release from reticuloendothelial cells. The associated microcytic anaemia is related to decrease in the availability of iron to the normoblasts and to a decrease mitochondrial production of haem. In human beings, the concentrations of iron in plasma are variable and the anaemia is not always microcytic. If a low plasma copper concentration is found in the presence of leukopenia and anaemia, 0.1 mg/kg of cupric sulphate orally, or 1-2 mg/daily may be administered along with nutrients for parenteral administration.

PYRIDOXINE

Pyridoxine may improve haematopoiesis in up to 50% of patients with either hereditary or idiopathic acquired sideroblastic anaemias. Patients suffering with sideroblastic anaemias show an impairment in haemoglobin synthesis and an accumulation of iron in the perinuclear mitochondria of erythroid precursor cells.

The oral therapy with pyridoxine is of proven benefit in correcting sideroblastic anaemias associated with the antituberculosis drugs INH and pyrazinamide, which act as vitamin B_6 antagonists.

RIBOFLAVIN

The appearance of red cell aplasia in human beings due to riboflavin deficiency is very rare, if it occur at all. However, it has been reported in combination with infection and protein deficiency, both of which can produce a hypoproliferative anaemia. Therefore it seems reasonable to include riboflavin in the nutritional management of patients with gross, generalized malnutrition.

HAEMOPOIETIC GROWTH FACTORS

Human being must generate regularly millions of granulocytes and millions of erythrocytes as well as numerous mononuclear cells and platelets. These are derived from a small number of self-renewing pluripotent stem cells which are laid down during embryogenesis.

The haemopoietic growth factors direct the division and maturation of the progeny of these various types of blood cells. These cytokine growth factors are glycoproteins. Erythropoietin is the factor that regulates the red cell line and the signal for production is blood loss and/or low tissue O_2 tension.

ERYTHROPOIETIN

It is a glycoprotein hormone produced by kidneys and released in response to tissue hypoxaemia. It is a primary regulator of erythropoiesis. The most important (although not the sole growth factor for erythropoiesis) regulator of the proliferation of committed progenitors (burst-forming units-E, BFU-E and colony forming units-E, CFU-E). It stimulates the proliferation of immature erythroid progenitor cells which give rise to marrow normoblasts, the immediate precursors of reticulocytes and mature red blood cells.

With anaemia due to hypoxaemia, renal synthesis and secretion of erythropoietin can increase rapidly by 100-fold, the released hormone acts on the late (CFU-E) progenitor cells to increase their survival and maturation. The feedback loop can be interrupted by renal disease, structural damage of the bone marrow; or deficiencies of iron, vitamin or mineral. Deficiency of iron will suppress the marrow's response to high concentration of erythropoietin. In the presence of infection or inflammation, erythropoietin secretion, iron delivery and erythroid precursor proliferation are suppressed by inflammatory cytokines [tumor necrosis factor (TNF), IL-1, and alpha and gamma interferons].

Uses

- Erythropoietin is very effective in the treatment of anaemias, especially those associated with a poor erythropoietic response.
- It is used routinely in the management of anaemia of chronic renal disease.
- Erythropoietin can ameliorate the anaemia associated with cancer chemotherapy (only when marrow-suppressive effect of chemotherapy is operative).
- Patients with a primary haematopoietic disorder.
- Patients with AIDS who are being treated with zidovudine (AZT). However, AIDS patients with high serum erythropoietin levels do not respond to erythropoietin therapy.
- Anaemia associated with prematurity.
- Patients undergoing elective surgery to decrease requirement for transfusion.
- Preoperatively to increase red cell production.

- Perioperatively to maintain a higher level of red cell production during immediate - postoperative period.

The therapy with erythropoietin is not intended for patients needing immediate correction of severe anaemias.

Erythropoietin has been produced by recombinant DNA technology as a 165-amino acid glycoprotein.

Recombinant human erythropoietin is available as epoetin alpha for IV or SC injection. To achieve adequate response it is given thrice a week, initial dose is 50-100 units/kg in patients with chronic renal failure. The haematocrit should be measured once each week. If there is increase of more than 4 g % in a 2-week period, the dose should be reduced.

In case after 2 months of therapy the haematocrit does not increase by at least 5% the dosage should be increased (increment of 25 units/kg at monthly intervals). The response is blunted in patients with reduced iron stores or iron deficiency, in that case it is necessary to give an oral iron supplement. However, oral iron alone may not meet the need of the rapidly proliferating marrow, iron dextran injection may be required. Inflammation may also delay or prevent a rise in haematocrit as it interferes with the supply of iron to the erythroid marrow. There are also other restricting factors such as aluminium intoxication, increased levels of parathormone, and osteitis fibrosa.

This drug is not given orally because it is broken down in the GIT.

Adverse effects

Patients with renal disease can experience worsening of their hypertension (due to rapidity of red cell mass and impact of such expansion on blood volume and viscosity). However, such adverse effects have not been significant problem when epoetin alpha is used in other clinical settings.

The colony - stimulating factors regulate the myeloid divisions of the white cell line and main stimulus of their production is infection.

CSFs (Colony stimulating factors): These stimulate particular committed progenitor cell to proliferate and cause irreversible differentiation. These are classified as cytokines.

GM-CSF is produced by many cell types and control at least five of the eight lines of blood cell development.

G-CSF is produced mainly by monocytes, fibroblasts and endothelial cells and controls development of neutrophils.

Recombinant G-CSF is available as **filgrastim** and **lenograstim.**

Recombinant GM-CSF is available as **molgramostin.**

Filgrastim

Filgrastim is a granulocyte colony-stimulating factor (G-CSF) and is also known as recombinant methionyl human granulocyte colony - stimulating factor (r-metHuG-CSF).

Filgrastim demonstrates first-order absorption and elimination. Following subcutaneous administration, peak serum levels are observed within 2 to 8 hours. Elimination half-life is about 3.5 hours.

Filgtrastim is indicated to lessen neutropenia associated with myelosuppressive chemotherapy. It may also be useful in preventing opportunistic diseases in patients infected with the human immunodeficiency virus.

Cautions: The most frequent adverse effect is bone pain; to avoid the potential complications of leucocytosis, monitor RBC twice per week during therapy. Filgrastim should not be given within 24 hours (before or after) chemotherapy administration. Simultaneous use of filgrastim with chemotherapy and radiation therapy should be avoided.

Lenograstim

Lenograstim is a glycosylated form of recombinant human granulocyte colony-stimulating factor (r HuG-CSF). It is derived from the Chinese hamster ovary cells. Filgrastim is non-glycosylated rHuG-CSF. Like filgrastim, lenograstim is a haematopoietic growth factor which stimulates the proliferation and differentiation of neutrophil precursor cells as well as some of the functional properties of mature neutrophil granulocytes.

Peak serum levels occur 6 hours following SC doses of 5 mcg/kg; the bioavailability with this dose is 30%. It is metabolized to peptides, with a small amount appearing unchanged in the urine (less than 1% of a dose). The elimination half-life of SC lenograstim is 2-8 hours in cancer patients.

The place in therapy of lenograstim is similar to that of filgrastim. It is effective in reducing the duration of neutropenia in cancer patients receiving chemotherapy and in those undergoing bone marrow transplantation.

Cautions: The most common adverse effects are bone pain and pain on SC injection. Other effects include nausea, vomiting, diarrhoea, headache, fever, alopecia. Thrombocytopenia has occurred after lenograstim.

Molgramostim

Molgramostim is an E. coli-derived non-glycosylated, recombinant human granulocyte-macrophage colony-stimulating factor (rh GM-CSF).

It is rapidly absorbed after SC injection, detectable after 5-10 minutes, reaches maximum serum concentrations after 2-6 hours, terminal half-life is 3 hours.

It is used in the treatment of chemotherapy-induced neutropenia.

Dose: Adults 5-10 mcg/kg/day subcutaneous for 7 to 10 days after chemotherapy.

Cautions: Pregnancy, lactation, myeloid conditions, pre-existing pulmonary diseases, autoimmune diseases.

Note: A "first-dose" reaction has been reported within 15 to 180 minutes of administration in doses greater than 1 mcg/kg. This reaction is characterized by the following symptoms: hypotension, tachycardia, rigor, fever, flushing, nausea, vomiting, back pain, leg spasms, and dyspnoea. The incidence for the first-dose reaction appears to be more common with I.V. administration than with SC.

VITAMIN B$_{12}$ AND FOLIC ACID

Deficiency of these maturation factors leads to megaloblastic anaemia.

Vitamin B$_{12}$

It is a water soluble cobalt containing compound produced by bacteria in alimentary canal or taken in food such as milk, cheese, egg yolk.

Box 7.1 : Haemopoietic Growth Factors

• Erythropoietin
  – regulates red cell production
  – available as epoietin
  – given by I.V./SC injection
  – can cause transient flu-like symptoms, hypertension, iron deficiency and increased blood viscosity.
• Granulocyte - macrophage colony-stimulating factor (GM-CSF):
  – stimulates many types of progenitor cells
  – available as molgramostim
  – given IV/SC injection
  – can cause fever, rashes, hypotension, bone pain, GIT symptoms.
• Granulocyte colony - stimulating factor (G-CSF)
  – stimulates neutrophil progenitors
  – available as filgrastim
  – given IV/SC injection

It is obtained commercially from *streptomyces griseus*. The daily human requirement is only 2 microgram and the daily diet has 5-30 microgram of vitamin B_{12}. Hence, its deficiency leads to pernicious anaemia if intrinsic factor (specific glycoprotein secreted from parietal cells of stomach) is absent or there is malabsorption from distal ileum e.g. in sprue. Normally the intrinsic factor forms a complex with extrinsic factor (vitamin B_{12}), which is absorbed from distal ileum.

Vitamin B_{12} is transported in blood in combination with a specific plasma globulin called transcobalamin.

Excess vitamin B_{12} is stored in liver (3-5 mg which can meet the requirement up to 5 years).

Hydroxycobalamin is more protein bound and hence it is better retained than cyanocobalamine.

The deficiency results in megaloblastic anaemia.

B_{12} deficiency affects both the haemopoeitic and nervous system.

Haemopoeitic : Megaloblastic anaemia characterised by neutrophils with hypersegmented nuclei, giant platelets, glossitis, GI dysfunction, damage to epithelial structure.

Neurological : Subacute degeneration of spinal cord, peripheral neuritis.

Conversion of methylmalonyl CoA to succinyl CoA is required for the synthesis of lipopro-teins in myelin tissue. This explains neurological compli-

cations such as peripheral neuritis, optic atrophy and sub-acute combined degeneration of spinal cord.

Mental changes : Poor memory, mood changes, hallucinations, etc. are late effects.

Vitamin B_{12} deficiency causes pernicious anaemia (Addisonian anaemia) which in turn causes retrobulbar neuritis with typical central scotomata. Vitamin B_{12} deficiency results in inadequate myelin synthesis affecting the optic, peripheral and cranial nerves.

Cyanocobalamin and hydroxocobalamin are mainly used clinically. Hydroxocobalamin in doses of 100 mg intramuscular is absorbed slowly. It is more protein bound, is excreted slowly and so higher blood levels are maintained for a longer period than cyanocobalamin.

Actions

Vitamin B_{12} is required for two essential enzymatic reactions in humans.

• Deoxyadenosylcobalamin is a required cofactor in the conversion of methylmalonyl - CoA to succinyl - CoA by the enzyme methylmalonyl - CoA mutase. This conversion can not occur if vitamin B_{12} is deficient.
• For conversion of 5-methyl tetrafolate and homocysteine methyl transferase.

Uses of Vitamin B_{12}

• Treatment of vitamin B_{12} deficiency
• Prophylaxis
• Tobacco amblyopia : Hydroxocobalamin is used. It traps cyanide derived from tobacco to form cyanocobalamin.
• Of doubtful value - mega doses used in neuropathies, cutaneous sarcoid, general tonic to allay fatigue, improve growth.

Uses: Pernicious anaemia.

Dose: 500-1000 microgram twice a week then 250 microgram weekly.

Folic acid (pteroylglutamic acid)

Its rich sources are green leafy vegetables, egg, liver, meat, fish, yeast. The daily requirement is 50-100 microgram and during pregnancy and lactation the requirement is 200-400 microgram daily.

The deficiency of folic acid results in megaloblastic anaemia. Deficiency of vitamin B_{12} also produces megaloblastic anaemia. The neurological symptoms such as peripheral neuritis, mental symptoms are present in vitamin B_{12} deficiency, but not in folic acid deficiency.

Preparations

- Oral 5 mg folic acid tablet/capsule.
- Parenterally 15 mg/ml.

Uses of folic acid

- For treatment of megaloblastic anaemia due to folate deficiency caused by:
  - poor diet (commonly in alcoholics)
  - malabsorption syndromes
  - use of some drugs such as phenytoin
- To treat or prevent toxicity from folate antagonist e.g. methotrexate.
- Prophylactically in persons at hazard from developing folate deficiency, e.g. pregnant women and patients with severe chronic haemolytic anaemia.

Contraindications

If given alone in pernicious anaemia, the haematological picture will improve but neurological complications are made worse because folic acid increases utilization of vitamin B_{12} including shift of B_{12} from neural tissue to bone marrow.

Vitamin B_{12} and not folic acid takes part in methylmalonyl CoA mutase reaction. When vitamin B_{12} is absent methylmanolyl CoA and deficiency of succinyl CoA results in synthesis of faulty fatty acids. These aberrant fatty acids incorporate into cell membranes of the CNS which produce neurological manifestations of vitamin B_{12} deficiency.

Table 7.3 shows comparison of haematinics.

HAEMOSTASIS

The circulating blood remains in a fluid state due to the fine balance maintained between coagulation and anticoagulant factors.

Bleeding and thrombosis are altered states of haemostasis. Impaired haemostasis results in bleeding, while stimulated haemostasis results in thrombus formation. A number of drugs are available to arrest bleeding and to inhibit thrombosis.

Mechanism of coagulation

There are two pathways in the cascade

- Extrinsic pathway which operates in vivo.
- Intrinsic or contact pathway which operates in vitro.

Both pathways result in activation of factors X which then converts prothrombin to thrombin.

Calcium and a negatively charged phospholipid (PL) are essential for three steps, namely the actions of –

- factor IX on X

Table 7.3. Comparison of haematinics

	Iron	Vitamin B_{12}	Folic acid
Source	Wheat, dry fruits, meat, egg yolk	Meat, egg, milk, liver	Green leafy vegetables, milk, egg, meat, liver
Daily requirement	0.5-1 mg	2 microgram	50 microgram
Absorption	Duodenum, proximal jejunum	Distal ileum	Jejunum
Deficiency	Microcytic hypochromic anaemia	Megaloblastic anaemia (neurological symptoms)	Megaloblastic anaemia
Store	Liver, spleen	Liver	Liver
Excretion	No specific system	Urine, stool	Urine, stool
Treatment	Ferrous sulphate 200-600 mg/d or iron dextran I.M./I.V.	0.1-1 mg I.M./d followed by once a month	1-5 mg/d, oral
Transport carrier	Transferrin	Transcobalamin	Plasma protein

- factor VIIa on X
- factor Xa on II

The clotting factors are given in Table 7.4.

Table 7.4. Clotting factors

Factor I	Fibrinogen
Factor II	Prothrombin
Factor III	Tissue thromboplastin
Factor IV	Calcium
Factor V	Proaccelerin
Factor VI	Not an independent factor
Factor VII	Proconvertin
Factor VIII	Antihaemophilic globulin (AHG-A)
Factor IX	Christmas factor
Factor X	Stuart-Power factor
Factor XI	Plasma thromboplastin
Factor XII	Hageman factor
Factor XIII	Fibrin stabilizing factor

The circulating platelets and the clotting factors do not adhere to the normal endothelium, vasospasm is the immediate haemostatic response of the damaged vessels, immediately followed by primary mechanism (of coagulation) where platelet plug is formed to stop bleeding.

Thrombin which is formed locally releases more ADP and stimulates prostaglandin synthesis from arachidonic acid of platelet membranes. Two groups with opposing effects are formed, viz. thromboxane A_2 synthesized within platelets induces thrombogenesis and prostacyclin synthesized within vessel wall inhibits thrombogenesis.

The extrinsic system in coagulation is activated by tissue fluid outside the blood vessels. Thromboplastin (III) is released from the damaged tissue into the circulating blood. Tissue thromboplastin converts factor X bound by calcium to phospholipid surfaces to Xa in the presence of factor VIIa. Fig. 7.2 shows blood coagulation mechanism.

VII°, IX°, X° and Prothrombin° are Vitamin K (coagulation vitamin) dependent in the liver. Heparin inactivates factors XIIa, XIa, IXa and Xa and increases the action of antithrombin III. Antithrombin III inhibits the conversion of prothrombin to thrombin and directly inactivates thrombin.

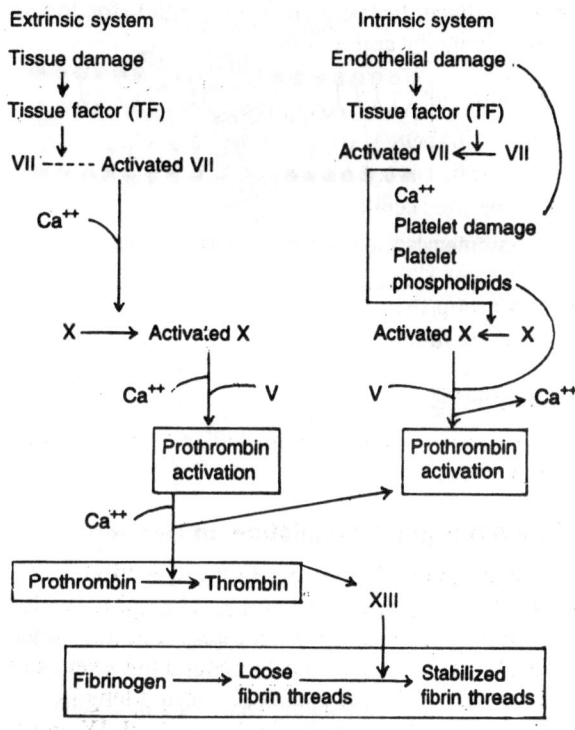

Fig. 7.2. Blood coagulation mechanism.

Local haemostatics

These stop bleeding from local site, e.g. local wounds, tooth socket etc. They promote coagulation by providing a network of fibrin. They stop oozing of blood from surfaces.

The use of alum, tannic acid and tincture of ferric chloride which were used in the past as local styptics are not commonly used now.

The substances now being used locally for checking haemorrhage are absorbable, and non-irritant.

Adrenaline soaked packs applied locally are used to stop epistaxis, nasal and facial bleeding during surgery.

Ethamsylate given systemically is useful in menorrhagia.

Carboprost (analogue of $PGF_{2\alpha}$) is useful in controlling postpartum haemorrhage in patients in whom oxytocin or ergometrine are not effective.

Oxidized cellulose is not recommended as a surface dressing, except for the immediate control of haemorrhage, because such application for longer time will inhibit epithelization.

Preparations

- Fibrin foam
- Gelatin sponge
- Oxidized cellulose
- Adrenaline
- Ethamsylate
- Carboprost
- Thrombin

Coagulants

These promote coagulation, indicated in haemorrhagic states.

Vitamin K (for 'Koagulation' in German)

It occurs naturally in two forms - as vitamin K_1 (phytonadione) in plants, and as Vitamin K_2 which is synthesised by bacteria in the gastrointestinal tract. Vitamin K_2 is not a single compound but a series of substances with side chains of varying lengths.

Clotting factors II (prothrombin), VII, IX and X are vitamin K dependent in the liver.

The daily requirement of Vitamin K is estimated to be 0.03 mcg/kg for adults.

Pharmacokinetic aspects

Natural vitamin K (phytonadione) can be administered orally as well as by IM or I.V. routes. If given orally, it requires bile salts for absorption. It is dispensed in 1 ml ampoules containing 50 mg of vitamin K.

A highly water soluble synthetic preparation, menadiol sodium diphosphate will not require bile salts for absorption. This compound takes longer to act than phytomenadione. It can be given orally, S.C., I.M. or I.V. like menadione.

There is very little storage of vitamin K in the body. It is metabolized to more polar substances which are excreted in urine and bile.

Preparations of vitamin K

- K_1 (from plants, fat soluble): Phytonadione
- K_2 (from bacteria): Menaquinones
- K_3 (synthetic):   i. Fat soluble: Menadione
  ii. Water soluble : Menadione sodium diphosphate

Uses of Vitamin K

- Vitamin K deficiencies
- Haemorrhagic disease of the new born
- Bleeding due to oral anticoagulant drugs

Synthetic variations

Naturally occurring vitamin K is a naphthoquinone derivative from plant and animal sources and is a product of bacterial fermentation in the gut. Synthetic variations, some oil soluble for I.M. injection, some water soluble for I.V. injection are available.

They may be given orally with 1-2 g of bile salts to facilitate absorption.

Menadione and menadione sodium bisulphite are oil soluble and water soluble, respectively.

Dose: 0.5-2 mg daily.

A highly water-soluble product is menadiol sodium diphosphate which can be given orally, S.C., I.M. or I.V. like menadione, it will hemolyze red blood cells in individuals deficient in glucose-6-phosphate dehydrogenase (G6PD) as well as in new born, especially premature infants. Vitamin K_5 is water soluble, and has actions and uses similar to those of phytonadione and menadione.

Aminocaproic acid inhibits fibrinolysis and is used in bleeding with excessive fibrinolytic activity such as occur in open heart surgery, bleeding of the urinary tract, neoplastic diseases, liver cirrhosis and abruptio placenta. This amino acid (related to lysine) inhibits conversion of plasminogen to plasmin and also to a lesser degree, directly inhibits the action of plasmin, which is the active fibrinolytic enzyme. It is given orally or I.V. It is excreted rapidly in the urine. It should not be used without definite diagnosis, indicative of hyperfibrinolysis.

Anticoagulants

These are used to reduce coagulability of blood.

Parenterally used: Heparin

Oral anticoagulants: Coumarin and Indanedione derivatives

Only for in vitro anticoagulation: Sodium citrate, sodium oxalate and sodium edetate.

The two most commonly used anticoagulants are heparin and warfarin.

HEPARIN

Heparin is so named because it was first extracted from liver. It is a mucopolysaccharide. It carries strong electronegative charge and is the strongest organic acid present in the body. It is present in the mast cells bound to granular proteins. Rich sources are lung, liver and intestinal mucosa.

It is commercially produced from bovine lung and porcine intestinal mucosa.

There are two types of heparin:

- High molecular weight heparin. It is a stronger anticoagulant.
- Low molecular weight heparin. Adverse effect of haemorrhage is less frequent with it.

Low molecular weight heparin (LMWHs 4000-6500), e.g. enoxaparin, are given by SC route and are commonly used because –

- Longer elimination half-life
- Effects are more predictable
- Dosing less frequent (once or twice a daily)
- Monitoring is not required routinely
- More convenient to use
- They do not prolong activated partial thromboplastin time (APTT).
- They have no effect on platelets
- Cause less bleeding complications
- At least as safe and effective as unfractionated heparin.
- Generally no need for blood tests and dose adjustments.

LMWHs increase the action of antithrombin-III on factor Xa but not its action on thrombin since the molecules are two small to bind to both enzyme and inhibitor, essential for inhibition of thrombin but not of factor Xa.

Enoxaparin

Enoxaparin, a low molecular weight heparin is formed by depolymerizing standard heparin. It is more bioavailable and has longer half-life than heparin. It has more anti-factor Xa activity than heparin. As it causes less inactivation of thrombin, less inhibition of platelets and less vascular permeability than heparin, bleeding complications are lower than with heparin.

Dose: SC 30mg/12hr for 7-10 days in thrombo-embolism, deep venous thrombosis and to reduce the risk of pulmonary embolism following hip or knee replacement surgery.

Pharmacokinetics and routes of administration

Heparin is a highly ionized molecule so it is not absorbed through the gastrointestinal mucosa. It is precipitated by gastric HCl and digested by enzymes. It also does not cross blood - brain barrier or placental barrier. Hence, it is given parenterally by continuous infusion, deep SC injection or intermittent I.V. injections. It is not administered by I.M. injection (produces painful haematomas).

Heparin is metabolized in liver by heparinase. Some quantity is extended in urine unaltered. Its half-life is 60-90 minutes upto < 100 units / kg. It increases with increase in dose.

Pharmacological actions

- Anticoagulant effect
- Antiplatelet effect in high doses, increase in bleeding time
- Lipemia clearing effect: Heparin in small doses activates lipoprotein lipase from vessel wall and tissues which hydrolyses triglycerides of chylomicrons and VLDL to FFA which then pass into tissues and plasma looks clear.

USP unit of heparin

One unit is the quantity that prevents 1.0ml of citrated sheep plasma from clotting for 1 hour after the addition of 0.2 ml of 1% calcium chloride.

Heparin sodium 1mg has 120-140 units of activity.

Monitoring of heparin therapy

Heparin therapy is monitored by whole blood clotting time (kept 2-3 times normal) and activated partial thromboplastin time (APTT) kept half-life to 2 times normal.

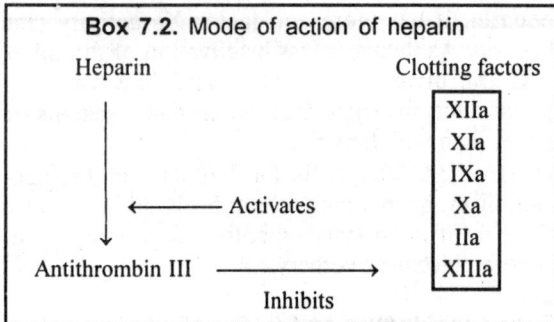

Box 7.2. Mode of action of heparin

Mechanism of action

Heparin acts indirectly by activating plasma antithrombin III. Plasma antithrombin III then inactivates activated coagulation factors including thrombin (IIa), Xa, IXa, XIa, XIIa and XIIIa, clotting factors.

The factors Xa and IIa are most sensitive to inhibition and so the anticoagulant actions are exerted mainly by inhibition of these clotting factors.

Heparin inhibits platelet aggregation due to its antithrombin effect (thrombin is a powerful platelet aggregator).

Uses

- To prevent postoperative deep venous thrombosis and pulmonary embolism. 5000 units S.C. every 8 to 12 hourly provides effective prophylaxis.
- To treat established venous thrombosis. Heparin initially for 8 to 10 days followed by warfarin should be given; I.V. injection of 12,500 units (bolus) followed by I.V. infusion of 9,000 units/hour or S.C. injection of 10,000 to 20,000 units every 12 hours.
- To prevent clotting in open heart surgery.
- To keep blood outside the body in fluid state.

Calcium complexing agents are used.

Heparin, sodium citrate are used for transfusion

Sodium oxalate is not used for transfusion being toxic but used for blood cell count.

Adverse reactions

- Bleeding (haematuria is generally the first sign). It results from excessive blockade of fibrin formation and interference with normal haemostasis.
- If used for long period (about 6 months) osteoporosis and spontaneous fracture of ribs and vertebrae may be produced.
- Alopecia (transient) on prolonged use
- Wound healing is slowed
- Depress cell-mediated immunity
- Allergic reactions include asthma, urticaria, fever, rhinitis
- Thrombocytopenia (less common with porcine heparin)
- Thrombocytoperia due to antibody formation may be serious in some cases. It can occur in upto 30% of patients resulting from heparin induced platelet aggregation.
- Hyperkalaemia due to inhibition of aldosterone.

A severe form of thrombocytopenia associated with the development of heparin dependent antiplatelet antibodies resulting in greatly increased platelet aggregation has been reported. It can occur in upto 30% of patients.

Contraindications

- Bleeding disorders
- Thrombcocytopenia
- Severe hypertension (patients are liable to bleed)
- GIT ulcers (patients are liable to bleed)
- Active tuberculosis
- History of hypersensitivity to heparin

Antagonist of heparin

Heparin is strongly electronegative. It is neutralized by highly basic peptide, protamine (obtained from fish sperm). Protamine sulphate 1% solution is given by I.V. infusion. For every 100 units of heparin 1mg protamine is given. Due consideration must be given to the amount of heparin that may have been degraded by the patient in the mean time.

An overdose of this antidote may itself inhibit blood clotting.

Hypersensitivity reactions are rare with heparin but more common with protamine.

Heparinoids

Certain sulphated mucopolysaccharides have

heparin like action e.g., dextran sulphate is a plasma expander, but dextran with 70,000 molecular weight interferes with platelet function and fibrin polymerization. It can be employed to prevent post operative venous thrombosis. However, it is quite weak anticoagulant as compared to heparin.

Newer thrombin - related agents

Dermatan sulphate is related to heparin, potentiates heparin cofactor II which inhibits thrombin selectively. Hence, it is likely to cause less bleeding than heparin. Its safety and efficacy remains to be compared with low molecular-weight-heparins.

Dose: IM 300mg once or twice daily for prophylaxis against post operative venous thromboembolism.

Antithrombin-III-independent anticoagulants

A number of direct inhibitors of thrombin are under trial. These include-hirudin, hirugen, argatroban. As these agents are immunologically quite distinct, they may have a niche in the treatment of patients who have developed immune thrombocytopenia/thrombosis during treatment with heparin.

ORAL ANTICOAGULANTS

- Coumarin derivatives: Dicoumarol, warfarin, phenprocoumon, acenocoumarol, nicoumalone
- Indandione derivatives: Phenindione, diphenadione, anisindione, bromindione

Mechanism of action of oral anticoagulants

They act indirectly by interfering with the synthesis of vitamin K dependent clotting factors in the liver. They act as competitive antagonists of vitamin K. They prevent the formation of active vitamin K hydroquinone resulting in reduced rate of formation of clotting factors prothrombin (II), VII, IX, X. Coumarin therapy increases plasma antithrombin levels.

Though the synthesis of these factors stops within 2-4 hours of administration of oral anticoagulants, the anticoagulant effect appears in 1-3 days, as these existing factors decline progressively.

Uses of anticoagulants

- To prevent extension of established deep vein thrombosis

- To prevent thrombosis on prosthetic heart valves
- To prevent thrombosis and embolisation in patients with atrial fibrillation.

Oral anticoagulants cross placenta, hence they should not be given during pregnancy. It they are given in the first months of pregnancy they are teratogenic (6-14 weeks is critical period); if given in later stages they cause intracranial haemorrhage during delivery.

Oral anticoagulants also appear in milk during lactation.

Factors that enhance actions of oral anticoagulants and thus increase the risk of unexpected haemorrhage:

- Disease
  Liver diseases interfere with the synthesis of clotting factors. Fever and thyrotoxicosis in which there is a high metabolic rate, increase degradation of clotting factors.
- Drugs
  Many drugs potentiate warfarin, including:
  - drugs that inhibit hepatic drug metabolism, e.g. co-trimoxazole, ciprofloxacin.
  - drugs that inhibit platelet function e.g. NSAIDs
  - drugs that displace warfarin from binding sites on plasma albumin, e.g. some of the NSAIDs and chloral hydrate
  - drugs that inhibit reduction of vitamin K, e.g. cephalosporins
  - drugs that decrease the availability of vitamin K, e.g. some sulphonamides and broad-spectrum antibiotics which depress the intestinal flora which normally synthesises vitamin K_2.

Factors that decrease the effect of oral anticoagulants (may result in ineffective treatment)

- Disease/Physiological state
  - hypothyroidism which is associated with reduced degradation of coagulantion factors.
  - pregnancy where there is increased coagulantion factor synthesis.
- Drugs
  - drugs that induce hepatic P450 enzymes

increase the degradation of oral anticoagulants, e.g. rifampicin, barbiturates, carbamazepine, griseofulvin
- drugs that reduce absorption, e.g. cholestyramine

WARFARIN

It is most commonly used oral anticoagulant. Warfarin (unlike heparin) is active only in vivo and not in vitro. The onset of action is after 8-12 hours and prolonged duration of action as compared to heparin.

Administration and pharmacokinetic aspects

Warfarin is promptly and totally absorbed from GIT after oral administration. It is strongly bound to plasma albumin. The effect of a single dose starts after 12-16 hours. The action lasts for 4-5 days. It is metabolised in liver. The elimination half-life is about 40 hours.

Table 7.5 summarizes comparison between warfarin and heparin.

Warfarin is used in established venous thromboembolism, initially 30-50 mg then 100 mg next day, there after 5-12 mg once a day (object is to lower the blood prothrombin activity to 25% of normal), followed by the maintenance dose of 5-7 mg/24 hours or 20-100 mg phenindione.

Adverse reactions

- Haemorrhage from GIT or urinary tract.
- Haemorrhagic disorders, bone formation and CNS abnormalities have been reported, because warfarin unlike heparin crosses placenta. Heparin may be given in pregnancy.
- Warfarin necrosis is a painful erythematous patch produced on the skin due to thrombi in affected tissue.
- A "purple toe" syndrome may be produced by cholesterol emboli from atheromatous plaques following bleeding into the plaques.

Side effects such as skin rashes, nausea, vomiting, pyrexia, jaundice are more common with phenindione.

Antidote: Phytomenadione.

Table 7.5. Comparison of warfarin and heparin

	Warfarin	*Heparin*
Source	Synthetic	Porcine intestinal mucosa, bovine lung
Nature	Coumarine derivative	Sulphated mucopolysaccharide
Activity	In vivo only	In vitro and in vivo
Route of administration	Oral	I.V./S.C. (Never I.M. due to danger of haematoma at site of injection)
Metabolism and excretion	Metabolized in liver	Metabolized by heparinase, excreted in urine
Plasma half-life	36 hours	90 minutes
Mode of action	Vit. K antagonist, inhibits synthesis of clotting factors II, VII, IX and X	Activates antithrombin III and inhibits clotting factors II, VII, IX and X. Blocks factor X and thrombin
Onset	8-12 hours	Immediate
Duration	4-7 days	1-5 hours
Test for controlling dose	PT to be raised 2 times of control value (12 seconds)	PT + to be raised 2 times of control value (30 seconds)
Adverse reactions	Haemorrhage, haemorrhage in foetus	Haemorrhage, on prolonged use osteoporosis, alopecia, thrombocytopenia
Antidote	Vitamin K	Protamine sulphate
Contraindications	Bleeding disorders, bleeding diathesis, pregnancy	Bleeding disorders, bleeding diathesis
Drug interaction	Many	Few

Contraindications

- Pregnancy
- Warfarin and heparin are both contraindicated in bleeding diathesis.
- Warfarin can be given as it is not excreted in milk.

Drug-drug interactions

- Metronidazole, chloramphenicol, ciprofloxacin, co-trimoxazole, phenylbutazone inhibit metabolism of warfarin and thus increase its activity.
- Phenylbutazone displaces it from plasma proteins and its activity is increased.
- On the other hand, barbiturates, rifampin through enzyme induction decrease warfarin action.
- Increased warfarin activity may result in unexpected haemorrhage, whereas its decreased activity will result in ineffective treatment.

FIBRINOLYTIC DRUGS

Heparin and oral anticoagulants do not affect fibrinolytic mechanism. The fibrinolytic system is shown in Fig. 7.3.

Thrombolytic or fibrinolytic agents are drugs that result in the dissolution of the blood clot by activation of plasminogen to active plasmin which degrades fibrin. The classical agents include streptokinase and urokinase. The newer agents are tissue plasmonigen activator (tPA), anisoylated plasminogen-streptokinase activator complex (APSAC) and single chain urokinase plasminogen activator (prourokinase).

- Streptokinase. It combines with proactivator plasminogen and this complex catalyses conversion of plasminogen to plasmin.
  Dose: loading dose 250,000 units, then 100,000 units per hour for 1-3 days.
- Urokinase directly converts plasminogen to plasmin.
  Dose: loading dose 300,000 units followed by 300,000 units per hour for 12 hours.
- Tissue plasminogen activator (tPA) 100 mg is administered I.V. in 3 hours. Compared to streptokinase and urokinase, it is fibrin-selective as it preferentially activates plasminogen bound to fibrin.

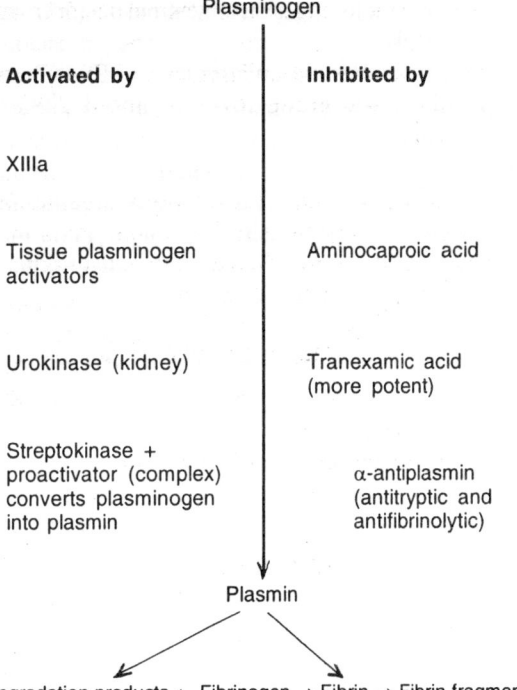

Fig. 7.3. Fibrinolytic system.

- Anistreplase [anisoylated (Anisoylated plasminogen-streptokinase activator complex (APSAC)] is given as a single I.V. injection over 4-5 minutes. The activity lasts for 4-6 hours.

Uses of fibrinolytic drugs

- In MI within 3-4 hours of onset, they reduce mortality in patients.
  However, efficacy has been reported 4 hours with therapy begun as late as 24 hours.
- Acute thrombotic stroke within 3 hours of onset.
- For deep vein thrombosis - in legs, pelvis, shoulder, etc.
- In pulmonary embolism
- For venous thromboembolism and local thrombosis in the anterior chamber of the eye.
- For peripheral arterial occlusion (small arteries).

Adverse effects of fibrinolytic agents

- The main hazard of all fibrinolytic agents is

bleeding including gastrointestinal haemorrhage and stroke.

- Streptokinase and anistreplase (APSAC) can produce low grade fever in about 25% of patients.
- Hypotension
- Streptokinase and APSAC are allergenic and antigenic (hypersensitivity, anaphylaxis may occur with them) whereas tPA and urokinase are not antigenic and allergenic.

Contraindications to fibrinolytic (thrombolytic) therapy

- Active internal bleeding
- Previous cerebrovascular accident
- Bleeding diathesis
- Pregnancy
- Uncontrolled hypertension
- Invasive procedures in which haemostasis is important
- Surgery within 10 days
- Recent cranial trauma
- Cerebral tumour

Treatment of overdose toxicity of fibrinolytic (thrombolytic) drugs

Antifibrinolytic drugs

Tranexamic acid inhibits plasminogen activation and thus prevents fibrinolysis. It is indicated in various conditions in which there is bleeding or risk of bleeding such as haemorrhage following dental extraction, in excessive menstrual blood loss (menorrhagia) and following thrombolytic overdose. It is given orally or intravenously.

Dose: 1-1.5 g orally 3-4 times/d for 3-4 days in menorrhagia.

Oral 25 mg/kg body weight every 6-8 hr beginning 1 day before dental procedure.

Aprotinin is used for hyperplasminaemia (caused by fibrinolytic drug overdose) and in patients at risk of major blood loss during coronary artery by pass graft. Aprotinin inhibits proteolytic enzymes. It is usually well tolerated but nausea, vomiting, diarrhoea, muscle pains, and B.P. changes have occurred.

Allergic reactions (erythema) urticaria, bronchospams have been reported. Anaphylaxis has also occurred.

Dose: 2 million KIU over 20-30 minutes (loading dose), then constant infusion of 5 lac KIU/hr. is begun.

Units

Potency is expressed in terms of Kallikrein inhibitory units. One unit inactivates about 500ng of trypsin.

Other drugs affecting blood flow:

Pentoxyfylline (methylxanthine derivative) reduces serum fibrinogen and platelet aggregation is inhibited.

Danazol (synthetic androgen) increases serum concentrations of clotting factors VIII and IX.

ANTIPLATELET DRUG THERAPY

Antiplatelet drugs play a critical oral in the management of patients with arterial vascular disease and thromboembolism. Platelets play an important role in thromboembolic process, as shown in fig. 7.4. Aspirin is most widely used, because of its unique pharmacology. A single dose of aspirin irreversibly acetylates and inactivates enzyme cyclooxygenase and thereby inhibits platelet thromboxane A_2 production. Although aspirin may also inactivate cyclooxygenase in other tissues including endothelial cells, such cells recover rapidly by synthesizing enzyme. Platelets, which are anuclear cannot synthesize new enzyme and remain inactive the rest of their life span (7 to 10 days). The resumption of TXA_2 production depends on the entry of new platelets into the circulation. Thus continuous antiplatelet effects is readily achieved with low doses.

Aspirin in low doses upto 320 mg/d, produces irreversible acetylation of platelet COX and in low doses the effect on vascular COX is nominal and short lived. No other NSAID has this ability.

As little as 150mg of aspirin daily or a 325mg tablet every other day inhibits platelet thromboxane production and aggregation.

Although aspirin is clearly the most efficacious antiplatelet agent in clinical use today, a number of other drugs are being tested. Ticlopidine, a potent inhibitor of platelet function, is effective as an alternative to aspirin in patients of cerebrovascular disease and is superior to aspirin or warfarin in maintaining coronary stent patency. It is more expensive than aspirin and causes some serious side effects including neutropenia and rare episodes of thrombocytopenia. A related drug, clopidogrel has been proposed, but rare cases of TTP have also being noted with this drug.

The uses of antithrombotic therapy are evolving rapidly. However, aspirin is the current mainstay for chronic therapy and should be used indefinitely in any patient who has had a coronary or cerebral thrombosis. It will reduce ischaemic events by 25% or more.

Antiplatelet Drugs

Aspirin inactivates cyclooxygenase acting mainly on the constitutive enzyme. COX-1. This reduces both TXA_2 synthesis in platelets and prostacyclin synthesis in endothelium. Vascular endothelial cells, however, can synthesise new enzyme whereas cohort of platelets is replaced in 7-10 days. Besides this, higher doses of aspirin are needed to inhibit cyclooxygenase in vascular endothelium than in platelets. This is because platelets are exposed to aspirin in the portal blood, and systemic vasculature is partly protected by presystemic metabolism of aspirin by esterase in the liver. Therefore low doses of aspirin decrease the synthesis of TXA_2 without drastically reducing prostacyclin synthesis. The balance between prostacyclin (an inhibitor of aggregation generated by vascular endothelium) and TXA_2 (a stimulant of aggregation generated by platelets) is altered, since the endothelium can synthesise more enzymes but platelets cannot. TXA_2 synthesis only recovers when new platelets are formed.

The effectiveness of aspirin is limited because there are several pathways to platelet activation which do not depend on thromboxane (TXA_2). In contrast, prostacyclin inhibits all pathways of platelet activation. Prostacyclin is available for clinical use as epoprostenol, but its use is very limited because it has very short half-life and needs to be given parenterally. Iloprost is a stable analogue but causes vasodilatation resulting in flushing and headache.

Dipyridamole by itself has little or no effect

The beneficial effect of aspirin and dipyridamole is additive. It increases platelet cAMP and may be used combined with low dose aspirin. It blocks phosphodiesterase and thus increases cAMP. It produces vasodilatation and inhibition of platelet aggregation.

Dose: 75-100 mg orally 4 times/d.

Headache is a common side effect of dipyridamole. However, unlike aspirin it causes no excess risk of bleeding.

Sulphinpyrazone is a COX-inhibitor but not selective for platelets, needs triple daily doses and is less effective than the single daily dose of aspirin.

Dazoxiben

Dazoxiben selectively decreases TXA_2. This drug in combination with aspirin produces appreciable effect but alone it is not very effective.

Ticlopidine is a thienopyridine derivative, acts slowly, takes 3-7 days to achieve peak effect. It works through an active metabolite. Its efficacy in reducing stroke is similar to that of aspirin. It is recommended for patients unable to take aspirin.

Dose: 250mg twice a day with meals.

Short-term use (for one month) with aspirin substantially reduce cardiac events and haemorrhagic and vascular complications compared with the conventional treatment.

Adverse effects include nausea and diarrhoea in about 10% of patients and severe neutropenia in about 1% of patients. The adverse effects particularly neutropenia have limited its long-term use.

Ticlopidine inhibits binding of fibrinogen to activated platelets, thus it inhibits platelet aggregation.

It inhibits platelet aggregation and platelet deposition on fibrin It is used in stroke prevention, TIAs, MI.

Clopidogrel is structurally related to ticlopidine having similar but more potent actions.

Dose: Loading dose 300mg followed by 75mg once a day.

Antiplatelet drugs which are under development include agents that either inhibit TXA_2, synthesis or block TXA_2 receptors or have both actions.

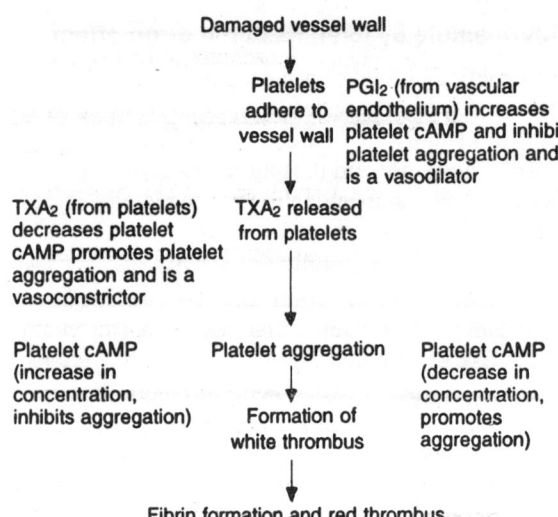

Fig. 7.4. Role of platelet thromboembolic process.

TXA$_2$ receptor antagonists e.g. GR32191 have been investigated. They are much more expensive than aspirin, unlikely to be more effective than low-dose aspirin but may be less toxic.

Compounds which have both TXA$_2$ synthetase inhibition as well as TXA$_2$ - receptor blocking activity seem better for inhibiting TXA$_2$ synthesis while increasing prostacyclin production. Drugs with this combination of activities e.g. ridogrel are being developed.

Uses of antiplatelet drugs

- Low dose of aspirin for prevention of high risk cases of MI, for prophylaxis of secondary MI.
- Coronary bypass.
- To prevent formation of microthrombin on prosthetic heart valves.

STUDY QUESTIONS

1. Define haematinics.
2. What are the different types of anaemias and how are they caused?
3. Name iron preparations, their pharmacokinetics, uses, adverse effects and treatment of acute and chronic toxicity of iron.
4. Describe the role of Vitamin B$_{12}$ and folic acid in the therapy of megaloblastic anaemia.
5. How the neurological symptoms in megalo-

blastic anaemia made worse if folic acid alone is given?
6. Describe the blood clotting mechanism.
7. Name the local haemostatics. What are their uses and limitations?
8. What is the role of vitamin K in blood clotting cascade?
9. Describe the uses, routes of administration, mode of action, and adverse effects of heparin.
10. Describe warfarin regarding its therapeutic uses, mode of action, route of administration, adverse effects, contraindications and drug-drug interactions.
11. Compare in tabulated form heparin and warfarin.
12. Name fibrinolytic agents. What are their uses?
13. Describe the role of platelets in thromboembolic process.
14. What are the uses of antiplatelet drugs? How does aspirin in low doses act as prophylactic for myocardial infarction?

GUIDE TO FURTHER READING

Dale D.C. 1995 where now for colony-stimulating factors? Lancet 346: 135-136.

Gomber, S., Kumar, S., Rusia, U., Gupta, P., Agarwal, K.N. and Sharma, S. Prevalence and etiology of nutritional anaemia in early childhood in an urban slum. Indian J. Med Res 107: 269, 1998.

Goodenough I.T. Monk T.G. et al 1997 Erythropoietin therapy N Engl. J. Med. 336: 933-938.

Grebe, G. et al: Effect of meals and ascorbic acid on the absorption of a therapeutic dose of iron as ferrous and ferric salts. Curr. Ther. Res., 1975; 17:382-397.

Hoelzer D 1997 Haemopoietic growth factors - not whether, but when and where. N Engl. J Med 336: 1822-1824

Levin J 1997 Thrombopoietin - Clinically realised ? N Engl. J Med 336: 434-436.

Lipschitz, D.A. et al: A clinical evaluation of serum ferritin as an index of iron stores. N. Engl. J. Med., 1974; 290:1213-1216.

Nutrient Requirements and Recommended Dietary Allowances for Indians (A Report of the Expert Group of the ICMR). Indian Council of Medical Research, New Delhi, p68, 1990.

Pritchard, J.A.: Hemoglobin regeneration in severe iron deficiency anemia. Response to orally and parenterally administered iron preparations. JMMA, 1966; 195:717-720.

Seshadri, S. Nutritional anaemia in South Asia. In: Malnutrition in South Asia. A Regional Profile. Ed. S. Gillespie, UNICEF Regional Office for South Asia, Kathmandu, Publication No. 5 p75, 1997.

Stebbins, R. et al: Drug-induced megaloblastic anemias. Semin. Hematol., 1973; 10:235-251.

Stebbins, R. et al: Megaloblastic anemia produced by drugs. Clin. Haematol., 1976; 5:619-630.

Sullivan, L.W. et al: Studies on the minimum daily requirement for vitamin B_{12}: hematopoietic responses to 0.1 microgm. of cyanocobalamin or coenzyme B_{12} and comparison of their relative potency. N. Engl. J. Med., 1965; 272:340-346.

Tamura, T. et al: The availability of food folate in man. Br. J. Haematol., 1973; 25:513-532.

Weir, D.G. et al: Interrelationships of folates and cobalamins. In, Nutrition in Hematology. (Lindenbaum, J. ed.) Contemporary Issues in Clinical Nutrition, Vol. 5. Churchill Livingstone, New York, 1983; pp. 121-142.

WHO Joint Meeting. Control of nutritional anaemia with special reference to iron deficiency. World Health Organization Technical Report Series No. 580, WHO, Geneva, 1975.

8

Drugs Affecting Gastrointestinal Function

Terminology associated with GIT

Cholecystitis	Inflammation of gallbladder
Cholelithiasis	Presence of gallstones
Enteritis	Inflammation of intestine
Dysphagia	Difficulty in swallowing
Nausea	Sensation of impending vomiting

DRUG THERAPY OF PEPTIC ULCER

Burning epigastric pain exacerbated by fasting and improved with meals is a symptom complex associated with peptic ulcer disease. An ulcer is defined as disruption of the mucosal integrity of the stomach and/or duodenum leading to a local defect or excavation due to active inflammation.

The drugs for the treatment of peptic ulcer can be better understood if the basic facts about the disease are known, i.e. how ulcer develops.

Previously it was thought that 'no acid no ulcer'. This view is no more held.

In gastric ulcer there is generally no increase in HCl, in duodenal ulcer in about 50% of patients HCl secretion is increased and in other 50% cases the rate of secretion is normal.

However, the gastric HCl is irritant and its neutralization by antacids will produce relief of pain in patients suffering from peptic ulcer.

Acid-pepsin have aggressive or offending (corrosive) effect.

The gastric epithelium is under a constant assault by a series of endogenous noxious factors including HCl, pepsinogen/pepsin, and bile acids. In addition, a steady flow of exogenous substances such as medications, alcohol and bacteria encounter the gastric mucosa. A biologic system is in place to provide defense from mucosal injury and to repair any injury that may occur.

Mucosal resistance or protection is provided by mucus in gastric juice present in a soluble phase and as an insoluble mucus gel which coats the mucosal surface of stomach. Mucosal prostaglandins also provide protection.

Ulcer develops when aggressive factors outweigh the mucosal resistance to ulceration.

Helicobacter pylori (*H. pylori*), a gram negative bacillus is a potential cause of ulcer formation. Besides this organism, the mucosal resistance is also lowered by nonsteroidal antiinflammatory drugs which may produce ulceration (iatrogenic) by inhibiting prostaglandin synthesis.

Effects of prostaglandin depletion

- $\uparrow$ HCl secretion
- $\downarrow$ Mucin secretion
- $\downarrow$ HCO_3 secretion
- $\downarrow$ Surface active phospholipid secretion
- $\downarrow$ Epithelial cell proliferation

Fig. 8.1 shows factors involved in maintaining acid balance.

The treatment of peptic ulcer is aimed at:

- Withdrawal of the offending agents such as NSAIDs and improve lifestyle (avoid smoking, alcohol, spicy food, caffeine containing beverages).
- Relief of pain.
- Acceleration of ulcer healing.

Drugs used to treat acid peptic diseases

The major categories of drugs are :

(i) antacids

(ii) H_2-receptor antagonists

(iii) proton pump inhibitors, and

(iv) drugs that enhance mucosal resistance

CLASSIFICATION OF DRUGS EMPLOYED IN THE TREATMENT OF PEPTIC ULCER

A. Drugs which reduce gastric acidity

- Antacids
- Antisecretory drugs
  - Anticholinergic (Pirenzepine)
  - H_2-receptor antagonists: Cimetidine, Ranitidine, Famotidine, Nizatidine
  - Prostaglandins (Misoprostol)
  - Anti-gastrin (Octreotide)
  - Proton pump inhibitor (Omeprazole)

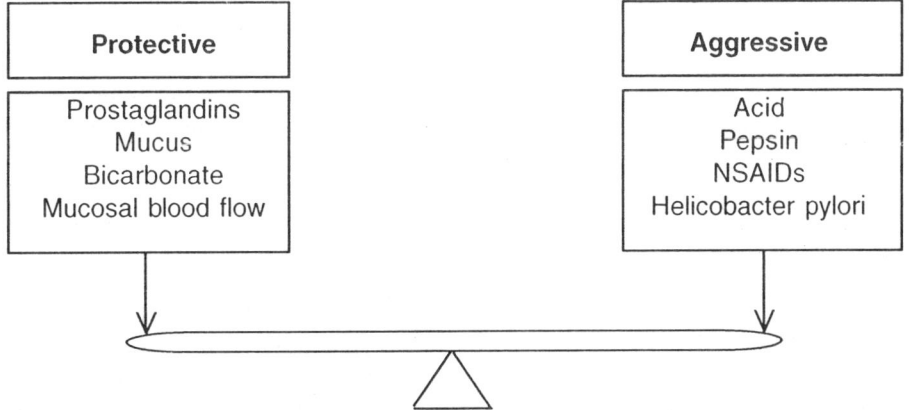

Fig. 8.1. Factors involved in maintaining acid balance.

B. Mucosal protective agents
 • Carbenoxolone
 • Sucralfate
 • Colloidal bismuth salts
 • Prostaglandins
C. Drugs acting by other mechanisms
 • Metoclopramide

A. DRUGS WHICH REDUCE GASTRIC ACIDITY

Gastric antacids (Table 8.1)

Antacids are drugs which on ingestion neutralize gastric HCl and prevent activation of pepsin. They react with the hydrochloric acid of the gastric contents to lower the acidity.

The following properties are required in an ideal antacid:
 • Rapid onset and prolonged action
 • Potent in neutralizing HCl
 • Not absorbed from GIT
 • No interference with gastrointestinal function i.e. no diarrhoea, no constipation
 • No acid rebound
 • Acid base balance should not be disturbed
 • No irritation to GIT
 • Should be neutral in aqueous suspension but capable of neutralizing acidity
 • Negligible amount of sodium
 • Palatable
 • Inexpensive
 • Free from side effects

The antacids act by :
 • Chemical neutralization e.g. sodium bicarbonate, calcium carbonate and phosphate, magnesium oxide and carbonate.
 • Physical mechanism (buffer action) e.g. gastric mucus, bismuth carbonate and subnitrate.
 • Both chemical neutralization and buffer action, e.g. aluminium hydroxide and phosphate, magnesium hydroxide and magnesium trisilicate.
 • Anion exchange resins e.g. polyaminostyrine.

Classification of antacids

1. Systemic antacids. Sodium bicarbonate, sodium citrate and acetate. These are absorbable and may produce alkalosis.

2. Nonsystemic and buffer antacids. Aluminium hydroxide gel, aluminium phosphate gel, magnesium trisilicate. These are buffer antacids that limit the rise in pH of gastric contents usually only to about pH 4. The non-buffer non systemic antacids e.g. magnesium oxide, magnesium hydroxide, calcium carbonate produce pH of gastric contents to 7 or less.

Uses of antacids

 • Gastric hyperacidity
 • Gastritis
 • Peptic ulcer

Individual antacids

Sodium bicarbonate

It acts by chemical neutralization of HCl and as it is absorbed it causes systemic alkalosis.

$$NaHCO_3 + HCl \xrightarrow{\text{Fast}} NaCl + CO_2 + H_2O$$

Sodium bicarbonate is potent, rapidly acting, inexpensive and easily available.

1 g neutralizes 120 ml of 0.1 N HCl.

Dose: 300 mg to 2 g, 1-4 times a day.

The disadvantages include short duration, systemic alkalosis, rebound acidity, inhibition of pepsin, liberation of carbon dioxide leading to epigastric distress and may result in perforation of ulcer.

Sodium bicarbonate is contraindicated in hypertension, cardiac disease.

Magnesium compounds

These are effective (magnesium carbonate is less potent and magnesium trisilicate is slow acting). These act by chemical neutralization and adsorption of gastric acid. Magnesium trisilicate also has demulcent action.

1 g of magnesium oxide neutralizes 500 ml of 0.1N HCl.

The dose is 250 mg-4 g/d or 250 mg four times a day.

Magnesium trisilicate, 1 g neutralizes 100 ml of 0.1 N HCl. It is a slow acting and weak antacid. The dose is 1 g four times a day.

The magnesium compounds are potent, nonsystemic antacids, without rebound acidity. They have

Table 8.1. Common antacids

Drug	Mode	Potency	Onset	Duration	HCl rebound	Demul-cent	Systemic alkalosis
Sodium bicarbonate	Chemical neutralization	Potent	Quick	Short	Yes	No	Yes
Calcium compounds (CaCO₃ and phosphate)	Chemical neutralization	Moderate	Quick	Prolonged	Yes yes	No	No
Magnesium compounds (oxide, hydroxide, trisilicate)	Chemical and physical (adsorbent/buffer action)	Potent	Slow	Prolonged	No	Yes	No
Aluminium compounds (hydroxide, phosphate)	Chemical and physical (adsorbent/buffer action)	Potent	Slow	Prolonged	No	Yes	No
Bismuth salts (carbonate, subnitrate)	Physical	Weak	Slow	Prolonged	No	Yes	No

slow but prolonged action. They can produce diarrhoea.

$$Mg(OH)_2 + 2HCl \xrightarrow{\text{Slow/moderate}} MgCl_2 + 2H_2O$$

Aluminium hydroxide reacts with HCl in stomach, forms aluminium chloride which further reacts in small intestine to form insoluble salts. Aluminium salts are not absorbed. They act by both chemical neutralization and adsorption of gastric acid; aluminium hydroxide has demulcent action like magnesium trisilicate. Aluminium hydroxide gel is available as suspension (dose 5-30 ml), chewable tablets, capsule 475 mg.

Aluminium salts are constipating. Aluminium binds phosphate within gut lumen and facilitates phosphate excretion so prolonged and regular use may produce systemic phosphate depletion resulting in muscular weakness, anorexia and malaise.

$$Al(OH)_3 + 3HCl \xrightarrow{\text{Slow}} AlCl_3 + 3H_2O$$

Calcium carbonate

Calcium carbonate and calcium hydroxide react with gastric acid to form calcium chloride, some of which is absorbed, absorbed calcium stimulates release of gastrin. Hence, Ca containing salt in larger amounts, and if frequently used, may lead to increased gastric acid production.

The calcium salts produce constipation as a side effect.

$$CaCO_3 + 2HCl \xrightarrow{\text{Fast}} CaCl_2 + H_2O + CO_2$$

1 g CaCO₃ neutralizes 200 ml of 0.1 N HCl.

Bismuth salts (carbonate, subnitrate) act by adsorbent action. Although these have prolonged effect and do not produce rebound acidity and alkalosis, but these may produce kidney damage. These are also slow acting and weak. They have constipating effect.

Gastric mucin acts by adsorption and demulcent action. It is weak and unpalatable, so rarely used.

Anion exchange resins are weak, bulky, having bad taste, costly and side effects like nausea, vomiting and diarrhoea are common.

Ca, Al and Bi salts are constipating. Magnesium salts are diarrhoea producing.

Magnesium hydroxide, magnesium oxide and calcium carbonate are rapidly acting.

Magnesium carbonate has intermediate onset of action.

Magnesium trisilicate, aluminium compounds have slow onset of action.

The concurrent use of magnesium hydroxide and aluminium hydroxide provides fast acting (15 minutes) and more sustained action. Such combination also counteracts the side effects (magnesium salts are laxative and aluminium salts are constipating).

Drug interactions

Calcium, aluminium and magnesium decrease the gastric absorption of tetracyclines and oral iron products.

Aluminium hydroxide decreases the absorption of digoxin, INH, phenytoin, quinidine, warfarin and corticosteroids.

Adverse effects due to excess use

- Sodium bicarbonate: alkalosis, sodium overload
- Magnesium salts: diarrhoea
- Aluminium hydroxide: constipation, phosphate depletion resulting in muscular weakness
- Calcium carbonate: hypercalcaemia

Many antacids contain large amount of sodium, hence, contraindicated in hypertension, and/or cardiac disease.

Antisecretory drugs

Anticholinergics

Pirenzepine: It is an anticholinergic which inhibits gastric acid secretion. It is more selective and more specific in inhibiting gastric acid secretion with fewer side effects. The other anticholinergics (atropine etc.) produce a number of side effects such as dryness of mouth, blurring of vision, urinary retention, cardiac arrhythmias.

Dose: 50 mg twice a day for 4-6 weeks promotes duodenal ulcer healing.

H₂-receptor antagonists

These are the most popular drugs for the treatment of peptic ulcer. They bring about symptomatic relief and promote ulcer healing.

Gastric acid secretion involves H_2-receptors which are blocked by H_2-blockers.

Cimetidine

It is a potent inhibitor of gastric acid secretion. It produces healing in 60% of patients of duodenal ulcer and after 8 weeks this figure exceeds 80%. Following oral administration 80% is absorbed and mostly excreted unchanged in urine, so caution should be exercised in renal failure.

Dose: 200 mg thrice a day or 400 mg twice a day with meals and at bed time.

The adverse effects include diarrhoea, drowsiness, itch and skin rashes. It has some antiandrogenic effect, but it is not known how far this property is responsible for the occasional occurrence of gynaecomastia and hyperlactinaemia.

Cimetidine also inhibits P450 and retards metabolism of oral anticoagulants, phenytoin and theophylline.

Drug interactions: cimetidine potentiates the effect of warfarin and phenytoin.

Ranitidine

It is a potent H_2 antagonist having the same indications as cimetidine.

It is entirely excreted unchanged in urine so the dosage should be reduced in renal failure. The half-life of ranitidine is longer than cimetidine, no serious side effects have been reported so far. Unlike cimetidine it does not interfere with the oxidative metabolism of other drugs and it also does not produce undesirable endocrine disturbance like gynaecomastia. It has less effect on androgen receptors and P450 systems. Ranitidine is 6 times more potent as antisecretory than cimetidine.

Dose: 150 mg twice a day or 300 mg at bed time.

Famotidine

It is a newly introduced H_2-receptor antagonist, about 20 times more potent than cimetidine and 8 times more potent than ranitidine in inhibiting gastric acid secretion. It has longer half-life.

Famotidine is well tolerated and possesses fewer side effects.

Dose: 40 mg once a day at bed time or 20 mg twice a day.

Nizatidine

After administration of 100 and 300mg., peak plasma concentration reaches within 0.5 to 3 hr plasma concentration after 10 hr are less than 10 μg/L. The elimination half-life is 1 to 2 hr., more than 90% of oral dose is excreted in urine within 12hr, 60% as unchanged drug. Therefore it should be used in reduced dosage in patients with severe renal insufficiency.

Adverse effects include somnolence, sweating, and urticaria. Hepatocellular injury, ventricular tachycardia, decreased libido, gynaecomastia and thrombocytopenia have been reported but are rare. Safety and efficacy in children have not been established.

Roxatidine

Roxatidine is similar to nizatidine but more potent. Its absorption is not decreased in the presence of food or antacids. Dose is 150 mg at bed time or 75 mg twice a day. The common side effects include headache, diarrhoea and skin rashes.

Ebrotidine

Ebrotidine is a new H_2-receptor blocking agent. It inhibits acid production as well as possesses gastro-protective action. It is under further trials.

Table 8.2 shows comparison of H_2-receptor antagonists.

Prostaglandins

PGE_2, PGI_2 maintain gastroduodenal mucosal integrity. They reduce gastric secretion mainly by increasing mucus and bicarbonate, mucosal blood flow, mucosal repair and increase in phospholipid content of surface epithelium so prevent acid assault.

Synthetic analogue of PG, misoprostol is given for 2-3 weeks.

It is contraindicated in pregnancy (stimulation of uterus causes abortion).

Fig. 8.2 shows the three principal agonists viz., gastrin, ACh and histamine which act on parietal cell and produce gastric HCl.

Fig. 8.3 shows antagonists of the three principal agonists.

Somatostatin is an antigastrin.

Octreotide, a long acting synthetic somatostatin analogue under trial.

Pirenzepine is an effective anticholinergic agent.

H_2-receptor antagonists are useful as antisecretory agents.

Proton Pump Inhibitors (H^+, K^+ – ATPase inhibitors)

The final common pathway in gastric acid secretion is the proton pump - an H^+/K^+ ATPase.

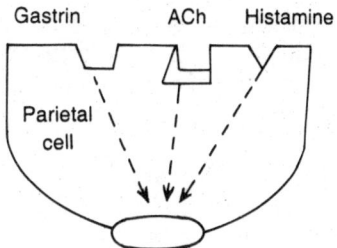

Fig. 8.2. Principal agonists.

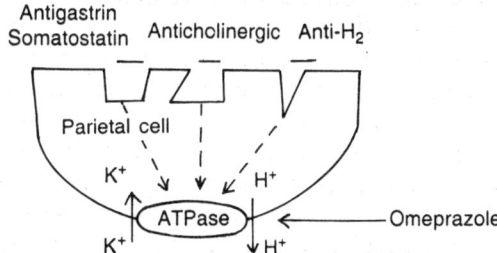

Fig. 8.3. Antagonists of the three principal agonists.

The physiological essence of this enzyme is the exchange of hydrogen ion for potassium ion. Thus, hydrogen is secreted by the parietal cell into the gastric lumen in exchange for potassium. The proton pump inhibitors omeprazole and lansoprazole belong to a new class of antisecretory drugs called substituted benzimidazoles. The prototype omeprazole, is an irreversible inhibitor of the proton pump. Its plasma half-life is 0.5 to 1 hr, but its duration of action is greater than 24hr, reflecting the time required to generate new H^+/K^+ AT Pase.

The proton inhibitors should be taken prior to meals. This is because in the resting state, the proton pump resides on the inner membrane of secretory vesicles within the parietal cell. When the cell is activated by eating (or by pharmacological stimulus),

Table 8.2. Comparison of H_2-receptor antagonists

Characteristic	Cimetidine	Famotidine	Nizatidine	Ranitidine
Relative potency	1	20-50	4-8	4-8
Equivalent dose	1600 mg	40 mg	300 mg	300 mg
Bioavailability	60-80%	40-50%	50-60%	90-100%
Time to peak concentration (hr)	1-2	1-3	1-3	1-3
Serum half-life (hr)	1.5-2.5	2.5-4	2-3	1-2

the inner membrane of the vesicle is externalised and becomes the outer, i.e. the secretory membrane, of the secretory villus. The proton pump inhibitors are prodrugs that need to be protonated and this can occur only when the proton pump is externalised and secreting acid. They are also absorbed more effectively in the morning and thus should be dosed about 20 minutes prior to breakfast.

The proton pump inhibitors are used for the short-term treatment of acid peptic disease, gastroesophageal reflex, gastric ulcer, duodenal ulcer, Zollinger-Ellison syndrome.

The therapeutic advantages of the proton pump inhibitors over the H_2-receptor antagonists are higher healing rate and the ability to heal patients who have not been helped by H_2-receptor antagonists therapy.

Although there are numerous side effects of proton pump inhibitors including headache, diarrhoea, abdominal pain and dizziness, but they occur infrequently.

Omeprazole is a substituted benzimidazole which irreversibly inhibits the proton-pump, the terminal step in the acid secretory pathway. It markedly inhibits both the basal and stimulated gastric acid secretion.

Lansoprazole has a similar mechanism of action, but some data suggest that its effect may be reversed by a mechanism that involves cellular glutathione. However, its effect also last longer than would be predicted from its plasma elimination half-life.

Omeprazole and lansoprazole are available for oral administration as delayed-release capsule.

Newer $H^+ - K^+ - ATPase$ inhibitors are being developed which do not covalently bind to the enzyme.

Table 8.3 shows duodenal healing rates and acid suppression with antisecretory drugs.

B. MUCOSAL PROTECTIVE AGENTS

Carbenoxolone

It is a derivative of glycyrrhizic acid (constituent of liquorice). It is a ulcer healing drug. It increases production of gastric mucus secretion, with no effect on gastric acidity and motility. It increases the life span of gastric mucosal epithelial cells, increases the secretion and viscosity of gastric mucus and increases endogenous PG levels and thereby increases mucosal defence.

The use is limited due to mineralocorticoid activity.

Dose: 100 mg twice or thrice a day.

The adverse effects include retention of sodium and water, oedema, weight gain, iatrogenic hypertension.

Caution is exercised in its use in elderly persons.

Sucralfate

It is an aluminium salt of sucrose octasulphate. It is a complex polyaluminium hydroxide salt of sucrose sulphate. It is an ulcer protective.

It has some acid neutralizing capacity, and is pepsin inhibitor.

The efficacy in healing duodenal and gastric ulcers is similar to that of cimetidine.

Table 8.3. Duodenal ulcer healing rates and acid suppression with antisecretory drugs

	4-wk Healing rate (%)	Suppression of	
		Nocturnal acidity	24-hr acidity
Lansoprazole, 30 mg qam	92-100	90	92
Omeprazole, 20 mg qam	75-97	88	90
Cimetidine, 800 mg qhs	80	79	48
Cimetidine, 300 mg qid	74	68	65
Famotidine, 40 mg qhs	82	94	64
Ranitidine, 300 mg qhs	84	90	68
Ranitidine, 150 mg bid	79	70	68

However, as it is not absorbed so it is almost free of side effects.

On oral administration, sucralfate adheres to ulcerated mucosa but not to healthy mucosa. The dense sticky layer in the crater (ulcer bed) acts as a physical barrier, separating acid and pepsin from ulcer base, thus facilitates healing of ulcer. It binds to ulcer bed for up to 12 hours and also binds bile acids and pepsin and reduces their injurious effect.

It is active only in acid medium so it should not be combined with antacids, H_2-blockers, omeprazole.

It reduces the absorption of a number of other drugs, including fluoroquinolone antibiotics, tetracycline, digoxin, theophylline and amitriptyline.

Unwanted effects are few. Constipation occurs in some patients. Other side effects (rare) include nausea, vomiting, dry mouth, headache and rashes.

Dose: 1 g four times a day or 2 g 12 hourly for 4-6 weeks.

Colloidal bismuth salts

These aid ulcer healing. They form (in an acid medium) a bismuth-protein coagulant which protects the ulcer from acid-pepsin digestion. They are also of value because of antibacterial effect on *H. pylori*.

Bismuth subsalicylate increases PG synthesis. The dose is 30-120 mg 6 hourly.

The adverse effects include black stool, discoloration of tongue and teeth.

Treatment of *H. pylori* infection

Helicobacter pylori is a gram-negative bacterium capable of producing urease, that lives in the mucous layer adjacent to the mucosa predominantly of gastric antrum and in areas of gastric metaplasia in the duodenum. The urease activity by which it splits urea, liberating ammonia, is required for the survival of the organism. Some patients with *H. pylori* infection remain totally asymptomatic, while others develop symptomatic disease, such as dyspepsia, duodenal or gastric ulcer, gastric cancer, or mucosa associated lymphoid tissue lymphoma and even lymphoma.

To eradicate *H. pylori* infection the following combinations of drugs are recommended :

Omeprazole, amoxycillin and metronidazole
or Omeprazole, clarithromycin and amoxycillin
or Tetracycline, metronidazole and bismuth chelates

Regimens used for eradication of *H.pylori* in patients of peptic ulcer are given in Table 8.4

Prostaglandins

These are mostly PGE_1 and PGE_2 analogues.

- Reduce basal and stimulated gastric acid secretion
- Enhance mucosal resistance to tissue injury as they stimulate gastric mucus secretion, stimulate bicarbonate secretion, maintain mucosal blood flow, maintain gastric mucosal barrier to back diffusion of H^+ and stimulate mucosal cellular renewal and regeneration.

Enprostil is a synthetic PGE_2 analogue claimed to have a healing rate more than 80% in a month in case of duodenal ulcer. However, it is somewhat inferior to ranitidine for the treatment of gastric ulcer. The oral dose is 35 mcg twice a day or 75 mcg once a day.

The adverse effects include diarrhoea which is the commonest side effect (20-50% patients), abdominal cramps, nausea, vomiting, flatulence, headache, backache, loss of appetite.

Misoprostol is a synthetic PGE_1 analogue. It inhibits secretion from gastric parietal cells and also shows cytoprotective activity. Gastric and duodenal ulcers heal in 4-6 weeks. The oral dose is 200 mcg four times a day.

The side effects are similar to that of enprostil.

Rioprostil is a synthetic PGE_1 analogue. The oral dose is 300-600 mcg at beg time.

Arbaprostil is a synthetic PGE_2 analogue which has activity and adverse effects similar to enprostil. The oral dose is 100 mcg four times a day.

The main beneficial effect of PGE_1 and PGE_2 analogues is their ability to prevent ulceration and bleeding from gastric mucosa in patients who take aspirin or other NSAIDs for chronic pain. These drugs may become useful for the treatment of duodenal ulcer in smokers because smoking slows the rate of healing and enhances rate of recurrence of duodenal ulcers. Smoking inhibits tissue

Table 8.4. Various regimens used for eradication of *H.pylori* in patients with peptic ulcer

Therapy	Comments
Monotherapy Bismuth, amoxycillin, clarithromycin or nitroimidazoles	Low cure rates High risk of developing drug resistance
Dual therapy Amoxycillin + proton pumps inhibitor	Cure rate less than clarithromycin + pump inhibitor High risk of developing drug resistance
Triple therapy Amoxycillin or Clarythromycin + nitroimidazole + proton-pump inhibitor	> 90% cure rate. However, resistance is a problem with clarythromycin-based regimens. Taste perversion with clarithromycin may result in non-compliance. Diarrhoea and rash may occur with amoxycillin. Incidence of diarrhoea may be reduced when amoxycillin is combined with nitroimidazole.
Regimens Recommended for eradication of H. Pylori Infection **Triple therapy** 1. Bismuth subsalicylate plus metronidazole plus tetracycline	2 tablets qid 250 mg qid 500 mg qid
2. Ranitidine, bismuth citrate plus tetracycline plus clarithromycin or metronidazole	400 mg bid 500 mg bid 500 mg bid
3. Omeprazole plus clarithromycin plus metronidazole or Amoxycillin	20 mg bid 250 or 500 mg bid 500 mg bid 1g bid
Quadriple therapy Omeprazole Bismuth subsalicylate Metronidazole Tetracycline	20 mg daily 525 mg qid 250 mg qid 500 mg qid

prostaglandin therapy resulting in inhibition of healing process. Prosta-glandin analogues reverse this imbalance.

Contraindications

These compounds have uterotonic property and are potential abortifacients so should not be prescribed in women who may become pregnant.

C. DRUGS ACTING BY OTHER MECHANISMS

Metoclopramide

It increases gastric motility and accelerates gastric emptying.

It is a prokinetic agent. It is rapidly and completely absorbed but undergoes about 75% first-pass effect.

It is available as 5 mg and 10 mg/ml injectable solution (iv/im), as syrup 5 mg/ml and as 5, 10 mg tablets.

Metoclopramide can cross placenta, and also reaches breast milk.

The adverse effects include extrapyramidal symptoms, anxiety, drowsiness and dizziness.

PURGATIVES (CATHARTICS)

These are drugs which promote to evacuate faeces. The term laxative is used for drugs which produce soft formed stool. Drastic purgatives produce severe action, watery stool. The term purgative is all embracing.

Classification

Purgatives hasten evacuation of bowel by several different methods:

1. Irritant purgatives: These stimulate the mucosa and reflexly increase peristalsis.
   - Castor oil
   - Anthracene (Senna, rhubarb, cascara, aloes)
   - Phenolphthalein
   - Sulphur
   - Resins (drastic purgatives such as colocynth, podophyllum - these are obsolete)
2. Nonirritant purgatives
   - Bulk purgatives:
     - Osmotic purgatives (magnesium sulphate, sodium sulphate, sodium potassium tartrate) increase the water content.
     - Hydrophilic purgatives (agar, methyl cellulose, indigestible vegetable fibres e.g. ispaghula) adsorb water and swell.
   - Lubricants or emollient purgative (liquid paraffin, olive oil).
   - Surface active agents or faecal softeners (dioctyl sodium sulfosuccinate) alter the consistency of faeces.

Irritant purgatives

Caster oil acts in small intestine, onset is 2-3 hours, dose is 5-20 ml. The other irritant purgatives act on large intestine and the onset of action is 6-8 hours.

Castor oil, obtained from seeds of ricinus communis, itself is nonirritant. In the small intestine it is hydrolysed by lipase into highly irritant ricinoleic acid and glycerol. Ricinoleic acid stimulates local nerve plexuses causing increased peristalsis and purgative action. The purgative action is followed by after constipation due to thorough purgation.

Anthracene purgatives (Cascara sagrada, senna)

The active principle is anthraquinone (emodin) which is a glycoside released by enzymatic hydrolysis in the ileum, absorbed and re-excreted in the colon where it acts as an irritant purgative (due to stimulation of mesenteric plexus resulting in contraction of colonic muscle). These are given late in the evening and exert effect the following morning.

The anthracene purgatives are not suitable for long term use as their repeated use may cause degeneration of the mesenteric plexus and impair normal physiological propulsive function.

Phenolphthalein

It is tasteless and odourless. Its duration of action is prolonged due to repeated absorption and re-excretion in bile (enterohepatic circulation). It acts in colon and takes 6-8 hours to act. Dose is 50-100 mg at bed time. Adverse effects include skin eruptions.

Bisacodyl

It is related structurally to phenolphthalein. It does not produce systemic effects as it is not absorbed. Oral administration of 2 tablets (5 mg each) in the night produces effect in 6 to 12 hours. One suppository (10 mg) acts in 15 minutes to 1 hour. The rectal administration is not common.

Saline purgatives

Magnesium sulphate 5-15 g before breakfast, sodium sulphate, milk of magnesia 30-60 ml and magnesium hydroxide 1.8-3.6 g are useful. Sodium potassium tartrate is now little used. Saline purgatives are retained in GIT and hold back water (by osmotic action) to keep these salts in solution, resulting in increase in the intestinal contents. The distension thus produced results in increased peristalsis and purgation.

Hydrophilic purgatives

Ispaghula 5-15 g, agar agar, methylcellulose 1 g four times a day, sodium carboxymethyl cellulose when given orally are neither absorbed nor digested. They adsorb water and swell. The increased bulk increases peristalsis resulting in purgation. These act on small and large intestines, take 12-24 hours. These have mild and unreliable effect.

Lubricant purgatives

These soften faecal mass. A mineral oil liquid paraffin (10-30 ml) has unpleasant taste, interferes with absorption of fat soluble vitamins and also due to

Table 8.5. Certain characteristics of purgatives

Drug	Dose	Active principle	Site	Onset (hours)	Effect	Remarks
Castor oil	5-10 ml	Ricinoleic acid	Ileum	2-4	Soft semi-solid stool	Colic, after constipation
Anthracenes Cascara Senna	100-250 mg 0.5-2 g	Emodin	Colon	8-10	Formed stool	No colic, no after constipation
Phenolphthalein	50-300 mg	Same	Colon	6-8		Mild but prolonged action
Osmotic or saline purgatives		Same	Ileum colon	10-12		Mild colic, after constipation, may cause dehydration
Magnesium sulphate	15 g	Same				
Hydrophilic purgatives	Same	Same	Ileum, colon	12-14		
Lubricants			Ileum, colon	12-24		Mild action, leakage
Dioctyl sulphosuccinate	50-100 mg	Same	Ileum, colon	12-24		Mild effect

leakage through anus it is not commonly employed. Olive oil also acts as a lubricant purgative. These act on small and large intestines.

Surface-active purgative such as dioctyl sodium sulphosuccinate lowers surface tension, increases water content of faeces. Dose is 50-400 mg.

Table 8.5 shows certain characteristics of purgatives.

Uses of purgatives

- Constipation
- To flush the intestines (with saline purgatives) in case of food or drug poisoning
- Prior to radiological examination of abdomen
- Preoperatively in abdominal surgery
- To minimise straining during defaecation in

Box 8.2 : Faecal consistency		
Softening of faeces 1-3 days	Soft or semifluid stool 6-8 hours	Watery evacuation 1-3 hours
Bulk forming Surfactant laxatives	Stimulant laxatives Phenolphthalein Bisacodyl Anthraquinones Senna Cascara sagrada	Osmotic laxatives Castor oil

conditions such as piles, fissures, cardiac disease

Contraindications of purgatives

- These are absolutely contraindicated in intestinal obstruction
- Undiagnosed constipation

Danger of purgative abuse

Malabsorption syndrome fluid and electrolyte imbalance, flaring of intestinal pathology, rupture of inflamed appendix.

General considerations

When constipation, is due to poor dietary habits i.e. lack of bulk-producing foods and inattention to stimulus for defaecation, the use of purgatives is not an answer to chronic constipation.

- Drugs acting only on colon produce formed stool and after constipation.
- Those which act on ileum produce semisolid or watery stools and after constipation.
- Drugs which take more than 6 hours are given at bed time and those whose onset is 1 to 4 hours are given in the morning.

Drugs which increase GI motility

These drugs increase GI motility without causing purgation. These are used for disorders of motility in GIT, some are also employed as antiemetic.

> **Box 8.3.** Some agents causing diarrhoea
> - Adrenergic neuron blockers (reserpine, guanethidine)
> - Antimicrobials (sulphonamides, tetracyclines and broad-spectrum antibiotics)
> - Cholinergic agonists and ChE inhibitors
> - Fatty acids
> - Osmotic and stimulant purgatives
> - Prokinetic agents (metoclopramide)
> - Prostaglandins
> - Quinidine

- Muscarinic agonists such as bethanechol and Anti-ChEs e.g. neostigmine.
- Domperidone (dopamine antagonist)
- Metoclopramide has central anti-emetic effect, also exerts local stimulant effect on gastric motility causing marked acceleration of gastric emptying.

It is rapidly and completely absorbed but undergoes about 75% first-pass effect.

Its adverse effects include extrapyramidal reaction in children and young adults, galactorrhoea (stimulates prolactin release) and disorders of menstruation.

ANTIDIARRHOEAL AGENTS

Diarrhoea is a frequent passage of faeces which are too liquid.

The rational management of diarrhoea is to find cause and give specific therapy, treat fluid and electrolyte depletion and maintain nutrition.

Antidiarrhoeal therapy

- Specific antimicrobial drugs such as metronidazole for amoebiasis.
- The use of antiinfective agents is usually not necessary in simple gastroenteritis.
- Nonspecific antidiarrhoeal drugs are:
  - Adsorbants for irritable bowel. Ispaghula adsorbs water.
  - Adsorbants like kaolin, pectin, activated charcoal.
  - Astringents like bismuth salts, tannic acid, methyl cellulose.
  - Antimotility drugs such as codeine, diphenoxylate and atropine, furazolidone, metronidazole, pectin, kaolin.

For rehydration; I.V. NaCl, KCl, $NaHCO_3$ in water or 5% glucose solution may be employed. Oral rehydration therapy (ORT) consists of NaCl, KCl, sodium citrate and glucose.

To maintain nutrition, boiled potatoes, rice, banana should be given as soon as the patient can eat.

Fasting is bad.

ANTISPASMODIC AGENTS

Drugs which reduce spasm in the gut are indicated in irritable bowel syndrome and diverticular disease. Muscarinic receptor antagonists decrease spasm by inhibiting parasympathetic activity.

Agents such as propantheline and dicyclomine are available for this purpose. Dicyclomine has additional direct relaxant action on the smooth muscle besides inhibition of parasympathetic activity. The unwanted effects due to parasympathetic inhibition in other tissues (dry mouth, blurred vision, tachycardia, dry skin, difficulty with urination) are less frequent and less marked.

Mebeverine (a derivative of reserpine) produces a direct relaxant action on GI smooth muscle. Side effects are few.

DRUGS FOR CHRONIC INFLAMMATORY BOWEL DISEASE

This disease comprises ulcerative colitis and Crohn's disease (a granulomatous condition affecting terminal ileum and the colon).

Following agents are used:

Glucocorticoids are of value as anti-inflammatory agents. Predinisolone is given locally in the bowel by enema or suppository.

EMETICS

These produce vomiting and are useful to expel poisons if ingested.

Vomiting may be triggered by a variety of stimuli as shown in Figs. 8.4 and 8.5.

The vomiting center (VC) has mainly muscarinic receptors.

CTZ lies adjacent to vomiting center (VC)

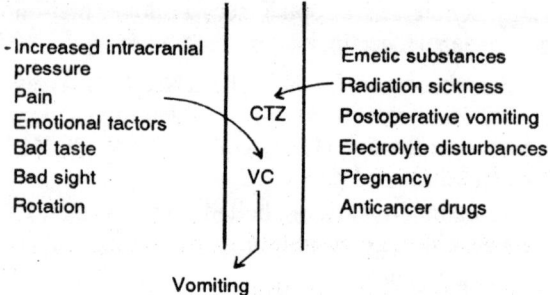

Fig. 8.4. Emetic substances and factors that trigger vomiting by acting directly on vomiting center (VC) and through chemoreceptor trigger zone (CTZ).

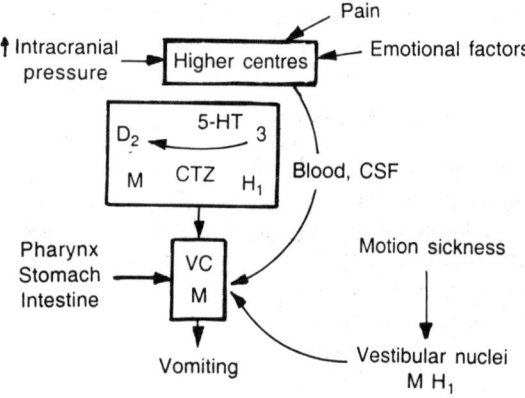

M = Muscarinic receptor
D_2 = Dopamine (D_2) receptor
H_1 = Histamine (H_1) receptor

Fig. 8.5. Dopamine 2,5-HT_3, muscarinic and H_1 receptors in CTZ.

CTZ is not implicated in motion sickness

Drugs which act directly on vomiting center (VC) are effective against all causes of vomiting including motion sickness.

Emetics may be classified as:
1. Centrally acting: Morphine, digitalis, apomorphine
2. Peripherally acting: Copper sulphate, concentrated solution of sodium chloride, ipecac.

Drinking of concentrated solution of common salt is direct irritant to gastric mucosa and vomiting is reflexly induced by vagus. It is simple procedure but not so reliable. Reflexly acting emetics are mustard, copper sulphate, ipecac, tartar emetic besides strong NaCl solution.

Apomorphine acts on the chemoreceptor trigger zone (CTZ) in the brain stem. It produces vomiting within few minutes following 4-8 mg s.c. injection.

ANTIEMETICS (Table 8.6)

These are drugs which oppose or counteract nausea and vomiting.

These are used for the prevention of treatment of nausea and vomiting associated with :
• motion sickness
• vestibular disorders
• uraemia
• after radiation treatment
• postoperative vomiting
• morning sickness of pregnancy
• gastrointestinal disorders
• anticancer drugs

Antiemetics belong to the following categories:
1. Centrally acting
   • Anticholinergic: Scopolamine (hyoscine)
   • Antihistaminics: Cyclizine, diphenhydramine
   • Phenothiazine derivatives: Chlorpromazine, prochlorperazine
2. Peripherally acting
   • Kaolin, bismuth salts, local anaesthetics, chlorbutanol (also acts centrally).

Antiemetics can also be grouped according to their antagonistic actions on receptors.

Phenothiazine derivatives e.g. chlorpromazine, perphenazine, prochlorperazine act as dopamine receptor antagonists in the chemoreceptor trigger zone. They are nonselective D_1 and D_2 antagonists, effective in most forms of vomiting. However, they are of no use in prevention of motion sickness. The antiemetic dose of chlorpromazine and prochlorperazine is about 20% of the antipsychotic doses. Perphenazine is used in similar doses for treating vomiting or psychosis.

Hyoscine is an antimuscarinic drug. It is very effective for prophylaxis of motion sickness. It is administered in a dose of 0.2-0.4 mg orally or intramuscularly. Transdermal patch of hyoscine (scopolamine) is now available and its action is prolonged for three days.

Antihistaminics e.g. promethazine, cyclizine, meclizine are H_1 receptor antagonists are antiemetics.

Cinnarizine is H_1-receptor antagonist which also blocks calcium channels. In addition to its use as a prophylactic agent against motion sickness, it is a useful drug in vertigo because it suppresses labyrinthine activity by inhibiting the passage of calcium ions from endolymph into the vestibular sensory cells or increasing blood flow to the vestibular nucleus. It is available as 25, 75 mg tablets.

Ondansetron is a $5-HT_3$ receptor antagonist. The dopamine activity in CTZ is decreased by blocking 5-HT receptors modulating dopamine synthesis and release. It is also a $5-HT_3$ receptor antagonist acting on the afferent vagal nerve terminals in upper GIT. Unlike metoclopramide or prochlorperazine it does not have antidopaminergic activity and will not cause extrapyramidal effects. It is effective orally in a dose of 8 mg thrice a day. Its half-life is 4.5 hours, extensively metabolised in liver and only about 1% is excreted unchanged in urine. It can also be given by i.v. route. It is not effective in motion sickness.

Metoclopramide is a dopamine receptor antagonist, blocks $5-HT_3$ in CTZ and also acts peripherally. It is useful in all types of vomiting except in motion sickness and labyrinthine disorders.

It has D_2 blocking activity in CTZ (effectiveness in many forms of vomiting) and agonistic action on $5-HT_4$. In high concentrations it inhibits $5-HT_3$ receptors (controls vomiting due to cytotoxic agents).

The peripheral gastrokinetic effect is due to its action on $5-HT_4$ receptors.

Metoclopramide can be given orally as well as by i.m. and i.v. routes. The dose is 10 mg thrice a day orally or intramuscularly. It is available as liq. 5 mg/5 ml and inj. 5 mg/ml.

Adverse effects :
- Dystonia (extrapyramidal effect) in about 1% of patients.
- Drowsiness and restlessness in about 20% of patients.
- Blockade of D_2-receptors in anterior pituitary

gland results in increased prolactin secretion and produce lactation.

Drug interaction : Metoclopramide increases bioavailability of drugs such as aspirin, diazepam by facilitating gastric emptying.

Domperidone is a potent D_2-receptor antagonist. It is a butyrophenone derivative. Its poor penetration of blood-brain barrier results in lack of drowsiness and a very low incidence of extrapyramidal side effects. The major indications include vomiting induced by drugs in parkinsonism and by cytotoxic agents.

The dose is 10-40 mg thrice a day in adults, in children the dose is 0.3-0.6 mg/kg. It should not be given i.v. as cardiac arrest and arrhythmias have been reported when administered by this route.

The adverse effects after oral administration include headache, dryness of mouth, and diarrhoea.

Antiemetics for cancer patients

Ondansetron is more effective than metoclopramide alone when administered intravenously. Adding dexamethasone increases the efficacy of ondansetron (how, unclear).

Granisetron is a $5-HT_3$ receptor antagonist. The mode of action is similar to that of ondansetron. It has a half-life of 9 hours.

It is metabolised in the liver and the metabolites are excreted in urine and faeces.

This drug is available both for oral administration as well as by i.v. route.

The adverse effects include headache, constipation.

Dronabinol is an oral tetrahydrocannabinol indicated in patients who do not respond to the conventional antiemetic agents.

Adverse effects include postural hypotension, sedation, ataxia, dysphoria, xerostomia.

Phenothiazines and butyrophenones are effective when administered intravenously.

Adverse effects include acute dystonic reactions, hypotension and extrapyramidal symptoms.

Sialagogues

These are drugs which increase secretion of saliva. These act by:

- Reflexly stimulating taste buds in mouth, e.g. bitters or vagal nerve endings in the stomach e.g. subemetic doses of emetics.
- Affecting cholinergic receptors of salivary gland, e.g. pilocarpine, carbachol.
- Direct action on salivary glands during excretion of drugs such as iodides.

Sialagogues were previously used for the treatment of dryness of mouth, now these are rarely used.

Box 8.4. Antiemetics

- Muscarinic receptor antagonists : Scopolamine (hyoscine), benztropine
- Histamine H_1-receptor antagonists : Promethazine, cyclizine, meclizine, diphenhydramine, cinnarizine
- Dopamine receptor antagonists : Nonselective D_1 and D_2 antagonists—Chlorpromazine, prochlorperazine, haloperidol, droperidol
- Selective D_2 antagonists : Metoclopramide, domperidone
- 5-HT_3-receptor antagonists : Ondansetron, granisectron, tropisetron, renzapride, zacopride
- Miscellaneous drugs : Pyridoxine (vitamin B_6) lorazepam

Table 8.6. Choice of antiemetics

Drug	Condition
Antimuscarinic	
Hyoscine	Motion sickness
H_1-antihistaminics	
Diphenhydramine	Motion sickness, hyperemesis
Promethazine	gravidarum
Dopamine antagonists	
Chlorpromazine	Uraemia, radiation sickness, cancer
Prochlorperazine	chemotherapy, postoperative vomiting, labyrinthine disorders
Metoclopramide	Gastrointestinal disorders, cancer chemotherapy

Antisialagogues are drugs which decrease secretion of saliva. These are anticholinergic drugs which may be used to check salivation in parkinsonism and heavy metal poisoning. These are rarely used now.

Stomachics are drugs which increase gastric secretion.

They act reflexly producing parasympathetic stimulation or directly by the presence of food, peptone, etc.

Bitters possess bitter taste and reflexly stimulate salivary and gastric secretions. These are:

- Simple bitters such as calumba, quassia, gentian, chirata.
- Aromatic bitters contain volatile oils besides bitter principles e.g. orange peel, lemon peel, cardamom.
- Astringent bitters contain tannins besides bitter principles, e.g. kalmegh.
- Alkaloidal bitters, e.g. quinine.

Bitters may be used as sialagogues, stomachics and appetizers.

Carminatives are drugs which expel gases from stomach and intestines.

These act by:

- Mild irritation resulting in increased gastrointestinal motility, e.g. ginger, coriander, cardamom, clove, peppermint. These contain volatile oils.
- Liberating carbon dioxide, e.g. sodium bicarbonate.

Carminatives are used in cases of flatulence. These produce relief and sense of comfort.

Digestants are agents which help in the digestive processes of the GIT. These agents are:

- Dilute HCl (10%) 4-6ml diluted with water sipped by straw (to prevent contact with teeth).
- Glutamic acid hydrochloride and betaine hydrochloride liberate HCl in stomach.
- Pepsin, papain have pepsin like activity, Pancreatin contains trypsin, amylase and lipase.
- Cholagogues increase bile secretion by the liver, the drugs used to dissolve non-calcified cholesterol gall-stones are chenodeoxycholic acid (CDCA) and ursodeoxycholic acid (UDCA).

CDCA and UDCA on oral administration are handled by the body in the same way as endogenous bile acids. They decrease hepatic synthesis and secretion of cholesterol.

CDCA is one of the two primary bile acids. UDCA, the β-hydroxy epimer of CDCA occurs in small quantity in human bile and is the main bile acid in the bear (hence "urso"). The adverse effect is mainly diarrhoea. The preferred treatment of gallstones is surgery in most cases when active intervention is indicated. CDCA or UDCA may be used only in selected patients.

Appetizers increase appetite. Bitters and digestants and drugs which stimulate feeding center such as cyproheptadine can act as appetizers. However, the cause of loss of appetite should be found and specific treatment should be given.

Anorexiants (appetite suppressants) reduce appetite. The appetite may be reduced by:

– Amphetamine, dextroamphetamine which stimulate satiety center, but they produce CNS stimulation and have liability to produce drug dependence.

– Bulk anorexiants e.g. methyl cellulose give sense of filling (fullness of stomach).

– Thyroid hormone stimulates metabolism.

STUDY QUESTIONS

1. What are the aims to be achieved in the treatment of Peptic ulcer? How are these achieved by various drugs.
2. Describe H_2 antagonists.
3. How does carbenoxolone promote ulcer healing?
4. What is sucralfate and how does it work?
5. Why ranitidine and famotidine are considered better than cimetidine?
6. Classify antacids giving proper examples. What are the properties required in an antacid? How do they act?
7. What are the advantages and disadvantages of (a) sodium bicarbonate (b) aluminium salts (c) magnesium salts as antacids?
8. Classify purgatives according to their mode of action and give suitable examples. What are the therapeutic indications and contraindications of purgatives?

9. What are the sites and mode of action of castor oil, anthracenes and saline purgatives and phenolphthalein?
10. What are the disadvantages of lubricant purgatives?
11. Describe nonspecific antidiarrhoeal agents. What is advocated for oral rehydration therapy (ORT)?
12. List centrally acting and peripherally acting antiemetics. What are the uses of antiemetics?
13. Give examples of emetics which act centrally and peripherally. Indicate which emetic substances or conditions trigger emetic action, and which of them act directly on vomiting center and which act through CTZ.
14. Categorize antiemetics on the basis of their antagonistic actions on dopamine, 5-HT, muscarinic and H1-receptors.
15. Define, give examples and uses of the following: (a) bitters (b) stomachics (c) anorexiants (d) appetizers (e) digestants (f) sialagogues (g) antisialagogues (h) carminatives (i) cholagogues.
16. List the drugs which increase GI motility. Describe the therapeutic uses, mode of action and adverse effects of metoclopramide.

GUIDE TO FURTHER READING

Albibi R.: Application of somatostatin and its analogue octerotide in the therapy of gastrointestinal disorders. In, Gastrointestinal Pharmacotherapy Saunders Co., Philadelphia, 1993; pp. 275-292.

Barradell, L.B. et al: Lansoprazole. A review of its pharmacodynamic and pharmacokinetic properties and its therapeutic efficacy in acid-related disorders. Drugs, 1992, 44:225-250.

Black, J. et al: Reflections on the analytical pharmacology of histamine H2-receptor antagonists. Gastroenterology, 1993, 105: 963-968.

Blaser, M.J. et al: Parasitism by the "slow" bacterium Helicobacter pylori leads to altered gastric homeostasis and neoplasia, J. Clin. Invest., 1994, 94:4-8.

Burkitt, D.P. et al:How to manage constipation with high-fiber diet. Geriatrics, 1979, 34:33-40.

Deakin, M. et al: Histamine H2-receptor antagonists in peptic ulcer disease, Drugs, 1992, 44: 709-719.

Devrodede, G.: Constipation. In, Gastrointestinal Disease, 5th ed. W.B. Saunders Co., Philadelphia,

1993; pp. 837-887.

DuPont, H.L. et al: Prevention and treatment of traveler's diarrhea. N. Engl. J. Med., 1993; 328:1821-1827.

Fine, K.D. et al: Diarrhea, In, Gastrointestinal Disease, 5th ed, W.B. Saunders Co., Philadelphia, 1993; pp. 1043-1072.

Gonzalez, E.R. et al: Management of stress-related mucosal damage and its consequences in the critically ill patient. In, A Pharmacologic Approach to Gastrointestinal Disorders. Williams & Wilkins, Baltimore, 1994, pp. 47-74.

Gorbach, S.L.: Infectious diarrhea and bacterial food poisoning. In, Gastrointestinal Disease, 5th ed. W.B. Saunders Co., Philadelphia, 1993; pp. 1128-1173.

Grunberg, S.J. et al: Control of chemotherapy-induced emesis. N. Engl. J. Med., 1993; 329:1790-1796.

Hansten, P.D. et al: Drug interactions of gastrointestinal drugs. In. A Pharmacologic Approach to Gastrointestinal Disorders. Williams & Wilkins, Baltimore, 1994, pp. 535-563.

Joss, R.A. et al: The antiemetic activity of high-dose alizapride and high-dose metoclopramide in patients receiving cancer chemotherapy: a prospective, randomized, double-blind trial. Clin. Pharmacol. Ther., 1986; 39:619-624.

Labenz, J. et al: Toward an optimal treatment of Helicobacter pylori-positive peptic ulcers, Am. J. Gastroenterology, 1995, 90:692-694.

Leng-Peschlow et al: Pharmacology, 1992; 44Suppl. I:1-52.

Lindberg, P. et al: the first proton pump inhibitor. Med. Res. Rev., 1990, 10:1-54.

Maton, P.N. et al: H+/K+ ATPase inhibitors, anticholinergic agents, antidepressants, and gastrin receptor antagonists as gastric acid antisecretory agents. In, Gastrointestinal Pharmacotherapy. Saunders, Philadelphia, 1993, pp. 85-112.

McCarthy, D.M. et al: Sucralfate. N. Engl. J. Med., 1991, 325:1017-1025.

McTavish, D. et al: An updated review of its pharmacology and therapeutic use in acid-related disorders. Drugs, 1991, 42: 138- 170.

Mitchelson, F.: Pharmacological agents affecting emesis: a review Drugs, 1992a; 43:295-315.

Mitchelson, F.: Pharmacological agents affecting emesis: a review Drugs, 1992b; 43:443-463.

Soll, A.H.: Gastric, duodenal, and stress ulcer., In, Gastrointestinal Disease: Pathophysiology, Diagnosis, Management, 5th ed. Saunders, Philadelphia, 1993, pp. 580-679.

Symposium. NIH Consensus Development Panel on Helicobacter pylori in peptic ulcer disease. J.A.M.A., 1994, 272:65-69.

Wormsley, K.G.: Safety profile of ranitidine. A review. Drugs, 1993, 46:976-985.

Yarker, Y.E. et al: Granisetron. An update of its therapeutic use in nausea and vomiting induced by antineoplastic therapy. Drugs, 1994; 48:761-793.

Yoshida, C.M. et al: Gastroduodenal mucosal protection. In, Gastrointestinal Pharmacotherapy. Saunders, Philadelphia, 1993, pp. 113-137.

CHAPTER

9

Drugs Affecting Uterine Motility

CHAPTER CONTENTS AT A GLANCE

- Oxytocics (ecbolics), directly acting and indirectly acting
- Oxytocin
  - Actions on uterine fundus, body and cervical segment, mammary gland and blood vessels
  - Routes of administration
  - Preparations and doses
  - Therapeutic uses
  - Adverse effects and contraindications
  - Differences between the two hormones oxytocin and vasopressin secreted from posterior pituitary
- Ergometrine
  - Difference between oxytocin and ergometrine actions on uterus and cervix
  - Mode of action
  - Preparations and routes of administration
  - Therapeutic uses
  - Adverse effects
- Prostaglandins
  - Preparations and routes of administration
  - E and F series
  - Actions on the fundus and body of uterus and cervix
  - Preparations
  - Uses
  - Adverse effects
  - Contraindications
- Uterine-relaxing (tocolytic) agents
  - Selective Beta2 adrenoceptor agonists
  - Salbutamol, terbutaline, isoxsuprine
  - Ritodrine
  - Magnesium sulphate
  - Uses

DRUGS THAT AFFECT UTERINE MOTILITY

1. Uterine stimulants (ecbolics or oxytocics)

- Oxytocin
- Methylergonovine
- Prostaglandins

2. Uterine relaxants (tocolytics)

- Progestins
- B_2 sympathomimetics
- Calcium antagonists
- Prostaglandin inhibitors
- Oxytocin antagonists - atosiban

Uterine stimulants of importance in obstetrics

- Oxytocin
- Ergometrine (Ergonovine)
- E and F type prostaglandins

These drugs contract myometrium. These are more effective at delivery time.

OXYTOCIN

Synthesis, storage and release of oxytocin :

It is synthesized in the supraoptic and paraventricular nuclei of the hypothalamus within neurons that are distinct from those that contain antidiuretic hormone (ADH). It is transported via supraopticohypophyseal tract and stored complexed with a protein in the posterior pituitary. Oxytocin is released from nerve terminals in posterior pituitary. Suckling, coitus and cervical dilatation stimulate release of oxytocin.

Oxytocin differs from vasopressin (antidiuretic hormone, ADH) in following respects :
- No effect on water diuresis
- It is a potent uterine stimulant
- It has little effect on smooth muscles and coronaries
- It is not a vasoconstrictor

Pharmacological properties

Uterus

The posterior pituitary secretes two hormones oxytocin and vasopressin. Oxytocin is released from nerve terminals in posterior pituitary. Suckling, coitus and child birth stimulate release of oxytocin.

Oxytocin stimulates both the frequency and force of contractile activity in uterine smooth muscle and dilatation of cervix. The responsiveness of the uterus to oxytocin roughly parallels the increase in spontaneous activity; in early pregnancy only very high doses elicit response. About eightfold increase in responsiveness occurs between the 20th and 39th week of gestation and most of this increase occurs during last 9 weeks.

Mammary gland

Oxytocin also contracts myoepithelial cells surrounding mammary alveoli resulting in milk ejection (milk let down).

Cardiovascular system

Oxytocin causes a marked though transient relaxation of vascular smooth muscle with large amounts in human beings. Systolic and particularly diastolic blood pressure fall with reflex tachycardia and increase in limb blood flow. The therapeutic doses do not produce any significant effect on blood pressure.

Other actions

Antidiuretic effect is observed with large doses.

Oxytocin can also suppress the action of ACTH.

Absorption, Fate, and Excretion

Oxytocin is effective after any parenteral route.

It is also readily absorbed from oral mucosa (buccal lozenges can be used). Intranasal application of a spray is less efficient but more convenient.

The elimination of oxytocin is largely by the kidney and the liver.

Mechanism of action of oxytocin

Specific receptors for oxytocin in human myometrium have been identified and differences in receptor density at various stages of labour have also been noted. Oxytocin has dual effects on the uterus. It regulates the contractile property on myometrial cells and elicits prostaglandin production by endometrial/decidual cells.

However, the exact signaling mechanism that mediates the diverse effects of oxytocin in the hypothalamus, pituitary, and the uterus are not yet known.

Preparations of oxytocin

Oxytocin injection (generic, pitocin, syntocinon) contains 10 IU/ml for injection, 1-5 IU/ml, oxytocin citrate as buccal tablet, and 40 IU/ml in the form of nasal spray.

Uses

- To induce and augment labour
- To remove uterine inertia
- To treat postpartum haemorrhage (PPH)
- Incomplete abortion
- To promote lactation in engorged breasts
- To promote milk ejection when this component (oxytocin) of lactation appears to be inefficient in nursing mothers.

Dose

1-3 milliunits/min by I.V. drip in 500 ml 5% glucose.

Oxytocin is not given orally as it is destroyed in GIT, usually given intravenously, buccal absorption is possible, oxytocin (syntocinon) nasal spray is also employed (less efficient but more convenient). The half-life of oxytocin varies from less than 5 to more than 12 minutes.

Unitage

Activity is expressed in terms of unit, each unit is equal to about 2 mcg of the pure hormone.

Adverse effects

- Nausea, vomiting
- Foetal distress
- Foetal hypoxia
- Uterine rupture
- Hypotension associated with tachycardia
- Fluid retention

Contraindications

- Cephalopelvic disproportion
- Abnormal foetal presentation
- Foetal distress
- Placental abnormalities
- Previous uterine surgery
- Sympathomimetics should not be used with oxytocin

ERGOT ALKALOIDS

Ergometrine

Ergot is the product of a fungus *Claviceps purpurea* which grows on rye and other grains. It has several alkaloids such as ergotoxine (mixture of 3 alkaloids ergocristine, ergocriptine and ergocornine), ergotamine (used in migraine), ergometrine (ergonovine) has oxytocic activity.

Ergometrine is preferred as an ecbolic compared to other ergot alkaloids because it has greater selectivity, and it is also less toxic. Its semisynthetic derivative methylergometrine is also employed. There is no relaxation in between the uterine contractions unlike oxytocin. They cause long sustained and powerful contraction of uterine fundus in later pregnancy which may result in rupture of uterus and foetal death. They produce non-rhythmic contractions of the uterus and cervical segment is also contracted. So they have no place in induction of labour or during labour.

Ergometrine and methylergometrine are rapidly and completely absorbed after oral administration. The half-life of methylergometrine in plasma ranges between 0.5 and 2 hours.

Mode of action

Ergometrine acts as an agonist at 5-HT receptors in uterine myometrium.

Uses

- To prevent and control postpartum haemorrhage (PPH). The uterine blood vessels get squeezed due to muscle contraction (nature's ligatures).
- To promote recovery of uterine tone. A uterotonic effect can be observed within 10 minutes after oral administration of 0.2 mg of ergometrine.
- In incomplete abortion.

Preparations

Ergometrine maleate, methylergometrine maleate are available orally as well as parenterally.

Syntometrine contains 5 units of oxytocin plus 500 mcg of ergometrine; I.M. at or after delivery is given for prevention and control of PPH. Oxytocin acts within 2 minutes and as its effect wears off, ergometrine action begins and is sustained.

Dose

125-250 mcg I.V. to control atonic PPH or bleeding due to incomplete abortion; 0.5-1.0 mg in divided doses are administered orally.

Adverse effects

Nausea, vomiting (stimulates CTZ), hypertension with headache and blurred vision, decrease in milk secretion (as prolactin activity is reduced). Existing angina pectoris or peripheral vascular disease may be aggravated as ergometrine has vasoconstrictor action.

Prostaglandins

In the female reproductive system, prostaglandins are found in the ovary, myometrium and menstrual fluid. At term and during labour, prostaglandin concentrations rise in amniotic fluid, umbilical cord blood, and maternal blood.

The prostaglandins can be considered to be local hormones (with few exceptions) since they exert their effects and are inactivated in the tissues or organs in which they are synthesized. E and F types of prostaglandins are found abundantly in the uterus and in the menstrual and amniotic fluid. Prostacyclin (PGI$_2$) is confined largely to the uterine, umbilical, and foetal circulation.

Effect on uterus

Those found abundantly in the uterus, and in the menstrual and amniotic fluid are of the E and F types, whereas prostacyclin (PGI_2) is found mainly in the uterine, umbilical, and foetal vasculature.

Prostaglandins used in obstetrical practice include PGE_2, $PGF_{2\alpha}$ and the synthetic derivative 15-methyl $PGF_{2\alpha}$. Recently, the PGE_1 analogue, misoprostol is under trial for use as an abortifacient and cervical ripening agent.

The administration of either PGE_2 or $PGF_{2\alpha}$ causes strong uterine contractions during the last two trimesters of pregnancy. As with oxytocin the sensitivity of the uterus increases as gestation progresses, though the change is less pronounced than for oxytocin. In the earlier months, prostaglandins are more effective than oxytocin in causing contractions.

Effect on cervix

These agents on local instillation can induce cervical ripening at doses that do not affect uterine motility.

Uses

- PGE_2 (dinoprostone) and 15-methyl $PGF_{2\alpha}$ (carboprost) for performance of midtrimester abortions.
- Locally applied PGE_2 is useful as a cervical ripening agent.
- Induction of labour in patients not responding to oxytocin.
- 15-methyl $PGF_{2\alpha}$ may be used as alternative to ergometrine or oxytocin in the treatment of postpartum haemorrhage (PPH).
- PGE_1 analogue (misoprostol) has been used as an abortifacient and cervical ripening agent. It appears to be more desirable choice than PGE_2, $PGF_{2\alpha}$ or 15-methyl $PGF_{2\alpha}$, as it produces less emesis, pyrexia and diarrhoea as side effect.

Preparations

Oral PGE_2 (Dinoprostone) 0.5 mg hourly is administered and dose is gradually increased to 2 mg. Vaginal administration of PGE_2 as a gel or pessaries can be used to prime the cervix. For second trimester termination, intrauterine route is used. The continu-ous infusion of PGE_2 (Dinoprostone) or PGF_2 alpha (carboprost) via a catheter through the cervix results in abortion within 48 hours in 90% of cases. For first trimester termination, prostaglandins are used to prime cervix before surgical termination by vacuum aspiration. This reduces risk of injury and haemorrhage.

Sulprostone ($PGF_{2\alpha}$ analogue), gemeprost (PGE_1 analogue) and carboprost ($PGF_{2\alpha}$ analogue) are available.

Adverse effects

- Nausea, vomiting, diarrhoea, intestinal colic
- Pyrexia due to action on thermoregulatory centre in the hypothalamus
- Uterine pain
- Headache, dizziness
- Phlebitis at the site of injection
- Hypertension in large doses due to constriction of vascular smooth muscle
- $PGF_{2\alpha}$ in large doses may cause vasodilatation resulting in hypotension

Intravaginal pessary may cause systemic toxicity.

Misoprostol (PGE_1 analogue) produces less vomiting, diarrhoea and pyrexia as side effect.

Contraindications

- $PGF_{2\alpha}$ should not be given to asthmatics as it is a bronchoconstrictor
- Hypersensitivity to PGs
- Patients with active cardiac, pulmonary, renal or hepatic disease.

UTERINE RELAXANTS (MYOMETRIAL RELAXANTS, TOCOLYTICS)

- Progestins
- β_2 sympathomimetics
- Calcium antagonists
- Prostaglandin inhibitors
- Oxytocin antagonist—atosiban

Tocolytic agents inhibit uterine motility

Progestins

They bind to myometrial receptors and inhibit myometrial excitability and contraction. This effect is slowly developed hence, they are ineffective to arrest labour.

They are used to prevent preterm labour (prophylactic) in predisposed persons.

Progesterone is a physiological uterine relaxant, used to prevent premature labour as it decreases sensitivity to oxytocin, But it is ineffective, if preterm labour has started.

Side effects

- Maternal: jaundice, postpartum haemorrhage.
- Foetal: premature closure of cranial sutures, strabismus.

β_2 sympathomimetic tocolytic agents (adrenergic agonists).

Innervation of the uterus and the effect of sympathomimetic amines: The nerve supply to the uterus includes both excitatory and inhibitory sympathetic fibers.

Selective β_2-adrenoceptor agonists (stimulants) such as terbutaline, salbutamol, orciprenaline, isoxsuprine relax uterine muscle with limited success.

Salbutamol or terbutaline initially 4 mcg/min. i.v. infusion then rate doubled 8 mcg/min. i.v. every 5-10 minutes till uterine contractions stop, usually 16-32 mcg/min. is needed, maintained for 12 hrs, followed by 2-5 mg 6 hourly orally.

Ritodrine hydrochloride has more predictable effect as uterine relaxant. It is a β_2 adrenergic agonist, relaxes uterus by stimulating the β_2 adrenergic receptors of uterine muscle. The half life is 1.7 - 2.6 hours.

Dose: Orally, 10-20 mg 4-6 hourly

Parenterally, 0.1mg/min. infusion, gradually increased, maximum 0.35 mg/min.

Adverse effects

β_2-adrenergic receptor agonists may produce a number of cardiovascular (lowered B.P.) and metabolic side effects (hyperglycaemia) in the mother. Hypokalaemia is another consequence of administration of these agents.

Contraindications

- Cardiac diseases
- Hyperthyroidism
- Uncontrolled hypertension
- Uncontrolled diabetics mellitus

Calcium antagonist tocolytics

Magnesium sulphate, nifedipine.

Magnesium sulphate

It competes with intracellular calcium and interferes with excitation-contraction coupling. It is used in conditions where beta sympathomimetics are contraindicated. Magnesium sulphate 10% solution i.v. infusion depresses uterine activity. Loading dose is 4 g i.v. over a period of 20 min, then infusion at the rate of 1-2 g/hr till uterine contractions are reduced to less than one every 10 minutes, followed by 1g/hr for 24-72 hours. It has low efficacy when cervix is more than 1 cm dilated.

Magnesium sulphate is given frequently to control eclamptic seizures during pregnancy.

Nifedipine

10 mg is given sublingually as a loading dose and repeated every 20 minutes for 2-3 doses, followed by 10-20 mg 4-6 hourly as maintenance dose.

Prostaglandin Inhibitors

Prostaglandin-synthetase inhibitors such as indomethacin have been used for the cessation of preterm labour. If they are to be used their use is limited to gestation period to 24 weeks.

A number of side effects have been reported including premature closure of ductus arteriosus, production of hypertension and oligohydramnios.

Dose: 50 mg initially, then 25 mg, 6 hourly for 2-3 days.

Indomethacin is combined with beta-sympathomimetics to:

- Reduce the risk of foetal vascular complications and
- To restore the beta-receptors thereby preventing tolerance to them

Atosiban

It significantly inhibits preterm uterine contractions.

A decline (not cessation) in uterine activity occurs within 60 minutes of initiation of a 300 mcg/min infusion. The elimination half life is 1.7 hours.

Adverse effects

Chest pain, tachycardia, headache, nausea, vomiting.

Contraindications

- Prior hypersensitivity to this drug
- Preeclampsia or eclampsia
- Undiagnosed vaginal bleeding
- Intrauterine foetal distress or foetal death

Uses of uterine relaxants

- To delay or prevent premature parturition in selected individuals, by decreasing uterine motility. It can prevent premature labour and threatened abortion.
  For successful result: (i) cervical dilatation should be < 4 cm, (ii) membranes not ruptured, (iii) absence of severe toxaemia of pregnancy and (iv) no intrauterine infection.
- To relieve foetal distress
- To treat hypertonus due to uterine stimulants
- Also useful in pains of dysmenorrhoea
- To slow or arrest delivery for brief periods in order to undertake other therapeutic measures.

STUDY QUESTIONS

1. Which oxytocics (ecbolics) are directly acting?
2. Describe the actions of oxytocin on the fundus and body of the uterus and cervix.
3. What are the actions of oxytocin on mammary gland and blood vessels?
4. What are the main differences in the actions of oxytocin and ergometrine on the uterus?
5. Describe the preparations, routes of administration and therapeutic uses of oxytocin. Identify the advantages of oxytocin as compared to ergometrine.
6. What are the main differences between oxytocin and vasopressin which are both secreted from posterior pituitary?
7. What is ergot? What are the main alkaloids of ergot? Why ergometrine is preferred as an ecbolic among them?
8. Describe the mode of action, uses and adverse effects of ergometrine.
9. Which prostaglandins are used as uterine stimulants? Name a few preparations, their routes of administration and therapeutic uses. What may be their adverse effects and contraindications?
10. Name important uterine relaxants, their routes of administration and therapeutic uses.

GUIDE TO FURTHER READING

Amico, J.A. et al: Studies of oxytocin in plasma of women during hypocontractile labor. J. Clin. Endocrinol. Metab., 1984; 58:274-279.

Bossmar, T. et al: Receptors for and myometrial responses to oxytocin and vasopressin in preterm and term human pregnancy: effects of the oxytocin antagonist atosiban. Am. J. Obstet. Gynecol., 1994; 171:1634-1642.

Bugalho, A. et al: The effectiveness of intravaginal misoprostol (Cytotec) in inducing abortion after eleven weeks of pregnancy. Stud. Fam. Plann., 1993; 24:319-323.

Chard, T. et al: Release of oxytocin and vasopressin by the human fetus during labour. Nature, 1971; 234:352-354.

Goodwin, T.M. et al: The effect of the oxytocin antagonist atosiban on preterm uterine activity in the human. Am. J. Obstet. Gynecol., 1994; 170:474-478.

Hausknecht. R.U.: Methotrexate and misoprostol to terminate early pregnancy, N. Engl. J. Med., 1995; 333:537-540.

Kimura. T. et al: Molecular characterization of a cloned human oxytocin receptor. Eur. J. Endocrinol., 1994; 131:385-390.

Murray, C. et al: Nifedipine for treatment of preterm labor: a historic prospective study. Am. J. Obstet. Gynecol., 1992; 167:52-56.

Pavo, I. et al: Enhanced selectivity of oxytocin antagonists containing sarcosine in position 7. J. Med. Chem., 1994; 37:255-259.

Peyron, R. et al: Early termination of pregnancy with mifepristone and the orally active prostaglandin misoprostol. N. Engl. J. Med., 1993; 328:1509-1513.

Petty, M.A. et al: The cardiovascular effects of the neurohypophysial hormone oxytocin. J. Auton. Pharmacol., 1987; 7:97-104.

10

Hormones and Hormone Antagonists

GENERAL ASPECTS

Endocrine dysfunction

Pituitary gland dysfunction

Anterior pituitary lobe disorders

- Pituitary dwarfism (in children)
- Hypersecretion of pituitary hormones
  - Acromegaly and gigantism (growth hormones)
  - Cushing's syndrome
  - Galactorrhoea (prolactin)

Posterior pituitary lobe disorders

- Diabetes insipidus due to insufficient production of vasopressin (ADH)

Thyroid dysfunction

- Hypothyroidism
  - Cretinism in children
  - Myxoedema in adults
- Hyperthyroidism
  - Thyrotoxicosis, Graves' disease
  - Thyroid storm or crisis
- Goiter
- Thyroiditis
  - Hashimoto's disease (autoimmune)
  - Subacute granulomatous thyroiditis
  - Riedel's (fibrous) thyroiditis
- Thyroid neoplasms

Parathyroid dysfunction

- Hypoparathyroidism (postoperative tetany)
- Hyperparathyroidism

Adrenal dysfunction

- Hyposecretion
  - Addison's disease (primary insufficiency)
  - Secondary adrenal insufficiency
- Hypersecretion
  - Cushing's syndrome
  - Congenital adrenal hyperplasia
  - Adrenal virilism (adrenogenital syndrome)
  - Hyperaldosteronism
- Pheochromocytoma
- Nonfunctional adrenal masses

Gonadal dysfunction

- Male hypogonadism
- Testicular feminization syndrome
- Precocious puberty

Terms associated with endocrine system

Cretinism : Infantile hypothyroidism resulting in stunting of bodily growth and of mental development.

Myxoedema : Hypothyroidism characterized by hard oedema of subcutaneous tissue.

Dwarfism : The condition of being markedly undersized.

Gigantism : Overgrowth of the entire body.

Acromegaly : A disorder marked by progressive enlargement of the head and face, hands and feet and thorax, due to excessive secretion of growth hormone by the anterior lobe of the pituitary gland.

Cushingoid : Resembling the signs and symptoms of Cushing's disease or syndrome.

Goiter : A chronic enlargement of the thyroid gland not due to a neoplasm.

Exophthalmic goiter : Any of the various forms of hyperthyroidism in which the thyroid gland is enlarged and exophthalmos is present.

Exophthalmos : Protrusion of the eye balls (marked prominence of the eyeball).

HYPOTHALAMIC REGULATORY HORMONES AND PITUITARY HORMONES

Hypothalamic and pituitary hormones

The peptidergic neurons in hypothalamus secrete factors which regulate anterior pituitary. These peptidergic neurons are themselves influenced by higher centers in the central nervous system through dopamine, noradrenaline and 5-hydroxytryptamine.

Several peptide hormones are secreted by hypothalamus which influence a number of secretions from anterior pituitary. These hypothalamic hormones are important mediators for the feedback mechanism. They have little clinical use.

The following are the hypothalamic regulatory hormones:

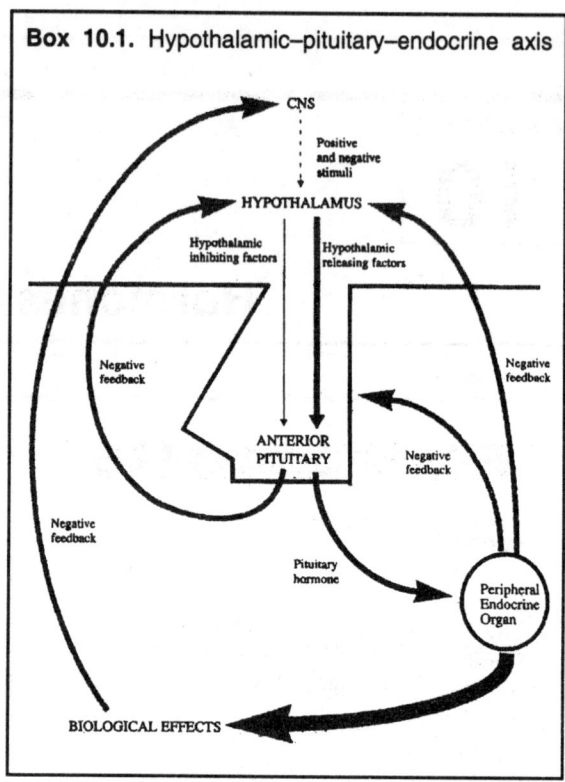

Box 10.1. Hypothalamic–pituitary–endocrine axis

- GHRH (growth hormone-releasing hormone) and GHRIH (growth hormone-inhibiting hormone, also called somatostatin)
- CRH (corticotropin-releasing hormone)
- TRH (thyrotrophin-releasing hormone)
- GnRH (gonadotrophin-releasing hormone)
- PRH (prolactin-releasing hormone) and PIH (prolactin-inhibiting hormone, now believed to be dopamine)
- MRF (melanocyte releasing hormone)
- MIF (melanocyte-inhibiting hormone)

The pituitary hormones which affect the peripheral endocrine organs is shown in Fig. 10.1.

Anterior pituitary hormones can be grouped as

(a) Somatomammotropins
  - Growth hormone (GH)
  - Prolactin
  - Placental lactogen
(b) Glycoproteins
  - LH (luteinizing hormone)

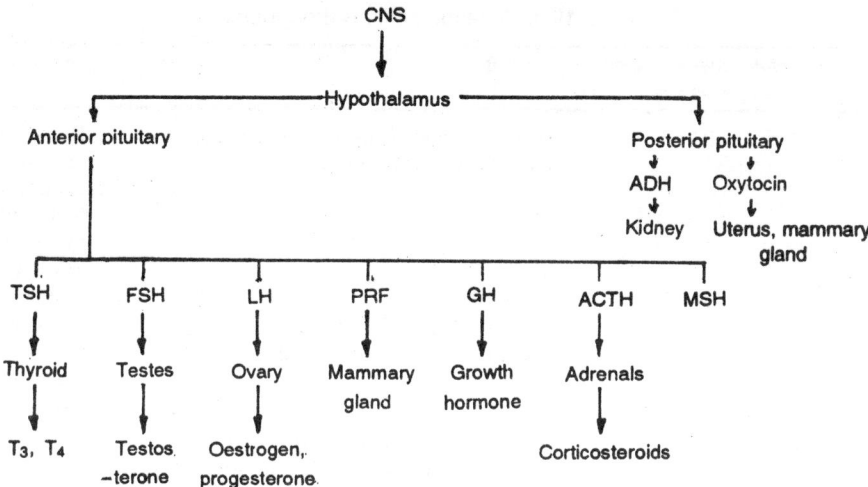

Fig. 10.1. Hypothalamus regulates release of pituitary hormones which affect peripheral endocrine organs.

- FSH (follicle-stimulating hormone)
- Human chorionic gonadotropin (hCG) hormone
- GRF (gonadal hormone releasing factor)
- TSH (thyroid-stimulating hormone, thyrotropin)

(c) Corticotropin and related peptides
- ACTH (adrenocorticotrophic hormone, adrenocorticotropin)
- α-MSH (melanosite stimulating hormone)
- β-MSH (melanosite stimulating hormone)
- β-lipoproteins (β-LPH)
- γ-lipoproteins (γ-LPH)

ANTERIOR PITUITARY (ADENOHYPOPHYSIS)

It releases several hormones, some are directly acting, e.g. growth hormone (GH) and prolactin and some act indirectly e.g. ACTH, TSH, FSH and LH. The hypothalamus regulates the release of anterior pituitary hormones.

Table 10.1 lists anterior pituitary hormones.

Growth hormone (GH, somatotropin) effects:

Growth hormone secretion is pulsatile with about 8.5 mg/d released in 6-8 irregular bursts. The secretion may be elicited by hypoglycaemia, stress, protein - rich diet and after the onset of deep sleep.

- Skeletal muscles—linear growth

- Helps entry of amino acids into the cells (anabolic effect)
- Antagonizes insulin effects
- Increases lipolysis
- Increases DNA replication and RNA synthesis
- Retention of Na, K, Ca and PO_4

Growth hormone may act by stimulating synthesis or release of somatomedins, which are identical to peptides known as insulin- like growth factors (IGF) 1 and 2. Low levels of IGF-1 are associated with dwarfism. Growth hormone deficiency may result in adult hypopituitarism (Sheehan's syndrome) which with low cortisol levels leads to hypoglycaemia.

Juvenile hypopituitarism results in pituitary dwarfism.

Growth hormone is available only at certain special centers. Its use is limited in hypopituitary dwarfism in children. Dose is 0.5-1.0 units I.M. There are two synthetic versions of growth hormones viz. (a) somatotropin and Humatrope (new brand of somatotropin) and (b) somatrem (protropin).

Growth hormone hypersecretion may result in acromegaly and gigantism.

The use of bromocriptine in acromegaly is paradoxical because dopamine stimulates growth hormone secretion in normal persons. Octreotide, an analogue of somatostatin offers promise in the treatment of acromegaly.

Table 10.1. Anterior pituitary hormones

Hormones	Associated hypothalamic regulating hormones	Actions	Selected disorders
Human growth hormone (hGH)	GHRH, GHIH	Growth of body cells, protein metabolism, elevation of blood glucose	Hyposecretion during growth years results in **dwarfism**, hypersecretion results in **gigantism**, hypersecretion during adulthood results in **acromegaly**
TSH	TRH	Controls secretion of thyroid hormones	Exophthalmic goiter
ACTH	CRH (corticotropin releasing hormones)	Controls hormones of adrenal cortex	Hyposecretion results in Addison's disease
FSH	GnRH	In females, initiates development of ova and secretion of oestrogen. In males, stimulates testes to produce sperm	
LH [also called interstitial cell stimulating hormone (ICSH) in male]	GnRH	In females, together with FSH stimulates ovulation and formation of progesterone-producing corpus luteum. In males, stimulates interstitial cells in testes to develop and produce testosterone.	
Prolactin (PRL)	PRF (prolactin releasing factor) PIF (prolactin inhibiting factor)	In female, together with other hormones initiates and maintains effects of LH in prompting milk secretion by mammary gland. In male, it enhances the production of testosterone.	

Adverse effects

Although there are no serious adverse effects, however, intracranial hypertension with papilloedema, mild hyperglycaemia and glycosuria may occur.

Contraindications

- Closed epiphyses
- Active neoplasia
- Active or unhealed intracranial lesions.

Prolactin

Prolactin is produced in anterior pituitary and resembles GH in structure to some extent. It promotes development of mammary tissue during pregnancy, stimulates milk production in postpartum period.

During pregnancy, high oestrogen and progestin levels inhibit prolactin activity, but after birth, these hormone levels drop, leaving the actions of prolactin unopposed. Breast-feeding elevates prolactin levels, which mediates an antigonadotropic effect, causing a lack of ovulation. This natural contraception diminishes over several months as the prolactin response to the sucking response wanes.

Dopamine antagonists are potent stimulants of prolactin release.

Dopamine agonists such as **bromocriptine** suppress prolactin release.

The main functions of prolactin in females is the control of milk production. Prolactin along with other hormones, is responsible for the proliferation and differentiation of mammary tissue during pregnancy. It inhibits gonadotrophin release and/or the response of the ovaries to these trophic hormones. This is one of the reasons why ovulation does not occur during breast feeding.

The high post-delivery concentration of prolactin reflects the biological function of 'parental' hormone. The 'parental' behaviour in mice and rabbits and nest building activity in birds can be induced by prolactin injections.

There may be similar action in humans, but this is conjectural.

Regarding the function of prolactin in males, one can only speculate.

Prolactin itself is not used clinically. The clinical need is to decrease its secretion.

The agent used for this purpose is bromocriptine.

Uses of bromocriptine

- To prevent as well as to suppress lactation
- To treat galactorrhoea i.e. non-puerperal lactation due to excessive prolactin secretion
- To treat prolactin - secreting pituitary tumours
- To treat parkinsonism
- To treat acromegaly

Bromocriptine is well absorbed orally, metabolised in liver and excreted in bile.

Adverse effects include nausea and vomiting (which may be ameliorated by taking the drug with meals). Postural hypotension, dizziness and constipation have also been reported.

ACTH (corticotropin, adrenocorticotrophic hormone) stimulates growth of adrenocortical cells and cortisol biosynthesis. It is used to investigate adrenocortical insufficiency.

ACTH, TSH, FSH, and LH regulate the functions of adrenal cortex, thyroid, and gonads respectively.

Gonadotropic hormones FSH and LH are produced and secreted by the gonadotropic cells of the pituitary. Their release is mediated by plasma steroid concentrations.

In men, FSH and LH plasma levels are quite stable; in women, plasma levels vary with the stage of the menstrual cycle.

POSTERIOR PITUITARY (NEUROHYPOPHYSIS)

It secretes two polypeptide hormones (Table 10.2)
1. Antidiuretic hormone (ADH, vasopressin)
2. Oxytocin

ADH is also called vasopressin due to its vasoconstrictory effect. It controls the water content of the body through its action on the cells of the distal tubule of nephron and the collecting tubules of the kidney. The antidiuretic effect is due to increased permeability in the renal collecting duct cells and increased reabsorption of water from the filtrate.

Higher concentrations produce non renal effects: It accelerates glycogen breakdown in liver cells, stimulates aggregation and degranulation of platelets and increases concentration of factor VIII of blood coagulation cascade (extra renal V_2-like receptors mediate release of this factor).

Vasopressin acts on two types of receptors (i) V_1 receptors on vascular smooth-muscle cells and mediate vasoconstriction and (ii) V_2 receptors on renal tubule cells and mediate antidiuresis as a result of increased water permeability and water reabsorption in the collecting tubules.

Vasopressin can be administered by S.C./I.M./I.V. and also by intranasal route.

Preparations

- Vasopressin: Antidiuretic hormone (ADH). The duration of action is short and has weak, selectivity for V_2-receptors. Given by SC/IM injection or I.V. infusion. It has 0.8 times the diuretic action of ADH and 60% of its vasopressor potency. Its $t\frac{1}{2}$ is 10 minutes and eliminated rapidly.

Table 10.2. Posterior pituitary hormones

Hormones	Principal actions	Control of secretion
Oxytocin	Stimulates contraction of smooth muscle cells of pregnant uterus during labour and stimulates contraction of contractile cells of mammary gland for milk ejection	Neurosecretory cells of hypothalamus secrete oxytocin in response to uterine distension and stimulation of nipples
Vasopressin (ADH)	Decreases urine volume, also raises B.P. by constricting arterioles during severe haemorrhage	Neurosecretory cells of hypothalamus secrete ADH in response to low water concentration of the blood, ACh, nicotine, morphine. Alcohol inhibits secretion. Hyposecretion of ADH results in diabetes insipidus.

- Desmopressin has longer duration of action and is V_2-receptor selective. Given as nasal spray. It has 12 times the diuretic action of ADH and 0.4% of its vasopressor potency. Its $t\frac{1}{2}$ is 75 minutes.
- Lypressin is similar to vasopressin but given as a nasal spray. Its half-life is 10 minutes and eliminated rapidly.
- Terlipressin has increased duration of action, is V_1-selective and is given by I.V. route. It has low vasopressor action and minimal antidiuretic property.
- Felypressin has short duration of action and is V_1-selective. It is used as a vasoconstrictor with local anaesthetics to prolong their action.

Dose

- Aqueous vasopressin 5-10 units S.C. or I.M./ 36 hours for transient diabetes insipidus; 0.1-0.5 units/min I.V. for gastrointestinal bleeding.
- Vasopressin tannate (pitressin tannate in oil) is long acting, suitable for I.M. injection only in 2.5-5 units/24-72 hours.
- Lypressin is short acting nasal spray, 2 units sprayed deeply in one or both nostrils every 4-6 hours. Inhalation of vasopressin may be ineffective when nasal congestion is present.
- Desmopressin acetate is preferred in chronic diabetes insipidus. It can be given parenterally as well as by transnasal route. The nasal dosage is 10-40 microgram in 2-3 divided doses.

Bedtime desmopressin therapy relieves nocturnal enuresis in dosage of 10-20 microgram intranasally.

Disorder of ADH secretion

Diabetes insipidus

It results from either reduced circulating ADH (called neurohypophyseal diabetes insipidus); or an impaired response of the nephron to normal ADH levels (called nephrogenic diabetes insipidus). Nephrogenic diabetes insipidus is due in many cases to defective V_2-receptors.

Uses of ADH

- As a replacement therapy in diabetes insipidus of pituitary origin but valueless in nephrogenic diabetes insipidus.

- In portal hypertension, it lowers portal venous pressure by causing splanchnic arteriolar constriction.
- To promote intestinal motility and expel gases.

Contraindications

Angina pectoris, myocardial infarction.

Drug interactions

Chlorpropamide, clofibrate and carbamazepine potentiate effects of vasopressin.

Adverse Effects

I.V. vasopressin may cause spasm of coronary arteries with resultant angina. It also frequently causes abdominal and uterine cramps.

Intranasal administration in therapeutic doses produces few adverse effects. Nausea and abdominal cramps and hypersensitivity reactions have been reported.

STUDY QUESTIONS

1. What are the different hypothalamic hormones (factors) that affect pituitary gland? Why these hormones are not important for clinical applications?
2. Name the various hormones elaborated by the anterior pituitary.
3. Describe the effects of prolactin, thyroid stimulating hormones, follicle stimulating hormones and luteinizing hormone.
4. What are the hormones secreted by posterior pituitary? Describe the mode of action, preparations, routes of administration and uses of ADH (vasopressin).
5. What are the contraindications, adverse effects and drug interactions of vasopressin?

GUIDE TO FURTHER READING

Bagatell, C.J. et al: Comparison of a gonadotropin releasing- hormone antagonist plus testosterone (T) versus T alone as potential male contraceptive regimens. J. Clin. Endocrinol. Metab., 1993; 77:427-432.

Carr, B.R.: Disorders of the ovary and female reproductive tract. In, Williams Textbook of Endocrinology. W.B. Saunders Co., Philadelphia, 1992; pp. 733-798.

Conn, P.M. et al: Gonadotropin-releasing hormone and its analogues. New Engl. J. Med., 1991; 324:93-103.

Jorgensen, J.O.L.: Human growth hormone replacement therapy: pharmacological and clinical aspects. Endocrine Rev., 1991; 12:189-207.

Lapthorn, A.J. et al: Crystal structure of human chorionic gonadotropin. Nature, 1994; 369:455-461.

Loy, R.A.: The pharmacology and the potential applications of GnRH antagonists. Curr. Opin. Obstet. Gynecol., 1994; 6:262-268.

Schlegel, P.N.: Medical management of prostatic diseases. Adv. Intern. Med., 1994; 39:569-601.

ADRENOCORTICAL STEROIDS AND THEIR SYNTHETIC ANALOGUES; INHIBITORS OF THE SYNTHESIS AND ACTION OF ADRENOCORTICAL HORMONES

ADRENOCORTICOTROPIC HORMONE (ACTH; CORTICOTROPIN)

A number of stimuli, e.g. trauma, chemicals and emotions can produce release of corticotropin - releasing factor (CRF) from hypothalamus which stimulates the anterior pituitary gland which in turn stimulates release of ACTH. ACTH circulates in the blood stream and stimulates the production of glucocorticoids from the adrenal cortex.

A negative feedback pathway maintains homeostasis. When the levels of endogenous corticosteroids increase, the pituitary- adrenal axis is suppressed and the production of ACTH and CRF is reduced (Fig. 10.2).

Endogenous corticosteroids released by the adrenal cortex chiefly affect carbohydrate and protein metabolism.

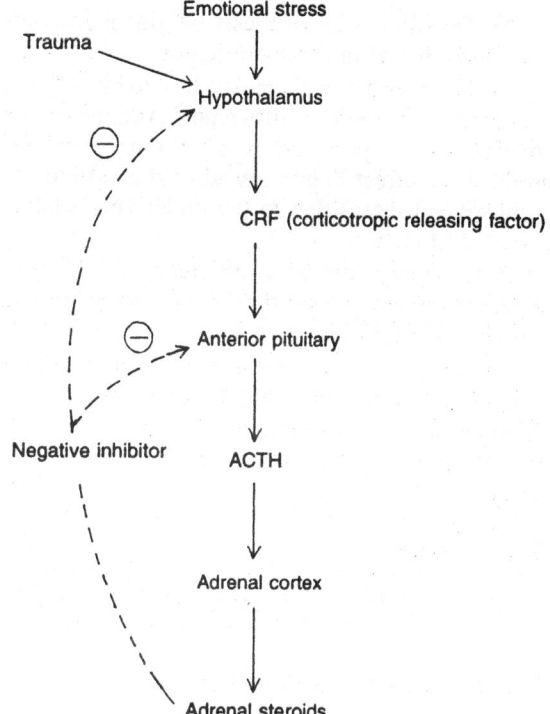

Fig. 10.2. Pituitary-adrenal axis.

Box 10.2. Normal daily production rates and circulatory levels of the predominant corticosteroids

	Cortisol	Aldosterone
Rate of secretion under normal condition	10 mg/d	0.125 mg/d
Concentration in peripheral plasma		
8 AM	16 mcg/100 ml	0.01 mcg/100 ml
4 PM	4 mcg/100 ml	0.01 mcg/100 ml

Sites of synthesis of adrenal corticosteroids

- Zona glomerulosa : Mineralocorticoids e.g., aldosterone (mainly), desoxycorticosterone
- Zona fasciculate : Glucocorticoids e.g., cortisol (mainly), cortisone, corticosterone
- Zona reticularis : Gonadocorticoids e.g., oestrogens and androgens
- Hydrocortisone 2- mg and aldosterone 0.125 mg are synthesized daily by an adult

Corticosteroids

- Cortisol (Hydrocortisone) 10-25 mg is secreted daily
- Cortisone, 0.5 - 2.0 mg is secreted daily
- Corticosterone, 30-150 mcg is secreted daily

ADRENOCORTICOTROPIC HORMONE (ACTH)

Human ACTH is a polypeptide hormone consisting of 39 amino acids. The number of amino acids is less in synthetic derivatives who possess similar activity of endogenous ACTH.

ACTH stimulates synthesis of glucocorticoids more than that of mineralocorticoids.

ACTH is used as a diagnostic tool to identify the two types of adrenal insufficiency. Administration (ACTH is given parenterally, often i.m.) of ACTH produces no effect in primary adrenal insufficiency (Addison's disease) due to the underlying adrenal cortex dysfunction.

In secondary adrenal insufficiency, ACTH produces response by synthesizing and releasing adrenocorticosteroids.

The adrenal cortex releases hormonal steroids which can be grouped as those having (i) effect on carbohydrate metabolism (glucocorticoids), (ii) salt-retaining property and (iii) androgenic or oestrogenic activity.

Glucocorticoids

The amount of endogenous corticosteroids secreted daily can increase tenfold in stressful conditions.

Structure-activity relationship

The general structure of adrenal corticosteroids is shown in Fig. 10.3.

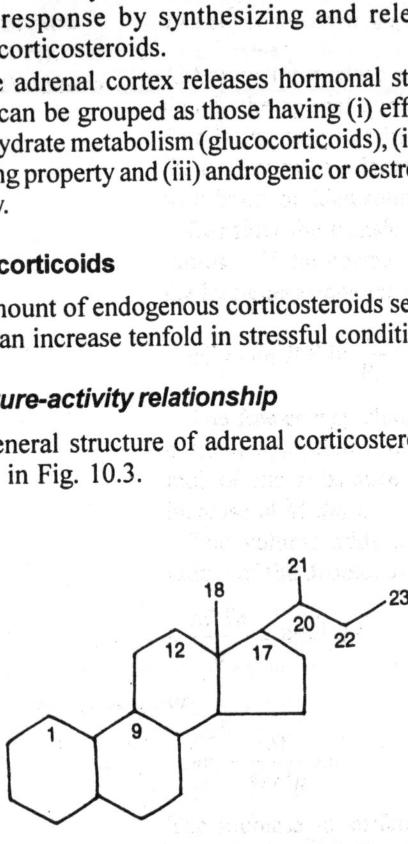

Fig. 10.3. General structure of adrenal corticosteroids.

- Position 11: Oxygen or halogen is essential for corticoid activity.
- Position 17: Presence of –OH or –C=O increases corticoid activity.
- A double bond at positions 1,2 increases glucocorticoid activity.
- Positions 6 or 9: Halogenation increases activity.
- Positions 6 or 16: Presence of alkyl group increases glucocorticoid activity.

Mode of action

Glucocorticoids are transported through cell membranes and bind to the cytoplasmic glucocorticoid receptor-heat-shock protein complex. The heat shock protein is released and the hormone- receptor complex is then transported into the nucleus where it interacts with glucocorticoid response elements (GREs) on various genes and other regulatory proteins and stimulates or inhibits their expression.

Metabolic effects

- Carbohydrate metabolism: These steroids have evolved to protect glucose-dependent functions by stimulating the formation of glucose, diminishing its peripheral utilization and promoting its storage. But the prolonged exposure to large doses results in exaggeration of these changes in glucose metabolism. Glucocorticoids produce
  - increase in gluconeogenesis
  - inhibition of peripheral glucose uptake
  - deposition of glycogen occurs in liver

  Thus hyperglycaemia may result or latent diabetes mellitus becomes overt as an adverse effect.
- Protein metabolism: Conversion of amino acids to proteins is decreased. The anabolic effect due to the large doses may produce a large number of adverse effects including wasting of muscles, weakness, osteoporosis, etc.
- Fat metabolism: Glucocorticoids inhibit uptake of glucose by fat cells leading to lipolysis. However, the increased insulin secretion induced by hyperglycaemia stimulates lipogenesis resulting in fat deposition. The fat deposition occurs on shoulders, face, back of neck and abdomen and there is loss of fat from the extremities. Adipocytes in the extremities, in contrast of the trunk are less sensitive to insulin and more sensitive to glucocorticoid facilitated lipolytic effect. There is lipolysis of triglycerides of adipose tissue.
- Calcium metabolism
  (i) inhibition of Ca^{2+} absorption from intestine and enhancement of its renal excretion,
  (ii) loss of calcium from bone due to loss of

osteoid (decreased formation due to protein catabolism),

(iii) spongy bones (vertebrae, ribs) are more sensitive,

(iv) in large doses they inhibit linear growth in children where new cells are being added but not in adults where these are replacing cells.

Other effects

Water excretion : In adrenal insufficiency water load occurs.

- Urinary system: Urinary calcium excretion is increased and renal stones may form. These have anti-vitamin D activity.
- Cardiovascular system: Glucocorticoid induced hypertension is due to (1) retention of sodium, (ii) plasma renin activity and (iii) ADH may be involved.
- Skeletal muscles: Weakness (in hypocorticism due to hypodynamic circulation) and muscle wasting and myopathy are due to excess of glucocorticoids.
- CNS: Euphoria, increased motor activity, anxiety, insomnia or depression. Euphoria or psychotic states may occur due to changes in the electrolytes in CNS.
- High doses lower seizure threshold - caution in epileptics.
- GIT: Increased secretion of gastric acid and pepsin may aggravate peptic ulcer.
- Lymphoid tissue:
  Destruction of lymphoid cells (T-cells more than B-cells) used in lymphomas. Lymphoid tissue is reduced.
- RBCs and other blood cells: Increase in number of RBCs and neutrophils, decrease in lymphocytes, eosinophils and basophils.

Antiinflammatory and immunosuppressive effects

They suppress all cardinal signs of inflammation. They reduce capillary permeability, local exudation, cellular infiltration, phagocytic activity and late responses like collagen deposition and scar formation.

Glucocorticoids inhibit inflammatory response whether the inciting agent is radiant, mechanical, chemical, infection or immunological.

These inhibit (i) early phenomenon of inflammation i.e. influence oedema, fibrin deposition, capillary dilation and migration of leukocytes into inflamed area, (ii) inhibit late manifestation i.e. proliferation of capillaries and fibroblasts, collagen deposition and (iii) still late manifestations i.e. cicatrization.

The antiinflammatory effect is useful but it is palliative because the underlying pathology continues which in some cases may be harmful.

They suppress all types of hypersensitization and allergic phenomenon.

Glucocorticoids reduce inflammation due to their action on concentration, distribution and function of leukocytes and inhibition of phospholipase A_2 activity.

The concentration of neutrophils is increased due to influx from bone marrow and decreased migration from blood vessels which reduce the number of cells at the site of inflammation, while the number of lymphocytes (T and B cells), monocytes, eosinophils and basophils in the circulation is decreased due to their movement from circulation to lymphoid tissue.

Glucocorticoids produce inhibition of function of leukocytes and tissue macrophages, resulting in less ability of these cells to respond to antigens. The effect on macrophages reduces their ability to phagocytose and kill microorganisms.

Besides the action on leukocytes, corticosteroids also influence the inflammatory response by reducing prostaglandin and leukotriene synthesis.

Thus inflammatory response is depressed, allergic responses are suppressed, lymphoid tissue is reduced, blood eosinophils are reduced in number, there is anti-vitamin D activity, urinary calcium excretion is increased (renal stones may form), euphoria or psychotic states may occur (due to changes in the electrolytes in CNS), antibody production is reduced (with high doses, growth in children slowed where new cells are being added but not in adults where there are replacing cells).

Pharmacokinetics

Absorption occurs when given by mouth, from parenteral sites and also from sites of local application such as synovial spaces, conjunctival sac and the skin.

Most of the hormone after absorption is bound to globulin.

Steroids are metabolized through conjugation reactions principally in liver and to some extent in kidney. These are conjugated with sulphate or with glucuronic acid to form water-soluble sulphate esters or glucuronides and excreted.

Routes of administration

They are available orally, parenterally and topically as well as some as aerosols. Water soluble preparations are given intravenously for rapid action. Suspensions are injected intramuscularly for more prolonged effects. Oral steroids are best taken around 8.00 am to mimic the natural secretion of adrenal cortex (corticosteroid secretion shows a diurnal rhythm, peak secretion occurs between 4.00 am and 8.00 am).

Mineralocorticoids

Electrolyte and water balance

Mineralocorticoids increase the reabsorption of sodium by acting on distal tubules and collecting ducts of the kidney. They increase excretion of both K^+ and H^+.

Fludrocortisone has both mineralocorticoid and glucocorticoid activity. It is given orally.

It has predominantly sodium retaining activity, 0.1 mg, 2-7 times weekly is used in the treatment of adrenocortical insufficiency.

Deoxycortone (DOCA): is predominantly a mineralocorticoid. Its normal secretion is 200 microgram per day. It is not effective when swallowed due to hepatic first-pass effect. It has been superseded by fludrocortisone.

Aldosterone

It is a naturally occurring salt-retaining hormone. It is secreted at the rate of 100-200 microgram daily normally. If given orally, it is rapidly eliminated due to hepatic first-pass effect. It can be given intramuscularly 0.5mg which can be repeated several times a day. Fludrocortisone has replaced it because it is equally effective and is active orally.

Clinical use of mineralocorticoids

• For replacement therapy. Fludrocortisone is given orally to produce mineralocorticoid effect. It increases Na^+ reabsorption in distal tubules and increases K^+ and H^+ efflux into the tubules.

Adverse effects

• Sodium and water retention, oedema
• Hypertension
• Hypokalaemic alkalosis

Individual adrenal steroids

• Hydrocortisone (cortisol) is a naturally occurring steroid, taken orally, hydrocortisone sodium succinate inj. (soluble salt) can be given intravenously; hydrocortisone acetate inj (suspension) can be given intramuscularly for longer action and also intra- articularly.
• Cortisone is a prodrug converted to active drug hydrocortisone in the liver. It is therefore not suitable for local application.
• Prednisone is a prodrug, converted to prednisolone in the liver.
• Prednisolone is mainly glucocorticoid (anti-inflammatory). It has little sodium retaining activity.
• Methylprednisolone has similarity to prednisolone.
• Triamcinolone has no sodium retaining activity. However, loss of appetite, CNS depression and severe muscle wasting may occur with high doses.
• Dexamethasone and betamethasone have potent antiinflammatory property.

Beclomethasone and budesonide are inactivated by hepatic first- pass effect. These are used for the treatment of bronchial asthma by inhalation.

Table 10.3 shows relative potencies of glucocorticoids. Table 10.4 shows potencies of topical steroids.

Precautions to be observed during glucocorticoid therapy

Before starting therapy : Enquire about history of peptic ulcer, watch for anaemia, diabetes, any infection including tuberculosis.

During therapy : Prescribe the drug with food, examine urine periodically for sugar, keep record of

Table 10.3. Relative potencies and equivalent doses of glucocorticoids

Drugs	Anti-inflammatory potency	Na⁺-retaining potency	Topical potency	Equivalent oral dose (mg)	Duration
Cortisol	1	1	1	20	Short
Cortisone	0.8	0.8	0	25	Short
Prednisone	4	0.8	0	5	Intermediate
Prednisolone	4	0.8	4	5	Intermediate
6-alpha-methylprednisolone	5	0	5	4	Intermediate
Triamcinolone	5	0	5	4	Intermediate
Fludrocortisone	10	125	7	1.5	Short
Betamethasone	25	0	10	0.75	Long
Dexamethasone	25	0	10	0.75	Long

Short = Biological half-life 8-12 hours; Intermediate = Biological half-life 12-36 hours; Long = Biological half-life 36-72 hours

Table 10.4. Potency of topical steroids

Lowest	Hydrocortisone 0.1%-0.5%
	Methylprednisolone 0.25%-1.0%
Low	Triamcinolone acetonide 0.025%
	Fluocinolone acetonide 0.01%
Intermediate	Triamcinolone acetonide 0.1%
	Betamethasone valerate 0.1%
	Fluocinolone acetonide 0.1%-0.025%
	Betamethasone benzoate 0.1%-0.025%
High	Triamcinolone acetonide 0.5%
	Desoximetasone 0.25%
	Betamethasone dipropionate 0.025%-0.2%
Highest	Betamethasone dipropionate 0.05%

weight and B.P. increase the dose in infections or during surgery.

Instruct the patient not to stop therapy abruptly While stopping therapy :

Taper off therapy

Some general principles

1. Except in adrenal insufficiency, the administration of corticosteroids are neither specific nor curative but only palliative by virtue of their anti-inflammatory and immunosuppressive effects.
2. A single dose even a large one is virtually without harmful effect.
3. A few days of therapy in the absence of contraindications is not likely to produce adverse effect except at the most extreme dosages.
4. If therapy is prolonged over periods of weeks or months, the incidence of toxicity increases.
5. When steroids are to be given for long periods, smallest dose should be used that will achieve the desired effect. This is found by trial and error. Of course, in life-threatening situation the initial dose should be a large one.
6. Abrupt withdrawal of prolonged, high dose corticosteroid therapy is associated with a risk of adrenal insufficiency which may be threatening to life. The doses must be tapered-off rather than stopped abruptly. The suppression of the pituitary-adrenal axis must be avoided because consequences can be fatal (adrenal cortex will not respond to stress). Once the axis is suppressed, it will take more than one year for normal function to return.

To minimize suppression of pituitary adrenal axis:
- Use shorter acting steroids e.g. prednisolone, hydrocotisone
- Use lowest possible dose
- Use for shortest possible time
- Give entire daily dose at one time in the morning
- Switch to alternate day therapy, if possible

However, less than 25 mg of prednisone per day or equivalent taken at 8.00 am for 5-10 days usually does not suppress the pituitary- adrenal axis.

Glucocorticoids with highest antiinflammatory activity and least sodium retaining potency:

Betamethasone > dexamethasone > triamcinolone

Glucocorticoids with high sodium retaining capacity:

Cortisol > Cortisone = prednisolone > methyl prednisolone

Glucocorticoids used as inhalational antiasthmatic agents:

Beclomethasone, budenoside, triamcinolone.

Glucocorticoids classified according to duration of action:

- Short acting (half-life 8-12 hours): Cortisone, hydrocortisone
- Intermediate acting (half-life 12-36 hours): Prednisone, prednisolone, methylprednisolone, triamcinolone
- Long acting (half-life 36-72 hours): Dexamethasone, betamethasone

Use in endocrine disease

- Replacement of hormone therapy
- To suppress inflammation
- As immunosuppressive (by inhibiting antibody synthesis)
- In acute adrenal insufficiency (Addisonian crisis)
- In chronic primary adrenocortical insufficiency (Addison's disease)
- In iatrogenic adrenocortical insufficiency

Use in nonendocrine diseases

- Collagen diseases e.g. rheumatoid arthritis, ankylosing spondylitis, polyarteritis nodosa, lupus erythematosus, polymyositis. But scleroderma is usually refractory.
- Severe allergic reactions of all kinds, e.g. hay fever, serum sickness, urticaria, drug reactions, contact dermatitis, allergic rhinitis, bee stings, angioneurotic oedema. In anaphylaxis immediate therapy should be given with adrenaline 0.3-1.0 ml of a 1: 1000 solution IM/SC because corticosteroids take some time to act.
- Bronchial asthma (not as a routine), useful in status asthmaticus.
- Eye diseases such as acute uveitis, allergic conjunctivitis, optic neuritis, choroiditis.
- Shock (particularly in septic vascular shock).

- Haematologic disorders such as acute lymphatic leukaemia, lymphomas and multiple myeloma.
- Inflammatory conditions of bones and joints e.g. arthritis, bursitis, tenosynovitis. In some patients intraarticular injection.
- Skin diseases e.g. atopic dermatitis, eczema.
- Diseases of intestinal tract e.g. celiac sprue.
- As immunosuppressive in organ transplants.
- Renal disease e.g. nephrotic syndrome.
- In cerebral oedema (but no convincing evidence).

Adverse effects

One or two doses do not produce any adverse effect. But prolonged use can produce a large number of unwanted effects, some of which are of serious nature.

The main problem in steroid withdrawal is flare-up of the underlying disease for which steroids were prescribed. Acute adrenal insufficiency results from too rapid withdrawal after prolonged therapy. In addition to this, a characteristic glucocorticoid withdrawal syndrome consists of fever, arthralgia, myalgia, and malaise.

In general, patients who have received supraphysiological doses of glucocorticoid for two weeks within the preceding year may have some degree of hypothalamus-pituitary-adrenal impairment in settings of acute stress and should be treated accordingly.

The adverse effects due to the prolonged therapy are :

- Cushing's syndrome characterized by 'moon' face, buffalo hump, oedema, hypertension, hirsutism, abnormal deposition of fat (back of neck, supraclavicular area, central obesity), muscle wasting, osteoporosis of the spine with fractures of ribs, vertebrae, femur.
- Hypertension.
- Weight gain due to fluid retention.
- Hyperglycaemia: Diabetes mellitus may occur. Glycosuria may be present.
- Susceptibility of infections including tuberculosis.
- Acne, hirsutism.
- Peptic ulceration. Large doses of gluco-

corticoids stimulate excessive production of acid and pepsin in the stomach and facilitate the development of peptic ulcer.

- Osteoporosis (due to reduction of bone protein matrix). It is due to catabolic effect on bone.
- Myopathy characterized by weakness of the proximal muscles of arms and legs and of their associated shoulder and pelvic muscles. Corticoids stimulate protein synthesis in liver but they have catabolic effects in lymphoid and connective tissue muscle, fats and skin, so decrease muscle mass and produce weakness.
- Glaucoma (also with prolonged use of eye drops).
- Postsubcapsular cataracts.
- Behavioral disturbances may take various forms including euphoria, insomnia, nervousness, changes in mood, suicidal tendencies are not uncommon. Depression and psychosis may occur.
- Healing of wounds is delayed.
- Growth in children is retarded. Growth and cell division is affected due to adverse effect on epiphyseal cartilage. Growth is reduced in children also due to catabolic effects. However, if alternate day therapy is given to children, normal growth pattern can be maintained and suppression of the pituitary-adrenal axis by negative feedback is less likely to occur.
- Striae, bruising occur due to increased capillary fragility.

Effects of prolonged glucocorticoid excess is depicted in Fig. 10.4.

Drug interactions with glucocorticoids

- Decrease the dose of glucocorticoids when they are administered with:
Erythromycin, cyclosporin, INH, ketoconazole – these reduce the metabolic clearance of corticosteroids.
- Increase the dose of glucocorticoids when they are administered with:
Phenytoin, carbamazepine, barbiturates,

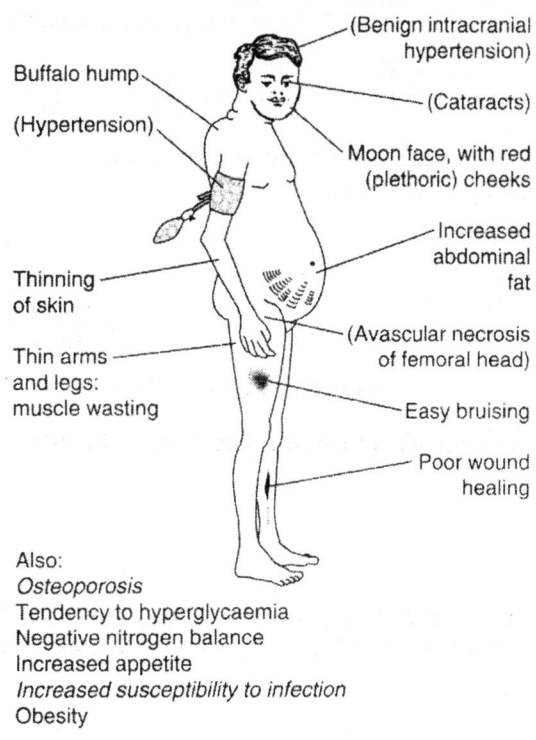

Euphoria
(though sometimes depression or psychotic symptoms, and emotional lability)

(Benign intracranial hypertension)

Buffalo hump

(Hypertension)

(Cataracts)

Moon face, with red (plethoric) cheeks

Increased abdominal fat

Thinning of skin

Thin arms and legs: muscle wasting

(Avascular necrosis of femoral head)

Easy bruising

Poor wound healing

Also:
Osteoporosis
Tendency to hyperglycaemia
Negative nitrogen balance
Increased appetite
Increased susceptibility to infection
Obesity

Fig. 10.4. Effects of prolonged glucocorticoid excess: iatrogenic Cushing's syndrome. Italicised effects are particularly common. Less frequent effects, related to dose and duration of therapy, are shown in brackets.

rifampicin - these increase the metabolism by enzyme induction.
Cholestyramine decreases absorption.
- Adjust the dose while using with:
Antianxiety and antipsychotic drugs (poor control of CNS symptoms because of inherent glucocorticoid effects), anticholinesterases (may precipitate myasthenia), anticoagulants, antihypertensives, hypoglycaemics, sympathomimetics, salicylates.

Contraindications

- Diabetes mellitus
- Hypertension
- Peptic ulcer

- Epilepsy
- Tuberculosis
- History of mental disorder
- Glaucoma
- Herpes simplex infection
- Osteoporosis

Inhibitors of the biosynthesis and actions of adrenocortical steroids

The following five pharmacological agents have been useful as inhibitors of adrenocortical secretion :
1. Mitotane (adrenocorticolytic)
2. Metyrapone
3. Aminoglutethimide
4. Ketoconazole
5. Trilostane

Mitotane

It is chemically similar to the insecticide DDT. It causes a prompt reduction in levels of adrenocorticoids in blood and urine. It is an adrenocorticolytic agent, used in the treatment of neoplasms derived from the adrenal cortex, as a palliative in inoperable adrenocortical carcinoma.

Dose: 2-6 g/d in 3-4 divided doses.

Adverse effects such as nausea, vomiting and diarrhoea may be complained by about 80% of the patients. About 30% may develop depression and lethargy. Skin problems like dermatitis occur in about 20% cases.

Metyrapone

It interferes in the biosynthesis of steroid hormones. It affects synthesis of aldosterone less than that of glucocorticoids. It has more selective effect at low doses than mitotane and also less toxic. It is used in the treatment of hypercortisolism due to adrenal neoplasms.

Dose: 750 mg/4 hourly for 6 doses to test adrenal function, 250 mg twice a day to 1g four times a day can reduce cortical production to normal levels.

Adverse effects include dizziness and gastro-intestinal disturbances. On long term use it may produce hypertension due to excessive secretion of desoxycorticosterone.

Aminoglutethimide

It blocks conversion of cholesterol to pregnenolone and thus causes reduction of all hormonally active steroids including hydrocortisone, sex hormones and aldosterone. It has been used (i) to decrease the excessive secretion of cortisol in adrenal tumors (autonomously functioning), (ii) hypersecretion of cortisol resulting from ectopic production of ACTH, (iii) with dexamethasone to decrease or eliminate oestrogen and androgen production in patients suffering from carcinoma of breast, and (iv) with ketoconazole to reduce steroid secretion in Cushing's syndrome due to adrenocortical cancer which don't respond to mitotane.

Dose: 250 mg/6 hourly, gradually increased but the daily dose should be less than 2 g.

Ketoconazole

It is an imidazole derivative which has important antifungal activity. In doses higher than required as antifungal, it inhibits the biosynthesis of steroids in the adrenal cortex and testes. It is a nonselective inhibitor of adrenal and gonadal steroid synthesis. It is a promising drug for the management of Cushing's syndrome and carcinoma of the prostate.

Dose: 200-1200 mg/d.

Trilostane

It decreases the synthesis of both cortisol and aldosterone. It has been used in Cushing's syndrome but its status in long term therapy is not yet established.

Dose: 30 mg 4 times a day, gradually increased, maximum daily dose 480 mg.

ANTIGLUCOCORTICOIDS

Mifepristone is a synthetic steroid which binds to glucocorticoid as well as to progesterone receptors.

It is a partial agonist at progesterone receptors, thus it has some inherent progestogen agonist properties but inhibits progesterone action. It is given orally and has a half-life of 21 hours. It sensitises the uterus to the action of prostaglandins.

Given within 49 days of the last menstrual period, in a single oral dose, followed 48 hours later by gemeprost (prostaglandin analogue) given as an intravaginal pessary, produces complete abortion in about 95% of cases.

Mifepristone inhibits ovulation if it is given in the last follicular phase of the menstrual cycle. Hence it has potential as a postcoital contraceptive agent.

Mifepristone also has antagonistic action at glucocorticoid receptor, in higher concentration.

Its therapeutic use in the treatment of Cushing's syndrome produced by adrenal tumors is being investigated. Not only the determination of appropriate doses is essential but there has to be a close follow up of the patients because excessive glucocorticoid receptor blockade is likely to produce acute adrenal insufficiency.

MINERALOCORTICOID ANTAGONISTS

Amphenone B interferes with aldosterone synthesis. It is more potent than mitotane and it does not possess the destructive effect on the tissues. The block of synthesis leads to excessive production of ACTH and hyperplasia of the gland.

It is very toxic. It cause CNS depression, gastrointestinal disturbances and skin disorders. It impairs liver and thyroid function. It is not a suitable drug for use in humans.

Spironolactone (Aldactone) is a potassium-sparing diuretic. It antagonizes the sodium-retaining action of mineralocorticoids including aldosterone. It is a competitive antagonism.

Spironolactone has been used (i) in the treatment of primary aldosteronism in doses of 50-100 mg/d, (ii) for diagnostic purpose to detect aldosteronism in doses of 400-500 mg/d for 4-8 days, (iii) for preparing patients for surgery (300-500 mg/d for 2 weeks) to reduce incidence of cardiac arrhythmias, (iv) to ameliorate signs and symptoms when surgical removal of an adenoma is delayed, and (v) in the treatment of hirsutism in women (dose 50-200 mg/d). It reduces growth of facial hair in patients with idiopathic hirsutism or due to androgen excess. The effect is due to inhibition of androgen production and also its action at the hair follicle.

The onset of action of spironolactone is slow but effect lasts for 2-3 days after the drug is discontinued.

In case of hirsutism, the effect starts appearing in 2 months and becomes maximum in about 6 months.

Adverse effects include hyperkalaemia, menstrual disorders, gynaecomastia, headache, sedation, gastrointestinal disturbances, and skin rashes.

There are also certain other steroids that compete with aldosterone for binding sites and decrease its activity peripherally, e.g. progesterone but it is mildly active in this respect.

STUDY QUESTIONS

1. How do glucocorticoids act? And what are their metabolic effects on carbohydrate, protein and fat.
2. Describe the pharmacokinetics and routes of administration of corticosteroids.
3. What are the general principles which should be kept in mind regarding the use of corticosteroids?
4. Explain, why abrupt withdrawal of prolonged, high dose corticosteroid therapy is dangerous?
5. Describe the various therapeutic uses of adrenocorticoids and give reasons for their beneficial effect in each condition.
6. How do glucocorticoids act as antiinflammatory and immunosuppressive agents?
7. Describe the adverse effects observed (i) after abrupt withdrawal and (ii) after prolonged therapy. Also give reasons for producing these adverse effects.
8. What is Cushing's syndrome? How is its treatment managed?
9. Explain how large doses of adrenocorticosteroids produce (i) osteoporosis, (ii) peptic ulceration, (iii) hypertension (iv) glaucoma, (v) myopathy, (vi) behavioral disturbances, (vii) hyperglycaemia, (viii) retardation of growth in children.
10. What are the contraindications of adrenocorticosteroids?
11. Give a comparison of relative antiinflammatory and salt-retaining properties of commonly used glucocorticoids and mineralocorticoids. Which among them are not effective on topical application?
12. What are the actions, uses and adverse effects of antagonists of adrenocortical agents?

13. Write short notes on:
    (a) Intraarticular injection of glucocorticoids
    (b) Ketoconazole as a inhibitor of biosynthesis in adrenal cortex
    (c) Mode of action and uses of aminoglutethimide
    (d) Spironolactone as an antagonist to sodium-retaining action of mineralocorticoids, including aldosterone
    (e) Aldosterone

GUIDE TO FURTHER READING

Adachi, J.D. et al: Corticosteroid-induced osteoporosis. Semin. Arthritis Rheum, 1993; 22:375-384.

Barnes, P.J.: Inhaled glucocorticoids for asthma. N. Engl. J. Med., 1995; 332:868-875.

Boumpas, D.T. et al: Glucocorticoid therapy for immune-mediated disease: basic and clinical correlates. Ann. Intern. Med., 1993; 119:1198-1208.

Byyny, R.L.: Withdrawal from glucocorticoid therapy. N. Engl. J. Med., 1976; 295:30-32.

Chrousos, G.P.: The hypothalamic-pituitary-adrenal axis and immune-mediated inflammation. N. Engl. J. Med., 1995; 332:1351-1362.

Honig, P.K. et al: Terfernadine-ketoconazole interaction. Pharmacokinetic and electrocardiographic consequences. JAMA, 1993; 269:1513-1518.

Imura, H.: Adrenocorticotropic hormone. In, Endocrinology. Saunders, Philadelphia, 1994; pp. 355-367.

Lin, D. et al: Role of steroidogenic acute regulatory protein in adrenal and gonadal steroidogenesis. Science, 1995; 267:1828-1831.

Lukert, B.P. et al: Glucocorticoid-induced osteoporosis. Rheum. Dis. Clin. North Am., 1994; 20:629-650.

Mankin, H.J.: Nontraumatic necrosis of bone (osteonecrosis). N. Engl. J. Med., 1992; 326:1473-1479.

McGowan, J.E. Jr. et al: Guidelines for the use of systemic glucocorticosteroids in the management of selected infections. J. Infect. Dis., 1992; 165:1-13.

Mellon, S.H.: Neurosteroids: biochemistry, modes of action, and clinical relevance, J. Clin. Endocrinol. Metab., 1994; 78:1003-1008.

Miller, J.W. et al: The medical treatment of Cushing's syndrome. Endocr. Rev., 1993; 14:443-458.

Masharnai, U. et al: The endocrine complications of the acquired immunodeficiency syndrome. Adv. Intern. Med., 1993; 38:323-336.

Orth, D.N.: Cushing's syndrome. N. Engl. J. Med., 1995; 332:791-803.

Parker, K.L. et al: Transcriptional regulation of the genes encoding the cytochrome P450 steroid hydroxylases. Vitam. Horm., 1996; 51:339-370.

Pearce, D. et al: Mineralocorticoid and glucocorticoid receptor activities distinguished by nonreceptor factors at a composite response element. Science, 1993; 259:1161-1165.

Piper, J.M. et al: Corticosteroid use and peptic ulcer disease: role of nonsteroidal anti-inflammatory drugs. Ann. Intern. Med., 1991; 114:735-740.

Reichlin, S.: Neuroendocrine-immune interactions. N. Engl. J. Med., 1993; 329:1246-1253.

Shimkets, R.A. et al: Liddle's syndrome: heritable human hypertension caused by mutations in the beta subunit of the epithelial sodium channel. Cell, 1994; 79:407-412.

Wehling, M.: Novel aldosterone receptors: specificity conferring mechanism at the level of the cell membrane. Steroids, 1994; 59:160-163.

White, P.C.: Genetic diseases of steroid metabolism. Vit. Horm., 1994; 49:131-195.

Young, M. et al: Mineralocorticoids, hypertension, and cardiac fibrosis. J. Clin. Invest., 1994; 93:2578-2583.

THYROID HORMONES, ANTITHYROID DRUGS AND PARATHYROID HORMONE

Abnormalities of Thyroid Function

Hyperthyroidism (thyrotoxicosis) results in high metabolic rate, an increase in temperature and sweating and a marked sensitivity to heat. Nervousness, tremor, tachycardia, fatiguability and increased appetite associated with loss of weight occurs.

Common types of hyperthyroidism are (i) diffuse toxic goiter (also called Graves' disease) or exophthalmic goiter and (ii) toxic nodular goiter.

Hypothyroidism results in decreased activity of the thyroid and in severe cases it results in myxoedema. There are low metabolic rate, slow speech, deep hoarse voice, lethargy, bradycardia, mental impairment and sensitivity to cold.

Thyroid deficiency during development, caused by congenital absence or incomplete development of the thyroid, causes cretinism which is manifested by gross retardation of growth and mental deficiency.

Simple non-toxic goiter

Prolonged dietary deficiency of iodine or ingestion of goitrogens produces a rise in plasma thyrotrophic hormone and eventually an increase in the size of the gland. This is known as simple non-toxic goiter. The enlarged thyroid usually produces normal quantity of thyroid hormones. But if the iodine deficiency is very severe, hypothyroidism supervenes.

Thyroid gland is situated on trachea in the neck having two lobes. The hormones secreted by thyroid gland are two, viz. Thyroxine (tetraiodothyronine, T_4) and Triiodothyronine (T_3). Thyroxine is relatively inactive and T_3 which is converted from T_4 (thyroxine) by the enzyme thyronine 5-deiodinase is the active hormone. The structure of thyroxine and triiodothyronine are given in Fig. 10.5.

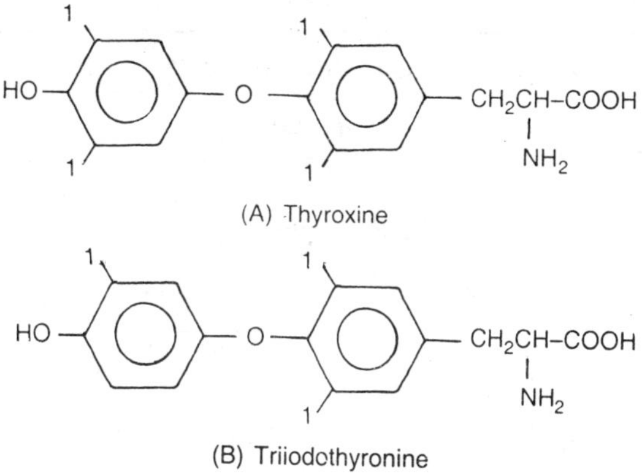

Biosynthesis, storage and release

The daily iodine requirement is 150-300 mcg supplied from food and water.

The functional unit of the thyroid is the follicle or acinus. Each follicle consists of a single layer of epithelial cells, around a cavity, the follicle lumen is filled with a thick colloid containing thyroglobulin. Thyroglobulin is a large protein of 600,000 molecular weight, synthesised in the thyroid gland.

Steps of synthesis, storage and release and site of action of inhibition by drugs is shown in Fig. 10.6.

1. Trapping of iodides: Thyroid gland has special affinity to take up iodides.

   Trapping is inhibited by thiocyanates and perchlorates; stimulated by thyroid stimulating hormone (TSH).

Fig. 10.5. Structures of thyroxine (A) and triiodothyronine (B).

2. Oxidation of iodide and iodination of tyrosine, brought about by an enzyme thyroperoxidase. Iodides are oxidized to iodine which rapidly iodinates tyrosine.

3. Iodination of tyrosine into Monoiodothyrosine (MIT) and Diiodothyrosine (DIT).

   It is inhibited by antithyroid drugs; stimulated by TSH.

4. Coupling of monoiodotyrosine results in diiodotyrosine (DIT); one molecule of MIT and 2 molecules of DIT form T_3; 2 molecules of DIT form T_4.

   Coupling is inhibited by antithyroid drugs; stimulated by TSH.

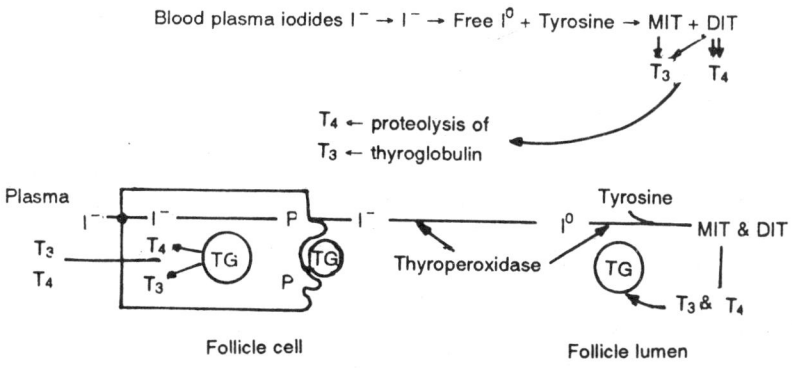

TG = Thyroglobulin; MIT = Monoiodothyrosine, DIT = Diiodothyrosine; T4 = Thyroxine; T_3 = Triiodothyronine, P = Pseudopod; • = Active transport; I^- = Plasma iodide; I^0 = Free iodine

Fig. 10.6. Thyroid hormone synthesis, storage and release.

Box 10.3. Thyroid hormone regulating loop

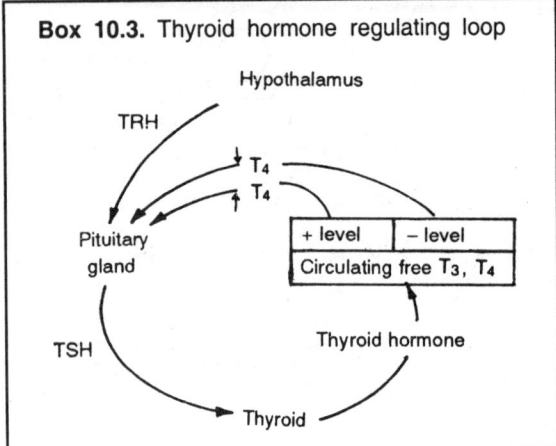

Ratio of T_4 to T_3 in thyroglobulin (TG) is 5 : 1.

5. Endocytosis of thyroglobulin (TG) into follicle cell, stimulated by TSH.
6. Proteolysis of thyroglobulin releases T_4 and T_3. It is inhibited by iodides; stimulated by TSH.
7. Peripheral deiodination of T_4 and T_3 is inhibited by propylthiouracil and propranolol.

Actions of thyroid hormones

Actions affecting metabolism

They increase in general the metabolism of carbohydrates, fats and proteins. The hormones are regulators of metabolism in most tissues.

Lipid metabolism - enhance lipolysis, produce hypocholesterolaemia - LDL is reduced

Carbohydrate metabolism - increase in BMR, increase in glycogenolysis and gluconeogenesis in liver producing hyperglycaemia.

Protein - synthesis of certain proteins is increased but overall effect is catabolism - tissue wasting. Weight loss is characteristic feature of hyperthyroidism.

Actions affecting growth and development: They have a critical effect on growth partly by a direct action on cells and partly indirectly by influencing growth hormone production and potentiating its effects.

They are important for a normal response to parathormone and calcitonin and for skeletal development.

CVS: increase in myocardial O_2 consumption, increase in heart rate, in contractility, palpitation and increase in systolic B.P.

GIT: Increased peristalsis (diarrhoea) in hyperthyroidism, and constipation in myxoedema. Achlorhydria seen in both the conditions.

Nervous system: Mental retardation in cretinism, sluggishness in myxoedema, in hyperthyroidism anxiety, nervousness, tremor.

Kidney: Retention of sodium and water in myxoedema

Calorigenesis: Increased BMR by stimulation of cellular metabolism (not in brain, gonads, uterus, lymph nodes and spleen), important for maintaining body temperature.

Haemopoiesis: T_4 facilitates erythropoiesis. In hypothyroidism - anaemia, megaloblastic anaemia also occurs.

Reproduction: Oligomenorrhoea and infertility seen in myxoedema, and menorrhagia in hyperthyoridism.

Skin: Deposition of mucopolysaccharides, connective tissue in skin in myxoedema results in rough skin.

Thyroid deficiency produces Cretinism in children and Myxoedema in adults. The dosage of thyroxine may vary from patient to patient due to variability in absorption. Serum TSH and the free thyroxine index should be measured at regular intervals and maintained within the normal range.

Transport and metabolism

Both hormones of the thyroid gland are strongly bound mainly to plasma proteins (thyroxine-binding globulin, TBG). Only 0.03% of T_4 and 0.2% T_3 is in free form. During pregnancy, thyroid binding globulin is increased.

T_4 is converted to T_3 in liver and kidney. Both are metabolized by deiodination and glucuronidation and sulphate conjugation. Part of it undergoes enterohepatic cycle. Plasma half-life of T_4 is 6-7 days and of T_3, 1-2 days.

These are degraded by deiodination, deamination and conjugation with glucuronic and sulphuric acids. This occurs mainly in liver. The free and conjugated forms are excreted partly in the bile and partly in the urine. The metabolic clearance of T_3 is 20 times faster than that of T_4 (which is about 6 days).

There is a large pool of T_4 in the body, it has a low turnover rate. It is found mainly in the circulation.

There is a small pool of T_3 in the body, it has a fast turnover rate. It is found mainly intracellularly.

T_3 is 3 to 5 times more active than T_4. T_4 may be regarded mainly as a prohormone.

Thyroid hormone kinetics :

	T_4	T_3
Daily production	70-80 µg	15-30 µg
Half-life (biologic)	7 days	1 day
Serum levels	5-11 µg/dL	95-190 ng/dL
Oral absorption	75-90%	95%

The differences between T_3 and T_4 are given in Table 10.5.

Table 10.5. Differences between T_3 and T_4

T_3	T_4
• Quicker onset of action, 6-8 hours	Delayed onset of action, 7-10 days
• Effective in small doses	Large doses needed
• Effect short-lived (t½ 1-2 days)	Effect lasts longer (t½ 6-7 days)
• More avidly bound to nuclear receptor	Less avidly bound to nuclear receptor
• Less tightly bound to plasma protein	More tightly bound to plasma proteins. About ¼ of T_4 is converted to T_3 in peripheral circulation.

Mechanism of Action

After entering the cell T_4 is converted to T_3 which binds with high affinity to specific receptors associated with DNA in the nucleus. When T_3 is bound, the receptors change conformation and activate transcription resulting in generation of mRNA and protein synthesis.

Therapeutic uses of thyroid hormone

Replacement therapy in deficiency states :
- Cretinism : 12.5 to 50 µg (6-8 µg/kg) started as early as possible because mental retardation is not reversible.

- Adult hypothyroidism : Initial dose 50 µg of l-thyroxine daily, increased every 2-3 weeks upto 100-150 µg/d.
- Myxoedema coma : Liothyronine 100 µg i.v. followed by 25 µg 6 hourly. Large doses of corticosteroids are given prophylactically.
- Nontoxic goiter (simple goiter) as well as nodular goiter
- After I^{131} therapy to treat post-radiation hypo-thyroidism.

Preparations

Thyroid tablets are not recommended as they vary in potency.

Eltroxin 0.025, 0.05, 0.1 mg tablets contain thyroxine, takes 10 days for full effect. The dose is given once a day because of the long half-life of thyroxine. The dosage changes should be made slowly as it takes 6-8 weeks to reach steady state in the blood stream.

Liothyronine 0.02 mg tablet, 0.02 mg ampoules contain triiodothyronine, acts more rapidly, 3-4 times more potent and full effect comes in 3 days. It is given as 0.1 mg by I.V. route in hypothyroid coma.

Levothyroxine sodium is sodium salt of L-thyroxine.

4 : 1 mixture of T_4 and T_3 is known as liotrix.

Thyroglobulin is a purified extract of pig thyroid.

Lugol's iodine 0.2-0.5 ml (5% iodine + 10% KI in water).

Equivalent clinical responses are obtained from the daily administration of about 60 mg of thyroid, 60 mg of thyroglobulin, 100 mcg of levothyroxine, or 25 mcg of liothyronine.

Adverse effects of thyroid hormones include insomnia, restlessness, palpitation, nervousness, weight loss, tachycardia, heat intolerance. Levothyroxine can produce thyrotoxicosis. During long term administration, serum T_4 levels may rise without a change in dose.

ANTITHYROID DRUGS

Classification of antithyroid drugs (Table 10.6)

- Inhibitors of hormone synthesis (thionamide, antithyroid agents) - block organification and interfere with coupling.

Table 10.6. Antithyroid drugs and other thyroid inhibitors

Class	Mode of action
Antithyroid agents	
Propylthiouracil	Inhibits peroxidase, thus inhibiting organification of iodine, inhibits peripheral conversion of T_4 to T_3
Methimazole	Inhibits peroxidase, thus inhibiting organification of iodine
Iodide/Iodine containing compounds	
Iodide	Large doses inhibit hormone secretion. However, the mechanism is not clear.
Lugol's iodine	Inhibits the release of T_3 and T_4
Beta adrenergic agonists	
Propranolol	Reduces activity of thyroid hormone on target tissues
Radioactive iodine	Cytotoxic effect
Ionic inhibitors (rarely used)	Competitively inhibit iodide uptake

Box 10.4. Mode of action of thyroid inhibitors

Inhibitor	Metabolic step
ClO_4^-, SCN^-	Iodide transport
Propylthiouracil, Methimazole	Iodination
Propylthiouracil, Methimazole	Coupling
Colchicine, Li^{2+}, I^-	Colloid resorption
I^-	Proteolysis
Propylthiouracil	Deiodination of T_4

Methylthiouracil, methimazole, carbimazole, propylthiouracil (in addition it also reduces conversion of T_4 to T_3).

- Inhibitors of hormone release (Antihyperthyroidism agents):
Iodine, iodide of sodium and potassium, organic iodide
- Destroyer of thyroid tissue (Antihyperthyroidism agents):
Radioactive iodine I^{131}, I^{125}, I^{123}
- Ionic inhibitors (inhibitors of iodide trapping):
Thiocyanate, perchlorate, nitrates

Mechanism of action of antithyroid drugs and other thyroid inhibitors :
- Inhibition of oxidation of iodide

- Inhibition of iodination of tyrosine residues
- Inhibition of coupling of iodotyrosine residues to form T_3 and T_4

These are reducing substances, they inhibit peroxidase/deplete the sources of hydrogen peroxide/reduce iodine. Thyroid colloid is depleted over time and blood levels of T_3 and T_4 are reduced.

Thionamides include carbimazole, methimazole and propylthiouracil. These are called antithyroid agents.

They reduce the synthesis of thyroid hormones. They inhibit iodination of tyrosine, block oxidation of iodides and interfere with coupling.

- Iodides in high doses. Lugol's solution contains 5% iodine and 10% potassium iodide (KI is used to dissolve iodine).
- Radioiodine I^{131}, emits β radiations
- Ionic inhibitors e.g., thiocyanate, perchlorate, nitrates. These are very toxic and hence not clinically used.

Thionamides (thioureylenes) antihyroid drugs

Pharmacokinetic aspects

Thioureylenes are given orally. Carbimazole is rapidly converted to methimazole which is the active compound.

Methimazole has t½ 6-15 hours.

Both methimazole and propylthiouracil cross placenta and appear in milk. However, this effect is less pronounced with propylthiouracil as it is more strongly bound to plasma proteins.

After degradation, the metabolites are excreted in the urine, propylthiouracil is excreted more quickly than methimazole.

Adverse effects include agranulocytosis (although most serious adverse effect but fortunately rare). It is reversible when the drug is stopped. This risk is lower with methimazole, it is preferred over propylthiouracil. Rashes (purpuric, urticarical papular) are more common (2-25%). The other adverse effects are headache, nausea, jaundice and pain in joints, fever, depigmentation of hair, lymphadenopathy.

Thionamide (Thioureylenes) antithyroid drugs are given orally and effects appear after 10-15 days.

- Carbimazole (neomercazole) 5-10 mg thrice a day.
- Methimazole (mercazole) 5-10 mg thrice a day.
- Propylthiouracil 50 mg tablet, 75-100 mg thrice a day.

These are related to thiourea. They inhibit the iodination of tyrosyl residues in thyroglobulin. They inhibit thyroperoxidase-catalysed oxidation reaction. Propylthiouracil has additional effect of reducing the de-iodination of T_4 to T_3, in peripheral tissues.

Advantages of thionamide antithyroid agents:
- Well tolerated
- Treatment induced hypothyroidism is reversible
- Safe in children
- Can be given during pregnancy
- Do not aggravate exophthalmos

Disadvantages of thionamides
- Prolonged treatment and follow-up
- Relapse is frequent
- Slow action, takes weeks to appear
- Common adverse effect is transient leukopenia, other adverse effects include rash, fever, arthralgia.
- Occasional serious toxicity (idiosyncratic agranulocytosis is most serious adverse effect, this risk is lower with methimazole).

Differences between propylthiouracil and carbimazole are shown in Table 10.7.

Table 10.7. Differences between propylthiouracil and carbimazole.

Propylthiouracil	Carbimazole
• Highly protein bound	Less protein bound
• Less transferred across placenta and milk	Larger amounts are transferred
• t½ 1-2 hours	t½ 6-10 hours
• Single dose acts for 4-8 hours	Acts for 12-24 hours
• No active metabolites	Has active metabolites
• Given in 2-3 daily doses	Given once daily
• Inhibits peripheral conversion of T_4 to T_3	Does not inhibit
• Less potent	More potent

Iodine/Iodide

Iodine is converted *in vivo* to iodide which temporarily inhibits the release of thyroid hormones. Over a period of 10-14 days, there is a marked reduction in vascularity of the gland, which becomes smaller and firmer and easier to operate. Iodine solution in potassium iodide (Lugol's iodine) is given orally. With continuous administration, maximum effect reaches in 10-15 days and then the action decreases (escape phenomenon for 2-3 months).

It is best to control hyperthyroidism first with an antithyroid drug such as propylthiouracil, iodide is then begun 10 days before the operation to avoid escape phenomenon.

Adverse effects

Allergic reactions can occur which include angioedema, rashes, drug fever, lacrimation, conjunctivitis, pain in the salivary glands and a cold-like syndrome, cutaneous haemorrhages, symptoms of serum sickness.

Chronic administration of iodides can result in iodism characterised by brassy taste, soreness of teeth and gums, increased salivation, swelling of eyelids, severe frontal headache, several types of skin lesions.

Radioiodine

Sodium iodide labelled with I^{131} or I^{125} is available as a solution and as capsule. It is given orally, used in one single dose. Its radioactivity disappears by 2 months.

I^{131} emits mainly β radiation (90%), which penetrates only 0.5 mm of tissue and thus allows therapeutic effect on the thyroid without damage to the surrounding structures, particularly the parathyroids. However, it also emits some of γ rays, which are more penetrating.

The half-life of I^{131} is 8 days. The cytotoxic effect of I^{131} on the gland is delayed for 1-2 months and does not reach its maximum for further 2 months.

It is very effective in the treatment of hyperthyroidism, specially in older patients with heart disease. It is also the treatment of choice for recurrent hyperthyrodism after antithyroid drug therapy. However, there is delayed onset in the control of hyperthyroidism.

Dose of I^{131} therapeutic: 4-10 millicuries (miCu) oral, once only.

I^{131} is best avoided in children for possible risk of cancer and in pregnant patients because of potential damage to the foetus.

Adverse effects include high incidence of hypothyroidism (though delayed).

Contraindications:

Pregnancy (I^{131} crosses placenta), lactation, damage to foetal thyroid after 16 weeks of pregnancy.

Ionic inhibitors such as thiocyanates and perchlorates block trapping. They are obsolete. They are not used as they are highly toxic and can cause aplastic anaemia, gastric irritation, fever, skin rashes, lymphadenopathy, agranulocytosis.

Other drugs used

Beta-adrenoceptor antagonists e.g. propranolol (not antithyroid drug, the synthesis and secretion of thyroid hormone are not effected). They decrease many signs and symptoms of hyperthyroidism (tachycardia, sweating, anxiety, tension, palpitation, agitation, tremor, dysrhythmias). Also used in preparation for surgery; for the initial treatment of hyperthyroid patients while the thioureylenes or I^{131} are taking effect and as part of treatment of thyroid storm.

The rationale of using beta adrenergic blockers e.g., propranolol in thyrotoxicosis:

The number of beta adrenergic receptors is increased in thyrotoxicosis and the heart is hypersensitive to catecholamines, therefore propranolol is used to reduce CVS manifestations. It is very useful in 'thyroid storm'.

Guanethidine, a postganglionic adrenergic blocking drug is used in eye drops to ameliorate the exophthalmos of hyperthyroidism. It acts by relaxing the sympathetically innervated smooth muscle that causes eyelid retraction.

Glucocorticoids may be needed for the exophthalmos of Graves' disease.

Thyrotoxic crisis (thyroid storm)

It is sudden acute exacerbation of all symptoms of thyrotoxicosis. The following drugs are indicated in this emergency condition :

- Propranolol I.V. 2-10mg repeated every 4 hours.
- Hydrocortisone (inhibits peripheral conversion of T_4 to T_3, 100 mg 6 hourly I.V.
- Antithyroid drugs in large doses, propylthiouracil 200mg or carbimazole 20mg 4 hourly.
- I.V. glucose infusion
- O_2 inhalation
- Digitalization if there is heart failure (not so effective)
- Vitamin B complex, antimicrobials
- Paracetamol and wet packs for hyperpyrexia (not aspirin because it displaces thyroxine from binding sites on plasma albumin).

Calcitonin

It is the hormone secreted by parafollicular C cells of the thyroid gland. It is a single chain polypeptide hormone with 32 amino acids and molecular weight of 3600. Parafollicular C cells are also found in parathyroid and thymus.

The action of calcitonin is opposite to that of parathormone.

It is secreted in higher amounts when serum calcium level rises. Calcitonin inhibits resorption by inhibiting the action on osteoclasts and enhancing action on osteoblasts. In the kidney, it decreases reabsorption of Ca and PO_4 in proximal tubules. The other effects are reduction in gastrin secretion, and gastric acid output.

Uses

1. To decrease hypercalcaemia and hyperphosphataemia in patients with
   - Hyperparathyroidism,
   - Vitamin D intoxication,
   - Osteolytic bone metastasis,
   - Idiopathic hypercalcaemia of pregnancy
2. To decrease the rate of bone loss in patients with postmenopausal osteoporosis
3. Calcitonin is effective in Paget's disease of bone but patient may become resistant within several months.

Preparations: Porcine (natural) calcitonin and salcalcitonin (salmon calcitonin) are given by S.C./ I.M. injection, 50 IU thrice a week or 100 IU by I.V. injection. It is available as porcine calcitonin in vials

160 international units (IU) for S.C. or I.M. injection. Salcalcitonin in vials 400 IU in 2 ml is available.

It is available as nasal solution containing 200/IU per metered spray/alternating nostrils daily.

Adverse effects

- Inflammation at the site of injection
- Facial flushing, urticaria
- Nausea, intestinal cramps
- Tingling sensations in the hands, hand swelling

Parathyroid hormone

There are four small endocrine glands close or embedded on the posterior surface of thyroid gland. They secrete parathormone (PTH).

Diseases of the parathyroid gland

Overproduction of hormone results in hyperparathyroidism. The symptoms and signs include hypercalciuria (renal calculi may be formed), nausea, vomiting, muscle weakness.

Treatment is by surgical resection of tumour, in poor surgical patients, neutral phosphate, low-calcium diet and fluids may be given.

Underproduction of hormone results in hypoparathyroidism which is one of the many causes of hypocalcaemia.

The symptoms and signs include paresthesias of the extremities, tetany, laryngospasm, generalized convulsions, tachycardia. The principal form of treatment is dietary supplementation of vitamin D and calcium.

Parathormone is a single chain polypeptide of 84 amino acids that regulates the concentration of calcium and phosphate levels in the extracellular fluid. Plasma calcium is the most important regulator of PTH secretion. For example, if blood calcium falls, the parathyroid glands are stimulated to produce more hormone which mobilizes calcium from bones by stimulating osteoclast activity, and inhibiting osteoblast activity. It increases the renal tubular reabsorption of calcium and the excretion of phosphate. The effects on both bone and kidney are probably mediated via cAMP.

It also stimulates synthesis of calcitriol which in turn increases calcium absorption from intestines. Thus the blood calcium level becomes normal. The

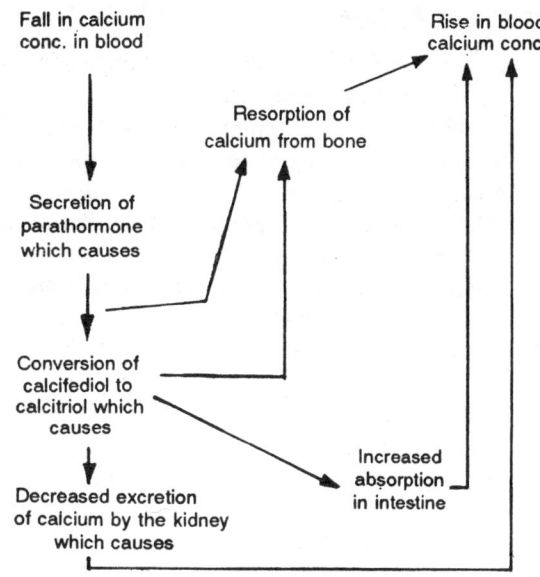

Fig. 10.7. Control of serum calcium levels.

control of serum calcium levels is shown in Fig. 10.7.

Parathormone has a plasma half-life 2-5 minutes, is destroyed in GIT so it is injected. The peak effect appears 6 hours after injection. It is rapidly removed by the liver and kidney.

Actions of Parathormone (PTH)

Parathormone increases plasma calcium levels by the following actions:

Bone: Increases resorption of calcium from older and stable part of the bone but not from the labile newly formed area. It is through activation of osteoclasts and inhibition of osteoblasts.

Kidney: In distal tubule, enhances reabsorption of Ca^{2+} and increases renal excretion of phosphate by decreasing reabsorption.

Intestines: By enhancing the formation of calcitriol in the kidney, it increases Ca^{2+} absorption from the intention.

Therefore, the net effect is to increase concentration of calcium in plasma and lower that of phosphate.

Uses

In tetany (carpo-pedal spasm, spasm of hands and feet).

STUDY QUESTIONS

1. Describe the steps of synthesis, storage and release of thyroid hormones.
2. At what sites the different drugs act which inhibit the synthesis and release of thyroid hormones?
3. What is the role of propranolol in the treatment of hyperthyroidism?
4. Describe antithyroid drugs. What is their mode of action and adverse effects?
5. What are the main differences between T3 and T4.
6. Write notes on (i) Lugol's iodine, (ii) Radioactive iodine, (iii) Thyrotoxic crisis (thyroid storm).
7. Describe actions, mode of action and uses of parathormone.
8. Describe calcitonin.

GUIDE TO FURTHER READING

Baran, D.T.: Thyroid hormone and bone mass: The clinician's dilemma Thyroid, 1994; 4:143-144.

Braverman, L.E. et al: Heart and Thyroid. Black-well-MZV, Vienna, 1994.

Braverman, L.E. et al: Clinical and Molecular Diseases of the Thyroid. Endocrine Society Press, Bethesda, 1994.

Brent, G.A.: The molecular basis of thyroid hormone action, N. Engl. J. Med., 1994; 331:847-853.

Chapuy, M.C. et al: Vitamin D3 and calcium to prevent hip fractures in the elderly women. New. Engl. J. Med., 1992; 327:1637-1642.

Coburn, J.W. et al: Control of serum phosphorous in uraemia. N. Engl. J. Med., 1989; 320:1140-1142.

Cooper, D.S.: Antithyroid drugs. N. Engl. J. Med., 1984; 311:1353-1362.

Farid, N.R. et al: Molecular basis of thyroid cancer. Endocr. Rev., 1994; 15:202-232.

Finch, J.L. et al: Differential effects of 1,25-$(OH)_2D_3$ and 22-oxacalcitriol on phosphate and calcium metabolism. Kidney Int., 1993; 43:561-566.

Glennon, J.A. et al: Hypothyroidism after low dose I^{131} treatment of hyperthyroidism. Ann. Intern. Med., 1972; 76:721-723.

Glinoer, D. et al: Risk of subclinical hypothyroidism in pregnant women with asymptomatic autoimmune thyroid disorders, J. Clin. Endocrinol. Metab., 1994; 79:197-204.

Grill, V. et al: Parathyroid hormone-related protein as a cause of hypercalcemia in malignancy. In, The Parathyroids: Basic and Clinical Concepts. Raven Press, Ltd., New York, 1994; pp. 295-310.

Hays, M.T. et al: Human thyroxine absorption: age effects and methodological analysis. thyroid, 1994; 4:55-64.

Kaplan, M.M. et al: Assessment of thyroid function during pregnancy. Thyroid, 1992; 2:57-61.

Kronenberg, H.M. et al: Parathyroid hormone biosynthesis and metabolism. In, The Parathyroids: Basic and Clinical Concepts. Raven Press, Ltd. New York, 1994; pp. 125-137.

Levine, M.A. et al: Pseudohypoparathyroidism: clinical, biochemical, and molecular features. In, The Parathyroids: Basic and Clinical Concepts. Raven Press, Ltd., New York, 1994, pp. 781-800.

Magner, J.A. et al: Methimazole-induced agranulocytosis treated with recombinant human granulocyte colony-stimulating factor (G-CSF) Thyroid, 1994; 4:295-296.

Martin, T.J.: Properties of parathyroid hormone-related protein and its role in malignant hypercalcemia. Q. J. Med., 1990; 76:771-786.

Mazzaferri, E.L.: Management of a solitary thyroid nodule. N. Engl. J. Med., 1993; 328:553-559.

Meier, C.A. et al: Diagnostic use of recombinant human thyrotropin in patients with thyroid carcinoma (Phase I/II study). J. Clin. Endocrinol. Metab., 1994; 78:188-196.

Nussbaum, S.R. et al: Advances in immunoassays for parathyroid hormone: clinical applications to skeletal disorders of bone and mineral metabolism. In, The Parathyroids: Basic and Clinical Concepts. Raven Press, Ltd. New York, 1994; pp. 157-170.

Roti, E. et al: The use and misuse of thyroid hormone. Endocr. Rev., 1993; 14:401-423.

Strewler, G.J. et al: Hypercalcemia in malignancy. West. J. Med., 1990; 153:635-640.

Takami, H.: Lithium in the preoperative preparation of Graves' disease. Int. Surg., 1994; 79:89-90.

Wilke, T.J.: Estimation of free thyroid hormone concentrations in the clinical laboratory. Clin. Chem., 1986; 32:585-592.

ANTIDIABETIC DRUGS

- Insulin
- Oral antidiabetic drugs

Diabetes mellitus is an endocrine disorder, deficiency of insulin secretion resulting in increased blood sugar level (hyperglycaemia). In this condition there are disturbances of carbohydrate, protein and lipid metabolism. Diabetes mellitus involves not only a deficiency of insulin but also an excess of certain other hormones, such as growth hormone, glucocorticoid, and glucagon. Thus, not only the pancreas is involved in glucose homeostasis but also the anterior pituitary gland and the adrenal cortex.

Underproduction deficiency or diminished action of endogenous insulin results in diabetes mellitus.

In type 1 (insulin dependent diabetes mellitus, IDDM, juvenile onset type) there is absolute insulin deficiency. There is no circulatory insulin in the plasma and thus insulin replacement is required. There is complete failure of pancreatic beta cell function. By contrast, alpha islet cells (secreting glucagon, delta cells (secreting somatostatin, and pancreatic polypeptide cells are preserved). The patient is both prone to hyperglycaemia and ketoacidosis.

Type 2 diabetes (maturity onset type, non-insulin dependent, NIDDM) is due to impaired secretion plus insulin resistance as there are less insulin receptors. The patient is not prone to ketoacidosis.

In both types of diabetes mellitus, plasma immunoreactive glucagon concentrations are increased. The normal suppression of glucagon by hyperglycaemia is also impaired.

In diabetes, capillary basement membrane thickening occurs. This change is responsible for the following major complications:

- Microangiopathy
- Neuropathy
- Nephropathy
- Retinopathy
- Atherosclerosis

Major hormones secreted from islets of Langerhans in pancreas:

- Beta cells (most abundant cells in the islets) secrete insulin
- Alpha islet cells secrete glucagon
- Delta cells secrete somatostatin
- Pancreatic polypeptide cells secrete pancreatic polypeptide

Insulin

It is secreted from beta cells of islets (about a mil-

lion islets) of Langerhans in pancreas. It is made of two polypeptide chains viz. (A) chain of 21 amino acids and (B) basic chain of 30 amino acids linked by two disulphide-S-S-bridges. The molecular weight is 6000. Normal pancreas secretes about 50 units daily.

Synthesis and secretion

Insulin is synthesised as a precursor (prepro-insulin) in the rough endoplasmic reticulum. It is transported to the Golgi apparatus where it is modified to proinsulin and then to insulin and C-peptide. These are stored in granules in the Beta-cells. Secretion normally occurs in pulses every 15-30 minutes.

The main factor controlling the synthesis and secretion of insulin is the blood glucose concentration and also the rate of change of blood glucose. There is a steady basal release of insulin and secretion is increased as a response to a rise in blood glucose. This response has 2 phases — an initial rapid rise (reflects release of stored hormone); and a slower, delayed phase (reflects both release of stored hormone and new synthesis. The response is abnormal in diabetes mellitus).

Overproduction: Insulin-secreting tumours (insulinomas) are rare, surgical removal of tumour is required. If surgery is not possible, diazoxide 50 mg thrice a day which inhibits insulin release gives symptomatic relief. Streptozocin (streptozotocin) is an antibiotic toxic to beta cells of pancreas and is of value in malignant insulinoma.

Pharmacological actions

1. Carbohydrate metabolism: Glucoregulatory effect: Insulin lowers blood sugar level by:
   - Increased glucose uptake by peripheral tissues
   - Inhibits glycogen breakdown so reduces hepatic glucose release. It favours storage of glucose as glycogen
   - Suppresses gluconeogenesis. It prevents glucose formation from proteins, amino acids and fat
2. Lipid regulatory effect: It decreases the release of free fatty acids from fat cells. Suppresses hepatic ketogenesis in the liver cells.
3. Protein regulatory effect: It increases muscle

Box 10.5. Role of alpha and beta cells of islet of Langerhans

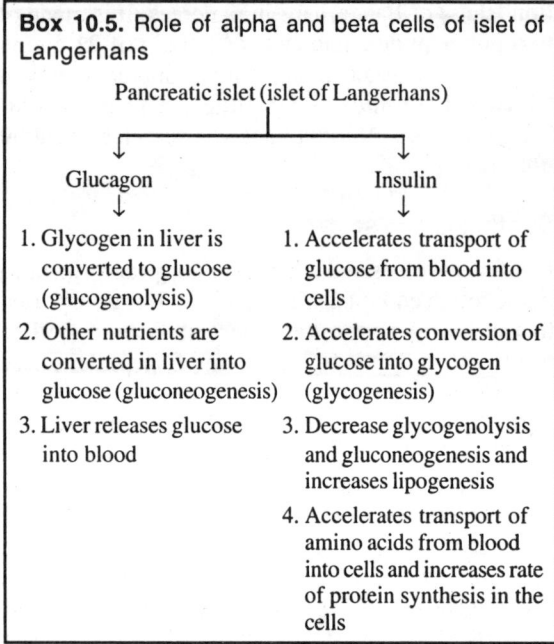

Pancreatic islet (islet of Langerhans)

Glucagon

1. Glycogen in liver is converted to glucose (glucogenolysis)
2. Other nutrients are converted in liver into glucose (gluconeogenesis)
3. Liver releases glucose into blood

Insulin

1. Accelerates transport of glucose from blood into cells
2. Accelerates conversion of glucose into glycogen (glycogenesis)
3. Decrease glycogenolysis and gluconeogenesis and increases lipogenesis
4. Accelerates transport of amino acids from blood into cells and increases rate of protein synthesis in the cells

amino acid uptake and protein synthesis i.e. it increases protein anabolism.

Preparations: These are available in 40 U or 80 U/ml. Regular insulin is also available in 100 U/ml and 500 U/ml. 1 mg of insulin contains 22 units. Highly purified insulin contains 25-30 units/mg. At present all insulin preparations are supplied at pH 7.2-7.4. Certain characteristics of insulins are shown in Table 10.8.

Regulation of insulin secretion

Insulin secretion is regulated by chemical, hormonal and neural mechanisms.

1. Chemical

- Glucose is the principal regulator of release and synthesis of insulin by the beta cells of pancreas
- Insulin secreting beta cells function as "fuel sensors" which secrete insulin in response to variation in plasma levels of glucose.
- Other nutrients are amino acids, fatty acids and ketone bodies.
- All these are more effective in release of insulin when given orally rather than I.V.
- These generate incretins (chemical signals) to release insulin

  The incretins are gut glucagon, secretin, gastrin, vasoactive intestinal polypeptide (VIP), gastric inhibitory polypeptide (GIP), pancreozymin - cholecystokinin.

2. Hormonal

- Growth hormone, corticosteroids, thyroxine: Modify insulin release
- Glucagon: Stimulates release of insulin and somatostatin
- Somatostatin: Inhibits insulin release
- PGE: Inhibits insulin release

Table 10.8. Certain characteristic, onset, peak effect and duration of action of insulins

	Appearance	Added protein	Zinc content (mg/100 units)	Buffer	Onset (hrs.)	Peak (hrs.)	Duration (hrs.)
1. Rapid							
Regular (crystalline) insulin	Clear	None	0.01-0.04	None	0.3-0.7	2-5	5-8
Semilente insulin	Cloudy	None	0.2-0.25	Acetate	0.5-1.0	2-8	12-16
2. Intermediate							
Lente	Cloudy	None	0.2-0.25	Acetate	1-2	6-12	18-24
Isophane insulin (NPH)	Cloudy	Protamine	0.016-0.04	Phosphate	1-2	6-12	18-24
3. Slow							
Ultralente	Cloudy	None	0.2-0.25	Acetate	4-6	16-18	20-36
Protamine zinc insulin suspension (PZI)	Cloudy	Protamine	0.2-0.25	Phosphate	4-6	14-20	24-36

3. Neural mechanisms

- Alpha$_2$ adrenergic receptor activation via NE or E: Inhibits insulin release (predominant)
- Beta$_2$ adrenergic receptor activation: Stimulates insulin release (less prominent)
- Cholinergic drugs via muscarinic receptors and vagal stimulation: Enhance insulin release

Factors altering insulin requirements

- Glucagon, adrenaline, and growth hormone all increase insulin requirements.
- Exercise decreases insulin requirements by making muscle more permeable to glucose and releasing muscle-bound insulin.
- Stress e.g. infection, fever, pregnancy and psychological stress increase insulin requirements due to adrenaline release.
- Obesity increases insulin requirements due to increase in the insulin-binding sites on the greater surface area of adipose tissue.
- Alteration in diet or change in eating time may increase or decrease insulin requirements.
- Effect of other drugs e.g. anticoagulants stimulate insulin secretion thus decrease insulin requirements.

Lente insulin is a mixture of 30% semilente which has rapid onset with 70% ultralente insulin which has delayed onset and prolonged duration. So it is widely used drug among lente series of insulins.

Newer insulins: Actrapid acts faster than regular insulin with greater action.

Rapitard: actrapid 1 part and 3 parts insoluble crystals of bovine insulin, acts similar to lente but the onset is rapid and blood sugar control is smoother.

Human insulin is now being manufactured either by genetic manipulation of *E. coli* or by chemical manipulation of porcine insulin.

The following are the merits of highly purified or human insulins:

- Allergy is very rare.
- Fat atrophy at the site of injection does not occur.
- Cases who show insulin resistance due to antibodies to bovine insulin and dose is more than 200 units per day, they respond to lower dose of highly purified or human insulin.

Pharmacokinetics

Insulin is rapidly proteolyzed (destroyed) and also not absorbed on oral administration so it is given by I.M. or S.C. injection; I.V. route is rarely employed in emergency. Only regular insulin can be given by I.V. injection. Insulin is metabolized by breakdown of disulphide linkages by enzyme insulinase present in liver and kidneys. It is excreted in bile and urine.

Mode of action

Insulin does not enter cells to produce effects but it binds to special protein molecules (receptors) on cell surface membrane of target cells. The insulin receptor complex elicits responses on liver, muscle and adipose tissue (Figs. 10.8).

Glucose enters β-cells, via a membrane transporter called Glut-2 and its subsequent metabolism via glucokinase (rate-limiting enzyme) that acts as the "glucose sensor" linking insulin secretion to extracellular glucose.

The main effect of insulin is to increase facilitated transport of glucose via a transporter called Glut-4.

Uses: Juvenile diabetes, diabetes with complications, diabetic coma, during pregnancy, when surgery is needed, primary or secondary failure to oral hypoglycaemics, insulin in schizophrenia (now rarely used), insulin, glucose and KCl in myocardial infarction, anorexia nervosa (insulin improves appetite), burns (insulin with glucose reduces nitrogen and potassium losses in severely burnt patients).

Dose: Potency is described in units. Preparations contain 40, 80, 100, 500 units/ml.

Adverse effects

- Local fat atrophy at site of injection (lipoatrophy due to irritation at the site of injection)

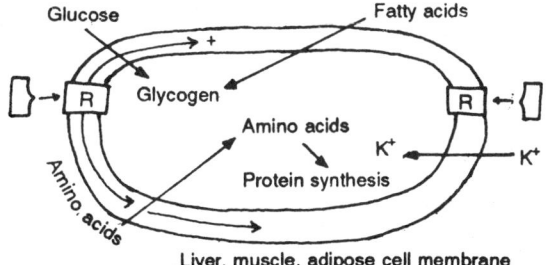

Fig. 10.8. Mode of action of insulin (insulin/receptor interaction).

Effects of insulin on carbohydrate, protein and fat metabolism

	Liver cells	Muscle	Fat cells
Carbohydrate metabolism	↑ glycolysis, ↓ glycogenolysis, ↓ gluconeogenesis, ↑ glycogenesis	↑ glycolysis, ↑ glucose uptake, ↑ glycogenesis	↑ glucose uptake, ↑ glycerol synthesis, ↑ synthesis of TG
Protein metabolism	↓ protein break down	↑ amino acid uptake, ↑ protein synthesis	—
Fat metabolism	↓ lipolysis, ↑ lipogenesis	—	↓ fatty acid synthesis, ↓ lipolysis, ↑ storage of TG

- Insulin resistance
- Hypoglycaemia due to overdose (its worst sequel is insulin shock including hypoglycaemic convulsions)
- Neuropathy
- Weight gain is an undesirable effect of intensive insulin therapy
- Growth promoting properties of insulin may be a factor in the macrovascular complications of diabetes.
- Hypersensitivity reactions may be in the form of local painful and itching lumps at the site of injection. In some cases there may be lymphadenopathy. The antigenic response is due to production of insulin antibodies. The hypersensitivity reactions are less of a problem with the development of new, more highly purified animal insulins and the advent of human insulin. The order of antigenic potency (in descending order) is beef > pork > highly purified pork > human insulin. Antigenicity increases as the duration of action of the insulin is increased.

Insulin Resistance

It is a state at which insulin produces less than normal response. It has been arbitrarily defined as the requirement of 200 or more units of insulin per day to control hyperglycaemia and prevent ketosis. Many conditions like hypertension, microvascular angina, glaucoma, cerebral venous thrombosis and diabetes nephropathy have been found to be associated with insulin resistance. "Insulin toxicity" may be more lethal than "glucose toxicity".

Causes of resistance

Insulin receptor defects:

- Reduced number of insulin receptors or the deficiency of target cells.
- Defects in receptor function
- Defects in genes responsible for insulin action
- Increased concentration of corticosteroids, growth hormone, catecholamines, glucagon, thyroid hormone etc.
- Anti-insulin antibodies
- Anti-insulin receptor antibodies.

Physiological e.g. during prolonged fasting and in 1st week of acute M.I. (protective response)

Pathological: When insulin resistance is present round the clock.

Management of insulin resistance

The aim is to restore normal insulin action by improving the body's sensitivity to endogenous insulin. This is achieved by the following:

- Weight loss and exercise
- Oral hypoglycaemic agents (biguanides)
- Insulin
  Exogenous insulin overcomes insulin resistance
- Substitution of omega fatty acids:

Diet high in saturated, monounsaturated (n9) or polyunsaturated (n6) fatty acids lead to severe insulin resistance. Subtituting a small proportion of fatty acids in the polyunsaturated fat diet with long chain (n3) fatty acids from fish oils, can completely prevent the development of insulin resistance in the liver and skeletal muscle.

Insulin resistance and compensatory hyperinsulinemia are primary events and enhanced sympathetic activity and diminished adreno-medullary activity are important links between the defective insulin action and the development of hypertension and associated metabolic abnormalities.

Newer more purified insulins

Single peak insulin

Purified preparations have been obtained by gel filtration (single peak insulins) or by ion-exchange chromatography (monocomponent insulins). These have been developed to overcome certain demerits of conventional insulin e.g. immunogenicity, instability at neutral pH and at room temperature.

Actrapid is neutral solution of highly purified porcine chromatographed insulin, injection 40 IU/ml.

Lentard is neutral suspension of porcine chromatographed insulin.

Actraphane is highly purified premixed suspension of 30% soluble porcine chromatographed insulin and 70% isophane porcine chromatographed insulin, injection 40 IU/ml.

Insulatard is highly, purified isophane (NPH) insulin, injection 40 IU/ml. It is recommended alone or in combination therapy in NIDDM.

Monosulin is highly purified neutral insulin (porcine), injection 40 IU/ml. It is suitable for use in split and mix regimens along with nordisulin.

Nordisulin is highly purified neutral insulin (porcine), injection 40 IU/ml. It is very suitable for quick metabolic control by i.v. route in patients with ketoacidosis and patients undergoing surgery, and labour.

Mixtard is highly purified biphasic insulin (porcine). It is a mixture of 30% nordisulin and 70% insulatard, injection 40 IU/ml. It is insulin of choice in elderly diabetics, patients with impaired eyesight and neurological handicaps.

Monocomponent insulins

Actrapid MC is highly purified monocomponent pork neutral insulin, injection 40 IU/ml.

Monotard MC is highly purified monocomponent pork zinc insulin suspension in 30% amorphous and 70% crystalline, injection 40 IU/ml.

Human insulins

Human insulins are effective, promptly absorbed and less immunogenic. However, they have slightly less duration of action than conventional insulins. They are more expensive and hypoglycaemia may be more frequently observed.

Human insulins have been prepared by inserting the human proinsulin gene into *E. coli* or yeast and treating the extracted proinsulin to form human insulin molecules (recombinant DNA method).

A semisynthetic human insulin has also been prepared by chemical modification of pork insulin in which carboxy terminal alanine of B chain is replaced by theonine.

Human insulins are dispensed as regular, NPH, lente or ultra lente insulins.

The premixed insulin is also available (70% NPH and 30% regular human insulin).

Human proinsulin having half-life 4-6 times longer than human insulin may be useful as an alternative to longer acting insulin.

Preparations of human insulins, injection 40 IU/ml, 100 IU/ml :

- Human actrapid
- Human actraphane
- Human monotard
- Human insulatard
- Human monosulin
- Human nordisulin
- Human isophane insulin

Merits of highly purified or human insulins

- Allergy is very rare
- Fat atrophy at the site of injection does not occur
- Cases who show insulin resistance due to antibodies to bovine insulin and dose is more than 200 units per day, they respond to lower doses of highly purified or human insulin.

Oral hypoglycaemics

Sulphonylureas

- First generation drugs
  - Tolbutamide
  - Chlorpropamide
  - Tolazamide
  - Acetohexamide
- Second generation drugs

  - Glibenclamide (Glynase)
  - Glipizide
  - Gliclazide
  - Glimepiride

Biguanides

  • Metformin (Glyciphage)
  • Buformin

Other agents

Meglitinide class: Repaglinide, used for NIDDM 0.5 to 4 mg before meals. Maximum daily dose not to exceed 16mg

Thiazolidinediones (Glitazones): Troglitazone, it should only be used in combination regimen. Dose: 200 mg/d

Rosiglitazone, 4 mg/d as single dose or in divided doses twice a day

Pioglitazone, for monotherapy initial dose 15-30 mg once a day without regard to meal. Its protein binding is > 99%.

Alpha-glucosidase inhibitor: Acarbose

Sulphonylureas

Pharmacokinetic aspects

Sulphonylureas are rapidly absorbed after oral administration. The onset of action is 1-2 hours and peak reaches in 4-6 hours.

They bind strongly to plasma albumin. The excretion occurs in urine.

They cross the placenta and stimulate foetal beta-cells to release insulin causing severe hypoglycaemia at the time of birth. Hence, the use of sulphonylureas is contraindicated in pregnancy.

Mode of action

Sulphonylureas stimulate beta cells, effective only in the presence of functioning pancreas. The presence of at least 30% beta cells is essential for their action. They are insulin secretagogues.

 (i) Pancreatic effect: stimulate pancreas to produce more insulin, and increase peripheral utilization of glucose.
(ii) Extra pancreatic effect: They inhibit gluconeo-genesis in liver.
(iii) They also produce post receptor intracellular

beneficial effects. They lower the elevated free fatty acid levels. Patients tend to gain weight.
(iv) They lower blood sugar both in normal and diabetic patients.

Uses

Useful in older (maturity onset) and non obese diabetics whose regular insulin requirement is less than 40 units per day and in the absence of complications. Sulphonylureas remain cornerstone of therapy. They are appealing in the treatment of type 2 diabetes mellitus because they are relatively inexpensive and are well tolerated. Hypoglycaemia, however is a major safety concern with the sulpho-nylureas.

It has been reported that 5% to 10% of patients per year who respond initially to a sulphonylurea become secondary failures (after months or a few years) due to decline β-cell functioning and due to increased insulin resistance. Changing to other oral agent will occasionally produce a satisfactory re-sponse, but most of these patients will eventually require insulin.

Sulphonylureas are ineffective in juvenile type of diabetes.

Contraindications

  • Diabetes mellitus (IDDM, Type-I)
  • Pregnancy and lactation
  • Hepatic and renal damage
  • In diabetic coma, severe trauma and stress, switch over to insulin

  Combination of insulin and sulphonylureas have been used in some patients with IDDM and NIDDM. The rationale is based on the potential of sulphonylureas to increase tissue sensitivity to insu-lin. This combination therapy has not shown im-provement in IDDM patients, but in NIDDM patients small improvement has been shown in the metabolic control.

Table 10.9 gives certain characteristics of sulpho-nylureas.

Adverse effects

  • Stimulate appetite and often cause weight gain as with insulin.
  • Severe hypoglycaemia may occur (but less than insulin) specially with chlorpropamide and

Table 10.9. Potency, peak effect and duration of action of sulphonylureas

Sulphonylureas	Potency	Peak effect (hrs.)	Duration (hrs.)	Tablet strength (mg)	Remarks
First generation					
Tolbutamide	1	5	6-12	500	Orally twice 30 min before breakfast and dinner; readily metabolized in the liver to inactive products; excretion occurs via the kidney
Acetohexamide		3	12-18	250-500	Not metabolized in liver; once a day
Tolazamide		6	10-18	100-250	Excreted renally
Chlorpropamide (diabinese)	6	2-4	24-72	100-500	Once at breakfast
Second generation					
Glyburide (Glibenclamide, Glynase)	150	4	18-24	5-15	Once a day; metabolized in liver
Glipizide (Glucotrol)	100	1-2	18-24	2.5-20	Once a day at breakfast; more active than talbutamide; both are metabolized by liver to products with little activity

glibenclamide. The incidence is lowest with tolbutamide.

- GI upsets (include nausea and vomiting) may occur in about 3% of patients
- Allergic reactions have been reported
- Bone marrow depression though very rare but can be severe (leukopenia, agranulocytosis, haemolytic anaemia).
- Adverse effect after 4-5 years of use of oral hypoglycaemic agents i.e. increase in cardio-vascular related deaths were suspected as compared with the patients treated with insulin, due to blockade of ATP sensitive K^+ channels in heart and vascular tissue. However, some studies do not support this view. But there is also no evidence that oral hypoglycaemic drugs reduce the cardiovascular complications of diabetes.
- Allergic rashes and photosensitivity have been reported.
- Increased CV mortality specially with tolbuta-mide
- Disulfiram - like reaction has been reported with the use of chlorpropamide. It can also cause hyponatraemia due to inappropriate secretion of ADH.
- Transient cholestatic jaundice occurs rarely

- Goitrogenic effect (due to inhibition of iodide uptake by thyroid).

Drug interactions with Sulfonylureas

Drugs which augment the hypoglycaemic effect of sulphonylureas:

NSAIDs, coumarins, sulphinpyrazone, alcohol, MAOIs, sulphonamides, trimethoprim, chloram-phenicol, some antifungal agents including mico-nazole and possibly fluconazole.

Drugs which decrease the hypoglycaemic effect:

Diuretics (thiazides and loop diuretics), cortico-steroids.

Biguanides

These have less clinical use as compared to sulphonylureas.

Phenformin has been withdrawn due to toxicity. Metformin is used.

Metformin (Glyciphage, Glucophage): 1-1.5 g in 2 or 3 divided doses (with meals) produces effect for 6 hours. It is available as 500 mg tablet. The GI upsets are more than sulphonylureas.

Unlike sulphonylureas, metformin does not lower normal blood sugar(antihyperglycaemic not hypoglycaemic).

It is effective even in the absence of functioning

pancreas. It is insulin sensitizer, requires presence of insulin for its action. It is useful in obese diabetics as it does not tend to increase weight, due to anorexia).

It does not produce significant effects on the secretion of glucagon, cortisol, growth hormone, or somatostatin.

Metformin often is given in combination with sulphonylurea.

Mode of action

- Stimulates peripheral utilization of glucose
- Decreases intestinal absorption of glucose
- Inhibits gluconeogenesis.
- Does not cause insulin release
- Does not cause hypokalaemia even in large doses

Contraindications: Cardiac failure, hepatic disease, chronic hypoxic lung disease, pregnancy.

Patients with renal impairment should not receive metformin.

Adverse effects: Acute side effects occur up to 20% of patients. The adverse effects include loss of appetite, metallic taste in mouth, weight loss, nausea, diarrhoea, allergy. Severe lactic acidosis is rare with metformin, Megaloblastic anaemia is also very rare with metformin, but still it is better to check serum folic acid and vitamin B_{12} levels yearly, as malabsorption of vitamin B_{12} and rarely foliate depletion have been observed with metformin.

Treatment with metformin should be stopped if the plasma lactate level exceeds 3 mmol/l. It should also be stopped if the patient is undergoing prolonged fast or is receiving very low caloric diet. It must be stopped immediately in MI or septicaemia.

Acarbose

Acarbose is an alpha-glucosidase inhibitor. It has been introduced for the treatment of noninsulin dependent diabetes mellitus patients who are inadequately controlled by diet and/or oral hypoglycaemic agents.

It has an antihyperglycaemic effect, but does not itself induce hypoglycaemia. If it is combined with sulphonylurea or metformin and if hypoglycaemia occurs, the dose of sulphonylurea, metformin or insulin should be decreased.

Dose is 50 mg once a day for one to two weeks, then 50 mg twice a day for one to two weeks followed by 50 mg thrice a day. The dose may be increased to 100 mg thrice a day depending on clinical response. The tablets should be swallowed whole with a little liquid directly before meal or be chewed with the first few mouthfuls of the meal.

Precautions

With higher dosages, asymptomatic liver enzyme elevations may occur in individual cases, therefore, liver enzyme monitoring may be done including the first 6-12 months of treatment. These changes are reversible on discontinuation of acarbose therapy.

Mode of action

Acarbose reduces intestinal absorption of starch, dextrin and disaccharides by inhibiting the action of intestinal brush border alpha-glucosidase. The postprandial rise in plasma glucose is blunted in both normal persons and diabetic patients.

It reduces postprandial plasma glucose level in IDDM and NIDDM subjects.

Acarbose is most effective when given with a starchy, high fibre diet with restricted amount of sucrose and glucose. Because of its different mode of action, it can be used as an adjunct with sulphonylureas, metformin and insulin.

Adverse effects

Adverse effects include abdominal bloating, flatulence and abdominal distention. Should symptoms of hypoglycaemia develop in the course of treatment with acarbose, glucose and not sucrose (cane sugar) should be taken.

Drug interactions

Sucrose (cane sugar) and foods containing sucrose often cause abdominal discomfort or even diarrhoea during treatment with acarbose due to increased carbohydrate fermentation in the colon.

Simultaneous administration with antacids, intestinal adsorbents and digestive enzymes should be avoided as these may influence the action of acarbose.

Contraindications

- Patients under 18 years of age.
- Pregnancy.
- Breast feeding.

- Chronic intestinal disorders associated with disturbances of digestion and absorption.
- Severe renal impairment.

Comments regarding oral hypoglycaemic agents are given in Table 10.10.

Glucagon

Glucagon is synthesized in Alpha (alpha-2) cells of islets of pancreas. It is a polypeptide single chain of 29 amino acids with mol. wt. 3485. It may also be synthesized by gastric cells. Glucagon also accelerates lipolysis with free fatty acid release from adipose tissue. It produces effects opposite to that of insulin.

Table 10.10. Oral Hypoglycaemic Agents.

Drug	Comments
First-generation sulphonylureas	
Tolbutamide	Short acting (6-12 hr)
Tolazamide	Similar to tolbutamide; intermediate acting (10-14 hr); has active metabolites
Acetohexamide	Similar to tolbutamide; intermediate acting (12-24 hr); has active metabolite
Chlorpropamide	Long acting (up to 60 hr); ADH-like acting, more serious toxicities
Second-generation sulphonylureas	
Glyburide	More potent than first-generation drugs; effects persist for 24 hours.
Glipizide	Shorter half-life (2-4hr); available as extended-release preparation
Glimepiride	Similar to glyburide and glipizide; more potent; longer half-life (5hr)
Biguanides	
Metformin	Actions do not involve stimulation of insulin secretion, some GI effects; rarely lactic acidosis
Meglitinide class	
Repaglinide	Similar in action to sulphonylureas; short acting (half-life 1 hr)
Thiazolidinediones (Glitazones)	
Troglitazone	Decreases insulin resistance by effects on target organs
Rosiglitazone	Similar to troglitazone
Pioglitazone	Similar to troglitazone

On GIT, it inhibits gastric secretion and secretion of pancreatic digestive enzymes. Glucagon has spasmolytic effect on smooth muscles.

On heart, glucagon produces positive inotropic and positive chronotropic effect which are not antagonized by beta blockers.

It mobilizes liver glycogen and thus release glucose in blood. After 0.5-1.0 mg S.C. or I.M. injection, effect appears in 10 minutes and may be used in insulin induced hypoglycaemic coma. I.V. glucose is the treatment of choice but I.V. glucose and glucagon can be given together, if needed, The other indication for glucagon is insulinoma.

Glucagon has been used in hypoglycaemia, and cardiogenic shock. However, it has limited use.

Somatostatin

It is released from the Alpha-1 or D cells of pancreas, provides local inhibition of the release of both insulin and glucagon. Glucagon stimulates the release of somatostatin which provides a negative feedback control loop between glucagon and somatostatin and between glucagon and insulin as shown in Fig. 10.9. Fig. 10.10 shows the factors (endogenous) that regulate insulin secretion.

The therapeutic uses of somatostatin are confined mainly to blocking hormone release in endocrine-secreting tumours including insulinomas, carcinoid tumours.

Octreotide (Sandostatin) is a longer acting analogue available for the treatment of carcinoid tumours, and acromegaly. Octreotide also can decrease blood flow to the GIT and hence it has been used to treat bleeding oesophageal varices, peptic ulcers, and postprandial orthostatic hypotension.

Adverse effects of chronic use of octreotide include gallbladder abnormalities (stones and biliary sludge), abnormal cardiac rhythm and gastrointestinal symptoms. Hyperglycaemia, hypothyroidism and goiter have been reported.

Amylin (Islet amyloid polypeptide)

This is stored with insulin in secretory granules in β-cells and released with insulin in response to glucose and other stimuli.

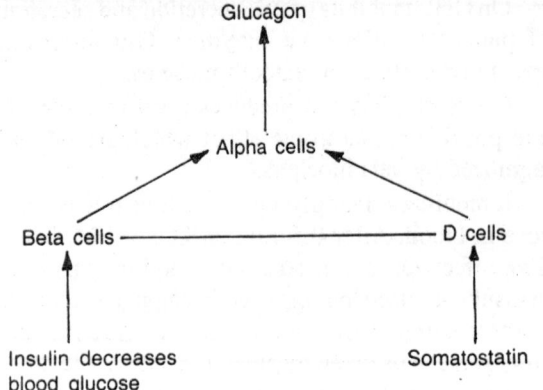

Fig. 10.9. Control loop between glucagon and somatostatin and between glucagon and insulin.

Amyloid is an amorphous protein (identified as a 37-amino acid peptide) that is deposited in different tissues in a number of diseases. Amyloid deposits occur in the pancreas of patients with diabetes mellitus. It is not known whether it is functionally important or a secondary phenomenon.

Amylin delays gastric emptying: Supraphysiological concentrations stimulate the breakdown of glycogen to lactate in striated muscle and subsequent rise in glucose concentration (reflects gluconeogenesis from lactate in liver).

Amylin also inhibits insulin secretion. It is structurally related to calcitonin and has weak calcitonin-like actions on calcium metabolism and osteoclast activity in Paget's disease.

It is not known whether amylin has a significant role in controlling glucose metabolism. However, an analogue of amylin such as pramlintide reduces its tendency to aggregate into insoluble fibrils. Trials show that pramlintide lowers glucose concentrations in type 1 diabetes mellitus.

STUDY QUESTIONS

1. Describe different types of insulin preparations along with their onset of action, time to reach peak effect and duration of action.

2. What are the indications of insulin, mode of action and adverse effects? How does insulin affect carbohydrate, protein and fat metabolism?

3. What are the different types of oral antidiabetic agents and how do they differ in their mode of

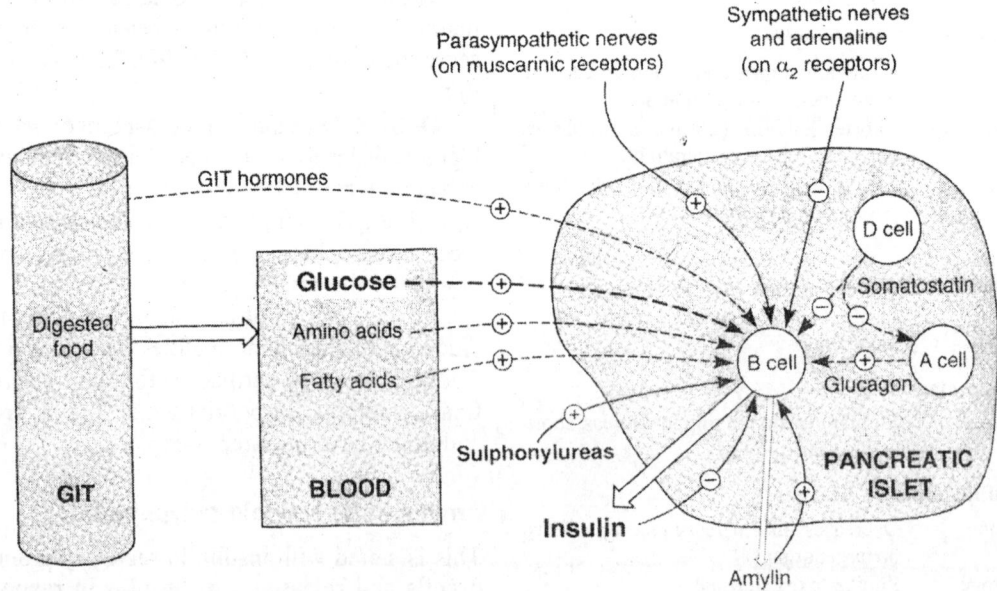

Fig. 10.10. Endogenous factors regulating insulin secretion of β-cells of the islets of Langerhans.

action? Name 3 oral antidiabetics along with their potency and duration of action.

4. Write short notes on (a) Glucagon, (b) Somatostatin

5. What are the advantages of purified or human insulin?

6. What factors influence requirement of insulin? Why insulin is not given orally?

GUIDE TO FURTHER READING

Alberti, D.G.M.M. et al: Inhibition of insulin secretion by somatostatin. Lancet, 1973; 2:1299-1301.

Bailey, C.J.: Biguanides and NIDDM. Diabetes Care, 1992; 15:755- 772.

Bingley, P.J. et al: Can we really predict IDDM? Diabetes, 1993; 42:213-220.

Blackard, W.G. et al: Morning insulin requirements: critique of dawn and meal phenomena. Diabetes, 1989; 38:273-277.

Boyd, A.E., III. Sulfonylurea receptors, ion channels, and fruit flies. Diabetes, 1988; 37:847-850.

Bressler, R. et al: New pharmacological approaches to therapy of NIDDM. Diabetes Care, 1992; 15:792-805.

Cheatham, B. et al: Insulin action and the insulin signaling network. Endocrine Rev., 1995; 16:117-142.

Cohick, W.S. et al: The insulin-like growth factors. Annu. Rev. Physiol., 1993; 55:131-153.

Cryer, P.E.: Hypoglycemia begets hypoglycemia in IDDM. Diabetes, 1993; 42:1691-1693.

DCCT Research Group. The effect of insentive treatment of diabetes on the development and progression of long-term complications in insulin-dependent diabetes mellitus. N. Engl. J. Med., 1993; 329:977-986.

DeFronzo, R.A. et al: Efficacy of metformin in patients with non- insulin-dependent diabetes mellitus. N. Engl. J. Med., 1995; 333:541-549.

De Meyts, P. et al: The structural basis of insulin and insulin- like growth factor-I receptor binding and negative cooperativity, and its relevance to mitogenic versus metabolic signalling. Diabetologia, 1994; 37: S135-S148.

Granner, D.D. et al: Molecular physiology and genetics of NIDDM. Diabetes Care, 1992; 15:369-395.

Meuckler, M.: Facilitative glucose transporters. Eur. J. Biochem., 1994; 219:713-725.

Myers, M.G. et al: The IRS-1 signaling system. Trends Biochem. Sci., 1994; 19:289-293.

Philipson, L.H. et al: Pas de deux or more: the sulfonylurea receptor and K^+ channels. Science, 1995; 268:372-373.

Rabkin, R. et al: The renal metabolism of insulin. Diabetologia, 1984; 27:351-357.

Robbins, D.C. et al: Biologic and clinical importance of proinsulin. N. Engl. J. Med., 1984; 310:1165-1175.

White, M.F. et al: The insulin signaling system. J. Biol. Chem., 1994; 269:1-4.

SEX HORMONES AND THEIR ANTAGONISTS

ANDROGENS AND ANTIANDROGENS

Androgens

The main natural androgen is testosterone. It is synthesized and secreted by the Leydig cells of testes in males and in small amount by ovary in females and adrenal cortex in both sexes. Testes also secrete small amounts of other androgens, viz. dihydrotestosterone (potent), androstenedione and dehydroepiandrosterone which are weak. Testes also release small amounts of pregnenolone and progesterone.

Mechanism of action

Testosterone is not the active form at many sites of action. It is converted to more active dihydrotestosterone by 5 alpha-reductases. About 65% of circulating testosterone or dihydrotestosterone binds in target tissues to the more active dihydrotestosterone. It binds to sex hormone binding globulin (SHBG) which is a specific protein produced by liver, rest is bound to albumin, 2% is in free form which enters cells and binds to intracellular receptors.

Pharmacokinetics

Testosterone given by mouth is readily absorbed but is less effective due to first-pass effect in liver. Testosterone injected as a solution in oil is quickly absorbed and metabolized, so the effect is small.

The esters of testosterone are less polar than the free steroid and when these are injected intramuscularly in oil, are absorbed more slowly. For example, testosterone propionate is more active testosterone; the cypionate and enanthate esters are fully effective when given at 1 to 3 weeks intervals.

Testosterone is inactivated primarily in the liver. Dihydrotestosterone and oestradiol are active metabolites whereas androsterone and etiocholanolone are inactive metabolites.

Dihydrotestosterone itself is converted in the liver to androsterone, androstanedione, and androstanediol.

The excretion as androsterone and etiocholanolone and also in small amounts of androstanediol and oestrogens also are excreted largely as glucuronide and sulphate conjugates.

The esters of testosterone are hydrolyzed to free testosterone and subsequently are metabolized in the same way as is testosterone. However, certain other changes in the molecule as in methyltestosterone and fluoxymesterone affect metabolic degradation resulting in longer half-lives (due to less rapid metabolism). The unchanged compounds, metabolites, and conjugate are excreted in urine and faeces.

Actions

Testosterone promotes growth of genitalia and development of male secondary sex characteristics. It is necessary for libido and potency. It has anabolic effect, promotes growth in height, is concerned in developing and maintaining muscle mass and prevents osteoporosis.

Box 10.6. Androgens used parenterally	
Testosterone	Aqueous suspension for I.M. use 10 to 50 mg 3 times weekly.
Testosterone propionate	Oily solution for I.M. use; 10 to 25 mg 2-3 times weekly.
Testosterone enanthate	Oily solution for I.M. use; 50-400 mg 2-4 weeks.
Testosterone cypionate	Oily solution for I.M. use; 50-400 mg every 2-4 weeks.

Box 10.7. Androgens used by oral and buccal route	
Danazol	Capsule: 200-800 mg/d
Fluoxymesterone	Tablets: 2.5 to 20 mg/d
Methyltestosterone	Tablets and capsules: 10-50 mg/d; Buccal tablets: 5 to 25 mg/d
Oxandrolone	Tablets: 2.5 to 25 mg/d

When given to males at the age of puberty, there is rapid development of the secondary sexual characteristics and a marked increase in muscular strength. Height increases gradually.

If given to males at the prepubertal age, there is premature closure of the epiphyses of the long bones and hence the individuals do not reach their full height.

If given to females, it results in masculinisation.

Preparations and routes of administration

Oral: Fluoxymesterone 10-20 mg/d is available orally. The other orally active androgens are danazol and methyltestosterone. Testosterone is rapidly absorbed on oral administration but mostly converted to inactive metabolites and only 1/6 of the dose is available in active form. Methyltestosterone and fluoxymesterone are active when given by mouth. I.M. Testosterone enanthate 250 mg/2-3 weeks is a depot preparation. Parenterally it has more prolonged absorption time. It has greater activity when esterified.

Implants: testosterone pellets 400-600 mg every 4-6 months are inserted S.C. into anterior abdominal wall by trocar and cannula under local anaesthesia.

Uses

- Male hypogonadism. As a replacement therapy in males, methyltestosterone orally 25-50 mg or 5-10 mg/d sublingually or testosterone propionate sublingually 5-20 mg/d or 10-50 mg by I.M. injection three times a week. Fluoxymesterone oral 2-10 mg/d. Testosterone pellets S.C. 450 mg every 4-6 months. The drug should be used very carefully otherwise there may be stunting of growth because of epiphyseal closure.

- To induce and maintain secondary sex characteristics and potency.

- To remove symptoms of testosterone deficiency e.g. tiredness, lack of concentration, depression, etc.

- To prevent osteoporosis.

- To treat mammary carcinoma in women because of antioesterogenic effect.

- As anabolic agents.

Adverse effects

Virilizing effects	Feminizing effects	Toxic effects in all patients
Women Acne, facial hair, deepening of voice, menstrual irregularities, male pattern baldness, hypertrophy of clitoris		Oedema, jaundice, hepatic carcinoma, cholestatic hepatitis
Children Premature closure of epiphyseal plates, altered bone development		
Men Inhibition of gonadotropin release, reduced spermatogenesis lasting months after discontinuation	Gynaecomastia	

Contraindications

Prostatic carcinoma, breast carcinoma, renal and cardiac disease.

The effect of FSH and LH on the testis is given in Fig. 10.11.

Anabolic steroids

Nandrolone, Stanozolol, etc.

These are synthetically modified structures of androgens having enhanced anabolic effects and less virilizing effects.

Actions

They increase protein synthesis and enhance muscle development resulting in weight gain.

Uses

- Debilitating and wasting conditions
- To promote growth in cases of delayed puberty
- May be employed in osteoporosis to speed healing of fractures
- To improve appetite and promote feeling of well being in terminal diseases

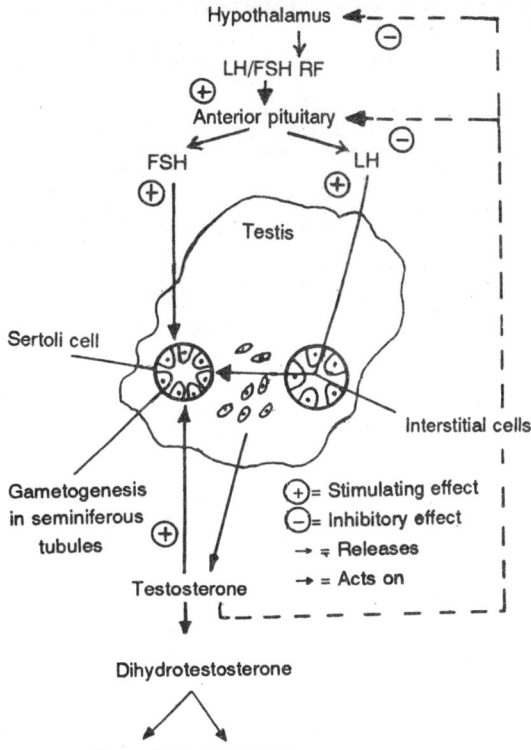

Fig. 10.11. LH/FSH RF controls secretion of gonadotropins by the anterior pituitary. FSH (follicle stimulating hormone) is responsible for the integrity of the seminiferous tubules and after puberty important in gametogenesis through an action on the Sertoli cells which nourish and support the developing spermatozoa. LH (luteinizing hormone) in male is also called interstitial cell stimulating hormone (ICSH), stimulates interstitial cells (Leydig cells) to secrete androgens in particular testosterone.

- Aplastic anaemia (erythropoiesis is stimulated)
- Breast cancer

But the anabolic steroids have limited applications as they have some androgenic activity. Their use by sportsmen to increase muscle bulk is illegal.

The relative androgenic and anabolic activity of some synthetic steroids is listed below:

Androgen/anabolic activity and routes of administration are given in Table 10.11.

Substitution in 17-beta position of testosterone affects lipid solubility and duration of action. In or-

Table 10.11. Androgen/anabolic activity and routes of administration.

	Androgen/ Anabolic Activity	Comments
Androgens		
Testosterone	1:1	Given IM/transdermally; inactive orally
Methyltestosterone	1:1	Orally active; short half-life (2.5 hr)
Fluoxymesterone	1:2	Orally active; long half-life (10 hr)
Danazol	—	Weak androgen; orally active
Anabolic steroids		
Oxymetholone	1:3	Orally active
Oxandrolone	1:3-1:13	Orally active
Nandrolone phen-propionate	1:3-1:6	Given IM
Stanozolol	1:3-1:6	Orally active

der of decreasing duration, the 17-beta esters of testosterone ethanate > cypionate > propionate > acetate.

The 17-alpha alkylated derivatives e.g. oxandrolone, norethindrone are orally active and less androgenic.

Preparations are available for oral, parenteral administration and transdermal (scrotal skin).

The maximum androgenic potency is with agents that are 17-beta esters of testosterone.

Unwanted effects of anabolic steroids

* Cholestatic jaundice
* Testicular atrophy
* Sterility
* Gynaecomastia in men
* Inhibition of ovulation
* Hirsutism.
* Alopecia, acne and deepening of voice in women

Antiandrogens

Antiandrogen receptor antagonists are cyproterone and flutamide.

These are indicated for the treatment of patients producing excessive amounts of testosterone. They are indicated to decrease excess sexual drive, in precocious puberty, and prostate cancer. These compounds have been used in the treatment of hirsutism in women, male-pattern baldness, acne, virilizing syndromes.

Cyproterone and cyproterone acetate (acetate is more effective) are synthetic progestogen having powerful antiandrogenic effect and mild glucocorticoid actions. These compete with testosterone and dihydrotestosterone for androgen receptor in target organs.

Besides this, they suppress pituitary LH and ACTH secretion so androgen production is reduced from both ovaries and adrenal glands.

Cyproterone acetate in a dose of 2 mg/d with an oestrogen is given for the treatment of hirsutism in women.

Side effects include weight gain, hypertension and loss of libido.

Flutamide is a potent antiandrogen. It is not a steroid but acts as a competitive antagonist at the androgen receptor. It has been found useful in the treatment of cancer of prostate. The dose is 250 mg thrice a day orally.

Adverse effects include mild gynaecomastia (due to increase in oestrogen production in testis) and hepatic toxicity (reversible).

5 alpha-reductase inhibitors

Finasteride does not interfere with testosterone-dependent functions, such as libido and potency. There may be impotance, decreased libido as delayed toxicity.

5α-reductase enzyme converts testosterone to more active dihydrotestosterone. Benign prostatic hypertrophy is androgen-dependent.

Finasteride is an aza steroid, preferentially active competitive inhibitor of type II 5α-reductase and thus inhibits the conversion of testosterone to its active metabolite dihydrotestosterone. This makes it a useful drug in the treatment of benign prostate hypertrophy. The agent causes a profound decrease in the concentration of dihydrotestosterone in plasma and in the prostate.

For the treatment of benign prostatic hypertrophy 5 mg of finasteride is given once daily for 6-12 months and if there is response the treatment is continued till prostate returns to its normal size. This drug may also be useful in the treatment of prostate cancer.

Finasteride is under trial for the treatment of male pattern baldness.

Certain antiandrogens such as nilutamide and bicalutamide (Casodex) are under investigation for the treatment of male pattern baldness.

5 alpha-reductase inhibitors, specific for 5 alpha-reductase type I are being developed.

Adverse effects

Finasteride may cause abnormal foetal development. Pregnant women should avoid contact with crushed tablets or the semen of men being treated with this drug.

Certain features of androgen hormone inhibitors and antiandrogens are given in Table 10.12.

Table 10.12. Certain features of androgen hormone inhibitors and antiandrogens.

	Comments
Androgen Hormone Inhibitor	
Finasteride	Inhibits 5-alpha-reductase in prostate
Leuprolide acetate	GnRH agonist injected SC; inhibits gonadotropin secretion resulting in decreased gonadal testosterone production
Goserelin	GnRH agonist similar to leuprolide in action
Antiandrogens	
Cyproterone acetate	Antagonist at androgen receptors
Flutamide	Competitive antagonist at androgen receptors

OESTROGENS, ANTIOESTROGENS, PROGESTINS, ANTIPROGESTINS

Oestrogens

These are synthesized mainly by the graafian follicle, stimulus being FSH, also synthesized in large amount by placenta and in small amount by testes in males and adrenal cortex in both sexes.

Steroidal natural oestrogens:
- Oestrone
- Oestriol
- Oestradiol
- Steroidal synthetic oestrogens:
- Ethinyloestradiol
- Mestranol
- Quinestrol

Non-steroidal synthetic oestrogens:
- Diethylstilbestrol (stilboestrol)
- Genistein

Table 10.13 lists some compounds with oestrogenic activity.

Certain major features of oestrogens are given in Table 10.14.

Actions

Given at the age 10 to 13 years, oestrogens are given with progesterone for primary hypogonadism. Oestrogens stimulate the development of the secondary sexual characteristics.

In amenorrhoea, oestrogens are given cyclically with a progestogen to induce an artificial cycle.

Its main use in adult women is for oral contraception and in postmenopausal hormone replacement therapy (HRT).

Oestrogens cause some degree of retention of salt and water and have mild anabolic actions.

The concentrations of triglycerides and of HDL are raised, and that of LDL is decreased.

An impairment of glucose tolerance can occur in some individuals.

Oestrogens affect bone in that they decrease resorption and can maintain bone mass in postmenopausal women, this effect may be indirect.

Oestrogens increase the coagulability of the blood, that is the risk of thromboembolism which may occur with contraceptive pill containing a high oestrogen content.

Low doses of oestrogens do not produce a significant change in clotting mechanisms.

Mechanism of action

Oestrogen receptors occur mainly in uterus, vagina, mammary gland and the anterior pituitary. These contain about 15,000-21,000 high-affinity oestrogen-binding sites per cell. There are also smaller numbers of sites in the liver, kidney, adrenal and ovary.

Table 10.13. Some clinically useful compounds with oestrogenic activity

Compound	Origin	Route of administration	Comments
Oestriol	Natural	I.M.	Very potent
Oestradiol	Natural	I.M.	Very potent
Ethinyloestradiol	Synthetic	Oral	
Mestranol	Synthetic	Oral	
Stilboestrol (diethylstilbestrol)	Synthetic	Oral	
Dienoestrol	Synthetic	Oral	
Chlorotrianisene	Synthetic	Oral	Stored in adipose tissue; prolonged weak action
Quinestrol	Synthetic	Oral	Inhibition of lactation

Table 10.14. Major features of oestrogens

Oestrogens	Comments
Natural oestrogens	
Oestradiol	Low oral bioavailability due to extensive first-pass hepatic metabolism; oral, IM, topical, and transdermal forms
Oestrone	Less active (1/12) metabolite of oestradiol; parenteral only
Conjugated Oestrogens	
Esterified Oestrogens	Mixture of sulfate esters of oestrogenic substances from pregnant mares; predominantly oestrone and equilin; used orally or topically
Synthetic Oestrogens	
Ethinyl oestradiol	Slower metabolism; half-life 13-27 hours
Mestranol	Metabolized to ethinyl oestradiol
Quinestrol	Slowly released from adipose tissue and metabolized to ethinyl oestradiol; used orally
Nonsteroidal Oestrogens	
Chlorotrianisene	Metabolized by liver to more active form after oral administration
Dienoestrol	Potent topical oestrogen
Diethylstilboestrol	Good oral absorption; slow inactivation

The effect of oestrogens on DNA is the induction of synthesis of progesterone receptors in tissues such as uterus, vagina, anterior pituitary and hypothalamus.

Prolactin increases the numbers of oestrogen receptors in the mammary gland and liver (but has no effect in the uterus).

Progesterone decreases oestrogen receptor expression in the reproductive tract by interfering with the de novo synthesis of the receptors.

Uses of oestrogens

- As replacement therapy in primary hypogonadism - oestrogen started at 11-13 years of age. It stimulates the development of secondary sexual characters and menstruation.

- As replacement therapy in postmenopausal syndrome. Due to decreased production of oestrogens at menopause, certain symptoms appear such as hot flushes, sweating, fatigue, anxiety, palpitation, muscle and joint pains, atrophic vaginitis.

  Hormone replacement therapy (HRT) is beneficial to relieve the above symptoms.

- Oestrogens are used for oral contraception.

- For dysmenorrhoea, oestrogens are combined with progestins to suppress ovulations and anovulatory cycles are painless. However, oestrogens are used only in severe dysmenorrhoea.

- As adjuvants to progesterone. Oestrogens are used for dysfunctional uterine bleeding.

- For palliative therapy of carcinoma prostate (androgen dependent tumour). Oestrogens antagonise androgens .

Hormone replacement therapy (HRT)

Benefits on general well being including a hoped - for reduction in facial wrinkles, to prevent osteoporosis (certainly) and to prevent ischaemic heart disease (possibly), due to falls in low density lipoprotein (LDL) and fibrinogen levels in blood, and rises in high density lipoprotein (HDL).

However, the unopposed oestrogen therapy if prolonged for years is associated with an increased incidence of endometrial carcinoma and gallbladder disease.

Addition of a progestogen ("opposed oestrogen therapy") reduces the risk but it is unnecessary in the absence of a uterus.

The risk of breast cancer is also increased by about 50% in older women after prolonged use (> 5 years). The risk should be weighed against the benefits in reducing risk of osteoporosis and IHD.

The indications and contraindications of HRT are given below:

Indications of HRT

- Symptomatic women
- High risk for osteoporosis
- High risk for ischaemic heart disease

Contraindications

Genital malignancy, carcinoma breast, pregnancy, severe liver disease, undiagnosed/suspected malignancy, vaginal bleeding, hypertension, arterial thromboembolic disease, diabetes mellitus, gall stones, migraine.

Benefits outweigh the risk

The benefits of HRT use on symptom relief, and on the prevention of osteoporosis, ischaemic heart disease and to a certain extent Alzheimer's disease far outweigh the risks of thromboembolic phenomenon and breast cancer risk. However, women with no risk factors for heart disease or hip fracture, but with two first degree relatives with breast cancer, should not receive HRT.

Preparations

Oestrogens are effective as replacement therapy, dose given is 0.2-1 mg once daily. It is best prescribed in cyclic manner with 3 weeks of drug and one week free of treatment.

Progestin is frequently used in combination so as to decrease the risk of endometrial carcinoma and induce prompt bleeding in the treatment free period.

Conjugated oestrogens (Premarin tablets 0.625 mg/1.25 mg; Conjugase tablets 0.625 mg) is a mixture of sodium oestrone sulphate and sodium equilin sulphate, derived wholly or in part from equine urine or synthetically from oestrone and equilin.

Use with caution: Epileptic patient, asthma, migraine, cardiac and renal failure, recurrent depression.

Adverse effects of oestrogens

Tenderness in breast, nausea, vomiting, loss of appetite, oedema (due to retention of salt and water), and increased risk of thromboembolism.

Carcinoma of the vagina and cervix in more common in young women whose mothers were given the synthetic oestrogen, stilboestrol in early pregnancy.

If oestrogen is given to pregnant women, there is a risk of producing nonmalignant genital abnormality in the offspring in both male and female.

Oestrogen in HRT frequently causes menstruation like bleeding. Endometrial hyperplasia can occur unless given cyclically with a progestogen.

Control of secretion of female sex hormones and effect of drugs are shown in Fig. 10.12.

FSH acts on ovaries promoting development of small groups of follicles each containing an ovum, one of them develops faster than others and forms graafian follicle and the rest degenerate. The cells of the ripening follicle secrete oestrogens which are responsible for the early proliferative phase of endometrial regeneration which occurs from day 5 or 6 until mid cycle. During this phase the endometrium thickens and the vascularity is increased, there is prolific cervical secretion of mucus of pH 8-9, rich in protein and carbohydrate which make the passage of sperm easier. The secreted oestrogens have a negative feedback on the anterior pituitary decreasing FSH release. In addition oestrogens sensitize LH releasing cells of anterior pituitary to

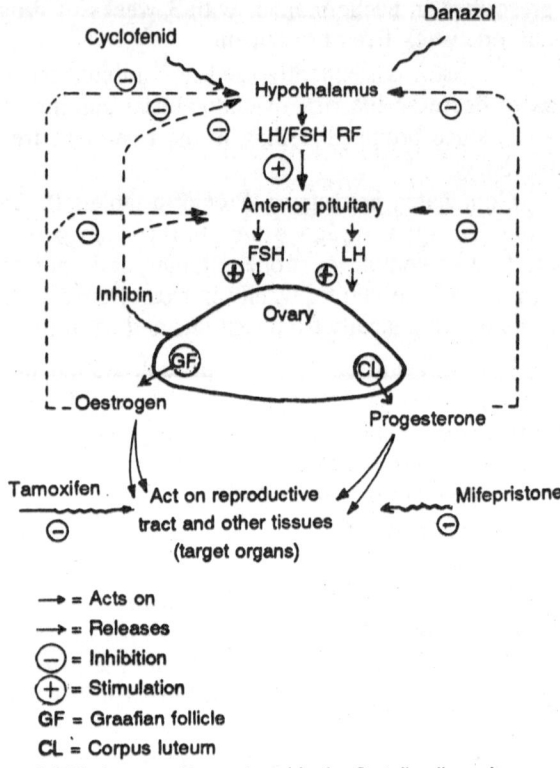

→ = Acts on
→ = Releases
⊖ = Inhibition
⊕ = Stimulation
GF = Graafian follicle
CL = Corpus luteum
Inhibin is a peptide produced in the Sertoli cells and ovary

Fig. 10.12. Female sex hormones and effects of certain drugs.

the action of the releasing factor and so determine the mid cycle surge of secretion of LH which causes rupture of main follicle resulting in ovulation. FSH stimulates the graafian follicle to secrete inhibin, a peptide of mol. wt. 20,000 which also has a negative feedback on FSH production.

LH influences the cells of the ruptured follicle and the follicle develops into corpus luteum which

---

Box 10.8. Role of oestrogen in decreasing risk of CHD in postmenopausal women

↑ HDL
↑ LDL receptors,
↓ LDL cholesterol
↓ Thromboxane effects on blood vessels
↑ PGI 2 production
↑ Cholesterol deposition in vessels

---

secretes progesterone which renders endometrium suitable for the implantation of a fertilized ovum. Progesterone has a negative feedback effect on the hypothalamus and anterior pituitary, decreasing release of LH. If the implantation of ovum does not occur progesterone secretion stops. Its sudden cessation is the main cause of onset of menstruation. If implantation occurs pregnancy results, the corpus luteum continues to secrete progesterone which by its feedback effect on hypothalamus and anterior pituitary prevents further ovulation.

Ovulation-inducing agents (Fertility drugs)

Clomiphene is a nonsteroidal partial antagonist that induces ovulation by blocking hypothalamic oestrogen receptors. The disturbed feed back inhibition produces enhanced gonadotropin secretion. In men, gametogenesis is also increased.

After clomiphene treatment, 80% of women ovulate, 30%-40% become pregnant and 10% of these pregnancies are multiple births.

Clomiphene has little or no effect in postmenopausal women.

Adverse effects include formation of ovarian cysts and ovarian hypertrophy, risk of ovarian tumours is also increased.

The other adverse effects include hot flushes, headache, constipation, hair loss, higher incidence of multiple pregnancies. Allergic skin reactions have also been reported.

Gonadotropins. Human menopausal gonadotropin (Pergonal) contains equal amounts of FSH and LH; Metrodin contains only FSH. These stimulate ovarian follicle development but require a sequential dose of hCG (human chorionic gonadotropin) to induce ovulation. These are given parenterally.

Treatment with these drugs is reserved for women who do not respond to clomiphene or cannot tolerate it. Multiple births may occur in about 10% of all treated pregnancies.

They may also be used in men to increase spermatogenesis (with hCG).

Contraindications

- Presence of primary ovarian failure
- Uncontrolled thyroid or adrenal dysfunction

- Presence of intracranial lesions e.g. pituitary tumour
- Pregnancy

Bromocriptine

It is an ergot derivative that binds to dopamine receptors in the pituitary and inhibits prolactin secretion. In amenorrheic women, treatment with bromocriptine leads to the onset of menses in 3-5 weeks when dosage of 2.5 mg 2-3 times a day are administered.

Antioesterogens (Clomiphene and Tamoxifen)

These inhibit or modify the action of oestrogens.

They belong to the following categories :
1. Competitive oestrogen antagonists
2. Oestrogen synthesis inhibitor

Competitive oestrogen antagonists

These act at oestrogen receptors in the anterior pituitary and hypothalamus. This disrupts the normal feedback inhibition of gonadotropin-releasing hormone (GnRH) and gonadotropin resulting in increased gametogenesis in the ovaries. The stimulation of ovaries results in ovulation. In some women the high incidence of multiple births (5-10%) may be produced, 75% of which are twins. In some women ovarian cysts may be produced.

Clomiphene

Clomiphene is a racemic mixture of both trans (enclomiphene) and cis isomer (zuclomiphene). Trans conformations have antioestrogenic activity, while the cis conformations show oestrogenic activity.

Clomiphene citrate and Tamoxifen are commonly used for the treatment of infertility and breast cancer.

Clomiphene citrate is readily absorbed following oral administration.

This drug and its metabolites are eliminated primarily in the faeces and to a lesser extent in the urine. Its plasma half-life is about 5-7 days.

The dose is 50 mg/d for 5 days.

Patients who do not ovulate even after 3 courses of 100 mg/d are not likely to respond.

Clomiphene is not useful in patients with ovarian or pituitary failure.

Tamoxifen

It is marketed as the pure transisomer.

The pharmacology of tamoxifen is similar to clomiphene. It is given orally like clomiphene. Due to the prolonged half-life, 3-4 weeks of treatment may be required to achieve steady-state plasma levels. The excretion is primarily in faeces. It blocks receptor sites in target organs. It is used in the palliative treatment of advanced oestrogen-dependent breast carcinoma. The effects of tamoxifen on proliferation of breast cancer cells appear to result largely from oestrogen receptor blockade.

Dose: 10-20 mg twice a day.

Adverse effects include hot flushes, nausea and vomiting.

Oestrogen synthesis inhibitors (GnRH and Aminoglutethimide)

Synthetic gonadotropin-releasing hormone (GnRH) is highly active in man, single i.v. dose of 10-100 microgram promptly increases concentrations of gonadotropins in the blood resulting in increased secretion of gonadal steroids. However, on continued administration over 2-4 weeks desensitize GnRH receptors in pituitary leading to suppression of secretion of both gonadotropins and gonadal steroids.

Leuprolide acetate injection 5 mg/ml for SC injection is available which is a synthetic GnRH.

Dose: 1 mg/d SC injection or 7.5 mg/monthly IM injection.

Its main use is in prostatic cancer.

Inhibition of aromatase blocks the conversion of androgens to oestrogens in all tissues. Aminoglutethimide and some imidazole derivatives are examples.

Certain agents decrease the effects of endogenous oestrogen by blocking their biosynthesis, e.g. continual administration of GnRH or use of long-acting GnRH agonists prevent ovarian synthesis of oestrogens, but not the peripheral synthesis of oestrogens from adrenal androgens.

Aminoglutethimide inhibits aromatase activity. It blocks oestrogen synthesis from all precursors. But it is not selective. It also inhibits other reactions involved in steroidogenesis.

Agents exerting opposing physiological actions

Examples: Progestins and androgens.

Progestins/progestational agents

The progestins include the naturally occurring hormone progesterone and a number of synthetic compounds that possess progestational activity.

Progesterone is most important progestin, serves as a precursor to oestrogens, androgens and adreno-cortical steroids. It is synthesized in ovary, testes and adrenals. During pregnancy large amounts are synthesized and released by placenta. Progesterone is rarely used therapeutically.

The various progestins are listed below:
  • Agents similar to progesterone: Hydroxypro-gesterone caproate, Medroxyprogesterone acetate.
  • Agents similar to 19-nortestosterone: Nore-thindrone, norethynodrel, norgestrel, deso-gestrel, norgestimate.

Synthetic progestational agents: These are active orally.

Medroxyprogesterone acetate

Megestrol acetate

Testosterone derivatives with progesterone like activity are:

Ethisterone, Norethisterone, Norgestrel, Ethyno-diol. These can be given orally.

Progestogens act on same tissues as oestrogens and modify their effects.

Box 10.9. Effects of progestins

• Increase in LDL
• Decrease in HDL
• Decrease in risk of endometrial cancer
• Decrease in endometrial hyperplasia

Table 10.15 lists compounds with progesterone-like activity.

The activity profile / major features of progestins are given in Table 10.16.

Uses

• As oral contraceptive, alone or in combination with oestrogen
• Dysfunctional uterine bleeding
• Endometriosis
• Primary dysmenorrhoea, combined oestrogen-progesterone preparation is more effective
• Habitual abortion (efficacy is doubtful)
• Malignancy (carcinoma of uterus, breast, pros-tate and rarely kidney and testes)
• Premenstrual syndrome
• Suppression of postpartum lactation

Adverse effects

Nausea, altered libido, weight gain, acne, urticaria, menstrual irregularity, virilization of foetus and gynaecomastia.

Antiprogestins

As abortifacients they are not superior to vacuum aspiration and prostaglandins in terminating early pregnancy.

Table 10.15. Compounds with mainly progesterone-like activity

Compound	Progesterone activity	Androgen activity	Route	Uses
Progesterone injection	High	+	Injection	Habitual abortion, amenorrhoea
Ethisterone	Delayed, prolonged	+	Oral	Uterine bleeding, dysmenorrhoea
Megestrol	High		Oral	Oral contraceptive
Medroxyprogesterone acetate	High		Oral	
Chlormadinone	Very high			Anti-oestrogen
Norethisterone	High, prolonged	+	Oral	Contraceptive
Norethynodrel	Oestrogen and progesterone	+	Oral	Contraceptive

Table 10.16. Activity profile/major features of progestins

Progestins	Activity Profile			
	Progestin	Oestrogen	Antioestrogen	Androgen
Progesterone and derivatives				
Progesterone	++++	0	+	0
Hydroxyprogesterone	+++	+	0	+
Megestrol acetate	+++	0	0	+
17Alpha-Ethinyl testosterone derivatives				
Dimethisterone	+	0	+	0
19-Nortestosterone derivatives				
L-Norgestrel	+++	0	++	+++
Desogestrel	+++	0/+	+++	0/+
Norgestimate	+++	0	+++	0
Ethynodiol diacetate	++	+	+	++
Norethindrone acetate	+	+	+++	++
Norethindrone	+	+	+	++
Norethynodrel	+	+++	0	0

+++ = High activity; ++ = Moderate; + = Low, 0 = Nil.

Mifepristone

It is a potent, competitive antagonist at both progesterone and glucocorticoid receptors binding to their respective receptors.

It is a 19-norsteroid, inhibits the action of progesterone by binding strongly to the progesterone receptor. It can be used to terminate early pregnancy and has been found useful for this purpose in about 80% cases with doses of 400-600 mg/d for four days or 800 mg/d for 2 days.

Combination of antiprogestin with a prostaglandin, sulprostone has been found very effective in early trials. If 600 mg of mifepristone single oral dose is given and a vaginal pessary containing 1 mg PGE_1 is administered during first 7 weeks of pregnancy, this combination can terminate pregnancy in 95% of patients.

Its adverse effects include nausea, vomiting, vaginal bleeding.

ORAL CONTRACEPTIVES (HORMONAL CONTRACEPTION)

There are three types of preparations :
1. Combination Oral Contraceptives (combination of oestrogen and progestin).

2. Sequential use of oestrogen followed by progestin.
3. Continuous use of progestin therapy without concomitant use of oestrogen.

Single-entity preparation
- Progestin-only contraceptives
- Postcoital contraceptives

The combined oestrogen-progestogen pill

Oestrogen employed is usually ethinyloestradiol 20-50 microgram or mestranol 50 microgram (in liver demethylated to ethinyloestradiol). Progestogen is norethisterone acetate 1-4 mg.

Combination tablet

Oestrogen		Progestin	
Ethinyloestradiol	0.02 mg	Norethindrone acetate	1.0 mg
Ethinyloestradiol	0.03 mg	Norethindrone acetate	1.5 mg
Ethinyloestradiol	0.03 mg	dl-norgestrel	0.3 mg
Mestranol	0.05 mg	Norethindrone	1.0 mg
Mestranol	0.1 mg	Norethindrone	2.0 mg

Dose: 1 tablet daily for 21 days taken at same time each day. 7 days interval given when withdrawal bleeding occurs. The course is started on 5th day of cycle till day 25 of menstrual cycle.

Mode of action

Central: Pituitary gonadotropins are suppressed by negative feedback. Ovulation in inhibited and maturation is impaired (Fig. 10.13).

Peripheral: cervical mucus becomes impenetrable to sperms, endometrium becomes unfavourable for implantation, gametal transport is impaired in fallopian tubes. Besides, oral contraception, these also produce following effects:

Menstrual flow is regulated. Dysmenorrhoea and premenstrual tension are alleviated, acne is improved and incidence of breast cancer is decreased. The hormonal contraception is a good choice in young women who do not smoke.

Advantages of the Combined Pill

- Safe and effective method of contraception
- Evidence indicates (but not proves conclusively) that after risk factors e.g. smoking, hypertension, and obesity have been identified, oral contraceptives are safe for most women.
- The use of combined pill markedly decreases the incidence of amenorrhoea, irregular periods and intermenstrual bleeding.

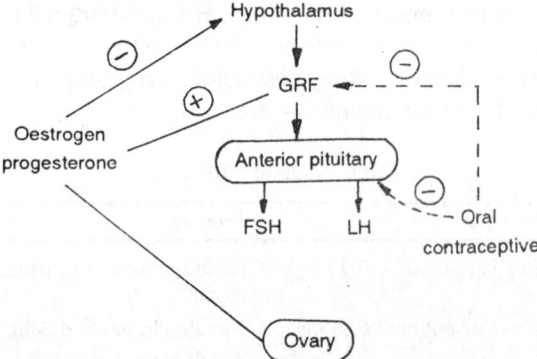

Fig. 10.13. Inhibition of hypothalamic gonadotropin releasing hormone by oral contraceptive (antiovulatory effect) exert direct inhibiting effect on anterior pituitary secretion of gonadotropins.

- The incidence of benign breast disease, uterine fibroids and cysts of the ovaries is reduced.
- There is less risk of thyroid disease.

Possible drawbacks (due to fluid retention or an anabolic effect or both)

- Weight gain, mood changes, nausea, flushing, skin changes such as acne and/or an increase in pigmentation, dizziness, depression or irritability in some individuals.
- Amenorrhoea on stopping the use of combined pill is sometimes seen. Permanent loss of fertility is rare. Normal cycles of menstruation usually start soon.

Contraindications

Absolute

- Cancer breast/uterus
- Abnormal undiagnosed genital bleeding
- History of myocardial infarction
- Acute or chronic hepatic disease
- Hyperlipidaemia
- Pregnancy

Relative

- Smoking
- Hypertension
- Diabetes
- Obesity
- Migraine
- Uterine fibroids

Drugs interactions

Oral contraceptives prolong half-life of phenylbutazone, pethidine.

Patients taking anticonvulsants such as phenytoin, phenobarbitone, carbamazepine increase binding of progesterone to sex hormone binding globulin thus lower free concentration of steroids. Such patients have to take high steroid dose.

Rifampicin increases rate of metabolism of both oestrogens and progestogens by inducing hepatic microsomal enzymes.

Adverse effects

Mild: nausea, flushing, dizziness, depression, irritability, breakthrough bleeding, oedema, headache.

Annoying side effects are breakthrough bleeding, weight gain (due to fluid retention, or anabolic effect or both), increased skin pigmentation, acne and hirsutism due to progestin.

Severe: Increased risk of thromboembolism (deep venous thrombosis and pulmonary embolism), due to increased coagulability of blood (due to high oestrogen content).

Hypertension occurs in about 5% cases after 5 years of use, probably by involving renin angiotensin system. The increase in B.P. is minimal but marked in some.

Gallstones occur about twice as commonly in women using the pill.

Pill may impair carbohydrate tolerance, thus may unmask latent diabetes and requirement of insulin is increased in diabetics.

Migraine may be precipitated.

Frequency of seizures is increased in epileptics.

Precaution: If nausea, breast tenderness and oedema are the complaints, oestrogen content should be reduced.

If mid cycle spotting, less flow or amenorrhoea are the complaints, the content of oestrogen should be increased or progestin content should be reduced or both.

If the patient gains weight, feels tiredness, depression, the progestin content should be decreased.

Oral contraceptives may cause birth defects if taken during the first trimester of pregnancy.

The development of certain types of cancer has been studied with oral contraceptives, but actual culpability is clouded by the long latency period and multiple risk factors.

Oestrogens are tumorigenic, causing tumours of the breast, testis, bone and other tissues.

Oral contraceptives are contraindicated in patients with known or suspected neoplasm.

Sequential regimen

Oestrogen for 15-16 days followed by 5-6 of combined oestrogen and progestin.

From day 5 to day 20, a single pill daily containing oestrogen alone is administered, followed by single oestrogen progestogen combination pill from day 21 to day 25 (16 + 5 = 21). There are 7 pill-free days during which withdrawal bleeding occurs.

There are reports of increased incidence of endometrial tumours with the use of sequential preparations.

Progestogen - only Pill

Norethisterone, levonorgestrel or ethynodiol are used.

The pill is taken daily without interruption.

The contraceptive effect is mainly due to the alteration of cervical mucus (which is made less suitable for the passage of sperm). The progestogen probably hinders implantation through its effect on the endometrium motility and secretion in the fallopian tubes.

Drawbacks

- The contraceptive effect of progestogen - only pill is less reliable than that of the combination pill.
- If a dose is missed, conception may result.
- Disturbances of menstruation are common.
- Irregular bleeding is likely to occur.

Advantage

Progestogen - only pill can be taken after parturition as unlike oestrogen-containing pills, it does not interfere with lactation.

Single-entity preparations

1. The "minipill" contains progestin alone. It acts by thickening the consistency of cervical mucus which serves as a barrier to sperm.

   It has higher failure rate than the other oral contraceptive and may cause irregular bleeding.

2. The "morning after" pill, or postcoital preparation contains diethylstilbestrol (DES). It should be started within 72 hours and continued (25 mg twice a day) for 5 days despite any nausea and vomiting. If DES fails, abortion is advised due to the increased risk of vaginal carcinoma in children exposed in utero to oestrogen and DES.

Ethinyloestradiol-norgestrel combination produces less side effects and is effective in about 95% cases if administration is initiated within 72 hours after coitus.

Mode of action: It acts on cervical mucus which

becomes inhospitable to sperm, also possibly affects the endometrium, motility and secretion in the fallopian tubes.

The contraceptive effect is less reliable than the combined pill or the sequential contraceptive schedule. However, the advantage is that they can be taken after parturition as unlike oestrogen containing pills they do not interfere with lactation.

Long-acting progestogen-only contraception

Medroxyprogesterone I.M. is safe and effective. But menstrual irregularities are common, and infertility may persist for many months after cessation of administration.

Levonorgestrel is impregnated subcutaneously in non-biodegradable capsules. The progestogen content is slowly released over 5 years. Irregular bleeding and headache are common adverse effects. Levonorgestrel - impregnated intrauterine device can prevent contraception for 3-5 years.

Adverse effects

- Cardiovascular side effects are increased in women who smoke.
- Thromboembolic disorders may require removal of the steroid implants.
- Bleeding irregularities diminish over time.
- Delayed follicular atresia and ectopic pregnancy are complications, although rare.

Dose-related side effects of oral contraceptives are summarized in Table 10.17.

Table 10.17. Summary of dose-related side effects of oral contraceptives

Oestrogen excess	Progestin excess
Nausea	Increased appetite
Patchy or generalized pigmentation of the skin (Melasma)	Weight gain
Migraine headache	Tiredness, fatigue
	Hypomenorrhoea
Hypertension	Acne, oily skin
Breast tenderness	Hair loss
Oedema	Depression
Oestrogen deficiency	**Progestin deficiency**
Early or midcycle breakthrough bleeding	Late breakthrough bleeding
Increased spotting	Amenorrhoea
Hypomenorrhoea	Hypermenorrhoea

Hormonal contraception in males

Various androgens including testosterone in doses of 400 mg orally produce azoospermia in less than half of persons treated.

Testosterone in combination with danazol is better tolerated but not more effective than testosterone alone. Danazol is a derivative of ethisterone (17 alpha-ethinyltestosterone).

Cyproterone acetate which is a powerful progestin also produces oligospermia but is not a reliable contraceptive.

Gossypol is a phenolic compound extract from the cotton plant of the genus gossypium; 20 mg/d for 2 months then 60 mg a week produces sperm count below 4 million/ml in 99.9% cases. It also impairs sperm motility. It is a potent azoospermic agent. The effects are reversible.

Adverse effects include hypokalaemia, weakness, oedema, dyspnoea, diarrhoea, neuritis and paralysis after higher doses.

STUDY QUESTIONS

1. What is the main natural androgen? Describe its uses and control of its secretion.
2. List the synthetic steroids with their relative androgenic and anabolic actions.
3. What are the therapeutic uses of androgens?
4. What do you understand by anabolic steroids? Give examples of such agents. What are their effects, uses and limitations?
5. What are the indications of antiandrogens? How do they act? What are their side effects? List a few antiandrogens.
6. What are (i) steroidal natural oestrogens, (ii) steroidal synthetic oestrogens and (iii) non-steroidal synthetic oestrogens?
7. How is the secretion of female sex hormones controlled?
8. Describe the actions, uses and adverse effects of oestrogens.
9. Write notes on: (i) antioestrogens (ii) antiprogestogens.
10. Describe progesterone. What are synthetic progestational agents? How do progestogens act and what are their uses? What are their adverse effects?

11. Describe the different types of preparations for hormonal contraception. What are the components of oestrogen and progestin in the combined oestrogen-progestogen pill?

12. What are the mechanisms of action of oral contraceptives? What are their adverse effects, contraindications and drug interactions?

13. Write notes on (i) progestin only pill, (ii) hormonal contraception in males (iii) sequential regimen and (iv) single-entity preparations.

14. Describe ovulation-inducing agents.

15. Describe the benefits, drawbacks, indications and contraindications of hormone replacement therapy (HRT).

GUIDE TO FURTHER READING

Archer, D.F.: Clinical and metabolic features of desogestrel: a new oral contraceptive preparation. Am. J. Obstet. Gynecol., 1994; 170:1550-1555.

Baird, D.T. et al: Hormonal contraception. N. Engl. J. Med., 1994; 328: 1543-1549.

Barrett-Connor, E. et al: Ischemic heart disease risk in postmenopausal women: effects of estrogen use on glucose and insulin levels. Arteriosclerosis, 1990; 10:531-534.

Belchetz, P.E. et al: Hormonal treatment of postmenopausal women. N. Engl. J. Med., 1994; 330:1062-1071.

Beller, F.K.: Cardiovascular system: coagulation, thrombosis, and contraceptive steroids—is there a link? In, Pharmacology of the Contraceptive Steroids. Raven Press, New York, 1994; pp. 309-333.

Beral et al. Breast cancer and hormone replacement therapy. Lancet 1997; 350:1047-1059.

Col-NF, Eckman-MH, Karas-RH, Pauker SG, Goldberg RG, Rose EM Orr RK, Wang JB. Patient specific Decisions about HRT in post menopausal women. JAMA 1997;277(14):1140-1147.

Collins P, Beale CM. The cardioprotective role of HRT: a clinical update. London: Partheon, 1996; 7-60.

Daly E, Vessey MP, Hawkins MM, Carson JL, Gough P, Marsh S. Risk of venous thrombo-embolism in users of hormone replacement therapy. Lancet, 1996, Oct. 12:348 (9033): 977-80.

Daly S.E. et al. HRT: An analysis of benefits, risks and costs. British Medical Buleetin (1992, Vol. 48, No. 2, pp 368-400).

Davidson, N.E.: Tamoxifen—panacea or Pandora's box. N. Engl. J. Med., 1992; 326:885-886.

Elking-Hirsch, K. et al: Metabolism: carbohydrate metabolism. In, Pharmacology of the Contraceptive Steroids. Raven Press, New York, 1994; pp. 345-356.

Eskin, B.A.: Sex hormones and aging. Adv. Exp. Med. Biol., 1978; 97:207-224.

Ettinger B. Grady D. Maximizing the benefit of estrogen therapy for prevention of osteoporosis. Menopause. 1994;1:19-24.

Felson DT.Zhang Y, Hannam MT, Kiel DP, Wilson PWF, Anderson JJ. The; effect of postmenopausal estrogen therapy on bone density in elderly women. N Engl J Med. 1993;329:1141-1146.

Fentiman, I.S.: Prospects for the prevention of breast cancer, Annu. Rev. Med., 1992; 43:181-194.

Fotherby, K.: Oral contraceptives and lipids. Br. Med. J., 1989; 298:1049-1050.

Gernstein, B.A. et al: Relationship of hormone use to cancer risk. J. Natl. Cancer Inst. Monograph, 1992; 12:137-147.

Glasier, A. et al: Mifepristone (RU-486) compared with high-dose estrogen and progestrogen for emergency postcoital contraception. N. Engl. J. Med., 1992; 327:1041-1044.

Goldzieher, J.W.: Are low dose contraceptive safer and better? Am. J. Obstet. Gynecol., 1994; 171:587-590.

Godsland, I.F. et al: Update on the metabolic effects of steroidal contraceptives and their relationship to cardiovascular disease risk. Am. J. Obstet. Gynecol., 1994; 170:1528-1536.

Grady D, Rubin SM, Diana B, Pettiti, Cary S, Dennis Black, Bruce Ettinger, Virgina L, Steven R, Cummings. Hormone therapy toprevent disease and prolong life in postmenopausal women. Ann Intern Med 1992;117:1016-2037.

Grimes, D.A.: The morbidity and mortality of pregnancy: still risky business. Am. J. Obstet. Gynecol., 1994; 170:1489-1494.

Grodstein F, stamfer MJ, Colditz GA, Willet WE, Manson JE, Jolfe M, Rosnee B, Fuchs C, Hankinson SE, Hunter DJ, Hennekens CH, Speizee FE. Postmenopausal hormone therapy and mortality. N. Eng. J. Med 1997 Jun 19;336:1769-75.

Jordan, V.C. et al: Endocrine pharmacology of antiestrogens as antitumor agents. Endocr. Rev., 1990; 11:578-610.

Kols, M. et al: Oral Contraceptives in the 1980s. Popul. Rev. A., 1982; 6:189-222.

Lobo, R.A. et al: New knowledge in the physiology of hormonal contraceptives. Am. J. Obstet. Gynecol., 1994; 170:1499-1507.

Massen T., Persson I, Adam; H, Bergstrom R, Bergkvist L. Hormone replacement therapy and the risk for first hip fracture. Ann intern Med. 1990; 113:95-103.

Miller K.L. Hormone replacement therapy in the elderly. Clin. obstel Gynecology 1996;39(4):912-932.

Miller-Bass, K. et al: Current status and future prospects for transdermal estrogen replacement therapy. Fertil. Steril., 1990; 53:961-974.

Paganini-Hill A, Henderson VW.Estrogen deficiency and risk of Alzheimer's disease in women. Am J Epidemiol. 1994;140:256-261.

Peyron, R. et al: Early termination of pregnancy with mifepristone (RU 486) and the orally active prostaglandin misoprostol. N. Engl. J. Med., 1993; 328:1509-1513.

Prince, R.L. et al: Prevention of postmenopausal osteoporosis. A comparative study of exercise, calcium supplementation, and hormone-replacement therapy. N. Engl. J. Med., 1991; 325:1189-1195.

Rebar, R.W.: et al: Characteristics of the new progestogens in combination oral contraceptives. Contraception, 1991; 44:1-10.

Samsioe, G.: Coagulation and anticoagulation effects of contraceptive steroids. Am. J. Obstet. Gynecol., 1994; 170:1523-1527.

Santen, R.J. et al: Endocrine treatment of breast cancer in women. Endocr. Rev., 1990; 11:221-265.

Shoupe, D.: New progestins-clinical experiences: gestodene. Am. J. Obstet. Gynecol., 1994; 170:1562-1568.

Spitz, I.M. et al: Mifepristone (RU 486)- a modulator of progestin and glucocorticoid action. N. Engl. J. Med., 1993;329:404-412.

Young, R.L. et al: Management of menopause when estrogen cannot be used. Drugs, 1990; 40:220-230.

Walsh, B.W. et al: Effects of postmenopausal hormone replacement with oral and transdermal estrogen on high density lipoprotein metabolism. J. Lipid Res., 1994; 35:2083-2093.

Chemotherapy of Different Types of Infections and Cancer Chemotherapy

ANTIMICROBIAL AGENTS

Chemotherapy denotes systemic treatment of specific infective diseases by drugs of known chemical structure which damage the invading organisms without injury to the host.

Antimicrobial agent designates synthetic as well as naturally (microbiologically) obtained drugs, e.g.

antibiotics, sulphonamides, trimethoprim, nitrofurans and quinolones. These are chemical substances that kill or suppress the growth of microorganisms.

Antibiotics are substances produced by microorganisms which suppress the growth and multiplication or kill other microorganisms at very low concentrations. The term antibiotic is now extended to include chemically related substances produced wholly or partially by chemical synthesis.

Classification of antibiotics on the basis of their molecular structure

1. Beta-lactam antibiotics: Penicillins, Cephalosporins
2. Tetracyclines and Chloramphenicol (Broad-spectrum antibiotics)
3. Aminoglycoside antibiotics: Streptomycin, Kanamycin, Neomycin, Gentamicin, Tobramycin, Amikacin, Netilmicin
4. Macrolide antibiotics: Erythromycin, Clarithromycin, Azithromycin
5. Polypeptide antibiotics: Polymyxin, Colistin, Bacitracin
6. Miscellaneous antibiotics: Clindamycin, Novobiocin, Lincomycin, Vancomycin

Classification based on mode of action

1. Inhibition of cell wall synthesis :
   Beta-lactams
      Penicillins
      Cephalosporins and cephamycins

Other categories of beta-lactams
　　Carbapenems e.g. meropenem
　　Monobactams e.g. aztreonam
　　Beta-lactamase inhibitors e.g. clavulanic acid
Other inhibitors of cell wall synthesis include –
　　vancomycin and teicoplanin

2. Inhibition of protein synthesis : Aminoglycosides. Those derived by streptomyces end in 'mycin' e.g. tobramycin. Others like gentamicin from micromonospora purpurea which is not a fungus, hence 'micin' and semisynthetic drug e.g. amikacin.
   - Tetracyclines
   - Macrolides e.g. erythromycin, clindamycin, other drugs include quinupristin, linezolid, chloramphenicol and sodium fusidate.

3. Inhibition of Nucleic acid synthesis : Sulphonamides. These drugs and trimethoprim with which these drugs are combined inhibit synthesis of nucleic acid precursors.

4. Quinolone, e.g. ciprofloxocin. They act by preventing DNA replication.

5. Azoles, e.g. metronidazole, they act by the production of short-lived intermediate compounds which are toxic to DNA of sensitive organisms. Rifampicin inhibits bacterial DNA-dependent RNA polymerase.

BETA-LACTAM ANTIBIOTICS

These contain beta-lactam ring.

The beta-lactam antibiotics are shown in Fig. 11.1.

PENICILLINS

All penicillins are derived from 6-aminopenicillanic acid which is a thiazolidine ring attached to beta-lactam ring to which the side chains are attached as shown below:

The ring marked 2 in the structure is the beta-lactam ring. The thiazolidine ring marked 1 is attached to beta-lactam ring. The structural integrity of the 6-aminopenicillanic acid nucleus is essential to the biologic activity of the nucleus. If the beta-lactam ring is enzymatically cleaved by bacterial beta-lactamase (penicillinases), the resulting product penicilloic acid, is devoid of antibacterial activity but is allergenic.

Acidic radicals (R, shown in Fig. 11.2) can be cleaved by bacterial and other amidases.

Structures of some penicillins

The following structures can each be substituted at the R to produce a new penicillin.

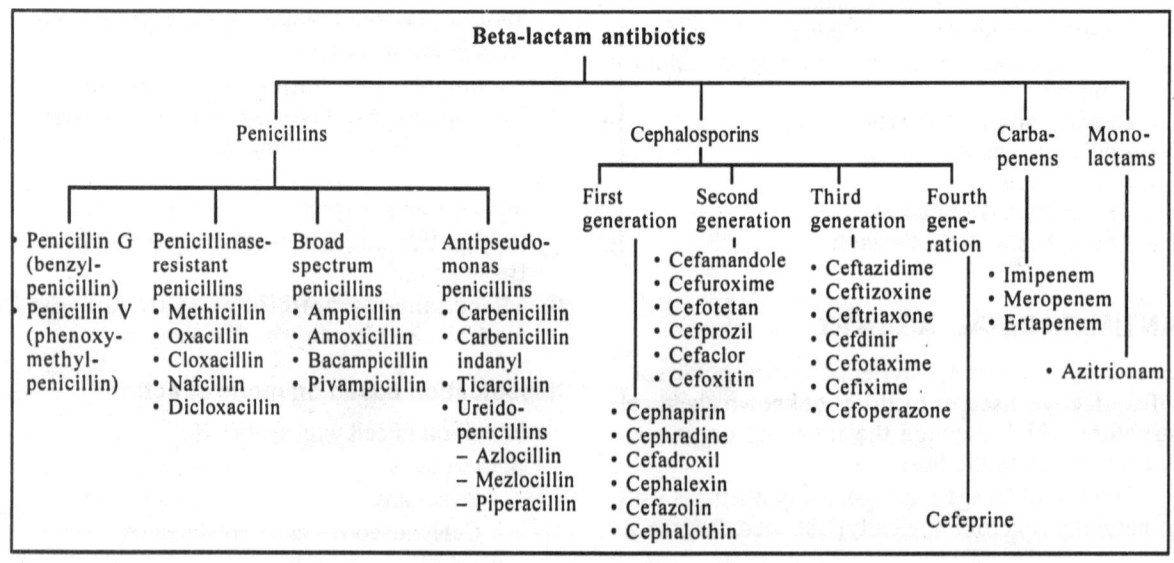

Fig. 11.1. Overview of the beta-lactam antibiotics which act by inhibiting cell wall synthesis.

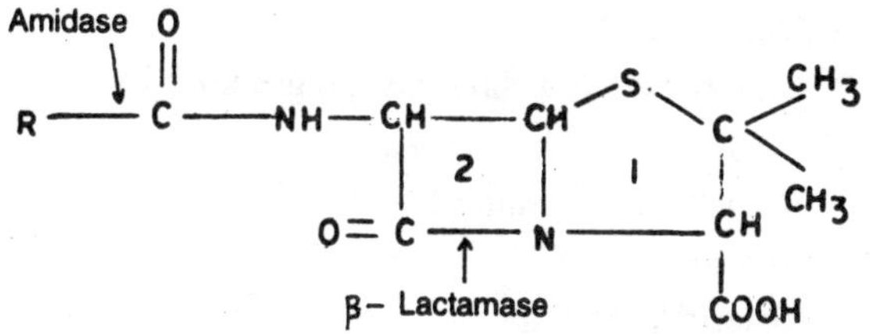

Fig. 11.2. Structure of penicillin.

Penicillin G (benzylpenicillin)

- Highly active against gram-positive bacteria.
- Less effective against gram-negative bacteria.
- Acid labile. Destroyed by β-lactamase.
- 60% protein bound.

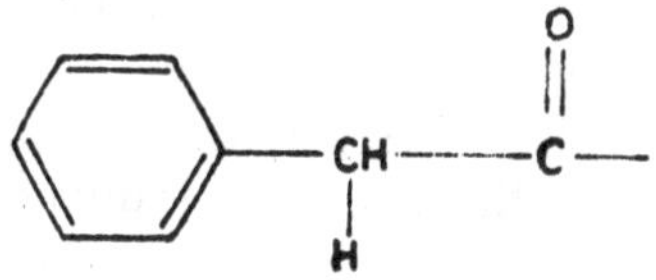

Structure of Penicillin G (benzylpenicillin)

Oxacillin (no Cl atom); Cloxacillin (one Cl atom)
Dicloxacillin (2 Cls); flucloxacillin (one Cl and one F in structure)

- Acid stable, can be taken orally.
- Highly protein-bound (95-98%).
- Similar to methicillin in β-lactamase resistance.

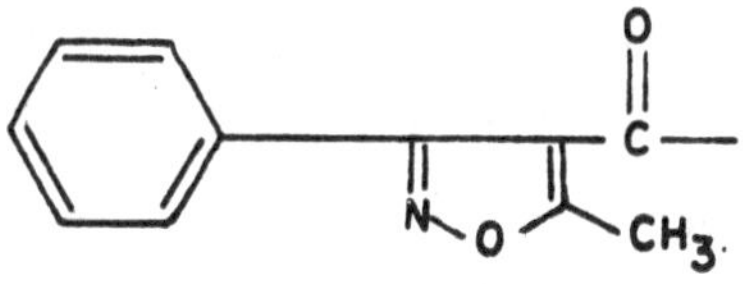

Structure of Oxacillin

Ampicillin

Similar to Penicillin G (destroyed by β-lactamase), but acid stable and more active against gram-negative bacteria.

Carbenicillin has –COONa in place of NH_2

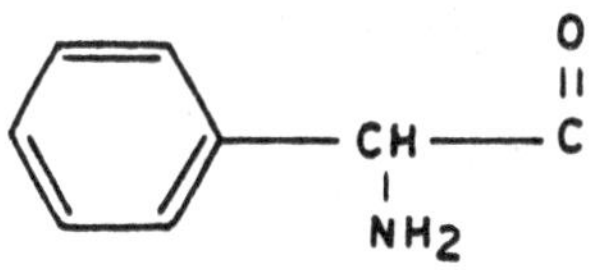

Structure of Ampicillin

Amoxicillin

Similar to ampicillin but better absorbed.

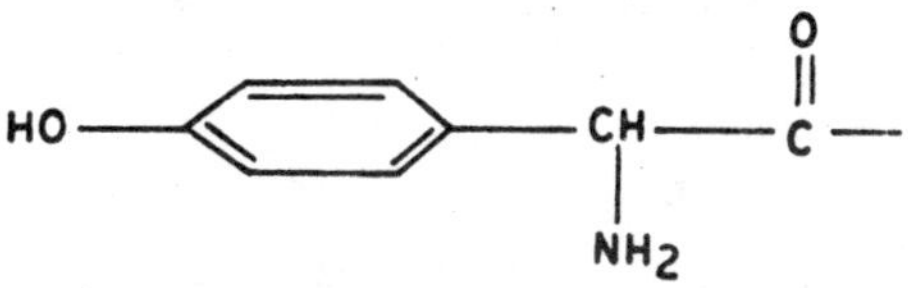

Structure of Amoxicillin

Nafcillin

- Can be given orally as well as parenterally.
- Resistant to staphylococcal β-lactamase

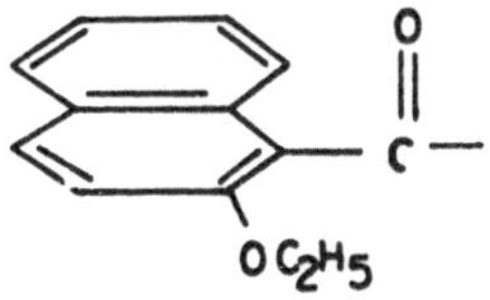

Structure of Nafcillin

Ticarcillin

Similar to carbenicillin but gives higher blood levels.

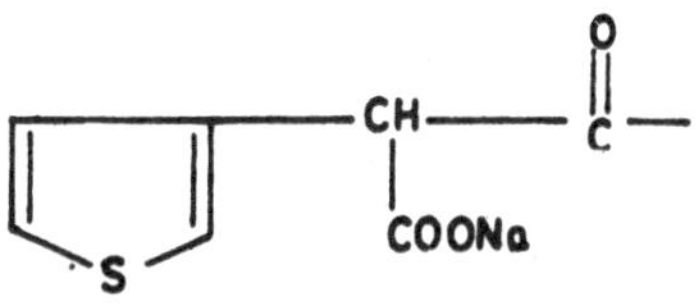

Structure of Ticarcillin

Piperacillin, Azlocillin, and Mezlocillin resemble ticarcillin in action against gram-negative aerobes.

Natural penicillins

There are four types of natural penicillins present in mould penicillium notatum, viz. penicillin G, K, F, X. Penicillin G is benzylpenicillin which is superior among these four types of penicillins. It is effective against gram-positive cocci but readily hydrolyzed by penicillinase and because of its instability in gastric acid, it is injected.

Natural penicillins are ineffective against most strains of *Staphylococcus aureus*.

Semisynthetic penicillins

(a) Penicillinase resistant

- Methicillin
- Oxacillin
- Cloxacillin
- Dicloxacillin

These are less potent antibacterial against microorganisms that are sensitive to penicillin G, but effective against penicillinase producing Staphylococcus aureus.

(b) Extended spectrum

1. Ampicillin, Amoxicillin, Cyclacillin, Bacampicillin and others comprise a group whose antimicrobial activity is extended to include such gram-negative microorganisms as *H. influenzae*, *E. coli* and *Proteus mirabilis*.
2. The antibacterial activity of Carbenicillin, Ticarcillin and azlocillin, is extended to include *Pseudomonas*, *Enterobacter* and *Proteus* species.
3. Other extended spectrum penicillins include mezlocillin and piperacillin which have useful antibacterial activity against *Pseudomonas*, *Klebsiella* and certain other gram-negative microorganisms.

The term penicillin is now used generically for the entire group of natural and semisynthetic penicillins.

Penicillins are still widely used, they are generally well tolerated and are bactericidal by virtue of their inhibitory action on the synthesis of the bacterial cell wall. Apart from hypersensitivity reactions penicillins are almost nontoxic.

Penicillin G (Benzylpenicillin) is the oldest member among the antibiotics. The following pathogenic organisms are usually sensitive to benzylpenicillin in the concentrations commonly achieved in the body during treatment.

Spectrum of activity of penicillin G and V

- Gram-positive coccal (streptococcal, staphylococcal) infections
- Gram-negative coccal (meningococcal, gonococcal) infections
- *Treponema pallidum*
- Oral anaerobes
- *Clostridium* (causing gas gangrene)
- *Corynebacterium diphtheriae*
- *B. anthracis* (anthrax)
- Actinomycosis
- Listeria infection

Among pathogenic microorganisms usually insensitive to benzylpenicillin are Acinetobacter species and most gram-negative bacilli including pseudomonas species and enterobacteriaceae, although some of these organisms e.g. some strains of *proteus mirabilis* may be inhibited by high concentrations of benzylpenicillin. Other organisms which are insensitive include mycobacteria, fungi (although not actinomyces), rickettsias and most viruses.

Benzylpenicillin is used as sodium or potassium salt. One international unit is equivalent to 0.6 microgram of the international standard sodium salt of penicillin. Long acting salt preparations include procaine penicillin and benzathine penicillin which slowly release benzylpenicillin after injection. The semisynthetic penicillins are expressed in weight and not in international units.

Benzylpenicillin is very safe except for allergy characterized by skin rashes, asthma like condition, angioneurotic oedema, arthralgia, anaphylactic shock. It is irritant to central nervous system on intrathecal injection. Anaphylactic shock is the most serious allergic reaction, the incidence is about 1 in 1000, and occurs within few minutes. There may be acute cardiovascular collapse and bronchospasm. The treatment of anaphylactic shock must be done immediately by intramuscular injection of 0.5-1 ml of 1: 1000 adrenaline solution, oxygen inhalation and administration of corticosteroids.

Semisynthetic penicillins have been developed to overcome the following drawbacks of benzylpenicillin (penicillin G):

- Poor oral efficacy
- Susceptibility to penicillinase
- Narrow spectrum of activity
- Short duration of action
- Allergy

1. Acid resistant penicillins (can be given orally)

- Phenoxymethyl penicillin (penicillin V)
- Phenoxyethyl penicillin
- Phenethicillin
- Propicillin

Phenoxymethyl penicillin is acid stable and therefore given by mouth but it is also inactivated by penicillinase. It is generally used for relatively mild infections.

2. Penicillinase resistant as well as acid resistant penicillins

- Cloxacillin
- Oxacillin
- Dicloxacillin
- Floxacillin
- Penicillinase resistant but only partially acid resistant (oral absorption not reliable): Nafcillin
- Penicillinase resistant but not acid resistant: Methicillin (it has to be injected).

Beta-lactamases are enzymes produced by many microbes which inactivate beta-lactam antibiotics.

Box 11.1. Microorganisms that are capable of producing penicillinase

- Staphylococcus aureus
- Bacillus species
- Becteroides species
- E. coli
- Proteus species
- Pseudomonas aeruginosa
- Mycobacterium tuberculosis

Box 11.2. β-lactamases

- Penicillinase and cephalosporinase are beta-lactamases. These are enzymes produced by many bacteria that render beta-lactam antibiotics ineffective.

Box 11.3. β-lactamase inhibitors

- Clavulanic acid
- Sulbactam

Beta-lactamase inhibitors

Enzymes that open the beta-lactam rings of penicillins, cephalosporins and related compounds at the beta-lactam bond are known as beta-lactamases.

Those that are excreted mainly from the bacterium and the genes which are located on plasmids are called penicillinase. They are type-II lactamases. They are mainly responsible for the penicillin resistance of gram-positive bacteria, gram-negative cocci and a number of gram-negative bacilli.

Clavulanate Potassium

It is absorbed well by the oral route but is also suitable for parenteral administration. The half-life is about 1 hour. In plasma about 30% is protein-bound, and about 25 to 50% is eliminated by renal tubular secretion and some is metabolized.

Sulbactam Sodium

It has greater activity against type-I beta-lactamases than clavulanate, but does not penetrate the cell walls of gram-negative bacteria as well.

It has weak antibacterial activity of its own.

It is absorbed by the oral route but is also suitable for parenteral administration. Its elimination is mainly by renal tubular secretion, however, it does not interfere significantly with the elimination of ampicillin, the only beta-lactam antibiotics with which it is combined. It is also secreted into milk.

The plasma half-life is about 1 hour.

Beta-Lactamase Combinations

Clavulanate potassium (125 mg) + Amoxicillin (500 mg): A combination given orally. It causes more diarrhoea than amoxicillin.

Clavulanate potassium (125 mg) + Ticarcillin (3 g): A combination given I.V. It is active versus more gram-negative bacilli.

Sulbactam sodium (0.5-1 g) + Ampicillin (1-2 g): A combination given I.V./I.M. It is active versus Staphylococcus and beta-lactamase producing H. influenzae and Strep. pneumoniae.

Tazobactam sodium (375 mg) + Piperacillin (3 g): A combination given IV. It is active versus more gram-negative bacilli.

3. Broad spectrum penicillins (extended spectrum) which are also acid resistant

- Ampicillin
- Amoxicillin
- Carbenicillin indanyl
- Broad-spectrum penicillin but not acid resistant: Carbenicillin

---

Box 11.4. Activity of broad spectrum penicillins
- Gram-positive organisms
- Some strains of E. coli, H. influenzae, Salmonella, Shigella and some Proteus species

---

Ampicillin

It is effective against all organisms sensitive to benzylpenicillin although generally less active against gram-positive bacteria. It is acid stable but destroyed by penicillinase. In addition many gram-negative bacilli e.g. *H. influenzae, E. coli, Proteus, Salmonella, Shigella* are sensitive. *Pseudomonas* is not sensitive. The dose is 500 mg orally, it is acid stable, and given 6-8 hourly. The commonest side effect is diarrhoea. A number of prodrugs including bacampicillin, metampicillin, pivampicillin and talampicillin are also said to be better absorbed and are hydrolyzed to ampicillin in vivo.

Amoxicillin

Amoxicillin is better absorbed, better tolerated and given thrice a day. The incidence of diarrhoea is less than with ampicillin. It has been reported to be slightly more active than ampicillin against streptococci and salmonella but is less active against shigella species.

Carbenicillin was the first penicillin with activity

Box 11.5. Activity against certain important micro-organisms

- Antipseudomonas penicillins (Carbenicillin, Carbenicillin indanyl, Ticarcillin, Azlocillin, Ureidopenicillins, Mezlocillin and Piperacillin)
- Gram-negative organisms, particularly *P. aeruginosa*, indole positive *Proteus* and *Enterobacter*
- Temocillin, a 6 alpha-methoxy derivative of ticarcillin is resistant to many β-lactamases and is active against most gram-negative aerobic bacteria except Pseudomonas aeruginosa and Acinetobacter species.

---

against *Pseudo. aeruginosa* and some *Proteus* strain that are resistant to ampicillin. It has been superseded by ticarcillin or piperacillin for most uses. Ticarcillin (semisynthetic penicillin is very similar to carbenicillin but it is 2-4 active against *Pseudo. aeruginosa.*

Carbenicillin indanyl is acid stable so it can be given orally. It resembles ampicillin but it is more active against pseudomonas and proteus.

The ureidopenicillins azlocillin and mezlocillin and the closely related piperacillin are more active than carbenicillin against *pseudomonas aeruginosa* and have a wider margin of activity.

Table 11.1 shows characteristics of penicillins.

4. Longer duration (Depository preparations)

Procaine penicillin G in oil with 2% aluminium mono-stearate (PAM) produces effects for 48-72 hours.

Benzathine penicillin effect lasts for about 14 days.

5. None is free from antigenicity

Preparations and dosage

1. Parenteral
   - Penicillin G sodium, intramuscularly 5000 units/4-6 hourly. Procaine penicillin G in oil with 2% Aluminium monostearate 1 or 1.2 mega units/48-72 hours.
   - Benzathine penicillin (Penidure) intramuscularly 2.4 mega units/14 days.
   - Ampicillin intramuscularly 1-2 g/6 hour.
   - Carbenicillin intramuscularly 1 g/6 hour.
   - Methicillin intravenously (less commonly used being more nephrotoxic than nafcillin).
2. Intrathecal in meningococcal meningitis 1000 units/ml, 10-20 ml/24 hours.
3. Oral
   - Penicillin V 250-500 mg/4 hour.
   - Oxacillin 0.75-0.5g/4-6 hours.
   - Cloxacillin 0.5-1.0 g/4-6 hour.
   - Dicloxacillin 0.25-0.5 g/4-6 hour.
   - Ampicillin 0.25-0.5g/6 hour.
   - Nafcillin 0.25-0.5g/4-6 hour.

Activity with other antimicrobial agents

Synergy between β-lactam compound and aminoglycosides has been attributed to enhanced

Table 11.1. Certain characteristics of penicillins regarding their absorption, resistance to penicillinase and antimicrobial spectrum

Name	Absorption after oral administration	Resistance to penicillinase	Useful anti-microbial spectrum
Penicillin G	Poor	No	Streptococcus, Neisseria, many anaerobes, spirochaetes
Methicillin Oxacillin Cloxacillin	Poor	Yes	Staphylococcus aureus
Dicloxacillin	Good	Yes	Staphylococcus aureus
Nafcillin	Variable	Yes	Staphylococcus aureus
Ampicillin	Good	No	Proteus mirabilis, E. coli
Amoxicillin	Excellent	No	Proteus mirabilis, E. coli
Carbenicillin	Poor	No	Above plus Pseudomonas species, Enterobacter species and Proteus
Carbenicillin indanyl	Good	No	Above plus Pseudomonas species, Enterobacter species and Proteus
Mezlocillin	Poor	No	Pseudomonas species, Enterobacter species, many Klebsiella
Piperacillin	Poor	No	Pseudomonas species, Enterobacter species, many Klebsiella

penetration of the aminoglycoside secondary to β-lactam induced cell wall destruction. Synergism has been demonstrated between benzylpenicillin and gentamicin, or other aminoglycosides, against some gram-positive organisms and some gram-negative anaerobic organisms including Lactobacilli, Bacteroides species and some streptococci, and also against enterococci.

Combinations of β-lactam antibiotics have shown both synergy and antagonism. Synergy may occur because each antibiotic binds to different target proteins. Antagonism of β-lactam combinations may result from induction of β-lactamases by one of the antimicrobials or because competition for, or alteration of, cell protein binding sites may occur.

Table 11.2 shows antibacterial spectrum, routes of administration of penicillins and beta-lactamase combination.

The final effect of β-lactam combinations depends on the particular combination used and the characteristics of the organism concerned. Since antagonism between penicillins and cephalosporins may have clinical importance, it has been suggested that β-lactam combinations should be avoided until clinical studies have shown a definite advantage over a single β-lactam or a β-lactam plus an aminoglycoside.

Antagonism has been reported between benzyl-penicillin and several other antibiotics including erythromycin against Listeria monocytogenes and polymyxin B against *Proteus mirabilis*.

Bacteriostatic drugs such as chloramphenicol might antagonize the bactericidal actions of penicillins, and clinical studies have demonstrated no benefit in giving chloramphenicol with benzylpenicillin compared with chloramphenicol alone to treat children with bacterial meningitis or severe pneumonia.

CEPHALOSPORINS

These are semisynthetic antibiotics derived from a fungus cephalosporium. The antibacterial spectrum is the same as penicillin but are highly resistant to penicillinase. They are bactericidal and act by inhibiting the synthesis of bacterial cell wall. They are generally well tolerated but are more toxic than penicillins.

Some bacteria elaborate a beta-lactamase called cephalosporinase which destroys antibacterial activity. However, many cephalosporins are resistant to the enzyme.

All cephalosporins are active against most gram-positive cocci, including penicillinase producing staphylococci and many strains of gram-negative organism such as *E. coli*, *Proteus* and *Pseudomonas*.

They are in general ineffective against enterococci.

Table 11.2. Antibacterial spectrum and routes of administration of penicillins and beta-lactamase combinations

Class	Comments
Natural Penicillins (best streptococcal and narrow spectrum)	
Penicillin G	Best narrow spectrum (streptococcal) IV, IM
Penicillin V	Same spectrum as penicillin G, oral only
Penicillinase-resistant Penicillins	
Cloxacillin	Oral
Dicloxacillin	Preferred oral
Methicillin	IV, interstitial nephritis may occur
Nafcillin	Preferred IV drug for staph
Oxacillin	Oral
Aminopenicillins (improved gram-neg., H. influenzae, Enterococcus, Shigella, Salmonella)	
Amoxacillin	Good oral absorption
Ampicillin	Preferred IV drug, incomplete oral absorb, diarrhoea, rash
Bacampicillin	Oral prodrug converted to ampicillin
Extended-spectrum (antipseudomonal) penicillins	
Carbenicillin	IV, high sodium, oral prodrug available
Ticarcillin	IV, similar to carbenicillin but less sodium
Mezlocillin	IV, similar to piperacillin
Piperacillin	Preferred IV, best gram-neg spectrum
Beta-Lactamase Combinations (expand spectrum to staph beta-lactamase producers)	
Clavulanate-Amoxicillin	Oral, more diarrhoea than amoxicillin
Sulbactam-Ampicillin	IV, active Vs staph and beta-lactamase producing H influenzae and strep. peneum.
Clavulanate-Ticarcillin	I.V., active versus more gram-neg bacilli.
Tazobactam-Piperacillin	IV active versus more gram-neg bacilli.

These drugs are used as alternative to benzyl-penicillin in persons who are allergic to benzyl-penicillin. Penicillinase producing staphylococci also respond to cephalosporins.

The most widely used system of classification of cephalosporins is by generations.

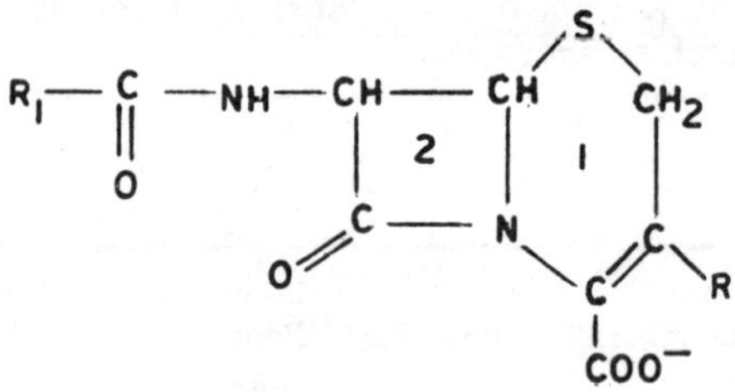

Fig. 11.3. Structure of cephalosporins.

The general structure of cephalosporins is shown in Fig. 11.3.

First generation cephalosporins

- Cephalothin
- Cefazolin
- Cephalexin
- Cephradine
- Cefadroxil
- Cephaloridine

The first generation agents generally penetrate the cerebrospinal fluid only poorly.

Cephalothin was one of the first cephalosporins to become available. It has good activity against a wide spectrum of gram-positive bacteria including penicillinase producing, but not methicillin resistant staphylococci. Enterococci are however resistant. Its activity against gram-negative bacteria is modest. It is not absorbed from the gastrointestinal tract and must be administered parenterally although intramuscular injection is painful.

Cephalothin should not be used in meningitis as it does not enter the cerebrospinal fluid; 6-12 grams daily is given intravenously to reach cerebrospinal fluid to a significant extent. I.V. injection 1 g produces 0.55 mcg/ml concentration in aqueous humour.

Cefazolin is a widely used parenteral first generation cephalosporin which is reported to be less painful on intramuscular injection than cephalothin. Although cefazolin is more active against E. coli and Klebsiella species, it is somewhat more sensitive to staphylococcal β lactamase than is cephalothin. Cefazolin is usually preferred among the first generation cephalosporins since it can be administered less frequently because of its longer half-life (1-8 hours) as compared to 0.5 hour for cephalothin.

The dose is 4 grams daily intramuscularly.

Cephaloridine is rarely used due to its nephrotoxicity.

Cefadroxil 1 gram 12 hourly and cephalexin 0.5 gram 6 hourly are administered only by mouth. The antimicrobial activity is similar to cephalothin. However, these are somewhat less active against penicillinase producing staphylococci.

Cephradine 0.5 gram 6 hourly can be given both by mouth and by injection.

Second generation cephalosporins

- Cefamandole
- Cefaclor
- Cefuroxime
- Cefoxitin
- Cefonicid
- Cefotetan
- Cefprozil

Cefamandole was the first available cephalosporin from this group. It has similar or slightly less activity than cephalothin against gram-positive bacteria. It has, however, greater stability to hydrolysis by β-lactamases produced by gram-negative bacteria and has enhanced activity against many of enterobacteriaceae and *H. influenzae*, *E. coli* and *Klebsiella* group. It is given by intramuscular injection.

Cefaclor is used orally. It has similar activity to cephalothin against gram-negative bacteria, particularly *H. influenzae*.

Cefuroxime is very similar to cefamandole in its spectrum of activity, although it is even more resistant to hydrolysis by beta-lactamases. The half-life of cefamandole (1.7 hour vs 0.8 hour). The concentrations in cerebrospinal fluid are about 10% of those in the plasma and the drug is effective for meningitis.

Cefuroxime axetil is the recently developed ester of cefuroxime which can be given by mouth.

Third generation cephalosporins

- Ceftizoxime
- Ceftriaxone
- Ceftazidime
- Cefotaxime
- Cefpodoxime
- Cefixime
- Cefoperazone

The third generation cephalosporins are even more stable than cefuroxime. Compared to the earlier generation of cephalosporins, they have a wider spectrum and greater potency of activity against gram-negative organisms including most clinically important Enterobacteriaceae; including beta-lactamase producing strains. Their activity against gram-positive organisms is however, generally less than that of the first generation agents.

Cefotaxime was the first of this group to become available and it has relatively modest activity against pseudomonas aeruginosa. However, activity against B. fragilis is poor as compared to agents such as clindamycin and metronidazole.

Ceftizoxime has a spectrum of activity very similar to that of cefotaxime. The half-life is longer (1.8 hour as against 1 hour) and thus can be administered somewhat less frequently.

Ceftriaxone has half-life of about 8 hours which is an outstanding feature. Administration of the drug once or twice daily has been effective for patients with meningitis and other infections.

A single dose of ceftriaxone (250 mg) is effective in the treatment of gonorrhoea and other diseases caused by penicillinase producing microorganisms.

Ceftazidime has half-life 1.5 hours, it is less active against gram-positive microorganisms than cefotaxime. Its activity against the Enterobacteriaceae is very similar, but its major distinguishing feature is good activity against Pseudomonas.

Fourth generation cephalosporin

Cefepime

It is stable to hydrolysis by many of the Beta-lactamases. It is a poor inducer of, and, relatively resistant to type 1 chromosomally encoded-beta-lactamases. It is more active against *H. influenzae*, *N. gonorrhoeae*, *N. meningitides* than cefotaxime. For *Ps aeroginosa* as effective as ceftazidime.

This drug is comparable to third-generation but more resistant to some β-lactamases.

Dose is I.V. 2 g every 12 hours ; half-life is 12 hours. It is 100% renally excreted and so doses should be adjusted in the presence of renal dysfunction.

Cefepime is stable to hydrolysis by many of the previously identified plasmid-encoded β-lactamases (TEM-1, TEM-2, SHV-1). It is a poor inducer of and relatively resistant to type 1 chromosomally encoded β$_2$-lactamases. It is thus active aganist cephalosporins via induction of type-1 β-lactamses. However, cefepime remains susceptible to many bacteria expressing extended-spectrum plasmid-mediated β-lactamses.

Cefepime has greater in vitro activity than cefotaxime against the fastidious gram-negative bacteria such as *H. influenzae*, *N. gonorrhoeae*, and *N. meningitides*. Against *P. aeruginosa*, cefepime has similar activity as ceftazidime but less active against other pseudomonas species.

Against streptococci and methicillin-sensitive staphlococcus aureus it has higher activity than ceftazidime and similar activity as cefotaxime.

Cefepime is inactive against penicillin-resistant *pneumococci*, *enterococci*, *B. fragilis*, *M. avian* complex or *M. tuberculosis*.

Table 11.3 shows certain characteristics of cephalosporins.

OTHER BETA-LACTAM ANTIBIOTICS

Carbapenems

Imipenem

It is a beta-lactam antibiotic derived from thienamycin. It is bactericidal. It acts by interfering with the synthesis of the bacterial cell wall. Its half-life is one hour.

If imipenem is given alone it is inactivated by a dipeptidase enzyme in the kidney, which opens the beta-lactam ring. Therefore, it is given in combination with cilastatin which is a dipeptidase inhibitor that inhibits the renal tubular metabolism of imipenem and prevents the formation of nephrotoxic compounds.

Table 11.3. Certain characteristics of cephalosporins

Class	Comments
First generation (Staph, some enteric gram-neg. bacilli)	
Cefadroxil	Oral, intermediate acting
Cefazolin	IM, IV intermediate duration, less painful
Cephalexin	Oral, short acting
Cephalothin	IM, IV, short acting, weakest spectrum
Cephapirin	IM, IV, short acting
Cephradine	IM, IV, oral, short acting
Second generation (more active vs gram-neg, some active vs H. influenzae and anaerobes)	
Cefaclor	Oral, short acting, active vs H. influenzae
Cefamandole	IM, IV, short acting
Cefmetazole	IV, short acting, good vs. anaerobes
Cefonicid	IM, IV, intermed-long acting
Ceforanid	IM, IV, intermedediate acting
Cefotetan	IM, IV, intermed-long acting, good vs anaerobes
Cefoxitin	IM, IV, short acting, good vs anaerobes
Cefprozil	Oral, short acting
Cefuroxime	IM, IV, oral, beta-lactamase resist., active vs H influenzae, good csf levels
Third generation (best gram-neg. spectrum, beta-lactamase resistant, poor vs staph.)	
Cefixime	Oral, intermed-long acting
Cefpodoxime	Oral, intermed acting, similar to cefixime
Cefoperazone	IM, IV, intermediate acting, good vs Pseudo
Cefotaxime	IM, IV, shortest acting, metabolised, good csf
Ceftazidime	IM, IV, short acting, good vs pseudo
Ceftizoxime	IM, IV, short acting, good csf levels
Ceftriaxone	IM, IV, long acting, good vs gonococci
Ceftibuten	Oral, similar to cefixime
Cefdinir	Oral, similar to cefixime
Fourth Generation	
Cefepime	I.V., better vs staph and strep than 3rd generation

Antibacterial spectrum

Imipenem has the broadest antibacterial spectrum among all the beta-lactam antibiotics. It is active against gram-positive and gram-negative cocci, except methicillin-resistant *staphylococci*, *enterobacteriaceae*, *Pseudomonas aeruginosa*, and anaerobic bacteria including *B. fragilis*.

Imipenem is effective against *gonococci* and *H. influenzae* strains which are resistant to penicillin and ampicillin. As it is partly broken down by dehydropeptidase it is given combined with cilastin, a dipeptidase inhibitor that inhibits the renal tubular metabolism of imipenem and prevents the formation of potentially nephrotoxic compounds.

Administration and uses

It is given by i.v. route and its use is mainly limited to the treatment of serious hospital-acquired infections due to susceptible organisms. Dose is 500 mg i.v.

Adverse effects

- *Pseudomonas* may acquire resistance.
- Nausea, vomiting and diarrhoea.
- Allergic reactions have occurred.
- Patients allergic to penicillin may be allergic to imipenem.

Aztreonam

It is a monobactam i.e. it has a monocyclic rather than bicyclic beta-lactam nucleus (unlike penicillins and cephalosporins).

It inhibits the synthesis of bacterial cell wall.

The half-life is 1.7 hours. Its bioavailability is 100%.

Antibacterial activity

It is markedly resistant to beta-lactamases. It is very active against aerobic gram-negative bacteria including *pseudomonas aeruginosa* and penicillinase-producing strains of *H. influenzae* and *gonococci*.

It has poor activity against gram-positive cocci and anaerobic bacteria.

Uses and administration

Aztreonam has narrow spectrum and should be used in combination with other antimicrobial agents.

This drug has been substituted for aminoglycoside antibiotics against the susceptible microorganisms. It shows little or no immunologic cross-activity with other beta-lactam antibiotics.

It is administered parenterally. Dose is 2 g 6-8 hourly.

Adverse effects

- Superinfection with gram-positive cocci.
- Pseudomembranous colitis.

Loracarbef

It is a beta-lactam, identical to cefaclor (chemically). But it is not classified as a cephalosporin because a methylene group replaces the sulphur atom.

It acts like other beta-lactams. Its half-life is 1 hour. It is well absorbed from GIT and excreted in an unaltered form in the urine. Its antibacterial activity is similar to that of cefaclor. The adverse effects are same as with similar spectrum anti-microbials.

BROAD-SPECTRUM ANTIBIOTICS (CHLORAMPHENICOL AND TETRACYCLINES)

Crystalline chloramphenicol is a neutral, very bitter in taste and stable compound with the following structure (Fig. 11.4).

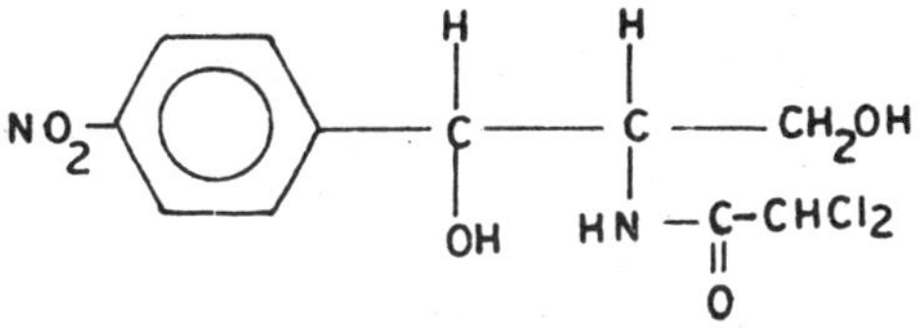

Fig. 11.4. Chloramphenicol.

Chloramphenicol is poorly soluble in water but highly soluble in alcohol. Chloramphenicol succinate is highly soluble in water and hydrolyzed in tissues with liberation of free chloramphenicol.

Antibacterial spectrum

The antibacterial spectrum is the same as tetracyclincs. However, it differs in being (i) highly effective in typhoid (ii) more effective in whooping cough and (iii) less active against gram-positive cocci.

Chloramphenicol is bacteriostatic for most gram-positive and many gram-negative bacteria. It may be bactericidal for those microorganisms which are highly susceptible such as *Haemophilus influenzae, Neisseria meningitidis* and some strains of Bacteroides.

Chloramphenicol acts by binding reversibly to a receptor site on the 50 S subunit of the bacterial ribosome resulting in inhibition of microbial protein synthesis. Chloramphenicol is also an inhibitor of mitochondrial protein synthesis in marrow cells.

Resistance to chloramphenicol is plasmid-mediated and results from production of chloramphenicol acetyltransferase which is bacterial enzyme that inactivates chloramphenicol. There is no cross-resistance between chloramphenicol and other antibiotics, but plasmids can transmit multiple drug resistance (chloramphenicol, tetracyclines and streptomycin, etc.) from one bacterium to another by conjugation.

Pharmacokinetics

Chloramphenicol is rapidly and completely absorbed after oral administration, widely distributed in all tissues and body fluids, including the CNS and CSF. Its concentration in brain tissue is almost equal to that in blood. It can be considered a unique property for the treatment of infection in the central nervous system. In blood, chloramphenicol is protein bound to about 30% extent. It is metabolized by conjugation with glucuronic acid in the liver or by reduction to inactive arylamines.

About 10% chloramphenicol in free (active) form and 90% as inactive degradation products are excreted in urine. Therefore the dose of chloramphenicol should be reduced in the presence of hepatic dysfunction and it need not be altered in renal insufficiency.

Dosage: Daily doses of 2g-3g orally for 14-21 days in adults produce blood levels of 8 mcg/ml. Prolonged treatment reduces the chances of relapse.

Chloramphenicol palmitate (dose 30-50 mg/kg/d orally) is hydrolyzed in intestine and liberates free drug.

Chloramphenicol succinate 25-50 mg/kg/d given by i.m. or i.v. injection yields free drug by hydrolysis.

Clinical Applications

Chloramphenicol is potentially toxic, hence it is a choice only in the following conditions:

- Salmonella infections (typhoid and paratyphoid fever). However, many strains are now showing resistance
- Serious infections with *H. influenzae* e.g. meningitis, 50-100 mg/kg/d orally or by I.V. injection for 8-14 days.
- Meningococcal or pneumococcal infections of the central nervous system (dose 50 mg/kg/d orally in 4 divided doses)
- Anaerobic or mixed infections in CNS e.g. brain abscess.
- Severe rickettsial infections as an alternative to tetracycline.

Chloramphenicol is also used topically in ophthalmic practice for eye infections because of its broad-spectrum activity and excellent penetration of ocular tissues and the aqueous humour. However, chlamydial infections do not respond.

Adverse Effects

GIT: nausea, vomiting and diarrhoea in 2-5 days. After 5-10 days due to alteration in microbial flora there may be candidiasis of mucous membranes.

Bone marrow depression: If chloramphenicol is taken in excess of 50 mg/kg/d, after 1-2 weeks, the blood levels become above 25-30 mcg/ml and defects in red cell maturation occurs. This disappears when the drug is discontinued. It is not related to aplastic anaemia.

Aplastic anaemia appears to be a specific genetically determined idiosyncrasy of an individual, not related to dose, route of administration and time of intake. However, it occurs more frequently after long term use and is irreversible and may be fatal. Aplastic anaemia probably occurs in one out of 25,000-50,000 patients.

Gray baby syndrome in new born infants

Due to lack of glucuronic acid conjugation mechanism, chloramphenicol accumulates, resulting in gray baby syndrome, manifested by vomiting, gray colour, hypothermia, flaccidity, shock and collapse. Therefore chloramphenicol should be used with great care in infants (dosage less than 50 mg/kg/d in full term infants and less than 30 mg/kg/d in premature infants).

Drug interactions

Chloramphenicol inhibits liver microsomal enzymes and thus raises blood concentrations of phenytoin, tolbutamide and warfarin.

Being a bacteriostatic it can antagonize the bactericidal actions of penicillins and aminoglycoside antibiotics.

Tetracyclines

Chlortetracycline was isolated from streptomyces aureofaciens and oxytetracycline from streptomyces rimosus; tetracycline was introduced by dehalogenation of chlortetracycline, and demeclocycline by demethylation of chlortetracycline. Recently more tetracyclines have been developed which are better absorbed and longer acting.

Free tetracyclines are crystalline substances with poor solubility but their hydrochloride salts are soluble.

Tetracyclines have a common polycyclic structure (Fig. 11.5).

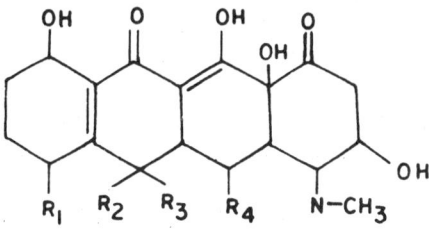

Fig. 11.5. General structure.

Antibacterial spectrum

Tetracyclines are broad-spectrum antibiotics for many gram-positive and gram-negative organisms and some anaerobes, for rickettsiae, chlamydia, mycoplasma, and for some protozoa e.g. amoeba. These are bacteriostatic. They act by binding reversibly on receptors on the 30 S subunit of bacterial ribosome that inhibits protein synthesis.

Resistance to tetracyclines is usually plasmid-mediated. Plasmids usually transmit resistance to multiple drugs. An organism resistant to one of the tetracyclines is usually resistant to all other members of the group. Although some tetracycline resistant staplylococci may be sensitive to minocycline and some resistant strains of Bacteroides may be sensitive to doxycycline.

Pharmacokinetics

About 30% of chlortetracycline, 60-80% of tetracycline, oxytetracycline and demeclocycline are absorbed from GIT on oral administration.

Minocycline and doxycycline are absorbed to about 90-100%. The absorption is impaired by chelation with Ca^{2+}, Mg^{2+}, Fe^{2+}, and Al^{3+}, specially in milk and antacids.

In the circulating blood, about 40-80% of various tetracycline is protein-bound.

The distribution is wide in tissues and body fluids except in CSF. Very high concentrations of minocycline are reached in tears and saliva (unique feature).

Tetracyclines cross placental barrier to reach foetus and are also excreted in milk. Tetracyclines are bound to growing bones and teeth as a result of chelation with calcium.

Excretion is mainly by way of bile and urine. 10-50% is excreted in urine and 10-40% is excreted in faeces.

Doxycycline and minocycline are almost completely absorbed and excreted more slowly. The serum levels persist longer. Doxycycline is not excreted in urine and so does not accumulate in renal failure.

	R_1	R_2	R_3	R_4	% protein binding	% absorption	$t_{1/2}$ (hr)
Tetracycline	H	CH_3	OH	H	77	50-65	8
Chlortetracycline	Cl	CH_3	OH	H		50-70	6
Oxytetracycline	H	CH_3	OH	OH	50	25-35	9
Doxycycline	H	CH_3	H	OH	93	80-95	11
Minocycline	$N(CH_3)_2$	H	H	H	98	80-95	16
Demeclocycline	Cl	H	OH	H	68	80-90	12

Clinical Applications

Tetracyclines are the drugs of choice in infections due to Mycoplasma pneumoniae, chlamydiae and rickettsiae and some spirochaetes, and vibrio infections. The other indications are acne, UTIs and bronchitis. They are sometimes given against protozoal infections due to *E. histolytica* or *Plasmodium falciparum*.

In combination with aminoglycoside, tetracyclines have been found useful in brucellosis, tularemia and plague.

Dosages (oral): Tetracycline hydrochloride 0.25 g 4 times a day for adults and 20 mg/kg/d for children. If infection is severe 3-4 times larger doses are to be given for 5 days. For the treatment of chlamydial infection the duration of treatment is 10-14 days. To suppress acne 250-500 mg daily is taken for many months. This suppresses lipase activity of propionibacteria.

Dosages (parenteral): 0.1-0.5g every 6-12 hourly in adults, and 10-15 mg/kg/d in children. I.M. injection is avoided due to pain and inflammatory reactions. It can be injected intravenously for which also there are very few situations such as an unconscious patient with rickettsial infection. I.V. injection may cause venous thrombosis.

Methacycline and Demeclocycline daily dose is 600 mg, 100 mg for doxycycline and 200 mg for minocycline.

Table 11.4 shows some charactericices of tetracyclines.

Table 11.4. Tetracyclines

Drugs	Comments
Chlortetracycline	Short acting, incomplete oral absorptions
Demeclocycline	Intermediate acting, more phototoxicity
Doxycycline	Long acting, good oral absorption, biliary excretion
Minocycline	Long acting, good oral absorption, dizziness, and vertigo, metabolized
Methacycline	Intermediate acting
Oxytetracycline	Short acting, incomplete oral absorption
Tetracycline	Short acting, incomplete oral absorption

Precautions

- Tetracyclines with the exception of doxycycline and minocycline are generally contraindicated in the presence of renal damage.
- To be avoided during pregnancy and to nursing mothers.
- To be avoided in patients with lupus erythematosus.
- Symptoms of myasthenia gravis may be exacerbated by tetracyclines.
- There is a possible antagonism of action of penicillin by predominantly bacteriostatic tetracycline.
- Absorption of tetracycline is diminished with concomitant use of milk, antacids, iron, magnesium and calcium.

Adverse reactions

GIT effects: nausea, vomiting and diarrhoea are very common during first few days, due to direct local irritation of GIT. After a few days, the normal flora is modified, and Proteus, staphylococci, Pseudomonas, resistant coliforms become dominant resulting in pruritis, GI disturbances and candidiasis. Even pseudomembranous enterocolitis with shock and death may be caused.

Effects on bones and teeth: Tetracyclines are bound to calcium in newly formed bones and teeth in young children. So tetracyclines are not given to children below 8 years of age. Children may develop yellow-brown discoloration of the teeth and suffer depressed bone growth.

Tetracyclines are not given during pregnancy as they can produce discoloration of teeth in the offspring.

Liver toxicity: Tetracyclines can impair hepatic function if high doses (more than 4 g daily) are administered intravenously. Tetracyclines can produce hepatic toxicity especially during pregnancy and in the presence of hepatic insufficiency.

Kidney damage: Tetracyclines (not doxycycline) may accumulate in the presence of kidney dysfunction resulting in renal tubular acidosis and nitrogen retention. This is more true if outdated tetracyclines are used. The ingestion of outdated and degraded tetracyclines can result in Fanconi's syndrome (renal tubular dysfunction which may lead to renal failure).

Local tissue toxicity: I.M injection produces pain and inflammatory reactions. I.V. injections may produce venous thrombosis.

Photosensitization: Demeclocycline, in particular can induce photosensitivity to sun light or ultraviolet light, especially in fair skinned persons.

Vestibular reactions: nausea, vomiting, dizziness, vertigo may be produced particularly with minocycline after 200-400 mg/d, in about 35-70% of patients. Table 11.5 lists comparison of tetracyclines and chloramphenicol.

AMINOGLYCOSIDES

A group of antibiotics including streptomycin, kanamycin, neomycin, gentamicin, tobramycin, amikacin and netilmicin are called aminoglycosides. They have similar chemical, antibacterial, pharmacologic and adverse characteristics.

The common features are:

- They are bactericidal for susceptible organisms. They are used primarily to treat infections caused by aerobic gram-negative bacilli. Their action against gram-positive bacteria is limited.
- They have a hexose nucleus, either streptidine (in streptomycin or deoxystreptamine (other aminoglycosides) to which amino sugars are attached by glycoside linkages and hence called aminoglycosides.

- They inhibit protein synthesis. They bind to receptors on the 30 S subunit of the bacterial ribosome.
- They are more active at alkaline than acidic pH.
- They are not absorbed from gastrointestinal tract. All oral dose is excreted in faeces.
- They are administered parenterally (IM/IV).
- Marked resistance may occur to their action from the acquisition of plasmids that contain genes that encode aminoglycoside metabolizing enzymes.
- Adverse effects include nephrotoxicity and ototoxicity (cochlear damage i.e. hearing loss or vestibular damage resulting in loss of balance, ataxia, and vertigo).
- They produce neuromuscular blockade (curare -like effect).

Streptomycin

Streptomycin was isolated from Streptomyces griseus by Waksman in 1944. Dihydrostreptomycin produced by reduction of streptomycin is more ototoxic hence no more used.

The antibacterial actions, routes of administration, mode of action and other characteristics are the same as with other aminoglycosides listed above.

Due to rapid emergence of drug resistance, streptomycin has now limited clinical usefulness e.g. in

Table 11.5. Comparison of tetracyclines and chloramphenicol

	Tetracyclines	Chloramphenicol
Antibacterial spectrum	Bacteriostatic broad-spectrum	Bacteriostatic broad-spectrum
Salmonella	Insensitive	Sensitive
Chlamydia	Sensitive	Insensitive
E.H.	Sensitive	Insensitive
Pharmacokinetics		
Absorption	Incomplete	Complete
Distribution	Good	Very good
Blood-brain barrier	Do not cross	Crosses
Placental barrier	Cross	Crosses
Excretion	Urine (bile, milk)	Metabolized 90% in liver
Resistance	Interference of cell envelope permeability barrier	Cell permeability barrier, and degraded by acetyl-transferase
Mode of action	Inhibit protein synthesis, act on 30 S subunit of bacterial ribosome	50 S

advanced tuberculosis and miliary tuberculosis. It is not given alone but in combination with other antimycobacterial drugs.

Streptomycin (I.M. injection) may also be given in certain non-tuberculous infections such as plague, tularemia, and brucellosis.

In certain diseases such as endocarditis caused by faecal streptococci or viridans streptococci and bacteremia due to gram-negative aerobic bacteria e.g. *Pseudomonas*, streptomycin combined with penicillin has been found effective.

Adverse effects include ototoxicity, nephrotoxicity and paralysis of neuromuscular function. Allergic reactions like fever, skin rashes etc. have also been reported.

Kanamycin and Neomycin

The pharmacokinetics and antibacterial spectrum, modification and adverse effects are similar to other aminoglycosides. These are effective against grampositive and gram-negative microorganisms and some mycobacteria. Pseudomonas and streptococci are generally resistant.

Due to ototoxicity these are not given parenterally. They are given orally or applied topically.

For topical use 1-5 mg/ml solution is used for application on topical surfaces or injected into joints. Ointment 1-5 mg/g is also available. Orally 1 g of neomycin is given 6-8 hourly for 1-2 days to reduce aerobic bowel flora prior to elective bowel surgery.

Allergy is uncommon but in few cases severe allergic reactions have occurred who used neomycin ointment for prolonged periods.

Gentamicin

Gentamicin is an aminoglycoside complex, isolated from Micromonospora purpurea.

Most of the properties are similar to other aminoglycosides. Sisomicin is similar to C_{1a} component of gentamicin.

The antibacterial activity is the same as with other aminoglycosides.

Resistance: Most streptococci are resistant. Organisms resistant to gentamicin are often resistant to tobramycin but not safer to amikacin.

Uses

Gentamicin and tobramycin (IM/IV) are used against severe infections due to gram-negative bacteria, especially *Pseudomonas*, *Enterobacter*, *Proteus*, *Klebsiella*.

Gentamicin and tobramycin are also effective in endocarditis due to *viridans streptococci* or *staphylococcus faecalis*.

Topical applications in the form of solution, cream or ointment (0.1%-0.3%) of gentamicin sulphate has been found useful for the treatment of infected wounds, and burns. It can also be administered subconjunctivally.

Intrathecal injection of gentamicin sulphate 1-10 mg/d may be given in meningitis due to gram-negative organisms.

Adverse effects include nephrotoxicity and ototoxicity as with other aminoglycosides. Allergic reactions are not common.

Tobramycin

The properties are identical to those of gentamicin. There is cross resistance in many cases. Nephrotoxicity of tobramycin is slightly less than that of gentamicin.

Dose: 5-7 mg/kg/d, IM/IV 8 hourly.

Amikacin

It is a semisynthetic derivative of kanamycin. It can be given against several enzymes that inactivate gentamicin and tobramycin.

Dose: 15 mg/kg/d, IM or 500 mg every 12 hourly.

Like other aminoglycosides it is nephrotoxic and ototoxic.

Netilmicin (Netromycin)

It is the latest of the aminoglycosides to be marketed which shares similarity with gentamicin and tobramycin in pharmacokinetic properties and dosage.

The dose is 5-7 mg/kg/d. It is also effective against certain gentamicin and tobramycin resistant bacteria, except enterococci. Like amikacin, it is not metabolized by the majority of the aminoglycoside-inactivating enzymes.

It is useful antibiotic for the treatment of serious

infections due to susceptible Enterobacteriaceae and other aerobic gram-negative bacilli.

Adverse effects

- Ototoxicity
- Nephrotoxicity

Studies in animals suggest that it is less toxic but this remains to be proven in human beings.

Adverse effects of aminoglycoside antibiotics

- Ototoxicity involves progressive damage and destruction of the sensory cells in the cochlea and vestibular organ of the ear. Vestibular damage produces vertigo, ataxia and loss of balance. Auditory disturbance produces deafness due to cochlear damage.
- Streptomycin, Gentamicin and Tobramycin affect more on vestibular component of the ear, whereas Kanamycin, Neomycin, and Amikacin affect hearing (cochlea) more than vestibular organ.
- Nephrotoxicity consists of damage of kidney tubules. Neomycin, Gentamicin and Amikacin are more nephrotoxic than Tobramycin and Netilmicin. Nephrotoxicity occurs more frequently in elderly persons, in the presence of pre-existing renal disease, low blood pressure and if loop diuretics are given concurrently. Table 11.6 shows the relative ototoxic and nephrotoxic risk potential.
- Neurotoxicity in the form of neuromuscular block (curare-like effect) which is observed if aminoglycosides (particularly streptomycin) are given with neuromuscular blockers. It is due to

Table 11.6. Relative ototoxic and nephrotoxic risk potential

	Ototoxic risk	Nephrotoxic risk
Streptomycin	+++++	
Gentamicin	++++	+
Kanamycin	++++	+++
Tobramycin	+++	+
Amikacin	+++	+++
Netilmicin	+	+

+, ++, +++, ++++ relative degree of toxicity

inhibition of Ca uptake necessary for exocytotic release of acetylcholine.

- Allergic reactions are not common with aminoglycoside antibiotics. However, allergic reactions may occur in some individual patients. The symptoms include drug fever, rashes, eosinophilia, haematological abnormalities including bone marrow depression, haemolytic anaemia and bleeding due to antagonism of clotting factor V.

MACROLIDE ANTIBIOTICS

Members of this group include erythromycin, azithromycin, clarithromycin, roxithromycin and spiramycin.

Erythromycin

Erythromycin was isolated in 1952 from Streptomyces erytherus.

It is considered as a prototype drug of this group.

Antibacterial spectrum

It is usually bacteriostatic but may be bactericidal in high concentrations against very susceptible organisms. Erythromycin is effective against gram-positive organisms, especially *pneumcococci*, *streptococci*, *staphylococci* and *corynebacteria* and *mycobacterium kansasii* etc.

It acts on the 50 S subunit of ribosomes. The receptor is a 23 S rRNA on the 50 S subunit. This receptor is close to the chloramphenicol receptor site.

Resistance develops from methylation of the rRNA-receptor on the 50 S unit of the ribosome under control of plasmid.

Cross-resistance among members of erythromycin group is complete. Some cross resistance to lincomycin may also occur.

The stearates and esters are acid resistant and well absorbed from the gastrointestinal tract. Erythromycin estolate is the best orally absorbed preparation but it imposes the greatest risk of adverse reaction and therefore the stearate or succinate salt is preferred. After absorption it is widely distributed in the body except in brain and CSF. It crosses placenta. The drug is excreted in bile, only 5% is excreted in urine.

Azithromycin and clarithromycin are newly introduced macrolides which have longer half-lives than erythromycin. Both of them have enhanced activity against mycobacterium avian-intracellulare as well as against some protozoa e.g. plasmodium spp. toxoplasma gondii and cryptosporidium.

Azithromycin

It is absorbed rapidly and distributed widely in the body except the brain and CSF.

It is currently indicated only for adult patients, the loading dose is 500 mg followed by 250 mg once a day. In AIDS patients the dose is 500 mg/d.

Azithromycin's unique pharmacokinetic properties include wide tissue distribution and high drug concentrations within cells (including phagocytes).

The bioavailability is decreased by 43% by food.

Azithromycin generally is less active than erythromycin against gram-positive organisms (*Streptococcus* spp. and *Enterococci*) and is more active than erythromycin or clarithromycin against *H. influenzae* and *Campylobacter* spp. It is active against *H. influenzae*, whereas erythromycin is not.

Clarithromycin

It is absorbed rapidly from GIT and undergoes first pass metabolism to its active metabolite, 14-hydroxyclarithromycin.

The usual dose is 250 mg twice a day, 500 mg twice a day for severe infections such as pneumonia, the dose for children less than 12 years 7.5 mg/kg twice a day.

AIDS patients require 1 g twice a day.

Clarithromycin is more potent than erythromycin-sensitive strains of *streptococci* and *staphylococci* but has only moderate activity against *H. influenzae* and *N. gonorrhoeae*. Strains resistant to erythromycin are also resistant to clarithromycin.

Roxithromycin

Roxithromycin has similar actions like erythromycin. Its $t_{1/2}$ is 12 hours. It is a long-acting drug and more resistant to acid hydrolysis and probably better absorbed and has good tissue penetration.

Dose : 150 mg twice a day.

Spiramycin

Spiramycin is a newer macrolide antibiotic with lesser side effects than erythromycin.

Dose : 6-9 million units/day in 2-3 divided doses.

Clinical applications

Erythromycins are most useful as penicillin substitutes in patients with streptococcal or pneumococcal infections which are hypersensitive to penicillin.

Erythromycins are the drugs of choice in diphtheria, in respiratory, neonatai, ocular, or genital chlamydial infections. Clarithromycin and Azithromycin are effective in suppressing disseminated/mycobacterium avium - intracellular infections in AIDS patients.

Dose: 0.25-0.5 g 6 hourly orally.

Erythromycin gluceptate and erythromycin lactobionate are available for i.v. administration which is usually given 6 hourly.

I.M. injection is painful so not recommended, i.v. administration is infrequent and reserved for severe infections.

Adverse reactions include loss of appetite, nausea, vomiting and diarrhoea. The more serious toxic effect particularly with estolate is acute cholestatic hepatitis which is probably allergic in nature. Other allergic reactions include rashes, eosinophilia and fever.

OTHER ANTIMICROBIALS

Lincomycin

Lincomycin is an antibiotic isolated from *streptomyces lincolnensis*. Its activity resembles erythromycin. There are only a few indications for its use because clindamycin which is a chlorine-substituted derivative of lincomycin has almost replaced it.

Clindamycin

Clindamycin is a chlorinated derivative of lincomycin. Its mode of action is like that of erythromycin and tetracyclines. Its antibacterial spectrum is like that of erythromycin but it is effective against *B. fragilis* in addition. Clindamycin is more active than erythromycin or clarithromycin against many anaerobes, especially *B. fragilis*.

Clindamycin is well absorbed, widely distributed including bone but penetrates poorly in the eye and CSF. The drug is metabolized in the liver and significant excretion occurs by the gut. The serum half-life is 3 hours.

Clinical applications

- Anaerobic infection caused by penicillin resistant organisms.
- Bone and joint infections, because the drug penetrates these tissues well.
- Intra-abdominal sepsis.

Preparations

Clindamycin palmitate, an oral preparation for paediatric use, is an inactive prodrug, but the ester is hydrolyzed rapidly.

The phosphate ester of clindamycin which is given parenterally is also hydrolyzed to active parent compound.

Dose: 150-300 mg 6 hourly.

Adverse effects

Diarrhoea is a common side effect (2%-20%), skin rashes in about 10% of patients.

Other less common side effects include exudative erythema multiforme (Stevens-Johnson syndrome), granulocytopenia, thrombocytopenia and anaphylactic reactions.

The most serious adverse effect of clindamycin is pseudomembranous colitis due to opportunistic infection of the bowel with *clostridium difficile* which produces an enterotoxin. If diarrhoea occurs the use of clindamycin should be stopped.

Local thrombophlebitis may follow i.v. administration.

Clindamycin can inhibit neuromuscular transmission and may potentiate the effect of neuromuscular blockers administered concurrently.

Vancomycin

It is an antibiotic produced by *Streptococcus orientalis*, an actinomycete isolated from soil samples obtained in Indonesia and India.

Vancomycin is bactericidal against several species of gram-positive and gram-negative cocci. It acts on multiplying organisms by inhibiting formation of the peptidoglycan component of the cell wall. It is given by I.V. route because of poor absorption by GIT and there is no suitable preparation for IM injection. Serum $t_{1/2}$ is 6 hours. Ototoxicity (auditory portion damage) limits its use.

Vancomycin should be given only to treat serious infections. It is particularly useful against methicillin-resistant staphylococci including pneumonia, empyema, endocarditis, oeteomyelitis. It is also very useful in severe stphylococcal infections in patients who are allergic to penicillins and cephalosporins.

Vancomycin can be administered orally to patients with pseudomembranous colitis, the dose for adults is 125-250 mg every 6 hours. Vancomycin hydrochloride oral solution is available for this purpose, as are capsules. The total daily dose for children is 40 mg/kg in 3-4 divided doses.

Vancomycin tends to cause thrombophlebitis so it is given diluted in isotonic saline 250 ml or glucose 5% and administered over 1 hour period to avoid infusion-related flushing.

Patients whose renal function is impaired are particularly at risk because the drug is excreted by the kidney.

Spectinomycin

It is produced by *streptomyces spectabilis*. The drug is an aminocyclitol. Its use is confined for the treatment of gonorrhoea caused by strains resistant to first-line drugs. It is also recommended as an alternative regimen in patients who are intolerant or allergic to beta-lactam antibiotics and quinolones.

Spectinomycin selectively inhibits protein synthesis in gram-negative bacteria. It binds to acts on the 30 S ribosomal subunit.

Its action has similarities to that of the aminoglycosides. However, it is not bactericidal.

A high degree bacterial resistance may develop as a result of mutation.

It is not active against *Chlamydia*.

Dose: Single deep I.M. injection of 2 g in adults.

Adverse effects include nausea, insomnia and dizziness.

Allergic reactions such as urticaria, chills and fever have occurred. The injection may be painful.

Sodium fusidate

It is a steroid antibiotic used almost exclusively against beta lactamase producing staphylococci.

The serum $t_{1/2}$ is 5 hours. It is readily absorbed from the gut and distributed widely including bone but not in CSF. The drug is metabolized, and very little is excreted unchanged in the urine.

It is an effective drug for the treatment of severe staphylococcal infections particularly for penicillin resistant organisms. As it penetrates well in bones it is effective in osteomyelitis.

Dose: 250-500 mg, 8 hourly orally; it can also be injected intravenously.

In the form of ointment or gel it is used topically for skin infections. Sodium fusidate is well tolerated.

The adverse effects include mild GI upsets, jaundice may appear with i.v. injection particularly with abnormal liver function. Oral route is preferable in-patients with abnormal liver function.

Novobiocin

Novobiocin is a bacteriostatic reserve drug for the treatment of resistant staphylococci.

Polymyxin B and colistin

Polypeptide group includes polymyxin B and colistin (polymyxin E) which are effective against gram-negative organisms, particularly *pseudomonas aeruginosa*. These are given topically for skin and external ear infection and bladder irrigation fluids.

Polymyxin B sulphate is available for ophthalmic, otic, and topical use in combination with a variety of other compounds. Colistin sulphate is marketed as a powder to be suspended in sterile water for injection.

Polymyxin B is similar in antibacterial spectrum to colistin. It is topically applied to skin, eye and ear infections and in bladder irrigation fluids. Other polymyxins are not used due to severe nephrotoxicity.

Polymyxins are a group of antibiotic substances elaborated by various strained of *Bacillus polymyxa*, an aerobic spore-forming rod found in soil. Colistin (polymyxin E) is produced by *Bacillus colistinus*.

Polymyxin B is a mixture of polymyxin B_1 and B_2.

The antibacterial activities of polymyxin B and colistin are similar and are restricted to gram-negative bacteria including *Enterobacter, E. coli, Klebsiella, Salmonella, Pasteurella, Bordetella* and *Shigella*. These are sensitive to concentrations of 0.05 to 2.0 mcg/ml. Most strains of *P. aeruginosa* are inhibited by less than 8 mcg/ml in vitro.

Owing to their significant toxicity with systemic administration, polymyxins are restricted to topical use. Ointments containing polymyxin B, 0.5 mg/g in mixtures with bacitracin or neomycin (or both) are commonly applied to infected superficial skin lesions. They are also poorly absorbed from skin (intact as well as denuded) and mucous membranes.

Polymyxin B and colistin are not absorbed when given orally.

Adverse effects

Due to complete lack of absorption from intact or denuded skin and mucous membranes, local application does not produce systemic reactions. Hypersensitivity is also uncommon. However, if large doses (600 mg) are taken orally, nausea, vomiting and diarrhoea may be produced.

Bacitracin

It is an antibiotic produced by Tracy-1 strain of *Bacillus subtilis*.

This antibiotic-producing bacillus was isolated from a compound fracture of tibia of a 7-year old girl named Tracy, hence named after her.

It is available in ophthalmic and dermatologic ointment, also available as powder for the preparation for topical solution. A number of topical preparations of bacitracin to which neomycin or polymyxin or both have been added are available, and some contain the three antibiotics with hydrocortisone.

Bacitracin is also nephrotoxic like other polypeptide antibiotics. It is used topically for skin, ocular and external ear infections and included in bladder irrigation fluids. However, bacitracin alone or in combination with other antimicrobial agents has no established value in the treatment of furunculosis, pyoderma, carbuncle, impetigo, and superficial and deep abscesses.

For open infections e.g. infected eczema and infected dermal ulcers, the local application is of some help in eradicating sensitive bacteria.

Suppurative conjunctivitis and infected corneal ulcer respond well to the topical use of bacitracin when they are caused by susceptible bacteria.

Oral bacitracin has been used with some success in case of antibiotic-induced diarrhoea caused by *Cl. difficile*.

Bacitracin is nephrotoxic like other polypeptide antibiotics.

Gramicidin

It has been used topically as creams and ointments for skin sepsis, combined with neomycin and framycetin.

Teicoplanin

It is a glycopeptide antibiotic produced by *Actinoplanes teichomycetius*. It is similar to vancomycin in chemical structure, mechanism of action, spectrum of activity and route of excretion (primarily renal).

It is an inhibitor of cell wall synthesis and it is active against only gram-positive bacteria. It is bactericidal.

Unlike vancomycin, teicoplanin can be given safely by i.m. injection, is highly bound to plasma proteins (95%) and has long elimination half-life (about 100 hours).

Dose: 6-30 mg/kg once a day.

Teicoplanin is used to treat a wide variety of infections including osteomyelitis and endocarditis caused by methicillin-resistant and methicillin-susceptible staphylococci, streptococci and enterococci. This drug is not as efficacious as antistaphylococcal penicillins for the treatment of bacteremia and endocarditis caused by methicillin-susceptible *S. aureus*.

Adverse effects

Skin rashes in higher dosages. Allergic reaction, drug fever, and neutropenia have been reported.

Ototoxicity has also been reported, though rarely.

STUDY QUESTIONS

1. Classify antibiotics on the basis of their molecular structure, giving suitable examples.
2. What are the drawbacks of benzylpenicillin and to what extent the semisynthetic penicillins have overcome these drawbacks?
3. Describe different penicillin preparations along with their doses.
4. Which antibiotics are bactericidal and which are bacteriostatic? What may happen if a bactericidal drug is combined with a bacteriostatic drug?
5. Describe the different cephalosporins (generation wise), their routes of administration, advantages and disadvantages.
6. What are broad spectrum antibiotics? Describe the pharmacology of tetracyclines and chloramphenicol. What are the main differences in their indications and adverse effects?
7. What is the mode of action of different antibiotics?
8. What are the contraindications and adverse effects of penicillin and tetracyclines?
9. What are the general properties of aminoglycoside antibiotics, their mode of action, therapeutic uses and adverse effects?
10. Write notes on (i) Vancomycin (ii) Clindamycin (iii) Polymyxins, and (iv) Metronidazole as antimicrobial.
11. Describe erythromycins—their indications, mode of action, antibacterial spectrum and adverse effects.
12. How do bacterial resistance develops to antibiotics? Give examples of cross-resistance among antibiotics.
13. Write notes on :
    (i) antimicrobial drug interactions,
    (ii) antimicrobial drug combinations and
    (iii) causes of failure of antimicrobial therapy and
    (iv) chemoprophylaxis.

GUIDE TO FURTHER READING

Beta-lactam antibiotics and cephalosporins

Barradell, L.B et al: A review of its antibacterial activity, pharmacokinetic properties and therapeutic use. Drugs, 1994; 47:471-505.

Barza, M et al: The nephrotoxicity of cephalosporins: an overview. J.Infect.Dis., 1978; 137:560-573.

Bennett, S et al: Pharmacokinetics and tissue penetration of ticarcillin combined with clavulanic acid. Antimicrob. Agents Chemother., 1983; 23:831-834.

Bryson, H.M et al: A review of its antibacterial activity, pharmacokinetic properties and therapeutic potential. Drugs, 1994; 47:506-535.

Catalan, M.J et al: Failure of cefotaxime in the treatment of meningitis due to relatively resistant Streptococcus pneumoniae. Clin. Infect. Dis., 1994; 18:766-769.

Centers for Disease Control and Prevention. Prevalence of penicillinresistant Streptococcus pneumoniae-Connecticut 1992-1993; MMWR, 1994; 43:216-217, 223.

Chambers, H.F et al: Penicillins. In, Mandell, Douglas, and Bennett's Principles and Practice of Infectious Diseases. 4th ed. John Wiley & Sons, Inc., New York, 1995; pp. 233-246.

Davies, J et al: Inactivation of antibiotics and the dissemination of resistance genes. Science, 1994; 264:375-382.

Durack, D.T et al: Prophylaxis in infective endocarditis. In, Mandell, Douglas, and Bennett's Principles and Practice of Infectious Diseases, 4th ed. Churchill Livingstone, Inc., New York, 1995; pp. 793-798.

John, C.C: Treatment failure with use of a third-generation cdphalosporin for penicillin-resistant pneumococcal meningitis:case report and review. Clin. Infect. Dis., 1994; 18:188-193.

Kancir, L.M et al: Adverse reactions to methicillin and nafcillin during treatment of serious Staphylococcus aureus infections. Arch. Intern. Med., 1978; 138:909-911.

Karchmer, A.W et al: Cephalosporins. In, Mandell, Douglas, and Bennett's Principles and Practice of Infectious Diseases, 4th ed. Churchill Livingstone, Inc., New York, 1995; pp. 247-263.

Levine, B.B et al: Antigenicity and cross reactivity of penicillins and cephalosporins. J. Infect. Dis., 1973; 128:S364-S366.

Nikaido, H et al: Prevention of drug access to bacterial targets: permeability barriers and active efflux. Science, 1994; 264:382-388.

Petz, L.D et al: Immunologic cross-reactivity between penicillins and cephalosporins: a review. J.Infect.Dis., 1978; 137:S74-S79.

Phillips, I et al: Cefotetan: a new cephamycin. J. Antimicrob. Chemother., 1983; 11 Suppl. A:1-303.

Spratt, B.G et al: Resistance to antibiotics mediated by target alterations. Science, 1994; 264:388-393.

Tomasz, A: Special report. Multiple-antibiotic-resistant pathogenic bacteria. A report on the Rockefeller University Workshop. New Engl. J. Med., 1994; 330:1247-1251.

Weiss, M.E et al: Beta-lactam allergy. In, Mandell, Douglas, and Bennett's Principles and Practice of Infectious Diseases, 4th ed. Churchill Livingstone, Inc., New York, 1995; pp. 272-277.

Broad spectrum antibiotics

al-Assi, M.T et al: Clarithromycin, tetracycline, and bismuth: a new non-metronidazole therapy for Helicobacter pylorei infection. Am.J.Gastroenterol., 1994; 89:1203-1205.

Black, J.R et al: Clindamycin and primaquine therapy for mild-to-moderate episodes of Pneumocystis cariniii pneumonia in patients with AIDS: AIDS clinical trials group 044. Clin. Infect. Dis., 1994; 18:905-913.

Centers for Disease Control. Sentinel surveillance for antimicrobial resistance in Neisseria gonorrhoeae-United States, 1988-1991., M.M.W.R., 1993a; 42:SS-3, 29-39.

Centers for Disease Control. Recommendations on prophylaxis and therapy for disseminated Mycobacterium avium complex for adults and adolescents infected with human immunodeficiency virus, 1988-M.M.W.R., 1993c; 42:RR-9, 17-20.

Centers for Disease Control. 1993 sexually transmitted diseases treatment guidelines, M.M.W.R., 1993b; 42:RR-14, 1-102.

Centers for Disease Control. Erythromycin-resistant Bordetella pertussis-Yuma County, Arizona, May-October 1994. M.M.W.R., 1994; 43:807-810.

Elmore, M.F et al: Tetracycline induced pancreatitis. Gastroenterology, 1981; 81:1134-1136.

Fraschini, F et al: Clarithromycin clinical pharmacokinetics. Clin. Pharmacokinet., 1993; 25:189-204.

Friedman, I.R et al: Management of infections caused by antibiotic-resistant Streptococcus pneumoniae. N. Engl. J. Med., 1994; 331:377-382.

Ji, B et al: Powerful bactericidal activities of clarithromycin and minocycline against Mycobacterium leprae in lepromatous leprosy. J. Infect. Dis., 1993; 168:188-190.

Jimenez, J.J et al: Chloramphenicol-induced bone marrow injury: possible role of bacterial metabolites of chloramphenicol. Blood, 1987; 70:1180-1185.

Periti, P et al: Pharmacokinetic drug interactions of macrolides. Clin. Pharmacokinet., 1992; 23:106-131.

Peters, D.H et al: Azethromycin- a review of its antimicrobial activity, pharmacokinetic properties, and clinical efficacy. Drugs., 1992; 44:750-799.

Saba, J et al: Pyrimethamine plus Azethromycin for treatment of acute toxoplasmic encephalitis in patients with AIDS. Eur.J.Clin.Microbiol. Infect.Dis., 1993; 12:853-856.

Speer, B.S et al: Bacterial resistance to tetracycline: mechanisms, transfer, and clinical significance. Clin. Microbiol. Rev., 1992; 5:387-399.

Standiford, N.H et al: Tetracyclines and chloramphenicol. In, Mandell, Douglas, and Bennett's Principles and Practice of Infections Diseases, 4th ed. Churchill Livingstone, New York, 1995; pp. 306-317.

Steigbigel, N.H et al: Macrolides and clindamycin.In, Mandell, Douglas, and Bennett's Principles and Practice of Infections Diseases, 4th ed. Churchill Livingstone, New York, 1995; pp. 334-346.

Walsh, C.T et al: Vancomycin resistance: decoding the molecular logic. Science, 1993; 261:308-309.

Yu, V.L. Legionella pneumophilla. In, Mandell, Douglas, and Bennett's Principles and Practice of Infections Diseases, 4th ed. Churchill Livingstone, New York, 1995; pp. 2087-2097.

Aminoglycosides

Blaser, J: Efficacy of once-and thrice-daily dosing of aminoglycosides in in-virto models on infection. J. Antimicrob. Chemother., 1991; 27:Suppl. C:21-28.

Bock, B.V et al: Prospective comparative study of efficacy and toxicity of netilmicin and amikacin. Antimicrob. Agents Chemother., 1980; 17:217-225.

Davies, J: Inactivation of antibiotics and the dissemination of resistance genes. Science, 1994; 264:375-382.

Fong, I.W et al: Comparative toxicity of gentamicin versus tobramycin: a randomized prospective study. J. Antimicrob. Chemother., 1981; 7:81-88.

McCormack, J.P et al: A critical reevaluation of the "therapeutic range" of aminoglycosides. Clin. Infect. Dis., 1992; 14:320-339.

Murray, B.E: New aspects of antimicrobial resistance and the resulting therapeutic dilemmas. J. Infect. Dis., 1991; 163:1184-1194.

Prins, J.M et al: Once versus thrice daily gentamicin in patients with serious infections. Lancet, 1993; 341:335-339.

Sanford, J.P et al: The Sanford Guide to Antimicrobial Therapy. Antimicrobial Therapy, Inc., Dallas, TX, 1994; p. 104.

ORGANIC SYNTHETIC ANTIMICROBIALS

SULPHONAMIDES

Sulphanilamide was the first antimicrobial agent effective against pyogenic bacterial infections. But it was soon found to possess narrow therapeutic index and therefore a number of its derivatives were synthesized which have higher potency and are safer than the parent compound.

The term sulphonamide is used as a generic name for the derivatives of sulphanilamide (paraaminobenzene sulphonamide).

Sulphonamides are described as a group as they have many similar properties. They are all poorly water soluble, white crystalline powders. These are weak acids and form salts with bases. Their sodium salts are readily soluble in water.

Antibacterial spectrum

Sulphonamides are effective against many gram-positive organisms and some gram-negative diplococci and bacilli. They are also effective against *Actinomyces*, *Nocardia*, *Chlamydia*, and some protozoa.

These drugs are effective in infections due to group A *streptococci*, *H. influenzae*, *Haemophilus ducreyi*, *pneumococci*, *E. coli*, *Brucella*, *P. pestis*, *B. anthracis*, *Corynebacterium diptheria*, *Cholera vibrio*, *Nocardia*, *Actinomycetes* and large viruses (producing psittacosis, lymphogranuloma inguinale and trachoma).

Gonococci, *meningococci* and *shigella* are variably sensitive. Many strains of *Klebsiella*, *Enterobacter* and *Proteus* are sensitive only with high concentrations obtained in the urine.

Many *staphylococci*, *enterococci*, *clostridia* and *pseudomonas* are highly resistant.

Acquired Bacterial Resistance

The main reason for the development of bacterial resistance is inadequate dosage. Resistance develops through 'variation by selection' which occurs slowly and is usually permanent.

The resistant mutants either (i) produce increased amounts of para amino benzoic acid (PABA), or (ii) their folates synthetase enzyme has low affinity for sulphonamides, or (iii) adopt an alternative pathway in folate metabolism.

Cross resistance occurs among sulphonamides, i.e. bacteria resistant to one sulphonamide is usually resistant to all sulphonamides.

Mode of Action

Sulphonamides are essentially bacteriostatic in the therapeutic doses. However, they act as bactericidal in the treatment of urinary tract infections as high concentrations are obtained in the urine.

Many bacteria synthesize their own folic acid of which PABA is a constituent and taken up from the medium. There is a close chemical similarity between PABA and sulphonamides. Therefore sulphonamides act as competitive inhibitors of the bacterial enzymes responsible for the incorporation of PABA into dihydropteric acid (immediate precursor of folic acid). Depletion of folic acid in bacteria inhibits formation of co-enzymes required for the formation of purines and pyrimidines which are essential for bacterial growth and reproduction. The bacteria which utilize preformed folic acid are not susceptible to sulphonamides.

The presence of any source of PABA e.g. pus, blood and tissue exudates at the site of infection diminishes the antibacterial activity of sulphonamides by displacing them from bacteria. However, sulphamylon (marfanil) activity is not diminished by PABA as it acts differently.

Sulphanilamide   PABA

Pharmacokinetics

The absorption of N′ substituted sulphonamides employed for systemic purposes is prompt and almost complete from small intestine. After absorption they are widely distributed in the body, enter serous cavities easily, pass through placental barrier and penetrate into cerebrospinal fluid in concentration of 35% to 75% of the concentration found in the blood. However, the free form of sulphadiazine, sulfisoxazole and sulphamerazine attain almost same concentration in CSF as in plasma.

In plasma, the sulphonamides are present both in free as well as in bound form with albumin. The free form is pharmacologically active. They are bound to serum proteins from 20% to 90%. Sulphadiazine, sulphamethoxazole and sulfisoxazole are bound to serum proteins to the extent of 50, 60 and 90% respectively. The long acting sulphonamides are highly protein bound, about 95%. The drug is released from bound form to the active free form in the blood. The optimum therapeutic blood level is about 10 mg/100 ml.

The primary and major pathway of biotransformation is acetylation in liver. The acetylated products are devoid of antibacterial activity but retain the toxic potentiality (crystalluria i.e. precipitation of acetylated metabolites in urine, the crystals formed may cause bleeding or obstruction of the kidney).

The acetylated (metabolites) products are less soluble in acidic urine. In order to avoid crystalluria, adequate amounts of water should be taken, urine made alkaline and employ mixture of sulphonamides as the presence of one sulphonamide does not affect the solubility of other sulphonamides in water or urine. A small amount of sulphonamides is conjugated with glucuronic acid.

Kidney filters the free fraction through glomeruli, a portion of the filtered drug is reabsorbed from renal tubules. The concentration in urine may be as much as 25 to 50 times higher than in plasma. This makes them particularly useful for the treatment of urinary tract infection.

Excretion is in both free and inactive acetylated forms, mainly in urine.

Classification according to pharmacokinetic properties

1. Promptly absorbed and excreted rapidly: employed to treat systemic infections:
   (a) Short acting sulphonamides (4-8 hours):
      - Sulphadiazine
      - Sulphamethizole
      - Sulphamethazine (Sulphadimidine)
      - Sulphamerazine
      - Sulphasomidine
      - Sulfisoxazole (Sulphafurazole).

      Dose: 2-3 g initial, 1 g/6 hourly.
      Half-life: 4-8 hrs.
   (b) Intermediate acting (8-16 hours):
      - Sulphamethoxazole
      - Sulphaphenazole.

Dose: 1-2 g initial, 0.5-1.0 g/12 hourly.

(c) Agents absorbed rapidly and excreted slowly i.e. long-acting (1-7 days):
  • Sulphamethoxypyridazine
  • Sulphamethopyrazine
  • Sulphadimethoxine
  • Sulphadoxine

Dose: 1 g initial, 0.5 g/12-24 hourly.

2. Agents absorbed poorly or not absorbed: employed as intestinal antiseptics. These are used for local action in GIT.
  • Sulphaguanidine
  • Succinylsulphathiazole
  • Phthalylsulphathiazole

Following oral administration and on reaching large intestine they are hydrolyzed by bacteria and sulphathiazole is liberated which is not well absorbed in the large intestine.

Dose: 2 g initial, 1 g/4 hourly.

3. Topically employed sulphonamides: Silver sulphadiazine and Mafenide (Sulphamylon) for infected wounds and burn dressings.

Sulphacetamide for infections in the eye, 1-2 drops of a 10-30% solution, 3-4 times a day.

4. Sulphonamides for special uses:
  • Sulphapyridine in dermatitis herpetiformis.
  • Sulphasalazine in ulcerative colitis.

Comparison of Sulphonamides/Choice

Sulphanilamide, sulphapyridine and sulphathiazole are not used now due to their greater toxicity and greater incidence of hypersensitivity reactions.

Among the commonly used sulphonamides, sulphadiazine crosses the blood-brain barrier more effectively than the others.

Sulphamethazine and Sulphamerazine are excreted more slowly by the kidney and bound to plasma protein to a greater extent than sulphadiazine.

Sulfisoxazole (Gantrisin) is about ten times more soluble at pH 6 than sulphadiazine and is not readily reabsorbed from the renal tubules. These factors make this drug superior in the treatment of urinary tract infections.

Sulfisomidine (Elkosin) is also very useful in urinary tract infections.

Sulphacetamide sodium is water soluble and its chief use is as a topical drug in ophthalmic infections as it is almost neutral (pH 7.4) and so non-irritant in contrast to the strong alkalinity of other sulphonamides. It penetrates into ocular fluids and tissues in high concentrations. The usual dose is 1-2 drops of a 10%-30% solution 3-4 times a day. An ophthalmic ointment may be used provided there is no wound in the cornea. Sulphacetamide is antagonistic to the inhibition of pseudomonas by gentamicin. Gentamicin inhibits pseudomonas growth at 7 mcg/ml levels, in the presence of sulphacetamide gentamicin levels of 15 mcg/ml are required for inhibition.

The intermediate acting systemic sulphonamides such as sulphamethoxazole is combined with trimethoprim. The combination product is bactericidal.

The long-acting sulphonamides such as sulphamethoxypyridazine and sulphadimethoxine are strongly bound to serum protein. These are rarely used due to greater incidence of hypersensitivity reactions. Sulphadoxine is a very long-acting drug (once a week) given with pyrimethamine for the prophylaxis of malaria.

The poorly absorbed or hardly absorbed sulphonamides such as sulphaguanidine, succinylsulphathiazole and phthalylsulphathiazole are used only for local effect in bowel lumen against Shigella infections (bacillary dysentery) and to sterilize the gut before bowel surgery. But *Proteus, Pseudomonas, Salmonella* and entercocci are usually resistant.

The structures of some sulphonamides are shown in Fig. 11.6 and certain characteristics in Table 11.7.

Table 11.7. Characteristics of some sulphonamides used systemically

	Serum half-life (hrs)	Protein binding (%)	Solubility in urine
Sulphadiazine	17	40-60	+
Sulphamethazine	7	60-80	+++
Sulfisoxazole	6	90	+++
Sulphamethoxazole	11	85-90	+
Sulphamethizole	2.5	90	+++
Sulphacetamide	12	20	+++

Short-acting sulphonamides

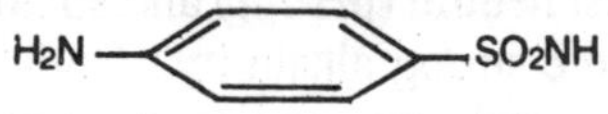

Sulphanilamide

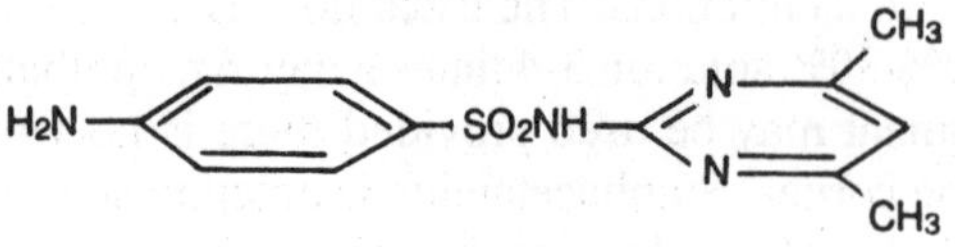

Sulphamethazine

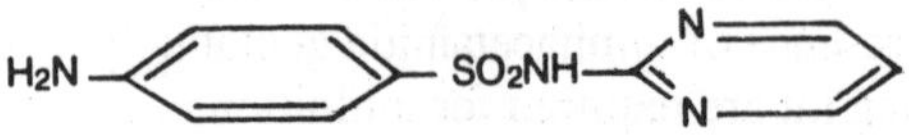

Sulphadiazine

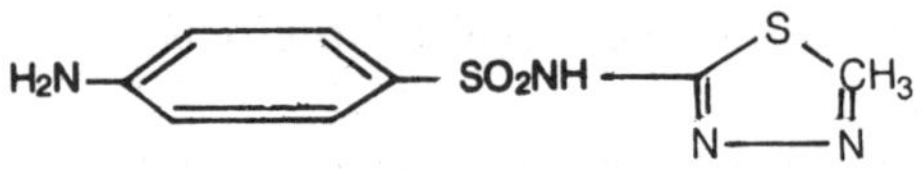

Sulphamethizole

Intermediate-acting sulphonamides

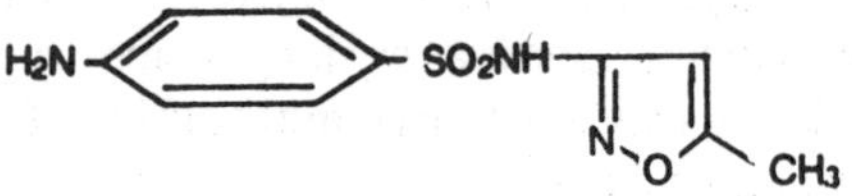

Sulphamethoxazole

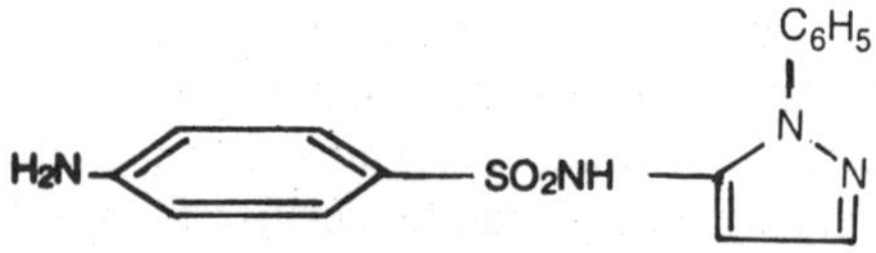

Sulphaphenazole

Topical sulphonamides

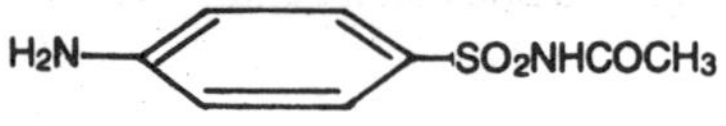

Sulphacetamide

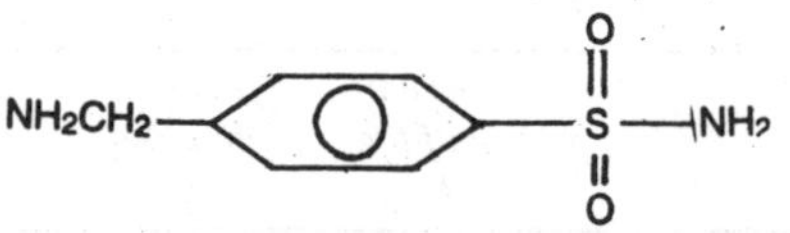

Mafenide

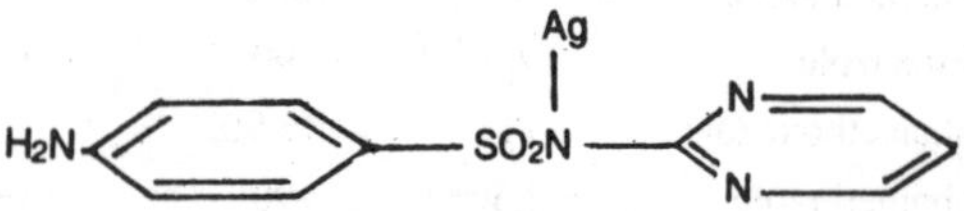

Silver sulphadiazine

Fig. 11.6. Structures of some sulphonamides.

Routes of administration

1. Oral: The systemic sulphonamides are generally given orally as they are promptly and completely absorbed from GIT. The poorly absorbed sulphonamides are given orally for their local action in the intestinal lumen.

2. Parenteral: If given parenterally, sodium salts e.g. sodium sulphadiazine can be given by I.V. injection (in about 10 min.). I.M or SC routes are not good as the salts are irritant to the tissues. They are never given intrathecally due to irritant effect.

3. Topical: Topical application is undesirable as the effectiveness is decreased by pus and sensitization is fairly common. However, there are certain exceptions, e.g. Mafenide acetate as cream or mafenide HCl solution are applied topically to infected wounds and for the treatment of burns. These are not inactivated by pus. Strictly speaking, mafenide is not a typical sulphonamide. It has CH_2 between the benzene ring and the amino group.

Sulphacetamide sodium salt is applied locally in infections of the eye.

Clinical uses

Due to availability of better antimicrobial agents, the usefulness of sulphonamides has decreased. However, they still continue to have some important role in the following conditions:

- Urinary tract infections (UTIs) caused by *E.coli* and some strains of *proteus* respond adequately. They are particularly useful in UTIs as bactericidal concentrations are reached in the urine. They are also useful in nocardiosis, trachoma and chancroid.

- Besides the use of promptly absorbed sulphonamides for systemic purposes, the poorly absorbed sulphonamides can be used as intestinal antiseptics. In bacillary dysentery they are of second choice to ampicillin.

- Their preoperative use before bowel surgery is of doubtful value.

- For topical application the sulphonamides used are (i) sulphacetamide sodium for ophthalmic infections such as trachoma and inclusion conjunctivitis, (ii) silver sulphadiazine in burns, mafenide topically is not inactivated by pus or PABA.

- For special use sulphapyridine has been found useful in dermatites herpetiformis (unrelated to antibacterial property).

Box 11.6. Sulphonamides

Clinical uses

Absolute indications are very few but may be used as follows:

- Combined with pyrimethamine for drug-resistant malaria and for toxoplasmosis.
- For infected burns, silverdiazine applied topically.
- Combined with trimethoprim (co-trimoxazole) as antimicrobial, for Pneumocystis carini.
- Inflammatory bowel disease and as an antiinflammatory drug—sulphasalazine.
- For certain respiratory infections e.g. infection with Nocardia.
- For some sexually transmitted infections.

Adverse effects

The common side effects are nausea, vomiting and anorexia. The serious toxic effects include nephrosis, crystalluria, haematuria, haemolytic anaemia in an individual with G-6-PD deficiency, other types of blood dyscrasias such as agranulocytosis, and thrombocytopenia may also occur. CNS disturbances (depression, ataxia, confusion), endocrinal disturbances (goiter) and hepatitis may also occur though rarely.

Kernicterus specially in premature neonates may occur by displacing bilirubin from plasma protein binding sites.

The hypersensitivity reactions may be in the form of rashes, urticaria, fever, contact dermatitis, serum sickness, Stevens-Johnson syndrome and polyarteritis nodosa (rare).

The bone marrow aplasia may be allergic in nature as well as due to myelotoxic effect of sulphonamides.

Interactions

Sulphonamides and methenamines should not be given simultaneously for the treatment of urinary tract infections. The formaldehyde liberated from methenamine in acid urine forms a precipitate with some of the sulphonamides.

The effects of oral hypoglycaemic agents such as tolbutamide and that of oral anticoagulants (coumarin derivatives) are enhanced as sulphonamides displace these from plasma binding sites.

The effect of dilantin (phenytoin sodium) is increased due to inhibition of its metabolism (breakdown) in the liver by sulphonamides.

Contraindications

- Avoid use of sulphonamides during pregnancy as folic acid antagonists are teratogenic in experimental animals.
- Sulphonamides should also not be used in infants to avoid kernicterus.
- They are also not recommended in the presence of hepatic and renal impairment.

Sulphonamide-antibiotic combinations

Sulphadiazine plus streptomycin or chloramphenicol are more effective against *Haemophilus influenzae*.

Sulphadiazine plus penicillin are more useful in actinomycosis and anthrax.

Sulphonamide-trimethoprim combination (Co-trimoxazole): The usefulness of sulphonamides has increased with the introduction of trimethoprim-sulphamethoxazole synergistic combintion of antibacterial agents.

Sulphamethoxazole 400 mg and Trimethoprim (pyrimidine derivative) 80 mg (5 : 1 ratio) combination has synergistic action. The combination is bactericidal while individually both have bacteriostatic activity, because they block two consecutive steps in bacterial metabolism as shown below. The sequential blockade produced by the combination of the two results in a synergistic inhibition of the folic acid biosynthetic pathway (Fig. 11.7). This converts the two bacteriostic compounds into a bactercidal combination.

Sulphamethoxazole is selected over other sulphonamides as both are absorbed and excreted almost at about same rate. The half-life (10 hours) of both in man is similar.

Co-trimoxazole is effective against a variety of gram-positive and gram-negative organisms.

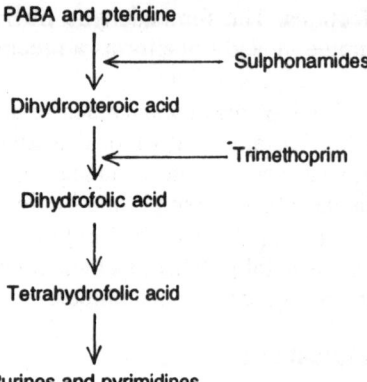

PABA and pteridine

     ←——————— Sulphonamides

Dihydropteroic acid

     ←——————— Trimethoprim

Dihydrofolic acid

Tetrahydrofolic acid

Purines and pyrimidines

Fig. 11.7. Site of action of sulphonamides and trimethoprim.

The absorption is rapid and produces effective concentration for 6 to 8 hours. Both the drugs are excreted unchanged mostly in urine.

Trimethoprim is about 50,000 times more active against bacterial dihydrofolate reductase enzyme compared to this enzyme from mammalian source. The human folate metabolism is thus unaffected by trimethoprim.

Structure of Trimethoprim

Trimethoprim 90 mg plus sulphadiazine 410 mg is another combination called co-trimazine.

Trimethoprim (diaminopyrimidine derivative) is related to antimalarial pyrimethamine.

Recently trimethoprim has been used alone and found as effective as the combination preparation in urinary tract and respiratory tract infections. This also avoids the adverse effects of sulphonamides. For acute conditions it is given in doses of 200 mg twice a day and for long time use 100 mg twice a day is recommended.

Trimethoprim is well absorbed from GIT and widely distributed including CSF. It crosses the blood-brain and placental barriers.

The excretion is mainly by the kidney.

Its half-life is 11 hours.

Trimethoprim concentrates in prostatic fluid and vaginal fluid, thereby exhibits more antibacterial action in these fluids as compared to other drugs.

Trimethoprim is an antifolate drug and therefore it can produce megaloblastic anaemia, leukopenia and granulocytopenia. Other adverse effects include nausea, vomiting, diarrhoea, skin rashes, anorexia. Long-term use can interfere with haematopoiesis. The simultaneous administration of folinic acid, 6 to 8 mg per day can prevent these adverse effects.

Indications and choice

The combination is indicated in urinary tract infections (*E. coli*, *B. proteus*), upper respiratory tract infections, shigellosis (bacterial diarrhoea and dysentery), cholera, enteric fever, gonorrhoea, *H. influenzae*, and vivax and falciparum malaria.

The prime indications are in the treatment of acute and chronic recurrent urinary tract infections and also very useful in upper respiratory tract infections including chronic bronchitis. In typhoid it is a second choice to chloramphenicol. It is effective in shigella and salmonella infections if these are resistant to ampicillin and chloramphenicol. In gonorrhoea it is of second choice to penicillin or ampicillin.

Dosage: 400 mg sulphamethoxazole plus 80 mg trimethoprim tablet, 1-2 tablets twice a day orally. The double strength tablets (800 mg + 160 mg) are also available.

200 mg sulphamethoxazole plus 40 mg trimethoprim/5 ml as suspension for oral route, 800 mg + 160 mg/3 ml for I.M. and 400 mg + 80 mg/5 ml for I.V. injection are available. The I.V. infusion is diluted in 125 ml of 5% dextrose solution given in 60 to 90 minutes.

The dose for children is 40 mg/kg sulphamethoxazole plus 8 mg/kg/trimethoprim, every 12 hourly.

The development of resistance seems to develop slowly to this combination.

Adverse effects

The combination preparations may show similar adverse effects as following the use of sulphonamides, such as mild CNS disturbances, skin rashes, blood dyscrasias, etc. Patients with AIDS have a particularly high frequency of adverse reactions to this combination, especially fever, rashes, diarrhoea and leukopenia.

Crystalluria is less likely to occur, but it has been reported that if diuretics are given along with co-trimoxazole, the incidence of thrombocytopenia is increased.

Caution

The combination preparation should be cautiously used in malnutrition states (low folic acid level) or in patients receiving phenytoin.

Contraindications

Patients with blood dyscrasias, hepatic damage, severe renal impairment, below one year of age and during pregnancy (folic acid inhibitors are teratogenic experimentally).

NITROFURANS

These are 5-nitro-2-furaldehyde derivatives used in the treatment of microbial infections.

The nitrofurans are broad-spectrum compounds that are active against gram-positive and gram-negative bacteria. They inhibit *E. coli*, *Klebsiella*, *Enterobacter*, *Salmonella*, *Shigella* and *Vibrio cholerae* as well as staphylococci and enterococci. However, most *Proteus* and *Pseudomonas aeruginosa* are resistant.

The three nitofuran derivatives are (i) nitrofurazone a local antiseptic for topical use (ii) furazolidone an intestinal antiseptic (not absorbed from GIT) and (iii) nitrofurantoin a urinary antiseptic.

Nitrofurantoin is used in the treatment of uncomplicated lower urinary tract infections although sulfonamides or antibiotics are generally the agents of choice. It is used prophylactically and for long term suppressive therapy. It is taken orally and plasma half-life is 0.3-1 hour. The absorption depends on crystal size.

The drug is absorbed from GIT and excreted in effective antimicrobial concentration in urine. The macrocrystalline form has slower absorption rates than the microcrystalline form. It is bacteriostatic and bacteriocidal according to the concentration attained in urine. It acts best in acidic medium at pH 5.5 or less.

Nitrofurazone is used topically and is not readily absorbed from the skin. It is occasionally used in the treatment of burns or skin grafts, in which bacterial contamination may cause rejection.

Dose: 400 mg orally in divided doses.

Contraindications : Severe renal insufficiency.

Structure of nitrofurazone

Adverse effects

They are dose related and generally include nausea, vomiting and anorexia.

Allergic reactions include skin rashes, urticaria, pruritis, fever and angioneurotic oedema. Acute pulmonary sensitive reactions characterised by sudden onset of fever, chills, cough, chest pain, dyspnoea, pulmonary infiltration, and pleural effusion associated with eosinophilia may occur within hours to a few days of beginning therapy, but these usually disappear with cessation of therapy. Chronic pulmonary symptoms including interstitial pneumonitis and pulmonary fibrosis may develop in patients on long term therapy and these are not always reversible.

Nitrofurantoin has also been associated with peripheral neuropathy, most notably in patients with impaired renal function.

Other adverse effects include megaloblastic anaemia, agranulocytosis, and haemolytic anaemia in persons with a genetic deficiency of glucose-6-phosphate dehydrogenase.

Nitrofurazone in a relatively safe topical agent, although skin sensitization has been reported.

Structure of Nitrofurantoin

QUINOLONES

A number of agents belong to this groups such as nalidixic acid, oxolinic acid, cinoxacin, enoxacin, norfloxacin, ciprofloxacin, pefloxacin, ofloxacin. All the agents available are 4-quinolones.

Nalidixic acid and oxolinic acid are synthetic chemicals useful against gram-negative bacteria but certain strains of *Enterobacter, Klebsiella, Proteus* and *Psuedomonas* are generally resistant. These are readily absorbed from GIT, 20% excreted in active form and 80% as glucuronide conjugate (inactive form) in urine.

Dose of nalidixic acid is 1 gm orally six hourly for 1-2 weeks, and the dose of oxalinic acid is 0.75 gm twice a day.

Resistance develops quickly but there is no cross resistance with other antibacterial agents.

Adverse effects include GI upsets, CNS stimulation and visual disturbances. CNS stimulation including convulsions appear to be more frequent with oxolinic acid. However, these older drugs are of relatively minor significance now because of their limited therapeutic utility and the rapid emergence of bacterial resistance.

The recently introduced fluorinated 4-quinolones such as ciprofloxacin are considered to be important advancement in antimicrobials. These agents have broad antimicrobial activity and are effective orally for the treatment of wide range of infections. Relatively few side effects are associated with these fluoroquinolones and microbial resistance does not develop rapidly.

Box 11.7. Effects of fluoroquinolones

- All are active against N. gonorrhea, H. influenzae, Moraxella catarrhalis, and against most organisms causing bacterial gastroenteritis.
- Ciprofloxacin is most active against P. aeruginosa among other fluoroquinolones.
- In general, penicillins and cephalosporins are more effective than fluoroquinolones against staphylocci and streptococci.
- Pneumococci and group A streptococci are resistent to enoxacin.
- Fluoroquinolones do not inhibit T. pallidum.

The antibacterial activity of nalidixic acid and the chemically related compounds cinoxacin and oxolinic acid includes most of the common gram-negative bacteria that cause urinary tract infections such as *E. coli, Klebsiella* and *Proteus. Pseudomonas aeruginosa* is resistant.

The newer agents, the fluoroquinolones are more potent than nalidixic acid against *E. coli* and various species of *Salmoella, Shigella, Enterobacter* and pneumococci. These agents have the additional advantage of possessing high activity against gonococci, staphylococci including methicillin resistant strains. These also have activity against *pseudomonas aeruginosa.* The quinolones have poor activity against anaerobic microorganisms.

The fluoroquinolones are all well tolerated when administered orally. Most clinical experience regarding the fluoroquinolones has been gained with ciprofloxacin. The bioavailability of ciprofloxacin is about 60%.

Ofloxacin and pefloxacin belong to the new generation of fluoroquinolones. The antimicrobial activity is similar to that of ciprofloxacin in general. Ofloxacin is also active in vitro, against some anaerobes like *Bacteroides fragilis, Clostridium* spp., *Gardnerella vaginitis. M. tuberculi* and *M. leprae* are also susciptible to it. These are less active than ciprofloxacin against *Pseudomonas aeruginosa.* These fluoroquinolones are superior to ciprofloxacin in their bioavailability and pharmacokinetic profile (Table 11.8). Among the commonly used fluoroquinolones, pefloxacin has the maximum bioavailability and longest half-life.

Mode of action of quinolones

The quinolines target bacterial gyrase and topoisomerase IV.

For many gram-negative bacteria, DNA gyrase is the primary quinolone target. For many gram-positive bacteria, quinolones block the decatenating activity of topoisomerase IV.

The individual stands of double-helical DNA must be separated for replication or transcription, which results in "overwinding" (excessive positive supercoiling). The bacterial DNA gyrase combats this mechanical obstacle by introducing negative supercoils in DNA. The DNA gyrase consists of two A and two B subunits. A subunits have strand-cutting

Table 11.8. Characterstics of clinically useful quinolones

Drug	Dose (mg)	Oral bioavailability in (%)	Max. blood level in (hrs)	Peak plasma concentration (mcg/ml)	Plasma half-life (hrs)	Plasma protein binding (%)
Ciprofloxacin	500	50-85	1-2	2.4	4	20-35
Norfloxacin	400	30-40	1	1.4	3	15
Pefloxacin	400	90-100	1-1.5	4.3	6-13	20-30
Ofloxacin	200	85-95	1-2	2.6	5-7	20
Nalidixic acid	1000	90-100	1-2	20-50	1.5	95

function and resealing the strands. The B submits introduce negative supercoils. This is an ATP dependent reaction requiring that both strands of the DNA be cut to permit passage of a segment of DNA through the break; the break is then sealed. Quinolones bind to subunits A and interfere with nicking and resealing function.

The schematic representation of mode of action is given in Fig. 11.8.

Table 11.9 shows spectrum of activity of certain fluoroquinlones.

Clinical applications of quinolones

Nalidixic acid and oxolinic acid are active against most gram-negative bacteria associated with urinary tract infections, but certain strains of *proteus* and *pseudomonas aeruginosa* are generally resistant. They are effective urinary tract antiseptic and this remains the main indicaton. Howver, bacteria can become resistant quickly to the drug if used for lengthy periods and so it is not recommended for long term chemoprophylaxis of urinary tract

Table 11.9. Fluroquinolones

Drugs	Comments
Classical Fluoroquinolones	
Ciprofloxacin	Intermediate spectrum, good distribution
Norfloxacin	Incomplete oral absorption, limited spectrum
Ofloxacin	Intermediate spectrum
Levofloxacin	More active than ofloxacin, long acting
Enoxacin	Limited spectrum
Lomefloxacin	Intermediate spectrum, photoxicity
Pefloxacin	Intermediate spectrum, long acting, phototoxicity
New Fluoroquinolones	
Sparfloxacin	Expanded spectrum, long acting, serious phototoxicity problems
Grepafloxacin	Expanded spectrum, long acting
Trovafloxacin	Expanded spectrum, no effect on drug metabolizing enzymes

infections. However, there is no cross resistance with other antibacterial agents.

Both oxolinic acid and cinoxacin are indicated for the treatment of urinary tract infections. They hardly appear to offer any advantage over nalidixic acid.

Among the new quinolones, the fluoroquinolones, most experience has been gained with ciprofloxacin. The primary uses of fluroquinolones are in urinary tract infections, enteric infections, respiratory infections including those in cystic fibrosis, gonorrhoea, obstetrical and gynaecological infections, bone and joint and skin and soft tissue infections. They are also indicated in typhoid fever and prophylaxis in granulocytopenic and immunocompromised patients, and in eye infections.

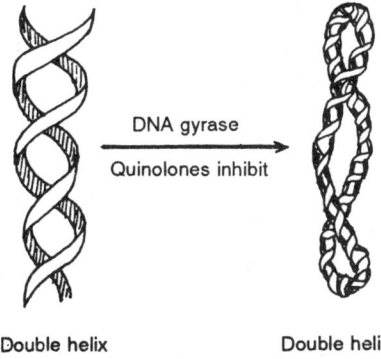

Double helix   Double helix in supercoiled form

DNA gyrase
Quinolones inhibit

Fig. 11.8.

Ciprofloxacin and norfloxacin are recommended for use in urinary tract infections, even those caused by *pseudomonas aeruginosa* or other multiple antibiotic resistant organisms. These drugs are active against most urinary pathogens. They also inhibit the growth of aerobic gram-negative faecal, vaginal, and periurethral flora which form the reservoir of pathogenic bacteria for reinfection and emergence of resistance during treatment.

Ciprofloxacin and ofloxacin given in single oral doses of 250-500 mg and 200 mg respectively are effective against uro-genital gonococcol infections, and probably also against rectal and pharyngeal infections. These are the drugs of choice in *Neisseria gonorrhoea* infections. These are also effective against *Chlamydia trachomatis*, ofloxacin being the most active among quinolones.

Ciprofloxacin and norfloxacin are highly effective in the treatment of enteric infections. Properties which make them highly effective are lack of plasmid mediated resistance, very low minimum inhibitory concentration (MIC) for pathogenic enteric bacteria. the high drug concentrations achieved in faeces and the preservation of the anaerobic bowel flora during treatment.

Ciprofloxacin is the drug of first choice against organisms such as *Campylobacter jejuni*, *Salmonella* and *Shigella*. Ciprofloxacin is effective for the treatment of typhoid fever, even in patients with chloramphenicol resistant strains.

Ciprofloxacin and ofloxacin levels in bones exceed 50% of the simultaneous serum levels. This offers sufficient drug concentrations to kill most strains of Enterobacteraceae, Staphylococci and *Pseudomonas aeruginosa* and makes them effective in osteomyelitis and chronic osteitis.

Ciprofloxacin and ofloxacin are effective in both upper and lower respiratory tract infections including those caused by pseudomonas in patients with cystic fibrosis. Pefloxacin is effective in the treatment of severe pulmonary infections. The susceptible organisms include *Strep. viridans*, *Pseudomonas aeruginosa*, *K. pneumoniae*, *S. aureus*, *Streptococcus* spp., *Proteus mirabilis*, *E. coli*, *Enterobacter*, *H. influenzae*, *Moraxella catarrhalis*, *Strep. pneumoniae*, *Providencia*, *Serratia marcescens* and beta-haemolytic streptococci.

Ciprofloxacin is recommended for selective decontamination of the gastrointestinal tract in granulocytopenic patients.

Ofloxacin and pefloxacin penetrate into tissues and body fluids better making them useful in variety of difficult infections. These agents are of value in treating immunocompromised patients.

Ofloxacin and ciprofloxacin are used in the treatment of eye infections. Ofloxacin is used as a 0.3% eye drops in a variety of eye infections including acute and subacute conjunctivitis, mucopurulent conjunctivitis, blepharitis, bacterial corneal ulcer, bacterial keratitis and keratoconjunctivitis, chronic dacryocystitis, prophylaxis in ocular surgery, postoperative infections and external ocular infections.

Most anaerobic microorganisms are resistant to fluoroquinolones except sparfloxacin.

Adverse effects

Quinolones and fluoroquinolones are generally well tolerated.

The most frequent adverse effects associated with the quinolones are nausea and other gastrointestinal disturbances. Allergic reactions have been reported, e.g., photosensitivity, rashes, urticaria and eosinophilia. CNS effects such as drowsiness, weakness, headache, dizziness and in severe cases convulsions and toxic psychosis, have also been reported. Crystalluria may occur with high doses of fluoroquinolones, which can be avoided by maintaining an adequate fluid intake during treatment.

It has been reported that all these agents can cause arthropathy and erosions of cartilage in several species of immature animals. Arthralgias and foot swelling have developed in children receiving fluoroquinolones. Hence, they are not recommended for use in patients younger than 18 years of age, or for pregnant or nursing mothers.

Emergence of resistance is occurring and is significant, especially concerning the treatment of infections caused by *S. aureus* and *P. aeruginosa*.

AGENTS FOR URINARY TRACT INFECTION (UTI)

Urinary tract infection is a common condition. About 95% cases are due to gram-negative organisms. *E. coli* is an invader in about 80% cases. Other organisms are *Proteus, Pseudomonas, Aerobacter aerogenes, Str. faecalis* and *staphylococci.*

Many systemic antimicrobial drugs are excreted in high concentration in urine. Doses much below those necessary to achieve systemic effects can therefore be of therapeutic value in infections of the urinary tract.

Systemically active drugs in urinary tract infection

Chemotherapeutic agents

(a) Sulphonamides: These are effective against most of the pathogens responsible for UTI especially *E. coli* and *Proteus.* Sulphasomidine (elkosin) and sulphamezathine are commonly employed, 2 g initially followed by 1 g every 6 hours orally. The combined sulphamethoxazole 400 mg with Trimethoprim 80 mg (co-trimoxazole) 2 tablets twice a day has bactericidal effect against majority of urinary pathogens.

(b) Broad spectrum antibiotics: Tetracyclines and chloramphenicol are effective against most of the UTI pathogens except *proteus* and *pseudomonas.* Tetracyclines should be preferred to chloramphenicol because of low toxicity.
Dose: 0.25 g/6houly.

(c) Aminoglycoside antibiotics: Most of the gram-negative bacillary infections respond to these drugs. Gentamicin is effective not only against *E. coli* and *Proteus* but also against *Pseudomonas.* It is preferred to streptomycin being less toxic.
Dose: 80 mg I.M.
Antibacterial activity is enhanced in alkaline urine.

(d) Ampicillin: Effective against *E. coli, Aerobacter* and *Proteus, staphylococci* and *streptococci,* but there is higher relapse rate than with co-trimoxazole.
Dose: 0.5 g/6 hourly
Methicillin, cloxacillin are advocated in resistant staphylococcal infection, cephalosporins for *Klebsiella* and *Proteus* infections, and carbenicillin is indicated in only serious *Pseudomonas* infection.

(e) Polymyxin B is indicated in resistant pseudomonas infection.
Urine should be acidified by ammonium chloride 2-6 g/d, or ascorbic acid for tetracycline, methicillin and cloxacillin.
Urine should be made alkaline by sodium bicarbonate 2 g 4 times a day for sulphonamides, co-trimoxazole, aminoglycosides and cephalosporins.
pH is immaterial for chloramphenicol, ampicillin and colistin.

(f) Cycloserine: It is an antibiotic derived from streptomyces and now synthesized. Its antibacterial spectrum includes coliforms, proteus, etc.
Dose: 0.25 g/6 hourly orally will inhibit mycobacters and gram-negative bacteria. As most of this drug is excreted in urine in active form it is useful in the treatment of urinary tract infections.

(g) Quinolones: *Nalidixic* acid and cinoxacin are useful only for the treatment of UTI caused by susceptible organisms.
The fluoroquinolones are more potent and have a much broader antimicrobial spectrum of activity.
Norfloxacin, ciprofloxacin, ofloxacin and co-trimoxazole are equally efficacious for the treatment of UTIs.

Adverse effects mainly include headache, vertigo, tremor, psychosis, convulsions.

Urinary antiseptics

These are drugs that exert antibacterial activity in the urine but have little or no systemic antibacterial effect. Their usefulness is limited to urinary tract infections.

Antibiotics and sulphonamides are now commonly used. Before their introduction and also occasionally now, drugs called urinary antiseptics are employed for the treatment of urinary tract infection.

The urinary antiseptics pass in urine in an active form and in an effective concentraction, as well as also reach tissues in effective concentration.

They do not have systemic antibacterial properties.

Choice of drugs

	I choice	II choice	III choice
E. coli	Co-trimoxazole, Ampicillin, Nitrofurantoin, Norfloxacin, Ciprofloxacin, Ofloxacin, Enoxacin	Tetracycline, Gentamicin, Mandelamine, Cephalosporin, Nalidixic acid	Chloramphenicol
Proteus	Co-trimoxazole, Ampicillin, Sulphonamides, Ciprofloxacin, Ofloxacin	Gentamicin, Cephalosprin	Chloramphenicol
Pseudomonas aeruginosa	Gentamicin, Carbenicillin, Norfloxacin, Ciprofloxacin	Polymyxin B	Chloramphenicol
Aerobacter	Gentamicin, Ciprofloxacin	Ampicillin Chloramphenicol	
Klebsiella	Cephalosporin, Norfloxacin, Gentamicin, Ciprofloxacin	Tetracycline	Chloroamphenicol
Str. faecalis	Ampicillin, Penicillin + streptomycin, Ciprofloxacin, Norfloxacin	Erythromycin	

Nitrofurantoin (Furadantin): It is a furan derivative.

The three nitrofuran derivatives are: Nitrofurazone (furacin) a local antiseptic for topical use; Furazolidine (Furoxone) as intestinal antiseptic (not absorbed from GIT); Nitrofurantoin a urinary antiseptic.

Nitrofuantoin is bacteriostatic and bactericidal according to the concentration attained in urine. It is effective against several Gram-positive and gram-negative organisms. It acts best in acidic medium at pH 5.5 or less. However, many strains of proteus and all strains of pseudomonas are insensitive to nitrofurantoin.

It does not possess systemic antimicrobial activity, even on I.V. administration.

Nitrofurantoin is absorbed from GIT and excreted in effective antimicrobial concentration in urine.

Dose: 400 mg orally in divided doses. For children 5-8 mg/kg/d with or after meals. I.V route may be employed to reduce incidence of GI upsets.

Contraindications: Severe renal insufficiency.

Adverse effects include anorexia, nausea and vomiting. Allergic reaction have been reported.

Quinolones

The earlier quinolones such as Nalidixic acid, Oxolinic acid and Cinoxacin did not achieve systemic anitbacterial levels and thus were useful only as urinary antiseptics.

These are synthetic chemicals useful against gram-negative bacteria on oral administration but certain strains of *Enterobacter, Klebsiella, Proteus* and *Psedomonas* are generally resistant. They do not have systemic antibacterial property as they are firmly bound to blood proteins. Possibly they inhibit DNA synthesis in *E. coli.*

These drugs are readily absorbed from GIT, 20% of the absorbed drug is excreted in active form in urine, and 80% in an inactive form as glucuronide conjuate.

Resistance develops fairly quickly during therapy but there is no cross resistance with other antibacterial agents.

Uses: Effective in UTIs due to coliform organisms. Nalidixic acid 1 g orally 6 hourly for 1-2 weeks; 30-60 mg/kg/d for children.

The dose of oxolinic acid is 0.75 g twice a day.

Adverse effects include GI upsets, CNS stimulation, visual disturbances. CNS stimulation including convulions appears to be more frequent with oxolinic acid and for that reason nalidixic acid is preferred.

Methenamine Mandelate (Mandelamine)

It is a salt of mandelic acid with methenamine. It is excreted in urine and breaks up mandelic acid, acidifies urine and methenamine liberates formaldehyde which has antimicrobial activity that is nonspecific against many diverse organisms. It is effective against most of urinary tract pathogens except *proteus* and *pseudomonas. Proteus* and others which make urine alkaline through release of ammonia from urea are not susceptible.

Dose: 1 g 6 hourly or 1 g twice a day methenamine hippurate.

Contraindication : Sulphonamides should not be given simultaneously otherwise they will form an insoluble compound with formaldehyde released by methenamine.

Adverse effects include gastric and bladder irritation.

STUDY QUESTIONS

1. Why sulphonamides have been replaced largely by antibiotics? In which diseases sulphonamides still retain their usefulness?

2. How do sulphonamides act? How does bacterial resistance develop with sulphonamides?

3. Give examples of sulphonamides which are (i) readily absorbed for systemic uses, (ii) very poorly absorbed, (iii) topically employed and (iv) used in the treatment of dermatitis herpetiformis (special use).

4. Describe the antibacterial spectrum of sulphonamides and their clinical uses.

5. Describe the pharmacokinetics, routes of administration and toxicity of sulphonamides.

6. Describe Co-trimoxazole. How does it become bactericidal while the individual drugs are bacteriostatic?

7. Write notes on (i) trimethoprim, (ii) cross resistance (iii) sulphacetamide.

8. Explain (i) how crystalluria can be prevented? (ii) the advantages of using trimethoprim alone; (iii) why sulphamethoxazole is combined with trimethoprim? (iv) why sulphonamides which are primarly bacteriostatic act as bactericidal in urinary tract infections?

9. Which are the systemically active drugs for the treatment of urinary tract infection? Why sulphonamides continue to play an important role in these infections?

10. What are the drugs of first choice and alternatives for the urinary tract infections caused by (i) E. coli, (ii) Proteus, (iii) Pseudomonas.

11. Define urinary antiseptics. Describe Nitrofurantoin.

12. Write short notes on (i) Nalidixic acid, (ii) Oxolinic acid, and (iii) Methenamine Mandelate regarding their effectiveness and adverse effects.

13. Name nitrofurans. What are their chief uses and adverse effects?

14. List different quinolones.

15. Describe the antibacterial spectrum, mode of action, therapeutic indications and adverse effects of Quinolones as antimicrobial agents.

GUIDE TO FURTHER READING

Andriole, V.T et al: The Quinolones. Academic Press, Inc., New York, 1988.

Andriole, V.T et al: The future of the quinolones. Drugs, 1993; 45 Suppl 3:1-7.

Beaman, M et al: Toxoplasma gondii. In, Mandell, Douglas, and Bennett's Principles and Practice of Infections Disease, 4th ed. Churchill Livingstone, inc., New York, 1995; pp. 2455-2474.

Bennish, M.L et al: Treatment of shigellosis. III. Comparison of one-or two-dose ciprofloxacin with standard 5 day therapy. A randomized blinded trial. Ann. Intern. Med., 1992; 117:727-734.

Bhattacharya, S.K et al: Double-blind, randomized, controlled clinical trial of norfloxacin for cholera. Antimicrob. Agents Chemother., 1990; 34:939-940.

Clement, J.J et al: In virto and in vivo evaluations of A-80556, a new fluoroquinolone. Antimicrob. Agents Chemother., 1994; 38:1071-1078.

Cruciani, M. et al: The fluoroquinolones as treatment for infections caused by gram-positive bacteria. J. Antimicrob. Chemother., 1994; 33:403-413.

Gallant, J.E et al: Prophylaxis for opportuinstic infections in patients with HIV infection. Ann. Intern. Med., 1994; 120:932-944.

Gentry, L.O et al: Ofloxacin versus parenteral therapy for chronic osteomyelitis. Antimicrob. Agents Chemother., 1991; 35:538-541.

Hooper, D.C: Quinolones. In, Mandell, Douglas, and Bennett's Principles and Practice of Infectious Diseases, 4th ed. Churchill Livingstone, Inc., New York, 1995a, pp. 364-375.

Hooper, D.C: Urinary tract agents: nitrofurantoin and methenamine. In, Mandell, Douglas, and Bennett's Principles and Practice of Infectious Diseases, 4th ed. Churchill Livingstone, Inc., New York, 1995b, pp. 376-380.

Hooper, D.C et al: Fluoroquinolone antimicrobial agents. N. Engl. J. Med., 1991; 324:384-394.

Lane, H.C et al: Recent advances in the management of AIDS-related opportunistic infections. Ann. Intern. Med., 1994; 120:945-955.

The GIMEMA Infection Program. Prevention of bacterial infection in neutropenic patients with hematologic malignancies. A randomized, muliticenter trial comparing norfloxacin with ciprofloxacin. Ann. Intern. Med., 1991; 115:7-12.

Medina, I et al: Oral therapy for Pneumocystis carinii pneumonia (PCP) in the acquired immune deficiency syndrome: a controlled trial of trimethoprim-sulfamethoxazole versus trimethoprimdapsone, N. Engl. J. Med., 1990; 323:776-782.

Sader, H.S et al: In vitro comparison of activity of OPC-17116, a new fluoroquinolone, against more than 5,000 recent clinical isolates from five medical centers. J. Chemotherapy, 1993; 5:283-288.

Stamm, A.M et al: Failure of sulfonamides and trimethoprim in the treatment of nocardiosis. Arch. Intern. Med., 1983; 143:383-385.

Stamm, W.E et al: Antimicrobial prophylaxis for recurrent urinary tract infections. Ann. Intern. Med., 1980; 92:770-775.

Stamm, W.E et al: Management of urinary tract infection in adults. N. Engl. J. Med., 1993; 329:1328-1334.

Stein, G.E et al: A multicenter comparative trial of three-day norfloxacin vs. ten-day sulfamethoxazole and trimethoprim for the treatment of uncomplicated urinary tract infections. Arch. Intern. Med., 1987; 147:1760-1762.

Zinner, S.H et al: Sulfonamides and trimethoprim. In, Mandell, Douglas, and Bennett's Principles and Practice of Infectious Diseases, 4th ed. Churchill Livingstone, Inc., New York, 1995, pp. 354-363.

Zitelli, B.J et al: Fatal hepatic necrosis due to pyrimethamine-sulfadoxine (FANSIDAR). Ann. Intern. Med., 1987; 106:393-395.

GENERAL ASPECTS OF ANTIMICROBIAL AGENTS

The term chemotherapy was coined by Ehrlich at the beginning of the century to describe the use of synthetic chemicals to destroy infective agents. Ehrlich hoped for maximally within "parasitotropic" and minimally "organotropic" agents i.e. highly selective agents. Now, some totally selective antibacterial agents have been produced.

The definition of the term has been broadened to include antibiotics as well as the use of other natural or synthetic substances which inhibit the growth or kill microorganisms. Chemotherapy also includes the use of antineoplastic agents.

The development of chemotherapy is one of the most important advances in the history of medicine. Chemotherapeutic agents are chemicals which are toxic for the parasitic cell but innocuous for the host. The selectivity of toxicity depends on the expolitable biochemical differences between the parasite and the host cell.

Parasitic cells may be prokaryotes (cell without nuclei—the bacteria) or eukaryotes (cell with nuclei). The eukaryotes include single-celled organisms, e.g. protozoa and multicellular organisma, e.g. helminths.

Viruses are not properly speaking, cells at all because they do not have their own biochemical machinery which presents problem for chemotherapeutic attack.

Cancer cells can be considerd as "foreign" or "parasitic" but these are host cells that have become malignant and are more similar to normal host cells than of the categories described above. Hence, selective toxicity is an especially difficult problem.

Mode of action (Fig. 11.9 and Table 11.10)

1. Competition for an essential metabolite:
   - Sulphonamides
2. Altered conformation of enzymes:
   - Sulphonamides
   - Co-trimoxazole
3. Inhibition of nucleic acid function:
   - Rifampicin
   - Actinomycin

   Inhibitors of DNA synthesis:
   - Fluoroquinolines such as ciprofloxacin, norfloxacin, ofloxacin
4. Inhibition of ribosome function: Ribosome is the site of protein synthesis. Bacteria have 70 S ribosomes (30 S and 50 S subunits), whereas mammalian cells have 80 S ribosomes (40 S and 60 S subunits).
   - Aminoglycosides and tetracyclines attach to 30 S subunit of microbial ribosome.

Box 11.8. Inhibitors of protein synthesis		
Aminoglycosides	*Tetracyclines*	*Macrolides*
Streptomycin, Neomycin, Kanamycin, Gentamicin, Tobramycin, Amikacin, Netilmicin	Tetracycline, Chlortetracycline, Oxytetracycline, Demeclocycline, Methacycline, Doxycycline, Minocycline	Erythromycin, Clarithromycin, Chloramphenicol, Clindamycin, Azithromycin

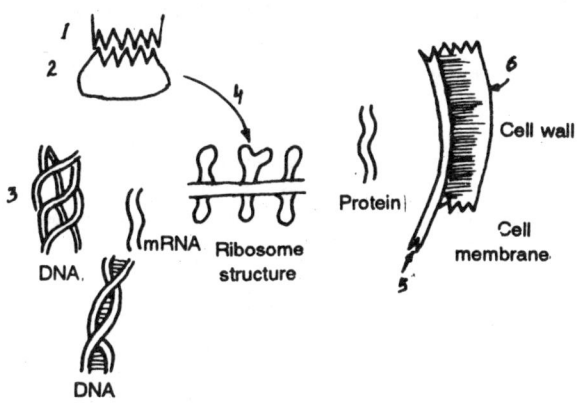

Fig. 11.9. Targets for chemotherapeutic attack in the bacterial cell.

• Macrolides and chloramphenicol bind to the 50 S subunit of microbial ribosome.

5. Increased permeability of cytoplasmic membrane:

Polymyxins selectively disrupt the cytoplasmic membrane of certain gram-negative bacteria.

6. Impairment of bacterial cell wall. If cell wall synthesis is imperfect, the bacterial cell absorbs water by osmosis and bursts. These are bactericidal.

   • Penicillins
   • Cephalosporins
   • Cycloserine
   • Bacitracin

The pharmacokinetic properties of some antimicrobial drugs is given in Table 11.10.

Table 11.10. Pharmacokinetic properties of some antimicrobial drugs with special indications

Drug	*Half-life (hrs)*	*Oral bioavailability*	*% protein bound in plasma*	*Major route of elimination*
Cell wall inhibitors				
Vancomycin	5-6	0%	< 10	Kidney, liver
Bacitracin	—	0%	—	Kidney
Novobiocin	< 6	High	> 90	Liver and bile
Protein synthesis inhibitors				
Erythromycin	1.4	18-45%	72	Bile
Azithromycin	40-60	40%	50	Bile
Clarithromycin	5-7	50%	—	Bile
Clindamycin	2.7	High	90	Bile (ative metabolite)
DNA synthesis inhibitors (Fluoroquinolones)				
Ciprofloxacin	3-4.5	50-80%	15	Kidney
Enoxacin	3-6	90%	40	Kidney
Lomefloxacin	8	95%	10	Kidney
Norfloxacin	3.5-5	30-40%	35	Kidney
Ofloxacin	5-7	> 90%	8	Kidney
Drugs with other mechanisms				
Metronidazole	6-11	80%	10	Metabolism in liver

Development of Bacterial Resistance

Resistance may be developed due to :
  A. Genetic determinants
  B. Biochemical mechanisms

A. Genetic determinants

1. Chromosomal mutation: The sensitive bacteria die, the resistant bacteria multiply resulting in selection of mutants.
2. Extrachromosomal plasmids: Many species of bacteria also have extra chromosomal elements called plasmids which exist free in cytoplasm. Plasmids which carry genes for resistance to antibiotics are called R-plasmids.
3. Transposons are bits of DNA which may carry one or more resistance genes found mainly in gram-negative bacteria.
4. Transfer of resistance genes between bacteria through conjugation, transduction and transformation. This is plasmid determined.

B. Biochemical mechanisms

1. Inactivation of antibiotics: The organisms can synthesize enzymes which can inactivate drug, e.g. beta-lactamases cleave beta-lactam ring and inactivate beta-lactam antibiotics.
2. Decreased drug accumulation in bacteria due to altered envelope permeability. There is failure of a drug to penetrate cell wall or bind to receptors. This form of resistance occurs with tetracyclines, aminoglycosides, chloramphenicol and polymyxins.
3. Alteration of a target or binding site, i.e. mutation of drug-binding sites. For example, resistance to aminoglycosides and erythromycin may also be due to mutation of binding sites on 30 S and 50 S subunits of bacterial ribosomes respectively.
4. Alternate metabolic pathway may be developed by the bacteria which become resistant to sulphonamides and trimethoprim.

Table 11.1 shows mode of development of resistance to antimicrobial drugs.

Cross-resistance

Chemically related drugs having similar mode of action show cross-resistance.

Table 11.11. Mode of development of resistance to antimicrobial drugs

Antimicrobial drug	Mechanism of action
Beta-lactams, Erythromycin, Lincomycin	Receptor modified, leading to reduced ability of the drug to bind to the receptor
Beta-lactams, Erythromycin	Hydrolysis of agent via enzymes produced by microorganisms
Beta-lactams, Fusidic acid	Sequestration of agent by protein binding
Tetracycline	Active transport out of microorganisms
Chloramphenicol	Reduced uptake by microorganisms
Bleomycin	Binding of specific immunity proteins to agent
Sulphonamides	Production of altered enzymes that are less affected by agent
Sulphonamides, Trimethoprim	Development of alternate metabolic pathway that renders reaction inhibited by the drug obsolete
Trimethoprim	Overproduction of the target

1. Between tetracyclines — Complete
2. Tetracycline-chloramphenicol
   • Gram-positive — None
   • Gram-negative — Fairly often
3. Methicillin-Cloxacillin — Complete
4. Erythromycin-Oleandomycin — Very often
5. Erythromycin-Chloramphenicol — Sometimes
6. Kanamycin-Neomycin — Often

Antimicrobial drug combinations

The following three main results may be observed due to interaction of two antimicrobial drugs:

1. Indifference or additive effect: Drugs A and B combined effect is equal to that of the single more active component of the mixture A + B or is equal to the arithmetic sum of the effect of the individual drugs.
2. Synergism: The combined effect of A + B drugs is far greater than that of either drug A or B alone. The effect is greater than expected from single addition of individual drug effects.

The mechanism of synergism may be as follows:

(a) Blocking successive steps in a metabolic sequence e.g. sulphonamide plus trimethoprim.

(b) One drug inhibits an enzyme that can destroy the second drug e.g. drug such as clavulanic acid which inhibits β-lactamases will protect penicillin G.

(c) One drug promotes entry of a second drug through microbial cell wall or cell membrane. For example, many streptococci exhibit a partial permeability barrier to aminoglycosides.

If a cell wall inhibitory drug is also present, it enhances the penetration of aminoglycoside which then acts on ribosomes and accelerates killing of the cell.

In the following conditions, combination of antimicrobials is advantageous.

- In the treatment of tuberculosis and leprosy, combination of drugs will delay or prevent emergence of resistant strains.
- Antimicrobial activity is enhanced in some cases (sulphonamides and trimethoprim), penicillin and gentamicin for enterococcal endocarditis, gentamicin and carbenicillin for pseudomonas infection. However, if combination is not chosen judiciously it will have certain disadvantages such as (i) superinfection, (ii) enhanced adverse effects and (iii) resistance may develop against both the drugs.

3. Antagonism: The bacteriostatic drugs (tetracycline, chloramphenicol, erythromycin) inhibit bacterial growth.

The bactericidal drug (penicillins, cephalosporins, aminoglycosides) require bacterial growth for killing (e.g. protein and cell wall synthesis).

In the case of cell wall active drugs, the inhibition of protein synthesis by chloramphenicol etc interfers with the production of some autolytic enzyme system which is probably an important final step in cell lysis.

Clinical importance

There are a larger number of instances of antimicrobial synergism and antagonism in vitro. Only a few well documented clinical examples are available.

Endocarditis due to enterococci (*E. faecalis*), streptococci and staphylococci is usually not cured by penicillin alone because penicillin is inhibitory and not bactericidal for enterococci, its or ampicillin use with aminoglycoside is an example of clinical synergism.

Beta-lactam antibiotics combined with aminoglycosides also appear to be synergistic in the treatment of endocarditis due to streptococci and staphylococci, as well as in the treatment of aerobic gram-negative rod infections.

For the treatment of cryptococcal meningitis, amphotericin B with flucytosine is superior to either drug alone.

Evidence for clinical antagonism

As in clinical practice, usually large doses of antimicrobial drugs are administered and hence antagonism is not observed frequently. However, there are a few documented examples of clinical antagonism e.g. combination of penicillin and chlortetracycline cured fewer patients suffering from pneumococcal meningitis than the same dose of penicillin alone. Another example is that of chloramphenicol plus ampicillin that resulted in more treatment failures than did ampicillin alone.

Chemoprophylaxis with Antimicrobial drugs

- Antimicrobials can not eradicate all microorganisms so prophylaxis should be directed against specific group of bacteria.
- The duration of prophylaxis should be short (as resistance is likely to develop with long term usage).
- Chemoprophylaxis is more successful if employed against pathogens which are poorly likely to develop resistance.
- The doses used for prophylaxis should be equal to those used for the treatment.
- Chemoprophylaxis should not be used indiscriminately due to cost, toxicity, superinfection and development of drug resistant organisms.
- Chemoprophylaxis should be used only in conditions where its efficacy is known both for non-surgical infections as well as in preoperative period to prevent postoperative complications.

Antimicrobial drug interactions

All broad-spectrum antimicrobials (other than rifampin) enhance the effect of coumarin anticoagulants.

Inhibition of sterol biotransformation by antimicrobial agents may decrease blood levels of contraceptive medication following oral administration, resulting in increased risk of pregnancy in women taking oral contraceptives.

Ampicillin produces interruption of enterohepatic circulation of oestrogen, possible reduction in oral contraceptive efficacy.

Chloramphenicol decreases dicumarol metabolism.

Erythromycin inhibits anticoagulant metabolism.

Ciprofloxacin probably also inhibits anticoagulant metabolism.

Rifampin increases oestrogen metabolism, possible reduction in oral contraceptive efficacy.

Iron decreases absorption of tetracycline.

Quinolone antimicrobials: Ciprofloxacin, and to a lesser extent norfloxacin inhibit caffeine metabolism

Sucralfate reduces GI absorption of ciprofloxacin, norfloxacin and probably other quinolones.

Common causes of failure of antimicrobial therapy

Causes related to drug

- Inappropriate drug
- Inadequate dose
- Improper route of administration
- Malabsorption
- Inactivation/ increased excretion
- Poor penetration at site of infection (e.g. brain, eye, prostate)

Causes related to patient

- Poor defences (e.g. leukopenia, granulocytopenia, AIDS etc.)
- Dead tissue (sequestrum)
- Retained infected foreign body
- Undrained pus (e.g. abscess)

Causes related to invading organism

- Development of drug resistance
- Superinfection by other pathogens

Laboratory error

- Errors in susceptibility testing (rare).

Bioterrorism

In recent years, the efforts of some governments and terrorist organizations to use biological weaponry have refocused public concern on the topic. The ability of infectious agents to inflict widespread illness and thus to cause societal disruption and panic, together with the low cost of these agents, has led to their being called a "poor man's nuclear arsenal".

Several pathogens have been considered likely candidates for biological warfare. *Bacillus anthracis* is widely viewed as a leading contender. The hardy spores of the bacillus can be distributed by bombardment or other dispersal mechanisms. Inhalation of this pathogen results in severe pneumonia with a mortality rate of 95% in untreated persons. A WHO report estimated that 50 kg of *B. anthracis* released upwind of a city with a population of 500,000 should result in up to 95,000 fatalities, with an additional 125,000 persons incapacitated.

The other bioweapons that combine the virulence and stability necessary for biological weapons include *Yersinia pestis*, the agent of plague, and *Francisella tularensis*, the agent of tularemia. Viral haemorrhagic fever agents such as the Ebola and Marburg viruses as well as toxins such as that from *Clostridium botulinum* have also been considered as biological weapons.

Smallpox, an ancient scourge, caused by vaccinia virus owing to its contagiousness and high mortality rate and to the declining population of immunized persons has also been considered as a bioweapon. Debate continues about whether to eradicate the two known existing stocks of the virus in U.S. and Russian government laboratories. Many investigators believe that additional undocumented stockpiles of the virus exist around the world.

STUDY QUESTIONS

1. Is there any difference between antibiotics and antimicrobials?
2. What are the different targets for chemotherapeutic attack in the bacterial cell? Give examples.

3. What are the different determinants/biochemical mechanisms for the development of resistance to antibiotics?

4. Explain cross tolerance among antibiotics.

5. What can result due to interaction of two antimicrobial drugs? Give examples of synergism and antagonism as a result of such combination. Describe the clinical advantages of such combination. What can be the disadvantages of irrational and unjudicious combinations?

6. Write notes on (i) Chemoprophylaxis with antimicrobial drugs (ii) common causes of failure of antimicrobial therapy.

GUIDE TO FURTHER READING

Anonymous: Antimicrobial prophylaxis in surgery. Med. Lett. Drugs Ther., 1993; 35:91-94.

Arthur, M et al: Genetics and mechanisms of glycopeptide resistance in enterococci. Antimicrob. Agents Chemother., 1993; 37:1563-1571.

Davies, J: Inactivation of antibiotics and the dissemination of resistance genes. Science, 1994; 264:375-382.

Gilbert, D.N et al: Once-daily aminoglycoside therapy. Antimicrob. Agents Chemother., 1991; 35:399-405.

Jawetz, E et al: Studies on antibiotic synergism and antagonism: the scheme of combined antimicrobial activity. Antibiot. Chemother., 1952; 2:243-248.

Kaiser, A: Postoperative infections and antimicrobial prophylaxis. In, Mandell, Douglas, and Bennett's Principles and Practice of Infectious Diseases, 4th ed. Churchill Livingstone, Inc., New York, 1990, pp. 2245-2257.

Lepper, M.H et al: Treatment of pneumococcic meningitis with penicillin plus Aureomycin: studies including observations on apparent antagonism between penicillin and Aureomycin. Arch. Intern. Med., 1951; 88:489-494.

Murray, A.W et al: Beta-lactamase-producing enterococci. Antimicrob. Agents Chemother., 1992; 36:2355-2359.

Nikaido, H: Prevention of drug access to bacterial targets: permeability barriers and active efflux. Science, 1994; 264:382-388.

Pratt, W.B et al: The Antimicrobial Drugs. Oxford University Press, New York, 1986.

Sande, M.A et al: Combination antibiotic therapy of bacterial endocarditis. Ann. Intern. Med., 1980; 92:390-395.

Spratt, B.G et al: Resistance to antibiotics mediated by target alterations. Science, 1994; 264:388-393.

Wehrli, W: Rifampin: mechanisms of action and resistance. Rev. Infect. Dis., 1983; 5: S407-S411.

CHEMOTHERAPY OF MALARIA

In order to understand the therapy and site of action of antimalarial drugs, it is essential to know the life cycle of malarial parasite.

Infected female anopheles mosquito needs blood meal for production of eggs. When it bites a person the sporozoites from its saliva reach man's blood and leave it soon (within an hour) and enter liver cells (pre-erythrocytic or primary tissue phase). During the next 10-15 days they undergo a pre-erythrocytic stage and at the end of this stage, liver cells rupture and merozoites are released into circulation. Merozoites reproduce asexually in red blood cells (erythrocytic stage or asexual cycle of malarial parasite), some merozoites again invade liver (secondary tissue phase), and some merozoites differentiate into male and female gametocytes in the erythrocytes, which can only develop further if ingested by a mosquito. The sexual cycle of malarial parasite takes place in mosquito.

Thus, the life cycle of malarial parasite consists of sporozoite phase, primary tissue phase, asexual or erythrocytic phase, secondary tissue phase, sexual phase (in mosquito).

In certain forms of malaria, some sporozoites on entering the liver cells form hyponozoites, or resting form of the parasite, which can be reactivated to continue as exoerythrocytic cycle of multiplication. The parasite may exist in a dormant hyponozoite form in liver and emerge after weeks or months to start the infection again.

The primary and secondary tissue phases together form exo-erythrocytic cycle which is responsible for relapses of malaria.

A single parasite of *P. vivax* is capable of giving rise to 250 million merozoites in 14 days.

The following are chief species of human malarial parasites:

1. *Plasmodium falciparum:* It has erythrocytic cycle of 48 hours and produces malignant tertian malaria ('tertian' refers to fever occurring every third day) and called 'malignant' as clinically it is the most severe form of the disease. *P. falciparum* does not

have a significant exo-erythrocytic stage so relapses do not occur after eradication of the erythrocytic stage.

2. *Plasmodium vivax:* Its erythrocytic cycle is of 48 hours and produces benign tertian malaria (benign as it is less severe). But exoerythrocytic forms persist for years and are responsible for relapses.

3. *Plasmodium ovale* has 48 hour cycle and exoerythrocytic stage occurs. It causes a rare form of malaria.

4. *Plasmodium malariae* has a 72 hour erythrocytic cycle and causes quartan malaria. Exoerythrocytic stage is absent.

Classification

The antimalarial drugs can be grouped (chemical groups) as under:

1. Cinchona alkaloids	Quinine
2. Acridine derivative	Mepacrine (atabrine)
3. 4-aminoquinolines	Chloroquine, hydroxychloroquine, amodiaquine
4. 8-aminoquinolines	Pamaquine, pentaquine, isopentaquine, primaquine
5. Diaminopyrimidines	Pyrimethamine (daraprim), trimethoprim
6. Biguanide	Proguanil (paludrine)
7. 4-Quinoline methanol	Mefloquine
8. Sulphonamides and Sulphones	Sulphadoxine, dapsone, sulphamethoxazole
9. Miscellaneous	Doxycycline, norfloxacin

Antimalarial drugs can also be classified by their selective actions on different phases of the parasite's life cycle:

1. True causal prophylactic should act on sporozoites, but no drug is available for this purpose.

2. Causal prophylactic drugs act on preerythrocytic stage: 8-aminoquinolines

3. Clinical prophylactic (for suppressive prophylaxis) act on erythrocytic cycle: 4-aminoquinolines and other clinical curative drugs

4. Clinical curatives act on erythrocytic forms: Chloroquine, hydroxychloroquine, amodiaquine, paludrine, daraprim

   These are blood schizonticidal drugs. Clinical attack of malaria with fever and rigor is due to bursting of red blood cells and release of parasites and debris.

5. Radical curative act on erythrocytic as well as on exoerythrocytic forms.

   For *P. vivax* — 8-aminoquinolines

   Exoerythrocytic forms do not persist in case of *P. falciparum*.

6. Gametocidal drugs destroy or inactivate gametocytes: 8-aminoquinolines destroy sexual forms

   Paludrine and pyrimethamine prevent fertilization of gametocytes.

Drugs which eliminate developing tissue schizonts or latent hypnozoites in the liver cycle i.e. 8-aminoquinolines (e.g. primaquine) are called tissue schizonticides.

These are used for (i) radical cure (attack on hypnozoites) (ii) causal prophylaxis (prevent hepatic cycle from becoming established).

Drugs which act on blood schizonts are blood schizonticides or suppressive agents e.g. chloroquine, amodiaquine, paludrine, daraprim, quinine and mefloquine.

These are used (i) to treat acute attack of malaria, (ii) as suppressive prophylaxis i.e. to prevent attacks by early destruction of the erythrocytic forms.

Drugs which act on the sexual forms (gametocides) are drugs that prevent infection by destroying gametocytes in the blood e.g. primaquine for *P. falciparum* and chloroquine for *P. vivax, P. ovale* and *P. malariae*.

Sporonticidal agents are drugs that render gametocytes noninfective in the mosquito e.g. pyrimethamine and paludrine.

Box 11.9. Choice of antimalarial agents

Malaria	Antimalarials	
	1st choice	*2nd choice*
P. falciparum		
Chloroquine-sensitive strains		
For prophylaxis, Chloroquine	—	
For treatment	Chloroquine	—
Chloroquine-resistant strains		
For prophylaxis	Mefloquin	Pyrimethamine-sulphadoxine or Doxycycline with or without chloroquine
For treatment	Mefloquin or Halofantrine	—
P. malariae		
For prophylaxis and treatment	Chloroquine	—
P. vivax, P. ovale		
For prophylaxis and treatment	Chloroquine plus primaquine	—

ANTIMALARIAL DRUGS

Drugs which affect clinical cure

These are blood schizonticidal agents : Quinine, mefloquine, chloro-quine, halofantrine, pyrimethamine, tetracycline doxycycline, artemether. These drugs act on the erythrocytic forms of the plasmodium. They can produce cure in infections with P. falciparum or *P. malariae*, which have no exoerythrocytic stage. With *P. vivax* or *P. ovale*, these drugs suppress the actual attack but the exoerythrocytic forms can cause later replapses.

Drugs which affect radical cure

These are tissue schizonticidal drugs. They act on the parasites in the liver. Only 8-aminoquinolines are effective in this regard (primaquine). They are also gametocidal drugs and thus reduce the spread of infection.

Drugs used for chemoprophylaxis (also known as causal prophylactic drugs):

True causal prophylaxis: prevention of infection by killing sporozoites on entry into the host: No such drug is available. Vaccines in the future may achieve it.

Prevention of the development of clinical attacks is possible by chemoprophylactic drugs that kill the parasites when they emerge from the liver after pre-erythrocytic stage. Chloroquine, meflo-quine, proguanil, pyrimethamine, dapsone and doxycycline are used in combination for chemoprophylaxis, administration of drugs should begin 1 week before entering the area, continued throughout stay and to 1 month afterwards.

Drugs used to prevent transmission: Primaquine, proguanil and pyrimethamine destroy gametocytes, thus preventing transmission by mosquito.

Cinchona alkaloids

Quinine

It is an alkaloid obtained from cinchona bark. Quinine has local irritant action, possesses weak analgesic and antipyretic systemic effect.

As an antimalarial drug, it acts on the erythrocytic phase of the parasite so it may be useful for the treatment of acute attack of malaria. But for this purpose chloroquine has almost replaced it because chloroquine is more effective, less toxic and better tolerated. The administration of quinine alone has no place now in the treatment of malaria. However, resistance to quinine has not been reported in severe falciparum infections like cerebral malaria, quinine is given parenterally in both chloroquine sensitive and resistant infections, given by rate-controlled infusion and not I.V. bolus injection.

Dose : 0.3 to 0.6 g/d as suppressant. 1.2 to 2 g/d in divided doses as curative.

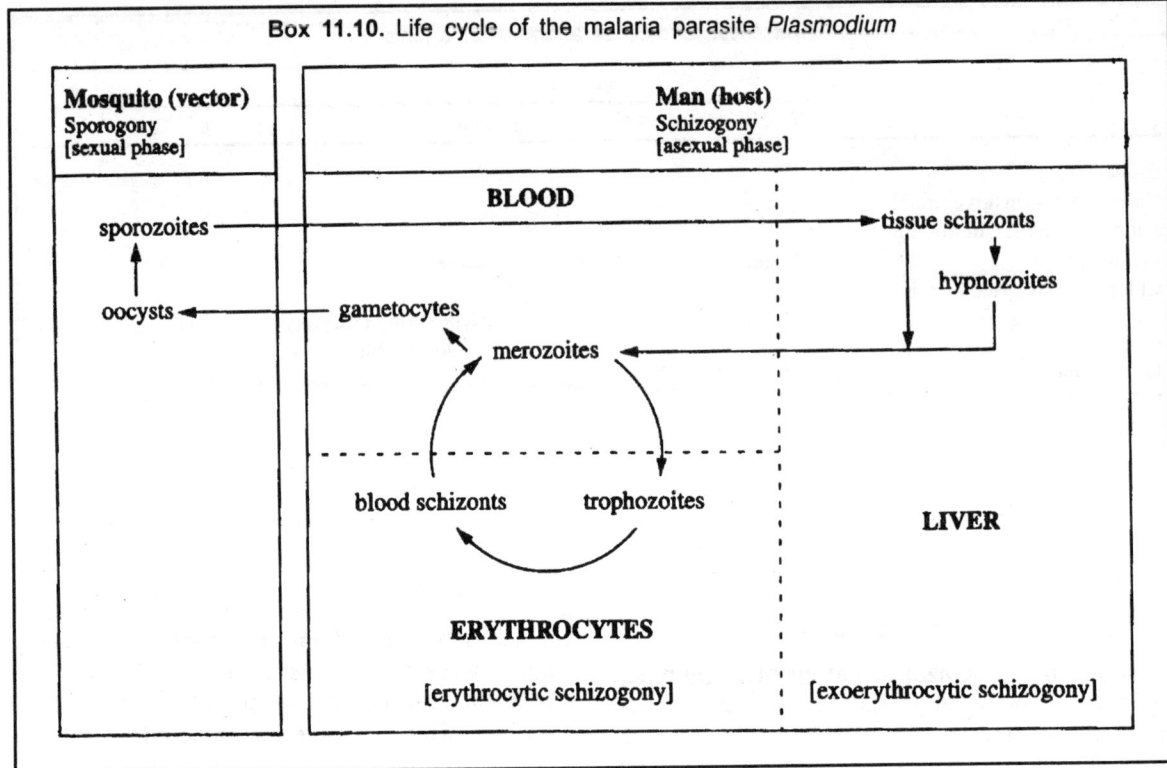

Box 11.10. Life cycle of the malaria parasite *Plasmodium*

Mosquito (vector)
Sporogony
[sexual phase]

Man (host)
Schizogony
[asexual phase]

BLOOD

sporozoites ──────────→ tissue schizonts

hypnozoites

oocysts ◄──── gametocytes

merozoites

blood schizonts   trophozoites

LIVER

ERYTHROCYTES

[erythrocytic schizogony]   [exoerythrocytic schizogony]

Quinine does not affect exoerythrocytic cycle.

Adverse effects are many and occur frequently. These include nausea, vomiting, vertigo, confusion, ringing in ears, visual defects and difficulty in hearing. These are collectively called cinchonism.

Besides the limited antimalarial property of quinine, it also has limited value in the treatment of myokymia due to its curare like effect. Oral administration of 0.32 g (repeated several times a day) relieves twitching of the orbicularis muscle. However, quinine produces many ocular adverse effects including blurred vision, constricted visual fields, scotomas, disturbed colour vision and even amblyopia. Quinine amblyopia may be sudden.

During pregnancy, if large dosage of quinine is taken (which induces tinnitus), it damages foetus resulting in congenital blindness. The eye finding in these cases are typical of quinine amblyopia.

Quinine poisoning can also damage iris resulting in a dilated irregular pupil with poor light reaction.

4-aminoquinolines

Chloroquine

Chloroquine is a very effective drug acting on asexual forms of the malarial parasite. It is available by all routes of administration and is well absorbed and a well tolerated drug. It has been the drug of choice as clinical suppressive and clinical curative drug. It has no action against exoerythrocytic forms.

Chloroquine has a quinoline ring like that of quinine with a side chain identical to that of quinacrine. The d- and l- isomers are equally potent, but the d-isomer is slightly less toxic.

For terminating acute attack, 1 g initially, after 6-8 hours 500 mg followed by 500 mg single dose daily for two days is adequate (total dose of 2.5 g given in 3 days).

For suppressive therapy 500 mg orally on same day of each week upto 6 weeks after last exposure is recommended.

Chloroquine is used for chemosuppression and

treatment of malaria, except for strains of P. falciparum that are partially or completely resistant to it.

The mode of antimalarial action is probably due to its ability to block the enzymatic synthesis of DNA and RNA in both mammalian and protozoal cells.

Besides the antimalarial effect for which it is mostly employed, chloroquine has a slight quinidine like effect on the cardiovascular system as well as it possesses antiinflammatory effect. The antiinflammatory effect is useful in the treatment of rheumatoid arthritis and discoid lupus erythematosus. Chloroquine is also a useful drug for the treatment of hepatic amoebiasis and giardiasis.

The *adverse effects* of chloroquine include ocular toxicity (blurred vision, corneal deposits which regress when chloroquine is discontinued). Besides ocular toxicity, the other side effects include vertigo, anorexia, malaise, headache, diarrhoea, urticaria and pruritus. Toxic psychosis with hallucinations and peripheral neuropathies may also occur. High doses can also produce ECG changes (flattening or inversion of T wave).

Chloroquine crosses the placenta and may damage the foetus resulting in congenital deafness and mental retardation in children born to mother who has been taking large doses during pregnancy.

Hydroxychloroquine is almost identical in its properties and can be used if chloroquine is not available.

Amodiaquine (camoquin) is almost similar to chloroquine.

Acridine derivative

Mepacrine (Quinacrine, Atabrine)

It acts only against erythrocytic cycle but chloroquine is a much better drug. It is a cumulative drug. Besides antimalarial property, it is also effective against tape worms and giardiasis but better drugs are now available for giardiasis e.g. metronidazole etc.

The *adverse effects* include dermatitis, hepatitis, psychosis, bone marrow depression, retinopathy.

8-aminoquinolines

8-aminoquinolines (pamaquine, pentaquine, isopentaquine and primaquine):

Among these primaquine is preferred being relatively less toxic.

8-aminoquinolines are highly effective against exoerythrocytic forms of the malarial parasite and also possess marked gametocidal property. However, they have weak effect on asexual (erythrocytic) forms.

Primaquine is mainly used as radical curative drug with chloroquine. Dose of primaquine is 15 mg once a day for 14 days.

8-aminoquinolines are very toxic. They may produce cyanosis, bone marrow depression, intravascular haemolysis, haemolytic anaemia and GIT upsets.

Diaminopyrimidine

Pyrimethamine (daraprim)

Its antimalarial action resembles that of paludrine but it is more potent. It prevents development of fertilized gametes (indirect gametocidal activity).

The dose for clinical cure is 300-600 mg, as prophylactic and suppressive 100 mg followed by 300 mg daily. Its chief use is as a suppressive prophylactic and for this purpose doses of 25 mg once a week for 6 weeks after leaving the malarious area is recommended. As a clinical curative, this drug is not valuable due to slow action.

Adverse effects are not common. However, nausea and rashes have been reported in some persons.

Trimethoprim

It is an antibacterial drug. As an antimalarial its activity resembles that of pyrimethamine but weaker.

Biguanides

Chloroquanide (paludrine)

Its antimalarial action is against asexual forms but acts more slowly than chloroquine. It also prevents development of gametocytes like daraprim. It does not affect exoerythrocytic forms.

Paludrine is a slowly absorbed and rapidly excreted drug.

Adverse effects include quick development of resistance, haematuria, bone marrow depression and GI upsets.

Quinoline-methanol (Mefloquine)

Mefloquine hydrochloride is a synthetic 4-quinoline methanol derivative, chemically related to quinine. As it produces marked local irritation so it is not given parenterally. It is given only orally. It is well absorbed, and widely distributed in the body, including the CNS. The drug is highly bound to plasma proteins and concentrated in red blood cells. It is metabolized in the liver and its metabolites are slowly excreted, mainly in the faeces.

Mefloquine has strong schizonticidal activity against *P. falciparum* and *P. vivax*, but it is not active against *P. falciparum* gametocytes or the hepatic stages of *P. vivax*. Besides the antimalarial property, mefloquine has quinidine-like effects on the heart.

Although mefloquine is effective against chloroquine sensitive *P. falciparum*, it should be reserved for use in malarious areas in which chloroquine is not effective. This drug is used in prophylaxis and treatment of chloroquine-resistant and multi-drug resistant (e.g. pyrimethamine-sulphadoxine resistance) falciparum malaria. It is also effective as prophylactic agent against *P. vivax, P. ovale* and *P. malariae*.

Single dose of 1 g every 4 weeks has prolonged suppressive effect. It can be given as 250 mg weekly or 500 mg every 2 weeks.

Adverse effects of mefloquine include GI upsets, confusion and dizziness. Sporadic and low levels of resistance have been reported from Asia and Africa. In some cases resistance may emerge rapidly.

Mefloquine is *contraindicated* if there is history of epilepsy or psychiatric disorder. It should also not be used in children below 2 years of age (due to poor absorption in this age group).

Concurrent administration of mefloquine with quinine, quinidine, beta-blockers or calcium channel blockers or any other drug which alters cardiac conduction is contraindicated. Concurrent administration of mefloquine and chloroquine or quinine increases the risk of convulsions. Patients taking anticonvulsant drugs particularly valproic acid may have breakthrough seizures.

Mefloquine should not be taken by persons whose work requires fine coordination e.g. airline pilots.

This drug should not be used in pregnancy.

Antibacterial agents in antimalarial chemotherapy

Sulphonamides and Sulphones

Sulphonamides and sulphones are not effective antimalarial when given alone, but when combined with pyrimethamine are useful for prevention and treatment of chloroquine resistant malaria. Pyrimethamine acts synergistically with sulphadoxine or dapsone to provide an effective treatment for drug resistant strains. This combination is slow acting schizonticide against certain strains of falciparum malaria. It is ineffective in *P. vivax*.

The sulphonamides used as antimalarial are sulphadoxine and sulphamethoxazole. The only sulphone used is dapsone.

The above combinations i.e. pyrimethamine-sulphadoxine or pyrimethamine-dapsone are effective only against erythrocytic forms.

The *adverse effects* are chiefly those associated with adverse effects of sulphonamides manifested by haematologic, gastrointestinal, dermatologic and renal systems.

This combination should not be used in patients who have had adverse side effects to sulphonamides. It should also not be used in pregnancy, in nursing mothers and in infants below 2 months of age. It should also not be used in patients with allergic disorders such as bronchial asthma.

Alternative Drugs

Doxycycline, a tetracycline drug is effective as prophylactic against multi-drug resistant *P. falciparum* in doses of 100 mg/d while staying in the endemic area and taken for four weeks after leaving that area. For the treatment of acute malaria it is effective when combined with quinine.

Halofantrine hydrochloride is a phenanthrene methanol compound effective against asexual forms of *P.vivax* and chloroquine sensitive as well as chloroquine resistant *P. falciparum*.

This drug is now employed primarily as an alternate to quinine and mefloquine to treat acute malarial attacks caused by chloroquine-resistant and multidrug resistant strains of *P. falciparum*, especially falciparum cerebral malaria.

This drug should not be used for prophylaxis

because its prolonged elimination may produce drug-resistance of *P. falciparum.*

The clinical responsiveness is unpredictable due to slow and erratic absorption. Fatty food can increase absorption and exacerbate adverse effects.

The drug is well distributed and metabolized to N-desbutyl halofantrine (a major active antimalarial metabolite). The metabolites are excreted with some quantity of unaltered drug in faeces.

Dose: 500 mg 6 hourly for 3 doses.

This drug is *contraindicated* in pregnancy because embryotoxicity has been reported with high doses in laboratory animals.

Adverse effects

- Halofantrine is well tolerated. Minor side effects include nausea, vomiting, diarrhoea and abdominal pain.
- High doses prolong QT interval like quinine.
- This drug has arrhythmogenic potential.

Tetrandrine is a new antimalarial drug particularly effective against chloroquine-resistant *P. falciparum.*

Tables 11.12 and 11.13 show properties and doses of antimalarial drugs respectively.

Potential new antimalarial drugs

Pyronaridine derived from mepacrine is a synthetic schizonticidal agent. Atovaquone is used for the treatment of Pneumocystis carinii pneumonia is under test as an antimalarial.

Qinghaosu (artemisinin) and related compounds:

These are derived from the herb, quing hao a traditional Chinese remedy for malaria. Artemisia is the scientific name given to this herb by Linnaeus.

Artemisinin is a chemical extract from Artemisia. It is poorly soluble in water, is a fast-acting blood schizonticide, effective against acute attack of both vivax and falciparum malaria, including chloroquine-resistant and cerebral malaria. It can be given orally, intramuscularly or by suppository. The t½ is about 4 hrs. Artesunate is a water soluble derivative, can be given by IM or IV injection. The half-life is 45 minutes. Artemether and artesunate are synthetic analogues, having higher activity and also better

absorbed, given orally or by IM injection. The half life of artemether is 4-11 hours.

These compounds are not effective against liver hypnozoites. They are also not useful for chemoprophylaxis.

The mode of action is not clearly known. It may damage the parasite membrane by free radicals or covalent alkylation of proteins.

They are rapidly absorbed and widely distributed. They are converted in the liver to the active metabolite, dihydroartemisinin.

Adverse effects

Few have been reported so far. Transient heart block, transient decrease in blood neutrophils and brief episodes of fever have been reported.

Antimalarial Schedules

As propylactic

Drugs should be given 1-2 weeks before going to an endemic area, continued during stay and for 6 weeks after return from that place.

Chloroquine 300 mg (base) once weekly or pyrimethamine 25 mg weekly is recommended.

In chloroquine-resistant *P. falciparum* area, pyrimethamine 25 mg plus sulphadoxine 500 mg or 100 mg dapsone are indicated.

For acute attack (excluding cerebral malaria): Chloroquine 600 mg (base) initially, then 300 mg (base) at 6 hours, then 300 mg (base) at 24 hours and 48 hours, thus total dose 1.5 g in 3 days should be administered. However, if patient does not respond in 24 hours it indicates chloroquine-resistant case for which quinine sulphate 650 mg thrice a day for 4-6 days with pyrimethamine 25 mg plus sulphadoxine 500 mg, 3 tablets on the first day or doxycycline 100 mg twice a day for 7 days are recommended.

In multi-drug resistant cases: Mefloquine 1-1.5 g orally in a single dose.

For radical treatment

Chloroquine 1.5 g in 3 days followed by primaquine 15 mg/24 hours for 15 days.

Table 11.12. Properties of antimalarial drugs

Drug(s)	Pharmacokinetic properties	Antimalarial activity	Toxicity	
			Minor	Major
Quinine	Good oral and IM absorption $t_{1/2}$:16 h in malaria, ll h in healthy persons	Acts mainly on trophozoites blood stage, kills gametocytes of *P. vivax*, *P. ovale*, and *P. malariae*; no action on liver stage by <1%	Cinchonism tinnitus, high-tone hearing loss, vomiting QT interval in ECG prolonged	Hypoglycaemia Rarely-hypotension, blidness, deafness
Chloroquine	Good oral absorption, very rapid IM/SC absorption $t_{1/2}$:1-2 months	As for quinine but acts slightly earlier in asexual cycle	Nausea, pruritus in dark skinned persons, postural hypotension	Acute: Neuropsychiatric reaction chronic: Retinopathy and cardiac myopathy
Mefloquine	Adequate oral absorption, no parenteral preparation $t_{1/2}$:14-20 days (shorter in malaria)	As for quinine	Nausea, giddiness, fuzzy thinking, sleeplessness, nightmares, sense of dissociation	Neuropsychiatric reactions, convulsions
Halofantrine	Highly variable absorption related to fat intake; $t_{1/2}$:1-3 days (active desbutyl metabolite $t_{1/2}$: 3-7 days)	As for quinine	Diarrhoea	Cardiac conduction disturbances QT interval prolongation in ECG, potentially lethal ventricular tachyarrhythmias
Artemisinin and derivatives (artemether artesunate)	Good oral absorption, variable absorption of IM artemether, artesunate and artemether biotransformed to active metabolites dihydroartemisinin; all drugs eliminated rapidly $t_{1/2}$: <1h	Broader stage specificity and more rapid than other drugs; no action on liver stages	Reduction in reticulocyte count; fever, allergy	Neurotoxicity of oil-based IM preparation reported in animal but no evidence in humans
Pyrimethamine	Good oral absorption, variable IM absorption; $t_{1/2}$: 4 days	For blood stages; causal prophylactic; not used alone for treatment	Well tolerated;	Megaloblastic anaemia, pancytopenia, pulmonary infiltration
Proguanil	Good oral absorption; biotransformed to active metabolite cycloguanil; $t_{1/2}$:16h	Causal prophylactic; not used alone for treatment	Well tolerated; mouth ulcers and rare alopecia	Megaloblastic anaemia
Primaquine	Complete oral absorption; active compound not known; $t_{1/2}$:7h	Radical cure; eradicates hepatic forms of P.vivax and *P. ovale*; kills gametocytes of *P. falciparum*	Nausea, vomiting, diarrhoea, abdominal pain, haemolysis methemoglobinemia	Massive haemolysis in subjects with severe G6PD deficiency
Atovaquone	Highly variable absorption related to fat intake; $t_{1/2}$:30-70h	Acts mainly on trophozoite blood stage	None indentified	—
Lumefantrine	- do - $t_{1/2}$:3-4 days	As for quinine	- do -	—

Table 11.13. Recommended therapeutic doses of antimalarial drugs

Drug	Uncomplicated malaria (oral)	Severe malaria (parenteral)
Chloroquine	10 mg of base/kg followed by 10 mg/kg at 24 h and 5 mg/kg of 12, 24 and 36 h (initial dose, 25 mg/kg); for *P. vivax* or *P. ovale*, primaquine (0.25 mg of base/kg per day for 14 days) added for radical cure	10 mg of base/kg by constant rate infusion over 8 h followed by 15 mg/kg over 24 h or by 3.5 mg of base/kg by IM or SC injection every 6 h (total dose, 25 mg/kg)
Sulphadoxine/ pyrimethamine	2.5/1.25 mg/kg single oral dose	—
Mefloquine	15 mg/kg followed by 8-12 h later by second dose of 10 mg/kg	—
Quinine	10 mg of salt/kg q8h for 7 days combined with tetracyclinc (4 mg/kg qid) or doxy-cycline (3 mg/kg OD) or clindamycin (10 mg/kg bid) for 7 days	20 mg of salt/kg by I.V. infusion over 4 h followed by 10 mg/kg infused over 2-8 h every 8 h.
Artesunate	In combination with 25 mg of mefloquine/kg. 12 mg/kg given in divided doses 3-5 days, if used alone given for 7 days	
Artemether	Same as for artesunate	3.2 mg/kg IM followed by 1.6 mg/kg per day
Atovaquone-proguanil	For adults 740 mg/kg each dose comprises 4 tablets (each containing 250 mg and proguanil 100 mg) taken once daily for 3 days with food.	
Artemether-lumefantrine	For adults ≥ 35 kg, each dose comprises 4 tablets (each containing artemether 20 mg and lumefantrine 120 mg) at 0, 8, 24 and 48 h (semi-immune) or at 0, 8, 24, 36, 48 and 60 h (nonimmune) taken after food	

Treatment of cerebral malaria

Quinine hydrochloride 650 mg (salt) diluted in 20 ml of normal saline is given slowly by I.V. injection in 10-15 minutes, which may be repeated after 8 hours (maximum dose 2 g in 24 hours).

STUDY QUESTIONS

1. What are the different types of malaria?
2. Describe the life-cycle of malarial parasite and indicate the site of action of various antimalarial drugs.
3. Classify antimalarials. Give a list based on their chemical nature. Also give a list based on their clinical uses i.e. for treatment of acute attack, as suppressive agents and to bring about radical cure.
4. Discuss quinine—its usefulness, limitations including adverse effects.
5. Describe uses and adverse effects of chloroquine.
6. Discuss 8-aminoquinolines regarding effectiveness, indications and adverse effects.
7. Write notes on (i) daraprim, (ii) paludrine, and (iii) sulphonamide-sulphone combination as antimalarial.
8. Describe the pharmacokinetics, route of administration, uses, doses and adverse effects of Mefloquine.

GUIDE TO FURTHER READING

Bateman, D.N et al: Quinine toxicity. Adverse Drug React. Acute Poisoning Rev., 1986; 5:215-233.

Bernstein, H.N et al: The ocular deposition of chloroquine. Invest. Ophthalmol. Visual Sci., 1963; 2:384-392.

Bitonti, A.J et al: Reversal of chloroquine resistance in malaria parasite Plasmodium falciparum by desipramine. Science, 1988; 242:1301-1303.

Cook, I.F et al: Haematological safety of long-term malarial prophylaxis with dapsone-pyrimethamine. Med. J. Aust., 1985; 143:139-141.

Dyson, E.H et al: Deatlh and blindness due to overdose of quinine. Br. Med. J (Clin. Res. Ed.), 1985; 291:31-33.

Easterbrook, M et al: Ocular effects and safety of antimalarial agents. Am.J.Med., 1988; 85 Suppl. 4A:23-29.

Edwards, G et al: Clinical pharmacokinetics in the treatment of tropical diseases. Some applications and limitations Clin. Pharmacokinet., 1994; 27:150-165.

Estes, M.L et al: chloroquine neuromyotoxicity: clinical and pathologic perspective. Am. J. Med., 1987; 82:447-455.

Ferrari, V et al: Simulation of kinetic data on the influx and efflux of chloroquine by erythrocytes infected with Plasmodium falciparum. Evidence for a drug-importer in chloroquine-sensitive strains. Biochem. Pharmacol., 1991; 42:S167-S179.

Heksby, N.A et al: The multiple dose pharmacokinetics of proguanil. Br. J. Clin. Pharmacol., 1993; 35:653-656.

Karle, J.M et al: Crystal structure and molecular structure of mefloquine methylsulfonate monohydrate: implications for a malaria receptor. Antimicrob. Agents Chemother., 1991; 35:2238-2245.

Palmer, K.J et al: Mefloquine: a review of its antimalarial activity, pharmacokinetic properties and therapeutic efficacy. Drugs, 1993; 45:430-475.

Rieckmann, K.H et al: Plasmodium vivax resistance to chloroquine? Lancet, 1989; 2:1183-1184.

Rynes, R.I et al: Ophthalmologic safety porfile of antimalarial drugs. Lupus, 1993; 2:S17-S19.

Slater, A.F et al: Inhibition by chloroquine of a novel haempolymerase enzyme activity in malaria trophozoites. Nature, 1992; 355:167-169.

Van Es, H.H et al: Chemotherapy of malaria: a battle against all odds? Clin. Invest. Med., 1993; 16:285-293.

Wellems, T.E et al: Genetic mapping of the chloroquine-resistance locus on Plasmodium falciparum chromosome 7. Proc. Natl. Acad. Sci. USA, 1991; 88:3382-3386.

White, N.J et al: Drug treatment and prevention of malaria. Eur. J. Clin. Pharmacol., 1988; 34:1-14.

White, N.J et al: Antimalarial pharmacokinetics and treatment regiments. Br. J. Clin. Pharmacol., 1992; 34:1-10.

Winstanley, P et al: Towards optimal regiments of parenteral quinine for young African children with cerebral malaria: importance of unbound quinine concentration. Trans. R. Soc. Trop. Med. Hyg., 1993; 87:201-206.

Zucker, J.R et al: Malaria: principles of prevention and treatment. Infect. Dis. Clinic North Am., 1993; 7:547-567.

CHEMOTHERAPY OF AMOEBIASIS

As the choice of drugs depends on the specific forms of amoebiasis and on the desired site of drug action, it is important to know that amoebiasis may be manifested as (i) asymptomatic intestinal infection, (ii) mild to moderate intestinal infection, (iii) severe intestinal infection (dysentery), (iv) amoeboma (an amoebic granuloma in the intestinal wall, (v) hepatic abscess.

The *Entamoeba histolytica* (EH), the causative amoeba exists in 2 forms, viz. trophozoites (active and motile form), and cysts.

Amoebiasis is produced by the ingestion of cysts which develop into trophozoites which invade intestinal mucosa and produce amoebic dysentery. The trophozoites may be carried to liver (more frequently), lungs, brain, and sites after producing ulceration in the intestinal mucosa. Under unfavourable conditions, the trophozoite undergoes cystic stage. Cysts are passed in faeces.

The trophozoites of EH may be found in the lumen of bowel, intestinal wall, in liver, lung, brain. Cysts remain only in intestinal lumen. The cysts can survive outside the body for about 7 days in a moist and cool environment.

Choice of amoebicide

In the intestine the cysts develop into trophozoites which adhere to colonic epithelial cells by means of a lectin on the parasite membrane that has similarity to host adherence protein. The trophozoite then lyses the host cell (hence histolytica) and invades the submucosa, where it may secrete a factor that inhibits gama-interferon-activated macrophages which would otherwise kill it. This process may result in dysentery and in many subjects a chronic intestinal infection occurs in the absence of dysentery. The parasite may invade the liver producing liver abscesses and in some subjects an amoebic granuloma (an amoeboma) develops in the intestinal wall. Some individuals are 'carriers', who harbour the parasite without manifestations of the disease, but cysts are present in their faeces and they can infect other individuals.

The choice depends whether the infection is in the intestinal lumen or in the tissues.

Drugs used to treat amoebiasis can be categorized as following :

1. Systemic amoebicides (tissue amoebicides): Chloroquine, Dehydroemetine, Emetine	Effective only against invasive forms of amoebiasis
2. Luminal amoebicides : Diloxanide furoate, Halogenated 8-hydroxyquinolines (Diiodohydroxyquin, Iodochlorhydroxyquin), Antibiotics (Paromomycin, Erythromycin, Tetracycline)	Effective against intestinal forms of amoebiasis
3. Mixed amoebicides are active against both intestinal and systemic forms of amoebiasis: Metronidazole (more effective against systemic than intestinal amoebiasis)	

SYSTEMIC AMOEBICIDES

Chloroquine

It is used as a systemic amoebicide to treat hepatic amoebiasis only when treatment with metronidazole is unsuccessful or contraindicated. The response is prompt and amoebae do not develop resistance to chloroquine.

Chloroquine is highly effective when administered with emetine or dehydroemetine in the treatment or prevention of amoebic abscess.

Chloroquine is effective against extraintestinal amoebiasis but almost ineffective against intestinal amoebiasis because it is almost completely absorbed from the small intestines and attains only low concentrations in intestinal wall.

Chloroquine is readily absorbed from the gut, is about 50% plasma protein bound, and is concentrated several fold in various tissues such as liver, spleen, heart, kidney and eyes.

For the treatment of extraintestinal amoebiasis, chloroquine phosphate 1 g daily for two days followed by 500 mg daily for 2-3 weeks is recommended. Because of low toxicity of chloroquine this dose schedule can be increased or repeated if required. Better results are achieved when used in combination with emetine/metronidazole.

Emetine and dehydroemetine

Emetine is an alkaloid derived from ipecac or synthesized.

Dehydroemetine is a synthetic substance. It is equally effective and probably less cardiotoxic than emetine.

These drugs are given by I.M. injection because their absorption on oral administration is erratic and due to irritant effect produce vomiting. After I.M. injection, absorption is good and they have selective storage in the liver, lungs, spleen and kidney.

These drugs have cummulative effect. The rate of excretion is slow.

Antiamoebic action

Emetine and dehydroemetine act only against trophozoites and not cystic stage. They are not given orally due to erratic absorption and irritant nature.

Dose: 60 mg once a day for 10 days by deep SC or I.M injection.

Clinical applications

- They rapidly alleviate severe intestinal symptoms but are rarely curative. Being highly toxic, they are given for 3-5 days to relieve severe symptoms.
- Emetine and dehydroemetine are curative for extraintestinal amoebiasis. They are administered for a period of 7-8 days.

Adverse effects

These are mild if given for 3-5 days, severe effects may appear if given upto 10 days; and serious effects are common if they are given for more than 10 days. They are cumulative drugs.

Pain at the site of injection, nausea, and vomiting (central in origin after parenteral use) and ECG changes occur. Minor paresthesias are reported. The serious toxicity includes hypotension, tachycardia, arrhythmias and congestive heart failure.

Contraindication and caution

- Inadvertent I.V. injection must be avoided
- These should not be used in the presence of cardiac or renal disease and in patients who give history of polyneuritis
- During pregnancy
- Extremes of age

LUMINAL AMOEBICIDES

Diloxanide Furoate

This drug is directly amoebicidal. In the intestine it is split into diloxanide and furoic acid. About 90% diloxanide is rapidly absorbed and rapidly excreted in urine as glucuronide conjugate. The unabsorbed diloxanide is the active amoebicidal substance.

It is mainly useful in eradicating the cystic forms from the intestinal lumen.

Uses

Diloxanide furoate is the drug of choice for asymptomatic and mild intestinal amoebiasis and in mild symptomatic intestinal amoebiasis, it is used with other drugs.

It is less effective in moderate to severe forms of intestinal amoebiasis.

In the treatment of liver abscess, diloxanide furoate is used to eradicate intestinal infection.

Dose: 500 mg thrice a day for 10 days.

It is not effective against extraluminal infection.

Adverse effects are uncommon. However, flatulence and nausea, vomiting, dryness of mouth, diarrhoea, urticaria may occur.

Its use is contraindicated in pregnancy and children under 2 years of age.

Halogenated 8-hydroxyquinolines

Among the halogenated hydroxyquinolines, diiodohydroxyquin (iodoquinol) is commonly used. It is effective against luminal amoebiasis but not against trophozites in the intestinal wall or extraintestinal tissues.

Diiodohydroxyquin (iodoquinol) is indicated as (i) an alternative drug for the treatment of asymptomatic or mild to moderate intestinal amoebiasis, (ii) to eradicate concurrent intestinal infection in patients suffering from extraintestinal forms of amoebiasis.

Halogenated hydroxyquinolines are effective against trophozoites as well as cysts.

Besides the use in amoebiasis, these are also useful for the treatment of giardiasis and *E.coli* infection.

Dose: Iodoquinol 650 mg thrice a day for 10 days, alone or with tetracycline 250 mg four times a day for 7 days.

Adverse effects of halogenated hydroxyquinolines are frequent and at times of serious nature if high doses are given for longer periods of time. The adverse effects include nausea, diarrhoea, gastritis, vomiting, fever, thyroid may be enlarged.

One of the halogenated hydroxyquinolines, iodochlorhydroxyquin (clioquinol) has been implicated in the production of neurotoxic syndrome (subacute myelo-optic neuropathy, SMON) characterized by optic atrophy, visual loss, and peripheral neuropathy. It is banned in U.S.A., Japan, India and other countries.

Iodoquinol is safer than clioquinol.

Diiodohydroxyquin has not been implicated in the production of neurotoxic effects with 650 mg administered thrice a day for 21 days.

Contraindications and caution

Diiodoquin should not be used for nonspecific diarrhoea.

For the treatment of amoebiasis only the recommended dosage for the prescribed duration should be taken.

It is contraindicated in patients with intolerance to iodine or in the presence of renal or thyroid disease.

It is more toxic to infants and young children so careful assessment should by made.

MIXED AMOEBICIDES

Metronidazole

It is one of the 5-nitroimidazole derivatives (Fig. 11.10). It is effective against both intestinal and extraintestinal amoebiasis (more effective in extraintestinal infection). It kills trophozoites but does not kill cysts of *E. histolytica*. It is not effective in chronic intestinal amoebiasis in which cystic forms persist in the bowel lumen.

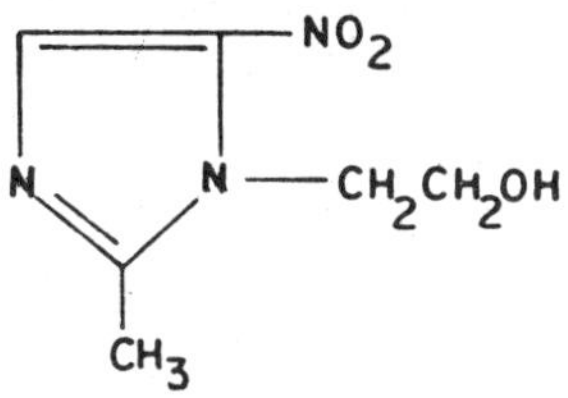

Fig. 11.10. Structure of metronidazole.

Metronidazole is well absorbed on oral administration, widely distributed including CSF, breast milk, and bones. The serum half-life is 7.5 hours. The drug is metabolized in liver. The drug and its metabolites are excreted in the urine.

Dose: In amoebiasis, 750 mg thrice a day for 5-10 days.

In giardiasis and trichomoniasis 250 mg thrice a day for 5-7 days.

Besides the use of metronidazole in amoebiasis, it is also the drug of choice in the treatment of giardiasis, bacterial anaerobes, and trichomoniasis.

Adverse effects

GIT disturbances are most common such as anorexia, nausea, vomiting, epigastric distress, abdominal cramps, unpleasant metallic taste, glossitis, stomatitis and furry tongue.

CNS serious adverse effects are peripheral neuropathy and seizures. The CNS less serious adverse effects include vertigo, ataxia, depression and insomnia.

Cardiac toxicity shows flattening of T-wave in ECG.

Renal/genitourinary side effects are in the form of deep red-brown colour of the urine, polyuria, dysuria, incontinence.

Haematological adverse effects include neutropenia (reversible).

Hypersensitivity reactions include fever, urticaria, etc.

Very uncomfortable symptoms and severe vomiting occur if metronidazole and alcohol are taken together because of its disulfiram like effect. All patients taking metronidazole should be warned not to use alcohol before starting the drug and for 48 hours after last dose.

Precautions and contraindications

The use of metronidazole should be avoided in pregnancy, in nursing women, and in young children. It should be used cautiously in patients with a history of blood dyscrasias.

Drug interactions

The effect of coumarin-type anticoagulants is potentiated by metronidazole. Phenytoin and phenobarbitone may increase excretion of metronidazole.

Box 11.11. Drugs of choice in amoebiasis			
Amoebiasis	Drug of choice		Remarks
	1st	2nd	
Asymptomatic and mild infection	Diloxanide furoate	Iodoquinol	Nephrotoxicity can be caused by excessive doses of iodoquinol
Moderate to severe intestinal infection (amoebic dysentery)	Metronidazole plus Diloxanide furoate	Paromomycin plus Diloxanide furoate	Iodoquinol may be given in place of diloxanide furoate
Systemic amoebiasis (including amoebic abscesses)	Metronidazole plus Diloxanide furoate	Chloroquine plus Diloxanide furoate	Emetine is effective but not frequently recommended due to potential toxicity

OTHER 5-NITROIMIDAZOLES

Tinidazole

Its duration of action is longer than metronidazole hence suited for once daily therapy.

2 gm per day for three days or 600 mg twice a day orally for 5 days is recommended for the treatment of amoebic dysentery; amoebic abscess requires 2 gm single oral dose for 5 days; for girdiasis single dose 2 gm or 600 mg once a day for 7 days. For amoebic infection prophylaxis the dose is 2 gm single dose before colorectal surgery, the therapeutic dose is 2 gm followed by 0.5 gm twice a day for 5 days.

Ornidazole

It is administered as 2 gm orally single dose for 10 days in amoebic dysentery.

Secnidazole

It is a 5-nitroimidazole with properties similar to those of metronidazole, apart from a much longer plasma half-life, it is effective in intestinal amoebiasis, girdiasis, trichomoniasis with single once only dose 2 gm orally in amoebic dysentery and girdiasis. In amoebic abscess, 1.5 gm orally daily for 5 days is recommended.

The side effects include epigastric pain, nausea, glossitis, headache, anorexia, diarrhoea, rash, leukopenia.

ANTIBIOTICS

Paromomycin sulphate is an aminoglycoside antibiotic obtained from *streptomyces rimosus*. It is an alternative drug in cases of mild to moderate intestinal amoebiasis. It is not absorbed from GIT. It acts directly as well as indirectly (inhibits bacterial flora in the bowel) as an amoebicidal drug.

It is effective against luminal amoebiasis only and not effective against extraintestinal amoebiasis.

The adverse effects include diarrhoea, ototoxicity and renal damage.

Tetracyclines

Tetracyclines particularly oxytetracycline, have weak direct amoebicidal effect, their indirect actions are by modifying the intestinal flora on which amoebae thrive in the bowel lumen. This makes tetracyclines useful as luminal amoebicide in cases of mild to severe infections. However, they should not be used in pregnancy and children under 8 years of age.

Erythromycin stearate (being less toxic than tetracyclines) can be used in place of tetracyclines, although it is less effective.

Suggested schedule of treatment

Asymptomatic intestinal	Diloxanide furoate 500 mg × 3/d for 10 days + Metronidazole 400 mg × 3/d for 4 days
Symptomatic intestinal,	Metronidazole 750 mg × 3/d for 5-10 days followed by Diloxanide 500 mg × 3/d for 10 days
Hepatic,	Metronidazole 750 mg × 3/d for 10 days followed by Diloxanide 500 mg × 3/d for 10 days followed by Chloroquine 300 mg for 14 days Hepatic abscess may require to be drained.
Carriers	Diloxanide furoate 500 mg × 3/d for 10 days (some patients harbour the parasite without developing disease but cysts are present in their faeces and may infect other individuals).

STUDY QUESTIONS

1. Discuss the choice of drugs for the treatment of specific forms of amoebiasis.
2. List (i) tissue amoebicides, (ii) luminal amoebicides, (iii) amoebicides which act both against intestinal and extraintestinal amoebiasis.
3. Discuss the therapeutic status of (i) emetine, (ii) chloroquine, (iii) diloxanide furoate.
4. Describe the pharmacokinetics, uses and adverse effects of halogenated hydroxyquinolines.
5. Write notes on: (i) paromomycin, (ii) tetracyclines as amoebicidal agents, (iii) tinidazole.
6. Describe metronidazole regarding its pharmacokinetics, uses, contraindications, precautions and adverse effects.

GUIDE TO FURTHER READING

Anonymous. Drugs for parasitic infections. Med. Lett. Drugs Ther., 1993; 35:111-122.

Bristow, N.W et al: Entamide, a new amoebicide; preliminary note. Trans, R. Soc. Trop. Med. Hyg., 1956; 50:182.

Burchard, G.D et al: Entamoeba histolytica: Virulence

potential and sensitivity to metronidazole and emetine of four isolates possessing nonpathogenic zymodemes. Exp. Parasitol., 1988; 66:231-242.

Diamond, L.S et al: A redescription of Entamoeba histo-lytica Schaudinn, 1903 separating it from Entamoeba dispar Brumpt, 1925. J. Euk. Miucrobiol., 1993; 40:340-344.

Fry, M et al: Mitocondria of mammalian Plasmodium spp. Parasitology; 1991; 102:17-26.

Fry, M et al: Site of action of the antimalarial hydroxy-naphthoquinone, 2-[trans-4-(4°-chlorophenyl) cyclohexyl]-3-hydroxy-1,4-naphthoquinone (566C80). Biochem. Pharmacol., 1992; 43:1545-1553.

Grogl, M et al: Characteristics of multidrug resistance in Plasmodium and Leishmania: detection of P-glycoprotein-like components. Am. J. Trop. Med. Hyg., 1991; 45:98-111.

Hopkins, R.J et al: Helicobacter pylori: the missing link in persepctive. Am. J. Med., 1994; 97:265-277.

Johnson, P.L et al: Metronidazole and drug resistance. Parasotp. Today, 1993; 9:183-186.

Krogstad, D.J et al: Amebiasis. N. Engl. J. Med., 1978; 298:262-265.

Lau, A.H et al: Clinical pharmacokinetics of metronidazole and other nitroimidazole anti-infectives. Clin. Pharmacokinet., 1992; 23:328-364.

Roe, F.J.C et al: Metronidazole: review of uses and toxicity. J. Antimicrob. Chemother., 1977; 3:205-212.

Woolfe, G et al: The chemotherapy of amoebiasis. In, Progress in Drug Research, Vol. 8. Birkhauser Verlag, Basel, 1965; pp. 11-52.

Wolfe, M.S et al: Nondysenteric intestinal amebiasis. Treatment with diloxamide furoate. JAMA, 1973; 224:1601-1604.

CHEMOTHERAPY OF LEISHMANIASIS, TRYPANOSOMIASIS, TRICHOMONIASIS, GIARDIASIS

HUMAN LEISHMANIASIS

Human leishmaniasis is caused by protozoal species and subspecies of the genus *Leishmania*. It can be classified into cutaneous, mucocutaneous, diffuse cutaneous and visceral forms (kala azar).

Only the cutaneous forms are self limiting.

Initial treatment with pentavalent antimonials appears safe and effective but resistance to these agents is increasing.

Second-line drugs such as pentamidine and amphotericin B are less satisfactory.

Drugs used for leishmaniasis

1. Pentavalent antimony compounds:
   - Urea stibamine intravenous 50-200 mg on alternate days for one month.
   - Sodium stibogluconate: It is the drug of choice for kala-azar; 20 mg/kg/day (maximum 850 mg); i.v./i.m. injection is painful.
   - For cutaneous forms, the duration of treatment is for 20 days and 30 days for visceral and mucocutaneous leishmaniasis.
   - Meglumine antimonate: It is least toxic among the members of this group. However, nausea, vomiting, metallic taste, kidney and liver damage have been reported as side effects.

   The dose is 20 mg/kg for 1-2 months.

2. Diamine derivatives: These are more potent and more toxic than pentavalent antimony compounds and hence used in cases resistant to pentavalent antimonials.
   - Pentamidine isethionate and lomidine mesylate are administered i.m. or slow i.v. 4 mg/kg thrice a week (12-15 injections). The adverse effects after injection include nausea, vomiting, hypotension, breathlessness, hepatotoxicity, thrombocytopenia and leukopenia (usually reversible). About 5% of patients develop insulin-dependent diabetes mellitus (IDDM) during pentamidine therapy.
   - Dihydroxystilbamidine isethionate is given i.v. 250 mg daily for 10 days.

3. Allopurinol may be added to antimony therapy, orally 300 mg in three divided doses for 15-30 days. It is beneficial in leishmaniasis, particularly in cutaneous form.

4. Antifungal agents such as amphotericin B (i.v. 0.1-1 mg/kg on alternate days, total dose 1.5-2 gm). Another antifungal agent ketoconazole 600 mg per day orally for one month has been found useful in cutaneous leishmaniasis.

5. Interferon shows promise as adjunctive therapy with pentavalent antimony in serious cases suffering from kala-azar.

Table 11.14 shows regimens for treatment of leishmaniasis

Table 11.14. Drug regimens for treatment of leish-maniasis

Clinical syndrome, drug	Route of administration	Regimen
Enteral Leishmaniasis		
Pentavalent antimony, (sod. stibogluconate)	IV, IM	20 mg/kg qid for 20 days
Amphotericin B (total 15-21 mg/kg)	IV	2-5 mg/kg qid
Paromomycin	IV, IM	15-20 mg/kg qid or thrice weekly for 21 days
Pentamidine isethionate	IV, IM	4 mg/kg qid or thrice weekly for 15-30 doses
Cutaneous Leishmaniasis		
Pentavalent isethionate	IV, IM	3 mg/kg qid for 4 doses or 2 mg/kg qid for 7 days
Amphotericin B	IV	0.5-1 mg/kg qid (total 30 mg/kg)
Alternatives		
Ketoconazole	per oral	600 mg/d for 28 days
Mucosal Leishmaniasis		
Pentamidine isethionate	IV, IM	2-4 mg/kg qid or thrice weekly for > 15 doses

Drugs for African sleeping sickness

- Suramin with pentamidine
- Melarsoprol (arsenical) for late stage with CNS involvement.

Drugs used in Chagas' disease

- Primaquine
- Puromycin
- Nifurtimox
- Benznidazole ⎫ in acute disease only

TRYPANOSOMIASIS

African trypanosomal 'sleeping sickness' and American or Chagas' disease affect many people.

Drugs for Trypanosomiasis

Suramin sodium

It is a naphthylamine-sulfonic acid derivative intro-duced for the therapy of trypanosomiasis. It is used to treat African trypanosomiasis but is of no value in South American trypanosomiasis (caused by T. cruzi).

It is given by slow I.V. injection as a 10% aqueous solution to avoid local inflammation and necrosis associated with subcutaneous or i.m injections.

Dose: 2-4 doses of 250-500 mg on alternate days 1, 3, 7, 14 and 21, weekly doses for additional 5 weeks are recommended.

Its main toxic effect is on kidney, other adverse effects include optic atrophy, adrenal insufficiency, haemolytic anaemia, rashes, and agranulocytosis.

The adverse effects are more severe in debilited persons. The serious immediate reaction consists of nausea, vomiting, shock, malaise, fatigue, convulsions and coma. Fortunately, the incidence is low (0.1% - 0.3%).

Although suramin is effective in clearing adult filariae in onchocerciasis, it has been replaced largely by ivermectin.

Melarsoprol

It is the arsenoxide form of an organic arsenical which has rapid lethal effect on African trypanosomes.

It is always administered intravenously. A small but therapeutically effective concentration reaches CSF which is lethal to trypanosomes infecting CNS.

It is a toxic drug hence, it is not recommended as a prophylactic agent against trypanosomes.

Nifurtimox

It is one of numerous congeners of nitrofurans. It is quite useful in American trypanosomiasis caused by *T. cruzi* (Chagas' disease). It reduces the severity of acute condition but ineffective in chronic stages.

This drug is well absorbed after oral administration.

Dose: 8-10 mg/kg/d in 4 divided doses for 120 days in adults and in children, 15-20 mg/kg/d in 4 divided doses for 90 days.

Ingestion of alcohol should be avoided otherwise the incidence of adverse effects will increase.

Adverse effects are common and include nausea, vomiting, myalgia, weight loss, headache, polyneuritis and psychic disturbances.

It may also cause leukopenia and decrease in sperm count.

Pentamidine isethionate

It is an alternative drug to suramin for the early stages of Trypanosomiasis. It can not be used when the central nervous system is involved as it does not cross the blood-brain barrier.

Dose: 4 mg/kg per day, usually given by i.m. injection or slow iv infusion over 60 minutes in a single daily doses of 4 mg base/kg.

Adverse effects include pain at the site of injection, rash, abnormal liver function tests, hypocalcaemia, hyperkalaemia, hypoglycaemia followed by hyperglycaemia.

Delayed nephrotoxicity has been reported. The other adverse effects (rare) include megaloblastic anaemia, acute pancreatitis, and thrombocytopenia. Deaths have occurred due to hypotension, hypoglycaemia, or arrhythmias.

Resuscitation facilities should be kept ready when pentamidine is injected because sometimes even after a single dose there may be severe hypotension.

Pentamidine should be carefully given in patients having low blood pressure, high blood pressure, latent or clinical diabetes mellitus, anaemia, renal or hepatic dysfunction.

Drugs for Trichomoniasis and Giardiasis

Trichomoniasis is caused by the flagellated protozoan *Trichyomonas vaginalis*. Giardiasis is caused by the flagellated protozoan *Giardia lamblia*.

Metronidazole is the treatment of choice for urogenital trichomoniasis, for which 250 mg orally thrice daily for 7 days or a single dose of 2 g or 1 g twice a day in one day are prescribed. The drug should be avoided in the first trimester of pregnancy.

The nitrogroup of metronidazole is chemically reduced by ferredoxin. The reduction products react with the intracellular macromolecules resulting in killing of the organisms (bactericidal effect).

Metronidazole-resistant strains of *Trichomonas vaginalis* have been reported.

For the treatment of giardiasis, 250 mg orally thrice a day (children 5 mg/kg thrice a day) for 5 days are recommended.

Besides the above, metronidazole has been found useful in many other conditions including amoebiasis.

Metronidazole is also useful against anaerobic infections following appendectomy, colorectal surgery, and abdominal surgery. Additionally infections due to *Bacteroides fragilis*, and clostridia which are refractory to other drugs, usually respond to metronidazole. Metronidazole can penetrate abscesses and necrotic tissues.

Metronidazole 250 mg orally 3 times a day with drug for aerobic infection and suitable topical treatment promotes healing, relieves pain, inflammation, swelling, and purulent discharge in phagedenic leg ulcers, acute ulcerative gingivitis, and decubitus ulcers.

Side effects only rarely are severe. The commonest side effects include headache, nausea, dry mouth, and metallic taste. Vomiting, diarrhoea may be occasionally experienced. Furry tongue, glossitis, and stomatitis may occur during therapy.

Dizziness, vertigo, encephalopathy, convulsions and ataxia (neurotoxic effects, rare) warrant discontinuation of metronidazole.

Quinacrine hydrochloride is an antimalarial drug which is effective in the treatment of giardiasis (cure rate about 90%).

Toxoplasmosis and Toxoplasmocidal drugs

Toxoplasma gondii is a protozoan that infects cats and other animals. Oocysts in the infected animal's faeces can infect humans. In most cases, toxoplasmosis is asymptomatic or self-limiting. However, infection during pregnancy can cause serious disease in the foetus.

Drugs used:

- Pyrimethamine - sulphadiazine (avoid in pregnancy)
- Trimethoprim- sulphamethoxazole
- Pentamidine parenterally
- Azithromycin

STUDY QUESTIONS

1. Which drugs are useful for the treatment of Leishmaniasis? Why the treatment is not generally satisfactory?

2. What are the uses and adverse effects of pentamidine?

3. Write notes on (i) suramin and (ii) amphotericin B
4. Describe in details the pharmacokinetics, doses, routes of administration, uses in various conditions, precautions and adverse effects of metronidazole.

GUIDE TO FURTHER READING

Bacchi, C.J et al: Effects of antagonists of polyamine metabolism on African trypanosomes. Acta Trop., 1993; 54:225-236.

Bacchi, C.J et al: Polyamine metabolism: a potential therapeutic target in trypanosomes. Science, 1980; 210:332-334.

Bacchi, C.J et al: Combination chemotherapy of drug-resistant Trypanosoma brucei rhodesiense infections in mice using DL-alpha-difluoromethylo-methylornithine and standard trypanocides. Antimicrob. Agents Chemother., 1994; 38:563-569.

Berger, J.D et al: Interactions between immunity and chemotherapy in the treatment of the trypanosomiases and leishmaniases. Parasitology, 1992; 105:S71-S78.

Berman, J.D et al: Biochemistry of Pentostam resistant leishmania. Am. J. Trop. Med. Hyg., 1989; 40:159-164.

Carter, N.S et al: Arsenical-resistant trypanosomes lack an unusual adenosine transporter. Nature, 1993; 361:173-176.

Chulay, J.D et al: Pharmacokinetics of antimony during treatment of viseral leishmaniasis with sodium stibogluconate or meglumine antimoniate. Trans. R. Soc. Trop. Med. Hyg., 1988; 82:69-72.

Chunge, C.N et al: Treatment of visceral leishmaniasis in Kenya by aminosidine alone or combined with sodium stibogluconate. Trans. R. Soc. Trop. Med. Hyg., 1990; 84:221-225.

Conte, J.E. jr.: Pharmacokinetics of intravenous pentamidine in patients with normal renal function or receiving hemodialysis. J. Infect. Dis., 1991; 163:169-175.

Donnelly, H et al: Distribution of pentamidine in patients with AIDS. J. Infect. Dis., 1988; 157:985-989.

Durel, P et al: Systemic treatment of human trichomoniasis with a derivative of nitroimidazole, 8823 R.P. Br. J. Vener. Dis., 1960; 36:21-26.

Dykstra, C.C et al: Inhibition of topoisomerases from Pneumocystis carinii by aromatic dicationic molecules. J. Protozool., 1991; 38:78S-81S.

Fairlamb, A.H et al: Characterisation of melarsen-resistant Trypanosoma brucei brucei with respect to cross-resistance ot other drugs and trypanothione metabolism. Mol. Biochem. Parasitol., 1992; 53:213-222.

Grogl, M et al: Drug resistance in leishmaniasis: its implications in systemic chemotherapy of cutaneous and mucocutaneous disease. Am. J. Trop. Med. Hyg., 1992; 47:117-126.

Hand, I.L et al: Aerosolized pentamidine for prophylaxis of Pneumocystis carinii pneumonia in infants with human immunodeficiency virus infection. Pediatr. Infect. Dis. J., 1994; 13:100-104.

Hill, D.R et al: Giardiasis: issues in diagnosis and management. Infect. Dis. Clin. North Am., 1993; 7:503-525.

Jokipii, L et al: In, vitro susceptibility of Giardia lamblia trophozoites to metronidazole and tinidazole. J. Infect. Dis., 1980; 141:317-325.

Navin, T.R et al: Placebo-controlled clinical trial of sodium stibogluconate versus ketoconazole for treating cutaneous leishmaniasis in Guatemala. J. Infect. Dis., 1992; 165:528-534.

Pepin, J et al: African trypanosomiasis and drug-induced encephalopathy: risk factors and pathogenesis. Trans. R. Soc. Trop. Med. Hyg., 1991; 85:222-224.

Ouellette, M et al: Mechansims of drug resistance in Leishmania. Parasitol. Today., 1993; 9:150-153.

Wolfe, M.S et al: Biology of Toxoplasma gondii. AIDS, 1993; 7:299-316.

Yarlett, N et al: Differential susceptibility of Trypanosoma brucei rhodesiense isolates to in vitro lysis by arsenicals. Exp. Parasitol., 1991; 72:205-215.

CHEMOTHERAPY OF HELMINTHIC INFECTIONS (HELMINTHIASIS)

Anthelmintics are drugs that act either locally to expel worms from GIT or systemically to remove adult helminths or development forms that invade organs and tissues. They can kill (vermicides) or expel (vermifuge) worms.

Some of these drugs paralyse the musculature of worms, e.g. piperazine, some of them inhibit the oxidative metabolism e.g. niclosamide and some inhibit the carbohydrate metabolism of the parasites e.g. niridazole. Benzimidazoles, exemplified by mebendazole and albendazole are versatile anthelmintics. They produce many biochemical changes in susceptible nematodes e.g. inhibition of mitochondrial fumarate reductase, reduced glucose transport, and uncoupling of oxidative phosphorylation. There is also strong evidence that the primary action of benzimidazoles is to inhibit microtubule polymerization by binding to beta-tubulin.

Brief descriptions of anthelmintics are presented in alphabetical order, without regard to their relative importance or therapeutic applications.

The main examples of worms that live in the hosts' GIT are:

- Intestinal roundworms (Nematodes):
  Ascaris lumbricoides (Common roundworm),
  Enterobius vermicularis (threadworm),
  Trichuris trichura (whipworm),
  Strongyloides stercoralis (threadworm is USA),
  Necator americanus,
  Ankylostoma duodenale (hookworms).
- Trematodes or flukes: These cause schisto-somiasis (bilharzia)
  Schistosoma haematobium,
  Schistosoma mansoni,
  Schistosoma japonicum
- Tapeworms (Cestodes):
  Taenia saginata
  Taenia solium
  Hymenolepis nana,
  Diphyllobothrium latum
- Tissue roundworms:
  Trichinella spiralis
  Dracunculus medinensis (guinea - worm)
  Filariae which include :
  Wuchereria bancrofti
  Loa loa
  Onchocerca Volvulus
  Brugia malayi
- Hydatid tapeworm:
  Echinococcus species

Albendazole

It is a broad spectrum oral anthelmintic, a congener of mebendazole with excellent tolerability. It is a benzimidazole carbamate.

In the treatment of roundworm and hookworm infection its single dose (400 mg) treatment is similar to 3 days treatment with mebendazole. For tapeworm it should be given for 3 days.

Albendazole is rapidly absorbed, the absorbed portion is metabolized and excreted in urine and only a small amount is excreted in faeces.

Anthelmintic actions: It blocks glucose uptake by larval and adult stages of susceptible parasites which are immobilized and die. It is effective against ascariasis, ancylostomiasis, and trichuriasis. It is also a drug of choice in hydated disease and cysticerosis.

It should be given on empty stomach when used against intraluminal parasites but with a fatty meal when used against tissue parasites (absorption is about four fold greater when taken with a fatty meal).

Adverse effects include GI upsets, insomnia and lassitude. It is contraindicated in the presence of cirrhosis.

Aspidium oleoresin (Extract of male fern)

It is no more used for tapeworms due to severe toxicity and unpredictable results.

Bephenium hydroxynaphthoate (Alcopar)

Previously it was used for the treatment of both species of hookworms and also for treating mixed infection of roundworms and hookworms.

There are no serious side effects, only nausea and vomiting may be produced due to bitter taste.

It is more effective in hookworms than mixed infection. It is seldom used now. Now there are better drugs available.

Bithionol

It is the drug of choice for sheep liver fluke. It is the alternative drug in the treatment of pulmonary paragonimiasis with 90% cure rate with a single dose.

Dose for fascioliasis is 30-50 mg/kg in 2 or 3 divided doses orally after meals on alternative days for 10-15 days.

Adverse effects include diarrhoea, abdominal cramps, nausea, vomiting, anorexia, headache, and dizziness.

Allergic reactions have also occurred resulting from release of antigens from dying worms.

Bithionol should not be used in small children.

Diethylcarbamazine citrate (Hetrazan)

It is a synthetic derivative of piperazine useful in some types of filariasis. It immobilizes microfilariae (results in displacement in tissues). It is the drug of choice against Wuchereria bancrofti, Loa loa. The drug has two types of action on susceptible microfilarae i.e. first to decrease the muscular activity and eventually immobilize the organisms which causes dislocation of the parasites from their normal habitats in the host. The second action is to produce alterations in the microfilarial surface membranes thereby rendering them more susceptible to destruction by defense mechanism.

Dose: 2 mg/kg 3 times a day for 3 weeks. Cure requires several courses of treatment.

Hetrazan is rapidly absorbed on oral administration, widely distributed except in fat, excreted in urine within 30 hours and it is not a cumulative drug.

Adverse reactions include anorexia, headache, malaise, insomnia and dizziness.

Hexylresorcinol has wide anthelmintic spectrum but less effective than other drugs.

Ivermectin

It is the drug of choice in onchocerciasis treatment and other forms of filariasis, strongyloidiasis, and cutaneous larva migrans.

It is well absorbed and widely distributed except that it enters the eye slowly and to a limited extent. The serum half-life is 28 hours. It is almost exclusively excreted in faeces.

Adverse effects are mainly due to killing of microfilariae, resulting in fever, dizziness, headache, rash, pruritus, myalgia, arthralgia, tachycardia, hypotension, lymphadenitis and bronchospasm.

Because of its effect on GABA receptors in the CNS, ivermectin in contraindicated in conditions associated with an impaired blood-brain barrier e.g. meningitis.

Care should also be taken about coadministration of ivermectin with other drugs that depress CNS activity.

This drug is not recommended for use in children less than 5 years old and in pregnant women.

It reduces secretion of milk in lactating women.

Contraindications include concomitant use of barbiturates, benzodiazepines and valproic acid because ivermectin enhances GABA activity. It should also not be used in pregnancy. Safety in children below 5 years is not established.

Levamisole

It is a levo-isomer of tetramisole, it produces neuromuscular inhibition resulting in paralysis leading to expulsion of worms. It is effective as 150 mg single dose in adults or 3 mg/kg single dose for children, available as 50-100 mg tablet and as syrup, for the treatment of roundworm infection. A single dose produces 90% cure rate. It is highly effective in eradicating ascaris and Trichostrongylus and moderately effective against both species of hookworm.

This drug should be used in combination with oxantel for the mixed infections with T. trichiura.

In the case of pinworm, it is wise to repeat the treatment after an interval of 2 weeks.

Adverse effects include nausea, fatigue, giddiness and drowsiness.

Mebendazole

It is a synthetic banzimidazole having a wide spectrum of anthelmintic activity and a low frequency of adverse effects.

This drug is effective and safe for:

- Trichuris trichura (whipworm, 90% cure rate with 100 mg tablet twice a day for 3-4 days).
- Pinworm (90% cure rate with single 100 mg dose).
- Ascaris and hookworm infection (90% cure rate with 100 mg twice a day for 3 days).

It is more effective and safer than quinacrine and aspidium oleoresin for tapeworms. It has no action on ova. It has a 75% cure rate in tapeworms.

Mebendazole inhibits uptake of exogenous glucose by nematodes resulting in glycogen depletion and decreased production of ATP for survival. the immobilizing and lethal action on worms is rather slow, takes 2-3 days.

It is poorly absorbed (10%) on oral administration. The tablets should be chewed before swallowing. It is well tolerated. It is excreted unchanged and as metabolites in urine.

Contraindication : Pregnancy.

Adverse effects are not common, only mild diarrhoea, nausea, and abdominal pain have been reported. Mebendazole should be used with caution in children under 1 year of age because of convulsions reported in this age group (though rare).

Concomitant use of carbamazepine reduces effectiveness of mebendazole, concomitant use of cimetidine may increase plasma levels.

Metrifonate

It is an organophosphate inhibitor of cholinesterase. It is less expensive and safe alternative drug against *Schistosoma haematobium* infection. It is useful against *Schistosoma mansoni* or *Schistosoma japonicum*.

It is used as an alternative to praziquantel only for the treatment of *S. haematobium* infection.

In vitro, the drug is equally potent as an inhibitor of acetylcholinesterases in S. mansoni and S. haematobium, yet clinically it is effective only against infection with *S. haematobium*.

Metrifonate acts through its biotransformation to dichlorvos through nonenzymatic transformation. Dichlorvos is the active metabolite. Dichlorvos is cholinesterase inhibitor and inhibition paralyzes the adult worms. However, it is not effective against eggs and the live eggs continue to pass in the urine.

Dose: 7.5-12.5 mg/kg orally 3 times at 14 days intervals.

Adverse effects are mild and include GI upsets, sweating, headache, vertigo and dizziness. In case of organophosphorus poisoning, atropine should be used.

The drug is *contraindicated* in pregnancy.

Niclosamide

It is a halogenated salicylamide derivative. It is tasteless, non-irritant, well tolerated, and safe drug during pregnancy. It acts against large and dwarf tapeworms. 4 tablets (2 g) are chewed and swallowed with water, saline purge is to be given after 2 hours. It is the drug of choice for the treatment of tapeworm infections.

This drug can be considered a second-choice drug to praziquantel for the treatment of *D. latum*, *H. nana*, *T. saginata* and most other cestode infections including *T. solium*.

The lethal action of the drug against the adult worm does not extend to the ova. Hence, its use in *T. solium* infections may expose the patients to the risk of cysticercosis because following digestion of the dead segments viable ova will be liberated into the lumen of the gut.

Adverse effects : Rarely nausea, vomiting and intestinal colic. There is no systemic toxicity as it is not absorbed.

Niridazole

It is useful in quineaworm infection. It has anti-infalmmatory action. It inhibits glucose uptake by parasites.

The drug is absorbed on oral administration, high first pass metabolism occurs in liver, and excreted in urine and faeces.

The *adverse effects* are manifested in cardiovascular and CNS systems, also has carcinogenic potential. Therefore it should be used only when there is a good reason for it.

Oxantel pamoate in combination with pyrantel

Oxantel is an analogue of pyrantel. It is effective for single-dose treatment of trichuriasis only against trichuriasis. It is also available in combination with pyrantel as pyrantel is effective against ascaris and hookworm infections and trichuriasis is frequently found along with ascaris and hookworms. But both oxantel and oxantel/pyrantel are not effective in strongyloidiasis.

Oxamniquine

It is an effective drug for the treatment of *Schistosoma mansoni* infections only. It is not effective against *S. haematobium* and *S. japonicum*. This drug is active against both mature and immature stages of *S. mansoni* and may act by DNA binding.

Oxamniquine has been used successfully in combination with metrifonate for the treatment of mixed infections with *S. mansoni*, *S. haematobium*.

Adverse effects are not frequent. But mild symptoms including dizziness, headache, drowsiness and GIT upsets may occur.

The drug is contraindicated in pregnancy.

Due to dizziness and drowsiness the patient should be instructed not to drive for a day or so.

Paromomycin (Humatin)

It is an aminoglycoside antibiotic indicated against large tapeworms and amoebiasis. It should not be used in *T. solium* because drug-induced vomiting results in cystocerosis.

Dose: 1 g every 15 minutes for 4 doses; after 2 hours, saline purge is given.

Piperazine (Antepar)

Particularly as citrate it is an alternative drug for roundworms. It is not useful for hookworms, trichuris trichura and strongyloides. It is no longer recommended for pinworm infections because of a 7-day course of treatment. Piperazine produces a reversible paralysis of the muscle of the worm, the myoneural blocking effect is produced by blocking the stimulating effect of acetylcholine at myoneural junction and the worms are expelled.

It is available as tablet or syrup.

Dose: 4.5 g once a day for 2 days for round worms.

Adverse effects include dizziness and urticaria, high doses may produce convulsions and neurotoxic adverse effects (seizures, ataxia and somnolence). Piperazine is potentially allergenic.

Contraindications: Renal or hepatic insufficiency, history of epilepsy (exacerbation of seizures). Piperazine and phenothiazines should not be given together.

Praziquantel

It is a synthetic pyrazinoisoquinoline derivative. It is the drug of choice for all forms of schistosomiasis in doses of 20 mg/kg 4-6 hourly for a total of 3 doses. For the treatment of *H. nana* infection it is highly effective for which a single dose of 25 mg/kg is used. It is useful against trematodes, cestodes, schistosomes. It has high efficacy and absence of toxicity Its use is increasing but cost is a limiting factor

It has two major effects on susceptible helminths. In lowest effective concentrations, it causes increased muscular activity followed by contractions and spastic paralysis. The affected worms detach from host tissues. At slightly higher therapeutic concentration it causes tegumental damage which activates host defense mechanisms resulting in destruction of the worms.

The membranes of affected helminths appear to be the primary target for praziquantel action. The drug causes increased membrane permeability to certain monovalent and divalent cations, particularly Ca^{++}.

It is rapidly absorbed on oral administration, high first pass metabolism occurs in liver, metabolites are excreted in urine.

Its efficacy is similar to niclosamide, brings about 90-100% cure rate after a single dose in tapeworm infestation.

The *adverse effects* include bitter taste (so not to be chewed), headache, drowsiness, dizziness, abdominal pain.

It should not be taken during pregnancy. As it causes dizziness and drowsiness, patient should not drive or engage in work which requires alertness.

Pyrantel pamoate

Pyrantel and its analogues are depolarizing neuromuscular blocking agents. They induce marked persistent activation of nicotinic receptors resulting in spastic paralysis of the worm. Pyrantel also inhibits cholinesterases.

Because pyrantel pamoate and piperazine are mutually antagonistic with respect to their neuromuscular effects on parasites, the two should not be used together.

It is a tetrahydropyrimidine, tasteless, non-irritant which induces spastic neuromuscular paralysis of worms.

It is a broad-spectrum anthelmintic, highly effective for the treatment of pinworms, ascariasis and trichostrongylus infections. It is moderately effective against hookworms.

It is an alternative to mebendazole in the treatment of ascariasis and enterobiasis.

Pyrvinium pamoate (viprynium embonate)

It is seldom used as its efficacy is low.

It is a cyanine dye available in suspension as a single dose treatment for pinworm infection (90-

100% cure rate) but considered as alternative drug to pyrantel and mebendazole as side effects are common.

The post-treatment stools are red for several days. The patient should be informed about it.

It has low activity against *trichuris trichura* and hookworm. It is ineffective against roundworms.

Dose: 5 mg/kg, maximum 35 mg. It can be repeated after 2-4 weeks.

Contraindications: children below 2 years of age.

Adverse effects: GI upsets, photosensitivity.

Oxantel pamoate

It is an analogue of pyrantel. It is useful against trichuriasis. In a single oral dose it produces 95% cure rate in pinworm infection, which can be repeated after 15 days.

It is also very effective (85-100% cure rate) in ascariasis and 90% cure rate in hookworm infections with single dose treatment. However, for severe hookworm cases it should be given for 3 days.

Dose: Single dose 10-15 mg/kg.

It is poorly absorbed, 50% is excreted unchanged in faeces and the rest in unchanged form and as metabolites in urine.

Adverse effects include anorexia, vomiting, dizziness, drowsiness, abdominal pain and rashes. However, these are not common.

Quinacrine (atabrine, mepacrine)

It was an alternative drug for the treatment of tapeworm infestations, it has to be preceded and followed by a purge. It is used only when niclosamide and mebendazole are not available, because of its toxicity.

Adverse effects include nausea, vomiting, diarrhoea, headache, euphoria, anxiety, confusion, restlessness, and aggressive behaviour.

Suramin

It is an alternative drug for the eradication of onchocerciasis and the drug of choice in the treatment of haemolymphatic stage of African trepanosomiasis.

Adverse effects are frequent and serious including peripheral neuritis, nephrotoxicity, anaemia, jaundice and exfoliative dermatitis. Some deaths have occurred. It should be given only by experts.

Tetrachloroethylene

It is an alternative drug for hookworms which are paralyzed. Other drugs with fewer adverse effects are now preferred, but it remains an effective inexpensive alternative drug, with mild adverse reactions.

In case of mixed infection, the treatment of roundworms should be given first otherwise they will migrate and due to large bulk may produce intestinal obstruction.

It does not kill or paralyze roundworms but stimulate them causing migration.

Adverse effects include GI upsets, nausea, vomiting, abdominal pain, CNS stimulation, headache, confusion.

It is *contraindicated* during pregnancy, gastroenteritis, severe constipation.

Thiabendazole

It was the first polyanthelmintic introduced for roundworm, hookworm and whipworm. It is a broad spectrum anthelmintic, available as mint-flavoured tablets used against nematodes (useful in roundworm and pinworm infestations, the results with hookworm and whipworm are not so favourable).

It may be applied locally in scabies.

It is rapidly absorbed, achieves 90% cure rate in strongyloides stercoralis and can be repeated after 7 days.

Dose: 25 mg/kg twice a day for 3 days, available as 500 mg tablet or suspension 100 mg/ml.

Its demerits include poor patient tolerability and frequent side effects such as anorexia, nausea, vomiting, headache, giddiness, hypotension, bradycardia, impaired alertness. Hypersensitivity reactions can also occur though rarely.

Table 11.15 lists choice of anthelmintics.

SOME GENERAL ASPECTS

Effective, and in some cases, broad spectrum agents are now available for cure or control most of human infections caused by flukes or intestinal helminths. But, cysticercosis, echinococcosis, filariasis and trichinosis are examples of systemic infections

Table 11.15. Choice of anthelmintics

Worm infestation	First choice	Alternatives
Nematodes (Roundworms)		
Ascaris lumbricoides	Mebendazole, Pyrantel pamoate	Piperazine, Albendazole, Levamisole, Bephenium
Hookworm (*Necator americanus/Ancylostoma duodenale*)	Pyrantel pamoate	Mebendazole, Albendazole, Levamisole, Bephenium
Pinworm (Enterobius vermicularis)	Mebendazole, Pyrantel pamoate	Albendazole
Combined infection with ascaris, trichuris and hookworm	Mebendazole, Albendazole	Oxantel, Pyrantel pamoate
Whipworm (*Trichuris trichura*)	Mebendazole	Albendazole, Oxantel
Threadworm or dwarf threadworm (*Strongyloides stercoralis*)	Ivermectin, Mebendazole	
Filarial worms (*Wuchereria bancrofti, Loa loa*)	Ivermectin	Diethylcarbamazine
Guineaworm (Medina worm) (*Dracunculus medinensis*)	No suitable anthelmintic therapy; Metronidazole provides symptomatic relief; traditional treatment is to draw adult female out-alive	Mebendazole, Thiabendazole
Flat worms		
Cestodes (tapeworm)		
Taenia solium (pork tapeworm)	Praziquantel, Albendazole	Niclosamide
Taenia saginata (beef tapeworm)	Niclosamide, Praziquantel	Mebendazole, Paromomycin, Dichlorophen, Quinacrine
Diphyllobothrium latum (fish tapeworm)	Praziquantel	Niclosamide
Hymenolepis nana (dwarf tapeworm)	Praziquantel	Niclosamide
Trematodes (flukes)		
Schistosoma (Blood flukes)		
S. haematobium, S. mansoni	Praziquantel	Metrifonate, Oxamniquine
S. japonicum	Praziquantel	None
Liver flukes	Praziquantel	Mebendazole
Lung flukes	Praziquantel	Bithionol
Intestinal flukes	Niclosamide	Hexylresorcinol, Tetracholorethylene

caused by tissue-dwelling helminths that respond only partially to currently available drugs.

- Unless otherwise indicated, oral drugs should be taken with water or after meals. Stool should be examined again after about a fortnight after giving the treatment in case of nemotade infection in intestines.
- Dosages for infants and children should be carefully calculated. In children below 2 years of age these drugs may not be given due to less experience in this age group or due to reported convulsions although rare.
- Pregnancy and ulcers of GIT are contraindi-

cations. Many anthelmintics are teratogenic in animal studies.

STUDY QUESTIONS

1. Describe the indications, mode of action, adverse effects and contraindications of Piperazine as an anthelmintic drug.
2. Write notes on (i) Tetrachloroethylene (ii) Levamisole, (iii) Albendazole and (iv) Thiabendazole.
3. Describe the merits and demerits of Mebendazole.
4. Describe in short:

(i)   Praziquantel
(ii) Metrifonate
(iii) Oxamniquine and
(iv) Niclosamide.

5. Describe the anthelmintic spectrum of :
(i)   Oxantel pamoate
(ii) Pyrantel pamoate
(iii) Diethylcarbamazine citrate (Hetrazan) and
(iv) Niridazole.

6. Discuss choice of anthelmintics. Give examples of drugs of first choice and alternatives for the following infection caused by:
(i)   Ascaris
(ii)   Hookworms
(iii) Threadworms
(iv)   Pinworms
(v)   Whipworms (Trichuris trichura)
(vi)   Tapeworms
(vii) Wucheresia bancrofti/Loa loa and Guinea worms
(vii) Blood flukes, Liver flukes, Lung flukes, and Intestinal flukes.

7. What are the mechanisms of action of anthelmintics? Give suitable examples.

GUIDE TO FURTHER READING

Albonico, M et al: A randomized controlled trial comparing mebendazole and albendazole against Ascaris, Trichuris, and hookworm infections. Trans. R. Soc. Trop. Med. Hyg., 1994; 88:585-589.

Andrews. P: Praziquantel: mechanisms of anti-schistosomal activity. Pharmacol. Ther., 1985; 29:129-156.

Arena, J.P et al: The mechanism of action of avermectins in Caenorhabditis elegans: correlation between activation of glutamatesensitive chloride current, membrane binding, and biological activity. J.Parasitol., 1995; 81:286-294.

Arjona, R et al: Fascioliasis in developed countries: a review of classic and aberrant forms of the disease. Medicine, 1995; 74:13-23.

Beech, R.N et al: Genetic variability of the beta-tubulin genes in benzimidazole-susceptible and resistant strains of Haemonchus contortus. Genetics, 1994; 138:103-110.

Bittencourt, P.R et al: Phenytoin and carbamazepine decreased oral bioavailability of praziquantel. Neurology, 1992; 42:492-496.

Blair, K.L., et al. Parziquantel: Physiological evidence for its site(s) of action in magnesium-paralysed Schistosoma mansoni. Parasitology, 1992; 104:59-66.

Botero, D., et al. Taeniasis and cysticercosis. Infect. Dis. Clin. North. Am., 1993; 7:683-897.

Brindley, P.J: Relationships between chemotherapy and immunity in schistosomiasis. Adv. Parasitol., 1994; 34:133-161.

Chodakewitz, J.A: Ivermectin and lymphatic filariasis: a clinical update. Parasitol. Today, 1995; 11: in press.

Cully, D.F et al: Cloning of an avermectin-sensitive glutamate-gated chloride channel from Caenorhabditis elegans. Nature, 1994; 371:707-711.

Dachman, W.D et al: Cimetidine-induced rise in praziquantel levels in a patient with neurocysticercosis being treated with anticonvulsants. J. Infect. Dis., 1994; 169:689-691.

Datry, a et al: Treatment of Strongyloides stercoralis infection with ivermectin compared with albendazole: results of an open study of 60 cases. Trans. R. Soc. Trop. Med. Hyg., 1994; 88:344-345.

Davies, H.D et al: Creeping eruption. A review of clinical presentation and management of 60 cases presenting to a tropical disease unit. Arch. Dermatol., 1993; 129:588-591.

Fisher, M.H et al: The chemistry and pharmacology of avermectins. Ann. Rev. Pharmacol. Toxicol., 1992; 32:537-553.

Gann, P.H et al: A randomized trial of single-and two-dose ivermectin versus thiabendazole for treatment of strongyloidiasis. J. Infect. Dis., 1994; 169:1076-1079.

Gelband, H: Diethylcarbamazine salt in the control of lymphatic filariasis. Am. J. Trop. Med. Hyg., 1994; 50:655-662.

Goa, K.L et al: Ivermectin. A review of its antifilarial activity, pharmacokinetic properties and clinical efficacy in onchocerciasis. Drugs, 1991; 42:640-658.

Gottshal, D.W et al: The metabolism of benzimidazole anthelmintics. Parasitol. Today., 1990; 6:115-124.

Hanjeet, K et al: The efficacy of treatment with albendazole. Acta. Tropica, 1991; 50:111-114.

Homeida, M et al: Pharmacoinetic interaction between praziquantel and albendazole in Sudanese men. Ann. Trop. Med. Parasitol., 1994; 88:551-559.

Kaye, B: Oxamniquine: metabolism, pharmacolinetics and mode of action. WHO Scientific Working Group on the Biochemistry and Chemotherapy of Schistosomiasis. WHO, Geneva, 1984; pp, 1-19.

Klotz, U et al: Ivermectin binds avidly to plasma proteins. Eur. J. Clin. Pharmacol., 1990; 39:607-608.

Krishna, D.R et al: Determination of ivermectin in human plasma by high-performance liquid chromatography. Arznemittelforshung, 1993; 43:609-611.

Kwa, M.S.G et al: Molecular characterisation of beta-tubulin genes present in benzimidazole-resistant populations of Haemonchus contortus. Mol. Biochem. Parasitol., 1994; 60:133-143.

Liu, L.X et al: Strongyloidiasis and other intestinal nematode infections. Infect. Dis. Clin. North. Am., 1993; 7:655-682.

Ottesen, E.A et al: Lymphatic filariasis infection and disease: control strategies. Parasitol. Today, 1995; 11:129-131.

Prichard, R et al: Anthelmintic resistance. Vet. Parasitol., 1994; 54:259-268.

Rohrer, S.P et al: Ivermectin interadtions with invertebrate ion channels. In, Molecular Action and Pharmaoclogy of Insecticides on Ion Channels. American Chemical Society, 1995; in press.

Shoop, W.L et al: Avermectins and milbemycins against Fasciola: in vivo drug efficacy and in virto receptor binding. Int. J. Parasitol., 1995; in press.

Wiest, P.M et al: Inhibition of phosphoinsositide turnover by praziquantel in Schistosoma mansoni. J. Parasitol., 1992; 78:753-755.

CHEMOTHERAPY OF TUBERCULOSIS AND MYCOBACTERIUM AVIUM COMPLEX DISEASE

Tuberculosis (Mycobacterium tuberculosis infection)

Tuberculosis was for centuries a major killer disease. With the introduction of effective antituberculosis drugs about 40 years back, this disease was regarded as an easily curable or treatable disease. However, the scenario has changed, because multidrug-resistant strains are now common and have rebounded with renewed ferocity. The WHO has declared tuberculosis to be a 'global emergency'. There is a synergy between *Mycobacterium tuberculosis*, *M. avium* and the AIDS virus.

It is a chronic disease caused by tubercle bacilli. It is a necrotizing bacterial infection. Lungs are most commonly affected but lesions may also occur in the kidneys, bones, lymph nodes or meninges or be disseminated throughout the body. Tuberculosis is now a 100% curable disease.

Tuberculosis has acquired a new dimension all over the world due to the spread of AIDS (acquired immuno-deficiency syndrome). HIV infection markedly reduces host defenses which are essential to combat tuberculosis.

Drugs used in tuberculosis can be categorized as:

Primary drugs or drugs of first choice	INH, Ethambutol, Rifampin, Streptomycin
Secondary drugs (alternative or reserve drugs) or drugs of second choice	PAS, Ethionamide, Kanamycin, Viomycin, Cycloserine, Capreomycin, Pyrazinamide, Amikacin, Thiacetazone
New secondary drugs	Rifabutin, Ofloxacin, Azithromycin

- Primary drugs are more effective and less toxic than the secondary drugs, hence these are the drugs of first choice. The majority of patients can be successfully treated with these drugs.
- Secondary drugs are alternate drugs employed when resistance has developed to primary drugs.

The main thing is that combination of at least two drugs is necessary to prevent the development of resistant tubercle bacilli. The other purpose of combining drugs is to enhance the antitubercular effect e.g. it is reported that combination of INH, ethambutol and streptomycin shows greater activity than that of each agent alone.

Isonicotinic acid hydrazide (INH, isoniazid)

- It is the most potent antitubercular drug.
- Rapidly absorbed after oral administration from gastrointestinal tract.
- Widely distributed and penetrates efficiently into CSF as well as caseous material.
- It is active against extracellular as well as intracellular tubercle bacilli.
- It can be given orally as well as by I.M. injection and intrathecally.
- It is tuberculostatic as well as tuberculocidal according to the concentrations. It is tuberculocidal only against actively growing tubercle bacilli.
- There is no cross resistance to other antitubercular drugs.

- This drugs is effective against the atypical mycobacterium kansasii, although less effective against many other atypical mycobacteria.

The main disadvantage of INH is that resistance develops within few weeks if taken alone.

INH is most important in the treatment of all types of tuberculosis.

Pharmacokinetics

INH is well absorbed from GIT, widely distributed in the body including CSF and enters cells. INH is inactivated by acetylation i.e. conjugation with acetyl group. 75 to 95% is excreted in urine in 24 hours as metabolites of the drug (enzymatic acetylation) acetylisoniazid, and (enzymatic hydrolysis) isonicotinic acid.

There is a bimodal distribution of slow and rapid acetylators due to differences in the activity of an acetyltransferase which depends on race and not on age or sex, e.g. fast acetylators in Eskimos and Japanese and slow acetylators in North African Caucasians.

Dose: 300 mg orally in single dose, may be given twice in divided doses. Pyridoxine (Vit. B_6) 20-30 mg/100 mg of INH should be given to prevent neuritis.

Mechanism of action

The primary action appears to be inhibition of biosynthesis of mycolic acids which are important constituents of mycobacterial cell wall. Mycolic acids are unique to mycobacteria.

INH interferes with pyridoxine metabolism and induces pyridoxine deficiency, pyridoxine output in urine is increased.

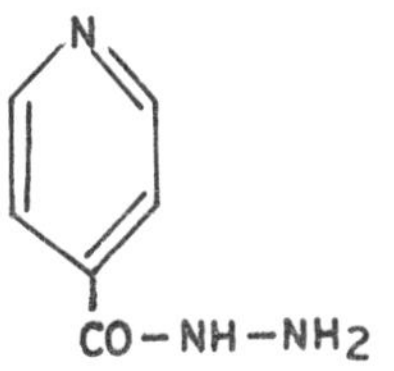

Isoniazid

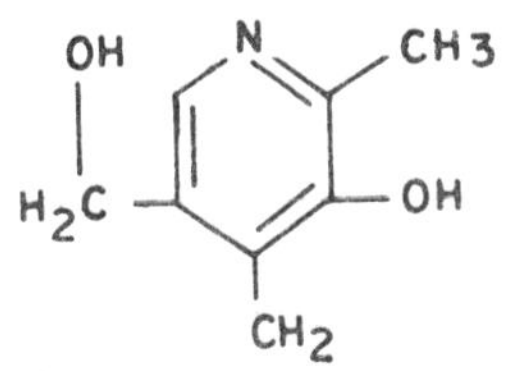

Pyridoxine

Adverse effects

- Neurotoxicity: The neurotoxicity is manifested as peripheral neuritis, muscle twitchings, convulsions and psychosis. Neurotoxicity is due to pyridoxine deficiency because there is structural similarity of INH to pyridoxine (vitamin B_6).
- INH and pyridoxine are structural analogues, and INH exerts competitive antagonism. The administration of large doses of pyridoxine to patients receiving INH does not interfere with the tuberculostatic action of INH, but it prevents neuritis.
- Neuritis can be avoided by giving 20-30 mg vitamin B_6 for every 100 mg of INH.
- Hepatotoxicity: It is manifested as jaundice.
- In glucose-6-phosphate dehydrogenase deficiency, INH may cause haemolysis.
- Allergic reactions include skin rashes, fever and hepatitis.

Interactions: Rifampin increases hepatic toxicity of INH; INH can reduce the metabolism of phenytoin, increasing its blood levels and toxicity.

PAS increases blood levels of INH as both are acetylated and there is competition for this pathway.

Contraindications: Epilepsy, psychosis.

Ethambutol

It is a synthetic, water-soluble and heat-stable antituberculosis drug.

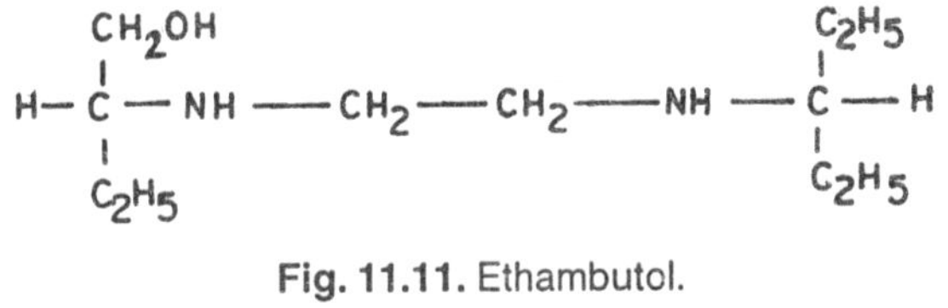

Fig. 11.11. Ethambutol.

- Its d-form is 200 times more potent than l-form.
- It is effective against nearly all strains of *M. tuberculosis* and *M. kansasii* but has no effect on other bacteria.
- It is tuberculostatic; mechanism of action is not clear.
- It is less active than INH and Rifampin.

Usually the dose is 25 mg/kg during first 2 months and then reduced to 15 mg/kg orally in one dose each day; 75 to 80% is absorbed from the gut on oral administration, half-life is 3-4 hours. About

50% is excreted unchanged in urine within 24 hours, and 15% as metabolites. The drug is excreted by glomerular filtration as well as tubular secretion and about 20% in unchanged form in faeces.

Resistance to ethambutol develops slowly and there is no cross-resistance. It is effective against INH and streptomycin-resistant tubercle bacilli.

Adverse effects are very few, the most important side effect is decrease of visual acuity and loss of ability to perceive green and red (red-green colour blindness) colours. It may be unilateral or bilateral. There is recovery after withdrawal of the drug. It is believed that zinc deficiency may increase ocular toxicity of ethambutol.

Symptoms of ocular toxicity typically develop several months after the initiation of therapy, but rapid-onset optic neuritis has been reported. The risk of optic neuritis depends on the dose and duration of therapy; this reaction develops in 5% of patients receiving a daily dose of 25 mg/kg but in fewer than 1% of patients given a daily dose of 15 mg/kg.

Optic neuritis with associated visual loss is usually reversible, but recovery may take 6 months or longer. Other adverse effects are infrequent.

Hyperuricaemia occurs but is usually asymptomatic.

Precaution: Vision should be tested at regular intervals. It also decreases renal excretion of uric acid.

Contraindication: It is not recommended in pregnancy.

Rifampin

It is a semisynthetic derivative of an antibiotic rifamycin produced by streptomyces mediterranei. It is the only important antitubercular drug which acts against a large number of gram-positive and gram-negative cocci, gram-negative bacilli. Mycobacterium leprae, chlamydia and pox viruses.

It is less active than penicillin but slightly more than erythromycin and cephalosporin against gram-positive organisms.

It is inferior to tetracycline and aminoglycosides and chloramphenicol against gram-negative bacilli. However, it is very effective against staphylococcus aureus and also highly effective in Neisseria meningitidis. It is a bactericidal drug against sensitive organisms. It inhibits RNA synthesis in bacteria.

It is also effective against intracellular tubercle bacilli.

Rifampin has both intracellular and extracellular bactericidal activity. It blocks RNA synthesis by specifically binding and inhibiting DNA-dependent RNA polymerase.

Combination with INH is highly effective. It is of great value in resistant infections. But resistance develops rapidly if given alone so it is used in tuberculosis in combination with other antitubercular drugs.

Dose: 600 mg orally once a day. The standard dose is 600 mg that achieves serum levels of 10 to 20 µg/ml. Rifampin turns body fluid (urine, saliva, sputum, tears) to a red-orange colour makes it simple and inexpensive to check on a patient's compliance with therapy. Excretion is through bile and urine.

It is well absorbed from GIT, widely distributed including CSF, metabolized in liver, excreted mostly in bile (3/4 is eliminated in bile) in deacetylated form. This metabolite retains full antibacterial activity, the half-life is 1.5 to 5 hours.

Adverse effects are not very frequent. Nausea, vomiting, diarrhoea, and hepatotoxicity have been reported. Some may show allergic reactions such as rash, fever, flu like syndrome.

Chronic liver disease, alcoholism and old age increases incidence of severe hepatic problems when rifampicin is given alone or with INH.

Contraindications: Hepatic dysfunction.

Interactions: PAS interferes with absorption of rifampicin, hepatotoxicity of INH is increased as it is an enzyme inducer.

Effectiveness of oral anticoagulants and oral contraceptives is decreased.

Streptomycin sulphate

It was the only effective antituberculosis drug from 1947 to 1952. Most 'atypical' mycobacteria are resistant to streptomycin.

It is the least used first-line supplemental drug for tuberculosis, because of its toxicity. It is bactericidal for rapidly dividing extracellular mycobacteria but is ineffective in the acidic environment within the macrophage. It diffuses poorly into the meninges.

It acts mainly against extracellular tubercle bacilli.

In vivo it suppresses and not eradicate tuberculosis. When used alone resistance develops in about 4 months in patients of tuberculosis.

It inhibits protein synthesis by disruption of ribosomal function.

Adverse effects: It has many toxic effects, serious among them is ototoxicity. It is not available orally in tuberculosis as it is not absorbed from GIT. It is not distributed to CSF.

Adverse effects occur in 10 to 20% of patients. Ototoxicity and renal toxicity are most common and the most serious ototoxicity involves both hearing loss and vestibular dysfunction. The latter is more common and involves loss of balance, vertigo and tinnitus. Less serious reactions include perioral paresthesia, eosinophilia, rash and drug fever.

Resistance develops after a few months if it is given alone.

Other antitubercular drugs are always given simultaneously to delay emergence of resistant strains.

Dose: 0.5-1 g i.m. injection once daily for 2-3 weeks, 0.5-1 g i.m. daily followed by 1 g i.m. 2-3 times weekly for several months.

It is bactericidal to extracellular bacilli, does not penetrate cell wall. It can not kill intracellular tubercle bacilli.

SECOND LINE DRUGS

Paraaminosalicylic acid (PAS)

It is tuberculostatic, much less effective than streptomycin, INH, rifampicin.

Microorganisms other than *M. tuberculosis* are not affected.

Development of resistance is slower than with streptomycin.

It is of little value alone.

Dose: 8-12 g in 3-4 equally spaced doses daily after meals. It is not recommended in renal dysfunction.

It is readily absorbed from GIT, widely distributed but little in CSF. 50% acetylated compound and rest as free acid are excreted in urine.

Adverse effects: GI disturbances, skin rashes, hepatic damage (rare), interference with thyroid function (hypothyroidism), crystalluria, agranulocytosis.

Allergic reactions include fever, rash, enlarged lymph glands.

Pyrazinamide

It is a relative of nicotinamide. It is tuberculostatic, less effective and more toxic than several other antituberculosis drugs. It penetrates cell wall of macrophages. It is bactericidal in acid intracellular milieu.

Dose: 20-35 mg/kg orally in 3-4 equally spaced doses, maximum 300 mg/day for one or two months.

The absorption is good from GIT, well distributed and excretion is through glomerular filtration.

It is hydrolysed to pyrazinoic acid and subsequently hydroxylated to 5-hydroxypyrazinoic acid which is the major excretory product.

Adverse effects: Diabetes may become difficult to control. It inhibits excretion of urates. It is hepatotoxic and may cause arthralgia, nausea, vomiting, fever, anorexia and hyperuricaemia.

Capreomycin sulphate

It is polypeptide antibiotic related to viomycin, elaborated by streptomyces capreolus.

Dose: I.M. 1 g/day or 15 mg/kg/day.

Chemical and pharmacological properties are similar to viomycin, resistance develops quickly when given alone. It is bactericidal to extracellular bacilli, but does not penetrate cell wall.

There is cross resistance with kanamycin and viomycin.

It is valuable in the treatment of 'resistant' or treatment failure tuberculosis when given with INH or ethambutol 20 mg/kg or 1 g for 60-170 days, then 1 g 2-3 times a week with these drugs.

Adverse effects include hearing loss, nitrogen retention, leukopenia, rashes, fever, eosinophilia. Injection is painful.

Amikacin

Amikacin is active against *M. tuberculosis* and several of the nontuberculous species, including *M. scrofulaceum*, *M. leprae*, the dose is 10 to 15 mg/kg IM/IV three to five times per week. It is bactericidal to extracellular organisms.

Cycloserine (seromycin)

It is a broad spectrum antibiotic produced by streptomyces orchida, inhibits cell wall synthesis, well absorbed from GIT, widely distributed including CSF, 50% is excreted unchanged, rest is metabolized. Dosage in tuberculosis is 0.5-1 g/d. It is used in re-treatment cases; resistance develops slowly.

Adverse effects: Nausea, vomiting, peripheral neuritis, headache, confusion, tremor, insomnia, irritability, suicidal tendencies. Adverse effects include CNS dysfunction and psychotic reactions. Some of these can be controlled by phenytoin 100 mg/d orally.

Contraindications : Epilepsy, history of psychosis.

Ethionamide

It is less effective than INH.

Dose: 0.5-1 g/day, 250 mg twice a day orally with meals.

It is given with other drugs only, when therapy with primary drugs is ineffective or contraindicated. It is active against INH resistant tubercle bacilli. It is a bacteriostatic agent. There is cross resistance between ethionamide and thiacetazone.

Prothionamide

It acts similar to ethionamide. It is more toxic than streptomycin. There is cross resistance to viomycin/ streptomycin and kanamycin but those resistant to streptomycin and kanamycin still respond to viomycin. However, those resistant to viomycin are resistant to both streptomycin and kanamycin.

Viomycin

It inhibits protein synthesis of *M. tuberculosis*. Mycobacterium insensitive to kanamycin are also resistant to viomycin. The absorption and excretion are similar to streptomycin, penetration into CSF is poor.

Dose: 2 injections of 1 g each 12 hours apart twice a week.

Kanamycin

It is administered parenterally i.m. 1 g 3-4 times/ week or 0.5 g daily.

Severe 8th nerve damage (largely hearing loss), vertigo is less common. It can also produce nephrotoxicity, neuromuscular block, drug fever, rashes.

Thiacetazone

It is not commonly used because of bone marrow depression and ototoxicity.

Cycloserine

It is produced by *Streptomyces orchidaceus* and is active against a broad spectrum of bacteria, including *M. tuberculosis*, well absorbed after oral administration and is widely distributed in body fluids, including the CSF.

Serious side effects limit its use and include psychosis (with suicide in some cases), seizure, peripheral neuropathy, headache, somnolence, and allergic reactions.

Contraindications :
  • epilepsy
  • severe renal insufficiency
  • history of depression or psychosis

Fluoroquinolones (ciprofloxacin, ofloxacin and sparfloxacin)

These are effective but reserved for selected cases only as alternate drugs for tuberculosis and lepromatous leprosy.

Regimens of treatment

1. Conventional drug therapy:
   • Initial triple drug therapy: INH 300 mg once a day orally. Rifampicin 600 mg once a day orally supplemented by ethambutol 25 mg/ kg once a day orally or streptomycin 1 g IM daily for first two months.
   • Continuation double drug therapy: INH 300 mg once a day orally. Rifampicin 600 mg once a day orally or ethambutol 15 mg/kg once a day orally or streptomycin 1 g IM twice a week. The duration of treatment

for this regimen is 18 months to 2 years. If properly treated tuberculosis is a curable disease.

2. Short course treatment (9 months): INH plus rifampicin for 9 months with 0.75 g streptomycin IM or ethambutol 25 mg/kg for first two months.

3. Short course (6 months): Streptomycin, INH, rifampicin plus pyrazinamide for 2 months then INH, Rifampicin and streptomycin IM twice a week for 4 months.

Chemoprophylaxix of tuberculosis

Household contacts or close associates of patients of tuberculosis should be given isoniazid for six months after the contact has been broken. In case the skin test becomes positive the prophylactic treatment should be continued for one year.

Persons infected with HIV who are exposed to multidrug-resistant tuberculosis should be administered high dose ethambutol and pyrazinamide, with or without a fluoroquinolone.

Anergic HIV-infected persons from populations at risk for tuberculosis should be given prophylaxis.

Prophylaxis with isoniazid is contraindicated in the presence of hepatic disease or who have had reactions to the drug.

In pregnant women, prophylaxis should be delayed until after delivery.

DRUGS FOR M. AVIUM COMPLEX (MAC)
(Table 11.16)

Rifabutin

It is a derivative of rifamycin. It inhibits mycobacterial RNA polymerase like rifampin.

It has better activity against the MAC organisms than rifampin. It is mainly indicated for the prevention of MAC infection in HIV-infected persons. The dose is 300 mg/d. It has significant activity against *M. avium intracellulare* and *M. fortuitum.*

Adverse effects

Rifabutin generally is well tolerated. The adverse effects include rash, GIT intolerance and neutopenia.

Rifabutin like rifampin can induce hepatic microsomal enzymes which can decrease the half-

life of several compounds including zidovudine, digitoxin, quinidine, propranolol, phenytoin, sulphonylureas, warfarin, prednisone and ketoconazole.

Rifapentine

It is a semisynthetic cyclopentyl rifamycin antibiotic.

It is the first new drug approved for tuberculosis in 25 years in USA. While similar to rifampin, rifapentine is lipophilic and longer acting.

Dose: 600 mg once or twice weekly.

$t_{1/2}$ is 13 h, bound to serum protein (93 to 97%).

Adverse effects are similar to that of rifampin.

Macrolides in the treatment of MAC infection

Clarithromycin is about 4 times more active than azithromycin against MAC bacteria in vitro. However, azithromycin has greater intracellular penetration in vivo.

Clarithromycin (500-1000 mg twice a day) or azithromycin (500 mg daily) is used in combination with at least one other drug such as rifampin, rifabutin, amikacin, clofazimine, ethambutol, ciprofloxacin.

Quinolones

Ofloxacin, ciprofloxacin, sparfloxacin and pefloxacin are active against many mycobacteria including *M. tuberculosis, M. leprae, M. marinum, M. kansasii* and *M. fortuitum.* While not approved for antituberculous therapy in USA, ofloxacin used in combination with isoniazid and refampin in pulmonary tuberculosis has been as active and safe as ethambutol in initial trials.

Adverse effects are uncommon. These include GI intolerance, rashes, dizziness and headache. However, more serious reactions are being reported and include confusion, seizures, interstitial nephritis and acute renal failure.

Resistance to fluoroquinolones develops rapidly. Fluoroquinolone-resistant tuberculosis is a source of growing concern.

Antituberculous therapy with quinolones should be reserved for patients with multidrug resistance or those who cannot tolerate first-line drugs.

Table 11.16. Drugs used in the treatment of tuberculosis and Mycobacterium avium complex

	First line	Alternate drugs
M. tuberculosis	Isoniazid + rifampin + pyrazinamide + ethambutol + streptomycin	Ciprofloxacin or ofloxacin, cycloserine, capreomycin, kanamycin, ethionamide, PAS, amikacin
M. avium complex	Clarithromycin + ethambutol or ciprofloxacin or amikacin	Rifampin, ethionamide, cycloserine, imipenem, azithromycin
M. kansasii	Isoniazid + rifampin + ethambutol	Ethionamide, cycloserine, clarithromycin, amikacin, streptomycin
M. fortuitum	Amikacin + doxycycline	Cefoxiten, rifampin, ciprofloxacin, ofloxacin, clarithromycin, imipenem, co-trimoxazole
M. marinum	Rifampin, ethambutol	Co-trimoxazole, clarithromycin, kanamycin, minocycline, doxycycline, amikacin

Clofazimine

It inhibits most MAC isolates in vitro. However, clinical experience in combination with other agents has not been encouraging.

Amikacin

It has a role as a third or fourth agent in a multiple-drug regimen for MAC treatment.

STUDY QUESTIONS

1. List drugs of first choice and drugs of second choice for the treatment of tuberculosis, and explain the reasons for designating them as drugs of first and second choice.
2. Why is it essential to give triple drug therapy initially followed by continuation double-drug therapy? Describe the regimen of treatment of one and half to 2 years duration as well as for short courses lasting for 9 months and 6 months.
3. Describe the advantages and disadvantages of INH as compared to streptomycin.
4. What are the toxic effects of (1) streptomycin, (ii) INH and (iii) ethambutol.
5. Write notes on (i) pyrazinamide, (ii) capreomycin, (iii) amikacin, (iv) rifampicin, (v) cycloserine and (vi) kanamycin and (viii) rifabutin.
6. What is the role of vitamin B6 in the treatment of tuberculosis with INH?
7. Describe the treatment possibilities of some 'atypical' mycobacteria.
8. Comment on chemoprophylaxis of tuberculosis.
9. What is the therapeutic status of macrolides and quinolones in the treatment of tuberculosis.
10. Name the drugs which are indicated in the treatment of certain 'atypical' mycobacteria such as M. kansasii, M. fortuitum and M. marinum.

GUIDE TO FURTHER READING

Banerjee, A et al: a gene encoding a target for isoniazid and ethionamide in Mycobacterium tuberculosis. Science, 1994; 263:227-230.

Barnes, P.F et al: Tuberculosis in the 1990s. Ann. Intern. Med., 1993; 119:400-410.

Bobrowitz, I.D et al: Ethambutol-isoniazid versus streptomycin-ethambutol-isoniazid in original treatment of cavitary tuberculosis. Am. Rev. Respir. Dis., 1974; 109:548-553.

Bowersox, D.W et al: Isoniazid dosage in patients with renal failure. N.Engl.J.Med., 1973; 289:84-87.

Centres for Disease Control. Initial therapy for tuberculosis in the era of multidrug resistance. Recommendations of the Advisory Committee for the Elimination of Tuberculosis. M.M.W.R., 1993; 42:1-18.

Edwards, P.O et al: Tuberculosis, now and the future: short-term therapy, preventive therapy, and bacillus Calmette-Guerin. Bull. N. Y. Acad. Med., 1977; 53:526-531.

Farr, B.F et al: In, Mandell, Douglas and Bennett's Principles and Practice of Infectious Diseases, 4th ed. Churchill Livingstone, Inc., New York, 1995; pp. 317-329.

Fox, H.H et al: The chemical attack on tuberculosis. Trans. N. Y. Acad. Sci., 1953; 15:234-242.

Gallant, J.E et al: Prohylaxis for opportunistic infections in patients with HIV infection. Ann. Intern. Med., 1994; 120:932-944.

Goldman, A.L et al: Isoniazid: a review with emphasis on adverse effects. Chest, 1972; 62:71-77.

Haas, D.W et al: Myocobacterium tuberculosis. In, Mandell, Douglas and Bennett's Principles and Practice of Infectious Diseases, 4th ed. Churchill Livingstone, Inc., New York, 1995; pp. 2213-2243.

Iseman, M.D: Treatment of multidrug-resistant tuberculosis. New Engl. J. Med., 1993; 329:784-791.

Lane, H.C et al: Recent advances in the management of AIDS-related opportunistic infections. Ann. Intern. Med., 1994; 120:945-955.

Nightingale, S.D et al: Two controlled trials of rifabutin prophylaxis against Mycobacterium avium complex infection in AIDS. New Engl. J. Med., 1993; 329:828-833.

Sanders, W.E et al: Other Mycobacterium species. In, Mandell, Douglas and Bennett's Principles and Practice of Infectious Diseases, 4th ed. Churchill Livingstone, Inc., New York, 1995; pp. 2264-2272.

Snider, D.E et al: Pyridoxine supplementation during isoniazid therapy. Tubercle, 1980; 61:191-196.

Snider, D.E et al: Preventive therapy with isoniazid for "inactive" tuberculosis. Chest, 1978; 73:4-5.

CHEMOTHERAPY OF LEPROSY (ANTILEPROSY DRUGS)

Leprosy (Hansen's disease) is a chronic granulomatous infection which attacks skin, peripheral nerves and nasal mucosa. Mycobacterium leprae is the causal organism. The two major types are (i) lepromatous leprosy (multi bacillary type with extensive involvement and (ii) tuberculoid type (paucibacillary) with few skin lesions.

Therapy for leprosy remains difficult because of:

- long course required
- high cost
- frequency of adverse reactions to drugs
- acquisition of drug resistance
- difficulty of determining a disease end point or cure
- difficulty of conducting susceptibility testing (M. leprae still cannot be grown in vitro).

Sulphones are most important drugs for the treatment of leprosy. They do possess some antibacterial activity as well and show limited value in tuberculosis but they are used only as antileprotic agents.

Dapsone is the parent substance.

Diaminodiphenyl sulphone (DDS) is most widely used. It inhibits folate synthesis.

Dapsone combined with rifampin is recommended for the initial treatment to avoid emergence of resistant strains.

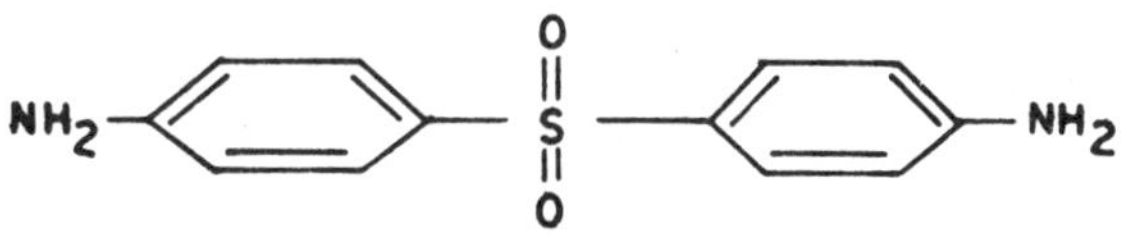

Fig. 11.12. Structure of dapsone.

Acedapsone (4,4-diacetamidodiphenyl sulphone) is a repository form of dapsone. A single IM injection of 300 mg maintains dapsone levels in tissues upto 3 months.

Other sulphones such as diasone, sulphetrone, promin and others are derivatives of dapsone, these are not superior to the parent substance.

All other sulphones are converted to DDS in the body, and none is superior. Sulphones are bacteriostatic for mycobacterium leprae.

Dapsone is slowly but nearly completely absorbed from GIT on oral administration, 50% is bound to plasma proteins, distributed throughout and tend to be retained in skin and muscle, especially in liver and kidney. Dapsone is acetylated in liver and degree of acetylation is genetically determined, 70% to 80% is excreted in urine as such. Its serum half-life is 1-2 days.

Dose: 50 mg daily gradually increased to 100 mg daily orally, 100-400 mg twice weekly is also effective. Duration of treatment is for 2-3 years or even life long.

Sulphones may be given safely for many years provided small doses are given initially and the dose is increased gradually and laboratory and clinical supervision is done periodically.

Dapsone is the drug of choice. It is safe and cheap.

Box 11.12. Drugs used in leprosy		
	First-line theory	*Alternative drugs*
Mycobacterium leprae	Dapsone rifampin clofazimine	Ofloxacin, clarithromycon, minocycline

Diasone may be given in place of depsone if latter drug causes gastric irritation. However, when intolerance develops, it is to all sulphones.

Sulphone resistance: Secondary resistance in 2 to 8% cases; recently primary resistance has been reported. Resistance develops if low doses are given and also due to irregular treatment. In such resistant cases other antileprotic drugs clofazimine and rifampin are effective.

Adverse reactions : anorexia, nausea, vomiting, headache, gastric upsets, fever, pruritus, allergic rashes, psychosis, hepatitis. Methaemoglobinaemia may occur. Sulphones may cause haemolytic anaemia in patients with glucose-6-phosphate dehydrogenase deficiency.

In lepromatous leprosy, erythema nodosum reaction may develop.

Rifampin

The rifamycins are a group of structurally similar, complex macrocyclic antibiotics produced by streptomyces mediterranei.

Rifampin is a semi-synthetic derivative of one of these rifamycin B.

It is bactericidal antibiotic. It is the most rapidly bactericidal drug for leprosy, kills bacteria in skin and upper respiratory tract within 3-4 days, so the patient becomes non-infective within 2 weeks. It is strikingly effective in lepromatous leprosy. However, it should not be given alone otherwise resistant strains develop fairly quickly. Its high cost also limits its use. It is usually given in combination with dapsone or another antileprosy drug.

It is effective against dapsone resistant strains. A single monthly dose of 600 mg is beneficial in combination therapy.

Clofazimine

It is a phenazine dye, leprostatic as well as marked anti-inflammatory and prevents the development of erythema nodosum leprosum. It is effective against sulphone-resistant leprosy or when patients are intolerant to sulphone. Clofazimine also is useful for the treatment of chronic skin ulcer produced by M.ulcerans, and it has some avitivity against the MAC.

Dose : 100-300 mg orally daily. In combination therapy a dose of 50-100 mg is satisfactory. Duration of treatment is for 50 days.

It is relatively nontoxic but causes red-brown to nearly black discoloration of skin. Eosinophilic enteritis has been reported. Gastrointestinal intolerance occurs occasionally.

Besides the use of clofazimine in leprosy, it has also been used in combination therapy to treat mycobacterium avium intracellular infection in patients with AIDS. It is weakly bactericidal against *M. intracellulare*.

MISCELLANEOUS AGENTS

Amithiozone (thiacetazone)

It is a thiosemicarbazone employed as a substitute for dapsone in intolerant patients. It is more effective in tuberculoid than in lepromatous leprosy. Dose 150 mg/d or 450 mg twice weekly is advocated. Resistance develops rapidly if given alone. Gastrointestinal intolerance occurs frequently. It is hepatotoxic in high dosages.

Ethionamide

It can be used as a substitute for clofazimine in oral doses of 250 to 375 mg/daily.

New promising drugs (so far limited experience in patients) include **minocycline, clarithromycin, pefloxacin,** and **ofloxacin.**

Drug combinations

In case of drug-resistant leprosy, multiple drug therapy is used: Rifampin 600 mg/o/monthly plus dapsone 100 mg/o/d plus clofazimine 50 mg/o/d (if skin pigmentation makes it unacceptable then ethionamide 250 mg/o/d) are employed.

- For tuberculoid leprosy (treatment for 6 months): Dapsone 100 mg/d + Rifampicin 600 mg/ monthly.

• For lepromatous leprosy (treatment for 2 years): Dapsone 50-100 mg/d + Rifampin 600 mg/ monthly + clofazimine 50 mg/d.

STUDY QUESTIONS

1. Describe the different antileprosy drugs.
2. Describe the pharmacokinetics of sulphones, doses, routes of administration and adverse effects.
3. What is the therapeutic status of (i) rifampin (ii) clofazimine and (iii) amithiozone as antileprosy drugs? What are their adverse effects?
4. Write short notes on: (i) multiple drug therapy in the treatment of leprosy; (ii) repository form of sulphone; (iii) erythema nodosum reaction.

GUIDE TO FURTHER READING

Bullock, W.E et al: Rifampin in the treatment of leprosy. Rev. Infect. Dis., 1983; 5:S606-S613.

Centres for Disease Control. Increase in prevalence of leprosy caused by dapsone-resistant Mycobacterium leprae. M.M.W.R., 1982; 30:637-638.

DeGowin, R.L et al: A review of the therapeutic and hemolytic effects of dapsone. Arch. Intern. Med., 1967; 120:242-248.

Gelber, R.H et al: Leprosy, In, Mandell, Douglas and Bennett's Principles and Practice of Infectious Diseases, 4th ed. Churchill Livingstone, Inc., New York, 1995; pp. 2243-2250.

Goodwin, C.S et al: Inhibition of dapsone excretion by probenecid. Lancet, 1969; 2:884-885.

Hastings, R.C et al: Chemotherapy of leprosy. Annu. Rev. Pharmacol. Toxicol., 1988; 28.231-245.

Medical Letter, Clofazimine for leprosy and Mycobacterium avium complex infections. 1987; 29:77-78.

Pengelly, C.D.R. et al: Dapsone-induced hemolysis. Br. Med. J., 1963; 2:662-664.

Rapoport, A.M et al: Dapsone-induced peripheral neuropathy. Arch. Neurol., 1972; 27:184-186.

Shepard, C.C et al: Experimental chemotherapy of leprosy. Bull. W.H.O., 1976; 53:425-433.

Shepard, C.C et al: Chemotherapy of leprosy. Ann. Rev. Pharmacol., 1969; 9:37-50.

Trautman, J.R et al: The management of leprosy and its complications. N.Engl.J.Med., 1965; 273:756-758.

WHO Study Group. Chemotherapy of leprosy for control programmes. WHO Technical Report Series No. 675, WHO, Geneva, 1982; 7-33.

ANTIFUNGAL AGENTS

There are only a few substances which exert an inhibitory effect on the fungi pathogenic for humans, and most of them are relatively more toxic. Antibacterial drugs do not possess antifungal property.

There are four categories of antifungal agents:
1. Antibiotics
   • Polyenes
     – Amphotericin B
     – Nystatin
     – Hamycin
     – Natamycin
   • Heterocyclic benzofuranes
     – Griseofulvin
2. Antimetabolites
   • Flucytosine
3. Azoles
   • Imidazoles
     – Clotrimazole
     – Miconazole
     – Econazole
     – Ketoconazole
   • Triazoles
     – Fluconazole
     – Itraconazole
4. Other topical agents
   • Tolnaftate
   • Benzoic acid
   • Undecylenic acid
   • Haloprogin
   • Buclosamide

The major antifungal agents can also be grouped under two headings (A) systemic and (B) topical. However, this division is becoming arbitrary because many fungal infections can be treated either systemically or topically.

Tables 11.17 and 11.18 give treatment of superficial and deep mycoses, respectively.

A. SYSTEMIC ANTIFUNGAL AGENTS

Amphotericin B

Amphotericin A and Amphotericin B are antifungal antibiotics. Amphotericin A is not used in therapy.

Amphotericin B is one of a family of some 200 polyene macrolide antibiotics.

Table 11.17. Treatment of superficial mycoses

Superficial mycoses	Drugs
Candidiasis	
Vulvovaginal	Topical: Clotrimazole, miconazole, butaconazole, nystatin, terconazole, tioconazole; Oral: Fluconazole
Oropharyngeal	Topical: Clotrimazole, nystatin; Oral (systemic): Fluconazole, ketoconazole
Cutaneous	Topical: Amphotericin B, clotrimazole, econazole, ketoconazole, miconazole, nystatin
Ringworm	Topical: Clotrimazole, econazole, haloprogin, ketoconazole, miconazole, neftifine, terbinafine, undecylenate Systemic: Griseofulvin, itraconazole, terbinafine

Table 11.18. Treatment of deep mycoses

Deep mycoses	Drugs
Aspergillosis	
Immunosuppressed	Amphotericin B
Nonimmunosuppressed	Amphotericin B, itraconazole
Blastomycosis	
Rapidly progressing	Amphotericin B
Indolent, non-CNS	Ketoconazole, itraconazole
Coccidioidomycosis	
Rapidly progressing	Amphotericin B
Indolent	Ketoconazole, itraconazole
Meningeal	Fluconazole, intrathecal amphotericin B
Cryptococcosis	
Non-AIDS and initial AIDS	Amphotericin B, flucytosine
Maintenance, AIDS	Fluconazole
Histoplasmosis	
Chronic pulmonary	Itraconazole
Dissemented	
Rapidly progressing	Amphotericin B
Indolent, non-CNS	Itraconazole
Maintenance, AIDS	Itraconazole
Sporotrichosis	
Cutaneous	Iodide, itraconazole
Extracutaneous	Amphotericin B

Antifungal activity

It is an antibiotic derived from streptomyces nodosus. Its spectrum of activity is wide against yeast like fungi. It is effective against infections caused by *Coccidioides immitis*, *Cryptococcus neoformans*, *Blastomyces dermatitidis*, *Candiada* species, *Histoplasma capsulatum* and *Aspergillus*.

Amphotericin B is ineffective against viruses, protozoa and bacteria.

Box. 11.13. Antifungals	
Class	Comments
Drugs for Systemic Mycoses	
Amphotericin B	IV only, broad spectrum, nephrotoxicity
Flucytosine	Narrow spectrum, bone marrow suppression
Fluconazole	IV or oral, good oral absorption, and distribution, long acting
Ketoconazole	Oral absorption good unless reduced gastric acid, limited distribution, inhibits CYP3A4
Iraconazole	Very lipophilie, so food improves per oral absorption, metabolized, inhibits CYP3A4
Oral Drugs for Cutaneous Mycoses	
Griseofulvin	Food improves oral absorption, fungistatic
Terbinafine	Good oral absorption, fungicidal, shorter therapy
Topical Drugs for Cutaneous Mycoses	
Clotrimazole	High efficacy Vs dermatophytes
Miconazole	Best efficacy Vs dermatophytes
Ciclopirox	High efficacy Vs dermatophytes
Tolnaftate	Good efficacy Vs dermatophytes
Haloprogin	Good efficacy Vs dermatophytes
Undecylenic acid	Lower efficacy Vs dermatophytes

Chemistry

Amphotericin B is an amphoteric polyene macrolide (polyene = containing many double bonds; macrolide = containing a large lactone ring of 12 or more atoms). It is insoluble in water and unstable at 37°C (stability for about 7 days only) but stable for longer period (several weeks) at 4°C. Microcrystalline preparations are available for topical application. However, the absorption is not significant. The parenteral preparation is a micellar (micelles are molecular aggregates) suspension with the bile salt desoxycholate from which the active drug separates in the body. The solution should be handled carefully to avoid contamination as it lacks antibacterial activity. Amphotericin B is both heat labile and light sensitive and therefore the dry powder should be refrigerated and protected from light.

Pharmacokinetics

Amphotericin B is a broad-spectrum antifungal antibiotic, not absorbed from the gastrointestinal tract. Its oral administration will be effective only against fungi present in the lumen of the gut and for systemic diseases, it is administered by I.V route. On intravenous injection the drug is more than 90% protein-bound. It penetrates well into tissues but poorly into body fluids and serous cavities. It is metabolized and little unchanged drug appears in the bile or urine. The half-life is about 15 days and hence after stopping the treatment, the drug persists in the body for several days.

Administration

As amphotericin B is insoluble in water, it is not absorbed when given orally. It has to be given by intravenous infusion for the treatment of systemic fungal infections, for which a solution of 0.1 mg/ml in a 5% solution of dextrose is used. Saline should not be added otherwise amphotericin B will precipitate. The rate of injection should be such that the total dose is infused over a period of 3 to 6 hours. The drug should be injected once a day or on alternate days. The dosage is individually adjusted because tolerance to this drug varies greatly among patients. Dosage of less than 1 mg/kg may not be effective (1 mg/kg produces blood levels of 1 to 2 microgram per milliliter). At times the dosage may have to be increased to 1.5 mg/kg/day. However, dose-related adverse reactions may result if this dose is exceeded. The object is to avoid renal damage and produce a prolonged fungistatic effect.

Clinical uses

Amphotericin B is most effective for severe systemic mycoses for which it is given by slow I.V. infusion. However, this drug is difficult to administer and can produce many adverse effect.

Amphotericin B is the drug of choice for majority of systemic fungal infections, e.g. candidiasis, aspergillosis, coccidioidomycosis and histoplas-

mosis. A usual course of treatment is for 6 to 12 weeks, in which time 2-3 gram of amphotericin B is infused intravenously daily.

Amphotericin B has been used in the sterilization of corneal ulcers due to fungi. For this topical instillation is effective. In case of lid infection e.g. Aspergillus granuloma of the lid 1 mg of this drug diluted in distilled water may be injected into the granuloma. Injection is given weekly for about 2 months.

For topical administration a 0.15% solution freshly prepared with sterile water is used. For the treatment of fungus keratitis drops are instilled every half an hour or at hourly intervals for 3 to 4 days after that drops are instilled four times a day for about a month. Topical concentration of 0.5% amphotericin B is more effective than 5% natamycin and 1% imidazoles in the treatment of candida albicans keratitis. The dose of 2-5 mg in 0.5 ml solution can be given subconjunctivally but it is painful. For the anterior chamber irrigation the dose is 500 microgram in 0.1 ml; 5 microgram in 0.1 ml for intravitreal injection.

In corneal ulcers caused by fungi, a solution (1 mg/ml) instilled on the conjunctiva every 30 minutes can be curative.

The clinical use of liposomal amphotericin B in a variety of fungal infections is under investigation.

Mechanism of action

Amphotericin B is bound firmly to the fungal cell membrane in the presence of ergosterol and disturbs the permeability and transport characteristics of the membrane. The basic structure of polyene is double bounded system linked to an amino acid. Larger polyenes such as amphotericin B and nystatin selectively bind to a sterol present in plasma membrane of susceptible fungi, resulting in loss of macromolecules and cation ions particularly K^+ loss from the cell.

The damage is irreversible. Bacteria are insusceptible to polyenes because they lack the ergosterol that is essential for attachment to the cell membrane. Resistance to amphotericin may develop due to decrease in membrane ergosterol or its modification in structure so that its combination with the drug is insufficient.

Adverse effects are not infrequent and hence amphotericin B should be used under close medical supervision.

Adverse effects of intravenous injection of amphotericin B include chills, fever, vomiting, headache, anorexia, abdominal pain, haemorrhagic gastroenteritis, azotemia and haematologic disturbances.

Amphotericin B can impair renal function, if high doses are given for prolonged periods.

Shock like fall in the blood pressure, hypokalaemia and several neurological symptoms may also occur commonly. Anaemia may also occur due to bone marrow depression and decreased red blood cell production. This anaemia is self limited and disappears when therapy is stopped.

Local chemical thrombophlebitis may be produced due to irritating nature of this drug.

Amphotericin B, being a toxic drug, should be reserved for severe infections.

Ocular penetration

The blood-eye barrier is very resistant to the passage of amphotericin B. That is the reason why intravenous administrations of this drug is not employed in ophthalmic practice.

Ocular tolerance

Topical application of amphotericin B is much safer than when injected intravenously. For the treatment of corneal infection, topical application is the route of choice, 0.1% solution topically or 1-2 mg injected subconjunctivally.

Topically applied 0.5% ointment is irritant and if 5% ointment is used it produces oedema of cornea and severe iritis persisting for a week or so.

Flucytosine

Flucytosine (5-fluorocytosine, 5-FC) is a fluorinated pyrimidine which was initially introduced as an antimetabolite for the treatment of leukaemia.

It is enzymatically converted to 5-fluorouridylic acid which is incorporated into RNA where it interferes with normal protein synthesis within fungal cell. Mammalian cells do not metabolize flucytosine and hence remain unaffected.

Flucytosine is well absorbed after oral adminis-

tration and widely distributed in tissues including the CSF. About 20% is protein bound.

It is largely excreted in urine. In the presence of renal failure, the drug may accumulate in the blood to toxic levels.

Orally 50 to 150 mg/kg/day in divided doses are usually administered. For topical application the concentration employed is 1%.

Resistance often develops rapidly and regularly which limits the usefulness of flucytosine. For this reason combined treatment with amphotericin B is being given with some success.

Flucytosine has synergistic action with amphotericin B, with increased antifungal activity against candida, cryptococcus, aspergillus and others

Adverse effects of flucytosine include depression of bone marrow, loss of hair, nausea, vomiting, skin rashes and abnormal liver function.

Imidazoles and trizoles

Azole antifungals include two broad classes, imidazoles and triazoles. Both classes share the same antifungal spectrum and mode of action.

Among imidazole group Clotrimazole and Miconazole are effective topical antifungals but toxic in systemic use. Similar topical azoles include econazole, oxiconazole and sulconazole. These are used mainly in oral, vaginal, or cutaneous candidiasis in the form of creams and troches. Terconazole, fluconazole and itraconazole are triazoles used in vulvovaginal candidiasis.

These are fungistatic in low concentrations and fungicidal in high concentrations.

Clotrimazole

It is slightly soluble in water and hence unsuitable for parenteral use, but it is effective on topical application against dermatophyte, yeast and other fungal infections. It is immediately metabolized on oral administration.

Topical clotrimazole 1% in arachis oil is a broad spectrum antifungal agent, having high efficacy in the treatment of Aspergillus infection.

It is well tolerated. However, the adverse effects include superficial punctate keratopathy and ocular irritation.

Miconazole

It possesses antifungal as well as mild antibacterial property. It has a broad spectrum of activity against yeast and filamentous fungi.

This drug must be given intravenously for systemic treatment of blastomycosis.

Subconjunctivally as well as topically 1% ophthalmic preparation in arachis oil or 2% cream are used where topical nystatin is ineffective. In blastomycosis it is given intravenously as it is incompletely absorbed from the gut.

Adverse effects include conjunctival congestion and punctate corneal erosions. The adverse effects after intravenous injection include thrombophlebitis, anaemia, vomiting and leukopenia.

Econazole

It is a similar broad-spectrum topical antifungal drug. It is more effective than miconazole against penicillium, aspergillus and fusarium. It is very slightly soluble in water. It readily penetrates into the stratum corneum. 1% cream is used topically for the skin.

Isoconazole is effective as a single-dose topical threapy for vaginal candidiasis.

Ketoconazole

It is well absorbed from the gut. The systemic antifungal treatment can be carried out by oral administration. It is water soluble. The half-life is 8 hours.

It is effective for the treatment of superficial mycoses. It is the drug of choice for chronic mucocutaneous candidiasis and for eradicating dermatophyte infections of skin, nails and hair.

The usual dose for this purpose is 200 mg daily.

It is available as 1% topical preparation which is well tolerated.

Mode of action

Ketoconazole blocks the fungal synthesis of ergosterol which is essential to the integrity of the cell membranes of nearly all the pathogenic fungi. It has a broad-spectrum of antifungal activity.

Ketoconazole has also been used for certain nonmycotic conditions such as prostatic cancer.

Adverse reactions following systemic use include photophobia, pruritus, giddiness, nausea and headache. It can damage liver which is of greater concern regarding its toxicity. There may be transient elevation of hepatic transaminases and alkaline phosphatase in some cases, but in other cases there may be severe impairment of liver function. Liver damage may cause death.

Itraconazole

This triazole is closely related to ketoconazole. It is administered orally. It has a wider spectrum of antifungal activity and appears to have fewer side effects.

It is preferred over ketoconazole for the treatment of nonmeningeal histoplasmycosis. It is given for the maintenance therapy of AIDS patients (200mg twice daily) with disseminated histoplasmosis whose disease has stabilized during amphotericin B therapy.

Itraconazole is useful for cutaneous sporotrichosis for patients unable to tolerate iodides.

Cryptococcosis may respond but amphotericin B or fluconazole are better.

Adverse effects include gastrointestinal distress, hypertriglyceridemia, hypokalaemia and rash. Occasionally hepatotoxicity may occur. Adrenal insufficiency, lower limb oedema, hypertension have also been reported. Doses above 400 mg per day are not recommended for long-term use.

Fluconazole

It is a fluorinated bitriazole. It is almost completely absorbed from GIT. Fluconazole 50-100 mg daily is effective in oropharyngeal candidiasis.

Fluconazole 200 mg daily is the drug of choice to prevent relapse of cryptococcal meningitis in AIDS patients whose infection has been controlled by amphotericin B.

It is the drug of choice for the treatment of coccidioidal meningitis. This drug is also active against histoplosmosis, blastomycosis, sporotrichosis and ringworm, but less effective than itraconazole.

Fluconazole does not appear to be effective in the prevention or treatment of aspergillosis.

Adverse effects include nausea, vomiting, headache, skin rash, alopecia, hepatic failure (rare).

Terbinafine

It is keratinophilic fungicidal agent having a broad spectrum of activity against a wide range of skin pathogens. It inhibits the enzyme, squalene epoxidase, which is involved in the synthesis of ergosterol from squalene in the fungal cell wall. The accumulation of squalene within the cell is toxic to the organism.

Terbinafine is used for the treatment of fungal infections of the nails. It is absorbed rapidly after oral administration and taken up by the skin, nails and adipose tissue. It penetrates skin and mucous, membranes after topical application.

Adverse effects include GI disturbances, pruritus, headache joint pains, myalgia dizziness. Hepatitis though rare, may occur.

Griseofulvin

It was isolated from *Penicillium griseofulvum*. It is very insoluble in water but quite stable at high temperature including autoclaving.

Antifungal activity

Griseofulvin inhibits the growth of dermatophytes including epidermophyton, microsporum and trichophyton affecting hair, skin and nails. The spectrum is limited to ringworm fungi. It is ineffective against superficial candidiasis and all systemic mycoses.

Pharmacokinetics

The absorption is aided by high-fat foods. The absorbed drug has affinity for diseased skin and is deposited there bound to keratin. The keratin is made resistant to fungal growth. Its half-life is 36 hours. It is metabolized in the liver. The drug is excreted mainly in faeces and only a small quantity in the urine.

Mode of action

Griseofulvin probably interferes with microtubule function or with nucleic acid synthesis and polymerization. The mode of action is still not fully understood. It is fungistatic and not fungicidal.

Dose: 0.5-1 g daily in divided doses orally if it is a microsize preparation; and 0.3-0.6 g in case of ultramicrosize preparation (physical state of drug influences rate of absorption).

Topical application is ineffective or has little effect.

Resistance can develop among susceptible dermatophytes

Clinical uses

Dermatophytoses involving skin, hair or nails: If only hair or skin is involved, treatment is given for 3-6 weeks. If nails are affected, the treatment is for longer period (3-6 months).

Adverse reactions include nausea, vomiting, diarrhoea, headache, confusion, photosensitivity and hepatotoxicity. Allergic skin reactions may occur but are not serious.

B. POLYENE TOPICAL ANTIFUNGAL ANTIBIOTICS

Nystatin (Mycostatin)

Nystatin is a polyene macrolide, slightly soluble in water. It decomposes quickly in the presence of water or plasma. This drug is stable in dry form. Nystatin is a streptomyces-derived antibiotic with broad spectrum activity against a variety of fungi, molds and yeasts.

Antifungal activity

In vivo it is effective on surfaces where the nonabsorbed drug comes in direct contact with the fungi, although in vitro it inhibits many fungi, including candida dermatophytes and fungi which produce deep seated mycoses. This agent is selected only when culture and sensitivity tests show indication for its use because it is toxic. Nystatin has no antibacterial or antiviral activity.

Pharmacokinetics

It is poorly absorbed from skin, mucous membranes, or gastrointestinal tract. After oral administration the entire quantity is excreted unaltered in faeces.

Administration

It is too toxic for systemic use. It is not absorbed from the alimentary canal.

It is employed for local action in the eye e.g. as ocular topical cream 100,000 units/gm, ointment 100,000/gm or suspension 100,000 units/gm.

The dose for candidiasis of the alimentary tract is one tablet (500,000 units) or 5 ml of the suspension four times a day (1 mg = 3500 units). It is effective against Candida albicans (moniliasis).

Clinical uses

Nystatin can be applied topically to the skin or mucous membranes (buccal, vaginal) in the form of creams, ointments, suppositories, suspensions or powders for the suppression of local candida infections. It has also been given orally for the suppression of candida in the lumen of the bowel.

Oral preparations are poorly absorbed; I.M injection is painful and I.V injections cause chills and fever. Hence Nystatin is given topically for the treatment of surface fungi infections.

It is valuable in the treatment of ocular infections caused by *Candida* or *Aspergillus*. However, the limitation is topical toxicity and poor ocular penetration. Topical nystatin therapy may become ineffective after 2 days because cornea blocks drug penetration. When *Candida* enter anterior chamber, topical nystatin does not reach there.

Mode of action

Nystatin binds to fungal membrane sterols, mainly ergosterol which disturbs membrane permeability and transport features. This produces leak of macromolecules and cations from the cells. Resistance may develop due to decrease in membrane sterols or a change in binding properties or change in their structure.

Nystatin is fungistatic and not fungicidal.

Adverse effects

Topical instillation of 100,000 units of nystatin/ml does not produce toxicity but the subconjunctival injection of 2,000 units or more may produce localized necrosis. If 800 units are given subconjunctivally, transitory conjunctivitis may result.

Adverse effects after oral administration are mild gastrointestinal upsets. Intramuscular injection is painful. Intravenous injection is too toxic, and haemolytic anaemia may be produced.

Natamycin

It is a small polyene antifungal antibiotic with a broad spectrum of activity. Its mode of action is similar to that of nystatin. It is less toxic after topical application. Topically it is given as 5% ophthalmic suspension. It is useful for the treatment of keratitis caused by *Fusarium*, *Cephalosporium* or *Aspergillus*. Its antifungal activity is against *Candida*, *Aspergillus*, *Cephalosporum*, *Fusarium* and *Penicillium*.

Natamycin 5% suspension is applied every 1-2 hours initially and then every 4 hourly for 2-3 weeks. It is well tolerated.

Adverse effects

Corneal toxicity is superficial punctate keratitis. Subconjunctival injections cause conjunctival necrosis. However, adverse effects are rare on local application.

Imidazoles and triazoles for topical use

These are synthetic antifungal agents that are used both topically and systemically.

For topical use the indications are ringworm, tinea versicolor and mucocutaneous candidiasis.

Cutaneous applications are indicated in tinea corporis, tinea pedis, tinea cruris, tinea versicolor and cutaneous candidiasis. The application is done twice a day for 3-6 weeks.

Vaginal applications in the form of creams, suppositories and tablets are the preparations of choice for vaginal candidiasis.

Oral use in the form of troche (10 mg) is indicated in oropharyngeal candidiasis. The patient should suck on the troche until it dissolves.

Clotrimazole is available as a 1% cream, lotion and solution, 1% vaginal cream or vaginal tablets and 10 mg troches are available.

On the skin, the preparation is applied twice a day; for vagina, 100 mg tablet once a day is given at bedtime for 7 days, one 500 mg tablet inserted only once, or 5 g of cream applied once a day for 7-14 days. Troches are to be dissolved in mouth 5 times a day for 14 days.

Econazole readily penetrates the stratum corneum.

Miconazole is a very close chemical congener of econazole.

Terconazole and butoconazole: Vaginal suppository of terconazole (80 mg) is inserted at bedtime for 3 days, while the 0.4% vaginal cream is applied for 7 days; butoconazole nitrate is available as a 2% vaginal cream used at bedtime for 2 days.

A single-dose of tioconazole (4.6 gm) ointment containing 6.5% of the drug is given at the bedtime for the treatment of candida vulvovaginitis.

Oxiconazole nitrate as a cream and sulconazole nitrate as a solution are used for the topical treatment of infections caused by dermatophytes.

Haloprogin

It is a halogenated phenolic ether, fungicidal to various species of Epidermophyton, Microsporum, Trichophyton, Pityrosporum and Candida.

It is active in vitro against many dermophytes and in vivo against tinea corporis. It is available as 1% cream or solution. About 15% of the topically applied drug may be absorbed. Sometimes it produces local irritation.

Tolnaftate

It is a topical antifungal drug used in cream, powder, solution in the treatment of dermatophytosis. Candida is resistant with topical application; there is no systemic absorption. Toxic and allergic reactions are minimal.

Tolnaftate is available as 1% solution, 1% powder, and 1% cream for topical application against dermatophytosis. However, candida is resistant. The drug is not absorbed. Side effects are rare.

Naftifine

Naftifine decreases synthesis of ergosterol. A 1% cream is useful in tinea cruris and tinea corporis.

MISCELLANEOUS TOPICAL ANTIFUNGAL DRUGS

Undecylenic acid

Undecylenic acid and its salts are effective topical antifungals. These are used as powders and creams against tinea pedis and corporis. Undecylenic acid is used as ointment or powder, 10% for skin and 15% for mucous membranes. Undecylenic preparations

are used in the treatment of various dermatomycoses, especially tinea pedis.

Benzoic acid, salicylic acid, also possess antifungal activity when applied topically on skin. An ointment containing benzoic and salicyclic acids in known as Whitfield's ointment. It combines the fungistatic action of benzoate and the keratolytic action of salicylate. It contains benzoic acid and salicyclic acid in ratio of 2: 1 (6%: 3%). It is mainly used in tinea pedis.

Propionic acid and caprylic acid can be used for the treatment of dermatomycoses but have low efficacy and high cost.

Selenium sulphide (selsun) may be used for skin fungal infection. It is also used for seborrheic dermatitis.

Potassium iodide 1 g/ml is useful in treating cutaneous sporotrichosis. Ten drops in small amount of water is taken thrice a day.

Potential new antifungal agents

- A new azole, voriconazol is under clinical trial. It is fungistatic against all fungi, including resistant strains. It is, fungicidal against *asperigillus*.
- Recombinant forms of human granulocyte-colony-stimulating factor; e.g. lenograstim and molgramostim can increase the neutrophil count in neutropenic patients, with fungal infection. This enhances the patient's ability to combat the fungal pathogens. This approach is under study.
- Some drugs are under development, such as echinocandin which is targeted at the fungal cell wall which has no human analogue.
- Fungal protein synthesis requires an elongation factor that is missing from human cells. It can be another target for antifungal drug development.

STUDY QUESTIONS

1. Why antibacterial antibiotics are not antifungal? And antifungal antibiotics are also not antibacterial, why?
2. List (i) polyenes, (ii) imidazoles and (iii) antimetabolites which possess antifungal activity.
3. Describe Amphotericin B regarding mode of action, uses and adverse effects.

4. Describe Griseofulvin—its source, mode of action, pharmacokinetics and adverse effects.
5. Discuss the uses and limitations of Nystatin.
6. Write notes on (i) Natamycin, (ii) Hamycin, (iii) Clotrimazole, (iv) Miconzole
7. Which drugs are used for topical antifungal activity?

GUIDE TO FURTHER READING

Aguado, J.M et al: Ventricular arrhythmias with conventional and liposomal amphotericin. Lancet, 1993; 342; 342:1239.

Balmaceda, C.M et al: Reversal of amphotericin-B-related encephalopathy. Neurology, 1994; 44:1183-1184.

Carlson, M.A et al: Nephrotoxicity of amphotericin B. J. Am. College Surg., 1994; 179:361-381.

Chavanet, P.Y et al: Trial of glucose versus fat emulsion in preparation of amphotericin for use in HIV infected patients with candidiasis. Br. Med. J., 1992; 305:921-925.

Daneshmend, T.K et al: Clinical pharmacokinetics of ketoconazole. Clin. Pharmacokinet., 1988; 14:13-34.

Debruyne, D et al: Clinical pharmacokinetics of fluconazole. Clin. Pharmacokinet., 1993; 24:10-27.

de Marie, S et al: Clinical use of liposomal and lipid-complexed amphotericin B. J. Antimicrob. Chemother., 1994; 33:907-916.

Drutz, D.J et al: Rapid infusion of amphotericin B: is it safe, effective and wise? Am. J. Med., 1992; 93:119-121.

Honig, P.K et al: Ketoconazole and fluconazole drug interactions. Arch. Intern. Med., 1994; 154:1038-1041.

Jacobson, M.A et al: Fatal acute hepatic necrosis due to fluconazole. Am.J.Med., 1994; 96:188-190.

Sachs, M.K et al: Interaction of itraconazole and digoxin. Clin. Infect. Dis., 1993; 16:400-403.

Sahai, J et al: Effect of fluconazole on zidovudine pharmacokinetics in patients infected with human immunodeficiency virus. J. Infect. Dis., 1994; 169:1103-1107.

Tolins, J.P et al: Adverse effect of amphotericin B administration on renal hemodynamics in the rat. Neurohumoral mechanisms and influence of calcium channel blockade. J. Pharmacol. Exp. Ther., 1988; 245:594-599.

Vanden Bossche, H et al: P450 inhibitors of use in medical treatment: focus on mechanisms of action. Pharmac. Ther., 1995; 67:1-22.

Vidal-Puig, A.J et al: Ketoconazole therapy: hormonal and clinical effects in non-tumoral hyperandrogensim. Eur. J. Endocrinol., 1994; 130:333-338.

Voss, A et al: Fluconazole in the mangement of fungal urinary tract infections. Infection, 1994; 22:247-251.

Zervos, M et al: Fluconazloe: a review . Int. J. Antimicrob. Agents, 1993; 3:147-170.

ANTIVIRAL AGENTS

Viruses are intracellular parasites and participate in the metabolism of host cells hence they present a more difficult problem of chemotherapy than do bacteria. However, some progress has been achieved in the development of antiviral agents because of differences between viral and human metabolism are being identified. Active search is under way for chemicals that inhibit virus-specific functions.

Viruses are of two types, viz. large viruses (chlamydia) cause diseases such as trachoma, rickettsial infections, psittacosis and lymphogranuloma venereum. Sulphonamides and antibiotics are effective against large viruses. The true viruses possess either DNA (herpes simplex, herpes zoster, chicken pox and small pox viruses) or RNA (mumps, measles, rabies and poliomyelitis).

Viruses are the smallest (17-300 nm) infecting agents consisting of a nucleic acid (RNA or DNA but not both) enclosed in protein.

Drugs that block viral replication must be administered before the onset of disease, i.e. as chemoprophylaxis, because in many viral infections, replication of the virus reaches a maximum near the time of the appearance of clinical symptoms or may be even earlier e.g. in case of influenza A and pox viruses. In some other infections such as herpes virus, virus replication continues for a time after the symptoms have appeared. In these cases inhibition of further virus replication may promote healing.

The antiviral drugs can be grouped as following:

1.	For herpes simplex	Idoxuridine, cytarabine, vidarabine, acyclovir
2.	For influenza A virus	Amantadine
3.	For pox viruses	Methisazone
4.	Nonspecific	Interferons

Antiviral agents can also be classified according to their mode of action:

A. Inhibition of adsorption and penetration of susceptible cells
  • Gamma globulin
  • Amantadine and rimantadine
B. Inhibition of nucleic acid synthesis
  (i) Ribavirin
  (ii) Pyrimidine and purine analogues
    • Fluorouracil (5-fluorouracil)
    • 5-bromouracil
    • Idoxuridine (5-iodo-2'-deoxyuridine, IDU, IUDR)
    • Cytarabine
    • Trifluridine
    • Vidarabine (ara-A, adenine arabinoside)
    • Acyclovir
    • Ganciclovir
    • Zidovudine (ATZ) and other dideoxynucleosides
  (iii) Other inhibitors of nucleic acid synthesis
    • Foscarnet
    • Phosphonoacetic acid (clinical potential unknown)
    • Interferons
  (iv) Inhibition of late protein synthesis
    • Fluorophenylalanine
    • Puromycin
    • Thiosemicarbazones
    • Methisazone
C. Inhibition of assembly or release of viral particles
    • Floxuridine
    • Rifampin

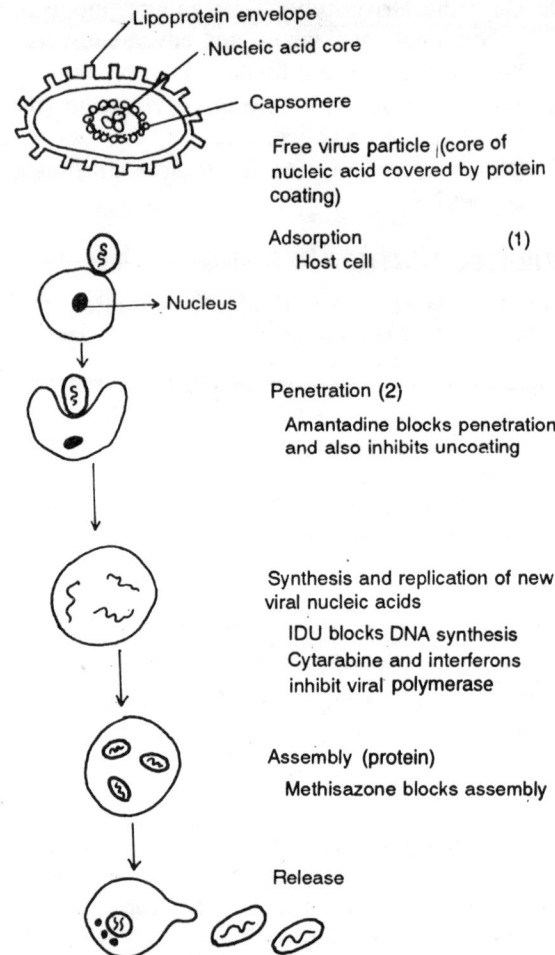

Fig. 11.13. Virus replication and sites of action of some antiviral drugs.

Stages of virus replication and possible targets of action of antiviral agents is shown in Fig. 11.13.

Viral replication involves the following steps: (i) Adsorption to and penetration of susceptible cells; (ii) Synthesis of early, nonstructural proteins, e.g. nucleic acid polymerase; (iii) Synthesis of RNA or DNA; (iv) Synthesis of late structural proteins; and (v) Assembly (maturation) of viral particles and their release from the cell.

Gamma globulin

If gamma globulin contains specific antibodies against antigens of a particular virus, it shall block entry of that virus particle (rather than adsorption). Pooled gamma globulin (immune globulin, 0.025-0.25 ml/kg injected intramuscularly during early incubation period can modify viral infections such as measles, rabies, hepatitis, poliomyelitis. This protective effect lasts for about 2-3 weeks. Special hyperimmune globulins given intravenously can protect against rabies, vaccinia, varicella, zoster, hepatitis B, and Rh disease.

Amantadine and Rimantadine

These inhibit the uncoating of certain viruses, e.g. influenza A (but not influenza B) virus, rubella after they have entered susceptible cells. These drugs may also inhibit virus particle release. A daily dose of 200 mg of either drug for 2-3 days before and 6-7 days after influenza A infection reduces the incidence and severity of the disease.

Amantadine is also beneficial in Parkinson's disease.

Amantadine is completely absorbed after oral administration. It is excreted in urine in unaltered form. Its half-life is about 12 hours.

Rimantidine is an analogue of amantadine. Ramitidine and amantadine are useful against influenza A virus.

The pharmacokinetics of rimantadine are similar to amantadine. Its half-life is longer (about 30 hours) and elimination is dependent on liver function. Rimantadine is as effective as amantadine. It does not require adjustment in dosage in renal insufficiency unlike amantadine. Adverse effects on CNS may be lower than for amantadine.

Adverse effects of these drugs include ataxia, insomnia, dizziness, slurred speech and other effects on the central nervous system such as headache, seizures, confusion, nervousness and coma. The GIT side effects include nausea and anorexia.

Contraindications: Nursing mothers, pregnancy.

Inhibition of intracellular synthesis

Effect (inhibition) on early protein synthesis

Guanidine is no doubt capable of inhibiting the replication of certain RNA entroviruses but not of others. It inhibits formation of RNA polymerase. Guanidine has no significant therapeutic activity in vivo.

Inhibition of nucleic acid synthesis

Ribavirin can inhibit the replication of both RNA and DNA viruses. A dose of 15 mg/kg gives some benefit against influenza A viruses. It also limits replication of respiratory syncytial virus in infants when given as an aerosol. It is effective against influenza A and B infections. This drug is not effective in rabies.

Idoxuridine (IDU, IUDR)

Idoxuridine is a halogenated pyrimidine where 5 methyl group thymidine is replaced by iodine. It is also called 5-iodo-2 deoxyuridine.

Mode of action

It is a thymidine analogue which competes with thymidine for phosphorylation by thymidine kinase. The viral DNA synthesis becomes defective because IDU is incorporated into DNA. Thymidines are fundamental building blocks of nucleic acids within the cells and IDU so much resembles thymidine that it can substitute thymidine in DNA synthesis. The effective metabolites block the final step of thymidine (nucleotide) DNA, and for this purpose the best drug so far known is IDU, 5-bromodeoxyuridine is also effective but produces chemical conjunctivitis and iritis.

Clinical use

Before the introduction of IDU, no medication was available to improve herpes simplex infection of the cornea without damage. Topical idoxuridine is useful for the treatment of infection due to herpes simplex and vaccinia keratitis. But being poorly soluble in water it does not penetrate the stroma and hence it is not effective in deeper infections.

It is available as 0.1% ophthalmic solution as well as 0.5% ointment. The solution is unstable in heat and light. It should be kept at cool place. The solution is instilled in the eye every hour during day and every two hours in the night for the first week. If ointment is applied 4 times daily or drops may be used in the day and ointment during night. In the second week the frequency of administration is reduced to every 2 hours during the day. If treatment is stopped before the herpetic lesion heals, lesions recur. If there is no response after giving treatment for 5-7 days, other drugs should be used as resistance to IDU may have developed. Topically applied IDU has no effect on skin lesions of herpes simplex or herpes zoster.

Adverse reactions

Adverse reactions on topical application in eye include local irritation and oedema of lids, photophobia and opacities of cornea on prolonged use, conjunctiva may show congestion and swelling and there may be reduced tear secretion. The systemic administration may cause depression of bone marrow, gastric ulcers, loss of finger nails and alopecia. Hepatotoxicity has also been reported.

Contraindications

Its use is not advisable during first few weeks after corneal transplantation or after penetrating corneal incisions because IDU inhibits corneal stromal healing. IDU is not antibacterial and erroneously prescribed antiviral therapy will worsen, bacterial keratitis has been reported.

Cytosine arbinoside (ara-C, cytarabine)

It inhibits DNA synthesis and interferes with replication of DNA viruses. By weight it is about 10 times more effective than IDU but also 10 times more toxic to host cells.

It is an inhibitor of nucleic acid synthesis compared to IDU, it is quite soluble and hence higher concentrations can be used topically. IDU resistant viruses respond to cytosine Arabinoside. Resistance develops to it more slowly.

1% ointment every 2 hours combined with topical corticosteroid and a cycloplegic has been found effective for the treatment of acute vaccinial blepharitis and keratitis.

In about 75% patients of severe ophthalmic herpes zoster, significant and quick improvement has been reported by injecting cytarabine intravenously (100 mg/ml/24 hours). In some cases doses 10-40 mg/ml/day are sufficient.

In high dosages such as 300 mg per day for about a week, the immunosuppressive effects may reduce host resistance more than the inhibition of the virus.

The corneal toxicity is comparable to IDU. Cytosine arabinoside toxicity includes punctate subepithelial opacities, punctate staining or progress to even corneal ulceration. The cellular metabolism of the epithelium of cornea and the stroma is inhibited to a greater extent than that produced by idoxuridine.

Methisazone

It was effective against small pox, which is now completely eradicated, hence, it has no indication.

Trifluridine (Trifluorothymidine, Viroptic)

It is a thymidine analogue which inhibits DNA

viruses. Its solubility in water is upto 1% concentration whereas IDU is soluble in water to 0.1%. This drug is also lipid soluble. Due to the biphasic solubility it has good corneal penetrability.

Clinical use

One drop of 1% trifluridine instilled five times daily for 2 weeks is used for the treatment of herpes simplex viruses induced corneal ulcers. In patients of dendritic or acute keratitis, 1% trifluridine instillations every 2 hours in the day time, the ulcers heal in about 6 days. It has been reported that successful healing occurred in 14 days in 96% cases with this drug and only 75% with IDU treatment. Herpetic relapses are not likely to recur when treatment with either IDU or trifluridine was continued for 2 weeks.

Trifluridine is better than IDU and vidarabine in the treatment of herpetic keratitis because it requires lesser frequency of administration, in whom other drugs have failed, it is relatively nontoxic, being a solution it does not blur vision and it is not antagonized by simultaneous corticosteroid therapy.

Trifluridine is much more active in the treatment of vaccinia than is IDU and also somewhat more active than is vidarabine.

0.1% solution instilled every 2 hours for 1 week or a 1% ointment applied 5 times a day for 3 weeks do not produce any toxicity on the cornea. Allergic reactions are much less common than to IDU.

Adverse reactions

Prolonged topical use may produce slight epithelial damage. It can cause conjunctival infection, superficial punctate keratopathy, occlusion of the lacrimal puncta, and conjunctival scarring. Anterior segment occlusion may be produced after prolonged use for about 4 months. Systemic administration may depress bone marrow.

Vidarabine (Adenine arabinoside, Vira A, ara-A)

Adenine arabinoside (Vidarabine) is a purine analogue. In inhibits DNA polymerase and ribonucleotide reductase, thus it blocks the DNA synthesis. Its mode of action is different from that of IDU and Trifluridine. Adenine Arabinoside does not incorporate into viral deoxynucleotide (DNA) chain. It arrests the growth of the viral DNA chain.

Adenine Arabinoside has better corneal penetration (i.e. more effective) than IDU and also less toxic. It has better ocular tolerance than IDU. It does not produce bone marrow depression. It can achieve better viricidal concentration in the aqueous humour after topical instillation, hence it has also been found useful in the treatment of stromal viral keratitis and iritis.

It can be used in patients who are allergic to IDU. It can be used in patients infected with herpetic strains resistant to IDU. The DNA viruses such as herpes simplex virus, varicella-zoster and vaccinia are also responsive to vidarabine. This antiviral drug can cross the blood-brain barrier and probably also the blood-ocular barrier. It is the least toxic and most effective of the purine analogues.

Hypoxanthine (ara-Hx) is a metabolite of vidarabine. It is 20% as active (as antiviral) as is vidarabine. Moreover it is 10 times as soluble as vidarabine. IDU is metabolized to uracil which does not have antiviral penetration power, which may be responsible for the beneficial effect of vidarabine against herpetic uveitis. It has been used to treat herpes simplex encephalitis in which case the mortality is reduced from 70% to 40%. Retinal viral infections are also likely to respond. Allergic reactions have been reported. Vidarabine does not interfere with the development of host immunity unlike cytosine arabinoside.

Vidarabine is available as 3% ointment, applied five times a day and if there is no response its use should be stopped after a week. Vidarabine can be given intravenously in doses of 20 mg/kg over an 8-12 hour period daily for 1 week in case of herpetic iridocyclitis. Topical vidarabine has no effect on skin or mucous membrane lesions of herpes simplex.

Vidarabine can also be given intravenously in doses of 10-15 mg/kg daily over a 12 hour period in the treatment of systemic herpes virus. If this systemic treatment is given for 10 days to a patient of herpetic encephalitis, there is significant reduction in the mortally rate. The results are very encouraging if the treatment is commenced before the onset of coma.

Adverse effects

The external ocular reactions are similar to IDU. Punctate staining and epithelial oedema occur less frequently than with IDU. However, it interferes with stromal healing to the same extent as IDU.

Acyclovir (Acycloguanosine)

It is a prodrug, converted in the body to acyclovir triphosphate that inhibits DNA synthesis. Acyclovir is a nucleoside analogue. It is more specific in affecting viral particle as it is activated by virus induced thymidine kinase and converted to an acyclomonophosphate form and then to triphosphate form which selectively inhibits virus induced DNA polymerase. It inhibits DNA synthesis, is effective in herpes simplex and varicella zoster virus infections. It has 30 times more affinity for virus DNA polymerase than for cellular polymerase. The introduction of acyclovir is remarkable as it has been the result of exploiting the suitable differences of viral and cellular enzyme function in the synthesis.

Acyclovir is available as 3% ophthalmic ointment, 200 mg capsules and 5% dermal cream. Acyclovir is more effective than IDU. IDU resistant viruses respond to acyclovir.

Clinical uses

For primary herpes simplex virus (HSV) blepharitis and orofacial lesions, 5% cream five times a day is effective.

For HSV superficial as well as deep corneal lesions, 3% ointment, five times a day is advocated till the lesions heal, thereafter it is applied 2-3 times a day for further few days. The therapy is for about a fortnight.

Advantages of acyclovir include
- better penetration into corneal epithelium;
- more selective and hence less toxic;
- it has wider spectrum; and
- crosses blood-brain barrier and probably also blood-ocular barrier.

For the treatment of herpes zoster virus infection (HZV), Acyclovir is not as effective as in case of herpes simplex virus infection (HSV). However, topically 3% ointment applied in eye 5 times daily and oral tablets 600 mg 5 times a day for 10 days have been found effective and give better results compared to topical application alone. The oral use of acyclovir is well tolerated and does not have the same potential for systemic complication, including renal impairment that I.V. use has. In herpes simplex and varicella zoster virus infection, the dose is 5 to 20 mg/kg i.v. 8 hourly for 5-10 days; 500 mg (1 tablet) 5 times a day for 5 days; cream 3% is applied on skin.

Acyclovir can be injected intravenously at dose of 1500 mg daily for 10-14 days for the treatment of acute retinal necrosis syndrome. But it has been seen that even after the lesions have been cured, patients develop retinal detachment. I.V. acyclovir is currently reserved for immunocompromised patients.

Adverse effects

These include gastrointestinal symptoms like nausea, vomiting on oral administration; stinging and burning sensation on topical application and fall in blood pressure on I.V. injection.

Penciclovir

Penciclovir is similar to acyclovir in its spectrum of activity and potency against herpes simplex virus (HSV) and herpes zoster virus (HZV). It is also inhibitory for hepatitis B virus (HBV).

Oral penciclovir has low bioavailability (5%).

Famciclovir

It is a diacetyl ester prodrug of penciclovir and lacks intrinsic antiviral activity. It is well absorbed orally and rapidly converted to penciclovir. Although it is absorbed poorly, the bioavailability of penciclovir is 65-77% following oral administration of famciclovir.

Oral famciclovir is well tolerated, however, adverse effects such as nausea, diarrhoea, headache may be experienced. Chronic administration may be tumorigenic and causes testicular toxicity in animals.

Oral famciclovir is used for the treatment of localized herpes zoster of less than 3 days duration in immunocompetent adults.

In treating acute zoster famciclovir 500 mg thrice a day for 7 days is as effective as acyclovir treatment.

Sorivudine

Sorivudine is a pyrimidine nucleoside analogue; it has potent and selective inhibitory activity against varicella-zoster virus infections. It inhibits viral DNA synthesis.

Valacyclovir

Valacyclovir is rapidly and almost completely converted to acyclovir after oral administration. It is useful in herpes zoster and is under trial for other conditions in which acyclovir is indicated.

This drug is well absorbed after oral administration; $t_{1/2}$ is 6 hours.

Adverse effects include nausea, vomiting and headache.

Uses of steroids in viral lesions of eye

Corticosteroids are contraindicated in ulcerative form where active multiplication of virus particles occur. Where there are stromal lesions (potential threat to vision), steroids are employed. When steroids are indicated, low doses which will produce therapeutic effect should be used, intraocular pressure should be regularly measured and the therapy should be tailed off and not stopped suddenly.

Combined corticosteroid and antiviral therapy

Patients of chronic herpetic keratitis become comfortable after topical application of corticosteroid therapy. However, these may reactivate dendritic keratitis in some cases. But if antiviral and corticosteroids are used together the reactivation is much less likely to occur. IDU protects cornea against corticosteroid reactivation of the disease.

Experimental and clinical observations indicate that if in case of superficial herpetic infection corticosteroids are given, the condition worsens and the infection spreads. IDU is beneficial in surface infections. If the two are combined, corticosteroid dose should be kept to minimum required for deep herpetic inflammation (1 drop of corticosteroid thrice a day). IDU 2 drops should be given every 2 hours during the day. IDU produces disappointing results in deeper forms of infection e.g. disciform keratitis or herpetic iritis because IDU has poor penetrating capacity. Deeper infections are benefited by corticosteroids. This is the rationale of the combination of corticosteroid and idoxuridine (IDU), although the efficacy of IDU for the treatment of epithelial disease is reduced from 85% to 70% when used with topical corticosteroid. Experimental evidences indicate that the efficacy of vidarabine, trifluridine and acyclovir does not drop due to simultaneous use of corticosteroid therapy. It has been recommended to employ one of these antivirals in place of IDU when corticosteroids are employed.

The duration of treatment is for 1-2 months. The corticosteroid drops should be gradually discontinued after deep infection improves but antiviral drug is given and dosage maintained constant till corticosteroid therapy is no more used. There is no need to taper off antiviral drug. IDU or other antiviral drug is stopped when the eye is quiet and comfortable without corticosteroid therapy.

Ganciclovir

It is a nucleoside analogue, a derivative of acyclovir. It enters cells infected into cytomegalovirus. It inhibits cytomegalovirus DNA polymerase.

Cytomegalovirus (CMV) retinitis occurs in several patients with AIDS resulting in retinal detachment and loss of vision.

This agent has inhibitory activity against all herpes viruses but is especially active against CMV.

Ganciclovir is given systemically at doses of 5 mg/kg twice a day initially for about 3 weeks and then the maintenance dose is given as 5 mg/kg once a day. The dosage has to be adjusted depending on the clinical course and renal function. In about 30% of patients recurrence occurs and 13% of patients develop neutropenia with white cell count of less than 1000 leukocytes cumm.

As the intravenous ganciclovir therapy produces marked myelosuppressive effect, intravitreal injection has been evaluated for the treatment of CMV retinitis. Intravitreal injection of 200-400 mg in 0.1 ml is given initially twice per week till retinal healing, then the maintenance therapy of one injection per week is given. Liposome encapsulation ganciclovir and ganciclovir- trifluridine combination give prolonged intravitreal concentrations of ganciclovir for about a month after a single injection. This delivery system is useful for the maintenance

therapy of cytomegalovirus retinitis. Ganciclovir is not used together with zidovudine otherwise the myelosuppressive effect will further exacerbate.

Ganciclovir is water soluble and can be given as a drop.

This drug does not offer any particular advantage over trifluridine. However, it is effective in resistant herpes simplex cases.

Resistant CMV may emerge to ganciclovir.

The most important adverse effects of ganciclovir are leukaemia, neutropenia, thrombocytopenia, renal impairment and seizures. Its excretion is reduced and its toxicity is increased in renal insufficiency.

Interferons (IFNs)

Interferons are a group of endogenous glycoproteins which exert virus nonspecific antiviral activities. There are three families viz Alpha, Beta and Gamma. These are antiviral proteins (protective glycoproteins) produced in host cells by viruses. These are extremely difficult to isolate even in semipurified form. They are nonspecific. Synthetic analogues such as polyinosinic acid, polycytidylic acid have been employed to act as interferon inducer. Inosine pranobex stimulates proliferation of lymphocyte-B and T cells and interferon. It is useful against mucocutaneous infections with herpes simplex.

Interferons may increase host resistance to herpes simplex virus and vaccinia but so far evidence for the same is lacking. Interferon alpha2 has been evaluated against adenoviral conjuctivitis but found not to produce any beneficial effect in keratoconjunctivitis. Interferon has also been evaluated against herpetic keratitis, combined with acyclovir. This combination has been found to produce quicker healing than with acyclovir alone. Similarly when interferon is combined with trifluridine healing is quicker. Interferon alone has little effect against herpetic keratitis.

Topical interferon alpha has been tried against HSV keratitis in patients with AIDS, in the dosage of 12 million units/ml given twice a day. The active epithelial disease was cured in 3 weeks time. Thus it is a topical adjuvant to the conventional antiviral therapy in resistant herpetic keratitis.

Dose-limiting toxicities of systemic interferons are bone marrow suppression, neurotoxicity, thyroid dysfunction, weight loss, cardiotoxicity and hepatotoxicity may occur.

Injection of interferon doses of 1 to 2 million units (MU) or more may produce acute influenza like syndrome (fever, chills, myalgia, arthralgia, nausea, vomiting, diarrhoea).

Foscarnet (Trisodium phosphonoformate)

It is a pyrophosphate analogue. It inhibits several viral RNA and DNA polymerase. It is a virustatic drug.

It is useful in the treatment of CMV retinitis and does not induce myelosuppression and for the same reason it can be used together with zidovudine.

Initially 20 mg/kg followed by infusion of 0.16 mg/kg/min is generally recommended for foscarnet. It is also preferred over ganciclovir for the treatment of CMV retinitis. However, it should not be given to patients with creatinine clearance less than 1.2 ml/min/kg.

Foscarnet's major dose-limiting toxicities are nephrotoxicity and symptomatic hypocalcaemia, CNS side effects include headache, tremor, irritability, seizures and hallucinations. The other reported side effects are fever, nausea, vomiting, anaemia, leukopenia, painful genital ulcerations.

Intravitreal Foscarnet

It has been employed in patients with AIDS and CMV retinitis, these cases gave history of previous acyclovir allergy and due to the presence of renal failure systemic foscarnet was considered contraindicated. Foscarnet is injected intravitreally, the injections are given every 3 days for about 2 weeks, followed by maintenance dose of one injection weekly. The treatment has been found effective in controlling CMV retinitis.

Tables 11.19 and 11.20 give antiviral targets and administration of antiviral drugs, respectively.

Agents used for the treatment of AIDS and related opportunistic infections

AIDS is caused by HIV. There are two types HIV-1 and HIV-2.

A large number of human cells can be infected by HIV, including macrophages and glial cells. HIC preferentially replicates in CD4+ helper T-lymphocytes.

ANTI-HIV DRUGS

Zidovudine (AZT, ZDV and azidothymidine)

Zidovudine formerly called azidothymidine (AZT)

Table 11.19. Antiviral targets and properties of antiviral substances

Agent	Viral target	Active against
Purine and pyrimidine analogues		
Acyclovir	DNA polymerase	Herpes simplex
Ganciclovir	DNA polymerase	Cytomegalovirus
Ribavirin	DNA polymerase	Respiratory syncytial
Vidarabine	DNA polymerase	Herpes simplex, zoster
Idoxuridine	DNA synthesis	Herpes (corneal)
Trifluridine	DNA synthesis	Herpes (corneal)
Dideoxynucleosides (AZT, ddI, ddC)	Reverse transcriptase, DNA synthesis	HIV
Other drugs		
Amantadine	Adsorption, penetration	Influenza A, rubella
Rimantadine	Adsorption, penetration	Influenza A, rubella
Foscarnet	DNA polymerase, reverse transcriptase	Cytomegalovirus, herpes simplex
Interferons	Protein synthesis	
Gamma globulins	Adsorption, penetration	Hepatitis B, rabies, small pox, other pox viruses
Methisazone	Protein synthesis	
Rifampin	Assembly of mature virus particle	Pox viruses

Table 11.20. Antivirals for topical, intravitreal and systemic administration

Drugs	Doses
Topical antivirals	
Idoxuridine	0.1% solution, 0.5% ointment
Acyclovir	5% dermal ointment, 3% ophthalmic ointment
Vidarabine	3% ointment
Trifluorothymidine	1% solution
Antiviral used intravitrealy	
Ganciclovir	200-400 mg/0.1 ml
Foscarnet	1,200 mg/0.05 ml
Antivirals for systemic administration	
Acyclovir	Oral: 600 mg 5 times a day; I.V: 1500 mg/m²/day
Ganciclovir	I.V.: initial 5 mg/kg 12 hourly for 2-3 weeks maintenance 5 mg/kg daily
Foscarnet	I.V.: 20 mg/kg bolus then 0.16 mg/min infusion
Zidovudine	Oral: 500-1500 mg/day; I.V.: 1-2 mg/kg four times a day

has been found beneficial in delaying the progression to AIDS in HIV infected persons who are asymptomatic or have very early symptoms.

It is a synthetic thymidine analogue. As the triphosphate, it inhibits the DNA polymerase (reverse transcriptase) of HIV; Zidovudine triphosphate is incorporated into viral DNA and terminate chain growth during DNA synthesis.

HIV can be inhibited by synthetic dideoxy-nucleosides. These analogues act on the viral DNA polymerase, so that synthesis of viral DNA is inhibited and virus replication markedly decreased. Zidovudine (AZT) is the most extensively studied drug among this group.

AZT is well absorbed from the gut and widely distributed in tissues and fluids. The serum half-life is 1.1 hours but the intracellular half-life is 3 hours, 75% of AZT is metabolized in liver by glucuronidation and 25% excreted unchanged in the urine.

It penetrates readily into the CSF.

Uses

Zidovudine increases survival from less than nine months to more than two years after diagnosis of AIDS.

It slows progression to AIDS in symptomatic HIV-infected persons and prolongs survival.

It slows progression to the symptomatic condition when used in asymptomatic HIV-infected patients but does not influence survival.

Zidovudine is administered orally every 4 hours around the clock. In the presence of anaemia, this drug is either stopped or dose reduced or the haematocrit is maintained with transfusion.

Dose: AZT 100-200 mg 3-5 times a day given orally daily.

Adverse effects

Haematologic adverse effects

- Aplastic and megaloblastic anaemia
- Neutrpenia
- Granulocytopenia and thrombocytopenia

Neurotoxicity

- Severe headache
- Insomnia
- Seizures

Other side effects

- Nausea, muscle pains

Resistance develops with continued use.

Drug interactions

Zidovudine is myelosuppressive and should not be given together with systemic ganciclovir. However, foscarnet can be given together with zidovudine but not in the presence of renal failure. Under these circumstances intraocular ganciclovir should be the choice.

Probenacid slows the metabolism and excretion of zidovudine, so risk of haematotoxicity is enhanced.

Acetaminophen interferes with glucuronidation.

Drugs that inhibit glucuronidation such as fluconazole, and/or renal excretion such as probencid may increase the risk of myelotoxicity. Clarithromycin decrease zidovudine absorption.

Rifabutin and rifampin decrease plasma concentrations of zidovudine.

Concomitant ganciclovir increases the risk of severe haematologic toxicity.

Severe somnolence may occur during combined use of zidovudine and acyclovir.

Didanosine

It is a reverse transcriptase inhibitor. Sequential use of zidovudine and didanosine, rather than continuing zidovudine is better as this delays deterioration in the clinical conditions.

AZT resistant strains respond to didanosine.

Dose: 125-300 mg twice a day orally.

Adverse effects include painful peripheral neuropathy, acute pancreatitis, hepatic failure and development of resistance. The other side effects include headache, seizures and bone marrow depression.

Zalcitabine (dideoxycytidine, ddC)

It is a reverse transcriptase inhibitor. It can be given concurrently with zidovudine in cases of advanced HIV infections.

Dose: 0.75 mg with 200 mg AZT thrice a day.

The main adverse effect is peripheral neuropathy.

Other side effects include GIT upsets, oedema of lower limbs, mouth ulcers and pancreatitis (rarely).

Stavudine

It is a thymidine nucleoside analogue that inhibits HIV-1 replication at concentrations similar to those of zidovudine.

Zidovudine-resistant strains of HIV-1 are susceptible to stavudine.

This drug is acid stable and well absorbed after oral administration.

Stavudine is indicated for treating adults with advanced HIV infections who are intolerant to other therapies.

Stavudine 40 mg twice daily is associated with more sustained elevations of CD4 counts than is zidovudine.

Adverse effects include painful sensory peripheral neuropathy in about 20% of patients, pancreatitis in about 1% of patients, arthralgia, rash, fever, anaemia in about 10% of patients.

Serious bone marrow toxicity is uncommon.

Safety in pregnancy is uncertain.

These drugs are reserved for treatment of AIDS and not recommended in asymptomatic HIV infected persons because (i) symptoms may develop after months or years, (ii) these drugs do not eliminate virus, (iii) HIV may develop resistance, and (iv) these drugs are very toxic.

The following are some newer antiviral agents (particularly for HIV infection) under clinical development.

Agents	Virus
Lamivudine, Adefovir	HIV-1
Lamivudine, Famciclovir, Fialuridine	Herpes B virus
Cidofovir, Lobucavir	Herpes viruses

Table 11.21 shows some characteristics of antiretroviral nucleosides.

PROTEASE INHIBITORS

It is a new class of agents for HIV infection.

In the process of replication, HIV produces protein and also a protease which cleaves the protein into component parts that are subsequently reassembled into virus particles; protease inhibitors disrupt this essential process.

These are metabolised by isoenzymes of the cytochrome P450 system notably by CYP3A4

The t½ is 2-4 hours

The drugs include amprenavir, indinavir, lopinavir, nelfinavir, retonavir and saquinavir.

The Adverse effects include GI disturbances, headache, dizziness, raised liver enzymes, neutropenia, pancreatitis and rashes.

Interactions

Protease inhibitors can interact with numerous drugs because of their involvement with the cytochrome P450 system. For example, drugs like rifampicin that induce P450 enzymes accelerate their metabolism and reduce plasma concentration; enzyme inhibitors such as ketoconazole raise their plasma concentration.

Table 11.21. Some characteristics of antiretroviral nucleosides

	Zidovudine	*Didanosine*	*Zalcitabine*	*Stavudine*
Oral bioavailability, %	70	40	80	75
Plasma $t_{1/2}$ elimination (hrs)	0.9-1.5	0.6-1.5	1.2-3	0.9-1.2
CSF/plasma ratio	0.3-0.5	0.2	0.2	0.5
% protein binding	30	< 5	< 4	—
Metabolism	Glucuronidation	Purine metabolism	Uncertain	Uncertain
Effect of meals on AUC (area under plasma conc.-time curve)	↓ (24%, high fat)	↓↓ (50%, acidity)	↓ (15%)	Negligible

Non-Nucleotide reverse transcriptase inhibitors

Efavirenz (t½ 52 h): It is taken once a day , rash is common during first two weeks of therapy. Adverse effects include GI disturbances, hepatitis, pancreatits. Neurological adverse effects may also occur.

Nevirapine (t½ 28 hours): It penetrates the CSF well. It is taken once daily. Rash and hepatitis are the commonest side effects.

Therapy of AIDS-related opportunistic infections

P. carinii pneumonia

It occurs in about 80% of patients with AIDS. If this infection is prevented, the AIDS-related illness is delayed by 6-12 months.

The treatment of choice for both pulmonary and extrapulmonary infections is co-trimoxazole 120 mg/kg/d by mouth or i.v. in 2 divided doses for 14 days or with pentamidine.

Pentamidine isethionate is administered parenterally to treat P. carinii pneumonia. This drug can produce severe adverse effects including hypoglycaemia (short term effect is insulin release, continuation use may cause secondary hypoinsulinemia), renal failure, postural hypotension and arrhythmias.

Dapsone with oral trimethoprim is also effective.

Atovaquone is better tolerated but less effective than trimethoprim against P. carinii pneumonia.

Mycobacterium infections

Tuberculosis caused ·by tubercle bacilli as well as mycobacterial disease caused by M.avium occur during HIV infection.

Tuberculosis responds to antituberculosis drugs. But it has been observed that AIDS patients infected with tuberculosis have a high mortality rate due to recent increase in multiple-drug-resistant tuberculosis.

Rifampin is useful against atypical mycobacterial disease caused by *M. avium*.

Cytomegalovirus infections

Ganciclovir and foscarnet are used to treat cytomegalovirus in AIDS cases.

Toxoplasmosis

Toxoplasma gondii produces intracranial mass lesions in AIDS patients. Trimethoprim-sulphamethoxazole is effective prophylactic.

For treatment, pyrimethamine and sulphadiazine or clindamycin with pyrimethamine are given.

Cryptococcosis

C. neoformans (a fungus) is acquired by inhaling the organism. About 80% of AIDS patients with cryptococcal disease develop cryptococcal meningitis.

Amphotericin B is useful.

Herpes simplex virus and varicella-zoster virus

Foscarnet is used to treat cytomegalovirus retinitis in AIDS patients, especially in the case of ganciclovir resistant cytomegalovirus.

It is the drug of choice for acyclovir resistant herpes simplex virus and varicella-zoster virus infections.

Possible future developments in antiviral therapy

Immune-directed approaches:

- Various approaches to changing the balance between HIV - suppressing and HIV-inducing host responses are under consideration. It is thought that the imbalance between different types of immune responses and the associated cytokines affects HIV replication and the progress to AIDS, for example, the primary pro-inflammatory cytokines TNF-Alpha and IL-I can induce HIV expression whereas IL-6 and IL-16 inhibit it. CD8 T cells release soluble factors that suppress HIV replication.
- Vaccines against the HIV coat protein are under phase 1 trial.
- Gene therapy, using genes encoding two HIV proteins, is under phase 1 trial.

Agents affecting early stages of viral replication:

- Ribonucleotide reductase inhibitors are being studied as antiviral agents.
- Integrase inhibitors are being investigated as potential antiviral agents.
- Antisense oligonucleotides (ANOs) are synthetic nucleotides which are in phase I trial for HIV treatment and anti-CMV (cytomegalovirus) is in phase-III clinical trial.

Agents affecting late stages of viral replication:

- Viral envelope formation occurs in late step of viral replication. The viral envelope formation involves glycosylation. Glycosylation inhibitors are being developed and studied.
- Certain processes are involved in assembly and release of virus particles. Agents which interfere with these processes are being studied.
- In influenza virus, neuraminidase is involved in the budding of new virus from infected cells. The inhibitor of neuraminidase, zanamivir is active against both influenza A and B viruses.

STUDY QUESTIONS

1. Classify antiviral drugs based on the mode of action.
2. What are the different sites or stages at which antiviral drugs act?
3. What are the differences between large viruses and true viruses as regards their responsiveness to drugs?
4. Which drugs are useful against (i) herpes simplex, (ii) influenza A virus (iii) HIV?. Why discovery of antiviral drugs has been more difficult than the introduction of antibacterial agents?
5. Describe the pharmacology of Idoxuridine.
6. Write notes on (i) Cytarabine (ii) Vidarabine.
7. Describe (i) Acyclovir (ii) Interferons
8. Describe the drugs which inhibit assembly and release of viral particles.
9. Describe the mode of action, uses, pharmacokinetics and adverse effects of Amantadine. In what respect Rimantadine differs from Amantadine?
10. Discuss the use of corticosteroids in combination with antiviral therapy.
11. Describe anti-HIV drugs. What are their uses and limitations?
12. Describe the therapy of AIDS-related opportunistic infections.

GUIDE TO FURTHER READING

Bangham CRM, Phillips, RE What is required of an HIV vaccine? Lancet 350: 1617-1621, 1997.

Beutner, K.R et al: Valaciclovir compared with acyclovir for improved therapy for herpes zoster in immunocompetent adults. Antimicrob. Agents Chemother., 1995; 39:1546-1553.

Cairns J.S., D, Souza M.P. Chumokines and HIV-I second receptors: the therapeutic connection. Nature Med. 4: 563-568, 1998.

Caliendo, A.M et al: Combination therapy for infection due to human immunodeficiency virus type 1. Clin. Infect. Dis., 1994; 18:516-524.

Chattha, G et al: Lactic acidosis complicating the acquired immunodeficiency syndrome. Ann. Intern. Med., 1993; 118:37-39.

Cohn J.A. Recent advances: HIV-I infection. Br. Med. J. 314:487-491, 1997.

Concorde Coordinating Committee. Concorde: MRC/ANRS randomised double-blind controlled trial of immediate and deferred zidovudine in symptom-free HIV infection. Lancet, 1994; 343:871-881.

Connor, E.M et al: Reduction of maternal-infant transmission of human immunodeficiency virus type 1 with zivovudine treatment. N. Engl. J. Med., 1994; 331:1173-1180.

Cooper, D.A et al: The efficacy and safety of zidovudine alone or as cotherapy with acyclovir for the treatment of patients with AIDS and AIDS-related complex: a double blind, randomized trial. AIDS, 1993; 7:197-207.

D'Aquila, R.T et al: Zidovudine resistance and HIV-I disease progressing during antiretroviral therapy. Ann. Intern. Med., 1995; 122:401-408.

Dieterich, D.T et al: Ganciclovir treatment of cytomegalovirus colitis in AIDS: a randomized, double-blind, placebo-controlled multicenter study. J. Infect. Dis., 1993; 167:278-282.

Drew, W.L et al: Cytomegalovirus infection in patients with AIDS. Clin. Infect. Dis., 1992; 14:608-615.

Dudley, M.N: Clinical pharmacokinetics of nucleoside antiretroviral agents. J. Infect. Dis., 1995; 171:S99-S112.

Englund, J.A et al: High-dose, short-duration ribavirin aerosol therapy compared with standard ribavirin therapy in children with suspected respiratory wyncytial virus infection. J. Pediatr., 1994; 125:635-641.

Erice, A et al: Brief report: primary infection with zidovudine-resistant hyman immunodeficiency virus type 1. N. Engl. J. Med., 1993; 328:1163-1165.

Field, A.K et al: "The end of innocence" revisited: resistance of herpesviruses to antiviral drugs. Clin. Microbiol. Rev., 1994; 7:1-13.

Fischl, M.A et al: Combination and monotherapy with zidovudine and zalcitabine in patients with advanced HIV disease. Ann. Intern. Med., 1995; 122:24-32.

Gill, P.S et al: Treatment of adult T-cell leukemia-lymphoma with a combination of interferon alfa and zidovudine. N.Engl.J.Med., 1995; 332:1744-1748.

Goldberg, L.H et al: Long-term suppression of recurrent genital herpes with acyclovir. Arch. Dermatol., 1993; 129:582-587.

Gu, Z et al: Identification of mutation at codon 65 in the IKKK motif of reverse transcriptase that encodes human immunodeficiency virus resistance to 2',3'-dideoxycytidine and 2',3'-dideoxy-3'-thiacytidine. Antimicrob. Agents Chemother., 1994; 38:275-281.

Havlir, D.N et al: Antiretroviral therapy. Curr. Opin. Infect. Dis., 1995; 8:66-73.

Haefeli, W.E et al: Acyclovir-induced neurotoxicity: concentration-side effect relationship in acyclovir overdose. Am. J. Med., 1993; 94:212-215.

Havlir, D el al: High-dose nevirapine: safety, pharmacokinetics, and antiviral effect in patients with human immunodeficiency virus infection. J. Infect. Dis., 1995; 171:537-545.

Hirsch, M.S et al: Therapy for human immunodeficiency virus infection. N.Engl.J.Med., 1993; 328:1686-1695.

Hirschel B, Francioli P. Progress and problems in t-fight against AIDS. N. Engl. J. Med. 338:906-908, 1998.

Jones, R.J et al: Minireview: nucleotide prodrugs. Antiviral Res., 1995; 27:1-17.

Kinoch-De Loes, S et al: A controlled trial of zidovudine in primary human immunodeficiency virus infection. N. Engl. J. Med., 1995; 333:408-413.

Marroni, M et al: Interferon-alfa is effective in the treatment of HIV-I, severe-related, zidovudine-resistant thrombocytopenia. Ann. Intern. Med., 1994; 121:423-429.

Pillay, D et al: HIV-I protease inhibitors: their development, mechanism of action, and clinical potential, Rev. Med. Virol., 1995 (in press).

Riddler, S.A et al: Antiretroviral activity of stavudine (2°,3°-didehydro-3°-deoxythymidine, D4T). Antiviral Res., 1995; 27:189-203.

Sen, G.C et al: Interferon-induced antiviral action and their regulation. Adv. Virus. Res., 1993; 42:57-102.

Stein, D.C et al: The effect of the interaction of acyclovir with zidovudine on progression to AIDS and survival. Ann. Intern. Med., 1994; 121:100-108.

Tokars, J.I et al: Surveillance of HIV infection and zidovudine use among health care workers after occupational exposure to HIV-infected blood. Ann. Intern. Med., 1993; 118:913-919.

Tudor-Williams, G et al: HIV-I sensitivity to zidovudine and clinical outcome in children. Lancet, 1992; 339:15-19.

Volberding, P.A et al: The duration of zidovudine benefit in persons with asymptomatic HIV infection. JAMA, 1994; 272:437-442.

Wagstaff, A.J et al: A reappraisal of its antiviral activity, pharmacokinetic properties and therapeutic efficacy. Drugs, 1994; 47:153-205.

Wei, X et al: Viral dynamics in human immunodeficiency virun type I infection. Nature, 1995; 373:117-122.

White, A et al: Birth outcomes following zidovudine therapy in pregnant women. MMWR, 1994; 43:409-416.

Wills, R.J: Clinical pharmacokinetics of interferons. Clin. Pharmacokinet., 1990; 19:390-399.

CHEMOTHERAPY OF CANCER

Whatever the cause, cancer is basically a disease of cells characterized by a shift in the control mechanisms that govern cell proliferation and differentiation. Hence, cancer (neoplastic disease) is a disease characterized by an unrestricted cell division, invasion and metastases.

The ability to migrate the cancer cell to distant sites in the body to colonize various organs is called metastasis.

Most of the anticancer agents act on the proliferating population of cells: none acts primarily to influence tumour cell invasion or metastases.

Most cells are clonal, arising from a single altered cell.

The term cytotoxic in restricted sense means drugs which inhibit cell division. They kill or damage cells.

The current therapy for cancer depends primarily on the use of surgery, irradiation, and chemotherapy.

Classification of anticancer drugs

1. Alkylating agents (cell cycle nonspecific)
   - Nitrogen mustards
     - Mechlorethamine
     - Cyclophosphamide
     - Chlorambucil (leukeran)
   - Ethylenimine derivatives
     - TEM (triethylene melamine)
     - Thiotepa (triethylenethiophosphoramide)
   - Alkyl sulphonate
     - Busulfan
   - Nitrosoureas
     - Carmustine
     - Lomustine
     - Semustine
   - Triazenes
     - Dacarbazine
2. Antimetabolites (cell cycle specific)
   - Folate antagonist:
     - Methotrexate
     - Purine antagonist
     - 6-MP
     - Pyrimidine antagonist
     - 5-FU
3. Natural products
   (a) Vinca alkaloids
   - Vincristine
   - Vinblastine
   (b) Antibiotics
     - Actinomycin D
     - Doxorubicin (adriamycin)
     - Daunorubicin
     - Bleomycin
     - Mithramycin
   (c) Enzyme
     - Asparaginase
4. Radioisotopes
   - I^{131}
   - P^{32}
   - Au^{198}
5. Drugs altering hormonal environment of malignant cells
   - Glucocorticoids
     - Prednisolone
   - Oestrogens
     - Diethylstilboestrol
     - Ethinyloestradiol
   - Androgens
     - Testosterone
   - Progestins
     - Hydroxyprogestrone acetate
     - Medroxyprogestrone acetate
6. Miscellaneous
   - Hydroxyurea
   - Cisplatin

In addition to these targeted drug discovery efforts, new efforts are in clinical trial exploring the possibility that the immune system can be harnessed to treat cancer. So far IL-2 therapy of renal cancer and melanoma is the only such approach which has shown promising results.

Cytotoxic agents

These drugs act directly on cells. These are alkylating agents, antimetabolites, vinca alkaloids and certain antibiotics.

Some drugs are *phase-specific* agents such as vinca alkaloids which act in mitosis, while drugs like methotrexate, mercaptopurine, and hydroxyurea act on S-phase.

Some drugs are *cell cycle-specific* (CCS) which act only against dividing cells at all stages of cell cycle and not on cells out of cycle (resting, Go cells). These include antimetabolites, bleomycin and plant alkaloids such as vincristine and vinblastine.

Some drugs are *cell cycle-nonspecific* (CCNS) i.e. act against cells in cycle (multiplying) as well as resting (Go) cells. These includes alkylating agents and nitrosoureas, cisplatin, antibiotics (daunorubicin, doxorubicin).

The cell cycle is shown in Fig. 11.14.

Some drugs are called cell cycle nonspecific agents as they can sterilize tumour cells whether cycling or resting in the compartment. They can kill both Go and cycling cells.

Cell cycle specific agents (CCS): These act on proliferating cells: Antimetabolites (5 FU, 6-MP, MTX), Bleomycin, Vinca alkaloids.

They do not act on Go phase.

Cell cycle-nonspecific (CCNS): Alkylating agents, antibiotics, nitrosoureas, cisplatin.

These act on cells regardless of their rate of proliferation.

These act on any phase of the cycle. They possess slight effect on Go phase.

Phase	Drugs
S	Antimetabolites, daunorubicin, actinomycin D
M	Vinca alkaloids, bleomycin
G1	Prednisolone, daunorubicin, asparaginase
G2	Bleomycin

ALKYLATING AGENTS

The major classes of alkylating agents are:
1. Nitrogen mustards
2. Nitrosoureas
3. Alkyl sulphonates
4. Triazines

These have cytotoxic and radiomimetic (like ionizing radiation) actions. As a class they exert cytotoxic effects via transfer of their alkyl groups to various cellular constituents. Alkylation of DNA within the nucleus leads to cell death.

Mechlorethamine HCl (Nitrogen mustard): It is given by I.V route for Hodgkin's disease. It can depress bone marrow and produce venous thrombosis, vomiting and ulceration of GI mucosa as adverse effects.

Cyclophosphamide I.V./oral: Indicated in myeloma, acute lymphatic leukaemia.

Chlorambucil (lukeran), is also available, orally for Hodgkin's disease and chronic lymphatic leukaemia.

Thiotepa is highly toxic, Busulfan (Myeleran) can produce pulmonary fibrosis (specific adverse effect).

Nitrosoureas e.g. carmustine, lomustine and semustine and streptozocin resemble alkylating agents

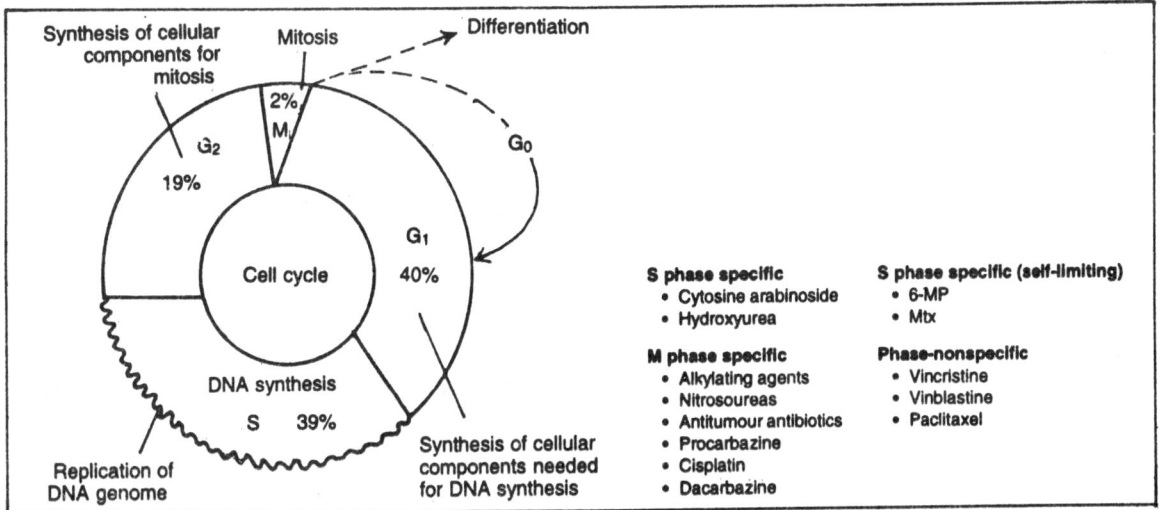

Fig. 11.14. Cell cycle phases that all cells—normal as well as malignant—must traverse before and during cell division. Percentages shown indicate the time spent in each phase.

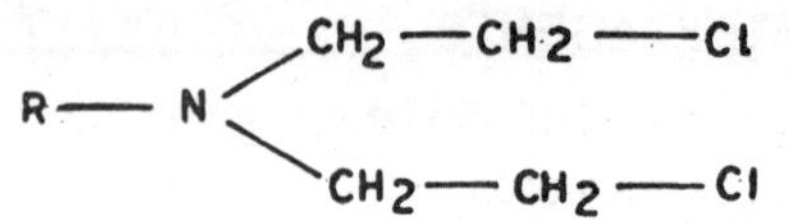

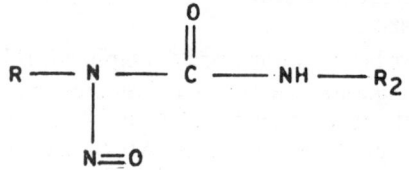

Fig. 11.15. Basic structure of nitrogen mustard.

$$R - N - C - NH - R_2$$

Fig. 11.16. Basic structure of nitrosoureas.

in mode of action. They are indicated in brain tumours, as they are highly lipid-soluble and cross the blood-brain barrier. They act by cross-linking through alkylation of DNA. One naturally occurring sugar containing nitrosourea is streptozocin that has minimal bone marrow toxicity and is effective in insulin-secreting islet cell carcinoma of pancreas and in Hodgkin's disease.

Alkylating agents are cytotoxic and radiomimetic or nucleotoxic agents (resemble effects of ionizing radiation or X-ray). These compounds are capable of displacing hydrogen atom in another molecule with an alkyl radical. They react to all constituents of the cell, effect on DNA is most critical, the cell loses ability to function.

Table 11.22 shows dosage and toxicity of alkylating agents and related drugs.

Doses of anticancer drugs are calculated on the basis of patients body surface area in m^2 rather than body weight.

Table 11.22. Dosage and toxicity of polyfunctional alkylating agents and related drugs

Alkylating agents	Dosage	Adverse effects
Nitrogen mustards		
Mechlorethamine	0.4 mg/kg I.V. in single or divided doses	Acute: nausea, vomiting with mechlorethamine and cyclo-phosphamide. No acute toxicity with other agents
Chlorambucil (Leukeral)	0.1-0.2 mg/kg/orally; 6-12 mg/d	
Cyclophosphamide	3.5-5 mg/kg/d/orally for 10 days, 1 g IV single dose	Acute: nausea, vomiting; Delayed: bone marrow depression with leukopenia, thrombocytopenia, bleeding, alopecia
Melphalan (Alkeran)	0.25 mg/kg/d/orally for 4 days, every 4-6 weeks	
Ethylenimines		
Thiotepa (triethylene thiophosphoramide)	0.2 mg/kg/i.v. for 5 days	Same as other alkylating agents
Alkyl sulphonates		
Busulfan (Myleran)	2-8 mg/d/orally 150-250 mg course	Skin pigmentation, pulmonary fibrosis and adrenal insufficiency
Nitrosoureas		
Carmustina (BCNU)	200 mg/M2 IV every 6 weeks	Leucopenia and thrombocytopenia, rarely hepatitis
Lomustina (CCNU)	150 mg/M2 orally every 6 weeks	
Semustine (Methyl-CCNU)	150 mg/M2 orally every 6 weeks	
Related drugs acting as alkylating agents		
Altretamine (Hexamethylmelamine)	10 mg/kg for 21 days	Leucopenia, thrombocytopenia, peripheral neuropathy
Procarbazine (Methylhy-drazine)	50-200 mg/d/orally	Bone marrow depression, CNS depression
Dacarbazine (Triazine)	300 mg/M2/d/IV for 5 days	Bone marrow depression
Platinum coordination complexes		
Cisplatin (Platinol)	20 mg/M2 IV for 5 days or 50-70 mg/M2 single dose every 3 weeks	Renal dysfunction, acoustic nerve dysfunction
Carboplatin (Paraplatin)	300 mg/M2/i.v. every 4 weeks	Leukopenia, thrombocytopenia; rarely neuropathy and hepatic dysfunction

Box 11.14. Anticancer drugs: Cytotoxic antibiotics

- Doxorubicin
- Bleomycin
- Dactinomycin
- Mitomycin

Box 11.15. Anticancer drugs: Plant derivaties

- Vicristine
- Etoposide

Box 11.16. Anticancer agents: Hormones or their antagonists and radioactive isotopes

- Glucocorticoids for leukaemias and lymphomas
- Oestrogens for prostate tumours
- Tamoxifen for breast tumours
- Gn RH analogues for prostate and breast tumours
- Antiandrogens for prostate cancer
- Inhibitor for sex hormone synthesis for postmenopausal breast cancer
- Radioactive isotopes, e.g. I^{131} for thyroid tumours

Box 11.17. Anticancer drugs: Miscellaneous agents

- Crisantaspase is active against acute lymphoblastic leukaemia cells which cannot synthesise asparagine
- Hydroxyurea
- Amsacrine acts on DNA-gyrase enzyme
- Mitozantrone causes DNA chain breakage
- Mitotane stops synthesis of adrenocortical steroids

Box 11.18. General toxic effects of anticancer drugs

- Severe nausea and vomiting
- Bone marrow toxicity with decreased leukocyte production and hence decreased resistance to infection
- Impaired wound healing
- Depression of growth in children
- Sterility
- Teratogenicity
- Alopecia
- Damage to gastrointestinal epithelium
- If there is a rapid cell distruction with extensive purine metabolism, urates may percipitate in the renal tubules and cause kidney damage
- They can also, in certain circumstances, be carcinogenic (i.e. they may themselves cause cancer)

Box 11.19. Dose-limiting extramedullary toxicities of alkylating agents

Alkylating agents	Major organ toxicities
Cyclophosphamide	Cardiac
Thiotepa	GI, CNS
Melphalan	GI
Busulfan	GI, Hepatic
Carmustine	Lung, hepatic
Cisplatin	Peripheral neuropathy, renal
Carboplatin	Peripheral neuropathy, renal, hepatic

Dacarbazine is N-demethylated by liver microsomal enzymes and then functions as an alkylating agent. It is one of the most active agents against malignant melanoma. It is also used for soft-tissue sarcomas and Hodgkin's disease.

Adverse effects include nausea, vomiting, myelosuppression and neurotoxicity.

ANTIMETABOLITES

- Folic acid analogues
  - Methotrexate (amethopterin)
- Pyrimidine analogues
  - Fluorouracil (5-fluorouracil, 5-FU)
  - Floxuridine (fluorodeoxyuridine)
  - Cytarabine (cytosine arabinoside)
- Purine analogues and related inhibitors
  - Mercaptopurine (6-MP)
  - Thioguanine (6-thioguanine)
  - Pentostatin

The site of action is shown in Fig. 11.17.

Methotrexate (MTX, Amethopterin)

It is a folic acid antagonist that binds to the active catalytic site of dihydrofolate reductase (DHFR), resulting in interfering with the formation of DNA and RNA.

Besides use in cancer, other applications of MTX are in the treatment of rheumatoid arthritis and psoriasis. It is being tried in asthma and with a prostaglandin as an abortificient.

MTX is administered by IV or oral route, 2.5-5 mg/d/orally; 10 mg intrathecally once or twice weekly.

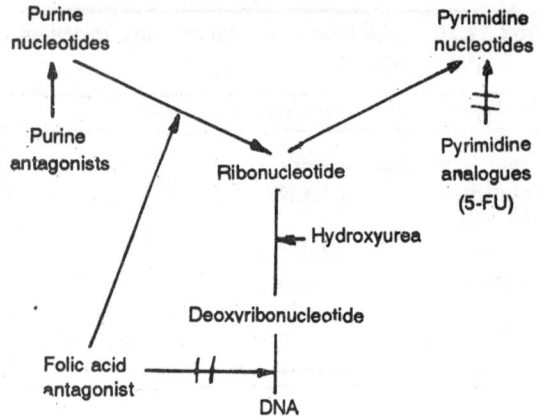

Fig. 11.17. Site of action of antimetabolites.

These drugs do not cause acute toxicity.

The delayed toxicity includes bone marrow depression, leukopenia, thrombocytopenia. The effects can be reversed by administration of leucovorin (Citrovorum factor).

Resistance may develop due to (i) decreased drug transport, (ii) altered DHRF with lower affinity for MTX and (iii) synthesis of increased DHRF.

Mercaptopurine (6-MP, Purinethol)

It is used primarily in the treatment of acute leukaemia in children. It is well tolerated but large dosages cause bone marrow depression.

Dose: 2.5 mg/kg/d orally.

Thioguanine (6-TG)

It inhibits several enzymes in the purine nucleotide pathway. It has a synergistic action when used with cytarabine in cases of adult acute leukaemia.

Dose: 2 mg/kg/d orally.

This drug is usually well tolerated, large dosages cause bone marrow depression. Resistance also occurs as with 6-MP.

PYRIMIDINE ANTAGONISTS

Fluorouracil (5-FU)

5-FU is converted to 5-fluorouridine triphosphate incorporated into RNA and interferes with RNA processing and function. It also inhibits DNA synthesis through 'thymineless death'.

Thus 5-FU is cytotoxic due to its effects on both DNA and RNA.

It can be given orally but as the bioavailability is erratic when given orally, IV injection is usually employed for the treatment of adenocarcinomas.

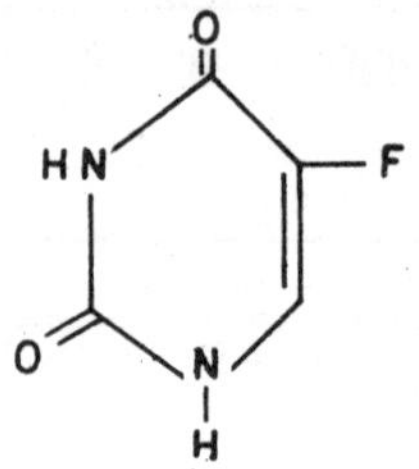

Fig. 11.18. Fluorouracil.

The adverse effects include mucositis and myelosuppression.

Florafur

Florafur is a recently introduced 5-FU congener, used orally in neoplasms of GIT and breast.

Cytosine arabinoside (Cytarabine, ara-C)

It is an S phase-specific antimetabolite that blocks DNA synthesis while RNA and protein synthesis continues resulting in an unbalanced growth. The drug is also incorporated into RNA and DNA. As cytosine arabinoside is S phase-specific, it is highly schedule-dependent so it should be given by continuous IV infusion or every 8-12 hours for 5-10 days. The dose is 100 mg/M2 for 5-10 days by continuous IV infusion or subcutaneously every 8 hours.

It is given for the treatment of acute myelogenous leukaemia.

Adverse effects include nausea, vomiting, stomatitis, alopecia, myelosuppression, leukopenia, thrombocytopenia, megaloblastosis.

Azacitidine

It is incorporated into DNA and RNA and inhibits DNA and RNA, and protein synthesis. It is an investigational drug.

Adverse effects include nausea, vomiting, diarrhoea, fever, hypotension, prolonged marrow hypoplasia.

NATURAL PRODUCTS

1. Vinca alkaloids (Vinblastine, Vincristine)
2. Antibiotics
   - Actinomycin D (Dactinomycin)
   - Anthracyclines (doxorubicin, daunorubicin, mitoxantrone)
   - Bleomycin
   - Mitomycin
   - Mithramycin
3. Biologic response modifiers
4. Enzymes
5. Epipodophyllotoxins
6. Western yew tree extract

Vinca alkaloids

Vinblastine

Vinblastine is an alkaloid obtained from vinca rosea.

Its mode of action involves depolymerization of microtubules, which are important part of mitotic spindle. The mitotic arrest occurs at metaphase.

This drug has been found useful in Hodgkin's disease and other lymphomas.

Dose: 0.1-0.2 mg/kg/IV weekly.

Acute toxic effects are nausea and vomiting.

Delayed toxicity includes alopecia, nausea, vomiting and bone marrow depression.

Desacetylvinblastine (Vindesine) and Vinzolidine are related drugs under investigation.

Vincristine (oncovin)

Vincristine is an alkaloid derived from vinca rosea, causes arrest of mitotic cycle (spindle poison) and although it is also closely related in structure to vinblastine but differs in clinical applications and toxicity.

This drug has been found useful in acute leukaemia in children, particularly in combination with prednisone.

Dose: 1.5 mg/m^2/IV (maximum 2 mg weekly).

Adverse effects

There is no acute toxic effect.

Delayed adverse effects include neurotoxicity (peripheral neuritis, paralytic ileus, muscle weakness) and occasionally mild bone marrow depression.

Antibiotics

The anticancer antibiotics include anthracyclines, actinomycin, bleomycin, mitomycin and plicamycin. These bind to DNA, block the synthesis of new RNA or DNA (or both).

They interfere with cell replication. These antibiotics are products of various strains of soil fungus, streptomyces.

Actinomycin D (dactinomycin)

It is isolated from streptomyces. It binds to DNA.

It inhibits DNA-dependent RNA synthesis.

It is useful as an adjuvant treatment of Wilm's tumour. It is also used with methotrexate in the treatment of choriocarcinoma.

Adverse effects include nausea, vomiting, diarrhoea, alopecia, skin eruptions, oral ulcers and all blood elements are affected profoundly, severe thrombocytopenia may occur. The drug is immunosuppressive.

Anthracycline antibiotics and their derivatives

These are produced by the fungus *Streptomyces peucetius* var. *caesius*. Two congeners **doxorubicin** and **daunorubicin** are in general use.

It is indicated in many different types of cancer and daunorubicin particularly for acute leukaemia. These are very useful cytotoxic anticancer drugs. These are given by IV route.

Doxorubicin (adriamycin) 60 mg/m^2/IV every 3 weeks (maximum total dose 550 mg/m^2) is recommended.

Acute toxicity includes nausea and red urine (not haematuria).

Delayed toxicity includes cardiotoxicity, alopecia, stomatitis, bone marrow depression.

The clinical value of anthracyclines is limited by an unusual cardiomyopathy.

In a search for agents with high antitumour activity but reduced cardiac toxicity, some related compounds including idarubucin, epirubicin and the synthetic compound mitoxantrone which is an anthracenedione have been developed. These have shown promise in clinical trials.

Idarabicin is a synthetic derivative. The recommended dosage is 12 mg/m2 daily for 3 days by IV injection in combination with cytarabine.

Daunorubicin and idarubicin are primarily indicated for acute leukaemias while doxorubicin is more effective in solid tumors.

Daunorubicin

It is similar to doxorubicin, lacks only hydroxyl moiety.

The dose 30-60 mg/m^2/d/IV for 3 days or 30-60 mg/m^2/IV weekly.

Acute toxicity includes nausea, fever, red urine (not haematuria).

Delayed toxicity includes cardiotoxicity, alopecia and bone marrow depression.

The mode of action of anthracyclines is due to (i) high affinity binding to DNA, (ii) binding to membranes that affects fluidity and ion transport, and (iii) generation of oxygen radicals (responsible for cardiac toxicity due to oxygen radical-mediated damage to membrane).

A new anthracycline analogue, idarubicin is under investigation in acute myeloid leukaemia.

Mitoxantrone

It is a synthetic anthracene related to anthracyclines.

It binds to DNA and inhibits both DNA and RNA synthesis. It is indicated in both childhood and adult acute myelogenous leukaemia, non-Hodgkin lymphomas and breast cancer.

Dose: 10-12 mg/m^2/IV every 3-4 weeks.

Adverse effects include nausea, bone marrow depression, occasional cardiac toxicity and alopecia.

Bleomycin

Streptomyces verticillus produces a series of bleomycins.

Bleomycin binds to DNA. It is a cycle cell specific drug that causes accumulation of cells in G2 and hence schedule-dependent.

It is synergistic with vinblastine, cisplatin for testicular cancer. It is also useful in squamous cell cancer of head and neck, cervix, skin, penis, rectum and in combination therapy for lymphomas.

A special use is for intracavitary therapy in cases of malignant effusions in ovarian and breast cancers.

The drug is available by SC, IM or IV route as well as by intracavitary route.

The adverse effects include fever, hypotension, lethal anaphylactoid reactions.

Pulmonary fibrosis is not common but seen sometimes in older patients. It is sometimes fatal. It does not produce significant myelosuppression.

Mitomycin (Mitomycin C)

It is 'bioreductive' alkylating agent that undergoes metabolic reductive activation to generate an alkylating agent which cross- links DNA. It is used with bleomycin and vincristine for squamous cell carcinoma of cervix and for adenocarcinomas of stomach, pancreas and lung (with doxorubicin and 5-FU). To some extent this drug is also useful for metastatic colon cancer.

A special use of mitomycin is in reducing the frequency of small bladder papillomas. For this purpose instillation of this drugs in distilled water (topical intravesical treatment) is held in bladder for 3 hours, repeated over a course of weeks. Very little is absorbed systemically when this procedure is employed.

Adverse effects include nausea and vomiting; anorexia occurs soon after injection; late toxicity includes severe myelosuppression. It is also nephrotoxic.

Plicamycin (mithramycin)

It is isolated from streptomyces plicatus. It interupts DNA-dependent RNA synthesis.

It has been found useful in testicular cancers and has few other indications only.

Plicamycin decreases plasma calcium level by acting on osteoclasts (independent of action on tumour cells). It has been useful in hypercaelcemia.

Adverse effects include nausea, vomiting, leukopaenia, hypocalcaemia, thrombocytopenia, bleeding disorders and hepatotoxicity.

Biologic response modifiers

These act directly on tumour cells or indirectly by enhancing the immunologic response to neoplastic cells, e.g. Interleukin-2 (IL-2). It is a cytokine secreted by T cells that enhance natural killer activity. It is being tried in melanoma and renal cell cancer.

Interferons (alpha, beta, gamma) have been used

in the treatment of hairy cell leukaemia and Kaposi's sarcoma in patients with AIDS.

Enzyme

L-asparaginase

L-asparaginase catalyzes the hydrolysis of asparagine to aspartic acid and ammonia. Due to deficiency of asparagine in malignant cells protein synthesis is inhibited resulting in cellular death.

It is an enzyme isolated from various bacteria. It is useful in childhood leukaemia. It produces catabolic depletion of serum asparagine to aspartic acid and ammonia.

It has modest success in acute lymphatic leukaemia.

Dose: 20,000 IU/m^2 daily IV for 5-10 days.

It is not usually given because it can give rise to acute toxicity including nausea, vomiting, fever and allergic reactions. Delayed toxicity include hepatotoxicity, pancreatitis and mental depression.

Crisantaspase

It is a preparation of the enzyme asparaginase. It is given by I.M. or I.V. injection.

It breaks down asparagine to aspartic acid and ammonia. It is active against tumour cells which are unable to synthesis asparagine and now require an exogenous supply of it, e.g. acute lymphoblastic leukaemia cells.

Adverse effects

Nausea, vomiting, CNS depression, liver damage.

Anaphylactic reactions have been reported.

However it has very little suppressive effect on the bone marrow or the mucosa of GIT or hair follicles.

Epipodophyllotoxins

Etoposide and teniposide are semisynthetic derivatives of podophyllotoxin, which is extracted from root of podophyllum.

These act in the late S-G2 phase of the cell cycle.

Etoposide is approved for use in USA for testicular cancer, oat cell carcinoma of lung and monocytic leukaemia.

Dose: 50-100 mg/m^2/d/IV for 5 days.

Adverse effects

Acute toxicity symptoms are nausea, vomiting and hypotension.

The delayed toxicity includes alopecia and bone marrow depression.

Western yew tree extract

Paclitaxel (Taxol)

It is an alkaloid ester obtained from Taxus brevifolia (Western yew), as Taxus baccata (European yew). It acts as a mitotic spindle poison. It is active against ovarian and advanced breast cancer.

Dose: 130-170 mg/m^2/IV over 3 or 4 hours every 3-4 weeks.

Acute toxicity includes nausea, vomiting, hypotension and arrhythmias.

Delayed toxicity includes bone marrow depression.

RADIOACTIVE ISOTOPES

These emit β-rays.

Radiophosphorous P^{32}, half-life of 14.3 days for polycythemia vera, chronic lymphocytic and chronic myeloid leukaemia, prostate cancer and for localizing brain tomours.

Radio gold Au^{198} has half-life 2.7 days for abdominal tumours, ascites and pleural effusion due to malignancy, carcinoma cervix.

Radio iodine I^{131} for diagnostic and therapeutic use in thyroid tumours. It has half-life of 8 days. It can be given orally or I.V.

HORMONES AND ANTAGONISTS

Adrenocorticosteroids

The glucocorticoids have been used in the treatment of acute leukaemia, myeloma, lymphomas, advanced breast cancer.

Steroid hormones bind to receptor proteins in cancer cells.

Specific receptors have been identified for oestrogens, progesterone, corticosteroids and androgens in certain neoplastic cells.

Most steroid-sensitive cancers have specific receptors. Measurment of oestrogen receptor (ER) and progesterone receptor (PR) proteins in breast cancer tissue is a standard clinical test. ER- or PR-positive results predict responsiveness to endocrine ablation.

Hydrocortisone 40-200 mg/d orally or predinsone 20-100 mg/d orally are advocated in the treatment of lymphoblastic and chronic lymphatic leukaemia, breast cancer, Hodgkin's disease, Non-Hodgkin's lymphomas and multiple myeloma.

Sex hormones

Oestrogen can stimulate breast and endometrial cancer growth and antioestrogens are useful in breast cancer; in prostate cancer androgens stimulate growth and oestrogen administration suppresses androgen production. Oestrogens, androgens and corticosteroids all can cause fluid retention due to their sodium-retaining effect; oestrogen may cause feminization and androgens may cause masculinization. Adrenocorticosteroids may cause hypertension, diabetes mellitus, increased susceptibility to infection and Cushingoid appearance.

Oestrogens

High doses of oestrogens diethylstilboestrol 1-5 mg orally 3 times a day or ethinyloestradiol 3 mg/d orally, are used in prostatic carcinoma, which is an androgen-dependent neoplasm.

Inoperable breast cancer in post-menopausal women may be sometimes favourably influenced temporarily by oestrogens and by an adrenal steroid.

Progestins as anticancer agents: medroxyprogesterone caproate 1 g IM twice weekly, megestrol 100-200 mg orally daily or 200-600 mg orally twice a week, megestrol acetate 40 mg orally 4 times daily are commonly employed.

These drugs are sometimes used in the therapy of metastatic endometrial carcinoma that can no longer be treated with surgery or radiation. These also have some limited use in metastatic renal cell carcinoma.

The adverse effects include mild fluid retention, vaginal bleeding.

Feminisation is inevitable and gynaecomastia is often painful.

Antioestrogen

Tamoxifen is oestrogen receptor antagonist, very

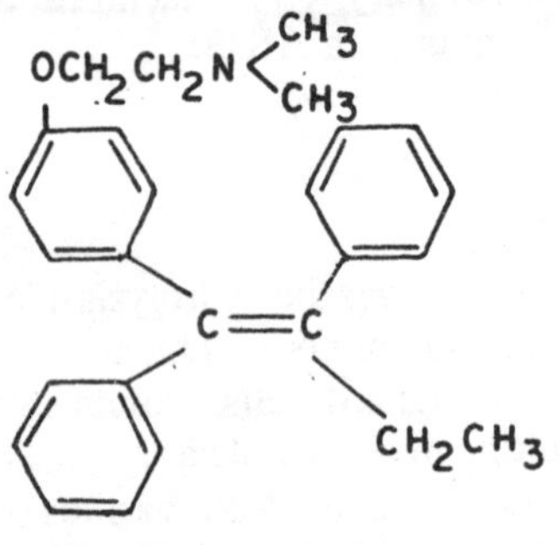

Fig. 11.19. Structure of tamoxifen.

useful in breast cancer. It binds to oestrogen receptors of oestrogen-sensitive tissues and tumours in women whose tumours contain oestrogen receptors.

Patients who benefit most are those who lack endogenous oestrogen (oophorectomy, or postmenopausal state), and in whom cytoplasmic ER or PR protein is demonstrable.

Dose: 10 mg twice daily.

Adverse effects include hot flushes, nausea, fluid retention, pruritis vulvae and dermatitis, menstrual irregularities and vaginal bleeding.

Androgens such as fluoxymesterone, dromostandone and testosterone propionate are indicated in breast cancer in post-menopausal women.

Antiandrogens

Androgen antagonists, flutamide and cyproterone are used in prostate tumours.

Flutamide is a non-steroidal anti-androgen, used with GnRH in the treatment of prostate cancer.

Cyproterone is a derivative of progesterone and has weak progestational activity. It is a partial against at androgen receptors, competing with dihydrotestosterone for receptors in androgen-sensitive target tissues. It depresses the synthesis of gonadotrophins through its action on hypothalamus.

Cyproterone is used as an adjunct in the treatment of prostate cancer during initiation of GnRH treatment. It is also used in the therapy of precocious puberty in males, and of masculinisation and acne in women. It also decreases libido by acting on CNS. It may be used in the treatment of severe hypersexuality in male sexual offenders.

Drugs which inhibit the enzymes which give rise to active steroids

Finasteride inhibits the enzyme 5 α-reductase that converts testosterone to dihydrotestosterone which has greater affinity for androgen receptors. It is used in the treatment of prostatic hyperplasia. However, terazosin (α_1-adrenoceptor antagonist) is more effective.

Tamsulosin is a selective α-1A-adrenoceptor antagonist that blocks the receptors in prostatic smooth muscle, but not in the vasculature. Hence, it produces less postural hypotension than with terazosin.

Other hormonally active agents

Gonadotropin-releasing hormone agonists:

- Goserelin acetate 3.6 mg by subcutaneous injection/monthly.
- Leuprolide 7.5 mg subcutaneous injection/monthly.

These are synthetic peptide analogues of naturally occurring gonadoropin-releasing hormone. When given continuously initial stimulation is followed by inhibition of the release of follicle-stimulating hormone and luteinizing hormone. This results in reduced testicular androgen synthesis. This makes them effective in the treatment of metastatic carcinoma of the prostate.

The endocrine effects of these drugs may prove useful in hormone receptor-positive breast cancer (still to be established).

MISCELLANEOUS AGENTS

Adrenocortical suppressant

Aminoglutethimide acts as an inhibitor of adrenal steroid synthesis at first step (conversion of cholesterol to pregnenolone), it also inhibits extraadrenal synthesis of oestrone and oestradiol.

It is also an inhibitor of aromatase enzyme that converts the adrenal androgen androstenedione to oestrone. This aromatization of androgenic precursor into oestrogen occurs in body fat.

Aminoglutethimide is effective in metastatic breast cancer which contains significant levels of oestrogen- or progesterone-receptors.

Dose: 250 mg orally twice daily with hydrocortisone 20 mg twice daily (to avoid adrenal insufficiency).

Adverse effects

Its acute toxicity includes dizziness, rash, lethargy and visual blurring.

This drug is somewhat more toxic than tamoxifen.

Mitotane

It is a derivative of the insecticide DDT. Its only indication is adrenal carcinoma.

Dose: 6-15 g/d orally.

Adverse effects include diarrhoea, mental depression, skin eruptions, nausea, anorexia and somnolence.

Peptide hormone inhibitor

Octreotide: 100-600 mcg/d SC in 2-4 divided doses.

Acute adverse effects are nausea and vomiting.

Cisplatin (*cis*-diamminedichloroplatinum [II])

Cisplatin is a heavy metal complex containing a central atom of platinum surrounded by two chloride atoms and two ammonia molecules in the cis position. It acts like alkylating agents (phase non-specific effect). It is the first totally inorganic compound to have a role in cancer chemotherapy.

It kills cells in all stages of the cell cycle, inhibits DNA biosynthesis and binds DNA through the formation of interstrand cross-links. Only the cis form is active.

Its major antitumour activity includes genitourinary cancer particularly testicular, ovarian and bladder cancer.

Combination of cisplatin with bleomycin and vinblastine is quite effective curative therapy for nonseminomatous testicular cancer.

Adverse effects

After IV injection, nausea and vomiting are quite common. Cisplatin has little effect on bone marrow but can produce significant nephrotoxicity, tinnitus and hearing loss.

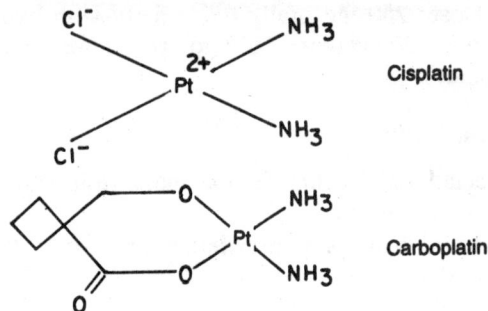

Fig. 11.20. Structure of cisplatin and carboplatin.

Carboplatin

A platinum analogue (carboplatin) produces less GI and renal toxicity.

The dose of carboplatin is 300 mg/m² I.V. every four weeks.

Acute toxicity includes nausea and vomiting. Delayed toxicity includes leukopenia, thrombopenia, neuropathy and renal dysfunction (rarely).

Substituted urea

Hydroxyurea is a derivative of urea.

It inhibits DNA synthesis acting in S-phase. It is useful in chronic myelogenous leukaemia. It is given orally.

Dose: 300 mg/m² orally for 5 days.

Adverse effects

Nausea, vomiting and diarrhoea are common.

Other adverse effects include bone marrow depression. Doses more than 40 mg/kg/d can produce megaloblastosis that does not respond to vitamin B_{12} or folic acid.

Retinoic acid derivatives

All-trans-Retinoic acid (etretinate) can be used as adjuvant in patients with head and neck squamous cell carcinoma.

Bone marrow growth factors

Granulocyte colony stimulating factor (G-CSF) and granulacyte-macrophage stimulating factor can reduce the incidence of infection associated with severe neutropenia.

Adverse effects

Retinoids can produces effect on mucocutaneous, skeletal and liver. Teratogenic effects are the most frequent toxic effects in animals.

Choice

- Acute leukaemia in children
  - Antimetabolites
  - Corticosteroids
  - Vincristine

Table 11.23. Treatment of choice

	Induction with
Acute lymphocytic leukaemia	Vincristine + predinsone; maintenance with 6-MP, methotrexate and cyclophosphamide
Acute myelocytic leukaemia	Cytarabine with daunorubicin
Chronic lymphocytic leukaemia	Busulfan
Hodgkin's disease	Mechlorethamine + vincristine, predinsone
Non-Hodgkin's lymphomas	Cyclophosphamide + doxorubicin, vincristine, predinsone
Multiple myeloma	Predinsone + melphalan
Polycythemia vera	Busulfan, chlorambucil or cyclophosphamide
Carcinoma of lung	Etoposide + cisplatin
Carcinoma of head and neck	5-FU + cisplatin
Carcinoma of ovary	Cyclophosphamide and cisplatin
Carcinoma of endometrium	Progestins or tamoxifen
Carcinoma of cervix	Cisplatin
Breast carcinoma	Tamoxifen after primary breast surgery; combination chemotherapy or hormonal manipulation for late recurrence
Carcinoma of testes	Cisplatin + bleomycin
Carcinoma of prostate	Oestrogens + flutamide
Carcinoma of thyroid	I^{131}, doxorubicin, cisplatin
Carcinoma of adrenal	Mitotane
Carcinoma of stomach, pancreas	5-FU + doxorubicin and mitomycin
Carcinoma of colon	5-FU + leucovorin
Neuroblastoma	Cyclophosphamide + doxorubicin and vincristine

- Hodgkin's disease
  - Chlorambucil
  - TEM
  - Mechlorethamine, methotrexate, vinblatine, corticosteroids
- Chronic lymphatic leukaemia
  - Chlorambucil, prednisolone

Combination therapies

Cyclophosphamide, vincristine, amethopterin, 5-FU and prednisone are effective in Hodgkin's disease (VAMP: vincristine i.v./week; methotraxate orally/d; 6-MP orally/d; prednisone orally/d is a useful combination. MOPP stands for mechlorethamine, vincristine (oncovin), procarbazine, and prednisolone.

Problems, hazards and obstacles with anticancer drugs

- Non-specific as cause of cancer is not known, hence these drugs lack specificity of action.
- Resistance develops. Some cells survive, some develop resistance and tumours finally become refractory to treatment.

  It can be primary, i.e. present when the drug is first given or

  Acquired (develop during drug treatment). It may be due to adaptation of the tumour cells or to mutation.
- These drugs are highly toxic agents.
- All anticancer drugs possess low therapeutic index.

Mechanisms of resistance may be:

1. Decrease in amount of drug taken up by the cell (methotrexate)
2. Insufficient activation of the drug (6-MP, 5-FU, Cytarabine)
3. Increase in inactivation (6-MP, Cytarabine)
4. Increased concentration of target enzyme (methotrexate)
5. Decreased requirement for substrate (crisantaspase).
6. Increased utilisation of alternative metabolic pathways (Antimetabolites).
7. Mutations in the p53 gene and over expres-

sion of the Bel-2 gene family (several cytotoxic drugs).
8. Altered activity of target, e.g. modified topoisomerase-II (doxorubicin).
9. Rapid repair of drug-induced lesions (alkylating agents).
10. Decreased accumulation of drugs in cells. It can be due to increased expression of a cell surface, energy-dependent drug transport protein, termed P-glycoprotein.

The physiological role of P-glycoprotein is to protect cells against environmental toxins, acts as a 'vacuum cleaner', picking up drugs as they enter the cell membrane and expelling then outside. The transporter is coded for by the mdr gene and is responsible for multidrug resistance (doxorubicin, vinblastine, dactinomycin, etc.).

Adverse effects of anticancer drugs

Immediate: Nausea and vomiting.

Delayed: Bone marrow depression (hypoplasia resulting in granulocytopenia, thrombocytopenia, lymphocytopenia, aplastic anaemia), gastrointestinal ulcers, alopecia, nerototoxicity, hepatotoxicity, reticuloendothelial system suppression (immuno-suppression), teratogenicity, impairment of fertility (effect on gonads), carcinogenicity (secondary cancer may develop after several years).

Vinca alkaloids are more likely to produce nausea, vomiting, alopecia, leukopaenia.

The antimetabolites particularly produce stomatitis, enteritis and bone marrow depression.

Specific adverse effects

Bleomycin and busulfan may produce pulmonary fibrosis.

Daunorubicin and doxorubicin are cardiotoxic and may produce hypotension and arrhythmias.

Present status

At present, chemotherapy provides palliative rather than curative therapy for many cancers resulting in prolongation of useful life. This is better achieved through combined therapy in which optimal combinations of surgery, radiotherapy, and chemotherapy are used.

Certain cancers can be cured by employing chemotherapy e.g. testicular cancer, diffused large cell lymphoma, Hodgkin's disease, choriocarcinoma, acute lymphoblastic leukaemia (in children), Burkitt's lymphoma, Wilm's tumour, and embryonal rhabdomyosarcoma. It has been shown that chemotherapy with initial surgery increases the cure rate in early-stage breast cancer and osteogenic carcinoma.

However, carcinomas of the lung and colon are usually refractory to presently available treatment.

Cancers in which drug therapy has an important place

- Hodgkin's disease
- Non-Hodgkin's lymphoma
- Chronic granulocytic leukaemia
- Acute lymphocytic leukaemia
- Hairy cell leukaemia
- Germ cell cancer (testis, ovary)
- Choriocarcinoma
- Prostate cancer

Future strategies

Current medicine knows only two ways in treating cancer—to kill the bad cells with chemotherapy or remove them with surgery. The major disadvantage has always been the destruction of healthy cells in the process.

Scientists have been working hard on finding a new way to treat cancer. Scientists who were looking for a specific chemical inside human cells that fights infectious disease, by accident stumbled upon an enzyme that has never been known before. Many months of experimentation led to the finding that this enzyme acts like a switch that controls a cancer cell's ability to produce energy.

This is explained on the basis of what is called as the "Warburg Paradox". More than 70 years ago, a German biochemist, Dr. Otto Warburg, discovered that cancer cells metabolize sugars without oxygen. What had not been discovered is how they are able to skip this requirement that normal, healthy cells have. With the discovery of this enzyme, however, it looks as though the answer is found. Because it appears that this enzyme—the 'molecular switch'—is always turned on in cancer cells, thus allowing them to produce energy without oxygen. Dr. Chesney displayed these results in an experimental cancer treatment in the laboratory, where two groups of cells were clearly identified. Untreated human cancer cells rapidly multiplied, whereas a second group of cells that was treated to turn off the switch stopped multiplying, which could be confirmed by observing a far fewer number of cells.

Attempts are being made to overcome the main drawbacks of the current chemotherapy:

- by developing new approaches based on the advances in knowledge of the biology of the cancer cell.
- by using selective targeting of anticancer compounds.
- by developing agents which reverse multidrug resistance.
- by boosting or enhancing the host's immune responses to the tumour.

STUDY QUESTIONS

1. What are the properties of ideal anticancer drugs? What is the present status?
2. Describe cell cycle. What is its importance in relation to administration of drugs? Give examples of drugs which are cell cycle specific and those which are cell cycle non-specific.
3. List classes of anticancer drugs with examples.
4. Describe alkylating agents; their mode of action, indications, dosage and adverse effects.
5. How do antimetabolites act? What are their major indications and toxic effects?
6. Which plant alkaloids possess cancer combating activity? Describe their mode of action, spectrum of activity and toxic effects.
7. Which antibiotics possess anticancer property? What are their indications and adverse effects?
8. Write notes on (i) combination chemotherapy in the treatment of cancer, (ii) differences in indications of vinblasting and vincristine, (iii) limitations of anticancer drugs in general, and (iv) cisplatin.
9. Give the current first choice of drugs in following conditions:
   (i) Acute leukaemia in childhood
   (ii) Cancer breast

(iii) Cancer prostate

(iv) Hodgkin's disease

(v) Carcinoma of colon

(vi) Carcinoma of cervix

10. Which anticancer drugs produce cardiac toxicity and how? Name the drugs which produce pulmonary fibrosis.

11. What is the relation of steroid hormones and sex hormones in stimulating growth of certain tumours and their inhibitors in the treatment of certain cancers? Give examples of oestrogens, antioestrogens, androgens and antiandrogens which are clinically used.

12. Describe radioactive isotopes useful in different cancers.

GUIDE TO FURTHER READING

Boccardo, F et al: Prophylaxis of superficial bladder cancer with mitomycin or interferon-alfa2b: results of a multicentric Italian Study. J. Clin. Oncol., 1994; 12:7-13.

Dabholkar, M et al: Messenger RNA levels of XPAC and ERCC1 in ovarian cancer tissue correlate with response to platinum-based chemotherapy. J. Clin. Invest., 1994; 94:703-708.

Dalgleish, A.G et al: Bleomycin pulmonary toxicity: its relationship to renal dysfunction. Med. Pediatr. Oncol., 1984; 12:313-317.

Dixon, K.H et al: A novel cDNA restores reduced folate carrier activity and methotrexate sensitivity to transport deficient cells. J. Biol. Chem., 1994; 269:17-20.

Feagan, B.G et al: Methotrexate for the treatment of Crohn's disease. N.Engl.J.Med., 1995; 332:292-297.

Fisher, D.E et al: Apoptosis in cancer therapy: crossing the threshold. Cell, 1994; 78:539-542.

Hausknecht, R.U: Methotrexate and misoprostol to terminate early pregnancy. N. Engl. J. Med., 1995; 333:537-540.

Love, R.R et al: Effects of tamoxifen on cardiovascular risk factors in postmenopausal women after 5 years of treatment. J. Natl. Cancer Inst., 1994; 86:1534-1539.

Lubitz, J.A. et al: Mitotane use in inoperable adrenal cortical carcinoma. JAMA, 1973; 223:1109-1112.

Meloni, G et al: Interleukin-2 may induce prolonged remissions in advanced acute myelogenous leukemia. Blood, 1994; 84:2158-2163.

Nicolaon, K.C et al: Total synthesis of taxol, Nature, 1994; 367:630-634.

Rosenberg, S.A et al: Treatment of patients with metastatic melanoma with autologous tumor-infiltrating lymphocytes and interleukin-2. J. Natl. Cancer. Inst., 1994; 86:1159-1166.

Takimoto, C.H et al: Challenges and promises of cancer therapy. In, Current Therapy in Hematology-Oncology, 5th ed. C.V. Mosby, Co., St. Louis, 1995; pp. 1-8.

Arbuck, S.G et al: Current dosage and schedule issues in the development of paclitaxel Semin. Oncol., 1993; 20 Suppl. 3:31-39.

Bukowski, R.M et al: Clinical pharmacokinetics of interleukin-1, interleukin-2, interleukin-3, tumor necrosis factor, and macrophage colony-stimulating factor. In, Cancer Chemotherapy: Principles and Practice, 2nd ed. J.B. Lippincott Co., Philadelphia, 1995 (in press).

Chabner, B.A: Cytidine analogues. In, Cancer Chemotherapy: Principles and Practice, 2nd ed. J.B. Lippincott Co., Philadelphia, 1995 (in press).

Chabner, B.A et al: Enzyme therapy: L-asparaginase. In, Cancer Chemotherapy: Principles and Practice, 2nd ed. J.B. Lippincott Co., Philadelphia, 1995 (in press).

Chabner, B.A et al: Pharmacology and toxicity of antineoplastic drugs. In, Williams' Hematology, 5th ed. McGraw-Hill, New York, 1994; pp. 143-154.

Cheson, B.D: The purine analogs- a therapeutic beauty contest. J.Clin. Oncol., 1992; 10:352-355.

Chu, E et al: Antimetabolites. In, Cancer Chemotherapy: Principles and Practice, 2nd ed. J.B. Lippincott Co., Philadelphia, 1995 (in press).

Donehower, R.C et al: Hydroxyurea. In, Cancer Chemotherapy: Principles and Practice, 2nd ed. J.B. Lippincott Co., Philadelphia, 1995 (in press).

Friedman, H.S et al: Nonclassic alkylating agents. In, Cancer Chemotherapy: Principles and Practice, 2nd ed. J.B. Lippincott Co., Philadelphia, 1995 (in press).

Grem, J.L et al: 5-Fluropyrimidines. In, Cancer Chemotherapy: Principles and Practice, 2nd ed. J.B. Lippincott Co., Philadelphia, 1995 (in press).

Keating, M.J et al: New platinum antitumor complexes. Crit. Rev. Oncol. Hematol., 1993; 15:191-219.

Lazo, J.S et al: Bleomycin. In, Cancer Chemotherapy: Principles and Practice, 2nd ed. J.B. Lippincott Co., Philadelphia, 1995 (in press).

McInnes, S et al: Infertility following cancer chemotherapy. In, Cancer Chemotherapy: Principles and Practice, 2nd ed. J.B. Lippincott Co., Philadelphia, 1995 (in press).

Rowinsky, E.K et al: The current status of Taxol. Prin. Pract. Gynecol. Oncol. Updates, 1993; I(1):1-16.

Rowinsky, E.K et al: Paclitaxel (Taxol). N.Engl.J.Med., 1995; 332:1004-1014.

Verweij, J et al: Antitumor antibiotics. In, Cancer Chemotherapy: Principles and Practice, 2nd ed. J.B. Lippincott Co., Philadelphia, 1995 (in press).

Zhou, X.J et al: Preclinical and clinical pharmacology of vinca alkaloids. Drugs, 1992; 44 Suppl. 4:1-16.

ANTISEPTICS AND DISINFECTANTS

The antiseptics and disinfectants are used to reduce the microbial population. They can be applied only topically, not systemically to humans.

The term antiseptic is applied to substances that inhibit bacterial growth both in vitro and in vivo when applied to the surface of living tissues.

The term disinfectant denotes a substance that kills microorganisms in an inanimate environment.

The term germicide includes both antiseptic as well as disinfectant. However, these terms have often been used interchangeably and definitions overlap in the literature.

Ideally germicide should be (i) lethal for micro-organisms in high dilution, (ii) noninjurious to living tissues or inanimate objects, (iii) stable, (iv) inexpensive, (v) odourless, (vi) nonstaining and (vii) rapid acting even in the presence of foreign proteins, exudates or fibres.

There is no preparation available that combines all the above properties to a high degree.

The antibacterial action of germicides depends on (i) concentration, (ii) temperature, and (iii) contact time. It has been noticed that very low concentration may stimulate bacterial growth, higher concentrations are inhibitory and still higher concentrations are lethal for certain microorganisms.

The choice of antiseptics to disinfect living tissues e.g. conjunctiva depends on the concentrations that can be safely applied to the tissues.

The efficacy to destroy bacteria by a germicide depends on the kind of organism, temperature, pH, and presence of organic matter. Another factor is that the progressive dilution by tears of the antiseptics may rapidly reduce the potency of germicidals introduced into the conjunctival sac.

Antiseptics and disinfectants can be grouped on chemical basis as follows:

Alcohol, Aldehydes, Acids, Oxidizing compounds. Heavy metals, Soaps, Phenols and related compounds, Cationic surface-active agents, Nitrofurans.

ALIPHATIC ALCOHOLS

Ethyl alcohol

It is bactericidal in 70% concentration in 1-2 minutes at 30 degree celsius but less potent at lower and higher concentrations. 70% alcohol as aerosol is effective disinfectant for mechanical respirators.

Isopropyl alcohol

It is more effective as antiseptic than ethyl alcohol. Ethyl alcohol and isopropyl alcohol are very satisfactory general antiseptics for skin surfaces. They are also useful for sterilizing instruments. However, they are not effective agaisnt spores.

Aliphatic alcohols are antibacterial by denaturing proteins.

ALDEHYDES

Concentration of 1-10% formaldehyde kills microorganisms and their spores in 1-6 hours. Formaldehyde combines with and precipitates protein. It is a good disinfectant for instruments but they are very irritating for use on tissues.

Methenamine

When given orally releases formaldehyde in acid urine (acts as urinary antiseptic).

Boric acid

5% in water or as powder acts as an antimicrobial agent which can be applied on skin lesions. However, boric acid can be absorbed and produce adverse effects.

Benzoic acid esters

These can be used as antiseptic preservatives of certain other drugs. Acetic acid 1% can be used in surgical dressings as a topical antibacterial substance. It is particularly effective against aerobic Gram-negative microorganisms e.g. *Pseudomonas*.

Mandelic acid

After oral administration it is excreted unchanged in

the urine, if 12 g of mandelic acid is taken orally it lowers the pH of urine to 5.0 (sufficient to be antibacterial).

HALOGEN-CONTAINING COMPOUNDS

Iodine

1 : 20,000 solution kills bacteria in 1 minute and spores in 15 minutes. The tissue toxicity is low. Tincture of iodine (2% iodine and 2.4% sodium iodide in alcohol) is a very effective antiseptic for intact skin. However, in hypersensitive persons, it may produce dermatitis. Solution of iodine (7% iodine and 5% potassium iodide in alcoholic solution) was previously employed for the treatment of acute herpetic keratitis. But the use of a strong solution of iodide has now been given up because of the danger of permanent stromal scarring. Mild solution of iodine is favoured. Now specific antiviral drugs are available such as topical IDU and vidarabine and therefore there is hardly any justification for the treatment of herpetic keratitis with iodides.

Iodine has been complexed with polyvinyl-pyrolidone (povidone-iodine). This water soluble solution is very effective as a skin antiseptic. It is a local antibacterial agent that kills bacteria in less than a minute as well as their spores but slowly.

Povidone-iodine is available as solution, ointment, surgical scrub, shampoo, individual cotton swabs, skin cleanser and vaginal gel. Povidone-iodine 0.1%, 1% and 5% exposure sterilizes herpes virus and *N. gonorrhoea*.

Chlorine

Chlorine concentrations of 0.25 ppm are bactericidal for many microorganisms except mycobacteria, which are 500 times more resistant. Presence of organic matter greatly reduces the antibacterial property of chlorine.

Chlorine exerts its antimicrobial activity in the form of undissociated hypochlorous acid (HOCl) that is formed when chlorine is dissolved in water at neutral or acid pH.

Chlorine is used for the disinfection of inanimate objects and particularly for the purification of water. Halazone is a chloramine in tablet form which is used for the sterilization of small volume of drinking water. If 4-8 mg of this substance is added per litre,

the drinking water will be sterilized in 15-60 minutes provided large amount of organic matter is not present. It may not inactivate cysts of *Entamoeba histolytica*.

OXIDIZING AGENTS

Hydrogen peroxide, sodium perborate and potassium permanganate are sometimes employed.

Hydrogen peroxide contains 3% H_2O_2 in water. When it comes in contact with tissues it releases molecular oxygen, producing antimicrobial action for a short period. It can be used as a mouth wash or for cleaning of wounds. It can also be used to disinfect soft contact lenses. Hydrogen peroxide does not penetrate the tissues.

Potassium permanganate 1 : 10,000 dilution in water kills many microorganisms in 1 hour. Higher concentrations irritate tissues.

METALLIC GERMICIDES

The topical use of most of these metallic germicides such as metallic salts and dyes are now obsolete because their use on the eye is limited by ocular tolerance, they delay healing of corneal epithelial defects resulting in permanent corneal opacity in some cases. They have been replaced by antibiotics.

Metallic germicides include 10% silver protein, 2% mercurochrome, 0.5% zinc sulphate, 1 : 3,000 benzalkonium chloride, 1 : 1,000 acriflavine, 1 : 2,000 nitromersol, 1 : 2,500 thiomersal and 1 : 5,000 mercuric oxycyanide. Mercury is a frequent allergen after 1-2 days of application of thimerosol, reddened and swollen allergic dermatitis around the eye develops. It hurts more than it itches.

Mercuric ion precipitates protein and inhibits sulphydryl enzymes. Mercurial antiseptics inhibit these enzymes or tissue cells as well as those of bacteria so they are very toxic if ingested.

Mercury bichloride 1 : 100 can be used as a disinfectant for instruments or unabraded skin.

Ammoniated mercury ointment 5% is a skin antiseptic in impetigo. Organic mercury compounds are less toxic than the inorganic salts. Nitromersol, thiomersal and phenylmercuric acetate (or nitrate) are available in liquid as well as solid forms. These are bacteriostatic antiseptics. They can also be used as preservative antiseptics in biologic products to inhibit accidental contamination. Mercurochrome 2% solution is a weak antiseptic. It stains tissues a brilliant red colour.

Other metal salts e.g. zinc sulphate, and copper sulphate are rarely employed in medicine for this purpose.

Copper

Copper ion has antimicrobial effect and it can be forced into cell membranes by iontophoresis. Copper sulphate iontophoresis is effective against herpes simplex keratitis (both epithelial and stromal). Systemic adverse effects have not been reported following ocular use of copper, although patients complain of burning sensation in the eye soon after iontophoresis, lasting for about 4 hours. The eye appears somewhat worse for a day after iontophoresis due to conjunctival hyperemia, loss of epithelium surrounding the ulcer, stromal oedema and anterior chamber flare.

Antiviral drug therapy is far superior and therefore copper sulphate iontophoresis is not popular now. Copper sulphate is not given systemically as copper is selectively deposited in liver and CNS, producing harmful effects.

Silver

Silver ions kill microorganisms but it is not selective because this effect is due to protein denaturation. Silver ions indiscrimately damage bacteria as well as conjunctiva and corneal epithelium.

Silver nitrate is an effective prophylactic against *gonococci* in eye, if used immediately after birth because it is very suitable to destroy surface organisms. However, the antibacterial effect lasts for short time and if instilled frequently it is very toxic. Sulphonamides and various antibiotics used systemically or topically applied are more effective than silver nitrate in gonorrheal prophylaxis. These are not only more effective but also much less irritating and also protect against eye infections from pyogenic organisms that are prevalent after the use of silver nitrate. Tissue chlorides precipitate insoluble silver chloride which prevents deep tissue penetration. This is the reason why deeper infections and established gonococcal infections are not cured by the silver preparation.

A 1% solution of silver nitrate is very irritating but not very destructive. A 2% solution should be followed by prompt irrigation with saline solution to avoid irritation. There should be no confusion of 10% silver protein solution (Argyrol) with 10% silver nitrate solution (child may become blind with 10% silver nitrate solution).

Silver nitrate applicator sticks for tissue cauterization has been used. One should be very careful in using this device. Its use within the eyelids does not seem prudent, because of dense scarring and extensive neovascularization may result from its application to the cornea.

Silverdiazine 1% cream slowly releases sulphadiazine and also silver and effectively suppresses bacterial flora. Collodial preparations have significant bacteriostatic activity and are less injurious to superficial tissues.

Prolonged use of any silver preparation can cause argyria.

Antiviral effects

A number of chemicals including silver nitrate, mercuric chloride, benzoquinone and iodine inactivate herpes virus in vitro but none of them is effective when applied topically to the infected cornea. The reason for this is that virus lies inside the epithelial cells and the effective concentration of these chemicals is very damaging to the cornea.

Antibacterial effects

Silver nitrate is very toxic to bacteria e.g. 1 mcg of its solution is able to kill 98.3% of *pseudomonas* in 5 minutes and 99.9% in 10 minutes. The chloride ions in the tissues reduce antibacterial activity due to the precipitaion of insoluble silver chloride.

There is a favourable therapeutic index for the topical use of silver as an antibacterial agent. A 0.5% silver nitrate solution applied as a soft compress is advised.

Argyrosis

It is bluish grey discolouration due to deposits of silver in tissues. Tissue chlorides are in intercellular spaces so silver staining is deposited outside the cells. This staining can be removed by subcutaneous or subconjunctival injection of a freshly prepared solution of 12% sodium thiosulphate and 0.5% potassium ferricyanide. The solution must be used within 30 minutes after preparing it. Deeper silver deposits are not removed in this way.

PHENOLS AND RELATED COMPOUNDS

Phenol was the first antiseptic employed during surgical procedures by Lister in 1867. Phenol denatures protein. The minimum effective concentration required for its antimicrobial action is 1-2% whereas 5% is strongly irritating to the tissues. It is mainly used as a disinfectant for inanimate objects and excreta.

Substituted phenols such as cresol and other alkyl substituted phenols e.g. lysol are commonly used. Some other phenol derivatives such as resorcinol, thymol and hexylresorcinol have also been used.

The chlorinated phenols are more active antimicrobial agents e.g. hexachlorophene which is insoluble in water but soluble in organic solvents, dilute alkalies and soaps. It is an effective bacteriostatic agent. Hexachlorophene liquid soap is commonly used in surgical scrub routines.

Soaps or detergents containing 3 % hexachlorophene may be used to prevent colonization of staphylcocci on newborn skin in the hospital. However, bathing the newborn and particularly premature infants with such preparations can be harmful (toxic effects to the nervous system) as hexachlorophene can be absorbed in sufficient quantity. Hence repeated bathing with such preparations should be discouraged.

Chlorhexidine is used as a skin cleanser, as a constituent of antiseptic soap and as a mouth wash. A 4% solution of chlorhexidine gluconate can be used to cleanse wounds, and as an antiseptic for surgical scrub and preparation of skin for operative procedures. Chlorhexidine is less effective against *pseudomonas* than gram-positive microbes. All antiseptic soaps may produce allergic reactions or photosensitization.

SURFACE-ACTIVE GERMICIDES

These are chemicals which alter the relationship of interfaces. These mey be anions e.g. sulfonate, cationic, e.g. quaternary ammonium compounds or nonionic e.g. alcoholic esters.

Surface-active agents are used as wetting agents, detergents and emulsifying substances. They also possess bactericidal activity which is in particular valuable in ophthalmic practice. The surface-active substances distrupt cell membrane which allows loss of vital intracellular constituents and thus antibacterial action. Its mode of action may also be due to direct toxic effect on enzymes and other bacterial protiens.

Soaps are anionic agents, usually sodium or potassium salts of various fatty acids. Most fatty acids are weak acids and NaOH and KOH are strong bases. Therefore most soaps when dissolved in water are alkaline (pH 8-10). The pH of skin is 5.5-6.5 and thus soaps irritate skin but are well tolerated. Excessive use of soaps dry normal skin.

Soaps remove dirt, surface secretions, desquamated epithelium and microorganisms contained in them. Certain disinfectant chemicals such as hexachlorophene. when added to certain soap provide additional antimicrobial property.

One of the surface-active agents which has been extensively studied for its antimicrobial activity is cetylpyridinium chloride aqueous solution. It has been found that many common microorganisms are killed by concentrations much more dilute than those used as germicidal. The germicidal activity of cetyl-pyridinium chloride aqueous solution has been reported against cocci. *E. coli, Proteus vulgaris, Shigella, Brucella, Candida albicans, Cryptococcus neoformans, Microsporum mycobacterium phlei, Cornyebacterium diptheriae, Klebseilla pneumoniae,* etc. However, *Pseudomonas* strains may be resistant.

Spores are resistant. Psittacosis virus is extremely resistant.

Quaternary ammonium compounds are useful to disinfect tissue surfaces as well as some instruments. These compounds are non- irritating, odourless, tasteless, stable, noncorrosive and neutral. But these compounds are inactivated by soap, protein, fats and other organic matter.

Benzalkonium

Benzalkonium chloride is a commonly used and popular cationic detergent. It is employed to preserve eye drops, for cleaning of skin and mucous membranes, and for sterilization of instruments.

As a preservative of eye drops a 1 : 5000 solution is well tolerated by the eye. Solution 1 : 7500 may irritate the eye and higher concentrations are not suited. Few cases have been reported when 12.8% concentrated solution for tonometer sterilization was accidently used in the eye which produced complete desquamation of the corneal epithelium.

The concentrations of preservative antiseptics in formulation for use in eye are such that they are bacteriostatic and not bactericidal and hence contaminations should be avoided during use. Benzalkonium chloride sterilizes in vitro cultures after only a few minutes but in vivo it takes much longer time for sterilization.

Benzalkonium is not compatible with some anions such as nitrate, salicylate, sulphonamides and fluorescein. Pilocarpine nitrate and physostigmine can not be preserved in benzalkonium but the hydrochloride salts of pilocarpine and physostigmine are compatible with benzalkonium.

Benzalkonium acting as a wetting agent enhances the transcorneal penetration of drugs, e.g. carbachol is unreliable pupillary constrictor in aqueous solution as it penetrates poorly into the cornea. Benzalkonium will enhance penetration.

Instrument disinfection

Benzalkonium can be used to sterilize equipment that would be damaged by heat. Such instruments can be immersed in 1: 750 aqueous solution of benzalkonium chloride for 30 minutes. Soap, blood clots, etc. should be removed from the instruments before immersion as these are inactivators of cationic detergents. Care should also be taken not to keep cotton gauze in sterilizing tray otherwise the germicidal effect of benzalkonium will be destroyed through its absorption on the cotton fibres. Soaking of cotton balls in benzalkonium chloride is of no use because the germicidal effect is quickly inactivated. Benzalkonium does not kill spores, fungi and viruses. So it is not a dependable chemical under these circumstances.

The solvent action of benzalkonium can damage optical instruments.

Skin preparation

Normal skin tolerates a 1 : 750 solution without irritation when benzalkonium is used for cleaning skin and mucous membranes.

As anionic detergents such as soap inactivate benzalkonium, it should be removed with water and alcohol prior to using benzalkonium.

Some reports have appeared which describe the failure of benzalkonium to sterilize as well as its being the source of infection. Inadequate disinfection bronchoscope with 1: 750 benzalkonium chloride was followed by *pseudomonas* infection in several cases because of infected benzalkonium solution.

Adverse effect

Benzalkonium chloride in 0.001% concentration is a safe dose for intraocular use. It is useless as a preservative in this concentration. Although 0.01% solution is nontoxic, a safety factor of 10× is believed to be the safe dose.

Thiomersal

Thiomersal-preserved solutions are surpassed by benzalkonium, chlorhexidine and chlorobutanol as a germicide. Thiomersal kills *S. aureus* in 24 hours and takes about 4 hours to kill *Pseudomonas* and benzalkonium takes only 15 minutes for similar effect. Thiomersal allergy has also been reported. The eye becomes red and irritated with epithelial changes ranging from mild irregularities to punctate keratopathy. Photophobia, lacrimation and reduced vision are a part of the syndrome which is not self limited rather it worsens. Bilaterity is the rule.

Chlorobutanol

A 0.5% solution of chlorobutanol is an effective and nonirritating preservative. Allergy to this chemical has not been reported so far.

Chlorobutanol is stable and can be autoclaved at pH 6 or even less, but alkaline solutions are hydrolysed by heat. Sodium fluorescein destroys the preservative.

Chlorobutanol is a good preservative for eye drops as 0.5% solution. It is bacteriostatic but if exposure is for about 24 hours it is usually bactericidal. In this concentration (0.5%) chlorobutanol inhibits gram-positive, gram-negative bacteria and many species of fungi. It has been instilled several times daily for years without producing ill effects.

Adverse effects

Chlorobutanol is safe as eye drops, but may not be tolerated as a continuous bath. A 0.4% chlorobutanol in isotonic saline solution produces diffuse epithelial damage of the cornea on bathing the eyes for 20 minutes. Chlorobutanol inhibits oxygen utilization by the cornea and loosens epithelial adhesion.

Chlorhexidine

As an ophthalmic preservative, chlorhexidine is similar to chlorobutanol and benzalkonium regarding efficacy and toxicity.

Table 11.24 shows activities of certain antiseptics.

NITROFURANS

Nitrofurazone is topical antiseptic, used on superficial wounds, or skin lesions and as a surgical dressing. The preparations contain 0.2% of the active drug.

Nitrofurantoin is a urinary antiseptic.

STERILIZING AGENTS

Cresol

It contains the following constituents:

Liquor cresol compound	8 ml
Oil of lavender	2 ml
Thymol crystals	2 g
Ethyl alcohol	88 ml

Table 11.24. Activities of certain antiseptics

	Activity						
	Bacteria			Viruses		Fungi	Use
	Gm+	Gm–	Spores	Lipophilic	Hydrophilic		
Alcohols							
Ethanol	HS	HS	R	S	V	–	Antiseptic
Isopropanol							
Aldehydes							
Formaldehyde	S	HS	S	S	MS	S	Disinfectant
Glutaraldehyde							
Chlorhexidine	HS	MS	R	V	R	–	Antiseptic
gluconate							
Chlorine sodium	HS	HS	S	S	S	MS	Disinfectant
hypochlorite							irrigant
Hexachlorophene	S	R	R	R	R	R	Soaps
							Shampoo
Iodine							
Povidone-iodine	HS	HS	S	S	R	S	Antiseptic
Phenols	HS	HS	R	R	R	–	Disinfectant
Oxidizing agents	HS	HS	S	V	V	S	Disinfectant
Hydrogen peroxide							irrigant
Quaternary							
Ammonium	HS	HS	R	S	R	–	Disinfectant
(benzalkonium							
chloride, cetyl-							
pyridinum							
chloride)							

Key: HS = highly susceptible, MS = moderately susceptible, S = susceptible, R = resistant, V = variable, - no data.

Cresol is not corrosive to metal instruments. If surgical instruments are immersed in this solution they are sterilized in 1-2 minutes and when solution is contaminated by 5% whole blood and when Bacillus subtilis is used gauze become sterile within 4 minutes. However, using *Bacillus subtilis* strains with high spore count and more rigid methods of evaluation, instruments are found contaminated after 30 minutes of immersion in cresol solution. It is now believed that no chemical method will sterilize instruments contaminated with spores, with the exception of ethylene oxide.

Ethylene oxide

Autoclaving dulls the sharp instruments. Ethylene oxide can be autoclaved as well as sharp instruments used in eye surgery, glass or plastic are not damaged. This gas is mixed with hydrocarbon gases to eliminate the explosive character of ethylene oxide.

Ethylene oxide gas is toxic.

Ultraviolet light

Ultraviolet light has germicidal properties. It is widely used for sterilization. The maximum germicidal activity is achieved at a wavelength of about 2537 Å against viruses, fungi and bacteria. The germicidal effect is due to nucleoprotein destruction. Actinic keratitis occurs at wavelength of 2,880 Å. At 2,537 Å the germicidal effect is 85% of maximum, whereas the keratitic effect is 20% of maximum, the discomfort of radiation keratitis can be reduced by the use of cycloplegics.

STUDY QUESTIONS

1. Define antiseptics and disinfectants. Classify them on chemical basis, giving suitable examples.
2. What are the properties of an ideal germicides? How do these agents differ from systemically employed antibacterial agents? Why antiseptics are not used systemically in humans?
3. Explain why (i) 70% ethanol is more effective as antiseptic than higher concentrations; (ii) povidone-iodine is better than iodine (iii) substituted phenols are better than phenol.
4. What are the uses of chlorine and oxidizing agents?
5. Describe the preparations and applications of metallic germicides.
6. Describe surface-active germicides.
7. Write notes on (i) benzalkonium (ii) chlorhexidine (iii) cresol and (iv) ultraviolet light as antiseptics.
8. Which factors determine the antibacterial action of germicides?
9. Write notes on (i) instrument disinfection and (ii) preoperative preparation of skin.

GUIDE TO FURTHER READING

Block, S.S: Disinfection, Sterilization and Preservation, 4th ed., Lea & Febiger 1991.

Brecx, M et al: Efficacy of Listerine, Meridol and chlorhexidine mouth rinses on plaque, gingivitis and plaque bacteria vitality. J.Clin. Periodontol, 1990; 17:292.

Burman, L.G et al: Prevention of excess neonatal morbidity associated with group B streptococci by vaginal chlorhexidine disinfection during labor. Lancet, 1992; 340:65.

Craven, D.E et al: Pseudobacteremia caused by povidone-iodine solution contaminated with pseudomonas cepacia. N Engl. J. Med., 1981; 305:621.

Dineen, P et al: Hand washing and degerming: a comparison of povidone-iodine and chlorhexidine. Clin. Pharmacol. Ther., 1978; 23:63.

Doebbeling, B.N et al: Comparative efficacy of alternative hand-washing agents in reducing infections in intensive care units. N. Engl. J. Med., 1992; 327:88.

Ducksbury, C.F.J et al: Contact dermatitis in home helps following use of detergents. Br. Med. J., 1970; 1:537.

Editorial. shingles: a belt of roses from Hell. Br. Med. J., 1979; 1:5.

Editorial. Out damned spot (disinfection). Lancet, 1978; 2:1349.

Editorial. Hexachlorophane—yes or no? Br. Med. J., 1977; 1-337 and subsequent correspondence.

Fraser, G.L et al: Leukopenia secondary to sulfadiazine silver. JAMA, 1979; 241:1928.

Gezon, H.M et al: Control of staphylococcal infections in the newborn through the use of hexachlorophene bathing. Pediatrics, 1973; 51:331.

Goutieres, F et al: Accidental percutaneous hexachlorophane intoxication in children. Br. Med. J., 1977; 2:663.

Hunter, J.A.A et al: Present and future trends in approaches to skin diseases. Br. Med. J., 1974; 1:283.

Kaul, F et al: Agents and techniques for disinfection of the skin. Surg Gynecol Obstet, 1981; 152:677.

Khan, J.S et al: A case of Dettol addiction. Br. Med. J., 1979; 1:791.

Koivisto, V.A et al: Is skin preparation necessary before insulin injection? Lancet, 1978; 1:1072.

Larson, E et al: Guidelines for use of topical antimicrobial agents. Am.J.Infect.Dis.Control, 1988; 16:233.

Lowbury, E.J.L et al: Preoperative disinfection of surgeons' hands: use of alcoholic solutions and effects of gloves on skin flora. Br. Med.J., 1974; 4:369.

Martin-Bouyer, G et al: Outbreak of accidental hexachlorophene poisoning in France. Lancet, 1982; 1:91.

Viljanto, J et al: Disinfection of surgical wounds without inhibition of normal wound healing. Arch Surg, 1980; 115:253.

Vitamins

On the basis of the belief that certain amines in diet were essential for life, this term "Vitamin" was introduced. Now it is known that they are not amines. These are chemical compounds that the human body needs in small amounts. Vitamins are organic substances required by the body for various metabolic processes.

Vitamin deficiency may result from inadequate absorption, increased excretion and increased requirements such as during pregnancy. Vitamin deficiency may also be induced by diseases or drugs.

Vitamins may be used clinically for the prevention and treatment of specific vitamin deficiency states. However, excessive intake of fat-soluble vitamins accumulate in the body and are therefore likely to cause serious toxicity. Excessive intake of most water soluble vitamins may be less toxic as they are rapidly excreted in the urine but several unwanted side effects have been reported.

The vitamins can be grouped in two categories :
1. Fat soluble vitamins: A, D, E, and K. These can be stored to massive degrees and therefore their toxicity potential exceeds that of the water-soluble vitamins.
2. Water soluble vitamins: B_1, B_2, B_3, B_6, B_{12}, folic acid and C. These are stored to only a limited extent, and frequent consumption is necessary.

VITAMIN A (ANTIXEROPHTHALMIC VITAMIN)

Although the term vitamin has been used to denote specific compounds, such as retinol or its esters, this term is now used more as a generic descriptor for compounds that show the biological properties of retinol.

The term retinoid refers to the chemical entity retinol or other closely related naturally occurring derivatives as well as related synthetic analogues which need not possess retinol-like (vitamin A) activity.

Vitamin A (also called retinol) is a fat-soluble vitamin that plays an important role in the maintenance of structure and function of the cornea and retina. It acts as oxidation reduction catalyst essential for epithelial cells. It is a component of rhodopsin.

Retinol (vitamin A_1) a primary alcohol is present in esterified form in the tissues of animals and saltwater fish, mainly in the liver.

The main sources of vitamin A are carotenoids

found in milk, fish liver oils, butter and green and yellow vegetables. Beta-carotenoid is the most active carotenoid that is rapidly absorbed from small intestine and stored in the liver. It can also be stored in the retinal pigment epithelium. Beta-carotenes are provitamins found in green vegetables and carrots, tomatoes, bananas and sweet potatoes.

Retinal is formed from retinol (vitamin A_1) by reversible oxidation. Vitamin A_2 is dehydroretinol present in butter, cheese, egg, milk, liver and fish liver oils.

Vitamin A and carotene are stable to mild cooking, unstable at high temperatures and in the presence of oxygen. Frying causes a considerable loss of vitamin A from ghee. Vitamin A should be stored in air tight containers.

Units and requirements

One international unit of vitamin A possesses the activity of 0.000344 mg of pure all-trans vitamin A acetate. It has the specific biological activity of 0.3 mcg of retinol and 0.6 mcg of β-carotene.

A daily dietary intake of about 750 mcg is recommended for healthy adults. Dietary vitamin A is derived from two sources, preformed retinol from liver, kidney, eggs and dairy products. Fish liver oil is the most concentrated natural source. Besides the animal source, the other source is from many plants, the provitamin carotenoids are converted to retinol in the body by an oxygenase present in the intestine and elsewhere. Some carotenoids like lutein cannot be converted to vitamin A but still possess antioxidant properties which make them important nutrients. They are less effectively utilized. Alpha, beta and gamma carotenes are major sources, and of these beta carotene has the maximum vitamin A activity and is the most plentiful in food. Beta-carotenes are found in carrots and dark green or yellow vegetables. Red palm oil is a good source of alpha and beta carotenes.

During pregnancy and lactation the daily requirement is 1000 retinol equivalents (RE). 1 RE represents 1 mcg of retinol.

Vitamin A is readily absorbed from the small intestine. Vitamin A esters are hydrolysed by pancreatic enzymes to retinol which is then absorbed. After absorption retinol is transported by chylo-micron to the liver. Some retinol is stored in the liver and the released retinol from the liver is bound to a specific alpha-1 globulin (retinol binding protein) in the blood. It can also be stored in retinal pigment epithelium. The retinol not stored in the liver undergoes glucuronide conjugation and subsequent oxidation to retinal and retinoic acid, these and other metabolites are excreted in urine and faeces.

Vitamin A does not readily diffuse across the placenta but is present in breast milk.

Visual Cycle

Stimulation of photoreceptors

Excitation of rods

The photo pigment in rods is called rhodopsin (visual purple) which is sensitive to low levels of illumination. Rhodopsin is composed of scotopsin (a protein) and retinal occurs as cis-retinal. In the presence of light, cis-retinal undergoes an immediate change in structure from a curved molecule to a straight molecule called all-trans-retinal (prelumirhodopsin) that rapidly decomposes sequentially to lumir-hodopsin, metarhodopsin I, metarhodopsin II, and parahodopsin. All these substances are loose combinations of scotopsin and all-trans-retinal. Ultimately, parahodopsin decomposes completely into scotopsin and all-trans-retinal. At the point where metarhodopsin I is converted to metarhodopsin II, the receptor potential develops in rods.

Following decomposition of rhodopsin into scotopsin and all- trans-retinal in the presence of light, rhodopsin is once again re-formed. In this process, which occurs in the absence of light, the all-trans-retinal is converted back to cis-retinal in the presence of an enzyme. Then cis-retinal combines with scotopsin to re-form rhodopsin. This compound is stable until its decomposition is again triggered by light energy.

Rhodopsin is highly light sensitive—even the light rays from the moon or a candle will break down some of it and thereby allow us to see. The rods, then, are specialized for night vision. However, they are of only limited help for daylight vision. In bright light, the rhodopsin is broken down faster than it can be manufactured. In dim light, production is able to keep pace with a slower rate of breakdown. These characteristics of rhodopsin are responsible for the experience of having to adjust to dark room after walking in from the sunshine. The normal period of adjustment is the time it takes for the completely dissociated rhodopsin to re-form. Nightblindness (nyctalopia) is the lack of normal night vision following the adjustment period. It is most often caused by vitamin A deficiency.

Excitation of cones

Cones are the receptors for bright light, colour, and visual acuity (sharpness). As in rods, photopigment decomposition produces receptor potentials as a result of hyperpolarization. The photopigments in cones are almost the same as those in rods. Both contain retinal, but the protein portions in cones are called photopsins, which are slightly different from the scotopsin in rods. Unlike rhodopsin the photopigments of the cones require bright light for their breakdown and they re-form quickly.

There are 3 types of cones, each containing a different combination of retinal and photopsin. Each of them has a different maximum absorption of light of different wavelenghts and thus each responds best to light of a given colour. One type of cone responds best to red light, the second to green light, and the third to blue light. Just as an artist can obtain almost any colour by mixing colours, cones can perceive any colour by differential stimulation.

If a single groups of colour receptive cones is missing from the retina, an individual can not distinguish some colours from others and is said to be colour blind.

Fig. 12.1 shows rhodopsin cycle.

Vitamin A and immunity

It has been known for many years that vitamin A deficiency is associated with increased susceptibility to bacterial, parasitic and viral infections.

Vitamin A and carcinogenesis

Vitamin A deficiency enhances susceptibility to carcinogenesis. The exact mechanism of the anticarcinogenic effects is unclear.

Symptoms of deficiency

Vitamin A deficiency has profound effect on the immune system. Beta-carotene may possess immune

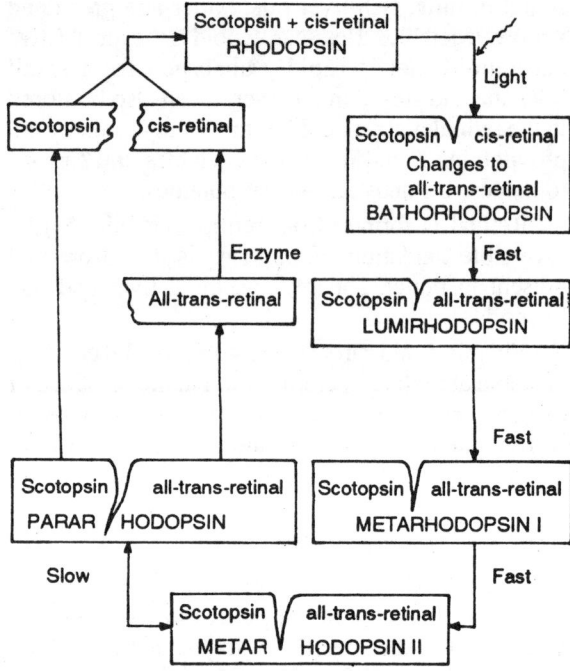

Fig. 12.1. Rhodopsin cycle.

enhancing effects in some vulnerable group of people, but its importance is not yet clear.

Nyctalopia (night blindness) is an early symptom of deficiency. Later on permanent structural changes occur in retina and retinal pigment epithelium. Yellow-white opacities in the cornea appear. About 68% of children who have vitamin A deficiency have abnormal corneal epithelial cell shape leading to xerophthalmia or dry eye, characterized by night blindness which may develop to severe eye lesions and blindness.

Bitot's spots are external signs of vitamin A deficiency, however, severe deficiency may exist without Bitot's spots. Chronic vitamin A deficiency may produce retinal damage.

Vitamin A deficient children tend to grow more slowly and become more anaemic and also have greater tendency towards infection.

Deficiency states may develop at plasma levels of 0.16 IU/ml due to inadequate intake in diet.

Clinical uses

The rational uses of retinol are in the treatment of

vitamin A deficiency and as prophylaxis in the high-risk subjects during periods of increased requirements, such as infancy, pregnancy and lactation.

During pregnancy and lactation it is recommended to increase the maternal intake of vitamin A by 25%.

It is given by mouth in an oil or water based form, or by i.m. injection in a water-miscible form.

There is a possibility that vitamin A and other retinoids may find important place in cancer chemoprevention and therapy. Recent clinical trials have produced encouraging results as chemoprophylactic of head and neck, skin, colon and cervical cancers and also modify the condition of established head and neck and lung cancers.

Vitamin A may be helpful in certain diseases of the skin such as acne and psoriasis.

In the treatment of xerophthalmia, vitamin A palmitate 110 mg or vitamin A acetate 66 mg (2,00,000 units) is given orally, repeated next day and later on 1-2 weekly additional doses.

Vitamin A ointment is used for the treatment of keratoconjuctivitis sicca. Topical vitamin A ointment also increases healing of cataract incisions.

Adverse effects and precautions

Hypervitaminosis A will result if excessive doses are given over long periods. The signs and symptoms of vitamin A toxicity are not very specific. It is characterised by irritability, fatigue, loss of weight, anorexla, low-grade fever, skin changes, hepatosplenomegaly, dry hair, alopecia, gastrointestinal disturbances, cracking and bleeding lips, hypercalcaemia, pain in bones and joints and subcutaneous swelling.

Excessive doses of vitamin A often affects children and rarely adults. It has been reported that large single doses e.g. 3,50,000 units for an infant causes an acute rise in cerebrospinal fluid pressure. The toxic manifestations include xerophthalmos, alopecia, rashes, exfoliative dermatitis and increased intracranial pressure with papilledema. Hepatomegaly, splenomegaly, hypoprothrombinemia and wide spread arthritic pains may also occur.

Topical retinoic acid employed for skin disorders may cause night blindness as a result of inhibition of ocular retinolol dehydrogenases leading to decrease in the formation of visual II cis-retinol.

Preparations

Halibut liver oil capsules 1-3 capsules/day
Vitamin A solution containing 50,000 units/g
Dose: 30,000-50,000 IU/day.

VITAMIN B-COMPLEX

Vitamin B$_1$ (Thiamine)

Vitamin B$_1$ is water soluble.

The main sources of vitamin B$_1$ are yeast, meat, cereals, nuts peas, potatoes, beans and most vegetables.

The daily intake of 1-1.3 mg is recommended for human requirements.

Vitamin B$_1$ is well absorbed from the gastro-intestinal tract and widely distributed in the body. It also appears in breast milk. Thiamine is not stored in the body to any appreciable amount.

Thiamine deficiency causes decreased central vision due to scotomas and are characteristic of thiamine amblyopia.

Vitamin B$_1$ deficiency may cause bilateral and often irreversible optic atrophy. The role of this vitamin in causing tobacco-alcohol amblyopia and nutritional amblyopia is not clear. But it has been reported that patients who suffer from nutritional amblyopia have reduced amount of transketolase which is thiamine dependent. Vitamin B$_1$ deficiency is also associated with Wernicke's encephalopathy which includes ophthalmoplegia and nystagmus. Vitamin B$_1$ deficiency is also associated with chronic alcoholism malnutrition.

Thiamine is an essential coenzyme for carbohydrate metabolism. Its deficiency leads to beri-beri. Chronic dry beri-beri is characterised by peripheral neuritis, muscle weakness, bradycardia and paralysis. Acute "wet" beri-beri is characterised by cardiac failure and oedema.

The only established therapeutic use of thiamine is for the treatment or prophylaxis of thiamine deficiency. Oral route is preferred but it can also be given by injection.

In mild deficiency, the dose is 5-30 mg daily and in severe conditions, doses as high as 300 mg have been administered.

The adverse effects of vitamin B_1 seldom occur. However, allergic reactions have been reported, particularly after parenteral administration which may be mild to very rarely, fatal anaphylactic shock.

Preparations

Thiamine hydrochloride 3 mg tablet for prophylaxis, 25-100 mg daily for treatment are given. It is also available for i.m./i.v. injection. Vitamin B complex (forte) contains thiamine HCl 5 mg, riboflavin 2 mg, nicotinamide 20 mg and pyridoxine HCl 2 mg.

Vitamin B_2 (Riboflavin)

Vitamin B_2 is very slightly soluble in water. It is stable to oxygen and acid conditions but not to light and alkali. Heat alone is not harmful.

The main sources are milk, meat, green leafy vegetables, egg white, fish, fruits, yeast, potatoes, cheese, liver and kidney.

A daily dietary intake of about 1 to 2 mg of riboflavin is recommended.

Vitamin B_2 is readily absorbed from the gastrointestinal tract, widely distributed in the body but little stored. It crosses the placenta.

Riboflavin is converted in the body to the coenzyme flavin mononucleotide (FMN) and then to another coenzyme flavine adenine dinucleotide (FAD). Riboflavin is excreted in urine as metabolites.

Riboflavin acts as an active prosthetic group of flavoproteins required for tissue oxidation in the control of cellular energy processes.

Deficiency of riboflavin interferes with cellular energy processes resulting in angular stomatitis, scrotal dermatitis, glossitis, photophobia, corneal opacities, burning feet syndrome, ulcer on buccal mucosa, tongue and lips, dry scaly skin and loss of hair.

Riboflavin is used for the prevention and treatment of the deficiency of riboflavin. Vitamin B_2 tablets 5 mg thrice a day are recommended.

No adverse effects have been reported with riboflavin. However, large doses produce bright yellow colour of the urine which may interfere with certain laboratory tests.

Vitamin B_3 (Nicotinic Acid)

The term niacin is a generic term used for nicotinic acid. It is a water soluble vitamin. it is stable and only some loss occurs from leaching with processing water.

The sources of vitamin B_3 are cereals, meat, potatoes and other vegetables, milk and fish. it is widely distributed in food stuffs.

Nicotinamide adenine dinucleotide (NAD) is used by most oxidative reactions in energy yielding metabolism, but NADP in a reduced form i.e. NADPH is utilized as the hydrogen donor for reductive reactions. such as the hexose monophosphate.

The deficiency of niacin causes pellagra characterized by diarrhoea, dermatitis, dementia, neurtitis and stomatitis. The deficiency also causes chilbains, peripheral vascular diseases and Meniere's syndrome.

Nicotinic acid is used for the prevention and treatment of deficiency of nicotinic acid. The dose recommended for prophylaxis is 15-20 mg daily and for the treatment 100 to 200 mg daily. Ampoules, for i.m./i.v. use, contain mixture of vitamins including nicotinamide.

Adverse effects of large doses are flushing (more with nicotinic acid), itching of skin, nausea, vomiting, dermatological lesions, tachycardia, hypotension, hyperglycaemia, exacerbation of peptic ulcer, jaundice and increased levels of liver enzyme transaminases.

Vitamin B_6 (Pyridoxine)

Pyridoxine is soluble in 1 in 5 of water. It should be kept in air tight containers and protected from light.

Vitamin B_6 is essential for metabolism of amino acids. It maintains healthy teeth, gums, vasculature, nervous system and haemopoietic system (haemoglobin formation). It is also involved in the carbohydrate and fat metabolism.

Pyridoxine is only one of the 3 similar compounds that may be referred to as vitamin B_6, the other two are pyridoxal and pyridoxamine.

The rich sources of vitamin B_6 are yeast, egg, liver, meat, fish, cereals and certain vegetables and fruits.

Human requirements are about 2 mg daily for adult males and 1.6 mg per day for adult females. This amount is present in most normal diets. The requirement for pyridoxine increases with the amount of protein in the diet. The minimum requirement is about 1.5 mg per day in individuals ingesting 100g of protein per day.

Pyridoxine, pyridoxal, and pyridoxamine are readily absorbed from the gastrointenstinal tract following oral intake and are converted to the active forms pyridoxal phosphate and pyridoxamine phosphate.

They are stored in the liver where these are oxidized to 4-pyridoxic acid which is excreted in the urine. Pyridoxol crosses the placenta and also appears in breast milk.

Pyridoxine deficiency is rare, however, it can be caused during isoniazid therapy.

Pyridoxine deficiency leads to the development of peripheral neuritis associated with carpal synovial swelling and tenderness. Pyridoxine deficiency also results in vascular congestion, hyperkeratosis and hair loss of eyelids. Corneal neovascularization may occur.

Pyridoxine is used in the treatment and prevention of pyridoxine deficiency states. It is usually given by mouth but can also be given parenterally; for pyridoxine deficiency anaemia 50-100mg daily and for pyridoxine -deficiency convulsions in infants, 4 mg/kg body weight is given for short periods.

Long-term administration of large doses (2-6 g per day) may cause severe peripheral sensory neuropathies, impairment of balance, weakness, damage to sensory and motor neurons.

An important drug interaction is that pyridoxine reduces the effects of levodopa.

Panthothenic acid

Its name, derived from Greek word signifying "from every where", is indicative of the distribution of the vitamin in nature particularly abundant in organ meats, beef and egg yolk. It is easily destroyed by heat and alkali. It has no outstanding pharmacological actions in normal persons, even in larger doses.

Its deficiency is manifested by symptoms of neuromuscular degeneration and adrenocortical deficiency. However, its deficiency has not been recognised in human beings consuming a normal diet. The daily requirement is 4-7 mg in adults.

There are no clearly defined uses for panthothenic acid, although it is commonly included in multivitamin preparations and in products for enteral and parenteral alimentation (nourishment).

Biotin

The food sources are organ meats, milk, egg yolk, fish and nuts. It is stable to cooking, but less so in alkali.

The daily requirement for adults is 100-200 mcg. Part of the biotin synthesised by the bacterial flora is available for absorption.

Biotin 5-10 mg may be given to babies with infantile seborrhea and to individuals with genetic alterations of biotin-dependent enzymes.

Vitamin B_{12} (Cyanocobalamin)

Vitamin B_{12} is the name generally used for a group of related cobalt-containing compounds, also known as cobalamines of which cyanocobalamin and hydroxocobalamin are mainly used clinically.

Vitamin B_{12} :

- Needs an 'intrinsic factor' (a glycoprotein) secreted by gastric parietal cells for absorption and forms a one-to-one complex with vitamin B_{12}.
- Vitamin B_{12} is absorbed by active transport, intrinsic factor being removed on the way.
- B_{12} is carried in the plasma by B_{12} binding proteins called transcobalamins.
- It is stored mainly in liver.
- Total amount in the body is about 4 mg.
- It is required for synthesis of purines and pyrimidines.
- It is used:
  - to treat pernicious anaemia and other causes of Vitamin B_{12} deficiency.
  - when used therapeutically, it is almost always given by I.M. injection, since its deficiency is virtually always due to malabsorption of the vitamin.

Vitamin B_{12} is soluble in water. It should be kept in air tight containers and protected from light.

Vitamin B_{12} occurs only in animal products. Meats, especially liver and kidney, eggs, milk and other dairy products and fish are good sources of vitamin B_{12}. It is not synthesized by animals or plants.

The chief dietary source of vitamin B_{12} is microbially derived.

Vitamin B_{12} is made up of a porphyrin-like ring with a central cobalt atom attached to a nucleotide.

For adults, daily 2 to 3 mcg is required and this amount is present in normal diets. The liver stores as much as 3000-5000 mcg, which is enough for 3-4 years. Hydroxocobalamin is better retained than cyanocobalamin; 90% of a 100 mcg dose is retained which is enough for 2-10 months.

Vitamin B_{12} in physiological amounts is absorbed only after it complexes with intrinsic factor. Intrinsic factor is a glycoporotein that is secreted by the parietal cells of gastric mucosa. The vitamin B_{12} intrinsic factor complex binds ileal mucosal cell receptors, from where it is transported into circulation. Once in the circulation, vitamin B_{12} is transported to the tissues by plasma beta-globulin transcobalamin II. It is preferentially stored in liver, excreted in the bile and undergoes enterohepatic recycling, part of a dose is excreted in the urine. Vitamin B_{12} diffuses across placenta and also appears in breast milk.

Vitamin B_{12} is essential for cell growth and for maintenance of normal myelin in the nervous system.

Vitamin B_{12} is necessary for the synthesis of thymidylate, which is the characteristic base of DNA. It is also important for the normal metabolic functions of folate.

Vitamin B_{12} is required for two essential enzymatic reactions in humans, (a) in one reaction deoxyadenosylcobalamine is a required cofactor in the conversion of methylmalanyl-CoA to succinyl-CoA by the enzyme methylmalanyl-CoA mutase. This conversion can not occur if vitamin B_{12} is deficient; (b) the other enzymatic reaction that requires vitamin B_{12} is conversion of 5-methyl tetrafolate and homocysteine methyl transferase.

The most common causes of vitamin B_{12} deficiency are pernicious anaemia (Addisonian anaemia), inflammatory bowel disease and diseases that affect the distal ileum, such as malabsorption syndrome.

The malabsorption of vitamin B_{12} is either due to lack of intrinsic factor or to loss or malfunction of the specific absorptive mechanism in the distal ileum. The dose for the treatment of pernicious anaemia is 500-1000 mcg thrice a week. The adverse effects of vitamin B_{12} are not serious.

Vitamin B_{12} preparations are used in the treatment and prevention of vitamin B_{12} deficiency. In the absence of neurological involvement it may be given in doses of 250-1000 mcg intramuscularly (never intravenously) on alternate days for 1-2 weeks, then 250 mcg weekly until the blood count returns to normal. Oral combination of vitamin B_{12} with intrinsic factor usually produces unreliable absorption and hence this route is not advisable.

Nutritional deficiency of vitamin B_{12} is rare. However, it may occur in strict vegetarians. Vitamin B_{12} deficiency causes pernicious anaemia which in turn causes retrobular neuritis with typical central scotomata. Vitamin B_{12} deficiency results in inadequate myelin synthesis affecting the optic, peripheral, and cranial nerves. Similar neurological syndrome is produced due to deficiency of thiamine, nicotinic acid, and riboflavin and by tobacco, amblyopia. The common mechanism is cyanide inhibition of cytochrome oxidase. It is due to deficiency in hydroxocobalamin which detoxifies cyanide.

Folic Acid (Pteroylglutamic Acid)

Folic acid is a yellow to orange brown, odorless crystalline powder, practically insoluble in water. It dissolves in dilute solutions of alkali hydroxides. It should be stored in air tight containers and protected from light.

Folic acid is a compound composed of a pteridine heterocycle, p-aminobenzoic acid, and glutamic acid. Various forms of folic acid are present in a wide variety of plants and animal tissues. The rich sources of folic acid are yeast, liver, kidney and leafy green vegetables. The daily requirement is 50-100 mcg. Pregnant or lactating women require 100-200 mcg/day. It is easily oxidized and destroyed during cooking. Folates present in food are in the reduced polyglutamate form. The mucosa of the duodenum and upper jejunum have dihydroreductase which methylates the reduced folate. After absorption folate is transported to tissues and stored inside the cells as polyglutamate. The ultimate role of the folates is the formation of folate cofactors essential for one-carbon transfer reactions necessary for DNA synthesis. Another essential reaction, in which a folate cofactor is essential, is the synthesis of thymidylic acid, an essential precursor of DNA.

Folic acid is a member of the vitamin B group. It is reduced in the body to tetrahydrofolate which is a coenzyme for various metabolic processes including the synthesis of purine and pyrimidine nucleotides, and hence in the synthesis of DNA.

Folic acid is rapidly and completely absorbed in the proximal third of the small intestine from normal diets and is distributed in the body tissues. It is mainly stored in liver. It is also distributed in breast milk. Oral folic acid is well absorbed and so its parenteral administration is rarely required.

Although folic acid stimulates haematopoiesis and can eliminate the megaloblastic anaemia associated with pernicious anaemia, it does not prevent the neurological complications of this disease.

Folic acid deficiency unlike vitamin B_{12} deficiency, is caused by inadequate dietary intake of folates. The deficiency of folic acid causes megaloblastic anaemia(its onset is more rapid than with vitamin B_{12} deficiency and there is no neurological abnormality associated with folate deficiency). It can be treated by giving orally initially 10-20 mg daily for 14 days. The daily maintenance dose is 2.5-10 mg. Folic acid can be given orally as well as parenterally. It is generally well tolerated, however, oral route is preferred.

Allergic reactions have been reported with parenteral administration (though rarely).

Larger amounts of oral folic acid may counteract the antiepileptic actions of phenytoin, primidone and phenobarbital.

Certain drugs can also cause folic acid deficiency which interfere with folate absorption or metabolism. Phenytoin, isoniazid and oral contraceptives interfere with folic acid absorption. Certain drugs such as methotrexate, trimethoprim and pyrimethamine inhibit dihydrofolate reductase.

Folic acid :

- Probably does not occur in nature as such.
- can be regarded as a parent component of a group of naturally occurring folates.
- folates are essential for DNA synthesis. They are cofactors in the synthesis of purines and pyrimidines and also necessary for reactions involved in amino acid metabolism.
- For activity, folate must be in the tetrahydro form, in which it is maintained by the enzyme dihydrofolate reductase.
- Dihydrofolate reductase enzyme reduces dietary folic acid to tetrahydrofolate (FH4).
- Folate antagonists act by inhibiting dihydrofolate reductase.
- Used to:
  - treat megaloblastic anaemia.
  - prevent or treat adverse effects from methotrexate (folate antagonist).
- usually given orally, preparations for parenteral use are available.

Vitamin B_{12} and Folic acid

- are needed for DNA synthesis.
- deficiencies affect mainly erythropoiesis.
- It is important to determine whether megaloblastic anaemia is due to vitamin B_{12} or folate deficiency, because if vitamin B_{12} deficiency is treated with folic acid, blood picture may improve while neurological lesions get worse.

Folinic Acid (Citrovorum factor, Leucovorin)

Folinic acid is a 5 formyl derivative of tetrahydrofolic acid, the active form of folic acid. It is mainly used as an antidote to folic acid antagonists, such as methotrexate. Leucovorin calcium (folinic acid) injection circumvents the action of dihydrofolate reductase inhibitor, such as methorexate. It is not used as a treatment for ordinary folate deficiency.

VITAMIN C (ASCORBIC ACID)

Vitamin C is colourless or white or slightly yellow crystalline powder. It is highly soluble in water. A 5% solution in water has a pH of 2.1 to 2.6. A 10% solution has a pH of 7 to 8. The solution for injection should have a pH of 5.5 to 7.0. Solutions of ascorbic acid deteriorate rapidly in air. These should be stored in air tight non-metallic containers and protected from light.

Ascorbic acid degradation depends on a number of interrelated factors. It is oxidized in aqueous solution by reaction with dissolved oxygen. The presence of catalysts, especially copper ions are also responsible for degradation. It is very labile in food stuffs. It is easily oxidized to dehydroascorbic acid.

The main sources of ascorbic acid are citrus fruits, tomatoes, raw cabbage green, and potatoes, fish and nuts. Pulses and cerels form it on germination. Only small amounts are present in milk and animal tissues.

Human beings and other primates as well as gunieapigs and some bats are the only mammals known to be unable to synthesize ascorbic acid.

Vitamin C is essential for normal tissue metabolism, bones, teeth and wound healing. Ascorbic acid enhances proline hydroxylation and hence a cofactor for collagen synthesis. Vitamin C is essential for the synthesis of collagen and intercellular material. Due to its reducing effect it helps in utilization of iron.

A daily dietary intake of about 30-60 mg of ascorbic acid is recommended for human adults, they are unable to form their own ascorbic acid so dietary source is necessary.

Ascorbic acid is rapidly absorbed from the gastrointestinal tract and widely distributed in the body tissues, some is metabolised to ascorbate-2-sulphate, which is inactive, and oxalic acid which are excreted in urine. Ascorbic acid in excess of body's needs is also rapidly eliminated in the urine. Normal body stores about 1500 mg vitamin C. Healthy adult human subjects lose 3% to 4% of their body store daily. To maintain a body store of 1500 mg of ascorbic acid or more, it will be necessary to absorb about 60 mg daily.

Ascorbic acid crosses the placenta and is distributed in breast milk.

Deficiency of vitamin C leads to scurvy characterized by capillary fragility, bleeding especially from small blood vessels and the gums, anaemias, cartilage and bone lesions and slow healing of wounds. When vitamin C is absent, normal fibrous collagen is replaced by non fibrous precursor.

Scurvy may occur in infants receiving formula diets with inadequate concentration of ascorbic acid. The infant is irritable and resents being touched due to pain (which is due to haemorrhages under the periosteum of the long bones), and hematomas may be visible as swelling on the shafts of these bones.

Vitamin C completely reverses symptoms of deficiency. It is usually given orally. It can also be given intramuscularly as sodium ascorbate. It can also be given subcutaneously and by intravenous route.

Doses of 0.25 to 1 gram daily in divided doses have been recommended for the treatment of scurvy. Eye drops containing potassium ascorbate have been used for the treatment of chemical burns.

Ascorbic acid and sodium ascorbate are used as antioxidants in pharmaceutical manufacturing and in food industries.

There is conflicting evidence regarding the use of vitamin C in common cold, asthma and improvement in atheletic performance.

In non-deficiency states, megadose therapy has been claimed to be beneficial in infective, allergic and toxic states of any kind, and infertility etc. but confirmation by controlled studies are required to substantiate these claims.

Vitamin C lowers intraocular pressure due to lowering of serum osmolarity. As it promptly crosses the blood-eye barrier so the ocular hypotensive effect is short-lived.

The aqueous concentration of vitamin C is lowered due to acid and alkali burns or mechanical injury to the eye. A 10% drops of ascorbic acid applied frequently for 6 weeks reduce the chances of corneal ulceration. Subcutaneous injections of vitamin C also reduce the incidence of corneal ulceration and perforation. The therapy must be commenced early as it will have little effect if ulceration has started.

Adverse effects due to overdosage include formation of oxalate stones in kidney. Ascorbic acid is mainly oxidized to oxalic acid so there is risk of provoking hyperoxaluria and oxalate stones. The minor side effects include diarrhoea.

VITAMIN D

The term vitamin D is used for a range of closely related sterol compounds which possess the property of preventing or curing rickets.

Even though it is termed 'vitamin D' it is a hormone that, together with parathormone, is a major regulator of the concentration of calcium in plasma. Vitamin D has hormonal nature.

Vitamin D is a prohormone which is converted in the body into a number of biologically active metabolites which function as true hormones. They maintain plasma calcium by increasing calcium absorption, mobilization from bone and decrease its renal excretion.

In humans, there are 2 sources of vitamin D:

1. Dietary ergocalciferol (D_2) derived from ergosterol in plants.

2. Cholecalciferol (D_3) is generated in the skin from 7-dehydrocholesterol by the action of ultraviolet irradiation (7-dehydrocholesterol formed from cholesterol in the wall of the intestine).

Vitamin D_1 is an impure mixture of sterols so it is to be ignored. Vitamin D_2 is ergocalciferol formed by the ultraviolet irradiation of ergosterol. It is plant-derived. Vitamin D_3 is cholecalciferol, a natural substance formed in skin from 7-dehydrocholesterol (oily secretion of mammalian skin) by action of ultraviolet light. There is no difference between the actions of vitamin D_2 and D_3. These are very stable and there is only little loss from processing.

Cholecalciferol and ergocalciferol are hydroxylated in the liver by the enzyme vitamin D 25-hydroxylase to form 25-hydroxycholecalciferol (calcifediol) and 25-hydroxyergocalciferol respectively. These compounds undergo further hydroxylation in the kidney by the enzyme vitamin D 1-hydroxylase to form the active metabolites 1,25-dihydroxycholecalciferol (calcitriol) and 1,25-dihydroxyergocalciferol respectively. Further metabolism also occurs in the kidney, including the formation of 1,24,25-trihydroxy derivatives.

Fig. 12.2 shows production and metabolism of vitamin D.

Many preparations containing vitamin D are marketed. Ergocalciferol (calciferol) is pure vitamin D_2, available for oral and i.m administration. Dihydrotachysterol (DHT) is the pure crystalline compound obtained by reduction of vitamin D_2 and is available for oral administration. Calcifediol (25-hydroxycholecalciferol) is also available for oral use. Calcitriol (1,25-dihydroxycholecalciferol) is available for oral administration or injection.

Vitamin D and its main derivatives:

- D_2 (Ergocalciferol, Calciferol) is formed in plants by ultraviolet radiation.

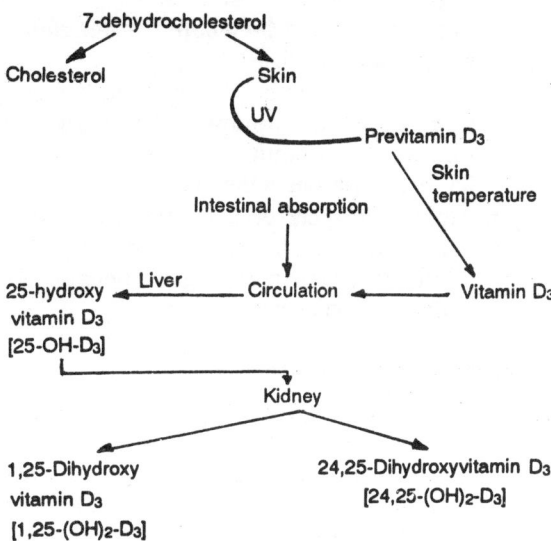

Fig. 12.2. Photosynthesis and metabolic pathways for vitamin D production and metabolism.

- D_3 (Cholecalciferol) is formed in skin from dehydrocholesterol by UV radiation.
- 25-hydroxy vitamin D_3 (calcifediol) is formed in the liver from cholecalciferol or ergosterol. It is the main storage form of vitamin D. It is important in reabsorbing calcium in the renal tubules and regulating calcium flux in muscle.
- 1,25-hydroxy-vitamin D_3 (calcitriol) is formed from calcifediol in kidney. It is most

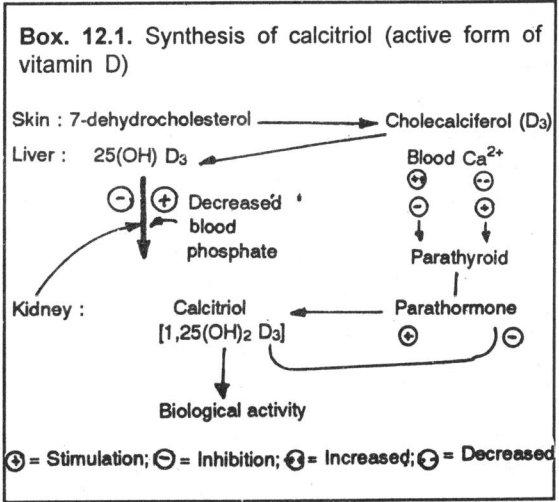

Box. 12.1. Synthesis of calcitriol (active form of vitamin D)

important potent metabolite in regulating plasma calcium (Ca^{2+}).

- Analogue of vitamin D_3 (dihydrotachysterol) is a crystalline compound prepared by reduction of vitamin D_2. It is activated by 25-hydroxylation in the liver.
- Alpha-hydroxycholecalciferol (alpha calcidiol) is a synthetic alpha-hydroxylated derivative of vitamin D_3. It undergoes hepatic 25-hydroxylation to calcitriol.

Modified forms of vitamin D

Dihydrotachysterol (DHT) is a vitamin D analogue which may be regarded as reduction product of vitamin D_2. It undergoes 25-hydroxylation to yield 25-hydroxydihydrotachysterol (25-OHDHT), which appear to be the active form in both intestine and bone.

1-alpha-hydroxycholecalciferol (1-OHD$_3$) is a synthetic derivative of vitamin D_3, it is hydroxylated in the liver to form 1,25-$(OH)_2D$.

Vitamin D_2 and D_3 occur in fatty fish and their oils, eggs, butter, some in cheese, very little in meat or white fish.

Vitamin D (cholecalciferol) is formed in the skin by photochemical conversion of a precursor, 7-dehydrocholesterol, via the energy of the shortest wave lengths of solar ultraviolet light (300-320 nm). It is also called vitamin D_3.

Vitamin D (ergocalciferol) is produced by ultraviolet irradiation of the fungal steriod ergosterol. As fungi tend to dislike sunlight, it is a rare form in nature. It is also called vitamin D_2.

The original antirachitic substance known as vitamin D_1 is a mixture of ergocalciferol and other sterols.

Vitamin D itself is biologically inactive. The functions are mediated by a trihydroxylated metabolite, 1,25-dihydroxy vitamin D or more correctly, 1,25-dihydroxycholecalciferol. The first step, the 25-hydroxylation takes place in the endoplasmic reticulum of liver cells and the product 25-hydroxycholecalciferol is secreted into the blood where it circulates in association with a specific vitamin D-binding globulin. Some of it is taken up by cells of the proximal convoluted tubule in the kidney where the second step, the 1-hydroxylation

occurs. The final product is 1,25-dihydroxy vitamin D as calcitriol is secreted back into blood and delivered to target cells where the function of vitamin D is expressed.

Vitamin D does not play an active role in bone formation but it ensures that calcium and phosphate are available when required. It plays important role for correct absorption of calcium from gut and for calcification of bones. The active metabolite of vitamin D (calcitriol) promotes the absorption of calcium from the intestine and also possibly of magnesium. It also promotes absorption of phosphate.

Of the natural metabolites of vitamin D, 25-hydroxy vitamin D as calcifediol, and 1,25-dihydroxy vitamin D as calcitriol are available for therapeutic use. Calcitriol is a very potent agent with respect to stimulation of intestinal calcium and phosphate transport and bone resorption.

A daily dietary intake of about 100-200 IU (2.5 to 5 mcg) of vitamin D is adequate for healthy adults. These small requirements are met mainly by exposure to sunlight and/or obtained from the diet. During pregnancy and lactation the requirement is about 400 IU per day.

The international unit is equivalent to the specific biological activity of 0.025 mcg of vitamin D_3 i.e. 1 mg equals 40,000 units.

Vitamin D substances are well absorbed from the gastrointestinal tract. The presence of bile is essential for intestinal absorption. Vitamin D and its metabolites circulate in the blood and bound to a specific alpha globulin. Vitamin D can be stored in adipose and muscle tissues for long time.

Cholecalciferol and ergocalciferol are hydroxylated in the liver by the enzyme vitamin D 25-hydroxylase to form 25 hydroxycholecalciferol and 25-hydroxyergocalciferol respectively. These are further hydroxylated in the kidney by the enzyme vitamin D_1 hydroxylase to form the active metabolites 1,25-dihydroxycholecalciferol (calcitriol). Further metabolism also occurs in kidneys, including the formation of 1,24,25-trihydroxy derivatives.

Vitamin D compounds and their metabolites are excreted in bile and faeces, only small amount appears in urine.

Certain vitamin D substances appear in breast milk.

Deficiency of vitamin D leads to the development of a syndrome characterized by hypocalcaemia, hypophosphataemia, bone softening, and osteomalacia. In osteomalacia there is defect in bone mineralisation with the accumulation of unmineralised osteoid on bone surfaces. This contrasts with osteoporosis where bone mineralisation is normal but there is a reduction in total bone mass. In children there may be skeletal deformity especially of long bones. It is known as rickets. Its deficiency also results in faulty dentition in children. Vitamin D deficiency affects eye growth, resulting in refractive error.

Therapeutic uses

- Prophylaxis and cure of neutritional rickets
- Treatment of metabolic rickets and osteomalacia
- Treatment of hyperparathyroidism
- Prevention and treatment of osteoporosis

Vitamin D compounds are involved in the regulation of calcium and phosphate homeostasis and bone mineralisation. These compounds are used in the treatment and prevention of vitamin D deficiency states. It is administered as cholecalciferol, or ergocalciferol or as an alpha calcidiol, calcifediol, calcitriol or dihydrotachysterol which do not require renal hydroxylation and hence useful in the presence of renal failure.

Dosage should be individualized for each patient. Cholecalciferol and ergocalciferol are generally given orally but can also be given intramuscularly. A dose of 1000 units daily is recommended for the treatment of rickets. Alpha calcidiol dose is 1-3 mcg daily orally, calcifediol (25-hydroxylated metabolite of cholecalciferol) dose is 50-100 mcg daily and calcitriol (1,25-dihydroxylated metabolite of cholecalciferol, it has highest antirachitic activity) is given in dose of 0.25-2 mcg daily.

Hypervitaminosis D

Adverse effects of vitamin D include pathologic calcification in many parts of the body. Conjunctival and corneal opacities appear in these patients. Scleral calcification may also occur. High doses given in infancy may result in narrowed optic foramina and optic atrophy may result.

Vitamin D toxicity occurs when synthetic vitamin D in milligram amounts are given by mouth for weeks or months. Excessive doses of 60,000 units (1.25 mg) daily can cause hypercalcaemia. Systemic adverse effects include anorexia, vomiting, dwarfism, mental retardation and renal damage with hypertension. Renal calculi may be formed and metastatic calcification may occur in renal tubules.

When excess vitamin D is consumed there is increased uncontrolled formation of 25 hydroxy vitamin D which is secreted from liver into blood. The specific vitamin D-binding sites on the circulating vitamin D-binding proteins, which normally are less than 5% saturated become mainly occupied with 25 hydroxy vitamin D. Because 1,25-dihydroxy vitamin D has a lower affinity for this protein than 25 hydroxy vitamin D, the functional hormone is displaced and circulates either in the unbound form or in a loose association with plasma albumin. Hence the availability of 1,25- dihydroxy vitamin D to its intracellular receptors is greatly increased.

The prolonged exposure of the skin to sunlight may induce sun burn but it does not produce excess of vitamin D, as the restricted accessibility of 7-dehydrocholesterol in skin to ultraviolet light and the slow rate of diffusion of vitamin D from skin limit the supply of this prohormone to its functional metabolism.

The treatment of hypervitaminosis D consists of immediate withdrawal of vitamin and administration of glucocorticoids.

VITAMIN K

The term vitamin K is used for a range of napthoquinone compounds which are necessary for the biosynthesis of blood clotting factors (factors II, VII, IX and X). An intake of about 2 mcg/kg body weight daily appears to be adequate which can be obtained from the average diet.

The daily requirement is 0.5 to 1 mcg/kg of body weight. Needs are satisfied by the average diet and in addition the vitamin synthesized by intestinal bacteria also is available to the host.

The fat-soluble vitamin K compounds, phytonadione and menadione require the presence of bile for their absorption from gut; the water soluble derivatives of menadion can be absorbed in the absence of bile. Vitamin K can be stored in the liver but for short periods. Vitamin K does not cross placenta and is poorly distributed in breast milk. Phytonadione is metabolised rapidly to more polar metabolites and is excreted in bile and urine as glucuronide and sulphate conjugates.

Vitamin K functions as an essential cofactor for a microsomal enzyme system in the hepatic synthesis of prothrombin (factor II) and other blood clotting factors (factors VII, IX and X). Thus vitamin K is essential for normal clot formation. It promotes hepatic biosynthesis of factor II (prothrombin), factor VII, factor IX and factor X.

Vitamin K activity is associated with two distinct natural substances, designated as vitamin K_1 and vitamin K_2. Vitamin K_1 or phytonadione is found in plants. Vitamin K_2 represents a series of compounds (menaquinones).

The natural vitamins K and menadione are lipid soluble.

Active water-soluble derivatives of menadione can be formulated by forming the sodium bisulphite salt or the tetrasodium salt of the diphosphoric acid ester. These compounds are converted in the body to menadione.

Menadione (vitamin K_3) is insoluble in water.

Water soluble preparations

Menadiol sodium diphosphate is marketed as 10 mg tablet or injection.

Fat soluble preparations

Phytonadione (vitamin K_1) is available as tablet (10 mg) and in a dispersion with buffered polysorbate and propylene glycol for i.m. injection (2 mg/ml). The fat soluble preparation is most rapidly effective whereas water soluble preparations take 24 hours to act but the action lasts for several days.

Phytonadione and the menaquinones are well absorbed from GIT only if bile salts are present; menadione and its water-soluble derivatives, however, are absorbed even in the absence of bile. Phytonadione and menaquinones are absorbed via lymph whereas soluble derivatives enter the bloodstream directly.

Deficiency states of vitamin K are rare. However, it may occur in patients with malabsorption syndrome, obstructive jaundice or in those receiving coumarin anticoagulants which interfere with vitamin K metabolism.

Deficiency leads to the development of hypoprothrombinaemia in which clotting time is prolonged and spontaneous bleeding may occur. Vitamin K compounds are used in the treatment and prevention of haemorrhage associated with vitamin K deficiency.

The dose of vitamin K is controlled by prothrombin time estimation.

Therapeutic uses

The rational use of vitamin K is to correct the bleeding tendency or haemorrhage associated with its deficiency.

Adverse effects

Excessive amounts of vitamin K cause pro-thrombin deficiency. Rapid intravenous administration of phytomenadion may cause facial flushing, chest constriction, chest pain, sweating, cyanosis and cardiovascular collapse. Administration of menadion and its water soluble derivatives such as menadiol sodium phosphate to neonates, especially premature infants, may cause haemolytic anaemia. These compounds may also produce haemolysis in subjects with glucose-6-phosphate dehydrogenase deficiency.

Allergic skin reactions have been reported following intramuscular injection.

VITAMIN E (TOCOPHEROLS)

Vitamin E is a fat soluble vitamin. It is clear slightly greenish yellow, viscous oily liquid, practically insoluble in water, freely soluble in ether, chloroform, acetone, fixed oils and alcohol.

Vitamin E includes d- or dl-alpha tocopheryl acid succinate. Vitamin E should be stored in air tight containers and protected from light. It is not destroyed by cooking processes.

Vitamin E is found in whole grain cereals, lettuce and vegetables and seed oils including soyabean, safflower, corn, sunflower, nuts and wheat germ. Animal products are poor sources of vitamin E. Vitamin E includes eight naturally occurring compounds in two classes designated as tocopherols and tocotrienols with different biological activity. The most active is alpha tocopherol.

One international unit (IU) of vitamin E is equivalent to the activity of 1 mg of dl-alpha tocopheryl acetate. d-alpha tocopheryl acetate has a potency of 1.36 IU/mg; d-alpha tocopherol, 1.49 IU/mg; and d-alpha tocopheryl succinate, 1.21 IU/mg.

The daily requirement is 2-3 mg, for which the recommended daily dietary allowance (RDA) for adults is 8 to 10 mg.

The absorption of vitamin E is dependent upon digestion and absorption of fat. It is absorbed from gastrointestinal tract. Free tocopherols are absorbed by passive process into the lymphatic circulation (about 45%), metabolites and small quantity of free vitamin E are absorbed through portal vein. Vitamin E is transported in blood mainly by low density lipoproteins and high density lipoproteins.

The absorption depends on the presence of bile. After absorption it enters the blood stream via lymph, widely distributed and stored in adipose tissues. It appears in breast milk. It is poorly transferred across the placenta. Some of vitamin E is metabolized in the liver to glucuronides and then to tocopheronic acid and excreted in urine.

Human requirements are about 3 to 15 mg daily, no supplementation is required in subjects on balanced diet, as vitamin E is widely distributed in food. Upto 2 mg/kg body weight of alpha tocopherol is the acceptable daily intake as an antioxidant.

Vitamin E deficiency is rare, but when it occurs it is characterized by peripheral neuropathy which can be prevented by supplemental vitamin E. Plasma vitamin E concentration can provide a good indication of recent vitamin E status of an individual and adipose concentration reflects long term vitamin E intake status. The normal plasma concentration of vitamin E is 23.2 micromol/L (1 mg/dl). When this value is below 11.6 micromol/L it is considered deficient state. Vitamin E deficiency can be produced by malabsorption syndrome which include extraocular muscle palsies, haemorrhagic retinopathy, and nystagmus.

Vitamin E is the most effective chain breaking lipid soluble antioxidant in the biological membrane, where it contributes to membrane stability. In addition to its antioxidant function, vitamin E influences cellular response through oxidative stress through modulation of signal transduction pathways. When cell growth is inhibited by lipid peroxidation, d-alpha-tocopherol may restimulate cell growth and proliferation by removing the inhibition. Conversely, it may also inhibit growth of cells through its non-oxidant properties: d-alpha-tocopherol inhibits protein kinase C activity which can regulate cell proliferation. The d-alpha-tocopherol has molecular specificity to inhibit proliferation of smooth muscle cell.

Vitamin E may modulate platelet adherence and aggregation; decreased vitamin E concentrations are associated with increased aggregation, which is reversible by improving vitamin E status. Data of various studies suggest that high dietary intake of vitamin E is associated with a reduced risk of cardiovascular diseases, but they do not prove a causal relation. Definitive conclusions should await the results of randomized trials. Vitamin E may participate in several events associated with the pathogenesis of cardiovascular diseases including LDL oxidation, adhesion of monocyte to endothelial cells, foam cell formation and fatty streak development, platelet adherence and aggregation and smooth muscle cell proliferation.

Vitamin E helps to prevent oxidation of polyunsaturated fatty acids in cell membranes and other body structures. It protects photoreceptor membranes from oxidative damage. It also retards the accumulation of cellular debris. it may prevent autooxidation induced by light in the eye reducing oxygen free radicals and thus limits retinal damage. The use of vitamin E in the prophylactic treatment of cataract has been suggested on the basis of reduction of free oxygen radicals. However, its use in this condition is controversial. Vitamin E has also been used in the treatment of intermittent claudication and some other conditions including angina pectoris, leg cramps, cancer but there is little evidence of beneficial effects. Dose in these conditions range from 300 to 600 mg daily by mouth for 3 months or longer.

Certain studies suggest that vitamin E may reduce the risk of cancer as it inhibits mutagenesis and cell transformation by eliminating oxygen free radicals and decreasing DNA damage. However, this role remains to be determined.

Vitamin E is also essential for normal functioning of the immune system. Immune cells are highly susceptible to harmful effects of free radical reactions. Few observations indicate that an increase in disease resistance can be expected. However, more studies are needed to find the immunostimulatory effect of vitamin E supplementation.

The list of therapeutic uses of vitamin E extends from minor skin ailments to schizophrenia.

Relative to other fat soluble vitamins, vitamin E is safe. It is well tolerated. Few side effects have been reported even with doses as high as 3200 mg daily. These minor side effects include fatigue, weakness, diarrhoea and abdominal pain. Topical application may produce contact dermatitis.

Vitamin E may antagonise the effects of vitamin K leading to an increase in clotting time in predisposed patients e.g. those taking anticoagulants.

FREE RADICALS AND ANTIOXIDANTS

There is a growing interest in the possible role of free radicals in the development of several diseases.

A free radical is defined as any atom, group of atoms or molecules in a particular state with one unpaired electron occupying an outer orbit. The unpaired electron of the free radicals accounts for the strong tendency of the radicals to interact with other electrons to form an electron pair and thus a chemical bond.

Free radical reactions are ubiquitous in living things. Studies on the origin and evolution of life provide a reasonable explanation for the prominent presence of this unruly class of chemical reactions. These reactions have been implicated in a large number of diseases which include inflammation, cancers, rheumatoid arthritis, Parkinson's disease, radiation injury, coronary artery disease, lung disease, cataract and a host of other diseases. Free radical reactions have also been implicated in the process of aging.

Free radicals include reactive oxygen species such as superoxide (O_2^-):

- Hydroxyl radicals (OH),
- Hydrogen peroxide (H_2O_2),
- Singlet oxygen ($^1O_2$),
- Hypochlorous acid (HOCl),
- Ozone (O_3), and

> **Box 12.2.** Ophthalmic effects of selected vitamin deficiencies
>
> A   Xerosis (dryness of conjunctiva); Conjunctiva (Bitot's spots); Cornea (keratomalacia is dryness with ulceration and perforation of cornea with absence of inflammatory reactions); Punctate keratopathy (which is noninflammatory dystrophy of cornea as distinct from keratitis)
> B_1 Optic nerve atrophy with visual field defect
> B_6 Cornea (Neovascularization)
> B_{12} Optic nerve atropyhy with visual field defects
> C   Lens (Cataract?)
> E   Macular degeneration?
> K   Conjunctiva (haemorrhage); Retina (haemorrhage)

- Nitric oxide (NO)
- RO Alkoxyl free radical
- ROO Peroxyl free radical
- LOOH Lipid peroxide

Free radical reactions arise upon exposure to ionizing radiation, from nonenzymatic reactions such as those with organic compounds and from enzymatic reactions particularly major energy gaining processes employed by living things such as photosynthesis.

The body's use of oxygen derived from food to fuel body processes is remarkable. Oxygen is moved around the body by red coloured particles of haemoglobin which contains iron. Oxygen is carried in blood stream to feed cells. This is called oxidation. However, oxygen also creates free radicals which cause problems when in excess. Free radicals are the by-product of oxidation. When oxygen is used by the body, it burns food to make energy; it also burns germs and toxic substances such as ozone and carbon monoxide. In the process free radicals are also produced. These free radicals damage the cell membrane, disturb chromosomes and genetic material and destroy valuable enzymes, causing a chained reaction of damage throughout the body. Thus free radicals are a cause of a large number of diseases.

Oxygen free radical (O_2) has also been found to be also generated by non-phagocytes like smooth muscle cells, human skin fibroblasts and endothelial cells. Free oxygen radical causes degradation of an endothelium derived vascular relaxation factor

(EDRF) which is possibly identical to nitric oxide (NO).

Oxygen in its ground state is a relatively weak oxidant. The complete reduction of oxygen by the univalent pathway results in the formation of superoxide anion radical, hydrogen peroxide and hydroxyl radical as the intermediates. These intermediates are too reactive to be tolerated by living tissues. Hence several protective and controlling mechanisms, which can be enzymatic, hydrophobic, hydrophilic and structural groups exist in the body. Cytochrome oxidase prevents the release of superoxide anion, hydrogen peroxide and hydroxyl radicals into the cellular milieu, superoxide dimutase is an enzyme which scavenges superoxide radical and catalyses and peroxidases can reduce hydrogen peroxide.

Vitamin E, intercalated in cellular membranes is probably the best hydrophobic scavenger known. Beta-carotenes and glutathione peroxidase, a selenium containing enzyme also play an important role in reducing hydrogen peroxide to water and also reduce lipid hydroperoxides.

Beta-carotene works in 2 ways: first it is converted to vitamin A by the body and the leftover beta carotene functions as an antioxidant.

There are 2 types of vitamin A. One is found in foods delivered from animals such as meat and milk, called retinol. The other are the carotenoids that are found in fruits and vegetables. There are many carotenoids but the most important one is beta carotene. The fruits and vegetables which are rich sources of beta carotene are melons, tomatoes, spinach and carrots (they were first found in carrots hence called carotenoids).

The damage of free radicals can be reduced by avoiding cigarette smoke and avoiding cooking oils heated to high temperatures. When fats are heated to high temperatures, their chemical structure breaks down to form peroxides which further break down to form the dangerous hydroxyl radical which is highly reactive and causes great damage to cells and DNA. The polyunsaturated fatty acids (PUFAs) are least stable at high temperatures, these become oxidized more quickly than monounsaturated fats such as olive oil.

Beta-carotene (precursor of vitamin A), vitamin C and vitamin E (ACE vitamins) form a base of good health. These are important antioxidants.

STUDY QUESTIONS

1. What factors may cause vitamin deficiency?
2. What are the main sources and functions of vitamin A? What may be caused by the deficiency of vitamin A? What are the adverse effects of hypervitaminosis A?
3. What is the essential role of thiamine (Vitamin B_1)?
4. What happens due to the deficiency of riboflavine (Vitamin B_2)?
5. What are the therapeutic uses and adverse effects of nicotinic acid?
6. What are the rich sources and therapeutic uses of pyridoxine (vitamin B_6)?
7. Which are cobalt containing compounds? Describe the pharmacokinetics and pharmacodynamics of Vitamin B_{12} (cyanocobalamin)?
8. What are the common causes of vitamin B_{12} and folic acid deficiencies? What is the line of treatment of megaloblastic anaemia in the presence of neurological complications?
9. What are the uses and adverse effect of ascorbic acid?
10. Describe the role, deficiency states, uses and toxicity of Vitamin D?
11. What are the claims of usefulness of vitamin E?
12. Describe the role, preparations, uses and adverse effects of vitamin K?
13. Define free radicals. What is their role in unruly class of chemical reactions? Give examples.
14. Name conditions in which free radicals are implicated.
15. What is the importance of the use of antioxidants? Name substances which possess antioxidant property.

GUIDE TO FURTHER READING

Achkar, C.C et al: Differences in the pharmacokinetic properties of orally administered all-trans-retinoic acid and 9-cis-retinoic acid in the plasma of nude mice. Drug Metab. Dispos., 1994; 22:451-458.

Alpha-Tocopherol, Beta-Carotene Cancer Prevention Study Group. The role effect of vitamin E and beta-carotene on the incidence of lung cancer and other cancers in male smokers. N. Engl. J. Med., 1994; 330:1029-1035.

Amento, E.P: Vitamin D and the immune system. Steroids, 1987; 49:55-72.

Anonymous, Vitamin A for measles [Editorial]. Lancet, 1987; 1:1067-1068.

Barash, P et al: Acute cardiovascular collapse after intervenous phytonadione. Anesth. Analg., 1976; 55:304-306.

Bendich, A et al: Safety of vitamin A. Am.J. Clin. Nutr., 1989; 49:358-371.

Bendich, A et al: Biological actions of carotenoids. FASEB J., 1989; 3:1927-1932.

Bernhardt, I.B et al: The use of vitamin K and bile in treatment of hemorrhagic diathesis in cases of jaundice. Proc. Staff Meet. Mayo Clin., 1938; 13:74-80.

Chopra, K et al: Involvement of oxygen free radicals in cardioprotective effect of rutin—a naturally occurring flavoncid. Ind. J. Pharmacol., 1994; 26:13-18.

Das, U.N et al: Free radicals: Biology and relevance to disease, JAPI Vol 38 no.7, 1990; 495-497.

Denham Harman: Free radical theory of aging, Mutation Research, 1992; 275:257-266.

Duthie, G.G et al: Arthur J.R. and James, W.P.T et al: Effects of smoking and vitamin E on blood antioxidant status. Am.J.Clin.Nutr., 1991; 53(Suppl):10615-10635.

Econs, M.J et al: Bone disease resulting from inherited disorders of renal tubule transport and vitamin D metabolism. In, Disorders of Bone and Mineral Metabolism. Raven Press Ltd., New York, 1992; pp. 935-950.

Finch, J.L et al: Differential effects of 1,25-(OH)$_2$D$_3$ and 22-oxacalcitriol on phosphate and calcium metabolism. Kidney Int., 1993; 43:561-566.

Fraser, D et al: Pathogenesis of hereditary vitamin-D-dependent rickets: an inborn error of vitamin D metabolism involving defective conversion of 25-hydroxyvitamin D to 1 alpha, 25-dihydroxyvitamin D. N. Engl.J. Med., 1973; 289:817-822.

Fraser, D.R: Regulation of the metabolism of vitamin D. Physiol. Rev., 1980; 60:551-613.

Fujita, T: Vitamin D in the treatment of osteoporosis. Proc. Soc. Exp. Biol. Med., 1992; 199:394-399.

Gallagher, J.C et al: Treatment of postmenopausal osteoporosis with high doses of synthetic calcitriol. A randomized controlled study. Ann. Int. Med., 1990; 113:649-655.

Greenberg, E.R et al: Preventation Study Group. A clinical trial of antioxidant vitamins to prevent colorectal adenoma. N. Engl. J. Med., 1994; 331:141-147.

Hahn, T.J et al: Effect if chronic anticonvulsant therapy on serum 25-hydroxycalciferol levels in adults. N. Engl. J. Med., 1972; 287:900-904.

Halliwell, B et al: Drug antioxidant effects—a basis for drug selection? Drugs, 1991; 42(4):569-605.

Haussler, M.R: Vitamin D receptors: nature and function. Annu. Rev. Nutr., 1986; 6:527-562.

Hertog, M.G.L et al: dietary antioxidant flaronoids and risk of coronary heart disease. Lancet, 1993; 342:1007-1011.

Hervert, V: The antioxidant supplement myth. Am. J. Clin. Nutr., 1994; 60:157-158.

Holick, M.F: Active vitamin D compounds and analogues: a new therapeutic era for dermatology in the 21st century. Mayo Clin. Proc., 1993; 68:925-927.

Hong, W.K. et al: Retinoids and human cancer. In, The Retinoids: Biology, Chemistry, and Medicine, 2nd ed. Raven Press, New York, 1994; pp. 597-630.

Hunter, D.J et al: A prospective study of the intake of vitamins C, E and A and the risk of breast cancer. N. Engl. J. Med., 1993; 329:234-240.

Hussey, G.D et al: A randomized controlled trial of vitamin A in children with severe measles. N. Engl. J. Med., 1990; 323:160-164.

Kaplan, L.A et al: Carotenoid composition, concentration and relationship in various human organs. Clin. Physiol. Biochem., 1990; 8:1-10.

Lippman, S.M et al: Cancer chemoprevention. J. Clin. Oncol., 1994; 12:851-873.

Love, J.H et al: Vitamin A, differentation and cancer. Curr. Opin. Cell Biol., 1994; 6:825-831.

Luine, V.N et al: Vitamin-D: is the brain a target? Steroids, 1987; 49:133-153.

Nemere, I et al: 1,25-Dihydroxyvitamin D3-mediated vesicular transport of calcium in intestine: time course studies. Endocrinology, 1988; 122:2962-2969.

Mangelsdorf, D.J. et al: The retinoid receptors in, The Retinoids: Biology, Chemistry, and Medicine, 2nd ed. Raven Press, New York, 1994; pp. 319-350.

Moon, R.C et al: Retinoids and cancer in experimental animals. In, The Retinoids: Biology, Chemistry, and Medicine, 2nd ed. Raven Press, New York, 1994; pp. 576-598.

Olson, J.A et al: The irresistible fascination of carotenoids and vitamin A: The 1992 Atwater Lecture. Am. J. Clin. Nutr., 1993; 57:833-839.

Ong, D et al: Cellular retinoid binding proteins. In, The retinoids: Biology, Chemistry, and Medicine, 2nd ed. Raven Press, New York, 1994; pp. 283-317.

Packer, L et al: Protective role of vitamin E in biological systems. Am. J. Clin. Nutr., 1991; 53(Suppl.): 10505-10555.

Puschett, J.B et al: Evidence for a direct action of cholecalciferol and 25-hydroxycholecalciferol on the renal transport of phosphate, sodium, and calcium. J. Clin. Invest., 1972; 51:373-385.

Reaven, P.D et al: Effect of dietary antioxidant combinations in humans. Protection of LDL by vitamin E but not by beta-carotene. Arteriosclerosis Thromb., 1993; 13:590-600.

Rimm, E.B. et al: Vitamin E consumption and the risk of coronary heart disease in men. N. Engl. J. Med., 1993; 328:1450-1556.

Ross, A.C: Vitamin A status: relationship to immunity and the antibody response. Minireview. Proc. Soc. Exp. Biol. Med., 1992; 200:303-320.

Shapiro, A.D et al: Vitamin K deficiency in the newborn infant: prevalence and perinatal risk factors. J. Pediatr., 1986; 109:675-680.

Simpson, K.L.: Relative value of carotenoids as precursors of vitamins A. Proc. Nutr. Soc., 1983; 42:7-17.

Sokol, R.J et al: Vitamin E deficiency and neurologic disease. Annu. Rev. Nutr., 1988; 8:351-373.

Stahl, W et al: Cis-trans isomers of lycopene and beta-carotene in human serum and tissues. Arch. Biochem. Biophys., 1992; 294:173-177.

Stamfer, M.J et al: Vitamin E consumption and the risk of coronary disease in women. N. Engl. J. Med., 1993; 328:1444-1449.

Steinberg, D: Antioxidants and atherosclerosis: A current assessment. Circulation, 1991; 84:1420-1425.

Steinberg, D (Editional): Antioxidants, Vitamins and coronary heart disease. N. Engl. J. Med., 1993; 328:1487-1489.

Stryer, L et al: Visual excitation and recovery. J. Biol. Chem., 1991; 266:10711-10714.

Symposium: Biological actions of carotenoids. J. Nutr., 1980a, 119:94-136.

Symposium: Retinoids. Pharmacol. Ther., 1989b, 40:1-169.

Van Poppel, G: Carotenoids and cancer: an update with emphasis on human intervention studies. Eur. J. Cancer., 1993; 29A:1335-1344.

Williams, M.L et al: Role of dietary iron and fat on vitamin E deficiency anemia of infancy. N. Engl. J. Med., 1975; 292:887-890.

CHAPTER
13

Autacoids and their Antagonists

AUTACOIDS (LOCAL HORMONES) AND THEIR ANTAGONISTS

The word autacoid is derived from Greek words: autos means self and akos means remedy. A large variety of cells in the body produce a variety of substances which exert pharmacological activity. Autacoids are also known as local hormones that originate from diffuse tissues rather than in glands, and act locally at the site of synthesis and release or at near tissues. They differ from hormones which are secreted by specific cells and act on distant tissues.

Autacoid can be divided into three categories on the basis of their structure:

Amines :
 Histamine, 5-Hydroxytryptamine

Peptides :
 Angiotensin, kinins

Phospholipid derived autacoids :
 Prostaglandins
 Leukotrienes
 Platelet activating factor (PAF)

HISTAMINE (Fig. 13.1)

Histamine is formed by the decarboxylation of histadine in almost all the tissues, largest amounts are present is mast cells, skin, lung, stomach, intestine, liver.

Histamine is stored chiefly in mast cells. The

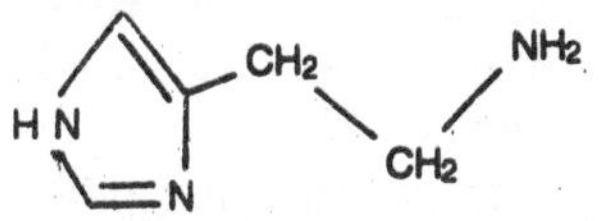

Fig. 13.1. Structure formula of histamine.

principal sites of storage are the lungs, skin and intestinal mucosa.

Histamine stored in the mucosal cells of the stomach can be released by food and vagal stimulation. The released gastric histamine regulates intestinal contraction and gastric secretion.

Histamine in the skin and lung tissue plays role in tissue growth and repair and in allergic responses.

Histamine is found in high concentrations in hypothalamus where it is released as a neurotransmitter.

Histamine acts on the following types of receptors:

1. H_1 receptors mediate allergic responses to histamine (bronchoconstriction, increased capillary permeability, vasodilatation and spasmodic contraction of GI smooth muscle).
2. H_2 receptors mediate other responses to histamine (increased secretion of gastric HCl, pepsin).
3. H_3 receptor stimulation may have negative modulatory effects.

All effects of histamine except those on gastric secretion are due to its action on H_1 receptors.

Main actions of histamine

- Stimulation of gastric secretion (H_2)
- Contraction of most smooth muscle other than that of blood vessels (H_1)
- Cardiac stimulation (H_2)
- Vasodilatation (H_1)
- Increased vascular permeability (H_1)

Pharmacologic effects

Cardiovascular system

Histamine produces vascular endothelium to release nitric oxide that stimulates the production of guanylate cyclase. The enhanced level of cGMP in vascular smooth muscle causes vasodilation.

Histamine dilates fine vessels of the micro-circulation resulting in oedema (effect on capillary permeability); due to capillary and arteriolar dilation, the systemic blood pressure falls; and unilateral cluster headaches (histamine headache) occurs due to dilation of cranial blood vessels.

Histamine produces positive inotropic and chronotropic effects which are mediated by both H_1 and H_2 receptors.

Extravascular smooth muscle

The H_1 receptor activation in smooth muscle causes contraction. It also increases intracellular levels of free Ca^{++} which helps to regulate contraction and secretion of histamine.

The contraction by H_1 receptors induces a rise in cyclic guanosine 3′,5′-monophosphate (cGMP) levels.

The activation of H_2 receptors produces relaxation of smooth muscle and a rise in cAMP levels.

Central nervous system

Little is known about the physiological role of histamine in the CNS. It does not cross blood-brain barrier.

Exocrine glands

Histamine when combines with H_2 receptors, it is a potent gastric secretagogue. It potentiates the release of gastric acid induced by gastrin and acetyl choline.

It can stimulate pancreatic, bronchiolar secretion and also produces salivation and lacrimation.

Skin

On intradermal injection, when histamine is introduced in skin, it produces triple response: (a) reddening at the site of injection (due to local vasodilation (b) wheal or disk of oedema (due to capillary permeability within 1-2 minutes (c) bright crimson flare or halo surrounding the wheal which may be about 5 cm and last for about 10 minutes.

Mode of action

Histamine is released from the storage cells by chemical or physical stimuli.

Histamine release

- The primary mechanism is immunologic during allergic reactions including anaphylaxis. Immunoglobulin E (IgE) antibody interacts with antigen on the surface of mast cells and basophils leading to histamine release without cell membrane disruption (immediate hypersensitivity reaction).
- Enzymes, venoms, organic bases such as morphine and polymers e.g. dextran liberate histamine without prior sensitization by disrupting the mast cell membrane.
- Tissue injury (trauma, burn) can release histamine from storage sites.

Inhibition of release of histamine can occur with high intracellular levels of cyclic AMP.

Role of histamine

- Histamine plays an important role in mediating HCl secretion in the stomach. Histamine occurs in gastric mucosa in cells which lie close to the parietal cells. The stimuli which produce gastric secretion (vagal stimulation, cholinergic drugs, gastrin, feeding) release histamine locally.
- Allergy: Histamine causes urticaria, bronchoconstriction and anaphylaxis. It mediates immediate type of hypersensitivity reactions. Following antigen antibody reaction, histamine is released from mast cells. The antibody coats mast cells and subsequent antigen-antibody interaction disrupts the cell, releasing vasoactive amines particularly histamine.
- Neurotransmission: Hypothalamus and midbrain have histamine. It is believed to act as a transmitter regulating body temperature, and cardiovascular function.
- Inflammation: Histamine acts as a mediator of vasodilatation that occurs during inflammation.
- Regulation of the microcirculation: Histamine plays a role in the regulation of the microcirculation through its vasoactive properties.
- Immunoreactivity:
  - H_1-receptor activation can suppress lymphocyte proliferation and the release of cytokines and on T lymphocytes inhibits suppressor cell function.
  - H_2-receptor activation activates levels of intracellular cAMP, blocking T-cell mediated cytotoxicity.
- Tissue repair/growth: In rapidly proliferating tissues such as liver, bone marrow and a variety of malignancies, a high histamine synthesizing capacity is found.

Preparations

Histamine phosphate is given intravenously to test for gastric acid secretion. However, the side effects limit its use.

Betazole (isomer of histamine) is 10 times more potent as stimulant of gastric secretion than as a vasodilator. It can be used to test gastric function as an alternative for histamine phosphate. It has a preferential effect on gastric secretion. It does not require premedication with an H_1 or H_2 receptor blocker.

Impromidine is a selective H_2 agonist; it stimulates the activity of H_2 recep-tors more than 10,000 times than at H_1 receptors.

Pentagastrin (pentapeptide) is a stimulant of gastric acid, pepsin and intrinsic factor secretion. It has few adverse effects and it is also short acting.

Betahistine is an orally active, selective H_1 agonist which produces vasodilatation in the internal ear. It is being tried in the treatment of vertigo.

Therapeutic uses

There are no established therapeutic uses for histamine and its analogues. However, they can be used diagnostically for :

Histamine and its analogues can be used to distinguish between pernicious anaemia and other forms of anaemia. The loss of gastric parietal cells in pernicious anaemia results from an inability to secrete gastric acid in response to histamine. More selective H_2-receptor agonist such as impromidine (stimulates H_2-receptor more than 10,000 times than at H_1 receptor), is also used to test for achlorhydria.

Phaeochromocytoma: histamine produces rise in blood pressure (due to release of catecholamines from the tumour) instead of fall in B.P.

Local neural and vascular integrity testing: if functional nerves and arterioles are absent, there will not be flare after intradermal injection of histamine.

Adverse effects

- Fall in blood pressure, flushing and tachycardia may be produced due to vasodilation by histamine.
- Visual disturbances, headache and rise in skin temperature may occur.
- Dyspnoea, diarrhoea and bronchoconstriction may occur due to smooth muscle stimulation.

Histamine antagonists

These fall into two categories i.e. H_1 or H_2 receptor blockers.

H_1-receptor receptor antagonists are antihistamine agents.

H_2-receptor receptor antagonists inhibit gastric acid secretion (Chapter 8). They do not have significant action on H_1-receptors.

Antihistamine agents

The term antihistaminic drugs usually refers to H_1-receptor antagonists, whereas H_2-receptor antagonists are referred as such and used for peptic ulcers. H_3-receptor antagonists such as thioperamide has no known therapeutic use as yet.

H_1-receptor antagonists competitively block H_1-receptors. They antagonize the effects of histamine on bronchial smooth muscle, gastrointestinal smooth muscle and capillaries. They also prevent (histamine induced) pain and itching of the skin and mucous membranes. They are useful to relieve allergic symptoms.

H_2-receptor antagonists produce competitive block of H_2-receptors and thus antagonize the effects of histamine induced gastric secretions. They are useful agents in the treatment of gastric hyper-secretory conditions.

H_1-receptor antagonists can be grouped as:

First-generation agents

- Ethanolamines (most sedating antihistaminics)
  - Diphenhydramine (25-50 mg)
  - Dimenhydrinate (50-100 mg)
- Ethylenediamines (less sedative, also less effective than ethanolamines)
  - Pyrilamine maleate (25-50 mg)
  - Tripelannamine hydrochloride (25-50 mg)
  - Tripelannamine citrate (37.5-75 mg)
- Alkylamines: (highly effective, less sedating than ethanolamines and ethylenediamines)
  - Chlorpheniramine maleate, 4 mg, 8-12 mg sustained release, 5-20 mg injection
  - Brompheniramine maleate, 4 mg, 8-12 mg sustained release, 5-20 mg injection
  - Triprolidine
- Piperazines (very effective antiemetics)
  - Cyclizine hydrochloride (50 mg)
  - Cyclizine lactate (50 mg)
  - Meclizine hydrochloride (12.5-50 mg)
  - Buclizine (50 mg)
- Phenothiazines
  - Promethazine hydrochloride (25 mg)

Second-generation agents

- Alkylamines
  - Acrivastine (8 mg)
- Piperazines
  - Cetirizine hydrochloride (5-10 mg)
- Piperidines
  - Astemizole (10 mg)
  - Loratadine (10 mg)
  - Terfenadine (60 mg)
  - Levocarbistine (0.5 mg/ml)

Miscellaneous

- Azatidine (1-2 mg)
- Mebhydroline (100-300 mg)

Pharmacokinetics

Absorption is complete from GIT, onset of action is within half an hour and the effect lasts for 3-4 hours. They are metabolized in liver by hydroxylation. The metabolites are excreted in the urine.

Actions

H_1-receptor antagonists competitively block histamine-induced effects.

These drugs also produce certain other following

pharmacological effects independent of their anti-histaminic activity.

- Sedation is a common side effect. However, certain drugs such as terfenadine, cetirizine, loratadine which do not cross the blood brain barrier have no sedative effect. They have slow onset but long duration of action. These are also free from anticholinergic action.
- Due to their anticholinergic action they may be useful in motion sickness and parkinsonism. However, dryness of mouth, blurred vision and retention of urine may be produced as side effects due to their anticholinergic action.
- Promethazine possesses weak antiadrenoceptor property.
- Cyproheptadine has anti 5-HT property.
- Local anaesthetic action is due to blockade of Na+ channels in excitable membranes.
- Antipruritic effect is due to prevention of histamine induced itching and pain.

In the immediate response type of allergy (such as hay fever), histamine-like substances released in the tissues are responsible for the symptoms. Drugs that are histamine antagonists will effectively relieve the allergic symptoms, including the ocular itching, redness, and tearing. The antihistaminics should be taken systemically because they are relatively ineffective when used topically. Contact drug allergies and eczema are not histamine mediated and do not respond to antihistaminic agents. In these cases, corticosteroids, which have a nonspecific blocking action against inflammation, are much more generally effective than antihistaminics. However, the mild local anesthetic effect of antihistamine drugs may give some symptomatic relief.

Therapeutic uses of H₁-receptor antagonists

Allergic disorders

Antihistamines are used therapeutically for palliative treatment in allergic reactions. Where the reaction is due to the release of histamine, antihistaminics will usually be of value; where other substances are involved in the allergic reaction, they may still be of value by virtue of their other actions. Most of them antagonize the actions of acetylcholine and produce local anaesthesia when applied locally.

Antihistamines improve and relieve the symptoms of seasonal hay fever in a high percentage of patients though a high dosage may be necessary in some individuals.

In vasomotor rhinitis, antihistamines are also beneficial. The nasal irritation and the watery discharge are most readily relieved but nasal obstruction is little affected.

Antihistamines are effective in abolishing the urticaria and skin irritations in serum sickness but the joint symptoms are little affected. Other itching skin conditions, including pruritus ani and pruritus vulvae, the pruritus of drug rashes and jaundice, contact dermatitis and insect bites, are often relieved by the oral administration of antihistamines. In patients with asthma, wheezing is not greatly improved by them, though coughing may be reduced. Some antihistamines have a powerful antiemetic action and are used for the prevention and treatment of motion sickness.

Antihistamines have also been used for the prevention and treatment of irradiation sickness, post operative vomiting, the nausea and vomiting of pregnancy, and drug induced nausea and vomiting; they have also been used for the symptomatic treatment of nausea and vertigo due to Meniere's disease and other labyrinthine disturbances.

Antihistamines with sedative and antiemetic properties are used for anaesthetic premedication. Although they may have some anticholinergic properties of their own they are usually given with an anticholinergic agent to provide more effective reduction of salivation.

Some antihistamines were formerly used in the treatment of Parkinson's syndrome, but more effective drugs are now preferred.

Diphenhydramine was used to reverse the extra-pyramidal side effects caused by phenothiazines but it is less effective than other agents such as artane.

Eye drops containing diphenhydramine have been used for ocular allergies.

Myokymia

The refractory period of muscle is prolonged by antihistamines. This property permits their use in the treatment of myokymia (twitching of the lids). The antihistaminic drug of choice may be given alone or together with quinine (0.32 g one to three times daily).

Cataract surgery

Constriction of the pupil occurs during cataract surgery despite the preoperative use of atropine and other mydriatics. This constriction is a result of liberation of histamine from injured tissue. It is suggested that preoperative antihistamine therapy can prevent pupilloconstriction. The antihistaminic may be administered orally (promethazine 25 mg 2 hours before surgery) or topically (pyrilamine maleate, 0.1% solution every 10 minutes three times).

Adverse effects of antihistamines (H₁-receptor antagonists)

The most common side effect is sedation, varying from slight drowsiness to deep sleep, and including inability to concentrate, lassitude, dizziness, hypotension, muscular weakness and incoordination. Sedative effects, when they occur, may diminish after a few days. Other side effects include nausea, vomiting, diarrhoea or constipation and gastro-intestinal disturbances such as epigastric pain. They may also produce headache, blurred vision, tinnitus, elation or depression, irritability, nightmares, anorexia, dryness of mouth, tightness of chest, tingling, heaviness, and weakness of the hands.

Administration of antihistamines may occasionally cause allergy. Local application of antihistamines carries a risk of skin sensitization with eczematous eruptions but dermatological reactions may also result from oral administration. Blood disorders, including agranulocytosis and haemolytic anaemia, though rare, have been reported.

Systemic side effects have been reported after topical application of antihistamines to large areas of the skin.

Narcotics and sedatives may be greatly potentiated by antihistamines; their effect is sometimes doubled.

Precautions

Antihistamines can lead to a wide range of adverse effects that may severely limit their use due to the following:

Hepatic enzyme induction

Because antihistamines induce the microsomal enzyme system and facilitate their own destruction, they become less effective with continued use. This commonly necessitates a change of product.

Anticholinergic effects

These are annoying but usually are manageable and do not warrant drug discontinuation. They include dry mouth, urinary retention, and blurred vision.

CNS depression

Drowsiness is a common side effect with all antihistamines and may be exacerbated (via synergism) by concurrent use of another CNS depressant.

Paradoxical effects

Antihistamines sometimes cause CNS stimulation instead of drowsiness. Flushing, hyperactivity, anorexia, and palpitations also may occur. Paradoxical effects are most common in children.

H₃-receptor agonists and antagonist

H₃-receptors are distributed in CNS (presynaptic, myenteric plexus); the representative agonist is (R)-α-CH₃-histamine. The representative antagonists are thioperamide and clobenpropit.

Based on the functions of H₃-receptors in the CNS, H₃-antagonists have potential use in improving attention and learning, in stimulating arousal, and as antiepileptic agents.

H₄-receptor agonists and antagonists

H₄-receptors are distributed in cells of haematopoietic origin; the representative agonist is clobenpropit (partial?); the representative antagonists are JNJ 7777120, thioperamide.

H₄-receptor is more similar to H₃-receptor; the availability of H₄-specific antagonists with anti-inflammatory properties should help to define the biological roles of the H₄-receptor.

Because of unique localization and function of H_4-receptors, H_4-antagonists are promising candidates to treat inflammatory conditions, such as allergic rhinitis, asthma, and rheumatoid arthritis.

H_3 and H_4 antihistamines are available only for research purposes.

5-HYDROXYTRYPTAMINE (5-HT, SEROTONIN)

About 90% 5-HT is present in the intestines and the rest in platelets and brain.

It is also found in scorpion sting. It is present in banana, pineapple, tomatoes, etc.

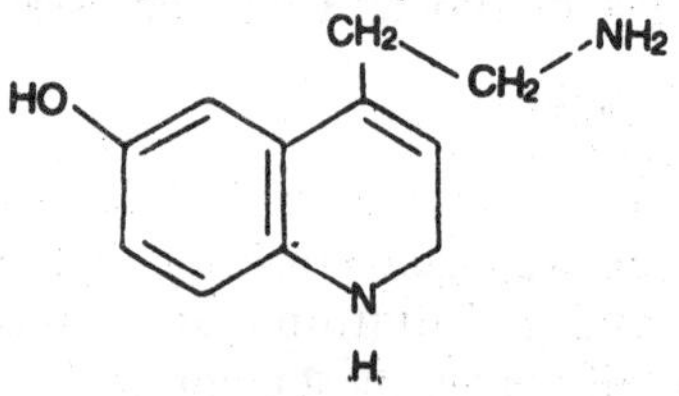

Fig. 13.2. Serotonin.

Pharmacologic effects

5-HT is a potent vasoconstrictor except in skeletal muscle and at coronary vessels that are dilated.

It produces positive inotropic and chronotropic effects on the heart. These effects may be masked by reflex responses.

It increases tone and motility of GIT, both by direct action and also through enteric plexuses.

It constricts bronchi (less than histamine).

It inhibits secretion of gastric HCl and pepsin but mucus production is enhanced.

5-HT is a weak platelet aggregator.

Effects of 5-HT injection are complex. Initially a brief depressor phase is observed due to transient reflex response to serotonin and vagus nerve stimulation. It is followed by increase in blood pressure due to increased cardiac output and reduction in peripheral resistance and finally prolonged depressor action occurs due to dilatation of blood vessels in skeletal muscles.

Role of 5-HT

• As neurotransmitter

– 5-HT is probably concerned in sleep, thought and mood, temperature regulation and perception of pain. Imbalance of 5-HT produces schizophrenia and affective disorders.
• Migraine
– 5-HT initiates initial stages of vasoconstrictor phase
• Raynaud's disease
– 5-HT released from platelets induce vasospasm of large arteries.
• Variant angina
– 5-HT released from platelets along with thromboxane A_2 may be involved in coronary spasm and variant angina.

Therapeutic uses

None.

5-HT RECEPTOR ANTAGONISTS

Ketanserin

It is relatively selective on $5-HT_2$ receptors. It has very little action on $5-HT_1$ and $5-HT_3$ receptors. The dosage for hypertension is 40-80 mg daily. This drug also acts as antagonist for α_1 adrenergic and dopamine receptors. It also inhibits serotonin-induced vasoconstriction, bronchoconstriction and platelet aggregation.

It is hypotensive by virtue of its $5-HT_2$ and α_1 adrenergic receptor antagonism.

The adverse effects include dry mouth, sedation, nausea, headache and dizziness.

Methysergide

It is an ergot derivative which blocks $5-HT_{2A}$ and $5-HT_{2C}$ receptors. It is useful as a prophylactic agent in migraine.

The adverse effects include GIT disturbances, drowsiness, confusion, hallucinations, psychosis, retroperitoneal fibrosis, pleuropulmonary fibrosis and coronary endothelial fibrosis.

Cyproheptadine

It resembles antihistamines in activity and uses. It is also secretogenic, antimuscarinic and calcium channel blocker.

It is used in allergic conditions, as appetite stimulant and for prophylaxis and treatment of vascular headache and migraine.

Dose is 12-16 mg per day orally.

The adverse effects are similar to antihistamines; it also stimulates appetite; the patient may gain weight.

POLYPEPTIDES

Plasma Kinins (bradykinin and kallidin)

These are polypeptides containing 8-12 amino acids. These are synthesized throughout the body. The kinins are vasodilating polypeptides.

The kinins produced from plasma proteins (alpha2-globulin precursors called kinitrogens) are known as plasma kinins which include bradykinin and kallidin which are inactivated by a group of enzymes known as kininases.

Synthesis and inactivation of plasma kinins

$$\text{Kininogen I} \xrightarrow{\text{Kininogenase}} \text{Kallidin}$$

$$\text{Kininogen II} \xrightarrow{\text{Kininogenase}} \text{bradykinin} \to \begin{array}{c}\text{Inactive} \\ \text{products}\end{array}$$

Kininogens are precursor to plasma proteins. The enzymes that release kinins are kininogenase (include kallikreins, pepsin, trypsin). Kininogenase enzymes are formed from inactive precursors (kallikreins) in secretory cells or plasma.

Two enzymes called kallikreins catalyze the formation of the plasma kinins bradykinin and kallidin.

High molecular weight kininogen is the precursor to bradykinin. The formation of bradykinin is catalyzed by plasma kallikrein. Plasma kallikrein is formed from prekallikrein.

Low molecular weight kininogen is the precursor of kallidin. Its formation is catalyzed by tissue kallikrein.

Pharmacologic effects

- Powerful algesic action caused by direct stimulation of nerve endings.
- Potent vasodilation, act directly on smooth muscles of fine resistance vessels.
- Constrict large arteries and most large and small veins.

- Constrict most nonvascular smooth muscles e.g. gastrointestinal and bronchiolar.

Bradykinin and kallidin are similar in potency and actions, they produce bronchoconstriction and contraction of GIT. As the arteriolar smooth muscles are dilated, blood pressure falls. They also increase the permeability of capillaries. In addition, there is intense pain.

Kinins are formed following damage which initiates inflammatory responses.

Role

Kinins are mediators of pain, inflammation and chronic inflammatory diseases.

Mode of action

It is not well understood, however, some responses may be mediated by PGs resulting from the stimulation of phospholipase A_2.

Uses

No therapeutic use exists for kinins.

Preliminary data exist for a few potential uses of kinins such as male infertility due to asthenozoospermia (weakness of sperms in semen) and oligospermia (deficiency of sperms in semen).

They may have potential value in enhancing the delivery of anticancer agents beyond the blood-brain barrier.

There are no specific antagonists of kinin activity but histamine and 5-HT antagonists sometimes show antibradykinin action.

Bradykinin receptors

There are 2 receptors for kinins designated as B_1 and B_2. The B_2 receptor selectively binds bradykinin and kallidin and is present in most normal tissues and mediate most of the effects of these kinins in the absence of inflammation. B_1 is less prevalent in most tissues. B_1 are present in normal vascular smooth muscle. B_1 receptors are upregulated by inflammation. During conditions such as tissue damage, injury or inflammation B_1 receptor effects predominate.

Bradykinin	Agonist, $B_2 > B_1$
Kallidin	Agonist, $B_2 \simeq B_1$
des-Arg^{10}-kallidin	Agonist B_1

Receptor Antagonists

These are being developed e.g. WIN 64338 (nonpeptide) and HOE 140 as B_2 antagonists and des-Arg9-[Leu8]-bradykinin as antagonists for B_1-kinin receptor.

These are available for research purposes. Some benefit has been reported with the use of kinin antagonist in septic shock, bronchoconstriction, inflammation and pain.

They are not available for clinical use.

Angiotensins

Angiotensin I (AI) is inactive, but the terminal two amino acids are split off by a peptidase called the converting enzyme to give highly active actapeptide angiotensin II(AII). The converting enzyme is widely distributed but particularly rich in lungs. AI gets activated during passage through pulmonary circulation to AII by converting enzyme.

Angiotensin II is a powerful smooth muscle stimulant, acting specially on the arterioles but also on gut and uterus. It is one of the most potent vasoconstrictors, it is about 40 times more potent than norepinephrine. It also has powerful action on the adrenal cortex causing release of aldosterone.

It stimulates the synthesis as well as secretion of aldosterone. It also stimulates sympathetic ganglion cells and enhances ganglionic transmission.

Role

Provides physiological stimulus for mineralocorticoid secretion, and electrolyte balance.

Uses

There are no approved therapeutic uses. A II amide if given as an infusion can produce sustained pressor response in shock but it may decrease tissue and organ perfusion due to vasoconstriction and may cause coronary spasm.

Angiotensinogen, a plasma alpha-globulin is the precursor for all angiotensins. Renin (juxtaglomerular enzyme controls formation of Angiotensin II) metabolizes angiotensinogen to form Angiotensin I. ACE which is present on capillary endothelial cells hydrolyzes A I to form the active A II. A II produces positive inotropic and positive chronotropic effects.

A II is metabolized to less active A III by aminopeptidase. ACE also inactivates bradykinin.

The formation of A II and relationship of kinin system to renin-angiotensin system is shown in Fig. 13.3.

The converting enzyme is a zinc containing enzyme. The angiotensin converting enzyme inhibitors have found important place in the treatment of hypertension.

Captopril inhibits conversion of the inactive angiotensin I to active angiotensin II but does not block angiotensin II receptors. Captopril decreases blood pressure which is more marked when sodium has been depleted by low sodium intake or by diuretics.

Dose: 25 mg thrice a day.

Enalapril is a recently introduced angiotensin converting enzyme inhibitor (ACE inhibitor), it is a prodrug which is converted in the body to enalaprilat acid (not used as such due to poor oral absorption). As compared to captopril this drug is more potent (dose 10-20 mg once or twice a day), longer acting and rashes are infrequent.

Antagonists of the renin-angiotensin system

1. Angiotensin II antagonists e.g. captopril, enalapril, lisinopril block the enzymatic

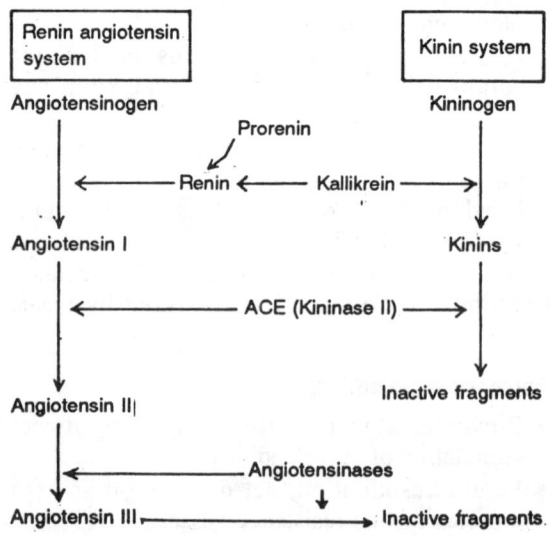

Fig. 13.3. Relationship of kinin system to renin-angiotensin system.

conversion of angiotensin I to Angiotensin II. The responsible enzyme is a peptidyl dipeptidase (it is ACE) hence drugs of this class are designated as ACE inhibitors.

General features of ACEIs:

- They do not antagonize angiotensin II
- They lower systemic blood pressure in hypertensive patients.
- They increase actions of bradykinin, which is inactivated by peptidyl dipeptidase.
- They can depress the secretion of aldosterone by lowering angiotensin II production

2. Inhibitors of enzyme peptidyl dipeptidase e.g. saralasin is a competitive inhibitor of angiotensin II receptors.

Eicosanoids (Fig. 13.4)

The arachidonate metabolites are 'eicosanoids'.

Eicosanoids (prostaglandins, thromboxanes, leukotrines) is the name given to a group of 20-carbon unsaturated fatty acids derived principally from arachidonic acid in cell walls. They are short-lived, extremely potent and formed in almost every tissue in the body. Eicosanoids are involved in most types of inflammation.

Arachidonic acid is stored mainly in phospholipids of cell walls. It is mobilised by the action of phospho-lipase A_2. Glucocorticoids prevent the formation of arachidonic acid by inducing the synthesis of an inhibitory polypeptide called lipocortin-1, inhibiting the subsequent formation of both-prostaglandins and leukotrienes.

Eicosanoids, unlike histamine, are not found preformed in the tissues; they are generated de nova from phospholipids. They are implicated in the control of many physiological processes and are among the most important mediators and modulators of the inflammatory reaction.

The main source of eicosanoids (PGs, TXs, LTs) is arachidonic acid, (component of membrane phospholipids) a 20-carbon unsaturated fatty acids containing 4 double bonds (hence 'eicosi' Greek-word referring to the 20 carbon atoms and 'tetra-enoic' referring to the 4 double bonds.

A variety of physical, chemical, hormonal, and neurochemical stimuli can initiate the release of arachidonic acid from lipid storage sites by phospholipases chiefly phospholipase A_2.

The metabolism of arachidonic acid involves certain oxidative pathways viz.,

(a) Cyclooxygenase (PG synthetase) pathway leading to the formation of prostaglandins (PGs) and thromboxanes (TXs).

(b) 5-lipoxygenase pathway leads to the formation of leukotrienes (LTs).

(c) Other lipoxygenase pathways lead to derivatives of eicosatetraenoic acid.

The PGs are named because they were thought to be originally obtained from seminal fluid.

LTs were first found in leukocytes. They are conjugated trienes.

TXs are synthesizes in thrombocytes (platelets) and contain an oxane ring.

Prostanoids

- The term prostanoids encampasses prosta-glandins (PGs) and thromboxanes (TXs).
- Cyclo-oxygenase (COX) acts on arachidonate to produce cyclic endoperoxides. There are two forms of cyclo-oxygenase: COX-1 a constitutive enzyme and COX-2, which is induced in inflammatory cells by inflammatory stimuli.
- These can give rise to:
  - PGI_2 (prostacyclin) predominently from vascular endothelium; It acts on IP-receptors. Main effects: vasodilation and inhibition of platelet aggregation.
  - TXA_2 predominently from platelets; it acts on TP-receptors. Main effects: platelet aggregation and vasoconstriction.
  - PGE_2 Main effects on EP_1-receptors - contraction of bronchial and GIT smooth muscle; on EP_2-receptors - relaxation of bronchial, vascular and GIT smooth muscle; on EP_3-receptors - inhibition of gastric acid secretion, increased gastric mucus secretion, contraction of pregnant uterus and of GIT smooth muscle, inhibition of lipolysis and of autonomic neuro-transmitter release, PGE_2 is a mediator of fever.

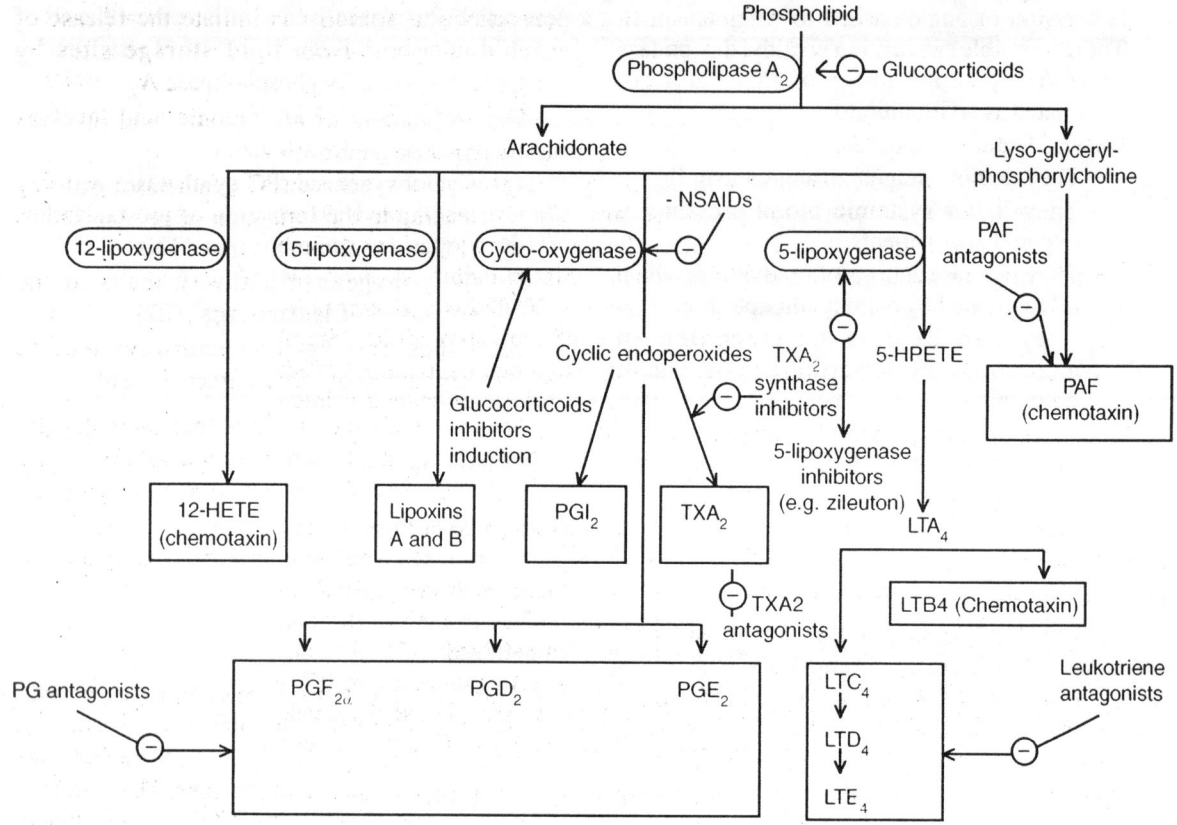

Fig. 13.4. Summary diagram of mediators derived from phospholipids and their actions, and the sites of action of anti-inflammatory drugs.

PG = prostaglandin; PGI_2 = prostacyclin; TX = thromboxane; LT = leukotriene; HETE = hydroxy-eicosatetraenoic acid; HPETE = hydroperoxy-eicosatetraenoic acid; PAF = platelet-activating factor; NSAIDs = non-steroidal anti-inflammatory drugs.

Properties

PGI_2	Vasodilator; hyperalgesic; stops platelet aggregation	LTB_4	Chemotaxin
PGF_{2a}	Bronchoconstrictor; myometrial contraction	LTC_4	Bronchoconstrictors
PGD_2	Inhibits platelet aggregation; vasodilator	LTD_4	Increase
PGE_2	Vasodilator; hyperalgesic	LTE_4	Vascular permeability
TXA_2	Thrombotic; vasoconstrictor	PAF	Vasodilator; increases vascular permeability; bronchoconstrictor; chemotaxin

- PGF_{2a} acts on FP-receptors which are found in smooth muscle and corpus luteum. Main effects in humans: contraction of uterus.
- PGD_2 derived particularly from mast cells, acts on DP-receptors. Main effects: vasodilation and inhibition of platelet aggregation.

Prostanoid receptors

Five main prostanoid receptors have been defined, one each for the natural prostanoids, PGD_2, PGF_{2a}, PGI_2 and PGE_2, termed DP-, FP-, IP-, TP- and EP-receptors respectively. It has been further proposed that there are three subgroups of receptors for PGE_2-termed EP_1, EP_2 and EP_3.

Actions of prostanoids

PGD_2 on DP-receptors

- Vasodilatation
- Inhibition of platelet aggregation
- Relaxation of GI muscle
- Uterine relaxation
- Modification of release of hypothalamic/pituitary hormones

Note: Its bronchoconstrictor effect is due to an action on TP receptors.

PGF_{2a} on FP-receptors

- Myometrial contraction in humans
- Luteolysis in some species (e.g., cattle)
- Bronchoconstriction in some species (e.g., cats and dogs)

Note: The receptors involved in PGF_{2a} mediated release of gonadotrophins and prolactin are not yet known.

PGI_2 (prostacyclin) on IP-receptors

- Vasodilatation
- Inhibition of platelet aggregation
- Renin release and natriuresis via effects on tubular reabsorption of Na^+

TXA_2 on TP-receptors

- Vasoconstriction
- Platelet aggregation
- Bronchoconstriction

PGE_2 on EP_1-receptors

- Contraction of bronchial and GI smooth muscle

PGE_2 on EP_2-receptors

- Bronchodilatation
- Vasodilatation
- Relaxation of GI smooth muscle
- Stimulation of interstitial fluid secretion

PGE_2 on EP_3 receptors

- Contraction of intestinal smooth muscle
- Inhibition of gastric acid secretion
- Increase of gastric mucus secretion
- Inhibition of lipolysis

- Inhibtion of autonomic transmitter release
- Stimulation of contraction of the pregnant human uterus

Prostaglandins

They are lipid acids which can be divided into 2 classes according to whether they are extractable by ether (E series) or not (F series). The letter after PG designates the state of the cyclopentane ring and the subscript refers to the number of double bonds in the side chain.

The principal prostaglandins (the '2' series) are formed from arachidonic acid via a cyclic peroxide intermediate, this intermediate can also be converted to thromboxane A_2 formed primarily by platelets which is a potent vasoconstrictor and platelet aggregating agent.

Prostacyclin (PGI_2) synthesized by vessel endothelium is a potent vasodilator and antiaggregating agent.

Prostaglandins are products of arachidonic acid which is most abundant fatty acid released from membrane lipids. Endoperoxides are formed after cyclization of arachidonic acid. Prostaglandins and TXA_2 are derived from endoperoxides.

The prostaglandins, unlike neurotransmitters are synthesized and released only when the occasion demands and they are not stored. Their actions tend to be prolonged.

Prostaglandins have important action as neuromodulators, particularly in the sympathetic nervous system. Stimulation of the ANS releases PGE_2 and PGF_2 alpha from postsynaptic sites; PGE_2 reduces noradrenaline release from sympathetic nerve terminals.

They do not exist free in tissues in appreciable amounts but are biosynthesized and released in response to many varied stimuli.

The major activity of prostaglandins is exerted on uterus, gonads, bronchi, kidney, CVS, platelets, GIT, nervous system, inflammatory and immune mechanisms.

Actions and role

CVS: PGE_2 is vasodilator to most vascular beds. $PGF_{2\alpha}$ constricts larger veins. Both are hypotensives.

Both increase cardiac output and stimulate heart by weak direct and prominent reflex action.

Bronchial muscle: $PGF_{2\alpha}$ and TXA_2 constrict; PGE_2 and PGI_2 dilate.

GIT: PGE_2 reduces acid secretion, produces colic and diarrhoea.

$PGF_{2\alpha}$ and PGI_2 have opposite effects.

Role: The E and F series are present in gut mucosa and control gut movements.

Uterus: PGE_2 and $PGF_{2\alpha}$ contract. Their role is initiation and progression of labour.

Table 13.1 shows the main differences in the activity of PGE_2 and $PGF_{2\alpha}$.

Table 13.1. Comparison between PGE_2 and $PGF_{2\alpha}$

	PGE₂	*PGF₂ₐ*
B.P.	↓ Due to peripheral vasodilation	–
Blood vessels	Dilated	Constricted
Gastric secretion	Inhibition of gastric acid secretion, increase in mucus secretion	–
GIT muscle	Contracts	Contracts
Uterus (non-pregnant)	Relax	Contract
Uterus (in pregnancy)	Contracts	Contracts
Bronchi	Relax	Contract

The plasma half-life of most of the prostaglandins, PGI_2 and TXA_2 is few seconds to few minutes. These are rapidly metabolized in most tissues, fastest metabolism occurs in lungs. These are excreted in urine.

Uses

- Induction of labour and abortion: $PGF_{2\alpha}$ or PGE_2 I.V. or orally induces labour which mimics the events of normal labour, although they are less reliable and their side effects are more than those of oxytocin. They may be used for the therapeutic abortion after the 12th week of pregnancy, they can be administered orally, intravaginally or by injection directly into the uterus (Dinoprostone, prostin E_2 20 mg vaginal suppository).

Dose: PGE_2 2-5 mg; PGF_{2a} (Dinoprost, prostin $PGF_{2\alpha}$ 5 mg/ml).

Some prostaglandins are now synthesized and used as abortifacients. Dinoprost tromethamine ($PGF_{2\alpha}$) is used for abortion between 16th and 20th weeks of gestation. Dinoprostone (PGE_2) is used between 12th and 20th weeks of gestation.

- For bronchodilatation (PGE_1 and PGE_2 by aerosol).
- For inhibition of gastric secretion (PGE_2).
- For vasodilation and diuresis.
- For inhibition of platelet aggregation.
- For erectile dysfunction PGE_1 (Alprostadil) produces relaxation of penile smooth muscle.

Side effects associated with PGE_1: diarrhoea, nausea, vomiting, fever, flushing, hypotension, uterine cramps, CNS irritability.

INDIVIDUAL DRUGS

Dinoprostone

It is an exogenous form of PGE_2. It can be administered i.v., orally, vaginally, intracervically or extraamniotically.

It possesses vasodilator and bronchodilatory effects.

It is used for ripening of the cervix. Its main use is for the induction of labour.

Dose is 0.5 mg tablet repeated hourly (maximum 1.5 mg).

The adverse effects are similar to dinoprost.

Dinoprost

It is exogenous $PGF_{2\alpha}$. It produces contractions of uterus. It is also vasoconstrictor and bronchoconstrictor.

It is mainly used for the termination of pregnancy and for the induction of labour.

The side effects include nausea, vomiting, diarrhoea, headache, flushing, dizziness, hypotension.

Contraindications : It should not be used in patients with history of caesarean section, cephalopelvic disproportion, malpresentation, hypertonic uterine contractions.

Misoprostol

It is a synthetic analogue of PGE_2. It is mainly used in the treatment of peptic ulcers and in prophylaxis of NSAIDs-induced ulcers.

Dose is 200 mcg four times or 400 mcg twice daily in the treatment of peptic ulcer.

The main *side effect* is diarrhoea.

Contraindications : Pregnancy, as it may produce abortion.

Alprostadil

It is an exogenous form of PGE_1. Its main use is to keep ductus arteriosus patent in children till surgery is undertaken.

Gemeprost

It is a synthetic analogue of alprostadil. Its main use is to soften and dilate cervix, to terminate pregnancy in first and second trimester.

It is used in the form of vaginal pessaries, 1 mg pessary in first trimester 3 hours before trying dilatation; for second trimester 1 pessary inserted every hour for termination of pregnancy (maximum 5 doses).

The *side effects* are less as it is given locally.

Carboprost

It is a synthetic analogue of dinoprost but action lasts longer. It is mainly used to control postpartum haemorrhage due to uterine atony; medical termination of pregnancy between 13th and 20th week.

Dose is 250 mcg/ml by deep i.m. injection for the treatment of postpartum haemorrhage (PPH); for medical termination of pregnancy 250 mcg by deep i.m. injection which is followed by 250 mcg after 2-3 hours (maximum 12 mg and not more than 2 days).

Trimoprostil and arbaprostil

These are synthetic analogues of dinoprostone which inhibit gastric acid secretion. The actions and indications are similar to that of misoprostol.

Epoprostenol

It is an exogenous form of prostacyclin (PGI_2). It inhibits aggregation of platelets. It is a vasodilator. The main use is to prevent platelet aggregation during hemodialysis and cardiac bypass. It has also been used in the treatment of peripheral vascular disease.

The *side effects* include hypotension, tachycardia, chest pain, nausea, vomiting, drowsiness and hyperglycaemia.

Ciprostone and iloprost

These are more stable analogues of epoprostenol. These are under investigation.

Inhibitors of PGs, prostacyclin and TXA_2

Aspirin and other nonsteroidal anti-inflammatory agents inhibit synthesis, whereas corticosteroids inhibit release of arachidonic acid from membrane lipids, thus indirectly reduce prostaglandin production.

LEUKOTRIENES : PRODUCTS OF THE LIPOXYGENASE PATHWAYS

The lipoxygenases, soluble enzymes are located in lung, platelets, mast cells and white blood cells. The main enzyme is 5-lipoxygenase which is the first enzyme in the biosynthesis of the leukotrienes 'leuko' as they are found in white cells and 'trienes' because they contain a conjugated triene system of double bonds.

LTB_4 is produced mainly by neutrophils.

LTC_4, LTD_4, LTE_4 and LTF_4 are referred to as the sulphidopeptide leukotrienes. These are cysteinyl - containing leukotrienes. These are mainly produced by eosinophils, mast cells, basophils and macrophages.

LTC_4, LTD_4 and LTE_4 are together known as slow - reacting substance of anaphylaxis (SRS-A).

The leukotriens are mediators of inflammation produced alongwith prostaglandins at site of injury and cause exudation of plasma.

They reduce B.P.; produce coronary constriction and reduce cardiac output.

They contract smooth muscles of GIT and bronchi.

LTC_4 and LTD_4 are mediators of allergic asthma.

Actions and receptors of leukotrienes

LTB_4 acts on specific LTB_4-receptors, transduction mechanism being IP_3 generation. It is a powerful chemotactic agent for both neutrophils and macrophages. On neutrophils, it also causes up regulation of the membrane adhesion molecules and increases the production of toxic oxygen products and the release of granule enzymes. On macrophages and lymphocytes it stimulates proliferation and cytokine release.

Cysteinyl - leukotrienes have specific receptors.

These leukotrienes have actions on:

- Respiratory system: They are potent spasmogens, causing contraction of bronchiolar muscle in vitro. LTE_4 is less potent than LTC_4 and LTD_4 but its effect is longer-lasting. All cause an increase in mucus secretion.
- Cardiovascular system. LTC_4 or LTD_4, given by I.V. route causes a short lived fall in BP and significant constriction of small coronary resistance vessels. Given by SC route, they cause wheal and flare like histamine. On topical use in the nose, LTD_4 increases nasal blood flow and increases local vascular permeability.

Role of leukotrienes in inflammation

LTB_4 can be found in inflammatory exudates and in tissues in many inflammatory conditions, including rheumatoid arthritis, ulcerative colitis and psoriasis (a chronic skin disease).

The cysteinyl-leukotrienes are present in the sputum of chronic bronchitis. In allergic rhinitis, on antigen challenge they are released into nasal lavage fluid. There is evidence that they contribute to the underlying bronchial hyper-reactivity in patients of asthma. It is also thought that they have a role in the cardiovascular changes of acute anaphylaxis.

Platelet-Activating Factor (PAF)

PAF is generated and released from most inflammatory cells when they are stimulated. Thus it is released from neutrophil polymorphs on phagocytosis, from activated macrophages and eosinophils, from mast cells and basophils on interaction with antigen and from platelets on stimulation with thrombin.

PAF is capable of producing local vasodilation resulting in oedema, hyperalgesia and wheal formation, increases vascular permeability, is chemotactic for leukocytes (especially eosinophils) activates and aggregates platelets and is spasmogenic for bronchial and intestinal smooth muscles.

PAF is an important mediator in acute and chronic allergic and inflammatory phenomena and is implicated in bronchial hyper-responsiveness and in the delayed phase of asthma.

General aspects of inflammation

Inflammation is the response of the body to a variety of stimuli, e.g. infection, trauma and allergy.

Inflammation is characterized by a reddening of the area due to vasodilatation, swelling and pain.

The processes involved in inflammation play an important role to attack and destroy the invading microorganisms but sometimes the body's own cells are attacked resulting in damage to tissues. The delicate structures of the eye are particularly susceptible to damage. The ocular inflammation if not treated properly may even produce permanent loss of vision.

The inflammatory response of the body involves the following processes:

- Prostaglandins are produced which have effect on smooth muscle and mediate inflammatory reactions.
- Release of histamine from mast cells is caused by the allergen-antigen reaction.
- Histamine produces pain and itch and also produces increased permeability of the capillaries resulting in loss of cells and proteins. The effect of proteins is to raise the osmotic pressure of the fluid. It causes increased loss of water into the tissues and consequent oedema.
- Vascular effects i.e. vasodilatation and increased capillary permeability are also produced by other locally active agents besides histamine.
- Increased leukocyte activity occurs at the site of inflammation in order to combat the invading cells. These contain lysosomal vacuoles which destroy the cells including the host inflamed cells.

- Fibroblastic activity e.g. fibroblast and collagen forming activity plays role in trauma. It is a part of the inflammatory response to stimulate wound healing. But it can sometimes result in scarring and in the cornea, opacity.
- Neutrophils and monocytes have an important role in defence against invading organisms and in the removal of debris from the site of inflammation. These cells act in part through release of cytokines which are peptides that regulate cell growth, differentiation and activation.
- Cytokines are peptides released from the inflammatory cells. They are also considered as autacoids. They are classified into 5 families.

Interleukins (ILs)

Colony-stimulating factors (CSFs)

Chemokines

Growth factor and tumour necrosis factor (TNF$_\alpha$)

Interferons

Primary pro-inflammatory cytokines are tumour necrosis factor-alpha (TNF-α) and interleukin-1 (IL-1). These are released from macrophages and many other cells and can start a cascade of secondary cytokines among which are the chemokines (a subfamily of cytokines) that attract and activate motile inflammatory cells. Chemokines are subdivided in two groups, viz. Alpha and Beta. The Alpha chemokines, mainly IL-8 act on neutrophils and are involved in acute inflammatory responses. The Beta chemokines, mainly monocyte chemoattractant protein-1 (MCP-1) act on monocytes, eosinophils and other cells and are involved in chronic inflammatory responses.

The anti-inflammatory cytokines include transforming growth factor (TGF-beta), IL-4, IL-10, IL-13. These can inhibit the production of chemokines.

IL-1 and TNF-α are pro-inflammatory cytokines.

Inflammation is usually divided into three phases:
1. Acute inflammation is the initial response to tissue injury mediated by the release of autacoids. This phase precedes the development of immune response.
2. Immune response occurs when immunologically competent cells are activated to foreign invading organisms or antigenic substances are liberated during the acute or chronic inflammatory response. The immune response is beneficial as it causes phagocytosis of the invading organisms. However, if it leads to the development of chronic inflammation without resolution of the injurious process, the outcome of immune response will be deleterious.
3. Chronic inflammation is characterized by the release of a number of mediators which are not prominent in acute inflammation.

The chief mediators of acute inflammation and chronic inflmmation and their effects are listed in Tables 13.2 and 13.3 respectively.

Table 13.2. Chief mediators of acute inflammation

Mediator	Vasodilation	Vascular permeability
Histamine	+	↑↑↑
Serotonin,	+/−	↑
Bradykinin	+++	↑
Prostaglandins	+++	↑
Leukotrines	−	↑↑↑

Table 13.3. Chief mediators of chronic inflammation

Mediator	Primary effects
Interleukins 1, 2 and 3	Lymphocyte activation, prostaglandin production
Granulocyte-macrophage colony-stimulating factor (GM-CSF)	Macrophage and granulocyte activation
Tumour necrosis factor alpha (TNF α)	Prostaglandin production
Interferons	Multiple
Platelet-derived growth factor (PDGF)	Fibroblast chemotaxis proliferation

STUDY QUESTIONS

1. Define autacoids. Which autacoids are (i) amines, (ii) lipid soluble organic acids and (iii) polypeptides. Give suitable examples.
2. How do autacoids differ from hormones?
3. What are the different types of histamine receptors? What are the effects mediated by these receptors?
4. Describe the formation of histamine, its receptors and the effects mediated by H_1 and H_2-receptors.
5. How H_1-receptor antagonists are grouped on chemical basis? Indicate the relative effectiveness and side effects of these groups.
6. What are the actions of histamine on (i) cardiovascular system, (ii) smooth-muscles, (iii) gastric secretion and (iv) skin.
7. Describe the role of histamine in (i) allergy and (ii) inflammation.
8. Describe the mode of action of antihistamines.
9. Describe the absorption, onset and duration of action, metabolism, excretion and routes of administration of antihistamines.
10. What are the actions of antihistamines, as those independent of the antihistaminic action?
11. What are the different uses of antihistamines? Explain the basis of their use.
12. Describe the adverse effects of antihistaminics. Explain how these are caused.
13. Which antihistamines do not cross blood brain barrier? Describe the onset and duration of their action and indications. Do they offer any advantage over the conventional antihistamines?
14. Describe the main sites where 5-HT is present and its role.
15. What are the different actions of serotonin?
16. Write short notes on (i) bradykinin, (ii) leukotrienes and (iii) angiotensin.
17. How are prostaglandins produced in the body? Draw a diagram to explain it.
18. Tabulate the main differences between PGE_2, and PGF_2 alpha.
19. Describe the major activity of prostaglandins exerted on (i) uterus, (ii) gonads, (iii) bronchi, (iv) platelets, (v) GIT, (vi) inflammatory mechanism, (vii) cardiovascular system.
20. Describe the therapeutic uses of prostaglandins and their possible adverse effects.
21. Describe the processes involved in inflammation.
22. List separately the mediators of acute and chronic inflammation.
23. Name different groups of drugs which act as antiinflammatory.
24. Draw a diagram to illustrate various steps that occur in producing inflammation and bronchospasm due to disturbance of cell membrane. Also indicate the site of action of antiinflammatory drugs.

GUIDE TO FURTHER READING

Arrang, J.M. et al: Highly potent and selective ligands for histamine H3-receptors. Nature, 327:117-123; 1987.

Barnes, C.L et al.: A new nonsedating antihistamine. Ann. Pharmacother., 1993; 27:464-470.

Black, J.W et al.: Definition and antagonism of histamine H2-receptors. Nature, 1972; 236:385-390.

Chen, X.S. et al.: Role of leukotrienes revealed by targeted disruption of the 5-lipoxygenasegene. Nature., 1994; 372:179-182.

Dray, A et al.: Bradykinin and inflammatory pain. Trends Neurosci., 1993; 16:99-104.

Farmer, S.G et al.: Effects of a novel nonpeptide bradykinin Beta-2 receptor antagonist on intestinal and airway smooth muscle: further evidence for the tracheal Beta-3 receptor. Br. J. Pharmacol., 1974; 112:461-464.

Food and Drug Administration. FDA reviews antihistamine mouse study. FDA TALKPaper, May 17, 1994.

Gaboury, J.P et al: Mechanisms underlying acute mast cell-induced leukocyte rolling and adhesion in vivo. J. Immunol., 1995; 154:804-813.

Galli, S.J et al: New concepts about the mast cell. N. Engl. J. Med., 1993; 328:257-265.

Gavras, I et al: Bradykinin-mediated effects of ACE inhibition. Kidney Int., 1992; 42:1020-1029.

Geppetti, P et al: Sensory neuropeptide release by bradykinin: mechanisms and pathophysiological implications. Reg. Peptides., 1993; 47:1-23.

Honig, P.K et al: Terfenadine-ketoconazole interaction: pharmacokinetic and electrocardiographic consequences. JAMA, 1993; 269:1513-1518.

Hausknecht, R.U. et al: Methotrexate and misoprostol to terminate early pregnancy. N. Engl. J. Med., 1995; 333:537-540.

Imamura, M et al: Unmasking of activated histamine H3 receptors in myocardial ischemia: their role as regulators of exocytotic norepinephrine release. J. Pharmacol. Exp. Ther., 1994; 271:1259-1266.

Israili, Z.H. et al: Cough and angioneurotic edema associated with angiotensin-converting enzyme inhibitor therapy: a review of the literature and pathophysiology. Ann. Intern Med., 1992; 117:234-242.

Lerner, U.H. et al: Regulation of bone metabolism by the kallikrein-kinin system, the coagulation cascade, and the acute-phase reactants. Oral Surg. Oral Med. Oral Pathol., 1994; 78:481-493.

Linz, W. et al: Role of bradykinin in the cardiac effects of angiotensin-converting enzyme inhibitors. J. Cardiovasc. Pharmacol., 1992; 20 Suppl. 9:S83-S90.

Madeddu, P et al: Receptor antagonists of bradykinin: a new tool to study the cardiovascular effects of endogenous kinins. Pharmacol. Toxicol. Res., 1993; 28:107-128.

Monti, J.E et al: Involvement of histamine in the control of the waking state. Life Sci., 1993; 53:1331-1338.

Patrono, C. et al: Aspirin as an antiplatelet drug. N. Engl. J. Med., 1994; 330:1287-1294.

Pellacani, A et al: Antagonizing and measurement: approaches to understanting of hemodynamic effects of kinins. J. Cardiovasc. Pharmacol., 1992; 20 Suppl. 9:S28-S34.

Piper, P.J. et al: Formation and actions of leukotrienes. Physiol. Rev., 1984; 64:744-761.

Raychowdhury, M.K et al: Alternative splicing produces a divergent cytoplasmic tail in the human endothelial thromboxane A2 receptor. J. Biol. Chem., 1994; 269:19256-19261.

RAPT Investigators. Randomized trial of ridogrel, a combined thromboxane A2 synthase inhibitor and thromboxane A2 prostaglandin endoperoxide receptor antagonist, versus aspirin as adjunct to thrombolysis in patients with acute myocardial infarction. Circulation., 1994; 89:588-595.

Regoli, D et al: Receptors for bradykinin and related kinins: a critical analysis. Can. J. Physiol. Pharmacol., 1993; 71:556-567.

Sale, M.E. et al: The electrocardiographic effects of cetirizine in normal subjects. Clin, Pharmacol. Ther., 1994; 56:295-301.

Sawutz, D.C. et al: The nonpeptide WIN 64338 is a bradykinin B2 receptor antagonist. Proc. Natl. Acad. Sci. U.S.A., 1994; 91:4693-4697.

Schror, K et al: Role of prostaglandins in the cardiovascular effects of bradykinin and angiotensin-converting enzyme inhibitors. J. Cardiovasc. Pharmacol., 1992; 20 Suppl. 9:S68-S73.

Schwartz, L.B et al: Mast cells: function and contents. Curr. Opin. Immunol., 1994; 6:91-97.

Simons, F.E.R. et al: The pharmacology and use of H1-receptor-antagonist drugs. N. Engl. J. Med., 1994; 330:1663-1670.

Spencer, C.M et al: Cetirizine: a reappraisal of its pharmacological properties and therapeutic use in selected allergic disorders. Drugs., 1993; 46:1055-1080.

Thurmond, R.L., Deais, P.J., Dunford, P.F. et al. A potent and selective histamine H_4 receptor antagonist with antiinflammatory properties. J. Pharmacol. Exp. Ther., 2004, 309 : 404-413.

Wachtfogel, Y.T et al: Structural biology, cellular interactions and pathophysiology of the contact system. Thrombosis Res., 1993; 72:1-21.

Waeber, B et al: Hemodynamic effects of a kinin antagonist. J. Cardiovasc. Pharmacol., 1990; 15 Suppl. S78-S82

Woosley, R et al: Analysis of potential adverse drug reactions—a case of mistaken identify. Am. J. Cardiol., 1994; 74:208-209.

CHAPTER
14

Heavy Metals and Heavy-Metal Antagonists

CHAPTER CONTENTS AT A GLANCE

- Manifestations of heavy metal poisoning
  GI disturbances, neuritis, blood disorders
- General principles of treatment
  Identification, maintenance of vital functions and elimination of drug
- Heavy metal antagonists
  Chelating agents, ideal properties of chelators
  Individual chelating agents : BAL, EDTA, penicillamine, desferrioxamine

The environmental metals of great concern are lead, mercury, arsenic, and cadmium.

Although iron is not an environmental poison, accidental intoxication with ferrous salts used to treat iron-deficiency anaemias has frequently resulted in poisoning and so included in this chapter.

Arsenic, mercury, copper and lead inhibit enzyme systems containing sulphydryl group even in low concentrations and thus interfere with cellular metabolism. They also bind to various macromolecules in membranes and cytosol and accumulate in the body because metal complexes are not metabolized.

Manifestations of heavy metal poisoning

- GI disturbances
- Peripheral neuritis
- Blood dyscrasias

General principles of treatment

- Identify the poison
- Maintain vital functions: Airway, circulation, fluid and electrolytes.
- Elimination of drug by gastric lavage, vomiting, forced diuresis, dialysis.

HEAVY METALS

Arsenic

Arsenic is present in soil, water and air. The main source of occupational exposure to arsenic-containing compounds is from the manufacture of arsenical herbicides and pesticides. Fruits and vegetables sprayed with arsenicals may also be a source of arsenic element.

The arsenic atom exists in the elemental form and in trivalent and pentavalent states. Their toxicity is related to rate of clearance from the body, i.e. in the degree of their accumulation in the tissues. In general, toxicity increases in the sequence of organic arsenicals < As^{5+} < As^{3+} < Arsine (AsH_3).

Inorganic preparations are not used clinically but poisoning with arsenious oxide as sodium and calcium arsenates sprinkled in ponds to check mosquito breeding has been reported.

Organic arsenicals are excreted more rapidly than inorganic forms. Pentavalent forms have low affinity for thiol groups and are less toxic than trivalent arsenicals. The mechanism of action of the pentavalent form is related to competitive substitution of arsenate for inorganic phosphate in the formation of adenosine triphosphate, with subsequent formation of an unstable arsenate ester which is rapidly hydrolyzed. Trivalent arsenicals inhibit enzymes containing -SH groups. The pyruvate dehydrogenase system is specially sensitive to trivalent arsenicals.

The toxicological effects of arsenic are manifested on many organ systems

CVS : Small doses of inorganic arsenic produces mild dilatation resulting in occult oedema, particularly facial (mistaken for healthy weight gain or a 'tonic effect'). Larger doses produce capillary dilatation and increased capillary permeability. Myocardial damage and hypotension may occur after prolonged exposure to arsenic. Prolongation of Q-T interval and abnormal T waves may persist for months after recovery from short-term intoxication.

GIT : Trivalent inorganic arsenicals in small doses produce mild splanchnic hyperemia. Large doses produce vesicles under the GI mucosa due to capillary transudation of plasma. These eventually rupture. The patient suffers from watery diarrhoea (rice - water stools). Faeces become bloody. Haematemesis occurs due to the damage of the upper GIT. Stomatitis may also be evident. The onset of GIT symptoms is usually very gradual.

Kidneys : Exposure to arsenic causes severe renal damage affecting renal capillaries, tubules and glomeruli. The patient complains of oliguria with proteinuria and haematuria.

Skin : In short term, there is vesicant effect resulting in necrosis and sloughing. Long term use of low doses of inorganic arsenicals causes cutaneous vasodilatation. Prolonged use causes hyperkeratosis (particularly of palms and soles), and hyperpigmentation of trunk and extremities. Eventually these effects possibly produce cancer.

Nervous system : Both short-and long-term exposure to arsenic can induce encephalopathy. The common neurological lesion is a peripheral neuropathy with a 'stocking-glove' distribution.

Blood : Inorganic arsenicals damage bone marrow. The patient has anaemia with slight-to-moderate leukopenia; eosinophilia is often present.

Organic arsenicals rarely produce serious, irreversible, blood and bone marrow disturbance.

Liver : Inorganic arsenicals are hepatotoxic resulting in fatty infiltration, central necrosis, and cirrhosis.

Carcinogenesis and Teratogenesis : Long-term exposure to arsenic predisposes to intraepidermal carcinoma of the skin as well as lung and liver cancer. Human studies which suggest carcinogenicity of arsenic have involved smelting operations where there is a co-exposure of other potential carcinogens.

Acute Arsenic Poisoning : Gastrointestinal disturbances may be produced within an hour or delayed about 12 hours if food is present in the stomach. The patient complains of difficulty in swallowing, burning sensation in lips, constriction of the throat, gastric pain, severe diarrhoea and projectile vomiting. Oliguria (eventually anuria) with haematuria is present. The patient also complains of severe thirst and marked skeletal muscle cramps. Due to marked loss of fluid, shock appears. There may be hypoxic convulsions, coma and death.

Chronic Arsenic Poisoning : The early symptoms include muscle weakness and aching, skin pigmentation, hyperkeratosis and oedema. Other symptoms are garlic odour of the breath, perspiration, excessive salivation and sweating, lacrimation, sore throat, numbness, dermatitis and alopecia. Subsequent symptoms are like that of coryza. Dermatitis and keratosis of the palms and soles are common. In the fingernails, white transverse lines (Mee's) of deposited arsenic usually appear 6 weeks after exposure. The liver may enlarge and jaundice appears. The hepatotoxicity leads to the development of cirrhosis. Renal damage is also produced. In advanced cases of chronic arsenic poisoning encephalopathy may develop. The bone marrow is damaged by arsenic and affect all haematological elements. Peripheral neuritis usually in legs is present (in contrast lead palsy affects the arms more).

Therapy of Arsenic Poisoning

After short-term exposure to arsenic, attention is directed to the status of the intravascular volume so that hypovolaemic shock does not occur.

Pharmacological support of blood pressure and pressor agents such as dopamine and fluid replacement may be necessary.

Chelation therapy with BAL (3 to 4 mg/kg IM every 4 to 12 hours) until abdominal symptoms subside is given initially and then penicillamine may be given orally for 4 days. Penicillamine is given in 4 divided doses to a maximum of 2 g per day. Succimer, a derivative of BAL (dimercaprol) appears a promising drug in the treatment of arsenic poisoning. However, succimer is approved currently by FDA only for lead chelation in children.

Dialysis may be necessary in case of severe arsenic-induced nephropathy.

Mercury

Mercury has a number of industrial uses (electrical equipments, paints and thermometers etc.). Poisoning from occupational exposure and environmental pollution can produce toxicity of mercury.

Mode of action

Mercury forms covalent bonds with sulphur. This property accounts for the biological properties of the metal. When sulphur is in sulphydryl groups, divalent mercury replaces the hydrogen atom to form mercaptides. Even in low concentrations mercurials inactivate sulphydryl enzymes and thus interferes with cellular metabolism and function.

There are 3 major forms of mercury: mercury vapour (elemental mercury), inorganic and organic mercurial preparations.

The upper limit of a nontoxic concentration of mercury in blood is 3 to 4 μg/dl.

The upper limit for excretion of mercury into urine is 5 μg/L. The concentration of mercury in hair is about 300 times that in blood.

Toxicity

Elemental Mercury: Short term exposure to vapour of elemental mercury produce metallic taste, weakness, chills, nausea, vomiting diarrhoea, dyspepsia, cough, tightness in the chest. Pulmonary toxicity may progress to pneumonitis.

Common features of mercury vapour poisoning are severe salivation and gingivitis. The major manifestations of exposure to mercury vapour are a triad of effects viz. increased excitability, tremor and gingivitis. Long - term exposure to mercury vapour also produces renal dysfunction.

Chronic exposure to mercury vapour produces neurological effects. Tremor and psychological changes (depression, irritability, insomnia, excessive shyness, forgetfulness, emotional instability, and confusion) may appear. Vasomotor disturbances such as excessive perspiration and uncontrolled blushing (together are referred to as erethism) are also produced.

Inorganic salts of mercury (mercuric chloride etc.): These can induce severe acute toxic effects resulting in ashen-gray colour of the mucosa of the mouth and pharynx, vomiting, intestinal pain. Hypovolaemic shock and death may occur unless proper treatment is given.

The systemic effect of inorganic mercury includes a strong metallic taste followed by stomatitis, gingival irritation, foul breath and loosening of the teeth. The most serious effect is renal toxicity.

Organic mercurials (methylmercury etc.): The symptoms include neurological disturbances (visual disturbances such as scotoma and visual-field constriction), ataxia, hearing loss, paresthesias, muscle tremor, mental deterioration and movement disorders. Severe exposure leads to paralysis and death.

Treatment of Mercury Poisoning

Elemental Mercury Vapour: Short-term respiratory support may be necessary. Chelation therapy for inorganic mercury should be initiated immediately.

Inorganic Mercury. After oral exposure, it is important to pay prompt attention to fluid and electrolyte balance and haematological status. Vomiting may be induced if the patient is awake and alert. However, emesis should not be induced in case there is corrosive injury. Emesis has little efficacy if the ingestion of mercury is more than 30 to 60 minutes before the treatment.

Chelation Therapy. Dimercaprol (5 mg/kg IM then 2.5 mg/kg every 12-24 h for 10 days) is indicated for high-level exposure or symptomatic patients. Penicillamine 250 mg orally every 6 hours is indicated for low-level exposure or asymptomatic patients. The new orally effective chelate, succimer is also effective for mercury.

Penicillamine-mercury chelate is excreted only in urine, hence extreme care should be taken in the presence of renal dysfunction. Haemodialysis may become necessary in' patient whose renal function declines.

Organic mercurials (short-chain organic mercurials) have poor reactivity with chelating agents. Dimercaprol is contraindicated, and clinical efficacy of penicillamine is also not impressive in the treatment of methylmercury poisoning (dose is 2 g/d, whereas in inorganic mercury poisoning dose is 1 g/d).

As methylmercury compounds undergo extensive enterohepatic recirculation in experimental animals, hence, a polythiol resin (non-absorbable mercury-binding substance) has been used in human beings. It appears effective.

Lead

It has no therapeutic use, but employed in industries (paints, batteries, rubber, shipyard).

Lead is of toxicological importance. The source may also be from cooking utensils, old water pipes, surma.

Absorption, distribution and excretion

Lead may be absorbed from the gastrointestinal tract and the respiratory system. Adults absorb about 10% of ingested lead, while children absorb upto 40%. Iron deficiency increases intestinal absorption of lead. There is a reciprocal relationship between the dietary content of Ca^{2+} and Pb^{2+} and it seems that they compete for a common transport mechanism.

The absorption of inhaled lead is determined by the form i.e. vapour versus particle, and also with concentration. Almost 90% of inhaled lead particles from ambient air are absorbed.

About 99% of the absorbed lead binds to haemoglobin in erythrocytes in the blood stream and only 1% to 3% of the circulating blood lead is in the serum available to the tissues. Initially the inorganic lead is distributed in the soft tissues, particularly the tubular epithelium of the kidney and in the liver. In time, lead is distributed and deposited in bone, teeth,

and hair. Eventually about 95% is found in bone. Only small amount of inorganic lead accumulates in the brain (mostly in grey matter and basal ganglia).

The half-life of lead in blood is 1 to 2 months, steady state reaches in 6 months. The half-life in bone is 20 to 30 years.

After the steady state is reached, the daily intake of lead approximates the output. The average daily intake of lead is 0.2 mg whereas positive lead balance begins at the daily dose of about 0.6 mg.

This amount ordinarily does not produce overt toxicity within a life time. But if the amount ingested daily is about 2.5 mg of lead, toxic burden is reached in nearly 4 years, daily intake of 3.5 mg produces toxic burden within a few months because deposition in bone is too slow to protect the soft tissues during rapid accumulation.

Acute lead poisoning

It is not common but may occur due to ingestion of acid-soluble lead compounds or inhalation of lead vapours. The symptoms include thirst, metallic taste, nausea, abdominal pain and vomiting. The vomitus may be milky due to presence of lead chloride. Stools are black due to lead sulphide. The patient may suffer from diarrhoea or constipation. In case large quantity of lead is absorbed rapidly, shock develops because of massive loss of gastrointestinal fluid.

Acute symptoms of CNS include paresthesia, pain and muscle weakness. Kidneys are damaged resulting in oliguria. An acute haemolytic crisis may occur which causes severe anaemia and haemoglobinuria. Death may occur in 1 or 2 days, if patient survies, the signs and symptoms of chronic lead poisoning may appear.

Chronic Lead Poisoning (Plumbism)

The **gastrointestinal effects** include anorexia, constipation (diarrhoea occasionally occurs), metallic taste. Severe abdominal pain (lead colic) due to intestinal spasm is a distressing feature. Calcium gluconate given intravenously produces relief of abdominal pain. The **neuromuscular effects** include muscle weakness or palsy. Wrist-drop and, to a lesser extent, foot-drop may occur. The **CNS** effects (lead encephalopathy) is more frequent in children. These include vertigo, ataxia, headache, insomnia, irritability and restlessness, followed by tonic-clonic convulsions. Vomiting and visual disturbances may also be present. **Haematological** effects (when blood lead concentration is near 80 µg/dl) include hypochromic microcytic anaemia due to decreased life span of the erythrocytes and an inhibition of heme synthesis. **Renal effects** are not frequent but some times nephropathy does occur. Clinically a **Fanconi-like syndrome** appears with proteinuria, haematuria and casts in the urine. Hyperuricaemia with gout occurs in the presence of lead nephropathy more frequently as compared to any other type of chronic renal disease. The **other effects** include ashen colour of the face, pallor of lips, poor muscle tone, black, grayish, or black lead line along the gingival margin (due to peridontal deposition of lead sulphide). There is a relationship between the blood level of lead and blood pressure (due to changes in calcium metabolism or renal function). Lead interferes with vitamin D metabolism. Lead-exposed males show decreased sperm count. Renal adenocarcinoma has been reported in several cases in lead workers, although human carcinogenicity of lead is not well established.

Treatment of lead poisoning

Initial treatment for acute phase needs supportive measures. Convulsions are treated with diazepam; cerebral oedema is treated with mannitol and dexamethasone. Chelation therapy is given to the patients who have symptoms of poisoning or in patients with a blood lead level in excess of 50 to 60 µg/dl. For this purpose, four chelators are indicated: edetate calcium disodium ($CaNa_2EDTA$) dimercaprol (BAL), d-penicillamine, and succimer. $CaNa_2EDTA$ and BAL are usually used in combination for lead encephalopathy.

$CaNa_2EDTA$ 30 to 50 mg/kg/daily is given in 2 divided doses by deep IM injection or slow IV infusion for upto 5 consecutive days (maximum total dose 500 mg/kg). The first dose of $CaNa_2EDTA$ should be delayed until 4 hours after the first dose of BAL.

Treatment with $CaNa_2EDTA$ produces relief from colic within 2 hours, paresthesia and tremor cease after 4 or 5 days, and gingival lead lines tend to decrease in 4 to 9 days.

Dimercaprol, 4 mg/kg is given IM every 4 hours

for 2 days, then every 6 hours for next 2 days and then every 6 to 12 hours for an additional 7 days.

d-penicillamine, 250 mg orally, four times daily for 5 days.

Succimer, 10 mg/kg every 8 hours for 5 days, then every 12 hours for an additional 2 weeks. It is orally active lead chelator available for children. It is more effective and safer than d-penicillamine.

Cadmium

Cadmium occurs in nature in association with zinc and lead. The extraction and processing of these metals often lead to environmental contamination with cadmium.

Cadmium is used in electroplating and in galvanization. It is also used in plastics, paint pigments and nickel-cadmium batteries. Coal and other fossil fuels contain cadmium, their combustion releases cadmium in the environment.

Those who are employed in smelters and other metal-processing industries are likely to be exposed to high concentration of cadmium in the air; for most of the population exposure to contaminated food is important. When foods such as rice and wheat are contaminated by cadmium in soil and water the metal concentration may be as high as 1 µg/g. Shellfish and animal liver and kidney may have cadmium concentration more than 0.05 µg/g. Cigarette smoking contributes significantly to cadmium intake. One cigarette contains 1 to 2 µg of cadmium and even with 10% pulmonary absorption, the smoking of one pack of cigarettes per day will produce a dose of about 1 mg of cadmium per year from smoking alone.

The half-life of cadmium in the body is 10 to 30 years.

Acute cadmium poisoning

The symptoms after oral intake include nausea, vomiting, diarrhoea, abdominal cramps. Cadmium is more toxic when inhaled and the signs and symptoms include chest pain, diarrhoea, dizziness, nausea, irritation of respiratory tract with severe pneumonitis. The toxicity may progress to fatal pulmonary oedema.

Chronic Cadmium Poisoning

The toxicity of long-term exposure to cadmium

produces kidney damage, dyspepsia, osteomalacia, testicular necrosis, and loss of ventilatory capacity in lungs. The effect of cadmium on the cardiovascular system is its role in hypertension (however, it is controversial). Epidemiological studies indicate that cadmium is a human carcinogen (more of the lungs and prostate, and to a lesser extent, kidney and stomach).

Treatment of cadmium poisoning

The patient must be removed from the source. Respiratory support and steroids may be necessary. Some recommend chelation therapy with $CaNa_2EDTA$, 75 mg/kg/o/d in 3 to 6 divided doses for 5 days (maximum not to excess 500 mg/kg per 5-day course). The use of dimercaprol appears promising in the treatment of chronic cadmium poisoning.

HEAVY METAL ANTAGONISTS

These are chelating agents. These agents bind metal ions, form stable, non-toxic complexes which are excreted by the kidneys. These are metal binding antidotal chemicals which bind the ions of heavy metals and render them biologically inactive. The process of complex formation is called chelation, 'chele', (Greek word) means 'claw'.

Chelate formation occurs when the legend forms coordination bonds with a central metal ion at more than one site (usually two sites are involved).

Properties of ideal chelating agent: It should be water soluble, resistant to metabolic degradation, able to retain chelating activity at pH of body fluids. Molecular structure and size should be such that will permit penetration to metal binding sites, storage sites and excretion, i.e. capable of distribution throughout the body, and readily excreted in urine. Chelates should be nontoxic, having low affinity for Ca to prevent hypocalcaemia.

However, no chelating agent is specific for a particular metal ion. All can remove Ca, and must be used quickly as prolonged exposure of the cell to metallic ions causes irreversible loss of enzymatic activity.

Therapeutic uses: Chelating agents are used mainly in the treatment of poisoning by heavy metals, cyanides, organophosphorus insecticides or in treating various physiological disorders like hypercalcaemia, iron storage disease, and Wilson's disease.

Main chelating agents

- Dimercaprol (BAL) chelates mercury, gold, antimony and lead.
- Ethylenediamine tetraacetic acid (EDTA, edetate) chelates calcium and lead.
- Penicillamine (Cuprimine) chelates copper.
- Desferrioxamine chelates iron.

Dimercaprol (British Anti-Lewisite, BAL)

It is a clear oily liquid with a pungent disagreeable odour. It is unstable in aqueous solutions and therefore peanut oil is the solvent used in pharmaceutical preparations. It is readily oxidized. It is effective against As, Hg, Au, Bi, Ni, Sb and Pb.

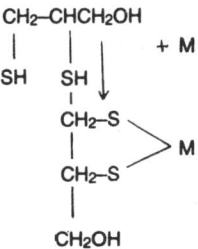

Fig. 14.1. BAL metal complex.

The chelate is excreted in urine.

Mechanism of action

Dimercaprol forms chelation complexes between its sulphydryl groups and metals. With metals like mercury, gold and arsenic, a stable complex is produced which is eliminated. However, the bond is labile in the acidic tubular urine which may increase the renal toxicity. Therefore concentration of dimercaprol in the plasma should be adequate to favour continuous formation of the more stable 2 : 1 (BAL : Metal) complex (Fig. 14.1) and its rapid excretion. This is maintained by repeated fractional dosage. Effect is more when given soon after exposure to metal.

Dimercaprol cannot be given orally. It is administered by deep IM injection as a 100 mg/ml solution in peanut oil. The half-life is short, metabolism and excretion occur in 4 hours.

Dose: 3-5 mg/kg deep I.M. injection 1-4 times a day.

Cal. disod. edetate is more effective than BAL in lead poisoning.

It is *contraindicated* in patients who are allergic to peanuts or peanut products. It is also not given in the presence of hepatic dysfunction except when it is due to arsenic poisoning.

Adverse effects may be produced in about 50% of patients who are administered 5 mg/kg intramuscularly. The adverse effects include pain at the site of injection, rise in both systolic and diastolic blood pressures along with tachycardia. The other side effects include nausea, vomiting, abdominal pain, feeling of constriction and pain in the chest, sterile painful abscess at the site of injection. Some times the patient complains of salivation, lacrimation, blepharospasm, sweating of forehead and hands. There may be unrest and feeling of anxiety. High doses lead to convulsions and coma.

Succimer

It is chemically similar to BAL which is an orally effective chelating agent useful in lead poisoning. It induces lead diuresis. It does not mobilize iron, copper and zinc.

Succimer is less toxic than BAL.

Adverse effects include anorexia, nausea, vomiting, diarrhoea. The drug should be discontinued if rashes appear.

EDTA (Ethylene diamine tetraacetic acid) and derivatives

EDTA is insoluble in water, hence not used therapeutically.

Disodium edetate is used for topical application for lime burns in eyes.

Cal. disod. edetate is primarily for Pb poisoning; it has strong affinity for Ca and Pb, more for Pb. Due to poor absorption from gut it is given intravenously.

It has insignificant effect against Zn, Cu.

It is ineffective for Hg, As, Au.

Dose: Not to exceed 50 mg/kg/d for adults and 30 mg/kg/d for children. Intramuscular injection

results in good absorption but causes pain at the injection site, so it is mixed with a local anaesthetic or given by slow intravenous drip by diluting in either 5% dextrose or 0.9% saline.

Adverse effects of EDTA

Rapid intravenous administration of Na_2EDTA causes hypocalcaemic tetany.

The principal toxic effect of $CaNa_2EDTA$ is on the kidney, eventually leading to degeneration of proximal tubular cells. Changes in distal tubule and glomeruli are less conspicuous.

The other side effects include malaise, fatigue excessive thirst, chills myalgia, frontal headache, anorexia, nausea and vomiting. Other possible undesirable effects include sneezing, nasal congestion and lacrimation, glycosuria, transitory lowering of B.P. and inversion of T wave of ECG.

Dicobalt edetate is useful in cyanide poisoning. The cobalt cyanide complex is nontoxic and stable.

Adverse effects include cobalt toxicity (chest pain, hypertension). The other adverse effects include sneezing, chills, muscle pain.

Dose: 1 g in 250-500 ml of 5% dextrose solution I.V. drip twice a day.

Penicillamine (Cuprimine)

It is a synthetic sulphydryl compound, inactive degradation product of penicillin.

It is effective in Cu, Zn, Fe, Hg, Pb and As poisoning.

It does not chelate Ca. It is well absorbed from gut. Antacids and iron reduce its absorption. Most of it is degraded by biotransformation in liver and very little is excreted in an unchanged form. The chelate is excreted by kidneys.

Dose: 250 mg capsule. The usual adult dose is 1-1.5 g per day in four divided doses. It should be given on empty stomach to avoid interference by metals in food.

Penicillamine is also used for the treatment of 'Wilson's disease. 'Wilson's disease (hepatolenticular disease due to an excess of copper), rheumatoid arthritis, cystinuria and scleroderma.

Penicillamine copper chelate is shown in Fig. 14.2.

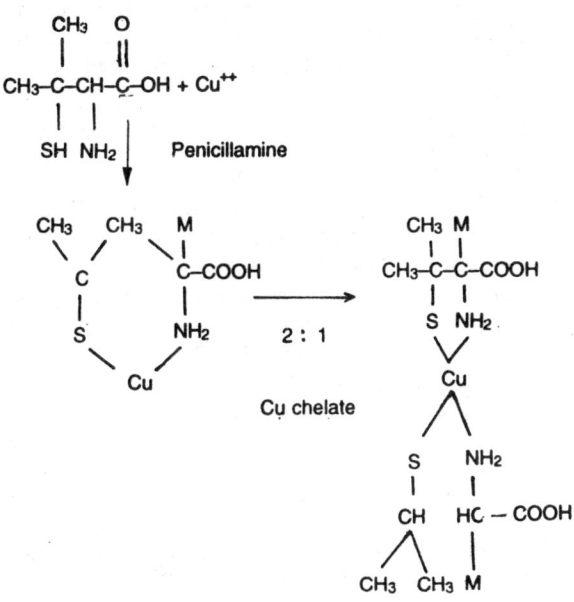

Fig. 14.2. Penicillamine copper chelate.

Box 14.1. Antidotes for heavy metal intoxication

Toxicant	Antidote
Arsenic	BAL
Antimony	BAL
Copper	Penicillamine
Gold	BAL
Iron	Deferoxamine
Lead	CaNa$_2$EDTA (Calcium disodium ethylene diamine tetraacetic acid), Penicillamine
Mercury	BAL
Zinc	Penicillamine
Nickel	BAL

Adverse effects of penicillamine for short term use as a chelating agent include anaphylactic reaction in patients allergic to penicillin. With long-term use, penicillamine produces cutaneous lesions. The haematological system may also be involved (leukopenia, aplastic anaemia, and agranulocytosis). Renal toxicity may also be induced (haematuria, proteinuria, nephrotic syndrome). Toxicity to the pulmonary system is not common. However, severe dyspnoea has been reported. Long-term therapy of penicillamine can induce myasthenia gravis.

Less serious side effects include nausea, vomiting, diarrhoea, dyspepsia, loss of appetite and a transient loss of taste for sweet and salt.

Contraindications

- Renal insufficiency
- Previous history of penicillamine induced reactions

Acetyl D-penicillamine

It is highly effective in mercury poisoning. Although it is less potent but also less toxic. The dose is 1 gm daily in 3-4 divided doses for 10 days.

Trientine

It has been found useful in patients who develop unwanted effects due to penicillamine. It is less potent than penicillium. The dose is 400 mg thrice a day orally. It may cause iron deficiency.

It has been reported to produce teratogenic effect in rats.

Treatment of acute and chronic iron toxicities

Stomach wash with 5% sodium bicarbonate solution; 8-12 g desferrioxamine is left in stomach by gastric tube and in severe cases 2 g i.v. twice a day (maximum 80 mg/kg in 24 hours) may be administered.

Desferrioxamine (Deferoxamine)

Desferrioxamine is obtained from streptomyces pilosus, is a potent and specific chelator of iron. It readily binds ferric iron to form ferrioxamine, a stable and water soluble chelate.

Desferrioxamine has 30 times more affinity for iron than for calcium. It has been found useful in the treatment of iron overload in thalassaemia (transfusion haemosiderosis). Iron in haemoglobin or cytochromes is not removed by deferoxamine. It has been used for chelation of aluminium in dialysis patients.

Dose: It is poorly absorbed after oral adminis-tration. For severe toxicity (serum iron > 500 mcg/dl), 10-15 mg/kg per hour is administered by constant intravenous infusion. In moderately toxic cases (serum iron 350-500 mcg/dl) a dose of 50 mg/kg with a maximum of 1g is given intramuscularly. For chronic intoxication (e.g. in thalassaemia) i.m. dose of 0.5-1.0 g/day is given. Blood transfusion is done with addition of 2.0 g deferoxamine per unit of blood by slow i.v. infusion.

Contraindications to the use of deferoxamine include renal dysfunction and pregnancy.

Deferiprone is under clinical investigation. It may be valuable in cases of thalassaemia major who are either unable to obtain or unwilling to use deferoxamine.

Adverse effects: GIT irritation, pruritus, skin rashes, anaphylaxis, hypotension, tachypnoea, hypoxemia, fever, eosinophilia, pain at the site of injection, and tachycardia.

A 'pulmonary syndrome' is produced by high doses (10-25 mg/kg per hour).

STUDY QUESTIONS

1. What are the general toxic effects of heavy metal poisoning?
2. Describe the general principles of treatment of heavy metal poisoning.
3. Describe the manifestations which are particularly produced by (i) mercury, (ii) arsenic, (iii) lead and (iv) iron poisoning.
4. What are the properties of an ideal chelating agent? What do you understand by chelate formation?
5. Name clinically used chelating agents. Describe the effectiveness and adverse effect of each of them.

GUIDE TO FURTHER READING

Alder F.H. et al: Pathologic study of ocular lesions due to lewisite (Beta-Chlorovinyldichloroarsine), Arch Ophthalmol, 1947; 38:89.

Ames, B.N et al: Ranking possible carcinogenic hazards. Science 1987; 236:271.

Baghurst, P.A et al: Environmental exposure to lead and children's intelligence at the age of seven years. The Port Piric Cohort Study. N.Engl.J.Med., 1992; 327:1279-1284.

Bell, C.L et al: The safety of administration of penicillamine to penicillin-sensitive individuals. Arthritis Rheum., 1983; 26:801-803.

Bellinger, D.C et al: Low-level lead exposure, intelligence and academic achievement: a long-term follow-up study. Pediatrics, 1992; 90:855-861.

Breinin G.M. et al: Chelation of calcium with edathamil calcium-disodium in band keratopathy and corneal calcium affection, Arch Ophthalmol, 1978; 10:355.

Clarkson, T.W et al: Metal toxicity in the central nervous system. Environ. Health Perspect., 1987; 75:59-64.

Eley, B.M et al: The release, absorption and possible health effects of mercury from dental amalgam: a review of recent findings. Br. Dent. J., 1993; 175:355-362.

Jarup, L et al: Arsenic exposure, smoking and lung cancer in smelter workers—a case-control study. Am. J. Epidemiol., 1992; 136:1174.

Lerda, D: Study of sperm characteristics in persons occupationally exposed to lead. Am. J. Industr. Med., 1992; 22:567-571.

Needleman, H.L et al: The long-term effects of exposure to low doses of lead in childhood: an 11 year follow-up report. N. Engl. J. Med., 1990; 322:83-88.

Olivieri, N.F et al: Iron-chelation therapy with oral deferiprone in patients with thalassaemia major. N. Engl. J. Med., 1995; 332:918-922.

Proctor, N.H et al: Chemical Hazards of the Workplace, 3rd ed. Lippincott, 1991.

Sarnet, J.M et al: The environment and the lung. JAMA, 1991; 266:670.

Schroeder, H.A et al: Cadmium as a factor in hypertension. J. Chronic Dis., 1965; 18:647-656.

Waalkes, M.P et al: Toxicological principles of metal carcinogenesis with special emphasis on cadmium. Crit. Rev. Toxicol., 1992; 22:175-201.

Wise J.B. et al: Treatment of experimental siderosis bulbi, vitreous hemorrhage and corneal bloodstaining with deferoxamine, Arch Ophthalmol, 1966; 75:698.

15

Nonmetallic Environmental Toxicants

Exposure to higher doses of chemicals in the environment can damage health.

The toxic effects of air pollutants, solvents and vapours, and pesticides are described in this chapter.

AIR POLLUTANTS

These are carbon monoxide, sulphur oxides, hydrocarbons, particulate matter and nitrogen oxides.

There are two kinds of pollution based on chemical nature: (i) reducing type of pollution characterized by sulphur dioxide and smoke from incomplete combustion of coal (ii) oxidizing type of pollution characterized by hydrocarbons, oxides of nitrogen, and photochemical oxidants. It is caused by automobile exhaust. Particulates, especially combustive adsorb gases or vapours and become more harmful.

Deposition of Toxicants by the Lungs

Particles of 5 μ or larger in diameter are usually deposited in the upper airways. Smaller particles of 1 to 5 μ are deposited in the terminal airways or alveoli.

Particles less than 1 μ in diameter remain suspended in the inhaled air and reach the alveolar zone of the lung, where they may be readily absorbed. The surface area of the alveolar zone is 50 to 100 M^2 the rate of blood flow is high; and the blood is in close proximity to the alveolar air (10 μ). These factors influence absorption.

Health Effects of Air Pollution

Acute effects on health are associated with the reducing type of pollution. There is less evidence to associate photochemical oxidant pollution with such effects on human health, there are significant correlations between levels of oxidants in the air and hospital admissions for allergic disorders, inflammatory diseases of the eye, acute upper respiratory infection, influenza, and bronchitis.

Ozone

Ozone (O_3) is an oxidant found in high concentrations in polluted atmosphere. Ozone is an irritant to lungs which causes chronic bronchitis, fibrosis, and emphysematous changes. The pulmonary injury due to ozone is due to the formation of reactive free-radical intermediates.

Nitrogen dioxide

It is a lung irritant that may cause pulmonary oedema, and other changes like those produced by ozone.

Aldehydes

Aldehydes are released as a result of incomplete combustion e.g. automobile exhaust, or by oxidation of hydrocarbons by sunlight.

About 50% of the aldehyde in polluted air is formaldehyde (HCHO) and about 5% is acrolein ($H_2C=CHCHO$).

Formaldehyde is irritant to the mucous membranes of nose, throat and eyes.

Acrolein is more irritating than formaldehyde.

Carbon monoxide (CO)

It is a colourless, tasteless, odourless and nonirritating gas.

The automobile exhaust system is the greatest source of CO. The other source of exposure to CO is smoking, and inadequate ventilation in houses.

Reaction of CO with haemoglobin

Carbon monoxide combines with the haemoglobin forming carboxyhaemoglobin (COHb) which is incapable for carrying on the usual oxygen transport. When 20% of Hb is thus combined, it results in headache and dizziness. With 40% combined produces collapse, with 60% combined leads to coma. High proportions of combined pigment is fatal. Carboxyhaemoglobin is a red pigment and cherry red, flushing of the skin may be a helpful diagnostic sign.

Affinity of carbon monoxide for Hb is 200-300 times greater than the affinity of O_2 for Hb hence exposure to CO concentration of as low as 0.1% can be fatal in about 2 hours.

CO is dangerous even at a very low concentration. 0.1% CO in air would result in about 50% carboxyhaemoglobinaemia as air contains 21% oxygen by volume.

CO toxicity

The toxicity is characterized by hypoxia. The maximum effects are observed on brain and heart as these organs need greatest oxygen demand. These organs are most sensitive to oxygen deprivation. The lesions are predominantly haemorrhagic. Severe headache is due to cerebral oedema and increased intracranial pressure. Ischaemic changes in heart have been reported.

The toxicity of CO is not due solely to the interference of CO with the delivery of oxygen by the blood. It also exerts a direct effect by binding to cellular cytochromes such as those in respiratory enzymes and myoglobin.

Signs and symptoms of CO toxicity

There is significant variation among individuals. There may be warning signs e.g. transient weakness and dizziness before consciousness is lost, but in others there may be no warning. In general, upto 10% of blood saturation with COHb does not produce any symptom, 10%-20% produce mild headache, dilatation of skin blood vessels, 20%-30% produces throbbing headache, 30%-40% produces severe headache, dizziness, dimness of vision, nausea, vomiting, collapse, 40%-50% increases respiratory rate and pulse rate, and there is possibility of syncope, 50%-60% results in syncope, coma, convulsions, 60%-70% leads to coma and possible death, 70%-80% causes respiratory failure and death.

The patient is cyanotic and pale and there is presence of COHb in the blood in case of acute CO poisoning.

Toxicity of prolonged and low-level exposure to CO

At 6%-12%, COHb metabolism shifts from aerobic to anaerobic.

When COHb is as low as 2%-5% vigilance is impaired but other behaviors are not affected (driving, reaction time, coordination, sensory processes and complex intellectual tasks).

CO crosses placenta. Persistent low levels of COHb in the foetus of a woman who has smoked during pregnancy may have effects on the development of CNS and display neurological sequelae.

Treatment

COHb is fully dissociable and once acute exposure is terminated CO is excreted via the lungs. Only a very small amount is oxidized to carbon dioxide.

CO cannot be excreted without active respiration.

The patients should be transferred to fresh air. If respiration has failed artificial respiration must be given.

Oxygen 100% reduces half-life of COHb from 5 hours to 1 hour. If poisoning is severe, hypobaric oxygen therapy at a pressure of 2-3 atm will reduce the half-life of COHb to 20 minutes. Oxygen should be given until the level of COHb decreases to at least 10%.

Supplementary care includes correction of hypotension and metabolic acidosis, and cardiac effects.

Generally, air pollution is associated with the contamination of air from automobile exhausts and industrial effluents. However, in developing countries, the problem of indoor air pollution is also important. There are four principal sources of pollutants of indoor air: (i) combustion, (ii) building material, (iii) the ground under the building, and (iv) bioaerosols. In developing countries the most important indoor air pollutants are the combustion products of unprocessed solid biomass fuels used by the poor urban and rural folk for cooking and heating.

A recent report of the World Health Organization (WHO) asserts the rule of 1000 which states that a pollutant released indoors is one thousand times more likely to reach people's lung than a pollutant released outdoors.

It has been estimated that more than half world's households cook their food on the unprocessed solid fuels that typically release at least 50 times more noxious pollutants than gas.

The fuels are not burned completely. The incomplete combustion of biomass releases complex mixture of organic compounds, which include suspended particulate matter, carbon monoxide, poly organic material (POM), poly aromatic hydrocarbons (PAH), formaldehyde, etc. The biomass may also contain intrinsic contaminants such as sulphur, trace metals etc.

Indoor air pollution caused by burning traditional fuels such as dung, wood and crop residues causes considerable damage to the health of particularly women and children. There is evidence associating the use of biomass fuel with acute respiratory tract infections, chronic obstructive lung diseases, and pneumoconiosis.

Radiation exposures

Doses of the order of 50,000 rads are followed by immediate injury and death due to damage to the CNS.

Exposure to about 1000 rads leads to death in several days due to loss of gut epithelium.

Total body irradiation with several hundred rads is followed by profound effects on the haematopoietic system with death in 2-4 weeks.

Smaller doses of 100 rads or less cause only acute symptomatology and may have long term effects such as cataracts, decreased life span or increased incidence of degenerative disease, tumours, long after the initial radiation insult.

Protection against radiation injury is difficult, some success may be achieved with SH-containing compound e.g. mercapto- ethylamine and cysteine in high almost toxic doses.

Cigarette smoke

Nicotine, CO, tars containing known carcinogenic hydrocarbons are related to cancer of lungs and larynx, mouth, oesophagus and urinary bladder. It is the most important cause of chronic bronchitis, has causative relation to pulmonary emphysema; also associated with peptic ulcer and myocardial infarction. Women who smoke during pregnancy have babies with smaller birth weights.

SOLVENTS AND VAPOURS

Aliphatic hydrocarbons

C1-C4 aliphatic hydrocarbons with 4 or fewer carbon

atoms are present in natural gas (methane, ethane) and in bottled gas (propane, butane). These are 'simple asphyxiants'.

C5-C8 aliphatic hydrocarbons like most organic solvents e.g. hexane depress CNS, produce polyneuropathy, symmetrical sensory dysfunction of the distal portions of the extremities.

Gasoline and kerosene

These contain aliphatic, aromatic, and a variety of branched and unsaturated hydrocarbons.

Intoxication by ingestion of gasoline and kerosene resembles that from ethanol. There is restlessness, confusion, excitement, ataxia, disorientation, delirium and finally unconsciousness.

There may be ventricular fibrillation as gasoline vapours sensitize the myocardium such that even small quantity of adrenaline in the circulation may precipitate this condition.

High concentration if inhaled over hours, may produce pneumonia.

High concentration depress CNS and death results due to respiratory arrest.

Treatment

Symptomatic and supportive care must be provided to the patients.

Gastric lavage or emesis should be avoided (to avoid aspiration).

Adrenaline and related substances should be avoided as they may induce cardiac arrhythmias.

Purgatives may be given with magnesium or sodium sulphate.

Antibiotics are indicated for the treatment of bacterial pneumonitis (if present).

Imbalance of fluid and electrolytes should be corrected.

Halogentated hydrocarbons

Carbon tetrachloride, chloroform, dichloromethane trichloro- ethane, tetrachloroethylene produce CNS depression, and sensitize the myocardium to catecholamines.

1,1,2-trichloroethane and chloroform have highest hepatotoxicity potential, whereas in case of trichloroethylene, tetrachloroethylene, 1,1,1- trichloroethane and dichloromethane hepatotoxicity potential is least.

Aromatic hydrocarbons

Benzene

Even short exposure to large amount by ingestion or by breathing is very toxic particularly on the CNS.

If there is mild exposure, euphoria, dizziness, nausea, vomiting, headache, tightness in chest are the usual complaints.

If exposure is severe, it produces blurred vision, tremors, rapid and shallow respiration, paralysis and coma.

The long term exposure produces drowsiness, pallor, anorexia, and headache. But the major toxic effect is aplastic anaemia and there is also danger of leukaemia.

Toluene

It is used as a solvent in paints, glues, and varnishes.

It produces CNS depression. However, unlike benzene it does not produce aplastic anaemia or leukaemia.

Pesticide Pollution

The term pesticide covers a wide range of compounds including insecticides, fungicides, herbicides, rodenticides and others. Among these, organo-chlorine (OC) insecticides are banned or restricted after 1960s. The other synthetic insecti-cides - organophosphate (OP) insecticides in the 1960s, carbamates in 1970s and pyrethroids in 1980s and the introduction of herbicides and fungicides in 1970s - 1980s helped greatly to achieve pest control and enhance agricultural output.

Ideally a pesticide must be lethal to the targeted pests, but not to non-target species, including man. Unfortunately, this is not so the use and abuse of these chemicals under the adage, "if little is good, a lot more will be better" has played havoc with human and other life forms.

Acute Pesticide Poisoning

Pesticides are toxic chemicals and as such they represent risks to the users.

Muscarinic manifestations such as vomiting

(96%), nausea (82%), miosis (64%), excessive salivation (61%) and blurred vision (54%) and CNS manifestation such as giddiness (93%), headache (84%), disturbances in consciousness (44%) were the major presenting symptoms.

Cardiac manifestations such as sinus tachycardia (25%), sinus bradycardia (6%) have also been observed.

INSECTICIDES

Organochlorine insecticides

These include DDT which is the most commonly used chlorinated ethane derivative (also known as chlorophenothane).

High doses of DDT cause paresthesias of the tongue, lips, and face, irritability, dizziness, tremors and convulsions.

The use of DDT has decreased now in many countries.

Another chlorinated ethane derivative is methoxychlor which has replaced DDT because it is less toxic than DDT.

This compound is not carcinogenic.

It is stored in adipose tissue to about 0.2% of the extent of DDT. It has shorter half-life.

Chlorinated cyclodienes (aldrin, heptachlor, chlordane) produce symptoms of poisoning like those of DDT.

Unlike DDT, cyclodiene insecticides have resulted in many fatalities due to acute poisoning. They are stored in adipose tissues and have carcinogenic potential.

Other chlorinated hydrocarbons

These include lindane, toxaphene, and chlordecone. They possess many properties which are similar to those of DDT.

The signs of poisoning of lindane are ataxia, tremors, and violent convulsions.

Toxaphene

Its major toxicity is stimulation of the CNS.

Chlordecone

It produces stimulation of the CNS and hepatic injury. It has oestrogenic effects which is responsible for testicular atrophy and reduced production of sperms. It is carcinogenic in laboratory animals.

Organophosphorus Insecticides

These have largely replaced the chlorinated hydrocarbons. These have very low carcinogenic potential, but higher acute toxicity in human beings.

The manifestations are colic, salivation, diarrhoea, tightness in chest due to bronchoconstriction, fall in blood pressure, tachycardia, respiratory paralysis, convulsions, coma, and death.

Treatment

Gastric lavage, atropine 2 mg i.v./10 min till pupils dilate, maximum 50 mg.

Pralidoxime 1 g i.v. is started early.

Insecticides used against ectoparasites

Ectoparasites are animal parasites.

Lindane is a miticide employed to treat scabies, as 1% cream, lotion, or shampoo as a thin layer which is not removed for 8 to 12 hours. If needed, second or third applications are made at weekly intervals.

This drug is also very useful in the treatment of pediculosis pubis, capitis, and corporis. It is also used (a single application of 1% lotion, or cream is sufficient) to treat the infestation by phthirum pubis (crab lice).

Malathion is an organophosphate insecticide. It is a very effective pediculocidal and niticidal, lice and their eggs (nits) are killed within 3-4 seconds b;y 0.003% and 0.06% malathion in acetone, respectively. For the treatment of head lice and nits it is gently applied onto the scalp and left for 8-12 hours, after that hair is shampooed. If necessary, second application is made after about a week.

Benzyl benzoate 26%-30% lotion is used in the treatment of scabies and also for pediculosis.

Crotamiton is an effective scabicide.

Thiabendazole can be applied on the skin for the treatment of cutaneous larva migrans. It has scabicidal activity. It also has mild antifungal activity.

Botanical Insecticides

Pyrethrum is a crude extract obtained from flowers of the pyrethrum plant, chrysanthemum cincerariae folium. Pyrethrin is a refined extract containing the six naturally occurring pyrethrins.

Pyrethrin 1 contains the maximum activity.

Pyrethroids are synthetic pyrethrin derivatives.

Pyrethrum is a very safe insecticide as its toxicity is low. However, the allergenic properties are marked. Preparations containing pyrethrins or synthetic pyrethroids are less allergenic than pyrethrum.

Rotenone is obtained from the roots of plants such as Derris and Lonchocarpus. It is applied directly to head lice, scabies, and other ectoparasites.

Local effects include pharyngitis, rhinitis, dermatitis, and conjunctivitis.

If ingested orally, it produces gastrointestinal irritation, nausea, and vomiting.

Its inhalation is more harmful, causes respiratory stimulation followed by depression and convulsions.

Human poisoning by rotenone is rare.

Nicotine is a very powerful insecticide. Its ganglionic stimulant property induces salivation and vomiting; due to stimulation followed by depression of the neuromuscular junction, there is muscular weakness and the effects on the CNS are manifested by convulsions and respiratory collapse.

RODENTICIDES

Warfarin as an oral anticoagulant (Chapter 7) is a very frequently used rodenticide. Daily intake of 1-2 mg/kg for 6 days can produce severe illness in humna beings.

Red squill

The selective rodenticidal usefulness is due to the inability of rats to vomit.

The active principles scillaren glycoside obtained from the bulbs of red squill (Urginea maritima) if injected in large doses will induce vomiting, abdominal pain, blurred vision, cardiac arrhythmias, convulsions and death from ventricular fibrillation. These glycosides like the digitals glycosides have cardiotonic effect. The treatment of overdoses is the same as for digitalis toxicity.

Sodium fluoroacetate

It is one of the most potent rodenticide and produces its toxic action by inhibiting citric acid cycle.

The signs and symptoms of poisoning are nausea and vomiting, cardiac arrhythmias, cyanosis, convulsions and death due to ventricular fibrillation or respiratory arrest.

Provision of large quantities of acetate appears to antagonize fluoro-acetate in a competitive manner, monkeys have been successfully protected from fluoroacetate poisoning by giving glycerol mono-acetate.

Strychnine

It is the main alkaloid present in the seeds of Strychnos nuxvomica tree.

In human beings, the first effect noticed is stiffness of the muscles of face and neck. Any sensory stimulus provoks a violent motor response. In later stages there is tetanic convulsions (body is arched in hyperextension i.e. opisthotonos so that only the head and heels touch the ground. Death results from medullary paralysis.

Treatment

Prevention of convulsions by administration of diazepam.

Anaesthesia or neuromuscular blockade will be required to control resistant convulsions.

Respiration must be supported including intubation and mechanical assistance.

All forms of sensory stimulation must be minimized.

Phosphorus

If ingested in human beings, it produces severe gastrointestinal irritation and if the dose is large the patient dies within 24 hours due to haemorrhage and cardiovascular collapse. The vomitus is luminescent and has garlic odour. The delayed sequelae of phosphorus poisoning is acute yellow atrophy of the liver that may be fatal.

Zinc phosphide

The gas phosphine is liberated due to the reaction of zinc phosphide with water and hydrochloric acid in the GIT. Phosphine gas produces severe gastrointestinal irritation. The signs and symptoms of toxicity resemble poisoning by yellow elemental phosphorus.

α-Naphthylthiourea

It has selective rodenticidal properties, the principal toxic effect in susceptible species is marked pulmonary oedema and pleural effusion.

Thallium Sulphate

It is very toxic. Acute poisoning leads to motor paralysis and death due to respiratory failure. However, small doses (sublethal doses), if taken over a period of time, produce alopecia, redness of skin, degenerative changes in the brain, liver and kidney, tremors, leg pains, polyneuritis in the legs and paresthesias of the hands and feet. Psychosis, convulsions and delirium may be observed.

Treatment

Administration of ferric ferrocyanide (Prussian blue) binds thallium in intestine and increases its faecal excretion.
- Haemodialysis
- Forced diuresis

Administration of systemic chelating agents should be avoided because they will increase the uptake of thallium in the brain.

FUNGICIDES

These are used to control fungal diseases on plants and seeds.

Dithiocarbamates

These do not seem to produce any injury in human beings except contact dermatitis. But carcinogenic and/or teratogenic effects have been reported in animals.

Dithiocarbamate fungicides are analogues of disulfiram so they can produce a disulfiram-like reaction when ethyl alcohol is ingested.

Hexachlorobenzene

The major toxic symptoms include skin lesions, and photosensitization, cutaneous porphyria, and porphyrinuria. Some deaths have also been reported.

Pentachlorophenol

It is an insecticide, herbicide as well as a fungicide.

In human beings, the signs and symptoms of acute poisoning are similar to those of nitrophenolic herbicides.

HERBICIDES

Chlorophenoxy compounds such as 2,4-dichlorophenoxyacetic acid and 2,4,5-trichlorophenoxyacetic acid, as their salts and esters are used to control weeds.

Poisoning in human beings is rare from chlorophenoxy herbicides. However, in the workers engaged in the manufacture of these compounds contact dermatitis may be produced.

Dinitrophenols

Substituted dinitrophenols are used in weed control.

In human beings, the signs and symptoms of acute poisoning are rapid respiration, cyanosis, tachycardia, nausea, restlessness, flushed skin, fever and finally coma and collapse.

Treatment

- Ice baths to reduce fever
- Oxygen inhalation
- Correction of fluid and electrolyte imbalances

Salicylates must be avoided as they contain phenolic group

Bipyridyl Compounds

Paraquat

Its toxicity includes damage to the lungs, liver and kidneys. Myocarditis has also been reported. It can also induce serious delayed pulmonary toxicity.

Treatment

- Gastric lavage
- Use of cathartics
- Removal of absorbed drug by haemodialysis

FUMIGANTS

Phosphine (PH_3) is a fumigant for grain. It is released gradually from tablets of aluminium phosphide.

The main toxic effects include severe pulmonary irritation and pulmonary oedema. It is also hepatotoxic and cardiotoxic.

Dibromochloropropane and ethylene dibromide are soil fumigants employed to control nematodes.

Inhalation in human beings produces pulmonary congestion and CNS depression. After ingestion acute gastrointestinal distress and pulmonary oedema are produced. They can produce sterility and/or abnormally low sperm counts.

These agents are carcinogenic (gastric carcinoma in laboratory animals).

Methyl bromide

It is a very toxic fumigant.

Methyl bromide poisoning produces malaise, nausea, vomiting, headache, visual disturbances. In severe cases, pulmonary oedema may be fatal.

Cyanide (hydrocyanic acid, HCN)

It causes a cytotoxic hypoxia. It is a highly toxic poison, death may result within few minutes of exposure. Cyanide has a very high affinity for iron (ferric state). After absorption it reacts with the trivalent iron of cytochrome oxidase in mitochondria resulting in inhibition of cellular respiration leading to lactic acidosis and cytotoxic hypoxia. Hypoxic convulsions occur and death is due to respiratory arrest.

Majority of patients die, few may recover fully, but in some surviving victims neurological sequelae (extrapyramidal syndrome, personality changes, and memory defects) may be observed.

Treatment

The treatment must be rapid to be effective.

The aim of the treatment is to prevent or reverse the cyanide-ferric ion binding in the cytochrome oxidase system.

Amyl nitrite is given by inhalation, followed by i.v. sodium nitrite(10ml of a 3% solution). Nitrite oxidizes a limited amount of haemoglobin to methaemoglobin, which has a greater affinity for cyanide resulting in dissociation of the cyanide-cytochrome complex. The i.v. use of thiosulphate converts cyanide to thiocyanate, which is relatively nontoxic.

If cyanide has been taken by mouth, gastric lavage should be followed by above lines of treatment and not precede.

Alternatively 4-dimethylaminophenol which also oxidizes Hb to methaemoglobin can be used (3 mg/kg i.v.).

Cobalt compounds also have high affinity for cyanide. Similarly hydroxocobalamin can be used to treat cyanide toxicity.

STUDY QUESTIONS

1. Name main air pollutants. Discuss carbon monoxide poisoning.
2. Describe the toxic effects of gasoline and kerosene.
3. Describe the treatment against ectoparasites.
4. What are the signs and symptoms of organophosphorus insecticides poisoning?
5. Describe some commonly used rodenticides.
6. Write short notes on (a) botanical insecticides (b) herbicides.
7. Describe the adverse effects and treatment of cyanide poisoning.

GUIDE TO FURTHER READING

Ames, B.N et al: Pollution, pesticides, and cancer., J AOAC Int., 1992; 75:1.

Ames, B.N et al: Ranking possible carcinogenic hazards. Science 1987; 236:271.

Behera, D. Health effects of indoor air pollution due to domestic cooking fuels. Indian J. Chest Dis Allied Sci 37:237,1995.

Bruce, N., Perez-padilla, R. and Albalak, R. Indoor air pollution in developing countries: A major environmental and public health challenge. Bull World Health Orga 78: 1078, 2000.

Folinsbee, L.J et al: Human health effects of air pollution. Environ Health Perspect, 1991.

ICMR Bulletin. Pesticides Pollution: Trends and Perspective Vol. 31, No. 9, Sept.-2001.

Johnson, E.S et al: Human exposure to 2,3,7,8-TCDD and risk of cancer, CRC Crit Rev Toxicol 1992; 21:451.

Mishra, V.K., Retherford, R.D. and Smith K.R. Biomass cooking fuels and prevalence of tuberculosis in India. Int. J. Infect Dis. 3: 119, 1999.

Penney, D.G et al: Is there a connection between carbon monoxide exposure and hypertension? Environ Health Perspect, 1991; 95:191.

Proctor, N.H et al: Chemical Hazards of the Workplace, 3rd ed. Lippincott, 1991.

Sarnet, J.M et al: The environment and the lung. JAMA, 1991; 266:670.

Seinfeld, J.H: Urban air pollution: State of the science. Science, 1989; 243:745.

Wright, E.S et al: Cellular, biochemical, and functional effects of ozone: New research and perspectives on ozone health effects. Toxicol Lett, 1990; 51:125.

Yardley-Jones A, et al: The toxicity of benzene and its metabolism and molecular pathology in human risk assessment. Brit J Indust Med, 1991; 48:437.

Immunomodulators

IMMUNE RESPONSE

There are two general types of lymphocytes involved in the immune responses: the B cells and T cells. The B lymphocytes get the designation B from the fact that in birds they derive from stem-cell cloned in the bursa of Fabricius; in man, the location of analogous clones may be in the intestinal mucosal Peyer's patches. The T cells get their designation from the fact that they are derived from stem cells cloned in the thymus gland.

From the physiological standpoint, immunological systems are evolved to provide protection against infections. This world is filled with a bewildering array of infectious agents of diverse shape, size, composition and subversive character which would very happily use host as rich sanctuaries for propagating their 'selfish genes', had the human beings not also developed a series of defense mechanisms which establish immunity (Latin immunitas, freedom from).

Immunity to infection involves a constant battle between the host defenses and the mutant microbes trying to evolve evasive strategies, bacteria try to avoid phagocytosis by surrounding themselves with capsules, secreting exotoxins which kill phagocytes or by colonizing relatively inaccessible locations. Antibody combacts these tricks.

Intracellular bacteria such as tubercle and leprosy bacilli grow within macrophages. They delay killing mechanisms by inhibiting lysosome fusion and by having strong outer coats. They are killed by cell-mediated immunity.

Viruses try to avoid the immune system by changes in the antigenicity of their surface antigens. Antibody neutralizes free virus and is particularly effective when the virus has to travel through the bloodstream before reaching its final target. "Budding" viruses which can invade lateral cells without becoming exposed to antibody are combated by cell-mediated immunity.

Diseases involving protozoal parasites and helminths affect hundreds of millions of people. Antibodies are usually effective against the blood-borne forms. 1gE production is notoriously increased in worm infestations. Organisms such as Leishmania spp; Trypanosome cruzi and toxoplasma gondii hide from antibodies inside macrophages. They are killed when the macrophages are activated by lymphokines produced during cell-mediated immune responses.

Immunity in the broadest sense may be defined simply as inborn or acquired resistance to disease and necessarily involves all of what may collectively be called the host defences.

The host defences are shown in Fig. 16.1.

Multipotential stem cells (Figs. 16.2 and 16.3) from the bone marrow give rise to all the formed elements of the blood. The differentiation of T-cells occurs within the micro-environment of the thymus. The thymus epithelial cells 'imprint' their MHC (major histocompatibility complex) haplotype on the developing T-cells, so they are restricted to the recognition of antigen in the context of that haplo-type. The initial step occurs in antigen presenting cells (APCs). The APCs regulate the proliferation of the cells of the immune system. A set of molecules on the surface of APCs is MHC. These bind antigen fragments and the resulting complex is recognized by helper T-cells.

B-cells differentiate in the foetal liver and then in the bone marrow to become immunocompetent B-cells after passing through pre-B and immature B-cell stages. The humoral immune response is brought about by B lymphocytes and their membrane immunoglobulins (cell surface receptors). These receptors recognize epitopes on the surface of intact protein molecules. The triggering of CD 4 helper T cells, interaction of CD 4 cells and their lymphokines with B cells are necessary for the generation of an antibody response. If this response occurs, B cells proliferate, and differentiate into plasma cells, and produce antibody molecules.

The key cells are the lymphocytes of which there are 3 main groups

- B-cells, these are responsible for antibody production (i.e. humoral immune response).
- T-cells, these are important in the induction phase of the immune response and are responsible for the cell-mediated immune reactions.

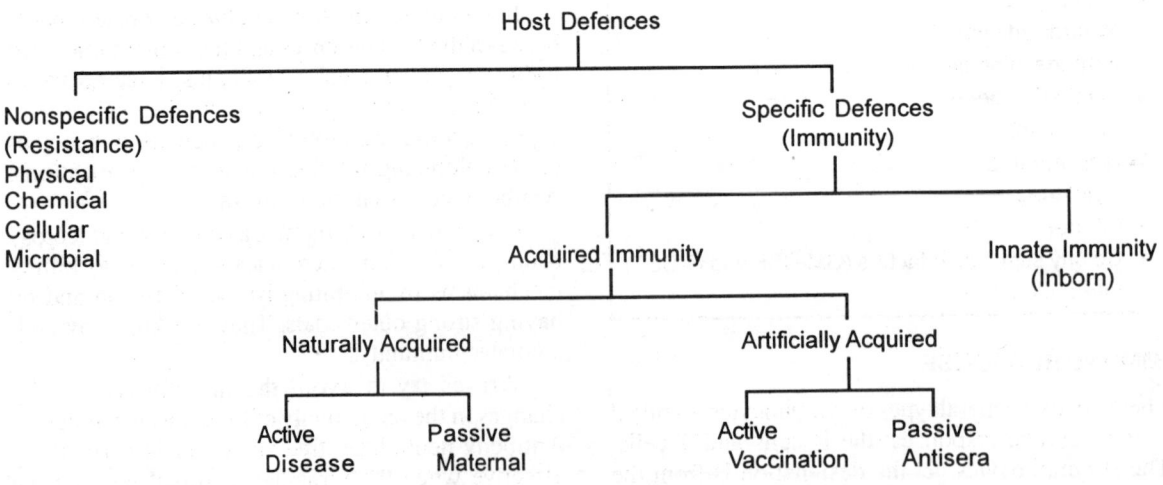

Fig. 16.1. Host defences.

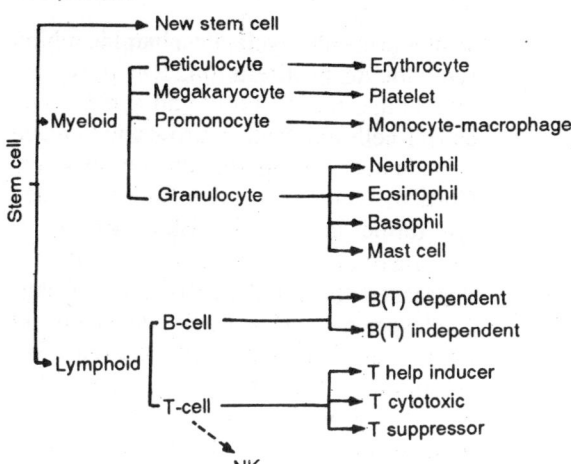

Fig. 16.2. Multipotential stem cell and its progeny.

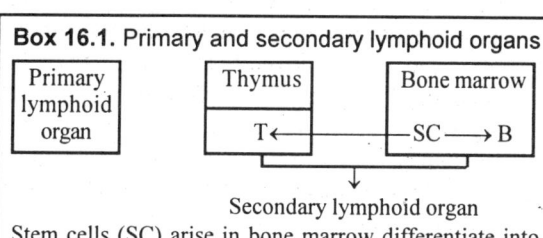

Box 16.1. Primary and secondary lymphoid organs

Stem cells (SC) arise in bone marrow differentiate into immunocompetent T- and B-cells in the primary lymphoid organs and then colonize the secondary lymphoid tissues where immune responses are organized.

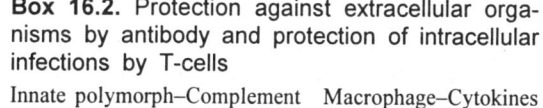

Box 16.2. Protection against extracellular organisms by antibody and protection of intracellular infections by T-cells

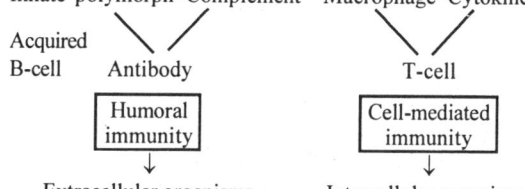

Antibody, complement and polymorphs give protection against most extracellular organisms while T-cells, soluble cytokines and macrophages deal with intracellular infections.

Box 16.3. Natural killer cells

Natural killer (NK) cells (CD 16, 56, 57+) play important role in tumour rejection and viral immunity. These cells are large lymphocytes which play an important role in host defence.

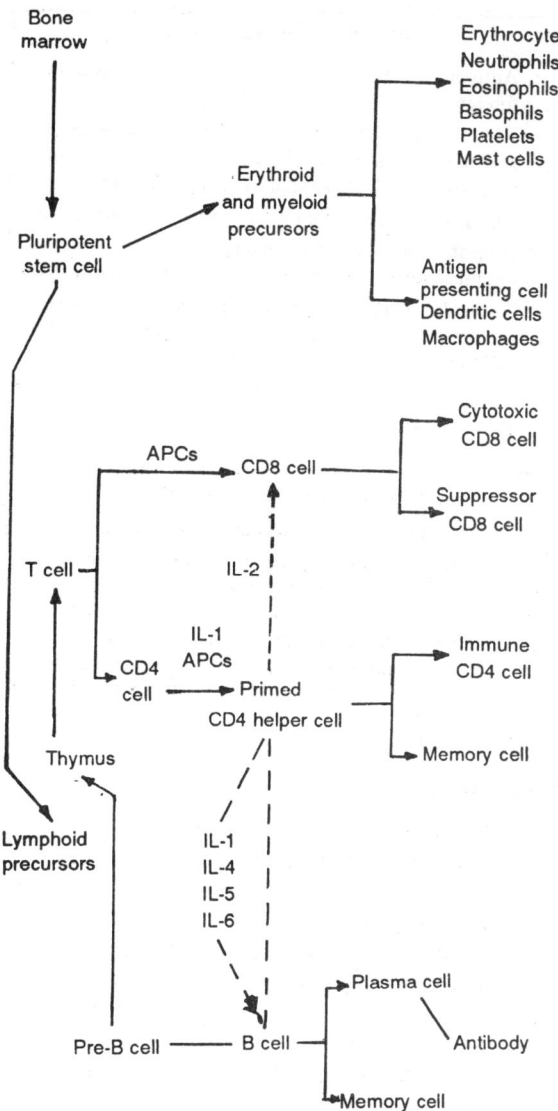

Fig. 16.3. Relationship of cells involved in the immune response.

• Natural killer cells (NK cells). These are specialised non-T and -B lymphoid cells that are active in the non-immunological innate reactions.

The specificity of cell-mediated and humoral immunity is directed to antigenic epitopes expressed on molecular components of infectious agents, or cancer (transformed cells), or transplant (foreign), or autologous cells (autoimmunity).

Box 16.4. Certain terms

- Antigen is any substance that the host considers it foreign.
- The region on the antibody which contacts the antigen is termed the paratope and the part of the antigen which is in contact with the paratope is designated the epitope.
- Autograft: tissue grafted back on to the original donor.
- Isograft: graft between syngeneic individuals i.e. of identical genetic constitution such as identical twins.
- Allograft (old term, homograft): graft between allogeneic individuals i.e. members of the same species but different genetic constitution, e.g. man to man.
- Xenograft (heterograft): graft between different species e.g. pig to man.

Box 16.5. Autoantibodies

When autoantibodies i.e. antibodies capable of reacting with 'self' components are produced resulting in autoimmune process, which contributes to the pathogenesis of the disease rather than situation where apparently harmless autoantibodies are formed following tissue damage e.g. heart antibodies appearing after a myocardial infarction.

IMMUNOSUPPRESSION

General Principles

For effective immunosuppression :
- The immunosuppressive therapy should be given before rather than after exposure to the immunogen.
- The immunosuppressive agents do not affect equally on all immuno responses. Hence doses will vary to produce inhibitory response on different antigens.
- The immunosuppressive therapy is more effective against primary (initial) immune responses than secondary immune responses.

Indications for immunosuppression

1. Organ transplantation: It is essential to suppress the normal immune response in the recipient to prevent rejection of the donor tissue.
   The drugs used for this purpose are:
   - Azathioprine, cyclophosphamide, prednisone, cyclosporin, tacrolimus and mycophenolate mofetil.
   - The non-specific cytotoxic agents e.g.

azathioprine and cyclophosphamide inhibit lymphocyte proliferation. But they also affect other rapidly proliferating cells such as GIT cells and bone marrow which result in bone marrow suppression and infection. Corticosteroids (e.g. prednisone) if added will further increase the risk of toxicity.
   - The use of cyclosporin and tacrolimus have decreased the incidence of side effects. Cyclosporin is being used extensively for organ transplantations. For acute rejection, lymphocyte immune globulin, antithymocyte, globulin and the monoclonal antibody muromonab-CD3 are often useful.

2. Selective immunosuppression for the prevention of Rh haemolytic disease of the newborn.
   The aim is to control selectively the immune response that develops in an Rh-negative mother who becomes sensitized to the D antigen on the foetal erythrocytes of her Rh-positive infant at the time of birth, miscarriage or ectopic pregnancy, when erythrocytes from the foetus may cross the placenta into mother's circulation. The antibodies against Rh- positive cells will transfer to the foetus during the third trimester in subsequent pregnancy resulting in haemolytic disease of the newborn.
   The primary antibody response to the foreign antigen (D antigen) can be blocked if specific anti-D antibody is given passively at the time of exposure to the antigen. Rh (D) immune globulin is a human IgG globulin solution that contains an enriched fraction of antibodies against D antigen. Rh (D) antibody should be received by the Rh-negative mother within 72 hours of the birth of an Rh- positive baby or after an abortion, miscarriage or ectopic pregnancy.

3. Immunosuppressive therapy in the treatment of autoimmune diseases :
   Autoimmune diseases occur when the immune system is sensitized by endogenous proteins which are treated as "foreign" antigens, resulting in the formation of antibodies or immune T cells which react with these antigens present in tissue leading to destructive changes.
   Immunosuppressives can suppress autoimmune reactions, but in general it is not so effective as

in organ transplantation or in the treatment of specific immune disorders such as Rh haemolytic disease of the newborn.

Certain autoimmune disorders such as idiopathic thrombocytopenic purpura, autoimmune haemolytic anaemia and acute glomerulonephritis respond well to immunosuppressives such as corticoids alone or with cytotoxic drugs.

Limitations to the general use of immunosuppressive agents

- Increased risk of infection of all types (bacterial, viral, fungal as well as unusual opportunistic infections)
- Increased risk of lymphomas and related malignancies.

Sites that can be manipulated to achieve immunosuppression

- Muromonab-CD3 (OKT3), antithymocyte globulin, or anti-CD4 deplete and inhibit the T-cell population.
- The relatively non-specific cytotoxic drugs such as azathioprine, cyclophosphamide or methotrexate inhibit the proliferation of T and B cells.

Mycophenolic acid is a cytotoxic drug which inhibits selectively de novo purine synthesis. It is more selective in inhibiting T and B cells.

INDIVIDUAL IMMUNOSUPPRESSIVE AGENTS

There are 4 classes of drugs:

1. T-Cell inhibitors: Cyclosporin, tacrolimus, rapamycin, (sirolimus), mycophenolate mofetil.
2. Glucocorticoids.
3. Cytotoxic drugs : Azathioprime, cyclophosphamide and other cytotoxic drugs.
4. Antibody reagents.
   Muromonab CD3
   Antithymocyte globulin

The sites of action of immunosuppressive agents on various stages in the immune response (from antigen recognition to proliferation and differentiation) are shown in Fig. 16.4.

Cyclosporin

Cyclosporin is the most important immunosupp-

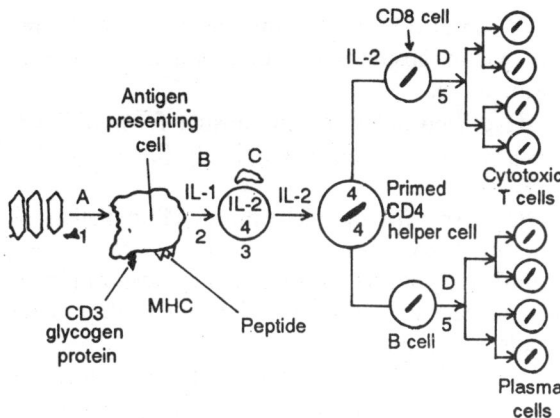

Fig. 16.4. Sites of action of specific immunosuppressive agents at various stages in the immune response.

Inhibitors at each step that act as immunosuppressive agents
A Antigen recognition
B Stimulation of IL-1
C Expression of IL-2 and other cytokines
D Proliferation and differentiation

Site	Drugs
1	Rh (D) immune globulin
2	Corticosteroids
3	Antithymocyte globulin, OK T3, anti-CD4
4	Cyclosporin, tacrolimus
5	Azathioprine, methotrexate, cyclophosphamide, rapamycin, mycophenolic acid

Abbreviations: CD = cluster differentiation; IL = interleukin; MHC = major histocompatibility complex

ressive drug used in transplantation and for the treatment of selected autoimmune disorders.

Cyclosporin is a fungal peptide. Cyclosporin is lipophilic and very hydrophobic. Hence, for use, it must be solubilised.

It is a very selective inhibitor of helper T cells. It inhibits the production of interleukin-2 (IL-2) by helper T cells and reduces the production and release of other lymphokines in response to an antigenic stimulus.

It also binds to lymphoid proteins called cyclophilins and to isomerase enzymes, which aid in the folding of certain proteins.

Routes of administration and pharmacokinetics

Cyclosporin is given by i.v. route as a 50 mg/ml solution made up in ethanol-polyoxyethylated castor oil mixture.

It can also be given orally as a 25- or 100 mg soft gelatin capsule or as a newer oral microemulsion formulation.

Cyclosporin in gelatin capsule formulation is absorbed slowly and incompletely (bioavailability 20% to 50%).

Cyclosporin in the microemulsion formulation has greater absorption. Ingestion of a fatty meal significantly delays absorption of cyclosporin in the gelatin capsule formulation but not in the microemulsion formulation.

After absorption, the drug distributes widely in the body. It disappears from the circulation with an elimination half-life of about 6 hours.

Cyclosporin is metabolized in the liver, there are more than 30 metabolites. Metabolism results in inactivation of the immunosuppressive properties, but it is possible that some metabolites may contribute to immunosuppression or toxicity.

Cyclosporin and its metabolites are excreted mainly through bile into the faeces and about 6% is excreted in the urine.

In the presence of hepatic dysfunction, it is necessary to adjust the dosage.

Therapeutic uses

- Cyclosporin is the most important immunosuppressive drug necessary for the prevention and treatment of transplant rejection. Its use has been responsible for graft survival (in renal transplantation) after 36 months in about 80% of patients. It has shown impressive efficacy in human organ transplantation.

  A dose of 15 mg/kg is given orally 4 to 24 hours prior to transplantation, this dose is continued once a day for 1-2 weeks postoperatively, subsequently the dose is reduced each week until the maintenance dose of 3-10 mg/kg daily is reached.

  If patient is unable to tolerate cyclosporin orally, the diluted i.v. formulation is infused slowly over a period of 2-6 hours. The daily dose is about one-third the oral dose. The i.v. administration should be discontinued when the patient is able to tolerate the oral medication.

- Cyclosporin is also effective in acute ocular Behçet's syndrome, endogenous uveitis,

psorisasis, atopic dermatitis, rheumatoid arthritis, active Crohn's disease, and nephrotic syndrome. This drug is used when standard therapy for these conditions is ineffective. In many cases cyclosporin is combined with a corticoid.

- Cyclosporin has been used as first line treatment in patients with moderate or severe aplastic anaemia who are not suitable for bone marrow transplantation.
- Some evidences suggest the use of cyclosporin in intractable pyoderma gangrenosum, polymyositis/dermatomyositis, and severe corticosteroid dependent asthma.

Adverse effects

The adverse effects are considerable, though less than those of corticosteroids and other cytotoxic agents.

Renal toxicity is the major toxic effect of cyclosporine. It may occur in 25%-75% of patients. Both the glomerular filtration rate and renal plasma flow are reduced, but these effects are usually reversible. The other adverse effects include hepatotoxicity, neurotoxicity, hypertension, hirsutism, gingival hyperplasia, GIT upsets (nausea, vomiting, diarrhoea, loss of appetite and abdominal pain), and increased incidence of infections.

Drug interactions

The clearance of cyclosporin is accelerated with coadministration of phenobarbitone, phenytoin, cotrimoxazole and rifampin due to induction of the hepatic P 450 systems, resulting in decreased cyclosporin levels leading to rejection of the transplanted organs.

The clearance of cyclosporin is decreased with coadministration of amphotericin B, erythromycin, or ketoconazole. This interaction may result in an increased risk of cyclosporin toxicity.

Tacrolimus

It is a macrolide antibiotic that was extracted from a fermentation broth of the soil microorganism *Streptomyces tsukubaensis*.

Cyclosporin and tacrolimus do not share similar chemical structure and react with different biochemical targets, but their mode of action is very similar on signal transduction in T lymphocytes resulting in a effective immunosuppressive action.

Tacrolimus, like cyclosporin, inhibits T-cell activation.

This drug can be given orally or intravenously. The oral dosage for adults is 150-200 mcg/kg daily; the i.v. dosage is 25-50 mcg/kg daily.

This drug is metabolized extensively in the liver and less than 1% of the drug is excreted in an unchanged form.

Therapeutic uses

Tacrolimus is about 100 times more potent than cyclosporin.

The clinical uses are similar to those of cyclosporin.

Adverse effects

The spectrum of toxicities is similar to that of cyclosporin.

Nephrotoxicity is the main problem. Besides this, neurotoxicity (headache, tremor, insomnia), GIT upsets, cardiovascular toxicity (hypertension) and metabolic toxicity (hyperglycaemia, hyperkalaemia) can develop.

Rapamycin (Sirolimus)

It is another new macrolide antibiotic which shows immunosuppressive effect. It blocks IL-2 receptor mediated signalling pathways by interfering with protein kinases. Unlike cyclosporin and tacrolimus, it does not inhibit IL-2 release or bind to phospho-protein phosphatase (calcineurin), therefore it can be combined with cyclosporin.

New immunosuppressant agents

An attempt has been made to obtain less toxic and more specific drugs.

Mycophenolate Mofetil

It is a semisynthetic derivative of mycophenolic acid, isolated from the mold penicillium *glaucum*.

It is used orally following renal transplantation. Its use in other conditions is under trial.

It is absorbed rapidly after oral administration. Its bioavailability is about 95%.

A dose of 1.0 g is given twice a day in combi-nation with cyclosporin and corticosteroids, within 72 hours following transplantation.

It has been used in kidney and liver transplantation patients. The results are promising.

Mycophenolate Mofetil and antacids containing aluminium and magnesium hydroxides should not be given together otherwise the absorption of mycophenolate mofetil will be decreased.

A closely related drug **mizoribine** is also effective in kidney transplantation.

Another drug **brequinar sodium** is under clinical trials.

15-deoxyspergualin isolated from *Bacillus laterosporus* has potent antimonocytic effects. It also has antilymphocytic actions. It is beneficial in the treatment of acute rejection in renal transplantation.

GLUCOCORTICOIDS

Prednisone and prednisolone are either used alone or in combination with other immunosuppressive drugs to prevent rejection of the transplant and to treat autoimmune diseases.

Corticosteroids inhibit T-cell proliferation, T-cell dependent immunity, and the expression of genes encoding cytokines (1L-1, 1L-2, 1L-6, alpha-interferon). Corticosteroids also produce non-specific antiinflammatory action as well as anti-adhesion effects which also contribute to immunosuppression.

The dosage range of prednisone for immunosuppression is 10-100 mg orally daily.

Uses

- To prevent transplant rejection. Corticosteroids are used liberally in the management of organ transplant recipients and are of particular value during rejection crisis because the dosage can be increased without fear of bone marrow toxicity.
- To minimize allergic reactions which may occur with the use of antilymphocytic globulin.
- To treat various autoimmune disorders such as autoimmune haemolytic anaemia, idiopathic thrombocytopenic purpura, inflammatory bowel disease, lupus erythematosus.

Adverse effects

In order to achieve immunosuppression, long-term use of corticosteroids is required and hence adverse effects are are more likely to occur. These include:

- Increased risk of infection (serious viral, bacterial, and fungal infections)
- Hyperglycaemia
- Ulcers
- Osteoporosis
- Adrenal suppression

CYTOTOXIC DRUGS

Azathioprine

It is a purine antimetabolite. It is a prodrug of 6-mercaptopurine (6-MP).

It can be administered both orally and intravenously.

Uses

Azathioprine is one of the major agents used to prevent transplant rejection. Daily doses of 3-10 mg/kg, 1 or 2 days before transplantation or on the day of operation are given. The maintenance dose is 1-3 mg/kg daily.

This drug is usually combined with cyclosporin and/or prednisone. At many places this drug is reserved for cases who do not respond to cyclosporin and prednisone. This drug has been of occasional use in prednisone -resistant antibody-mediated idiopathic thrombocytopenic purpura and autoimmune haemolytic anaemias.

Adverse effects

The risk of infection is increased; chief toxicity is bone marrow depression manifested as leukopenia, thrombocytopenia. Gastrointestinal toxicity, and hepatotoxicity also occur.

There is some evidence for mutagenicity and carcinogenicity.

Coadministration of allopurinol with azathioprine may result in enhanced toxicity, since, much of its inactivation depends on xanthine oxidase. To prevent excessive toxicity and if it is necessary to use both drugs together, the dose of azathioprine should be reduced to one-fourth the usual dose.

Cyclophosphamide

It is a nitrogen mustard (subclass of alkylating agents). It is one of the most potent immunosuppressive agents.

It affects both B and T cells. This drug has a greater effect through suppressing humoral immunity. It has more variable effect on T-cell mediated immunity (i.e. some cell-mediated responses are inhibited while others are stimulated). It destroys proliferating lymphoid cells.

Therapeutic uses

It is used in large doses in as an immunosuppressive agent. It has suppressive effect on the lymphoid elements of patients who are to receive bone marrow transplants.

For immunosuppression the drug is administered in a dose of 1.5-3 mg/kg/d.

In smaller doses, cyclophosphamide is administered for the treatment of autoimmune diseases such as systemic lupus erythematosus, idiopathic thrombocytopenic purpura and rheumatoid arthritis.

Leukopenia below 2,500 and platelet count below 100,000 mm^3 are indications for stoppage of the drug.

Adverse effects include haemorrhagic cystitis, cardiotoxicity and pancytopenia (simultaneous decrease in number of red cells, white cells and platelets).

Other cytotoxic drugs

Methotrexate, chlorambucil, vincristine, vinblastine and dactinomycin have been employed as immunosuppressive agents.

Methotrexate (which can be given orally) has been used more commonly among these agents for immunosuppression. It has been used in the treatment of rheumatoid arthritis and psoriasis.

ANTIBODIES AS IMMUNOSUPPRESSIVE AGENTS (ANTIBODY REAGENTS)

After repeatedly injecting the human cells into a nonhuman such as horses, the antilymphocyte or antithymocyte globulin has been prepared as an antiserum against lymphocytes or thymocytes. The antiserum or IgG or gamma globulin (purified

Table 16.1. Uses of immunosuppressive agents

Disease	Agents	Beneficial response
Organ transplantation		
Renal	Cyclosporin, azathioprine	Very good
Heart	Prednisolone, dactinomycin	Good
Liver	Cyclosporin, prednisolone	Fair
Bone marrow	Cyclosporin, prednisolone, cyclophosphamide, methotrexate	Very good
Autoimmune		
Idiopathic thrombocytopenic purpura	Prednisone, vincristine, azathioprine, high dose gamma globulin	Good
Haemolytic anaemia	Prednisolone, cyclosporin, azathioprine, 6-MP	Good
Acute glomerulonephritis	Prednisolone, 6-MP cyclophosphamide	Good
Isoimmune		
Haemolytic anaemia of the newborn	Rho (D) immune globulin	Excellent
Miscellaneous		
Systemic lupus erythematosus, rheumatoid arthritis, hepatitis, inflammatory bowel disease	Prednisolone, azathioprine, cyclosporin, cyclophosphamide	Very good

immunoglobulin fraction) can produce immuno-suppression.

Antithymocyte globulin

It binds to the surface of T lymphocytes in the circulation. It leads to lymphopenia and suppressed T-cell immune responses.

It is injected intravenouly daily at the dose of 10-30 mg/kg in saline over several hours. Its half-life is 3-9 days.

Therapeutic uses

• To treat allograft rejection during acute rejection.
• To prevent rejection.

Adverse effects

Serum sickness, nephritis, chills, fever, leukopenia, thrombocytopenia, rashes, and anaphylaxis (rarely).

Muromonab-CD3

Being monoclonal it acts as a more consistent immunosuppressant as compared to antithymocyte globulin (polyclonal antibodies).

Muromonab-CD3 inhibits T-cell participation in the immune response.

Therapeutic uses

• To prevent acute rejection of organ transplants
• To deplete T cells from donor bone marrow before bone marrow transplantation

Adverse effects include cytokine release syndrome characterized by flu-like symptoms and in severe cases shock-like reactions. This can be prevented by prior administration of large doses of steroids administered 1-4 hours before the first dose of this antibody. The other adverse effects are CNS toxicities which include cerebral oedema, seizures, headache and aseptic meningitis. The adverse effects due to immunosuppression include high risk of infection and neoplasia.

Hazards of life on immunosuppressive drugs

• Decreased immune responses render the patient more liable to secondary infections (bacterial and viral infection). All infections should be treated early and vigorously. If there is exposure to virus infection e.g. measles etc. human gamma globulin should be given for protection.
• Carcinogenicity is also a hazard after prolonged therapy.
• Leukaemias, lymphonas, skin cancers are more likely to occur.

- Where cytotoxics are used there is additional hazard of mutagenicity, which may induce cancer.
- Hazards also include those of longterm corticosteroid therapy and of cytotoxic agents in general (bonemarrow depression, infertility and terato-genesis).

Patients who have grave endangering disease may accept these hazards but it is a matter of great concern if immunosuppression regimens are proposed for younger patients with less serious disease e.g. rheumatoid arthritis.

Rho (D) Immune Globulin

Rho (D) immune globulin is a concentrated (15%) solution of human IgG globulin containing a higher titre of antibodies against the Rho (D) antigen of the red cell.

Its half-life is 21-29 days.

If Rho (D) antibody is administered within 72 hours after the birth of an Rh-positive baby, the mother's own antibody response to the foreign Rho (D)-positive cells is suppressed. In order that this prophylactic treatment is successful, the mother must be Rho (D)-negative and must not already be immunized to the Rho (D) factor.

The dose of Rho (D) immune globulin is 2 ml administered intramuscularly. It is used in Rh-negative mothers to prevent sensitization to Rh (D) antigen.

Rho (D) immune globulin is given to the mother and must not be administered to the infant.

IMMUNOSTIMULANTS

These can produce effect either through cellular, humoral immunity, or both.

These have potential role in three clinical settings:
- Immunodeficiency disorders such as AIDS. The AIDS epidemic has greatly increased interest in developing more effective immunostimulatory drugs. The HIV organism resides in and destroys CD 4+ helper cells leading to progressive immunologic paralysis.
- Chronic infectious diseases
- Cancer involving lymphatic system

Natural adjuvants

BCG (bacillus Calmette-Guérin) and its active component, muramyl dipeptide (derived from BCG) are bacterial products.

These possess immunostimulant action. BCG acts primarily on the T cells. It can also stimulate killer cells. It has shown effectiveness when given as an intravesicular agent in the patients of bladder cancer.

Adverse effects include hypersensitivity, shock, malaise, fever, chills.

Immune Globulin

It is prepared from pooled human plasma obtained from donors. It is used in immunodeficiency conditions, haematologic disorders, autoimmune haemolytic anaemia, measles and hepatitis.

The immune globulin is administered by i.v. or i.m. injection. Its half-life is 3 weeks.

The adverse effects include allergic reactions including anaphylaxis. A potential danger is exposure to HIV and hepatitis.

Synthetic agents

Levamisol (anthelmintic) can increase delayed hypersensitivity and/or T-cell mediated immunity. It has been used in Hodgkin's disease, rheumatoid arthritis and in adjuvant therapy of colorectal cancer.

Isoprinosine increases natural killer cell cytotoxicity. It also increases the activity of T cells and monocytes. It is minimally beneficial to patients with AIDS.

Cytokines

Leukocytes and related cells produce cytokines (a group of heterogenous proteins with diverse functions). Cytokines are a variety of soluble growth and activation factors released from various cell populations involved in the immune response and have a vital role in the initiation and regulation of immune responses.

Cytokines include:
- Interleukins (ILs)
- Cytotoxic factors
- Interferons
- Colony stimulating factors (CSFs)

Interleukins

These are produced by a variety of cells including T-cells, monocytes and macrophages. Interleukins stimulate proliferation of T-lymphocytes and activate natural killer cells.

IL-1 may play part in conditions such as sepsis syndrome and rheumatoid arthritis. IL-1 is pro-inflammatory.

IL-2 (aldesleukin) is used to treat metastatic renal cell carcinoma and malignant melanoma.

Interleukin-2 (IL-2) has the ability to stimulate the production of T helper and T-cytotoxic cells.

It is administered as i.v. bolus, i.v. infusion, sub-cutaneously, and intramuscularly.

IL-2 produces antitumour activity in metastatic melanoma and renal cell carcinoma.

Adverse effects include CNS toxicity (delirium) and skin toxicity. The other adverse effects include severe hypotension, pulmonary oedema, bone marrow suppression.

If the rate of infusion is slow, many adverse effects are minimized.

IL-3, IL-10, IL-13 inhibit inflammatory activity.

Cytotoxic factor

Tumour necrosis factor (TNF-alpha) is similar to IL-1 as pro-inflammatory. Monoclonal antibody to TNF-alpha shows improvement in patients of rheumatoid arthritis. It suggests that specific cytokine blockade offers hope for the treatment of this condition.

Interferons (IFNs)

These are cytokines with antiviral and immuno-modulatory properties. These are so named because they were found to interfere with the replication of live virus in some culture. IF-alpha is used for a variety of neoplastic conditions (hairy cell leukaemia and Kaposi's sarcoma). and for chronic active hepatitis. IF-alpha and IF-beta have mainly antiviral activity; IF-g has immunomodulating effect, used in multiple sclerosis.

Colony-stimulating factors

These have been deve-loped to treat neutropenic conditions, for example filgrastim (recombinant human granulocyte colony-stimulating factor, reHuG-CSF) and molgramostim (recombinant granulocyte macrophage-colony-stimulating factor reHuGM-CSF).

The above two drugs can be administered subcutaneously or intravenously.

Therapeutic uses

- To reduce severity and duration of neutropenia induced by intensive cancer chemotherapy.
- For persistent neutropenia in advanced HIV infection or that induced by zidovidine.
- To shorten duration of neutropenia in patients undergoing bone marrow transplantation after high dose intensive chemotherapy

Adverse effects

Molgramostim : Transient hypotension, flushing, bone pain, fever, musculoskeletal pain and GIT disturbances.

Filgrastim : Bone pain, splenomegaly, musculo-skeletal pain thrombocytopenia, anaemia, epistaxis.

The selected cytokine effects in the immune response are shown in Table 16.2.

Table 16.2. Selected cytokine effects in the immune response

Interleukin-1 (IL-1)	Stimulation of early bone marrow stem cells and lymphocyte precursors
Interleukin-2 (IL-2)	T cell proliferation and generation of cytolytic "killer" cells
Interleukin-3 (IL-3)	Proliferation of bone marrow lineage cells, B and T cells
Interleukin-4 (IL-4)	Activation of B and T cells and macrophages
Interleukin-5 (IL-5)	Generation of eosinophils by bone marrow
Interleukin-6 (IL-6)	Proliferation of bone marrow and plasma cells
Interleukin-7 (IL-7)	Stimulation of B and T cells; synergistic with IL-2
Interleukin-8 (IL-8)	Chemotactic for neutrophils, B and T cells
Interleukin-9 (IL-9)	Proliferation of mast cells
Interleukin-10 (IL-10)	Inhibition of T cells
Interleukin-11 (IL-11)	Synergistic with IL-3

(Contd.)

Interleukin-12 (IL-12)	Synergistic with IL-2
Alpha interferon	Activation of macrophages, T lymphocytes and natural killer cell activity
Interferon-Gamma (IFN-Gamma)	Activation of macrophages and T cells, enhanced MHC expression
Granulocyte macrophage colony Stimulating factor (GM-CSF)	Bone marrow proliferation and activation of antigen-presenting cells
Tumor necrosis factor (TNF α, β)	Cytotoxic effect on tumour cells; stimulation of inflammation

STUDY QUESTIONS

1. Describe the role of T and B cells in mediating cellular and humoral immunity respectively.
2. What are the different sites of action of immunosuppressive agents?
3. Describe the indications of immunosuppression.
4. What are the limitations of the use of immunosuppressive agents?
5. Describe the therapeutic status and adverse effects of the following immunosuppressive agents (a) cyclosporin, (b) azathioprine, (c) cyclophosphamide.
6. Write notes on antibodies as immunosuppressive agents.
7. Describe the uses, mode of action and adverse effects of corticosteroids as immunosuppressive agents.
8. Describe the following immunostimulants (a) Levamisole, (b) Cytokines, (c) Interleukins, (d) immuneglobulin, (e) BCG.

GUIDE TO FURTHER READING

Adorini L, Sinigaglia F; Pathogenesis and immunotherapy of autoimmune disease. Trends Immunol. 1997. 18: 209-211.

Akira S et al: Biology of multifunctional cytokines:IL6 and related molecules (IL1 and TNF). FASEB J 1990;4:2860.

Audibert FM, Lise LD: Adjuvants: current status, clinical perspectives and future prospects. Immunol Today 1993;14:281.

Bach, J.F et al: Immunosuppressive therapy of autoimmune diseases. Trends Pharmacol. Sci., 1993; 14:213-216.

Banchereau J, Steinman R M: Dendritic cells and the control of immunity. Nature. 1998; 392: 245-352 (Good coverage of important cells).

Banchereau J et al: Human B lymphocytes: Phenotype, proliferation and differentiation. Adv Immunol 1992;52:125.

Barry, J.M: Immunosuppressive drugs in renal transplantation. A review of the regimens. Drugs., 1992; 44:554-566.

Bellanti, J.A et al: Cytokines and the immune response. Pediatr. Clin. North Am., 1994; 41:597-621.

Benson, E.M et al: Immune modulation in HIV infection: fact or fantasy? J.Acquir. Immune Defic. Syndr., 1993; 6:S61-S67.

Blaese RM: Development of gene therapy for immunodeficiency: Adenosine deaminase deficiency. Pediatr Res 1993;33(Suppl):S49.

Borden E C: Interferons - expanding therapeutic roles. N Engl J Med. 1992 326: 1491-1493.

Bumgardner GL, Roberts JP: New immunosuppressive agents. Gastroenterol Clin North Am 1993;22:421.

Burke, J.E et al: Long-term efficacy and safety of cyclosporine in renal-transplant recipients. N. Engl. J. Med., 1994; 331:358-363.

Christians, U et al: Cyclosporin metabolism in transplant patients. Pharmacol. Ther., 1993; 57:291-345.

Contreras, M et al: The prevention and management of haemolytic disease of the newborn. J.R.Soc.Med., 1994; 87:256-258.

Dinarelo CA: Interleukin-1. Cytokine and Growth Factor Rev. 1997; 8: 232-265

Dinarello CA et al: Anticytokine strategies in the treatment of systemic inflammatory response syndrome. JAMA 1993;14:1829.

Dinarello, C.A et al: Modalities for reducing interleukin 1 activity in disease. Immunol Today 1993; 14:260.

Featherstone C: Anti-integrin drugs developed to treat inflammation. Lancet. 1996 347: 1106-1107.

Ferrara JLM, Deeg HJ: Graft-versus-host disease. N Engl J Med 1991;324:667.

Hooks, M.A et al: Tacrolimus, a new immunosuppressant—a review of the literature. Ann. Pharmacother., 1994; 28:501-511.

Hayes JM: The immunobiology and clinical use of current immunosuppressive therapy for renal transplantation. J Urol 1993;149:437.

Johnson, H.M et al: How interferons fight disease. Sci. Am., 1994; 270:68-75.

Kumar V, Sercarz E: Genetic Vaccination: the advantages of going naked. Nature Med, 1996 2: 857-859.

Kurman, M.R et al: Recent clinical trials with levamisole. Ann. N.Y. Acad. Sci., 1993; 685:269-277.

Lee B, Ciardelli TL: Clinical applications of cytokines for immunostimulation and immunosuppression. Prog Drug Res 1992;39:167.

Rieder MJ: Immunopharmacology and adverse drug reactions. J Clin Pharmacol 1993;33:316.

Schulak, J.A et al: Steroid withdrawal after renal transplantation. Clin. Transplant., 1994; 8:211-216.

Stites DP, Terr AI(editors): Basic and Clinical Immunology, 7th ed. Appleton & Lange, 1991.

Suthanthiran, M et al: Renal transplantation. N. Engl. J. Med., 1994; 331:365-376.

Vitetta, E.S et al: Immunotoxins: Magic bullets or misguided missiles? Immunol Today 1993; 14:252.

Wilkin TJ: Receptor autoimmunity in endocrine disorders. N. Engl. J. Med., 1990;323:1318.

Whittington, R et al: Interleukin-2, A review of its pharmacological properties and therapeutic use in patients with cancer. Drugs, 1993; 46:446-514.

Drug Use in Special Populations

DRUG USE DURING PREGNANCY
(Tables 17.1-17.3)

Drug use during pregnancy is of great concern. The effects of drug therapy depend on the stage of foetal development. The foetus develops in 3 stages viz.

1. Blastogenesis: During this stage (first 15-21 days after fertilization) germ layer formation occurs. Embryo cells are undifferentiated.

2. Organogenesis (from day 21 to day 90 after fertilization): The foetal organs undergo rapid growth and differentiation.

3. Foetogenesis: This stage begins 90 days after fertilization and lasts till birth. There is overall foetal growth. All major organs are now formed and functioning.

Table 17.1. Some safe drugs, some unsafe drugs during pregnancy and drugs which endanger continuation of pregnancy

Safe drugs during pregnancy : Penicillin, Cephalosporins, Antitubercular drugs, Proguanil, Pyrimethamine, Metronidazole, Carbamazepine, Thiazides, Methyldopa, Clonidine, Atenolol, ACEIs, Labetalol, Prazocin, Diazoxide, Frusemide

Unsafe drugs during pregnancy : Sulphonamides, Tetracycline, Chloramphenicol, Fluoroquinolones, Carbenicillin, Nitrofurantoin, Quinine, Primaquine, Chloroquine, Emetine, Aminoglycosides, Phenytoin, Trimethadione, Valproic acid

Drugs endangering continuation of pregnancy : Ergot alkaloids, Oxytocin, Quinine, Quinidine, Cholinergic drugs, Alpha-adrenergic agonists, Drastic purgatives.

The foetus is most vulnerable to the effects of maternal drug therapy during the first and third trimesters of pregnancy.

The placental drug transfer is affected by

- Molecular size: Drugs with very large molecules (e.g. heparin) do not cross the placental membrane as readily as those with smaller molecules
- pH: Weakly acidic and weakly basic drugs are transferred rapidly.
- Lipid solubility: Highly-lipid soluble compounds diffuse across the placental membrane easily.
- Physical characteristics of the placenta:

Table 17.2. Some drugs which should be avoided as they cross placental barrier

Drugs which may produce malformation: if given during first trimester:
- Penicillamine, Barbiturates, Lithium, Warfarin, Corticosteroids.

Drugs which should be avoided in all trimesters to avoid malformations:
- Anticancer agents, Phenytoin, Trimethadione, Valproic acid, Progestins.

Drugs can also produce certain effects other than malformations in neonates.

Drugs to be avoided in all trimesters:
- Aminoglycosides (ototoxicity), barbiturates, amphetamines, NSAIDs (delayed labour), chlorpropamide, opoids, alcohol, diazepam, tetracyclines (discoloration and defects of teeth and altered bone growth), ciprofloxacin (arthropathy, haemolytic anaemia)
- Chloramphenicol (gray-baby syndrome), androgens, oestrogens
- Morphine and pethidine in high doses (neonatal drug dependence)

Table 17.3. Significant adverse effects on the foetus by some commonly used drugs

Drugs	Trimester	Adverse effects
ACE inhibitors	All, specially second and third	Kidney damage
Aminoglycosides	All	Ototoxicity
Androgens	Second and third	Masculinization of female foetus
Barbiturates	All	Chronic use leads to neonatal dependence
Chloramphenicol	Third	Increased risk of gray baby syndrome
Diazepam	All	Chronic use leads to neonatal dependence
Ethanol	All	High risk of foetal alcohol syndrome
Iodide	All	Congenital goiter, hypothyroidism
Phenytoin	All	Cleft lip and palate
Progestins	All	Cardiovascular defects, ambiguous genitalia
Tetracyclines	All	Discoloration and defects of teeth and altered bone growth
Valproic acid	All	Spinal bifida
Warfarin	First	Hypoplastic nasal bridge
	Third	Risk of bleeding

Placental drug transfer becomes less efficient as the pregnancy advances and placenta ages. The presence of placental enzymes and as the thickness of the placenta changes during the course of the pregnancy, the placental transfer is reduced.

Drugs that cross the placenta may have (i) embryocidal, (ii) teratogenic, or (iii) foetotoxic effects.

- Embryocidal drug effects: Embryocidal effects are those that harm the developing embryo. Drugs that harm the developing embryo result in termination of pregnancy. Drugs administered during blastogenesis are embryocidal e.g. ACEIs, antidepressants, hormones and certain anti-infectives.

- Teratogenic drug effects: These cause physical defects in the foetus. Physical and mental defects are produced in the embryo. This risk is maximum during first trimester when organs are differentiating. Organ systems develop at different times e.g. CNS develops between day 18 and 38 of gestation and genitals form after day 45. Hence a drug taken before day 38 will affect the CNS and may not produce genital defects.

The potentially teratogenic drugs include vitamin A derivatives, oral antihyperglycaemic agents (insulin does not cross the placental membrane), Warfarin (heparin poorly crosses the placenta), oestrogen and oral contraceptives, cortisone, thyroid preparations, tetracycline (if taken after week 18 of gestation, the effect is evident later in childhood when tooth eruption occurs).

- Foetotoxic drug effects (physiological effects in the developing foetus) during foetogenesis. These effects include:
  - CNS depression with barbiturates, narcotics, analgesics, anaesthetics.
  - Neonatal bleeding may result due to mother's ingestion of NSAIDs, certain antidepressants and certain antianxiety agents.
  - Neonates may show withdrawal syndrome if mother has drug dependence on barbiturates or narcotics.
  - Underweight infant may be born to the

pregnant woman who smokes cigarettes or takes large amounts of alcohol.

DRUG USE IN LACTATING MOTHERS

Most maternal drugs are secreted in at least small quantities in the breast milk of a lactating woman. The concentrations are so small that these is no clinical response in the nursing infant.

However, there are some drugs that readily enter the breast milk and may adversely affect the nursing infant. These drugs should be avoided by nursing mothers, the following are some examples :

Most antibiotics taken by nursing mothers can be detected in breast milk. The concentrations of tetracyclines in breast milk are about 70% of maternal serum concentrations. These is risk of permanent tooth staining in the infant.

Chloramphenicol should also be avoided during lactation because of the remote possibility of bone marrow suppression (not sufficient concentration to cause gray baby syndrome).

Isoniazid reaches a rapid equilibrium between maternal blood and breast milk and pyridoxine deficiency may result in infant unless the mother gets vitamin B_6 supplements.

Most sedatives and hypnotics achieve concentrations in breast milk which can produce pharmacologic effects in infants.

Lithium enters breast milk in sufficient concentrations.

Drugs such as propylthiouracil and tolbutamide enter breast milk in concentrations that may affect endocrine function in the infant.

Radioactive substances such as radioiodine can cause thyroid suppression in infants and the chances of thyroid cancer may increase 10-fold in later life.

Anticholinergic drugs may produce adverse effects on CNS in infant, as well as reduce lactation in the mother.

Drugs like cimetidine, atenolol, metoprolol, nadolol, meprobamate, naproxen, metronidazole and ergot alkaloids are concentrated in breast milk and should be avoided in nursing mothers.

Drugs like reserpine and cascara may cause nasal congestion and diarrhoea respectively.

DRUG USE IN PAEDIATRIC PATIENTS

Special precautions must be taken when calculating paediatric dosages.

The average body surface area for an adult is taken as 1.7 sq meters. Table 17.4 indicates the fraction of adult dose for a child based on surface area of average adult (1.7 m²).

Table 17.4. Relationship between age, surface area and percent of adult dose.

Weight in kg	Age Approx.	Surface area m²	Percent of adult dose
2		0.15	09
4		0.25	14
6	3 Months	0.33	19
8		0.40	23
10	1 Year	0.46	27
15		0.63	36
20	5 Year	0.83	48
25		0.95	55
30	9 Year	1.08	62
35		1.20	69
40	12 Year	1.30	75
60	adult	1.07	100
70	adult	1.76	100

As patient has to rely on others for medication, the therapeutic or dosing compliance poses a challenge.

The poor compliance can also be due to unpalatable or hard-to-swallow medications and due to spillage or spitting of oral medications.

Pharmacokinetics (ADME) markedly influence drug response in paediatric patients due to the age-related characteristics.

Box 17.1. Drugs to be avoided in lactating mothers

Drugs which should not be given to lactating mothers as toxic effects may be produced in infants:
- Opiates, Alcohol, Benzodiazepines, Phenobarbitone, Chloramphenicol, INH, Sulphonamides, Anticancer drugs.
- Oral contraceptives and Bromocriptine suppress lactation.

Absorption

Due to reduced secretion of gastric acid and prolonged gastric emptying time, the absorption of oral drugs in neonates is usually erratic. The underdeveloped digestive enzymes also impair absorption of orally administered drugs.

Infants also have low concentrations of bile acids and lipase, which may decrease the absorption of lipid soluble drugs. Trypsin secretion is decreased during early infancy and hence, a drug (e.g., chloramphenicol palmitate) that requires cleavage from its salt by pancreatic enzymes prior to absorption, may demonstrate variable bioavailability in first 3 months. The gastrointestinal microflora and its metabolic abilities develop over few months. This can influence the absorption profile of many drugs, such as digoxin.

Topical agents get absorbed promptly in children due to thinner epidermis.

Drugs should be given carefully by parenteral route as the therapeutic index may be narrow in paediatric patients.

Distribution

In children, total body fluids (particularly extracellular fluid) is more compared to adults, hence the volume of distribution of water soluble drugs is greater in paediatric patients.

Children have less fat in proportion to body mass, hence lipid soluble drugs are distributed more slowly.

As children have few protein binding sites than adults, more free drug is available for receptor sites.

Metabolism

Liver is the primary organ for drug metabolism and different hepatic enzyme systems mature at different age. The cytochrome P-450 mono-oxygenase system appears to mature rapidly, with metabolic activity similar to adult value being achieved by 6 months of age. In contrast, glucuronide formation reaches adult values between third and fourth years of life. Although infants are regularly characterized as being slow metabolizers of drugs, there are examples of drugs (theophylline, phenytoin, phenobarbitone) that are more rapidly metabolized by infants than adults. There are qualitative differences, too. A drug may be preferentially metabolized by one pathway during the neonatal period (e.g. theophylline) as compared to adulthood. All these have practical implications. While determining dosages of drugs that undergo hepatic biotransformation, sequence of maturation of processes of drug metabolism has to be taken into account. The drugs that are metabolized at a rapid rate require higher doses. Thus, theophylline is administered at much higher doses and frequency during infancy than in adulthood.

Excretion

Kidney is the predominant organ concerned with drug excretion. Drugs are also excreted through the gastrointestinal tract, biliary tract, respiratory tract and sweat glands, but these are important routes of excretion only for an extremely small minority of drugs. Renal excretion is dependent upon glomerular filtration rate (GFR), renal blood flow (RBF) and rate of active tubular secretion. These are dependent on age and maturity. A term infant has GFR and RBF that approximates 30 percent of adult value. In the premature neonate, these renal capabilities are only 15 percent or less, depending on the degree of prematurity. The renal capacity to excrete solutes improves quickly to reach 50 percent of adult value by 4th week and equals that of adults by 9-12 months of age.

Special Aspects of Paediatric Pharmacology

Children develop and grow, and their response to drug therapy is conditioned by age, size and stage of development. Physiologic processes that influence pharmacokinetic variables in children change significantly during the first few months. Pharmacodynamic differences between paediatric and other patients are probably small.

Pharmacologic response in paediatric patients

- There may be enhanced CNS response due to greater permeability of the blood-brain barrier, for example, infants are especially sensitive to narcotics, barbiturates and antiemetics.
- Tetracyclines cause permanent tooth discoloration, enamel defects, mottling teeth, retarded bone growth in children under age 8 years.
- Corticosteroids or other drugs that affect growth

and development may produce suppression of growth.

- Due to erratic temperature controlling mechanism administration of NSAIDs or chlorpromazine, or topically applied alcohol may produce low temperature.

Adverse reactions to drugs administered to infants are given in Table 17.5.

Table 17.5. Adverse Reactions to Drugs Administered to Infants

Drug	Reaction
Sulfisoxazole	Kernicterus
Chloramphenicol	Gray baby-shock, bone marrow suppression
Vitamin K analogs	Jaundice
Novobiocin	Encephalopathy
Phenolic detergents	Jaundice
Amphotericin	Anuric renal failure
Tetracycline	Enamel hypoplasia
Aminoglycosides	Deafness, renal toxicity
Enteric gentamicin	Resistant bacteria
Phenobarbital	Drowsiness
Morphine	Hypotension, urine retention
Dexamethasone	Gastrointestinal bleeding, hypertension, infection, hyperglycaemia
Furosemide	Deafness, hyponatraemia, hypokalaemia, hypochloraemia, nephrocalcinosis, biliary stones
Heparin	Bleeding, intraventricular haemorrhage, thrombocytopenia

DRUG USE IN GERIATRIC PATIENTS

The elderly consume more drugs than any other age group. They are also more susceptible than younger people to adverse drug reactions. This is because elderly patients have several illnesses and take multiple medication. The drug-related problems increase when a physician prescribes a medication without knowledge of other medication which the patient may be taking.

Some elderly patients may inappropriately self-medicate which increases the chance for adverse drug reactions.

Pharmacokinetics in geriatric patients

Absorption

Age-related changes in the stomach and intestine may decrease the rate of absorption or produce erratic absorption.

The longer gastric emptying time in the elderly may result in irritation from prolonged mucosal contact with irritant drugs, absorption of poorly water-soluble drugs may increase, weakly basic drugs (levodopa, anxiolytics, analgesics, anticonvulsants) may have delayed onset of action.

Reduced gastrointestinal motility may cause erratic absorption.

Elevated gastric pH may effect dissolution of weakly acidic drugs and delay their onset of action.

Reduced blood flow in intestines may cause incomplete drug absorption.

Distribution

In elderly persons, plasma albumin level is decreased leading to fewer protein-binding sites. So dosages of highly-bound drugs should be decreased.

In elderly persons, the percentage of body water and protein falls and the percentage of body fat increases, therefore the onset of action is faster and higher and therefore higher blood concentration is achieved in case of water soluble drugs, while lipid soluble drugs have a slower onset and prolonged duration of action.

Metabolism

In elderly persons due to decreased hepatic blood flow and reduced liver enzyme function there is slower drug metabolism resulting in higher plasma levels of active drug (thus an increased risk of adverse effects).

Excretion

Renal excretion is dependent upon the renal blood flow, glomerular filtration rate, and tubular function, all of which decline with age. Between the ages of 20 and 90 years, there is an average decline of 35% in glomerular filtration rate. However, muscle mass causes a decrease in endogenous creatinine production so that serum creatinine concentrations remain within normal ranges and do not reflect the decrease in creatinine clearance. Renal tubular function deteriorates with age as the absolute number of nephrons decline and may affect in particular the elimination of drugs which are actively secreted in the nephron. In addition to the physiological decline in renal function, the elderly patient is particularly liable to renal impairment due to dehydration, congestive heart failure, hypotension and urinary retention, or to intrinsic renal involvement, e.g. diabetic nephropathy or pyelonephritis.

In elderly patients due to reduced renal function, the drugs which are excreted unchanged in urine (digoxin, aminoglycosides, cimetidine and some cephalosporins) may achieve toxic blood levels.

For drugs with substantial renal elimination, dosages should be individualised in the presence of renal dysfunction. As GFR indicates the status of renal function, it may be calculated by the following formula:

$$\text{GFR (ml/min)} = \frac{[140 \text{ minus age}] \times \text{body wt. in kg}}{72 \times \text{serum creatinine mg/dl}}$$

Table 17.6 shows some changes in protein-binding, metabolism and excretion of drugs in elderly.

Pharmacologic responses in geriatric patients

Most of the changes result from altered pharmaco-kinetics or diminished homeostatic responses.

Due to change in end-organ sensitivity there may be heightened or diminished response, for example, beta-adrenergic receptors may be less responsive (dosage of beta-blockers may have to be increased).

As a person ages, CNS neurotransmitters become depleted, leading to increased effects of drugs such as antidepressants, barbiturates, benzodiazepines, and antiparkinsonian drugs.

Due to decreased protein-binding, heparin and warfarin produce greater response in elderly (thus more likely to produce adverse effects).

Some examples of altered drug responses are given below:

The elderly are more sensitive to some sedative-hypnotics and analgesics.

The half-lives of many barbiturates and benzodiazepines increase 50-150% between age 30 and age 70 (most of this change occurs from 60 to

Table 17.6. Alteration of plasma protein-binding, metabolism and renal elimination of drugs in elderly

Reduction in protein binding	
Warfarin	Diazepam
Lorazepam	Phenytoin
Tolbutamide	Phenylbutazone
Meperidine	
Reduction in hepatic metabolism	
Alprazolam	Barbiturates
Carbamazepine	Ibuprofen
Imipramine	Phenytoin
Nortriptyline	Propranolol
Warfarin	Quinidine
Diazepam	Lidocaine
Diphenylhydramine	Meperidine
Theophylline	Chlordiazepoxide
Nitrazepam	
Renal elimination reduced	
Penicillin	Tetracycline
Digoxin	Cimetidine
Aminoglycosie antibiotics	Clonidine
Diuretics	Lithium
Atenolol	Nadolol
Ranitidine	Famotidine
NSAIDs	Enalapril
Lisinopril	Procainamide
Cephalosporins	

70). The age-relate decline in the functioning of the kidneys and liver result in reducing the elimination of these drugs.

The elderly patients are markedly more sensitive to respiratory effects of analgesics, particularly opoids. This is due to the age-related changes in pulmonary function.

There is also an increased responsiveness to antipsychotic and antidepressant drugs. The half-lives of some phenothiazines are increased in elderly people, e.g. the half-life of thioridazine is more than doubled.

There is relatively high incidence of infections in geriatric patients due to the various age-related changes. The antimicrobials are very useful. However, in the elderly, the major pharmacokinetic changes produce decreased renal function and hence beta-lactam antibiotics, aminoglycosides and fluoro-quinolones which are excreted by kidneys will change the expected half-lives of these drugs.

Osteoarthritis is very common in elderly persons. For treating this condition, the non-steroidal antiinflammatory agents are commonly used. However, in these patients, special care must be taken to avoid toxicities to which they are very susceptible. These drugs may produce renal damage, which may be irreversible. As theses drugs are eliminated by the kidneys, they accumulate more rapidly in elderly people. A vicious cycle is set up i.e. cumulation of the NSAIDs cause renal damage which further cause more renal damage, and so on.

Those elderly patients who do not tolerate NSAIDs, corticosteroids are given. However, osteoporosis specially hazardous toxic effect in these patients may be produced (dose- and duration-related). These drugs should be used with special care.

The other effects due to the pharmacodynamic changes are:

- The average blood pressure specially systolic goes up with age, and the incidence of symptomatic or postural hypotension also increases markedly.
- Temperature regulation is impaired, and hypothermia is poorly tolerated in the elderly.

Four golden rules apply in prescribing for the elderly viz., the smallest number of drugs, in the lowest dosages, for the shortest period, in the simplest regimen, should be given.

STUDY QUESTIONS

1. Describe the factors that affect placental transfer of drugs. Name drugs which cross placental barrier.
2. Name the drugs which should be avoided by the breast-feeding woman.
3. Name some drugs which can be (a) safely administered during pregnancy; (b) unsafe drugs during pregnancy.
4. Name some drugs which should be avoided in all trimesters of pregnancy.
5. Which drugs can endanger continuation of pregnancy?
6. Comment on (a) embryocidal drug effects, (b) teratogenic drug effects, (c) foetotoxic drug effects. Give proper examples of drugs which may produce the above effects.
7. Describe the age-related effects of drug therapy on pharmacokinetics and pharmacologic responses in (a) paediatric and (b) geriatric patients.

GUIDE TO FURTHER READING

Abrans, W.B et al: Cardiovascular drugs in the elderly. Chest 1990; 98:980.

Ashburn, M.A et al: Management of pain in the cancer patient. Anesth Analg 1993; 76:402.

Briggs, G.G et al: Drugs in Pregnancy and Lactation. Williams & Wilkins, 1990.

Brinbaum, L.S et al: Pharmacokinetic basis of age-related changes in sensitivity of toxicants. Annu Rev Pharmacol Toxicol 1991; 31:101.

Carlsson, A et al: Brain neurotransmitters in aging and dementia: Similar changes across diagnostic dementia groups. Gerontology 1987; 33:159.

Cody, R.J et al: Physiologic changes due to age: Implications for drug therapy of congestive heart failure. Drugs Aging. 1993; 3:320.

Eisen, S.A et al: The effect of prescribed daily dose frequency on patient mendication compliance. Arch Intern Med. 1990; 150:1881.

Gifford, R.W Jr: Myths about hypertension in the elderly. Med Clin North Am., 1987; 71:1003.

Gilman, J.T et al: Therapeutic drug monitoring in the neonate and paediatric age group: Problems and clinical pharmacokinetic implications. Clin. Pharmacokinet, 1990; 19-1.

Greenblatt, D.J et al: Implications of altered drug disposition in the elderly: Studies of benzodiazepines. J Clin Pharmacol, 1989; 29:866.

Gurwitz, J.H et al: The ambiguous relationship between aging and adverse drug reactions. Ann. Intern. Med., 1991; 114:956.

Heymann, M.A et al: Non-narcotic analgesics: use in pregnancy and fetal and prenatal effects. Drugs. 1986; 32(Suppl 4): 164.

Hyams, D.E et al: The elderly patient: A special case for diuretic therapy. Drugs, 1986; 31(Suppl 4): 138.

Koren, G et al: Maternal-Fetal Toxicology; A Clinician's Guide. Dekker, 1990.

Lebel, M et al: Pharmacokinetics in the elderly. Studies on ciprofloxacin. Am J Med; 1987; 82: (Suppl 4A):108.

Lindeman, R.D et al: Longitudinal studies on the rate of decline in renal function with age. J Am Geriatr Soc., 1985; 33; 278.

Loi, C.M et al: Drug metabolism in the elderly. Pharmacol Ther, 1988; 36:131.

Massoro, E.J et al: Biology of aging: Facts, thoughts, and experimental approaches. Lab Invest, 1991; 65:500.

Meyers, B.R et al: Clinical pharmacology of antibacterial drugs in the elderly. Implications for selection and dosage. Clin Pharmacokinet, 1989; 17:385.

Morselli, P.L et al: Clinical pharmacology of the perinatal period and early infancy. Clin Pharmacokinet. 1989; 17 (Suppl 1):13.

Nottarianni, L.J et al: Plasma protein binding of drugs in pregnancy and in neonates. Clin Pharmacokinet. 1990; 18:20.

Paap, C.M et al: Clinical pharmacokinetics of antibacterial drugs in neonates. Clin Pharmacokinet, 1990; 19:280.

Pan, H.Y et al: Decline in beta-adrenergic receptor-mediated vascular relaxation with aging in man. J Pharmacol Exp Ther., 1986; 239:802.

Preskorn, S.H et al: Recent advances in antidepressant therapy for the elderly. Am J Med, 1993; 95 (Suppl 5): 2S.

Prinz, P.N et al: Geriatrics: Sleep disorders and aging. N Engl J Med., 1990; 323:520.

Ray, W.A et al: Psychotropic drugs and injuries among the elderly: A review. J Clin Psychopharmacol, 1992; 12:386.

Roberts, J et al: Age and diet effects on drug action. Pharmacol Ther., 1988; 37:111.

Rowe, J.W et al: Health care of the elderly. N Engl J Med., 1985; 312:827.

Safety of antimicrobial drugs in pregnancy. Med Lett Drugs Ther 1987; 29:61.

Salzman, C: Geriatric psychopharmacology. Annu Rev Med., 1985; 36:217.

Schmucker, D.L et al: Aging and drug disposition: An update. Pharmacol Rev., 1985; 37:133.

Schug, S.A et al: Pharmacologic management of cancer pain. Drugs., 1992; 43:44.

Schwartz, J.B et al: Cardiac drugs: Adjusting their use in aging patients. Geriatrics., 1987; 42:31.

Tonkin, A et al: Aging and susceptibility to drug-induced orthostatic hypotension. Clin Pharmacol Ther., 1992; 52:277.

Tsujimoto, G et al: Pharmacokinetic and pharmaco-dynamic principles of drug therapy in old age. Int J Clin Pharmacol Therap Toxicol., 1989; 27:13, 102.

Tumer, N et al: Geriatric pharmacology: Basic and clinical considerations. Annu Rev Pharmacol Toxicol., 1992; 32:271.

Vestal, R.E et al: Reduced beta-adrenoceptor sensitivity in the elderly. Clin Pharmacol Ther., 1979; 26:181.

Gene Therapy

TERMS ASSOCIATED WITH GENE THERAPY

Chromosomes : Structure present in the nucleus of a cell containing a condensed DNA double helix.

Codon : Three consecutive nucleotides in DNA and RNA that specify a particular amino acid or the beginning or end of a coding region.

DNA : Deoxyribonucleic acid; composed of four deoxyribonucleotides A, G, C, T and containing genetic information.

Gene : A segment of DNA or RNA that constitutes a unit of inherited information.

Gene expression : The process whereby the information in a gene is used to produce a cellular component.

Genetic map : A depiction of the linear order of genes along a chromosome.

Genome : The total genetic information of the cells including genes and other DNA sequences.

Germ cells : Egg cells and sperm cells.

Somatic cells : All the cells of the body except the germ cells.

Plasmid : A double-helical DNA that can replicate independently of the genome within a cell.

Recombinant DNA : A DNA molecule containing DNA segments from different sources, either biologically or chemically synthesised and formed by joining the diverse segments together by laboratory procedures.

DNA resulting from the insertion into the chain of a sequence not originally present in that chain.

Recombinant : A microbe or strain that has received chromosomal parts from different strains.

Replication : The process in which DNA or RNA directs its own duplication.

Transcription : Process of RNA synthesis from a double stranded DNA as template.

Transduction : To transfer the genetic material from one bacterium to another by the mediation of bacteriophage.

Transgene : A gene that has been introduced experimentally into an organism's genome and is passed onto the offspring.

Translation : The process by which genetic code in mRNA is decoded into a polypeptide.

Vector : An organism carrying a DNA molecule that can be joined to a foreign DNA segment so that the recombinant DNA can then be introduced into a cell where it can be replicated.

Retrovirus : A virus with RNA genome that

reproduces by first copying its RNA in DNA through reverse transcription.

Mutation : An alteration in DNA structure.

Transgenesis: Gene manipulation to modify germ cells of animals permanently is called transgenesis. As a result the gene manipulation is inherited by offspring of these animals. All cells of these off-springs inherit the introduced gene as a part of their genetic make-up. Such animals are said to be transgenic. The whole animal thus becomes an ultimate assay system for manipulated genes which govern complex biological processes. Furthermore, the transgenic animals provide possibility for expressing useful recombinant proteins and for generating precise animal models of human genetic disorders.

Organoids : Resembling in superficial appearance or in structure any of the organs or glands of the body.

Complexion : A combination.

GENERAL ASPECTS

If one takes journey of the history of medicine, three major revolutions are encountered viz., first being establishing public sanitation systems, second was surgery with anaesthesia and the third was concerned with vaccines and antibiotics. A beginning of the next important revolution is underway. The new technology of gene therapy promises to revolutionise medicine. Gene therapy will constitute a fourth revolution, because delivery of selected genes into patient's cells can potentially cure or ease majority of diseases, including many that have so far resisted treatment.

The unprecedented advances in understanding of the genetic basis of human diseases are based on the application of molecular biology to clinical medicine. Techniques derived from virology, bacteriology, biochemistry, cell biology and molecular biology permit the rapid identification of gene loci that cause or contribute to diseases in humans.

The human body has about 100 trillion cells. The nucleus of each cell has 46 chromosomes and each chromosome is made of coils of DNA molecules. DNA is organised in the form of genes. Genes are bits of DNA. The entire set of genetic material in a living creature is termed as "genome". Genome has gene as well as "junk" DNA. The human genome is made of an estimated 30,000 genes.

All hereditary information is transmitted from parent to offspring through the inheritance of deoxyribonucleic acid (DNA). DNA is a linear polymer composed of purine (adenine and guanine) and pyrimidine (thymine and cytosine) bases whose sequence ultimately determines the sequence of amino acids in every protein made by the body. The four types of bases in DNA are arranged in groups of three, each triplet forming a code word, or codon, that signifies a particular amino acid. A gene represents the total sequence of bases in DNA that specifies the amino acid sequence of a single polypeptide chain of a protein molecule.

The so-called "Central dogma" of molecular biology can be stated as following: Genetic information flows from DNA to RNA to protein.

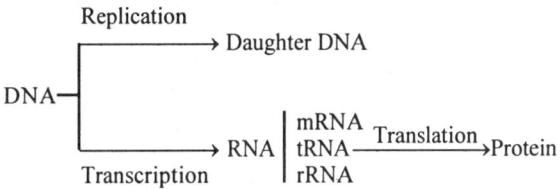

In nucleus:

$$DNA\ (a\ gene) \xrightarrow{Transcription} mRNA$$

At ribosome :

$$mRNA,\ tRNA\ and\ rRNA \xrightarrow{Translation} Protein$$

Genes are coded to produce proteins, they carry all the necessary information for making the proteins required by an organism. Genetic instructions are carried out by proteins. This knowledge will help us crack the human protein code, the proteome. Proteins (including enzymes) are versatile chemicals, determined by genes. They obey gene commands and carry out cellular functions.

A gene is a linear sequence of DNA that codes for a particular protein. On rare occasion, usually during the division of cell, the nucleotide sequence (the order of DNA pairs) of a gene can get jumbled up and mutated, so that the resultant protein is faulty. Such a mutation is the root cause of many diseases.

A defective gene leads to the failure, to synthesize a particular protein or to the synthesis of an abnormal protein. In either case, the absence of the normal protein can lead to a variety of clinical manifestations depending on the structural or enzymatic role that protein normally plays in the cell. Faulty protein may produce conditions which may range from mild disorders that require no treatment (e.g. colour blindness) to life-threatening diseases (e.g. haemophilia, cystic fibrosis). These diseases are in general, inadequately treated by conventional pharmacological means.

Therapy based on the replacement of the missing or defective protein (such as factor VIII for haemophilia, transfusions for sickle cell disease and adenosine deaminase for severe combined immuno- deficiency syndrome) is available for only a few of these disorders. Furthermore, these therapies are only partially effective in ameliorating the manifestations of the disease and are accompanied by significant complications.

For most genetic diseases, providing the missing protein in a therapeutic fashion is not feasible due to the complex and fragile nature of the protein and need to deliver it to a specific sub-cellular location (i.e. cell surface expression, lysosomal localization, etc.).

Transplantation of the major affected organ has been done in some instances (e.g. bone marrow transplantation for sickle cell disease, or liver transplantation for hyperlipidaemias), but this also has severe limitations of organ availability and adverse consequences arising from the immune suppression required to prevent rejection of an allogenic tissue.

Gene therapy overcomes these barriers by the selective introduction of recombinant DNA into tissues so that the biologically active proteins can be synthesized within the cells whose function is to be altered.

Gene therapy is a novel approach to treating diseases based on modifying the expression of a person's genes towards a therapeutic goal. Gene therapy is the genetic modification of cells to prevent, alleviate or cure disease. It involves transfer of recombinant DNA, transiently or permanently, into human cells for correction of disease.

The rationale for gene therapy lies in our understanding of the genetic basis of human diseases. It is probably safe to say that genes we inherit from our parents influence virtually every human disease.

The premise of gene therapy is based on cor-

recting disease at its root, i.e. the abnormal genes. There are essentially two forms of gene therapy: somatic gene therapy and germline gene therapy. Somatic gene therapy involves the manipulation of gene expression in cells that will be corrective to the patient but not inherited to the next generation. Germline gene therapy involves the genetic modification of germ cells that will pass the change onto the next generation.

Although the defective gene is present in all cells of an individual with an inherited disorder, only a few tissues or organs actually express the gene and therefore are affected. The limited number of tissues affected by most inherited disorders greatly simplifies the requirements for effective gene therapy, since a functional copy of the gene needs to be provided only to those tissues that actually require it.

Currently used drugs are estimated to interact with only about 400 genes or gene products to produce their therapeutic effects. However, the number of genes possibly involved in the disease processes would range anywhere from 3,000 to 10,000. Identification of new genes and their proteins may lead to development of new therapeutic targets.

The earliest human gene transfer experiments began in 1989 with lymphocyte marking studies. While offering no therapeutic benefit, these initial studies showed that gene transfer could be safely carried out and provided insight into many of the technical difficulties of human gene transfer. In September 1990, the first human gene therapy trial with therapeutic potential began. The ex vivo gene transfer of adenosine deaminase (ADA) gene into the lymphocytes of a child was carried out at the National Institutes of Health, USA. The results of this trial were encouraging.

Gene therapy has found therapeutic application in hereditary genetic disorders, cardiovascular diseases, cancer, infectious diseases and degenerative disorders, particularly those of the nervous system.

The main limitations that influence the success of gene therapy for inherited diseases are low efficiency of transduction, poor targeting, and adverse host immune response that often determine a low and short-term expression of the transgene.

The delivery of recombinant DNA in the target cell is critical to the success of gene therapy. A variety of DNA delivery systems have been developed based on viral life cycle pathways, liposome encapsulation, direct injection, complexion with proteins, DNA- ligand conjugates, plasmids and micro-carriers etc.

APPROACHES FOR GENE THERAPY

Various approaches have been tried for effective transfer of genes to appropriate target site. These approaches can be discussed under three categories. They are:

1. Gene modification
    (a) Replacement therapy
    (b) Corrective gene therapy
2. Gene transfer
    (a) Physical (Gene gun, Naked DNA etc.)
    (b) Chemical (CaPO$_4$ transfection)
    (c) Biological (Viral vectors)
3. Gene transfer in specific cell lines
    (a) Somatic gene therapy
    (b) Germline gene therapy

GENE MODIFICATION

The ultimate goal of gene therapy is either replacement therapy or corrective gene therapy.

In replacement therapy, a gene is inserted somewhere in the genome so that its product could replace that of a defective gene. This approach may be suitable for recessive disorders, which are marked by deficiency of an enzyme or other proteins. Though the gene functions in the genome provide an appropriate regulatory sequence, this approach may not be successful in treating dominant disorders associated with the production of an abnormal gene product which interferes with the product of a normal gene.

Corrective gene therapy requires replacement of a mutant gene or a part of it with a normal sequence. This can be achieved by using recombinant technology. Another form of corrective therapy involves the suppression of a particular mutation by a transfer RNA that is introduced into a cell.

Techniques of Gene Transfer

The transfer of DNA in the target cells is critical to the success of gene therapy. An ideal gene delivery system would be:

- capable of accommodating a broad size range of inserted DNA;
- available in a concentrated form;
- easy to produce;
- easy to target to specific types of cells;
- capable of not permitting replication of DNA;
- able to provide long-term gene expression;
- non-toxic and non-immunogenic.

An ideal gene delivery system does not exist. Various approaches have been developed most of which involve inserting the therapeutic gene into a delivery system called a "vector". These vectors can be grouped into 2 categories: (1) Viral vectors and (2) Non-viral.

There are two main strategies for delivering genes into patients: in vivo and ex vivo. The in vivo strategy is to inject a suspension of a vector containing the therapeutic gene directly into the patient (e.g., into a malignant tumour). The ex vivo strategy is to remove cells from the patient (e.g., stem cells from bone marrow), treating them with the vector, and injecting the genetically altered cells back into the patient.

Viral Vectors

A virus consists of genetic material (either DNA or RNA) encapsulated in a protein coat. Viruses can be taken up by the target cell, leading to the expression of virally encoded genes. Viruses take over the metabolic machinery of the cells they invade and may fuse with their nucleic acid. Most strategies for gene transfer utilise these properties, but for viral vectors to be useful, several viral functions must be altered. The virus must be rendered replication-incompetent to prevent uncontrolled spread of transgene (the newly introduced gene). Additional modification depends on the specific virus.

An ideal viral vector would be:

- cell specific and capable of delivering the therapeutic gene for particular clinical application;
- capable of regulated gene expression for the appropriate time duration to achieve the desired clinical response;

- capable of avoiding host defense system and would not induce immunogenic or inflammatory response;
- able to infect non-dividing cells;
- able to be handled easily, manipulated and grown on high titres in vitro.

There are five main categories of viral vectors currently undergoing clinical trials in gene therapy. These are:

1. Retroviruses
2. Adenoviruses
3. Adeno-associated viruses
4. Herpes simplex viruses
5. Vaccinia viruses

Each category has its own inherent set of advantages and limitations. The choice of viral vector depends on:

- the type of target tissue;
- the size of exogenous DNA;
- the nature of gene products;
- the required duration of expression of the gene product.

Retroviruses

A retrovirus contains two identical strands of RNA. After entering the host cell, the retrovirus releases an enzyme, reverse transcriptase, which makes a DNA copy of the viral RNA using building blocks present in the host cell.

Advantage of Retrovirus

Retroviral vectors have the greatest clinical use so far. Their effects are persistent because they become incorporated into and replicate with host DNA. So they are passed down to each daughter cell during division. They lack irrelevant and potentially immunogenic proteins.

Limitations

The application of retrovirus is limited to dividing cells because they are unable to penetrate the nuclear envelope. The nuclear envelope dissolves during cell division.

Application of retroviral approach

The approach using retroviruses has been used in trials to modify lymphocytes and haematopoietic cells, and to express immuno-modulatory agents in tumour cells. Retroviruses are being tested as potential agents to treat brain tumours. They are also being tried in the treatment of adenosine deaminase deficiency and hyperlipidaemia.

Adenoviruses

These are non-enveloped, double-stranded DNA viruses. They are not incorporated into the genome of the target cell but remain as an extrachromosomal entity in the nucleus of the host cell.

Advantages

Adenoviruses are the second most popular vehicle for gene transfer after retroviral vectors. In contrast to retroviruses, adenoviruses can efficiently infect non-proliferative cells. They do not integrate into the host cell genome, so they do not induce insertional mutagenesis. Furthermore, genes inserted into appropriate places are well expressed. They can be grown in vitro to high titres, are easy to handle and relatively easy for vector construction, all of which lower vector preparation cost.

Disadvantages

It may stimulate the host immune response, which can lead to destruction of vector transduced cells, local tissue damage and inflammation. The period of expression of an adenovirus-encoded transgene is very short. Treatment cannot be repeated because of neutralising antibodies.

Application

Adenoviral gene delivery is ideally suited to those situations that require only a one-off delivery of a transgene, for example, in growth factor therapy in which transient expression is required.

Routes of administration which can be used are I.V., intrabiliary, intraperitoneal, intravascular, intracranial and intrathecal injection and direct injection of the target organ parenchyma.

Adeno-Associated Virus (AAV)

These are single-stranded DNA, non-autonomous parvovirus which are able to integrate efficiently into the genome of non-dividing cells.

Advantages

AAV vectors offer many of the same advantages as adenovirus vectors including a wide host-cell range. In addition, unlike adenovirus, which can cause a high degree of cell-death (cytopathogenicity), AAV causes little damage in target cells.

Disadvantages

AAV vectors are significantly less efficient than retroviral vectors at transducing primary cell cultures. These are hard to mass produce and have a small capacity, so they cannot be used to carry large transgenes.

Herpes Simplex Virus (HSV)

It is a large, double-stranded DNA virus that replicates in the nucleus of infected cells. It has a broad host cell range, and can infect dividing and non-dividing cells as well as remain in a non-integrated state.

Applications

HSV vectors are being developed for several applications, particularly targeted at neuronal tissue. These include Parkinson's disease, malignant gliomas (a type of brain tumour) and cerebral ischaemia (starving of brain tissue from essential nutrients).

Advantages

HSV is maintained as an extrachromosomal DNA element in the nucleus of host cells, and has an excellent ability to establish long-lived asymptomatic infection in the nervous tissue. This provides the opportunity for long-term gene expression in neuronal target tissue.

Disadvantages

The main problem associated with the use of HSV as a gene therapy vector is the concern about its safety for clinical use owing to reports of wild-type virus replicating lytically in the human brain and resulting in potentially serious encephalitis.

Disabled version of human immunodeficiency virus (HIV): Unlike most other retroviruses, it infects non-dividing cells including neurons.

Non-Viral Gene Transfer

The potential limitations of viral vectors have led the investigators to examine the use of non-viral agents to mediate cellular uptake of exogenous DNA. These DNA delivery systems are constructed from known components and therefore their composition is well defined. Their formulation technically is much easier than that of viruses and in many cases these DNA delivery systems can be produced without the need for cell culture.

There can be two approaches for non-viral gene transfer. One approach is that the non-essential genes are removed from viral vectors to make more room for transgenes, to reduce inflammatory responses or to increase their safety. This involves the virus being simplified, sometimes to an extreme. What remains is an artificial 'vector shell', which has been designed to allow the gene of interest to be expressed at high levels in a highly regulated specific manner and for a controlled period of time (either short-term or long- term).

Another approach is to produce a system that can simply introduce genetic material to the nucleus of cells. This has been the focus of intensive research over the past few years, and has resulted in the development of several non-viral vector systems.

Liposomes

The basic challenge in in-vivo gene therapy is to deliver a transgene, a large hydrophilic molecule, across the plasma membrane and into the nucleus where it can have access to the cell's transcription machinery. Liposome delivery technology appears well suited to this task.

Liposomes, in their most basic form, consist of two lipid species, a cationic amphiphile and a neutral phospholipid. Liposomes bind to and condense DNA spontaneously to form complexes that have a high affinity for the plasma membranes of cells; this results in the uptake of liposomes to the cytoplasm by the process of endocytosis. Many modifications of this basic protocol have been tested and have resulted in varying levels of gene expression.

Plasmids

Plasmids are relatively small, double-stranded, closed- circular DNA molecules that exist apart from the chromosomes of their hosts. Plasmids present in a number of species of bacteria and yeast. Plasmids do not integrate into the actual hereditary material of the bacterial cells but float freely in the cytoplasm.

The most important property of a plasmid is that it bears DNA capable of replication that allows it to multiply within and independently of its host. If foreign sequences are combined with the plasmid, it still replicates and produces many copies of itself and its accompanying passenger.

Plasmids can permeate membranes and thus be transferred from donor cell through the membrane of the recipient cell. Protein structures on the surface of bacterial cells are a must for the docking of donor and recipient cells. The technique for achieving this transfer lies in equipping the plasmids with transfer (tra) and mobilising (mob) genes. Tra genes code for the protein structures while mob genes provide for the transfer of the plasmids genetic information.

Most of the genetic engineering research and industrial production is done using E. coli plasmid as a vehicle.

However, despite the simplicity of this approach, the transfection efficiency has been found to be low, limiting its application.

CaPO$_4$ Transfection

CaPO$_4$ transfection is a chemical method. It has been successfully used by molecular biologists to introduce transgenes into cells in vitro with a relatively good efficiency (10%). This method is not suitable for in vivo application.

Alternative Strategies for Gene Therapy

Implantation of genetically altered cells that secrete therapeutic gene products systemically or locally is another approach to gene therapy. This approach involves the development of 'organoids'. Cells that are genetically altered to produce high levels of a secretable gene product are expanded ex vivo. These cells are transplanted back into the recipient so that the gene product is secreted or delivered locally or systemically to a variety of cell types. Organoids have advantages for disorders that can be treated by a secreted protein that functions at distant cellular sites. Examples of this approach include expression

of factor VIII for haemophilia, β-glucuronidase for correction of mucopolysaccharidosis (MPS) type VII, and various cytokines for treatment of cancer.

DISEASE TARGETS FOR GENE THERAPY

I. Organ-directed gene therapy
1. Liver diseases e.g. familial hypercholesterolaemia.
2. Lung diseases e.g. familial emphysema, cystic fibrosis.
3. Cardiovascular diseases e.g. atherosclerosis, autoimmune vasculitis, restenosis, thrombolysis, hypertension, IHD. factor IX deficiency, anaemia, sickle cell disease.
4. Nervous system disorders e.g. Alzheimer's disease, Parkinson's disease, inherited metabolic brain diseases, neuro-degenerative disorders, brain injury.
II. Cancer.
III. Gene transfer into haematopoietic stem cells e.g. SCID, lysosomal storage disease.
IV. Gene therapy for infectious diseases e.g. AIDS, immunization.
V. Gene therapy applied to transplantation.

Liver Diseases

Liver can be afflicted with many kinds of metabolic, infectious and neoplastic diseases. Gene transfer methods might be used to deliver interferon alfa for the treatment of hepatitis B, cytotoxic therapy for hepatic carcinomas, or to provide a missing gene to correct an inherited metabolic defect.

There are multiple methods for targeting gene transfer to the liver. These methods are molecular conjugates, adenoviral vectors, liposomes and retroviral vectors.

For in vivo gene transfer, the liver is accessible by the routes like direct injection and intravenous and intra-biliary administration of vectors. Ex vivo strategies can be implemented by partial surgical resection of the liver, isolation of hepatocytes and in vitro hepatocyte transduction. The genetically modified cells can be reimplanted into the liver. This approach has been used experimentally to treat familial hypercholesterolaemia in which there is an inherited deficiency of LDL receptors.

Lung Diseases

The most common inherited lung diseases are familial emphysema and cystic fibrosis.

Familial emphysema is a consequence of a defect in the gene encoding the principal endogenous antiprotease, alpha-antitrypsin. This deficiency renders the lungs vulnerable to injury by neutrophil proteases released at sites of inflammation. The human gene has been cloned and delivered to the lungs in experimental studies.

Cystic fibrosis is the most common inherited disorder in the Caucasian population. Removal and reimplantation of airway cells is not technically feasible for therapy, because the target cells in the airway turnover very slowly and retroviral gene transfer requires cell division, is very inefficient. Hence, only in vivo approach remains. Adenoviral vectors are suited as they have tropism for respiratory epithelium.

Transient gene expression, low transfection efficiency and uncertainty of readministration due to inflammatory response are certain drawbacks of adenovirus.

Gene Therapy for Cardiovascular Diseases

Cardiovascular diseases have emerged as the most common cause of morbidity and mortality in most societies, especially the industrialised ones. The reason behind this seems to be that no effective therapy is available in case of diagnosis of certain defects like familial hypercholesterolaemia (FH) and restenosis after angioplasty. But now the molecular and pathophysiology of the cardiovascular system has been well understood. Researches have been diversified towards the use of gene therapy as a tool for the management of cardiovascular disorders.

Gene therapy towards cardiovascular diseases can be brought about by gene transfer. Gene transfer can be carried by 3 methods of gene modification i.e. gene replacement, gene correction and gene augmentation (addition of genetic material). Of these, gene augmentation is the most promising technique used in cardiovascular therapy. Gene transfer techniques most appropriate for cardiovascular application include:

(i) Viral-vector mediated gene transfer. These include viruses like retrovirus, adenovirus, sendai virus or haemagglutinating virus of Japan (HVJ).

(ii) Liposomal gene transfer e.g., cationic liposomes.

(iii) Reimplantation of cells modified in vitro.

Both the endothelial cells that line the blood vessels and the smooth muscle cells beneath the endothelium might be used to deliver transgene products into the blood stream. Genetic alteration of these cells might be useful to: (i) alter or prevent the process of atherosclerosis, (ii) deliver vasodilating agents locally, or (iii) provide local delivery of anti- coagulants.

Gene therapy approach may be utilized for a number of vascular disease conditions.

Atherosclerosis

Vascular cell proliferation and extracellular matrix protein deposition are associated with atherosclerotic narrowing of arteries. Factors that potentially contribute to this process can be studied by overexpressing their genes in arterial segments. For example,

(i) When acidic fibroblast growth factor (FGF-1) is ectopically expressed in porcine arteries, the vessel wall becomes thickened as a result of smooth muscle cell proliferation.

(ii) When TGF-β_1 is expressed ectopically in the vessel, extracellular matrix synthesis and intimal thickening result.

(iii) Platelet-derived growth factor B also has been shown to induce intimal hyperplasia following in vivo gene transfer.

These experimentally induced changes in the vessel wall mimic the changes found in atherosclerotic lesions. Gene transfer thus provides a useful tool to study the effects of agents that may be part of a complex disease process.

Autoimmune Vasculitis

When a foreign histocompatibility gene was delivered to vessel walls by liposome-mediated gene transfer it resulted in a focal immune response at the site of gene transfer that histologically resembles Takayasu arteritis. These experiments demonstrate that models of human disease can be developed by

604   Essentials of Pharmacology

introducing specific molecular changes in the blood vessel. These models may be useful in evaluating agents that can block these processes and alter the progression of the disease.

Restenosis

Prevention of local intimal hyperplasia and clinical restenosis after coronary angioplasty may be possible by introducing endothelial cells expressing genes for growth inhibitor proteins.

Thrombolysis

This may be possible by use of mutant forms of tissue type plasminogen activator (tPA) that can be delivered by an adenovirus to specific clot sites and quickly lyse a clot.

Hypertension

There is a possibility of treatment of hypertension using human tissue kallikrein genes.

Ischaemic Heart Disease

In ischaemic heart disease, administration of genes coding for angiogenic factors may result in enhanced growth of collateral vessels in areas of ischaemia.

Factor IX Deficiency

Patients have been treated with implants of autologous fibroblasts modified with a retroviral vector containing the gene for human factor IX.

Anaemia

Gene therapy may provide a means of augmenting the circulating red cell mass in the body. This may be done using recombinant adenovirus containing the human erythropoietin gene.

Sickle Cell Disease

A human beta globin and delta globin hybrid gene, namely, beta/delta sickle cell inhibitor (SCI), was transduced successfully by retroviral-mediated gene transfer.

Gene Therapy for Nervous System Disorders

Disorders of CNS have not gained due attention of researchers for the reason being a structurally and functionally complicated organ. The CNS involves differentiated cells which have different function and different anatomical connections. Similarly, the neurons are also much complicated both functionally and anatomically.

Despite these difficulties, a number of neurological disorders have emerged as promising gene therapy models. This advancement offered the realization that gene therapy for certain disorders, may not require the brain cells. Instead "surrogate" cells, such as autologous fibroblast, may be useful for delivery of therapeutic gene products after gene manipulation and transplantation to the brain. A new class of gene transfer vectors have been discovered which are capable of transferring the gene directly into neurons and glia in vivo. Herpes simplex virus (HSV-1) and retroviruses have properties of delivering foreign genes into neurons.

The application of gene therapy to neurological diseases has been possible with the increased understanding of the genetic basis of such diseases. Neurological disease where gene therapy may be useful are:

    (i) inherited metabolic brain disorder; and
    (ii) neurodegenerative disorders

Alzheimer's Disease

It is a neurodegenerative disorder in which there is a progressive loss of cholinergic neurons in the basal forebrain, with associated profound cognitive impairment. Treatment of this disease involves the delivery of nerve growth factor (NGF) which prevents the neuronal loss in addition to ameliorating deficits in learning and memory associated cells. The intercerebral transplantation of genetically modified fibrinoblasts has been applied to an animal model wherein a sparingly small amount of cholinergic neurons has been observed to produce NGF.

Parkinson's Disease

It is a disorder in which degeneration of dopaminergic neurons of the nigrastriatal pathways associated with a severe impairment of voluntary movement. Studies involving grafts of fetal substantia nigra dopamine neurons into the dopamine-depleted brain indicated that delivery of dopamine from grafted cells could lessen the movement disturbances.

Inherited Metabolic Brain Diseases

Diseases due to specific, single gene defect may be amenable to gene therapy e.g., Lesch Nyhan syndrome due to deficiency of enzyme hypoxanthine-guanine- phosphoribosyl transferases (HPRT) leading to severe behavioural and nervous system deficits.

Neurodegenerative Disorders

These have multifactorial causes and hence single gene replacement approach may not be effective. However, gene therapy may be useful for treatment of Alzheimer's disease, Huntington's chorea, Machado Joseph disease, dominantly inherited ataxia, familial amylotrophic lateral sclerosis and neurofibromatosis in which the defective genes have been identified.

Brain Injury

Gene therapy may be used to deliver the gene coding for an enzyme or growth factor, e.g., nerve growth factor (NGF) to enhance tissue healing. Diseases such as head trauma, stroke or multiple sclerosis may benefit with such therapy.

Cancer

Activation of oncogenes and mutation in tumour suppressor genes are common features of human malignancies.

Molecular processes that regulate cell-growth, although fundamental to tumour progression, are difficult to target with current gene transfer methods. One problem is that particular oncogenes are not uniformly present in all tumours of a given histological type. Another problem is related to metastasis. As most cancers exert their morbidity and mortality through metastatic spread, one is faced with not only targeting every cancer cell, but also targeting cancer cells in widespread anatomical locations. Furthermore, many lesions are microscopic metastatic deposits, undetectable by current diagnostic imaging methods.

Many tumours acquire a series of genetic defects as they progress. In addition, some tumours (e.g., chronic myelogenous leukaemia) arise as a consequence of mutations that result in a gain of function and thus require ablation of the new action.

Since 100% efficiency of gene-transfer has not been possible to achieve, following alternative strategies have been evolved which may be effective:

Cell-Targeted Suicide

The tumour cell may be genetically engineered to produce such an enzyme that will convert a particular drug to a toxic metabolite. Thus, a difference will be created between normal and tumour cells. A variety of enzymes are capable of performing such a function and kill cells by activation of a relatively non-toxic prodrug to a cytotoxic form. Insertion of the HSV-thymidine kinase gene into malignant cells in conjunction with systemic administration of ganciclovir has become a prototype gene therapy system that uses the enzyme-producing approach.

Ectopic Cytokine Expressions

Many types of cytokines decrease tumour growth when ectopically expressed on tumour cells or in their microenvironment. Tumour cells may be engineered to secrete such cytokines. A cytokine may have different effects in different types of tumours, e.g., interleukin-6 can have direct antiproliferative effects, recruit natural killer cells, or serve as an autocrine growth factor depending on the type of tumour investigated. In contrast, granulocyte macrophage colony stimulating factor (GM-CSF) has little effect on the tumourigenicity, but evokes a potent anti-tumour immunity.

Interleukin-2, interleukin-4, TNF-alpha, interferon gamma, and GM-CSF have shown promise in trials using tumour cells genetically engineered to secrete the cytokine.

Immune Enhancement

Approaches aimed at increasing the immune response to cancer cells have been developed. One such approach is to express highly immunogenic molecules on the surface of cancer cells, such as expression of allotypic major histocompatibility complex (MHC) antigens.

The immunogenic molecules engage specific receptors (e.g. CD-28, CTLA-4, etc.) on the T-cell surface in concert with antigen binding to the T-cell receptor. Subsequently, T-cell activation, cell proliferation, and cytokine production ensure and can lead to the elaboration of antitumour immunity.

Other promising approaches include restoring protective mechanisms such as p53; inactivating oncogene expression; delivery of proteins to healthy host cells in order to protect them (e.g., addition of multidrug resistance channel to bone marrow cells, ex vivo thereby rendering them resistant to drugs used in chemotherapy and protecting the patient from neutropenia and thrombocytopenia that may otherwise be caused by chemotherapy).

Gene Transfer into Haematopoietic Stem Cells

Because bone marrow can be removed easily and re- implanted, it provides an ideal setting for ex vivo gene therapy strategies. The ultimate goal is to be able to transfer genes into haematopoietic stem cells and allow these cells to reconstitute the bone marrow with the selective expression of the transferred gene in a specific haematopoietic cell lineage. Some of the diseases for which this strategy has been tried are:

Severe Combined Immunodeficiency Disease (SCID)

It is a single gene disorder in which there is deficiency of the enzyme adenosine deaminase (ADA). In children with this disorder, the absence of ADA leads to accumulation of deoxyadenosine triphosphate, which is toxic to lymphocytes.

Current standard therapy includes bone marrow transplantation. Intravenous ADA is used in patients who do not find a suitable marrow donor.

Clinical trials of gene therapy has resulted in clinical improvement. In this approach, haematopoietic stem cells are removed from an affected individual and transfected with functional genes. The engineered stem cells are then reinjected into the individual.

Lysosomal Storage Diseases

These result from the lysosomal accumulation of cellular material that cannot be degraded, or degraded material cannot be further processed. The absence of a particular lysosomal enzyme (a single gene defect) involved in the breakdown of glycolipids and sphingo- lipids leads to an increase in lysosome size and number. Gaucher's disease is a typical disorder

in which abnormal lipids or mucopolysaccharides accumulate in various organs. Gene transfer methods that may overcome the limitations of bone marrow transplant are being developed. These involve engineering the patients marrow to express the desired enzyme, so that patient's own leukocytes could deliver normal enzyme.

Gene Therapy for Infectious Diseases

The conventional antibiotics have failed to treat many serious pathogenic agents effectively, for example, HIV. The availability of unique molecular targets in these pathogens have encouraged the gene therapy studies for infectious diseases.

AIDS

Most of the current approaches are directed at stopping the replication of HIV in infected cells and preventing it from spreading to uninfected cells, ideally by rendering stem cells resistant to HIV before they mature.

In designing a gene transfer strategy for the treatment of AIDS, a dominant negative mutant protein has been used. The rev protein, produced by HIV virus, is a regulatory protein necessary for viral replication. Experimental studies have shown that by introducing a mutant rev gene, the HIV-infected cell produces an altered rev protein. This altered protein is not functional in promoting the synthesis of new viral proteins and ultimately attenuates HIV replication.

Immunization

An entirely different approach is immunization using gene transfer. Cells can be genetically engineered to synthesize an antibody with predetermined specificity. This would eliminate the need to rely on a variable or unpredictable immune response to a vaccine and could be used to direct the synthesis of the antibody to a specific site.

An antibody with specificity for the gp 120 HIV protein, that can be delivered by gene transfer, has been studied. It has been shown that human CD4+T lymphocytes can be transduced to express this antibody intracellularly.

Gene Therapy Applied to Transplantation

Organ transplantation is considered as an established

therapy for end-stage organ failure. Although advances in the development of immunosuppressive drugs (e.g., cyclosporin, corticosteroids etc.) have increased the survival rates of grafts, healthy grafts can still be rejected. Moreover, the use of systemic immunosuppressive agents is associated with significant risks, such as cancers, infection and ischaemic heart disease, even in patients with long-term functioning grafts.

Gene therapy is a good strategy for approaching existing problems associated with transplantation, but will most likely be used as a complementary approach. For example, grafts themselves could be targeted to reduce their immunogenicity by the introduction of genes to flock T-cell activation, or donor-specific MHC antigens could be introduced into the recipient before transplantation to induce transplantation tolerance.

Gene Transfer-Mediated Vaccination

It is a rapidly expanding field that is applicable to the treatment of both noninfectious and infectious diseases.

1. **Vaccination against noninfectious diseases:** Gene therapy for neoplastic diseases includes attempts to engineer an immune response to tumour cells. This idea came from the discovery of tumour-associated antigens on many different tumour types which suggests that tumour cells can be used to elicit an antitumour response.

   The strategies in this regard include: (1) transducing autologous tumour cells or tumour infiltrating lymphocytes to secrete a specific cytokine, for example, tumour necrosis factor, IL-2, IL-4, interferon gamma, etc.; (2) inducing tumour cell expression of a strong rejection antigen, for example, MHC molecules; and (3) inducing tumour cell expression of lymphocyte co-stimulatory molecules.

   The approaches have provided a limited data of phase-1 studies which is insufficient to indicate therapeutic effectiveness.

2. **Vaccination against infectious diseases:** The use of gene transfer to stimulate immunity to infectious agents is under trial. Insertion of DNA sequences that encode key antigens from patho-

genic agents would result in the cellular synthesis and presentation of these antigens which will mimic their presentation during infections, without risks of actual exposure to the infecting organisms. Such an approach will be of great importance in the development an HIV vaccine where the safety implications of a live, attenuated HIV vaccine are awesome.

ETHICAL AND SAFETY CONSIDERATIONS

As with any new technology, much attention has been directed toward ethical issues in gene therapy. Gene therapy can be subdivided into somatic cell gene transfer (that is, transfer to normal diploid cells), and germ-line gene transfer. In germ-line gene transfer, normal gene is inserted into haploid sperm, egg or one-celled embryo to correct the defect which is transmitted from generation to generation. The ethical issues associated with germ-line gene therapy are more complex, because the genes are transferred not only to treated individuals but also to their future generation.

There is currently no effective gene therapy in use. By knowing that a person carries a defective gene for a disease, has no use in cure. However, this knowledge raises numerous ethical and moral questions:

- If a mother finds out that her unborn child has a genetic abnormality, will she feel pressure to abort?
- If a person finds out he is susceptible to cancer because of a flawed gene, should life and health insurance agencies be given that information?
- Privacy of a person may be breached. In normal drug urine analysis test, urine may contain residual cells with complete DNA molecule intact. They may be screened for genetic abnormality. This information may be passed on to health and insurance agencies.
- The screening of individuals for genetic abnormalities have a potential for its misuse. About 4,000 genetically related diseases afflict humans. Once human genome is completely sequenced, it will be possible to screen embryos, foetus and adults for genetic diseases or pre- disposition to diseases.

- Treating human genetic diseases by intentionally altering the genes that are passed on to succeeding generations seems potentially dangerous. There is always the possibility of some unknown interactions between the introduced gene and the remaining genome. And the consequences of this ignorance would fall onto the foetus and innocent children in the succeeding generations. Here, there is no possibility of an informed consent.

There are safety concerns specific to particular therapy, e.g. polycythemia from over-expression of erythropoietin. There are also additional general concerns relating to viral vectors e.g.

- Vectors might acquire virulence during use.
- Viral proteins may be immunogenic.
- Can elicit an inflammatory response.
- Could damage the host genome and interfere with the cell cycle, can increase the risk of malignancy.

Ownership of human genes is the most intriguing ethical argument to date. Whether or not a person can receive a patent for a specific gene that everyone has? The United States patent office has already allowed patents for newly created species but has not yet given a judgment on the ownership of human genes. Although a person may not be the property of another, their genetic structure might be.

Several researchers have suggested that the human species could be "improved" by genetic alteration. The idea of re-engineering the human species has been gaining greater and greater attention throughout the world. Many ethicists and biologists are more concerned about the human drive for perfection. They worry that simple repair of genetic damage will lead to more radical re-engineering of the species. Almost everyone has some genetic trait or characteristic that is superior to everyone else. Some people have a photographic memory, the ability to function normally on only a few hours of sleep, or even a better emotional stability, what would be the result if all these traits, along with many others, could be isolated and engineered into a single individual? Would we have the perfect human? What are the moral and ethical implications of such research? What traits would science feel are undesirable?

The individuals born with genetic abnormalities are unfit and unwanted. What effect would a new wave of eugenics have on the countries that are made up of many hundreds of different cultures, races and ethnic backgrounds. Germany has the history of eugenic research and its consequences are known to the world. Nazi Germany justified their action by stating that, "the state was justified in demanding the sacrifice of the minority to advance the interests of the majority ...."

There is also concern about the possibility that gene transfer techniques would be used for trivial purposes such as cosmetic alterations e.g., alteration of normal characteristics like physical appearance, personality, intelligence and physical ability.

The new DNA diagnostics can be achieved using procedures such as Polymerase Chain Reaction (PCR), Restriction Fragment Length Polymorphisms (RFLPs), mapping, blotting and DNA sequencing. But these can also be used to discriminate among people. These diagnostics can be used by the prospective employers to select the candidates for the job. If a person's DNA data shows that he has an increased risk for certain disease, e.g. Alzheimer's disease, he might not be selected. Insurance companies, school authorities and even government, too can use similar arguments.

Prospects of the new diagnostics can be equally disturbing when the genetic component of behaviour is considered. Some forms of manic depression, schizophrenia and mental illnesses are thought to be, in part, to have a genetic basis. Intelligence is also partially genetically determined. Knowing DNA sequence can be of critical importance. In prenatal diagnosis of a birth defect or an enzyme deficiency, DNA diagnosis could be of immediate beneficial use. However, the issue of abortion is already explosive.

Although the medical potential for gene therapy is bright, the possibility of its misuse has to be kept in mind. There is a general consensus that somatic cell gene therapy for the purpose of treating a serious disease is an ethical option. Therefore, it is indispensable to ensure that gene therapy is used only ethically. Future research is inherently unpredictable in outcome. Deep thought and cautious analysis are required if we are to use the new technique.

OBSTACLES IN GENE THERAPY

Duration of Expression of Transgene

The main, real obstacle to the development of Gene Therapy as a powerful therapeutic tool remains the targeted and long-term regulated expression of the transgene. In the treatment of inherited diseases, it would be desirable to have stable gene expression over many years. In contrast, in the treatment of malignancy, it is possible that the long-term production of the therapeutic protein could have deleterious consequences.

Durable gene expression has yet to be conclusively demonstrated by any of the human trials to date.

DNA Delivery and Pharmacokinetics

Gene delivery is one of the main hurdles to making therapy practicable. The delivery of exogenous DNA and its processing by target cells require the introduction of new pharmacokinetic paradigms beyond those that describe the conventional medicines in use today.

With in vivo gene transfer, one must account for the fate of the DNA vector itself (volume of distribution, rate of clearance into tissues, etc.), as well as for the consequences of altered gene expression and protein function. A multicompartmental model is needed to describe it.

Processes that must be considered include the distribution of the DNA vector following in vivo administration; the fraction of vector taken up by the target cell population; the trafficking of the genetic material within cellular organelles; the rate of degradation of the DNA; the level of mRNA produced, the stability of the protein produced; and the protein's compartmentalization within the cell, or its secretory fate, once produced. It is conceivable, although yet to be realized, that each of these events may be incorporated into the design of the gene transfer system in a rational way so as to tailor the gene transfer to the specific requirements of the disease being treated.

Adverse Consequences of Heterologous Gene Expression

Because, in most circumstances, gene transfer will result in the synthesis of a new protein, the possibility of an immune response must be considered. A severe immune response could inactivate a secreted product (as is seen in haemophilia patients receiving factor VIII replacement therapy) or lead to an "autoimmune" response to transduced tissues.

In some circumstances, the DNA vector itself may be immunogenic, as has been demonstrated for adenovirus vectors. An immune response to the vector may preclude its readministration or limit the duration of its effectiveness. Pathological events may arise from viral vector replication.

Multiple Genetic Factor (Polygenic Defects)

Most diseases involve multiple genetic factors (they are polygenic). Until the precise involvement of different genes (their regulation and expression) in the disease process and the protein they encode is established, gene therapy is most likely to be clinically effective as a preventive or curative treatment for single-gene defects such as adenosine deaminase (ADA) deficiency, familial hypercholesterolaemia and cystic fibrosis.

Philosophical, Ethical and Theological Concerns

The limited clinical experience to date has generally been reassuring and has not so far provided evidence of insurmountable general problems. Besides the medical concerns, there are a number of philosophical, ethical and theological concerns. Though there is a general consensus that somatic cell gene therapy for the purpose of treating a serious disease is an ethical therapeutic option, considerable controversy exists as to whether or not germline gene therapy would be ethical.

In conclusion, the main limitations that influence the success of gene therapy for inherited diseases are: low efficiency of transduction, poor targeting and adverse host-immune response. These often determine a low and short-term expression of the transgene.

FUTURE PROSPECTS

The new technology of Gene Therapy promises to revolutionise medicine because delivery of selected genes into patient's cells can potentially cure or ease majority of diseases, including many that have so far resisted treatment. Genes give rise to proteins and defective genes can yield disease when they cause cells to make wrong protein.

Gene Therapy brings an entirely new approach for the treatment of disorders stemming from missing or defective genes, whether they are inherited or acquired.

Human Gene Therapy, although still in the infant stages of development, offers the possibility for major advances in prevention and treatment of a great number of diseases.

Moreover, this technology is likely to be evolved for the treatment of "non-genetic" illnesses, where the tissue-specific synthesis of a protein can be used for therapeutic benefit. The identification of new genes related to specific diseases will broaden the scope of application.

Currently, however, the clinical application of Gene Therapy is more limited by the availability of suitable gene transfer methodology than by the identification of suitable targets for genetic alteration.

Moreover, a better understanding of the pathophysiological processes will permit the design of physiologically appropriate interventions. It is to be hoped that increased collaboration among physicians, molecular biologists, and cell biologists will result in the development of highly integrated approaches to this new form of therapy.

STUDY QUESTIONS

1. Define the following: (i) Genome, (ii) Viral vectors, (iii) Non-viral vector, (iv) Retroviruses.
2. Discuss the rationale of gene therapy.
3. Describe the main approaches for gene therapy.
4. What will be an ideal gene delivery system?
5. Describe an ideal viral vector.
6. Describe some important disease targets for gene therapy.
7. What are the ethical considerations regarding gene therapy?
8. Discuss the obstacles in the development of gene therapy.

GUIDE TO FURTHER READING

Askari F.K., McDonnell, W.M. 1996: Antisense-oligonucleotide therapy. N Engl J Med, 334:316-318.

Blau, H.M., Springer, M.L. 1995: Gene therapy—A novel form of drug delivery. N Engl J Med, 333: 1204-1207.

Brenner, M.K. 1996: Gene transfer to hematopoietic cells. N Engl J Med, 335:337-339.

Chen, S.Y. Bagley, J. et al: Intracellular antibodies as a new class of therapeutic molecules for gene therapy. Hum. Gene Ther; 5:595-601, 1994.

Chen, S.Y., Bagley, J. et al: Intracellular antibodies as a new class of therapeutic molecules for gene therapy. Hum. Gene Ther; 5:595-601, 1994.

Docherty, K. 1997: Gene therapy for diabetes mellitus. Clin Sci, 92:321-330.

Gotesman, M.M., Germann, U.A. et al: Gene transfer of drug resistance genes; implications for cancer therapy. Ann N.Y. Acad. Sci. 716:126-138, 1994.

Gottesman, M.M., Germann, U.A. et al: Gene transfer of drug resistance genes; implications for cancer therapy. Ann N.Y. Acad. Sci. 716:126-138, 1994.

Hauck, W., Stanners. C.P., 1995: Transcriptional regulation of the carcinoembryonic antigen gene. J. Biol. Chem. 270:3602-3610.

Hill, A., Jugovic, P., York. I. Russ. G Bennink, J. Yewdell, J., Ploegh, H., Johnson, D., 1995: Herpes virus turns off the TAP to evade host immunity. Nature, 375:411-415.

Ido, A., Nakata, K., Kato, Y., Nakao, K., Murata, K., Fujita, M., Ishii, N., Tamaoki, T., Shiku, H., Nagataki, S., 1995: Gene therapy for hepatoma cells using a retrovirus vector carrying herpes simplex virus thymidine kinase gene under the control of human a-fetoprotein gene promoter. Cancer Res. 55:3105-3109.

Ilan, Y., Droguett, G, Chowdhury, N., Li. Y., Sengupta, K., Thummala, N.R. Davidson, A., Chowdhury, J.R., Horwitz, M.S., 1997: Insertion of the adenoviral E3 region into a recombinant viral vector prevents antiviral humoral and cellular immune responses and permits long-term gene expression. Proc. Natl. Acd. Sci. USA, 94:2587-2595.

Jolly, D: Viral vector systems for gene therapy. Cancer Gene Therapy, 1:51-64, 1994.

Jolly, D: Viral vector systems for gene therapy. Cancer Gene Therapy. 1:5-1-64, 1994.

Kaneko, S., Hallembeck, P., Kotani, T., Nakabayashi, H., McGarrity, G., Tamaoki, T., Anderson, W.F., Chiang, Y.L., 1995: Adenovirus-mediated gene therapy of hepatocellular carcinoma using cancer-specific gene expression. Cancer Res. 55:5283-5287.

Kennedy, P.G.E. and Steiner, I: The use of herpes simplex virus vectors for gene therapy in neurological diseases, Q. J. Med., 86:697-702, 1993.

Kennedy, P.G.E., and Steiner, L: The use of herpes simplex virus vectors for gene therapy in neurological diseases, Q.J. Med., 86:697-702, 1993.

Kotin, R.M: Prospects for the use of adeno-associated virus as a vector for gene therapy, Hum. Gene Ther. 5:793-801, 1994.

Kotin, R.M: Prospects for the use of adeno-associated virus as a vector for gene therapy. Hum. Gene Ther, 5:793-801, 1994.

Lachmann, R.H., Efstathiou, S., 1997: Utilization of the herpes simplex virus type 1 latency associated regulatory region to drive stable reporter gene expression in the nervous system. J. Virol. 71:3197-3207.

Lee, C. H. Liu, M., Sie, K.L., Lee, M.S. 1996: Prostate-specific antigen promoter driven gene therapy targeting DNA polymerase-a and topoisomerase Ila in prostate cancer. Anticancer Res. 16:1805-1812.

Leiden, J.M. 1995: Gene therapy—Promise, pitfalls and prognosis. N Engl. J. Med, 333:871-872.

Manca, F., Fenoglio, D., Franchin, E., Saverino, D., Li Pira, G., Buffa, F., Bignardi, D., Del Pup, L., Palu, G., 1997: Anti-HIV genetic treatment of antigen-specific CD4 lymphocytes for adoptive immunotherapy of opportunistic infections in AIDS. Gene Ther. 4:1216-1224.

Miyoshi, H., Takahashi, M., Gage, F.H., Verma, I.M. 1997: Stable and efficient gene transfer into the retina using an HIV-based lentiviral vector. Proc. Natl. Acad. Sci., USA, 94:10319-10323.

Neicfeld, E.F: Lysosomal storagee diseases. Annu. Rev. Biochem. 60:257-280, 1991.

Neufeld, E.F: Lysosomal storage diseases, Annu. Rev. Biochem. 60:257-280, 1991.

Nienhuis, A.W., McDonagh, K.T. et al: Gene transfer into hematopoietic stem cells. Cancer, 67:2700-2704, 1991.

Nienhuis, A.W., McDonagh, K.T. et al: Gene transfer into hematopoietics stem cells. Cancer, 67:2700-2704, 1991.

Ohno, T., Gordon, D. et al: Gene therapy for vascular smooth muscle cell proliferation after arterial injury. Science, 265:781-784, 1994.

Ohno, T., Gordon, D. et al: Gene therapy for vascular smooth muscle cell proliferation after arterial injury. Science, 265:781-784, 1994.

Palu, G., 1997: Combined strategies for gene therapy of AIDS. Gene Ther. 4:179-180.

Peng. K.W., Morling, F.J., Murphy, G., Russell, S.J., 1997: A gene delivery system activatable by disease-associated matrix metalloproteinases. Hum. Gene Ther. 8(6):729-738.

Pizzato, M., Franchin, E., Calvi, P., Boschetto R., Ferrini, S., Colombo, M., Palu, G., 1998: Production and characterization of a bicistronic Moloney-based retro- viral vector expressing human interleukin 2 and herpes simplex thymidine kinase for gene therapy of cancer. Gene Ther, 5:1003-1007.

Raper, S.E., Grossman, M., Rader, D.J., Thoene, J.G. Clark, B.J. Kolansky, D.M. Muller, D.W. Wilson. J.M., 1997: Safety and feasibility of liver-directed ex vivo gene therapy for homozygous familial hyper-cholesteromia. Ann. Surg. 225(4):442-443.

Riddell, S.R., Elliott, M., Lewinsohn, D.A., Gilbert, M.J., Wilson, L., Manley, S.A., et al., 1996: T-cell mediated rejection of gene-modified HIV-specific cytotoxic T lymphocytes in HIV-infected patients. Nat. Med. 2:216-223.

Schnierle, B.S. Groner, B., 1996: Retroviral targeted delivery. Gene Ther, 3:334-342.

Verma, I.M., Somia, N. 1997: Gene therapy—Promises, problems and prospects. Nature, 389:239-242.

Weichselbaum, R.R., Kufe, D. 1997: Gene therapy of cancer. Lancet 349 (Suppl II):10-12.

Wilson, J.M. 1996: Adenoviruses as gene-delivery vehicles. N Engl J Med, 334:1185-1187.

Wolff, J.A., and Lederberg, J: An early history of gene transfer and therapy. Hum. Gene Ther., 5:469-480, 1994.

Wolff, J.A., and Lederbery, J: An early history of gene transfer and therapy. Hum. Gene Ther., 5: 69-480, 1994.

York, I.A., Roop, C., Andrews, D.W., Riddell, S.R., Graham, F.L., Johnson, D.C. 1994: A cytosolic herpes simplex virus protein inhibits antigen presentation to CD8+ T lymphocytes, Cell, 77:525-535.

Zhou, S.Z., Li, Q., Stamatoyannopoulos, G., Srivastava, A., 1996: Adeno-associated virus 2-mediated trans-duction and erythroid cell-specific expression of human B-globin gene. Gene Ther., 3:223-229.

Zufferey, R.., Nagy, D., Mandel, R.J., Naldini, L., Trono, D., 1997: Multiple attenuated lentiviral vector achieves efficient gene delivery in vivo. Nature Biotech. 15:871-875.

CHAPTER

19

Vaccines and Sera

CHAPTER CONTENTS AT A GLANCE

- Types of immunity
  Natural
  - Species
  - Racial
  - Individual
  Acquired
    Active
    - Natural
    - Acquired
    Passive
    - Natural
    - Acquired
- Comparison between active and passive immunization
- Types of immunizing agents
  For active immunity
    Vaccines
    - Bacterial vaccines
    - Viral vaccines
    Toxoids
  For passive immunity
    Human immune sera
    - Immune globulin
    - Hyperimmune serum
    Animal immune serum
    - Antitoxin
    - Antiviral serum
    - Antivenin
- Immunization schedules
- A step ahead
- Adverse reactions
- Contraindications
- Chemical interactions of vaccines
- Immunologic interference
- Immunologic memory
- Points regarding maintenance
- Future

IMMUNITY

Immunity in the broadest sense may be defined simply as inborn or acquired resistance to disease. It is the resistance to possible attack of an infectious agent i.e. resistance to invasion and multiplication of a disease producing organism.

TYPES OF IMMUNITY

I. **Innate Immunity (Natural Immunity) :** It can be specific or non-specific in nature.
   (a) Specific : It can be :
      (i) Species specific
      (ii) Racial specific
      (iii) Individual specific
   (b) Nonspecific defence mechanisms

II. **Acquired Immunity**
   (a) Active : It can be
      (i) Natural
      (ii) Artificial
   (b) Passive : It can be :
      (i) Natural
      (ii) Artificial

Innate Immunity

Resistance to certain infections is a natural gift and is seen is all forms of life. This natural non-susceptibility to infections is called innate immunity. Innate immunity may be specific and nonspecific. When specific, it may be species specific, race specific or individual specific.

Species specific immunity : Certain infections occur only in particular species e.g. syphillis, gonorrhoea, leprosy, measles, diptheria, cholera, and many other diseases, occur only in man but not in lower animals. Birds are immune to tetanus, a disease affecting man and certain lower animals. Conversely some diseases occurring in animal are not found in man e.g. rinderpest, chicken cholera etc. It seems that the tissue of one or some other species are unsuitable to serve as host to certain parasites but those of others provide congenial home for them.

Race specific immunity : All races of same species are not found to exhibit the same degree of susceptibility or resistance to infection e.g. Negroes have a high resistance to yellow fever but white men are susceptible. The Caucasion race is more resistant to tuberculosis than negroes or American Indians.

Individual Specific : Some differences in susceptibility to certain infections do occur in individuals of same species e.g. individual of heterozygous traits of sickle cell anaemia, thalassaemia, haemoglobin 'C' disease, and deficiency of glucose-6-phosphate dehydrogenase are resistant to some types of malaria. Individuals of blood group 'O' and 'B' are more resistant to small pox than those of blood group 'A'.

Individual : Individuals in good health are endowed with high level of natural immunity.

Non-specific Defence Mechanisms : A number of defence mechanisms are operative non-specifically against a large number of microorganisms. They are (i) Mechanical barriers, (ii) Antagonisms of indigenous flora, (iii) Microbicidal substances of body fluids and those liberated by damaged cells, (iv) Phagocytosis by microphages and macrophages, (v) Natural killer cells and soluble factors, (vi) Acquired non-specific defence mechanisms.

Mechanical barriers : Access of many organisms to deeper tissues is prevented by skin and mucous membranes. Ciliary movements in epithelial cells of respiratory mucosa and peristaltic movements of intestine push the organisms away before they could invade.

Antagonism by indigenous flora : The normal microbial flora of mucous membranes prevent the proliferation of pathogenic organisms on account of substrate competition, or by producing inhibitory substances e.g. H_2O_2 or by altering the pH to make it unsuitable for the growth.

Bactericidal substances : Some substances present in blood and body fluids have microbicidal activity e.g. long chain fatty acids present in skin, Lactenin of milk (bactericidal for Strept. pyogenes), HCl of gastric juice, Lysozyme (muramidase), basic polypeptides e.g. spermine, spermidine, protamine for damaged blood cells and tissue (bactericidal in nature) etc.

Some metabolites like lactic acid, CO_2 which accumulate in an inflamed area and the depletion of O_2 by the inflammatory cells provide unfavourable conditions for growth of pathogenic organisms.

A number of plasma components like c-reative protein, α-1 antitrypsin, α-2 microgloblulin, fibrinogen, ceruloplasmin, C_9 factor B, collectively termed acute phase proteins show a marked increase in response to infection or tissue injury.

Nasal secretions and serum of normal human beings have the ability to neutralize certain viruses e.g. influenza A & B, vaccinia, mumps and newcastle viruses. This is due to the presence of certain enzymes like alkaline and acid phosphatases in serum and secretions which have the virucidal activities. Interferon, a non specific antiviral agent is synthesized by the cells in response to viral infection. It inhibits intracellular replication of viruses.

Phagocytosis : Microphages and macrophages which are phagocytic cells, migrate under the influence of chemotaxins to the site of infection and phagocytose the infective agents. Within the phagocytes the organisms are killed and disintegrated finally.

Natural killer (N.K.) cells and soluble factors: The N.K. cells (leukocytes), bind to the target cells and can kill them. These are activated by interferons which are themselves component of innate immune system.

The two extremes of life carry higher susceptibility to infectious diseases as compared to adults. The foetus in utero is normally protected from maternal infection by the placental barrier. Severe endocrine disorders such as diabetes mellitus, hypothyroidism and adrenal dysfunctions are associated with an enhanced susceptibility to infections.

Acquired Immunity

The resistance that an individual acquires during his life is known as acquired immunity (or adaptive immunity), as distinct from the inborn innate immunity.

Natural immunity is inadequate for protection against many microbial diseases and the additional immunity is acquired either actively, due to stimulation of the individual's antibody producing cells (active immunity) or passively, as a result of the introduction of antibodies from another person or animal (passive immunity).

Naturally acquired active immunity

This occurs when antigen results in a disease and antibodies are produced in sufficient amount to protect the individual from possible future infections by the same species of microorganisms. The infections which are produced may or may not result in clinical recognizable disease.

When a patient recovers from certain disease he is left with a high degree of immunity e.g. in case of diptheria, smallpox, etc.

Some times the invading organisms do not produce clearly distinguishable signs of the disease but the individual becomes immune, presumably because the antibody producing cells have received an adequate stimulus. Children in slum area because of more frequent exposure to sub-infection, often develop immunity to a variety of diseases more quickly than children in more affluent areas.

Artificially acquired active immunity

This involves the use of avirulent antigens in the form of biologics such as vaccines and toxoids, that are so modified as to be incapable of producing the disease state, yet at the same time, when introduced in the body will elicit the production of specific protective antibodies against the disease.

Passive immunity : Passive immunity can be acquired naturally or artificially similar to active immunity.

Naturally acquired passive immunity

This occurs on account of transplacental transfer of antibodies (IgG) from mother to foetus and it lasts for nearly six months after birth. Secretory antibodies (IgA) present in the milk also provide local immunity in g.i.t. of breast fed infants e.g. babies show high resistance to chickenpox, diptheria, measles, and scarlet fever, but usually this is lost after six months of age of child.

Artificially acquired passive immunity

Several biologics are involved in providing antibodies including antitoxins and sera of animal origin and immunoglobulin and hyperimmune sera derived from human plasma.

In passive acquired immunity, the antibodies are produced in another individual (human or lower animal). The immunity is acquired by the introduction of these antibodies and the host is not "actively" involved in antibody production but is "passively" receiving antibodies. Passive immunization is useful (i) for individuals unable to form antibodies e.g., congenital agammaglobulinemia; (ii) acutely ill, debilitated and immunocompromised individuals who may not be able to generate sufficient antibody response; (iii) for prevention of disease when time does not permit active immunization, e.g. post-exposure; (iv) for treatment of certain diseases normally prevented by immunization e.g., tetanus; and (v) for treatment of conditions for which active immunization is unavailable or impractical e.g., snakebite.

The passive immunity lasts for a short time and also associated with serious side effects, such as fatal anaphylaxis and serum sickness. However, the main advantage is the immediate availability of ready made antibodies against microorganisms.

Local immunity : The concept of local immunity has gained importance in the treatment of infections which are either localised or where it is operative in combating infections at the site of primary entry of the pathogens. In poliomyelitis, for instance, systemic immunity provided by active immunization with the killed vaccine neutralises the virus when it enters the blood stream. But it does not prevent multiplication of the virus at the site of entry (the gut mucosa) and its shedding. This is achieved by the local intestinal immunity acquired as a result of either natural infection or immunization with live oral vaccine.

Herd immunity means that a group of people or a community as a whole automatically develops immunity in the entire population if more than 85% of the targeted population is immunized. It is relevant in the control of epidemic diseases. When the herd immunity is low, epidemics are likely to occur on the introduction of a suitable pathogen, due to the presence of large number of susceptible individuals in the community. Eradication of communicable diseases depends on the development of a high level of herd immunity rather than on the development of a high level of immunity in individuals.

The effects of antigen-containing and antibody-containing preparations are shown in Table 19.1 and the comparison between active and passive immunization is given in Table 19.2.

Table 19.1. Effects of antigen-containing and antibody-containing preparations

Antigen-containing preparations	Antibody containing preparations
• Stimulate active immunity	• Give passive immunity
• Patient produces antibodies	• Patient receives antibodies
• Immunity develops slowly	• Immunity produced quickly
• Lasting effect	• Temporary effect
• Used for long-term effect	• Used for short-term prophylaxis and therapeutically

Table 19.2. Comparison between Active and Passive Immunization

Active Immunization	Passive Immunization
More efficacious	Less effective
Longer lasting	Shorter duration
Needs latent period of one to many weeks	Effective immediately after injection
Vaccines are only prophylactic	Prophylactic as well as curative
Avoided during corticosteroid or immunosuppressant medication as active immunization with vaccine may fail to "take"	

VACCINATION

Nearly 200 years ago, Edward Jenner carried out the remarkable studies which mark the beginning of immunology as a systematic subject. Noting the pretty pox-free skin of the milk maids, he reasoned that deliberate exposure to the pox virus of the cow, which is not virulent for the human, might confer protection against the related human smallpox organism. Accordingly, he inoculated a small boy with cowpox and was delighted and relieved to observe that he was now protected against a subsequent exposure to smallpox (what would today's ethical committees have said about that ?). This marked the beginning of modern vaccination (Latin Vacca, cow).

Immunization plays a very important role in control of infectious diseases. They help to build up immunity in the immunized individuals against specific diseases and thus help to decrease the transmission of diseases from one person to another.

Immunization can be active or passive, while vaccination is always active.

Immunizing agents and allergens (inciting agents of allergy) are two of the main groups of drugs that are classified as biologics.

Immunologists are also aggressively studying the relationship between the aging process and a progressive decline in immune system performance. If it can be understood how and why the immune system becomes less effective with aging, perhaps the process can be slowed or stopped and then one may expect to approach genetically programmed life span, which many people believe to be 110 to 120 years. It now appears certain that the immune system is an extremely important player along with how one thinks and acts.

Primary Immunization

When antigen first comes in contact of the body, it results in formation of antibodies after a variable 'lag phase' of about 2-6 weeks (sometimes as short as few hours like with pneumococcal polysaccharide). The titre of antibodies is low and response short lived. The antibodies formed in the primary response are predominantly IgM.

Secondary Immunization

When the same antigen i.e. the antigen which

produced the primary response again comes in contact with the body, the response is prompt, powerful and prolonged. The 'lag phase' is short or negligible. The titre of antibodies is much higher and last for long periods. The antibodies formed in the secondary response are IgG.

Types of Immunizing Agents

- Active Immunizing Agents (Vaccines)
- Passive Immunizing Agents (Antibody products)

For Active Immunity

Vaccine is a suspension of attenuated (live) or inactivated (killed) microorganisms or fractions thereof administered to induce immunity and thus prevent infectious disease.

Vaccine means any immunological product used in active immunization of humans and animals.

Vaccine can be defined as suspension or solution of an immunogenic substance or compound(s) that is intended to induce active immunity, and the process of active immunization is called vaccination.

The majority of vaccines consist of entire microorganisms that may be either inactivated (killed) or live attenuated. Attenuated refers to strains of organisms that have a reduced disease-causing capacity but that retain the major immunogenic characteristics of the so-called wild strains that circulate in the community. It can be seen that viral vaccines comprise most of the live attenuated viruses while most of the bacterial vaccines contain killed bacteria or their components.

Toxoids are protein toxins that have been modified (e.g. by treatment with formalin) to reduce the toxicity without significantly altering the immunogenicity. Two of the best known active immunizing agents are diphtheria toxoid and tetanus toxoid.

Generally speaking, live vaccines provide better immunity than killed and the natural route of administration is even better, for example, the inactivated poliovirus vaccines provide an excellent antibody response that protects well against systemic disease but produce little local immunity in the gut that is necessary to prevent infection and transmission of the wild virus. The live, oral poliovirus vaccines provide excellent antibody and cell-mediated immunity both systemically and locally in the gut.

How are vaccines produced?

For the production of vaccines against viral disease, strains of virus are often grown by using embryonated eggs. Individuals who are allergic to eggs cannot be given such vaccine preparation. Viral vaccines may also be produced by using tissue culture. For example, the older rabies vaccine, which was produced in embryonated duck eggs and had painful side effects, has been replaced with a vaccine produced in human fibroblast tissue cultures which has far fewer side effects. The production of the vaccines by bacteria, fungi and protozoa generaly involves growing the microbial strain on an antificial medium which minimises problem with allergic response. Vaccines should be tested and standardised before use.

Due to failure in creating effective vaccines against diseases such as German measles, diptheria, whooping cough, tetanus, smallpox, and poliomyelitus, new technologies are now available for producing new vaccines, like Recombinat DNA technology for influenza, AIDS. Reassortants for influenza, mutations for polio, genetic deletions for herpes, etc.

There are a number of limitations to the current mode of vaccine production :

Not all infectious agents can be grown in culture, so no vaccination has been developed for a number of diseases.

Production of animal and human viruses requires animal cell culture, which is expensive.

Extensive safety precautions are necessary to protect production personnel in the laboratory.

Batches of vaccine may be harmful, if insufficiently killed or attenuated.

Not all diseases (e.g. AIDS) are preventable through the use of traditional vaccines.

Most current vaccines have a limited shelf-life and often require refrigeration to maintain potency which creates stoage problems in countires with large rural, unelectrified areas. Hence, newer technologies should be adopted.

Live nonpathogenic carrier systems that carry discrete antigenic determinants of an unrelated pathogenic agent can be created. This helps in induction of strong immunological response directed against the pathogenic agent.

For those infections, agents that can not be maintained in culture, the genes for the proteins that have critical antigentic determinants can be isolated, cloned and expressed in an alternative host system such as E.coli or a mammalian cell line.

There are 3 types of vaccines (Table 19.3):

(1) Inactivated (killed) vaccine

The efficacy is less but are also less toxic. They are usually given by S.C. or I.M. injection. Examples : Vaccines against pertussis, rabies, hepatitis B, typhoid, influenza.

(2) Live attenuated vaccines

Live vaccines are prepared from attenuated organisms which have been made incapable of producing full blown disease but their immunogenic potential remains intact. Examples : BCG, oral polio vaccine, etc.

The live vaccines are more potent and more durable immunizing agents. Another advantage of live vaccine is that a single dose is sufficient for immunization, unlike killed vaccines which are required to be given in multiple doses. Live vaccines are contraindicated in leukaemia, lymphoma, in patients receiving corticosteroids and anticancer drugs.

(3) Toxoids

These are prepared by adding formalin to toxins of microorganisms and incubated at $37^{\circ}C$ for 3-4 weeks. This treatment completely destroys their toxic properties without causing significant loss of antigenic qualities. These elicit antibody response when administered.

Note : Toxoids are described separately sometimes, and the term vaccines is restricted to Killed vaccines and Live attenuated vaccines. Table 19.3 shows types of vaccines.

Table 19.3. Types of vaccines

Live attenuated vaccines

	Bacterial	Viral
	BCG	Polio
		Measles
		Mumps
		Rubella
		Varicella - zoster
		Hepatitis A, B

Inactivated or killed vaccines

	Bacterial	Viral
	Pertussis (whooping cough)	Polio
	Typhoid	Rabies
	Cholera	Influenza
	Plague	Hepatitis A

Combined Vaccines

Double antigen (DT-DA)	**Toxoids**
Triple antigen (DPT)	Tetanus
Typhoid-paratyphoid-cholera (TABC)	Diphtheria
Measles, Mumps, Rubella (MMR)	

Comparison between live attenuated and killed vaccines

Live attenuated vaccines are extremely potent and usually produce life long immunity even with one injection (measles, mumps, rubella). But there is a potential danger of transmitting vaccine virus to a susceptible immunocompromised person. Contact of the vaccine can cause vaccine virus induced disease (e.g., OPV). Thus live attenuated vaccines have theoretical risk of possible activation in the host and thereby causing the disease. Another disadvantage is that these vaccines need stringent storage and transport conditions.

Killed or inactivated vaccines are by and large safe. But they make comparatively poor immunogenic agents, usually requiring multiple doses for adequate protection.

The materials commonly used for active immunization are given in Table 19.4.

Immunizing Agents for Active Immunization

Active immunizing agents are immunogenic drugs that are usually administered to a patient prior to their exposure to a disease with the intention of providing long-term, even permanent, protection against the disease.

BACTERIAL VACCINES

Anthrax Vaccine Adsorbed

Uses : Recommended for active immunization of individuals who come in contact with animal hides, furs, bonemeal, wool, hair (especially goat hair) and for individuals contemplating investigational studies involving bacillus anthracis.

Dose : SC 3 injections of 0.5 ml., 2 weeks apart followed by 3 more 0.5 ml doses, 6,12 and 18 months after the initial injection.

Booster : 0.5 ml at 1 year intervals.

BCG Vaccine

BCG is a freeze dried live attenuated Calmette Guerin strain of bovine mycobacterium tuberculosis 0.1 to 0.4 million viable bacilli per dose.

Storage :
(a) Vaccine not in use : 2°C–8°C in middle compartment of refrigerator
(b) During immunization
   (i) Keep away from light.
   (ii) Use within 3 hours.
(c) If electricity fails : Can be left in the refrigerator. It is viable for 1 month even at 37 degree C.

Efficacy : Tuberculin conversion in almost 100%; clinical protective efficacy variable 0-80% in different studies.

Instruction to the mother after vaccination :
   (i) Raised wheal will disappear in about 1 hour.
   (ii) No reaction like fever, etc.
   (iii) Local reaction after 3-6 weeks with a nodule formation which ulcerates and heals by scarring.

Uses : BCG vaccine should be seriously considered for persons who have negative tuberculin skin tests and repeated exposure to untreated or ineffectively treated cases of pulmonary tuberculosis.

Route of administration : Intradermal in left upper arm at deltoid insertion. It should not be given by SC or I.M. route as small abscesses are most likely to occur if injection is given by these routes.

Dose : Intradermal, 0.1ml.

In 7 to 10 days after injection a red painless papule occurs at the site of injection which attains a size of 7-9 mm in 5 weeks, dries in 3 months and totally heals in 6 months.

Booster : Protection from tuberculosis by BCG vaccination is not permanent or entirely predictable. If the tuberculin test again becomes negative and the risk of infection continues then a booster shot may need to be given.

Side effects : Non healing ulcer and regional suppurative lymphadenitis.

Preparation of site of injection : None required (do not use antiseptics).

Complication: Risk of tuberculous disease in immune compromised host.

Contraindications : None (possibly avoid after measles infection or vaccination and in immunocompromised individuals.

Table 19.4. Materials commonly used for active immunization.[1]

Vaccine	Type of Agent	Route of admn.	Primary	Booster[2]	Indications
Diphtheria-tetanus-acellular pertussis (DTaP)	Toxoids and inactivated bacterial components	Intramuscular	one dose 2, 12-18 months	11-12 years	For all children
Haemophilus influenzae type b conjugate (Hib)	Bacterial poly-saccharide conju-gated to protein	Intramuscular	One dose 2 months	Not recommended	1. For all children 2. Asplenia and other conditions.
Hepatitis A	Inactivated virus	Intramuscular	One dose (administer at least 2-4 weeks before travel to endemic areas)	At 6-12 months for long-term immunity	1. Travellers to hepatitis A endemic areas 2. Homosexual and bisexual men 3. Illicit drug users 4. Chronic liver disease or clotting factor disorders 5. Persons with occupational risk for infection 6. Persons living in, or relocating to, endemic ares 7. Household and sexual contacts of individuals with acute hepatitis A
Hepatitis B	Inactive viral antigen, recombinant	Intramuscular (subcutaneous injection is acceptable in individuals with bleeding disorders)	Three doses at 0,1 and 6 months	Not routinely recommended	1. For all infants 2. Preadolescents, adolescents, and young adults 3. Persons with occupational lifestyle, or environmental risk 4. Hemophiliacs 5. Hemodialysis patients 6. Postexposur prophylaxis
Influenza	Inactivated virus or viral components	Intramuscular	One dose (children $\leq$ 12 yrs. of age should receive split virus vaccine only; children < 9 who are receiving influenza vaccine for the first time should receive two doses administered at least 1 month apart	Yearly with current vaccine	1. Adults $\geq$ 50 years of age 2. Persons with high risk conditions (eg, asthma) 3. Health care workers and others in contact with high-risk groups 4. Residents of nursing homes and other residential chronic care facilities
Measles	Live virus	Subcutaneous	Two doses at least 1 month apart	None	1. Adults and adolescents born after 1956 without a history of measles or live virus vaccination on or after their first birthday.

(Contd.)

Vaccine	Type of Agent	Route of admn.	Primary	Booster[2]	Indications
					2. Postexposure prophylaxis in unimmunized persons.
Measles-mumps-rubella (MMR)	Live virus	Subcutaneous	12-15 months	None	For all children
Menningococcal vaccine	Bacterial polysaccharides of serotypes A/C/Y/W-135	Subcutaneous	One dose	Every 3 to 5 years if there is continuing high risk of exposure	1. Military recruits 2. Travellers to areas with epidemic meningococcal disease 3. Individuals with asplenia, complement deficiency, or properdin deficiency 4. Control of outbreaks in closed populations 5. College freshmen who live in dormitories
Mumps	Live virus	Subcutaneous	One dose	None	Adults born after 1956 without a history of mumps or live virus vaccination on or after their first birthday.
Pneumococcal vaccine	Bacterial polysaccharides of 23 serotypes	Intramuscular or subcutaneous	One dose	Repeat after 5 years in patients at high risk	1. Adults $\geq$ 65 years of age 2. Persons at increased risk for pneumococcal disease or its complications
Poliovirus vaccine, inactivated (IPV)	Inactivated viruses of all three serotypes	Subcutaneous	2 months Adults : Two doses 4 to 8 weeks apart, and a third dose 6 to 12 months after the second.	One-time booster dose for adults at increased risk of exposure	1. For all children 2. Previously unvaccinated adults at increased risk for occupational or travel exposure to polioviruses
Rabies	Inactivated virus	Intramuscular (IM) or intradermal (ID)	Preexposure : Three doses (IM or ID) at days 0,7,and 21 or 28 Postexposure : Five-doses (IM only) at days 0, 3,7,14, and 28	Serologic testing every 6 months to 2 years in persons at high risk	1. Preexposure prophylaxis in persons at risk for contact with rabies virus 2. Postexposure prophylaxis (administer with rabies immune globulin)
Rubella	Live virus	Subcutaneous	One or two doses (at least 28 days apart)	None	Adults born after 1956 without a history of rubella or live virus vaccination on or after their first birthday

(Contd.)

Vaccine	Type of Agent	Route of admn.	Primary	Booster[2]	Indications
Tetanus-diphtheria (Td or DT)[3]	Toxoids	Intramuscular	Two doses 4-8 weeks apart, and a third dose 6-12 months after the second	Every 10 years	1. All adults who have not been immunized as children 2. Postexposure prophylaxis if > 5 years has passed since last dose
Typhoid, Ty21a oral	Live bacteria	Oral	Four doses administered every other day	Four doses every 5 years	Risk of exposure to typhoid fever
Typhoid, Vi capsular polysaccharide	Bacterial polysaccharide	Intramuscular	One dose	Every 2 years	Risk of expousre to typhoid fever
Varicella	Live virus	Subcutaneous	Two doses 4-8 weeks apart in persons past their 13th birthday	Unknown	1. For all children 2. Persons (at high risk for exposure) past their 13th birthday without a history of varicella infection of immunization 3. Postexposure prophylaxis in susceptible persons
Yellow Fever	Live virus	Subcutaneous	One dose 10 days to 10 years before travel	Every 10 years	1. Laboratory personnel who may be exposed to yellow fever virus 2. Travellers to areas where yellow fever occurs

1   Dosages for the specific product, including variations for age, are best obtained from the manufactuer's package insert.
2   One dose unless otherwise indicated.
3   Td = Tetanus and diphtheria toxoids for use in persons > 7 years of age (contains less diphtheria toxoid that DPT and DT).
    DT = Tetanus and diphtheria toxoids for use in persons < 7 years of age (contains the same amount of diphtheria toxoid as DPT).

Cholera Vaccine

(i)   It contains 6000 million killed bacteria of ogawa serotype of classical vibrio cholerae.

(ii) 6000 million killed bacteria of inaba serotype of classical vibrio cholerae.

Dose : Ideal age of primary vaccination : Not recommended. 0.25ml < 10 years; 0.5ml 10 years

SC, 2 injections of 0.5 ml., 1 week to 1 month or more apart.

Site of administration : Deltoid or anterolateral aspect of thigh.

Booster : Not recommended.

Preparation of site of administration : Clean with antiseptic (spirit).

Protection efficacy : Immunity develops in 7-10 days and lasts for 3-6 months. It provides about 50% protection

Contraindications : None

Side effects : Fever and local soreness, aches for 1 to 2 days.

Complication : None

Storage :

(i)   When not in use - keep in lower most compartment of fridge (DO NOT Freeze)

(ii) During immunization session - can be kept at room temperature.

(iii) In case of electricity failure - keep in cool and dark places.

Pertussis Vaccine

Uses : Available in the multiple antigen form of Diphtheria and Tetanus Toxoids and Pertussis Vaccine, Adsorbed (DPT) recommended for active immunization of infants and children through 6 years of age against diphtheria, tetanus and pertussis simultaneously. Injections should be completed no later than the age of 6 years. It is to be noted that Pertussis Vaccine is not recommended for immunizing persons 7 years of age and older because the severity of adverse reactions to pertussis vaccine increases with age, whereas the severity of pertussis infection decreases. It is seldom given separately. It is a component of triple antigen.

Dose : IM, 3 injections of 0.5ml given 4 to 8 weeks apart followed by a fourth dose of 0.5ml 1 year later. This fourth reinforcing dose is an integral part of the basic immunizing course.

Booster : 0.5ml between 4 and 6 years of age. Side effects include local pain and induration, severe systemic reactions such as high fever, shock like state and convulsions.

It is contraindicated in children with history of convulsions or other neurological disorders.

Plague Vaccine

It is a sterile, whitish suspension of formaldehyde killed Yersinia pestis.

Uses : Indicated for active immunization of persons at particularly high risk to plague including persons engaged in laboratory work involving Y. pestis organisms.

Dose : Intramuscular, for adults and children over 10 years of age, 1.0 ml i.m. twice 2-4 weeks apart or 2ml single done followed by 0.2 ml, 1 to 3 months later. A third injection of 0.2 ml, 3 to 6 months after the second injection is strongly recommended for children less than 10 years old.

Immunity lasts for 6-8 months.

Booster : Injection (0.1 to 0.2ml) every 6 months for individuals living in a known plague area.

Typhoid - Ty 21a Vaccine

TY21a strain of S. typhi is nonpathogenic but highly immunogenic. Typhoid - TY21a oral vaccine is prepared from this strain.

It has protective efficacy of 78% for 3 years. It is available as enteric coated capsules.

Dose : one capsule on days 1, 3 and 5 taken 1 hour before meals.

Side effects : diarrhoea, low grade fever, skin rash.

Typhoid - Paratyphoid A, B (TAB Vaccine) :

It is a sterile suspension of killed S. typhi and S. paratyphi A and B. One ml contains 1×10^9 S.typhi and 7.5×10^8 each of S. paratyphi A and B organisms in 5, 10 ml vials.

Dose : 0.5 ml SC followed by 1ml at 2 to 4 weeks intervals. Booster dose once in 3 years in endemic areas.

It is 70% to 90% protective for 1 year. Booster doses may be given every 1-3 years.

Side effects : Local pain, swelling and fever.

Typhoid Vaccine

It is prepared from purified Vi capsular polysaccharide of S. typhi.

Immunity develops after 7 to 15 days after injection, and lasts for 3 years. Its protective efficacy is about 60%, but does not protect against S. paratyphi A or B.

Dose : 0.5ml S.C. injection.

For children less than 10 years old 2 injections of 0.25 ml at least 4 weeks apart, adults and children over 10 years old 2 injections of 0.5 ml at least 4 weeks apart.

Uses : Indicated for active immunization against typhoid fever. Vaccine is estimated to be 70% or more effective in preventing typhoid fever depending in part on the degree of exposure.

Booster : Under conditions of continued or repeated exposure, a single booster injection of 0.5 ml or 0.25 ml (according to age) every 3 years.

Side effects : Fever, swelling, local pain.

VIRAL VACCINES

Rubella Virus Vaccine Live

It is given subcutaneously

Uses : Indicated for active immunization against rubella (German measles) in children from 12 months of age to puberty.

Dose : SC 1 - 0.5ml injection of reconstituted vaccine.

Booster - Not needed.

Influenza Virus Vaccine

It is formalin killed influenza virus consisting of antigens from inactivated influenza virus A and B Two doses are administered 4 to 8 weeks apart.

Uses : Indicated only for immunization against those strains of viruses from which the vaccine is prepared or against closely related strains.

The influenza vaccine is not recommended for individuals with a known anaphylactic hypersensitivity to chicken or egg protein.

Adverse effects include local tenderness and induration in 30%, allergic reactions and polyneuritis. Fever, malaise and myalgia for 1-2 days is less frequent.

Dose : SC or I.M. (I.M. preferred), 1 injection of 0.5 ml.

Booster : A single yearly dose for high risk individuals.

Hepatitis B Vaccine

The preparation (inactivated) contains hepatitis B surface antigen protein. It is given by i.m. injection in deltoid region in adults and in anterolateral thigh in neonates and infants.

Dose : 10 mcg in 0.4 ml suspension for neonates and children above 10 years of age. 20 mcg of antigen protein is given in adults. Three doses are recommended. The first dose at elected date, second dose 1 month later and third dose after 6 months from the date of first dose.

Side effects include erythema and induration at the site of injection, fever, headache, dizziness and nausea.

Hepatitis B vaccine can be given subcutaneously to persons at risk of haemorrhage following i.m. injections.

The new hepatitis B vaccine is prepared in yeast cells by recombinant DNA technique and contains Aluminium adsorbed hepatitis B virus surface antigen 20 mcg in 1 ml suspension.

Dose : IM 3 injections of 1.0 ml with the second and third injections given 1 month and 6 months

after the first dose. For younger children (birth to 10 years of age) dose is 0.5 ml.

A single booster may be necessary every 5 years. Available data suggest that immunity will last about 5 years in patients who have received all 3 doses.

Mumps Virus Vaccine live attenuated

It is prepared from mumps virus grown in cell culture of chick embryo.

A single dose of 5000 TCID 50 (tissue culture infectious dose 50%) administered subcutaneously. The protective antibodies persist for 12 years after inoculation.

Recommended for active immunization against mumps in children 12 months of age or older and adults.

Dose : SC, 1 injection.

Booster : Not recommended.

Contraindications : Fever, cancer patients receiving immunosuppressive therapy, pregnancy.

Measles Vaccine (Live attenuated)

It is a preparation of highly attenuated strain of measles virus (Schwarz or Edmonston-Zagreb strain), obtained by propagation of the live virus in chick embryo tissue cultures.

The vaccine may provide some protection if given within 72 hours after exposure to natural measles. However, better protection is provided if the vaccine is given a few days before exposure.

Uses : Recommended for active immunization against measles (rubella) in children 15 months of age or older.

The optimum age for vaccination is 9 months. It is given by S.C. injection.

Dose : Single dose vials contain 1000 TCID 50 of schwarz (RIME VAX) or Edmonston strain (M-VAC). The dose is 0.5 ml S.C.

Booster : Not recommended.

Caution in persons with history or family history of allergic diseases, those with the family history of epilepsy.

Side effects include fever with or without rash between 5th and 12th day after vaccination. Cough and headache may also occur. Children with fever may (though rarely) exhibit convulsions.

The dose is 0.5 ml S.C.

Poliomyelitis Vaccine

It is of two types viz. (i) Inactivated poliomyelitis vaccine and (ii) live oral vaccine.

(i) Inactivated Poliomyelitis Vaccine (Salk Vaccine)

Suspension of approved strains of poliomyelitis virus type 1, 2 and 3 grown in cultured kidney tissue of monkey. It is inactivated by formalin.

Dose : 1 ml S.C. / I.M. injection in deltoid region. Three doses are given at an interval of 4-8 weeks between first and second dose and 12 months between second and third dose.

Booster : dose is recommended at 18 months.

Further booster does of 1.0ml should be given every 5 years until age 18.

Side effects include fever, local pain and erythema.

Poliovirus Vaccine Inactivated (IPV) has been largely replaced by Oral Polio virus vaccine Live (OPV). It is used for adult immunization because there is less risk of vaccine associated paralysis than with OPV for adults.

(ii) Live Oral Poliomyelitis Vaccine (Sabin Vaccine)

It employs live virus. It is given orally.

Uses : Indicated for active immunization against infections of poliomyelitis caused by Poliovirus types 1, 2 and 3 in infants.

Dose : 0.5ml dropped directly in the month. First dose is given at birth and subsequently at 6, 10 and 14 weeks of birth. The booster dose is given at 18 months. Second booster is recommended at the age of 4-5 years.

Immunity develops in 80% or more.

Pulse Immunization

It is a programme which refers to intermittent polio immunization drive in a community or a region to vaccinate all susceptible children irrespective of their previous immunization status.

Rabies Vaccine

Rabies is a zoonotic infection caused by RNA rhabdovirus which is neurotropic and causes encephalitis (universally fatal).

Four vaccines are available :

(i) Inactivated Rabies Vaccine prepared on vero cells

Preparation of Vaccine

Brain of sheep is inoculated subdurally with brain substance of rabies infected rabbit.

Vaccine is available as sterile suspension of brain substance containing fixed virus of rabies, inactivated by phenol.

Uses : Indicated for active immunization in pre-exposure situations for animal handlers, researchers and other similar personnel.

The vaccine is also recommended for post-exposure treatment of animal bites with a potential risk of rabies.

Dose : IM, Pre-exposure : 3 injections of 1.0 ml of reconstituted vaccine on each of days 0,7 and 21 or 28.

Post - exposure : 5 injection of 1.0ml. of reconstituted vaccine on each of days 0, 3, 7, 14 and 28.

Booster : Every 2 years to persons with continuing risk of exposure.

The wound of the dog-bite should be thoroughly cleaned with soap and water (this eliminates large part of virus particles) and kept open. For post-dog bite cases 2-5ml is injected in the anterior abdominal wall below the costal margin daily for 14 days. Immunity is achieved for about 3 months.

Adverse effects include erythema and induration at the site of injection. Neuroparalysis may occur though rarely.

(ii) Purified chick embryo-cell Rabies Vaccine

One dose contains not less than 2.5 IU of inactivated rabies antigen of the virus multiplied in chicken fibroblast cell cultures having stabilizer. After exposure, to induce immunization against rabies, six injections are to be given.

One dose on each of day 0, 3, 7, 14, 39 and 90.

Adverse effects include pain, swelling and reddening at the site of injection, enlarged lymph nodes, GI complaints and pain in joints may occur.

(iii) Human Diploid Cell Rabies Vaccine

It is a preparation from human diploid cell culture, containing not less than 2.5 IU per ml vaccine.

Indication

Pre- and post-exposure prophylaxis against rabies.

For post-exposure cases, 5 does of 1ml each are given by SC or IM injection on day 0, 3, 7, 14 and 28. Some recommend an optional dose on day-90.

For prophylaxis, 4 dose of 1ml each by SC or I.M. injection are administered on day 0, 7, 21 and 365. Booster dose 1ml every 3 years is recommended.

(iv) Antirabic Vaccines Carbolized

It is a 5% suspension of brain substance containing carbolic acid fixed rabies virus for prophylaxis for 14days. It does not protect all who are vaccinated. Encephalitis has been reported as adverse effect. Neuroparalytic complications occur in 1 in 300 to 1 in 7000 recipients.

Yellow Fever Vaccine

It is a bacterially sterile light orange lyophilized preparation of the live 17D strain of yellow fever virus prepared in chicken embryos.

Uses : For active immunization of travellers planning a trip to countries primarily in Africa and South America which require a certificate of vaccination against yellow fever.

Dose : SC, 1 injection of 0.5ml of reconstituted vaccine.

Booster : Every 10 years.

MIXED VACCINES (Combined Vaccines)

When more than one type of immunizing agent is included, it is known as combined vaccine. Examples: DPT, MMR.

(i) Measles, Mumps, and Rubella Vaccine Live (MMR Vaccine)

Uses : It is indicated for simultaneous active immunization against measles (rubella), mumps and rubella (German measles) in children 15 months of age or older, or in adults.

Dose : SC, 1 injection of 0.5ml

Booster : Not recommended.

Side effects include hyperthermia and respiratory symptoms (of short duration).

(ii) Measles and Rubella Virus Vaccine Live (MR Vaccine)

Uses : Indicated for simultaneous active immunization against measles (rubella) and rubella (German measles) in children 15 months of age or older and adults.

Dose : SC, 1 injection of 0.5ml

Booster : Not recommended.

(iii) Rubella and Mumps Virus Vaccine Live

Uses : Indicated for simultaneous active immunization against rubella (German measles) and mumps in children 12 months of age or older and adults.

Dose : SC, 1 injection of 0.5ml

Booster : Not recommended.

Combination Vaccines offer the following benefits:

Benefit to patient and parents
    Decreased number of injections
    Decreased number of visits
Tangible public health benefits
    Decreased cost of administration
    Increased compliance
    Ease of storage
    Improved record keeping and tracking

TOXOIDS

Tetanus Toxoid

Tetanus toxoid is a formaldehyde detoxified bacteria free filtrate of Cl. tetani. It may be used for active immunization against tetanus. However, Tetanus Toxoid Adsorbed is preferred for all basic immunization because of more persistent antitoxin titre induction.

Dose : IM or SC, 3 injections of 0.5ml, 4-8 weeks apart followed by the fourth dose of 0.5ml, 6-12 months later.

Tetanus Toxoid Adsorbed

It is a sterile suspension of purified tetanus toxoid

(formaldehyde treated toxin of Cl. tetani alum precipitated or adsorbed onto aluminium hydroxide or aluminium phosphate.

Uses : For active immunization against tetanus.

Dose : IM, 2 injections of 0.5ml, 4-5 weeks apart, followed by a third reinforcing dose of 0.5ml, every 10 years.

Diphtheria Toxoid Adsorbed

It contains diphtheria toxin treated with formaldehyde.

Uses : Recommended for active immunization against diphtheria in infants and children under 6 years of age for whom products containing tetanus toxoid and/or pertussis vaccine would not be available.

Dose : IM, 2 injections of 0.5ml 6-8 weeks apart, and a third reinforcing dose of 0.5ml about a year later.

Booster : 1 injection at 5 to 10 years interval.

MIXED TOXOIDS AND BIOLOGICS

Tetanus and Diphtheria Toxoid Adsorbed for adult use

Uses : For active immunization of adults and children 7 years of age and older.

Dose : IM, 2 injections of 0.5ml., 4-8 weeks apart followed by a third reinforcing dose of 0.5ml, 1 year later.

Booster : 0.5 ml every 10 years.

Diphtheria and Tetanus Toxoids Adsorbed for children under 6 years of age

Uses : Recommended for active immunization against diphtheria and tetanus in infants and children through 6 years of age when it is undesirable or contra-indicated to give a triple antigen (DPT) containing the pertussis component.

Dose : IM, 2 injections of 0.5ml, 4-8 weeks apart, followed by a third reinforcing dose of 0.5 ml 1 year later. The reinforcing dose is an integral part of the basic immunizing course.

Booster : If active immunization is initiated during the first year of life, booster dose of 0.5 ml is given during 4-6 years of age. Over age 6, Tetanus and

Diphtheria Toxoids Adsorbed (for adult use) is recommended every 10 years.

Triple antigen (DPT)

Diphtheria and Tetanus Toxoids and Pertussis Vaccine Adsorbed :

It is a sterile suspension of purified diphtheria and tetanus toxoids alum precipitated or aluminium phosphate adsorbed and phase 1 pertussis vaccine.

Uses : For active immunization of infants and children 6 years of age against diphtheria, tetanus and pertussis simultaneously. Injection should be started at 2-3 months of age and completed not later than the age of 6 years. This vaccine should not be given to children over 6 years of age.

Dose : IM, 3 injections of 0.5 ml, 4-8 weeks apart followed by a fourth reinforcing dose of 0.5 ml, 1 year later. The reinforcing dose is an integral part of the basic immunizing course.

Booster : For children between 4 and 6 years of age, 0.5ml. For persons 7 years of age and older, Tetanus and Diphtheria Toxoids Adsorbed for Adult use is recommended every 10 years.

Side effects: Fever, swelling, local pain, irritability.

Mixed toxoids and biologics have the advantage of providing broad immunization coverage with a reduced number of injections.

Passive immunity

Passive immunization in the broadest sense involves the administration of any immune effector antibody or effector T cells. In practice it has been restricted to the use of antibody.

Box 19.1. For Passive Immunity

Immunoglobulin (Human) is prepared from pooled human plasma. It has high level of antibody titre.

Immunoglobulins (Human)

Immunoglobulins (IGs) are separated human gamma globulins which carry the antibodies. These may be nonspecific (normal) or specific (hyper immune) against a particular antigen. These are more efficacious than the corresponding antisera.

    Normal human gamma globulin

    Anti-D immunoglobulin

    Tetanus immunoglobulin

    Rabies immunoglobulin

    Hepatitis - B immunoglobulin

Antisera and **Immunoglobulins** impart passive immunity. Ready-made antibodies are transferred. These antibodies are produced by another person or animal who has been actively immunized.

Antibodies are the substances formed in the body in response to the presence of foreign proteins and certain other materials in the tissues. They are highly specific and attack only the specific substances i.e. microorganisms or toxins that stimulate their production. Materials when introduced into the body lead to antibody production are called antigens.

Antibodies are immunoglobulin molecules (serum proteins) 1gA, 1gD, 1gE, 1gG and 1gM.

Chemically, antibodies belong to a class of proteins known as globulins (alpha, beta and gamma). Most globulins are gamma globulins.

Antibodies are produced, particularly in the lymph nodes, by cells of the reticulo-endothelial system.

Animal Immune Serum

Antitoxin - a solution of antibodies derived from the serum of animals (usually a horse) immunized with specific toxins (toxoids) e.g., botulism, diphtheria and tetanus can achieve a passive immunity or to effect a treatment.

Antiviral Serum is a solution of antibodies derived from the serum of animals (usually a horse) immunized with a specific viral vaccine. For example, antirabies serum (equine). This is only one commercially important biologic available.

Antivenin is a preparation of antibodies derived from the serum of animals (usually horses) immunized with specific venoms e.g., rattle snakes, coral snakes and black widow spider, used to neutralize the venoms produced by the specific organisms.

BACTERIAL TOXINS

Characteristics of bacterial toxins

There are two kinds of bacterial toxins :
- Exotoxins diffuse freely through the bacterial wall into the medium in which the organisms are growing.
- Endotoxins are retained within the bacteria and are freed only when the cells die or disintegrate.

Exotoxins - characteristics

They are water soluble products of the metabolism of actively growing bacteria (produced mainly by gram-positive bacteria). Chemically they are high molecular weight proteins and some are enzymes which are thermolabile and lose activity at about 60°C. They are usually very toxic to the body. Botulinus toxin (produced by Cl. botulinum, an organism responsible for a dangerous type of food poisoning) is so toxic that 1mg is enough to kill about 20 million mice.

Endotoxins - characteristics

They are structured elements of bacteria (large amounts are found in Gram-negative bacteria), liberated only when the cells die or disintegrate. They are much less toxic. Chemically they are complexes of phospholipid, polysaccharide and protein, most of these are thermostable.

The exotoxin producing, endotoxin producing bacteria and antitoxins are shown below.

Exotoxin - Producing Bacteria

Clostridium botulinum, Clostridium tetani, Clostridium perfringens, Septicum and Welchii (gas gangrene) and Corynebacterium diphtheria (diphtheria).

Endotoxin - Producing Bacteria

Vibrio cholerae (cholera), Pasteurella pestis (plague), Salmonella typhi (typhoid) Salmonella paratyphi. (paratyphoid) and Bordetella pertussis (whooping cough).

Antitoxins

Products containing antibodies that neutralize exotoxins are generally called antitoxins, e.g.
> Botulinum antitoxin
> Diphtheria antitoxin
> Gas-gangrene antitoxin (oedematiens)
> Gas-gangrene antitoxin (septicum)
> Gas-gangrene antitoxin (welchii)
> Mixed gas-gangrene antitoxin
> Staphylococcus antitoxin
> Tetanus antitoxin

Passive Immunizing Agents

In the broadest sense passive immunization involves the administration of any specific immune effector, antibody or effector T-cell. But in practice it has been restricted to the use of antibodies since effector T-cells are limited in number, difficult to harvest, and, perhaps most importantly, MHC-restricted and not usually effective when transferred from one individual to another. Recently, attempts are being made to harvest the T-cells of the individual patient, expand their number in vitro with colony - stimulating factors, and reintroduce the cells into the patient.

The currently employed passive immunizing agents are all derived from immunoglobulins and the majority of these consist mainly of IgG isotypes.

Agents for Passive Immunization

Human Immune Sera (Homologous Sera)
    Immune Globulin
    Hepatitis B Immune Globulin (Human)
    Pertussis Immune Globulin (Human)
    Rabies Immune Globulin (Human)
    Rho(D) Immune Globulin (Human)
    Tetanus Immune Globulin (Human)
    Varicella-zoster Immune Globulin (Human)

Animal Immune Sera (Heterologous Sera)

Antitoxins (Equine)
    Botulism Antitoxin (Equine)
    Diphtheria Antitoxin (Equine)
    Tetanus Antitoxin (Equine)
Antiviral Serum (Equine)
    Antirabies serum
    Antivenins (Equine)

The agents for passive immunization are given below and the materials available for passive immunization are shown in Table 19.5. The major classes of immunoglobulins and antisera from horse are given below. The heterologous antitoxins are listed above.

Immunoglobulins

There are 5 major classes
- IgG is the only one which crosses placenta. Antibodies to gram positive bacteria, antitoxin antibodies and antiviral antibodies are found exclusively in IgG globulin.
- IgA is found predominantly in external secretions e.g., saliva, tears and bronchial secretions. It exhibits antibody activity to viral and bacterial antigens and toxins. Its half-life is 6-8 days. It comprises of 15% of total serum immunoglobulins.
- IgM comprises of 10% of serum immunoglobulins. Half-life is about immune globulin 120 days.
- IgD : Half-life is 2.8 days. Function is not yet clear.
- IgE is mainly bound to basophils and mast cells. Histamine, serotonin and SRS-A are released when specific antigen combines with IgE. Thus it is involved in mediating immediate hypersensitivity reactions (Type 1).

Biologics for Passive Immunization

Type of Products

It is useful to think three dichotomies when immunoglobulin containing products are considered : human or animal, IM or IV, polyclonal or monoclonal.

Human immune sera (Homologous sera)

These include immune globulin and hyperimmune (including Rho(D) immune globulin for specific diseases.

Five major classes of immunoglobulins are shown below.

The source of homologous sera is the pooled plasma (free of hepatitis B antigen) of adult donors either from the general population (for immunoglobulin) or from hyperimmunized donors (for immune globulins for specific diseases).

Immune Globulin (Gamma Globulin)

Immune Serum Globulin (Gamma Globulin) contains many antibodies normally present in adult human blood. It is recommended for passive prevention or modification of measles (rubella) and viral hepatitis A and for the routine maintenance of certain immunodeficient persons.

It is also known as Human Normal Immunoglobulin which contains primarily IgG antibodies. It

Table 19.5. Materials available for passive immunization

Indication	Product	Dosage	Comments
Black widow spider bite	Antivenin (Latrodectus Mactans), equine	One vial (6000 units) IV or IM	For persons with hypertensive cardiovascular disease or age < 16 or > 60 years.
Bone marrow transplantation	Immune globulin (intravenous)	500 mg/kg IV on days 7 and 2 prior to transplantation and then once weekly though day 90 after transplantation	Prophylaxis to decrease the risk of infection, interstitial pneumonia, and acute graft-versus-host disease in adults undergoing bone marrow transplantation.
Botulism	Botulism antitoxin (trivalent, type A, B and E), equine	According to CDC	Treatment and prophylaxis of botulism. Available from the CDC. Ten to 20 percent incidence of serum reactions.
Chronic lymphocytic leukaemia (CLL)	Immune globulin (intravenous)	Initial dose of 400 mg/kg IV every 3-4 weeks. Dosage should be adjusted ypward infection. if bacterial infections occur.	CLL patients with hypogammaglobulinemia anda history of at least one serious bacterial infection
Cytomegalovirus (CMV)	Cytomegalovirus immune globulin (intravenous)	Consult the manufacturer's dosing recommendations.	Prophylaxis of CMV infection in bone marrow, kidney, liver, lung, pancreas, heart transplant recipients.
Diphtheria	Diphtheria antitoxin, equine	20,000-120,000 units IV or IM depending on the severity reactions and duration of illness	Early treatment of respiratory diphtheria. Available from the CDC. Anaphylactic in ≥ 7% of adults and serum reactions in ≥ 5-10% of adults.
Hepatitis A	Immune globulin (intramuscular)	Preexposure prophylaxis : 0.02 mL/kg IM for anticipated risk of ≤ 3 months, 0.06 mL/kg for anticipated risk of > 3 months, repea-ted every 4-6 months for continued exposure. Post-exposure : 0.02 mL/kg IM as soon as possible after exposure up to 2 weeks.	Preexposure and postexposure hepatitis A prophylaxis. The availability of hepatitis A vaccine has greatly reduced the need for preexposure prophylaxis.
Hepatitis B	Hepatitis B immune globulin (HBIG)	0.06 mL/kg IM as soon as possible after exposure up to 1 week for percutaneous exposure or 2 weeks for sexual exposure. 0.5 mL IM within 12 hours after birth for perinatal exposure	Postexposure prophylaxis in nonimmune persons following percutaneous, mucosal, sexual, or perinatal exposure. Hepatitis B vaccine should also be administered.
HIV-infected children	Immune globulin (intravenous)	400 mg/kg IV every 28 days	HIV-infected children with recurrent serious bacterial infections or hypogammaglobulinema.
Kawasaki disease	Immune globulin (intravenous)	400 mg/kg IV daily for 4 consecutive days within 4 days after the onset of illness. A single dose of 2 g/kg IV over 10 hours is also effective.	Effective in the prevention of coronary aneurysms. For use in patients who meet strict criteria for Kawasaki disease.
Measles	Immune globulin (intramuscular)	Normal hosts : 0.25mL/kg IM. Immunocompromised hosts: 0.5 mL/kg IM (maximum 15 mL for all patients)	Postexposure prophylaxis (within 6 days after exposure) in nonimmune contacts of acute cases.

(Contd.)

Indication	Product	Dosage	Comments
Idiopathic thrombocyto penic purpura (ITP)	Immune globulin (intravenous)	Consult the manufacturer's dosing recommendations for the specific product being used.	Response in children with ITP is greater than in adults. Corticosteroids are the treatment of choice in adults, except for severe pregnancy-associated ITP.
Primary immuno-deficiency disorders	Immune globulin (intravenous)	Consult the manufacturer's dosing recommendations for the specific product being used.	Primary immunodeficiency disorders include specific antibody deficiencies (e.g., X-linked agammaglobulinemia) and combined deficiencies (e.g. severe combined immunodeficiencies).
Rabies	Rabies immune globulin	20 IU/kg. The full dose should be infiltrated around the wound and any remaining volume should be given IM at an anta-omic site distant from vaccine administration.	Postexposure rabies prophylaxis in persons not previously immunized with rabies vaccine. be combined with rabies vaccine.
Respiratory syncytial virus (RSV)	Palivizumab	15 mg/kg IM once prior to the beginning of the RSV season and once monthly until the end of the season.	For use in infants and children younger than 24 months with chronic lung disease or a history of premature birth ($\leq$ 35 week's gestation).
	RSV immune globulin	750 mg/kg IV once prior to the beginning of the RSV season may and once monthly until the end of the season.	As for palivizumab. Palivizumab is preferred for selected high-risk children, but RSV-IGIV be preferred for selected high-risk children.
Rubella	Immune globulin (intramuscular)	0.55mL/kg IM.	Nonimmune pregnant women exposed to rubella who will not consider therapeutic abortion. Administration does not prevent rubella in the fetus of an exposed mother.
Snake bite (coral snake)	Antivenin (Micrurus fulvius), equine	At least 3-5 vials (30-50 mL) IV initially within 4 hours after the bite. Additional doses may be required.	Neutralizes venom of eastern coral snake and Texas coral snake. Serum sickness occurs in almost all patients who who receive > 7 vials.
Snake bite (pit vipers)	Antivenin (Crotalidae) polyvalent, equine	The entire dose should be given within 4 hours after the bite by the IV or IM route (1 vial = 10 mL): Minimal envenomation: 2-4 vials Moderate envenomation : 5-9 vials Severe envenomation: 10-15 vials. Additional doses may be required.	Neutralizes the venom of rattlesnakes, copperheads, cottonmouths, water moccasins, and tropical and Asiatic crotalids. Serum sickness occurs in almost all patients who receive > 7 vials.
Tetanus	Tetanus immune globulin	Postexposure prophylaxis: 250 units IM. For severe wounds or when there has been a delay in administration, 500 units is recommended. Treatment: 3000-6000 units IM.	Treatment of tetanus and postexposure prophylaxis of nonclean, nonminor wounds in inadequately immunized persons (less than two doses of tetanus toxoid or less than three doses if wound is more than 24 hours old).
Vaccinia	Vaccinia immune globulin	According to CDC.	Treatment of severe reactions to vaccinia vaccination, including eczema vaccinatum, vaccinia necrosum, and ocular vaccinia. Available from the CDC.

(Contd.)

Indication	Product	Dosage		Comments
Varicella	Varicella-zoster immune globulin	Weight (kg)	Dose (units)	Postexpousre prophylaxis (preferably within
		≤ 10	125 IM	48 hours but no later than within 96 hours
		10.1-20	250 IM	after exposure) in susceptible immunocompro-
		20.1-30	375 IM	mised hosts, selected pregnant women, and
		30.1-40	500 IM	perinatally exposed newborns.
		> 40	625 IM	

CDC = Centres for Disease Control and Prevention.

also contains small quantities of IgM and IgA along with other serum proteins.

Human specific immunoglobulin is derived from blood of individuals who have been recently immunized against that disease.

It is given by IM injection for prophylactic as well as therapeutic uses.

Uses :

(i) For passive immunization. It provides temporary protection in measles, rubella, infective hepatitis, mumps, diphtheria and poliomyelitis.

(ii) For the treatment of patients suffering from hypogammaglobulinemia (serum gamma-globulin 200 mg or less).

Dose : 10% 1ml injection.

Side effects include pain at site of injection, fever, joint pains, hypotension, bronchospasm. Collapse may occur (rarely).

Human immune globulin products are derived from pooled plasma from 1000 or more donors. The antibody content of all these products is primarily IgG (90 to 98%) and the four isotypes are generally within the range of their natural distribution, IgG1 (60-70%), IgG2 (23-29%), IgG3 (4-8%) and IgG4 (2-6%). The composition of the products for both preparations (normal immune globulin as well as hyperimmune globulin) is very similar.

Hyperimmune serum (specific immune globulin): A special preparation obtained from human donor pools selected for high antibody titre against a specific disease, e.g., Hepatitis B Immune Globulin (HBIG) and Rabies Immune Globulin (RIG).

Intramuscular human immune globulin (IGIM) is the prototype for the specific human globulins that is administered by this route. The limitation is that, even with painful injections at several sites, the desired blood levels of 1gG are not always achieved. These products should not be injected intravascularly, for they contain immunoglobulin aggregates, that can activate the complement system and cause serious anaphylactic reactions.

The IGIM products are aqueous solutions containing 15 to 18% protein of which more than 90% is 1gG and each lot represents the pooled plasma of more than 1000 donors. They are standardized for antibody to measles, diphtheria and poliovirus.

Intravenous human immune globulin (IGIV) is the prototype for the specific human globulins that are administered by this route. Intravenous preparations are treated to prevent aggregation of the immunoglobulin and there is no limitation with respect to attainable blood levels.

The IGIV products are aqueous solutions or lyophilized powders that are reconstituted to provide 5% to 10% protein solutions. The IgG content ranges from greater than 90 to 99%. Each lot represents the pooled plasma of more than 1000 to 50,000 donors.

IGIM and IGIV are polyclonal antibody preparations.

Hepatitis B Immune Globulin (Human)

The product is derived from blood plasma of human donors who have high titres of antibodies against hepatitis B surface antigens. It is used for post-exposure passive immunization following exposure to materials involving HBs Ag such as blood plasma or serum.

It is also indicated for passive immunizations of infants born to HBs Ag-positive mothers.

Dose : IM, adult 0.06 ml/kg of body weight, preferably given within 7 days of exposure and repeated 28-30 days after initial dose. It is better prophylactic than normal gamma globulin.

Dose : 1000-2000 IU for adults 32-48 IU/kg for children.

Pertussis Immune Globulin (Human)

It is a solution of globulins derived from the blood plasma of adult human donors who have been immunized with pertussis vaccine. It is indicated for the passive prevention or attenuation or treatment of pertussis.

Dose : IM, Prophylactic, 1.25 to 2.5 ml depending on the age of the child, 1 or 2 times at 1-2 week intervals; Therapeutic, 1.25 to 2.5 ml depending on the severity of disease, repeated 1 or 2 times at 1 to 2 intervals depending on the clinical response.

Rabies immunoglobulin Human

Rabies Immune Globulin (Human) : It is a solution of globulins derived from the blood plasma of individuals immunized with rabies vaccine. It is indicated for individuals suspected of exposure to rabies. It is preferred over rabies antiserum.

Dose : IM 20 IU/kg body weight.

Human Anti-D Immunoglobulin

It is obtained from pooled plasma of naturally immunized women who have high titre of anti-D antibodies.

If the mother is Rh negative and if foetus is Rh positive, foetal erythrocytes may enter maternal circulation causing Rhesus immunization. This antigen on RBC may cause erythroblastosis foetalis in subsequent pregnancy. Hence, to prevent this 250-300mcg of Rho(D) 1g is administered within 72 hours of delivery.

Rho(D) Immune Globulin (Human) : It is a solution of globulin derived from human blood plasma containing the erythrocytic factor Rho(D). It is indicated for an Rh negative female who delivers an Rho(D) positive baby or for the Rh negative female after abortion or ectopic pregnancy unless the products of conception or father are conclusively shown to be Rh negative. The administration of Rho(D) immune globulin within 72 hours reduces the incidence of Rh isoimmunization from 12-13% to 1-2%, thus offering protection to the next infant of born Rho(D) positive.

Tetanus Immune Globulin (Human)

It contains gamma globulin prepared from the human plasma having high tetanus antitoxin titre. The half-life is 3-4 weeks. The prophylactic dose is 250-500 IU by IM injection. In case of tetanus neonatorium 500-10,000 IU, IM or 250 IU intrathecally. In children and adults, 500-10,000 IU, IM or 250 IU intrathecally.

It is a solution of globulins derived from the blood plasma of adult human donors who have been immunized with tetanus toxoid. It is indicated for immediate immunization against tetanus toxin. It is also used in the regimen of treatment of active cases of tetanus. It is more efficacious and longer acting than the equine antitoxin (ATS).

Tetanus immunoglobulin (human). It is more efficacious and longer acting than the equine antitoxin (ATS).

Dose : Prophylactic 250-500 IU

Varicella - Zoster Immune Globulin (Human)

It is a 10 to 18% solution of globulins (primarily IgG) derived from the blood plasma of adult human volunteers selected for high titers of varicella-zoster antibodies. It is indicated for passive immunization of susceptible immunodeficient children following exposure to varicella.

Dose : IM, the dosage if given within 96 hours after exposure modifies significantly the severity, and if given after 96 hours of exposure the value is uncertain and there is no evidence that it can modify the established varicella infection.

Animal Immune Sera (Heterogenous Sera)

Antiserum is defined as materials prepared in animals.

Antiserum from horses who have been given vaccine, toxin or toxoid contain antibody against microorganisms or their toxin.

Animal immune sera or heterogenous sera include antitoxins, antiviral serum and antivenins.

These preparation are obtained from the plasma of horses that have been immunized against the specific antigen (toxin, virus or venom). The finished biologic is in the form of solution or if an antivenin, lyophilized.

The horse was chosen because it has a large blood volume and is rarely used as a food animal which lessens the chance for sensitization.

There is little functional difference between human and animal antibodies but there is sufficient structural difference that allergy is a major problem with heterologous sera.

Serum sickness is a systemic immune complex disease that occurs 5 to 14 days after administration of foreign antibodies.

Patients should always be skin-tested for anaphylactic sensitivity prior to receiving heterogenous products; it is also notable that most of these products are administered by slow IV infusion since the onset of activity with IM administration is too slow to deal effectively with a serious intoxication.

Box 19.2. Antisera

- Antisera (from horse)
  Antisera are purified and concentrated preparations of serum of horses actively immunized against a specific antigen.
  – Tetanus Antitoxin
  – Gas gangrene - Antitoxin
  – Diphtheria Antitoxin
  – Rabies Antitoxin
  – Antisnake venom Polyvalent
- Heterologous Antisera
  – Antitoxins
  – Botulism Antitoxin Types A, B and E (Equine)
  – Botulism Antitoxin Monovalent Type E (Equine)
  – Diphtheria Antitoxin (Equine)
  – Antivenins

Antitoxins (Equine)

Botulism antisera (Equine)

Uses : Indicated for the passive prevention and treatment of botulism. This antitoxin only neutralizes the circulating toxins of Cl. botulinum type A and B and does not counteract the effect of toxin already bound to receptor cells in tissues.

Dose : Prophylactic, IM, 10,000 IU of each type.

Therapeutic, IV and IM, 1 vial IV diluted 1:10 followed by 1 vial IM. Further doses are indicated in 2-4 hours if signs and symptoms worsen.

Botulism : 10,000 IU of polyvalent antitoxin every 3-4 hourly.

Diphtheria Antitoxin

It is a serum preparation obtained from horses who are actively immunized with Cl. diphtheriae. It is available as 10,000 and 20,000 IU in 5,10ml ampoules.

Uses : Indicated for passive prevention and treatment of diphtheria. It neutralizes diphtheria toxin locally at the site of infection. But it does not neutralize the toxin which is bound to tissues.

Dose : Prophylactic, IM, 1500-3000 IU, to contacts immediately after exposure. It provides protection for 2-3 weeks.

Therapeutic, IV or IM 50,000 to 1,00,000 IU (partly IM, partly IV).

Adverse effects include anaphylactic shock, serum sickness and fever.

Tetanus Antitoxin (Equine) (Antitetanic serum, ATS)

It is a solution containing the refined and concentrated antitoxic antibodies, obtained from the blood of healthy horses that have been immunized against tetanus toxin. Cl. tetani toxins are given to horses for immunization and antitoxin globulins are obtained which neutralize tetanus toxin.

Uses : Indicated for passive prevention or treatment of tetanus, when tetanus immune globulin is not available.

Dose : Prophylactic, IM or SC, 1500-5000 units according to body weight. Therapeutic, IM and IV 50,000-1,00,000 units, half of it by IV route.

Antiviral Serum (Equine)

Antirabies Serum (Equine)

It is a solution containing the antiviral substances obtained from the blood plasma of healthy sources that have been immunised against rabies by means of vaccine. It contains globulins which neutralize rabies virus. It is a hyperimmune horse serum. In patients who are severely bitten it is recommended to give it with rabies vaccine.

Dose : IM, Post-exposure, Prophylactic 40 IU/Kg of body weight and infiltrated around the wound in a single dose with rabies vaccine.

Antisnake Venom Serum Polyvalent

Skin sensitivity testing is mandatory by 0.02 to 0.1ml of 1:10 diluted antivenom because some times antisnake venom causes anaphylactic or allergic reaction.

Lyophilized Polyvalent Antisnake Venom Serum contains antitoxin globulin, derived from immunized horses. It neutralizes toxins present in venom of krait, viper, cobra and Russel's viper.

Dose : 20ml, I.V. 1ml/min is given slowly and repeated at 1 to 4 hour interval till symptoms of poisoning disappear (Viper Venom is cardiotoxic and elapid venom is from snakes of the family Elapidae, including cobras, kraits, mambas, coral, tiger, and Australian snakes. The elipid venoms contain polypeptide toxins of various kinds, cytolytic, haemolytic, and neurotoxic factors, but fewer enzymes than viper of crotalid venoms).

After reconstitution each ml neutralizes :

0.6 mg of standard Cobra (Naja naja) Venom

0.6 mg of Russel's viper venom, 0.45 mg of standard Sawscaled viper venom, 0.45mg standard Krait Venom.

To avoid anaphylactic reaction, adrenaline is given subcutaneously simultaneously.

Glucocorticoid and antihistamine may be injected prophylactically.

Gas Gangrene Antitoxin

The mixed gas gangrene antitoxin is enzyme refined equine antitoxin against toxins of Cl. welchii, Cl. septicum and Cl. oedematiens. It is available in 4000, 6000 and 10,000 IU (ampoules).

Dose : Prophylactic, 10,000 IU, IM given immediately after injury. Therapeutic dose is 30,000-75,000 IU SC, IM or IV (only in urgent cases).

Schedules

Immunization schedule of any country or community depends on the disease epidemiology, availability of vaccine, economic constraints, logistic problems and advent of newer vaccines. As many of these factors differ from country to country and from time to time in the same country, the immunization schedule needs to be revised periodically.

The time table of the Universal Immunization Programme (UIP) is given in table 19.6 and the Indian Academy of Paediatrics is given in Table 19.7.

Table 19.6. Universal immunization programme (UIP schedule)

	Govt. of India
• BCG	Birth or 6 weeks
• OPV	Birth, 6, 10, 14 weeks
	15-18 months
• DPT	6, 10, 14 weeks
	15-18 months
• Measles	9 months
• DT	5 years
• TT**	10 and 16 years

** if given for the first time at this age give 2 doses at 4 weeks interval.

** for pregnant mothers 2 doses of TT at 4 weeks interval.

Table 19.7. Indian Academy of Paediatrics (IAP) immunization time table

Vaccine	Age recommended	Route
BCG	Birth to 2 weeks	Intradermal
OPV	Birth, 6, 10, 14 weeks, 9 months 15-18 months, 5 years	Oral
HB	Birth, 6 weeks, 6-9 months, 10 years	Intramuscular
DPT	6,10,14 weeks, 9 months	Intramuscular
MSL	9 months plus (earlier to 12 months)	Subcutaneous
MMR	15-18 months	Subcutaneous
TT	10, 16 years	Intramuscular

Routine Paediatric Immunizations

It is recommended that all normal children be immunized against 10 infectious diseases and for hepatitis A in areas of high incidence. Paediatric immunization remains one of the most important public health measures. Simultaneous immunization for diphtheria, tetanus and pertussis (DTP) has resulted in dramatic reductions in the incidence of all of these diseases.

Immunization of Adolescents (age 11-21)

It is recommended that at this age screening for

immunization deficiencies should be done and indicated vaccines administered. It is possible that in some persons of this age group vaccines were not available when they were younger or due to presence of chronic diseases, which makes them candidates for certain selective immunization. Additionally, adolescence is a time of risks for new infections for many because of travel, experimentation with drugs, sexual activity etc.

In a number of persons, infection with hepatitis B virus is acquired as an adolescent or young adult; the virus is transmitted primarily through sexual contact, IV drug use, household contacts or occupational exposure.

Many cases of measles occur in individuals over age 10 and this shift in the epidemiological pattern is due largely to the failure of primary immunization. Those adolescents who have not received two does of MMR beginning at or after 12 months of age should be immunized at this time.

Booster doses of adult diphtheria and tetanus toxoids are recommended every 10 years.

Immunization of Adults under age 65

Pertussis vaccine is not recommended for adults but the other 9 vaccines are indicated if there is not evidence of immunity. The only routine immunizations that is recommended for all normal adults between the ages of 18 and 65 years is a booster dose of adult diphtheria and tetanus toxoid every 10 years.

Immunization of Adults Age 65 and over

Older age is often thought of as being synonymous with declining immunity although there is little objective evidence to indicate that most older persons suffer from major immunodeficiency.

Evaluation of immune status and appropriate vaccination at age 65 is important to the quality of the later years. If adult diphtheria and tetanus toxoid boosters every 10 years have not been given, it is important to update their vaccinations at age 65. All individuals age 65 and over should receive annual influenza immunization and a single dose of pneumococcal vaccine. Those who received pneumococcal vaccine prior to age 65 should receive a booster dose if it has been 5 or more years since the first dose.

A Step Ahead

Infant protection through maternal Immunization :

The prevention of severe infectious diseases in children through immunization is a well recognised, beneficial, and cost-effective strategy worldwide.

Current Recommendation

Vaccines for use in pregnant women to protect newborn infants include -

Tetanus - diphtheria toxoid

Influenza virus inactivated

Immunization of pregnant women with tetanus toxoid atleast 6 weeks before delivery effectively provides protection of newborns against tetanus neonatorium by stimulating the production of specific IgG antibodies that cross the placenta while also protecting these women against puerperal tetanus with no adverse effects to mothers or foetuses.

Adverse Reactions

The most common adverse effects of vaccines are mild toxic and/or allergic reactions. These tend to be more common with the inactivated products than with live vaccines since they usually contain more antigen and require booster doses.

The products containing whole, killed, gram negative bacteria such as the cholera, plaque, and killed typhoid vaccines frequently cause minor inflammation at the site of injection as well as mild systemic febrile responses. These are direct toxic reactions.

That vaccines may cause allergic reactions is also quite predictable considering their immunogenic character. This is an uncommon problem with live virus vaccines that are administered locally and/or boosted less frequently. Symptoms of serum sickness are expected to occur within several hours of administration, especially following booster vaccination with an inactivated products.

IgE-mediated or anaphylactic sensitivity is more cause for concern and may take the form of urticaria, angioedema, wheezing or even life-threatening shock. These reactions usually occur soon (0 to 60 minutes) after administration and, if due to the vaccine antigen will generally occur after a booster dose. Reactions to components of the production medium (e.g., eggs), antibiotics (e.g., neomycin) or preservatives (e.g., thimerosal) are very rare today but are likely to occur on the first dose in previously sensitized persons who are strongly allergic.

It is worth noting that in case fresh Measles Vaccine is not used or which has not been stored properly or syringe needle is not properly sterilized, infective organisms may enter vial which will lead to symptoms of Toxic Shock Syndrome. If this occurs and it is not vigorously treated at the earliest, it may cause death.

Inactivated vaccines pose little infectious hazard if they are manufactured properly.

Live vaccines are unique in that infection of the patient receiving the product is intentional.

Contraindications

Contraindications associated with adverse reactions to Vaccination :
- Anaphylactic sensitivity to a vaccine or component is generally a contraindication to vaccination.
- Live vaccines generally are contraindicated in pregnancy but the risk atleast with the current vaccines, is largely theoretical and the benefits merit vaccinating a pregnant woman who is at serious risk of disease. However, the medico-legal aspects of vaccinating a pregnant woman also must be considered, particularly in the light of the relatively high incidence of miscarriages and birth defects during usual pregnancies.
- Commonly immunocompromised individuals should generally not receive vaccines that have the potential to cause serious disease in such individuals. Serious immunosuppression can result from congenital immunodeficiency, HIV infection, malignancy (e.g., leukemia, lymphoma, generalized malignancy, chemotherapy and/or immunosuppressive therapy. The immuno-suppressive effects of corticosteroids are poorly defined but most steroid therapy is not a contraindication for live vaccines including the following: therapy of less than 2 weeks, replacement therapy, alternate day therapy, and topically or locally administered steroids and intra-articular injections. However the best practice is to vaccinate prior to the immunosupp-

ression. Severely immunocompromised indivi-duals can be safely administered inactivated vaccines, although the immune response may be poor.

Contraindications related to achieving a poor immune response :
- Active immunization should generally not be conducted in infants under 1 or 2 years of age unless there is a special risk. Maternal antibodies can persist for 6 or more months in a neonate and it takes several years for the immune system to develop completely. Infants usually respond poorly to any immunizing agent, and there may be a risk of vaccine-induced illness if live vaccines are administered too early. Those paediatric immunizations recommended before 1 year of age all require completion of a primary series of doses to assure effectiveness. When other vaccines must be given early, revaccination at a later age is virtually always indicated.
- Serious febrile illness is a contraindication to active immunization, especially with live virus vaccines. Most acute febrile illnesses are caused by viruses that induce interferon and can interfere with virus replication and the response to the vaccine.
- Live vaccines are contraindicated for varying periods after administration of immunoglobulin containing preparations because specific antibodies can interfere with the immune response; this is not usually a problem with killed vaccines that contain sufficient immunogens to overcome any inhibition.
- The effect of immune globulin on virus vaccines varies with the vaccine. For example, Oral Poliovirus and yellow fever vaccines can be administered without regard to immune globulin administration. It is recommended to wait 6 weeks to 3 months before administering most live vaccines such as MMR. But this interval is not sufficient for measles vaccine when high doses of IV immune globulin are administered and vaccination may have to be delayed for up to 11 months.

However, the above recommended intervals have to be viewed with respect to the urgency of vaccination in the individual case.

Chemical Interactions of Vaccines

The combination of vaccines may produce decreased immunogenicity of the individual components because of physical interactions among the vaccine components. Buffers from one vaccine may not prove compatible with those of other vaccine. Also inherent incompatibility may exist between vaccine preservatives. For example, thimerosal, included in some diphtheria-tetanus-pertussis and Haemophilus influenzae type b (Hib) vaccines, destroys the potency of inactivated poliovirus vaccine. Aluminum hydroxide and phosphate are common adjuvants in vaccines, binding to inactivated vaccines by noncovalent ionic forces. After combination, some components of a vaccine that are normally adjuvants adsorbed may be displaced from the adjuvant.

Immunologic Interference

It has been observed that chloroquine interferes in the development of adequate antibody response to antirabies vaccine during pre-exposure prophylaxis. In the light of this observation it would be preferable to avoid chloroquine therapy during post exposure treatment also.

Immunologic interaction between different vaccine components of combination vaccines occur. The interaction can enhance the immune response to individual components as occurs with whole cell pertussis vaccine when combined with diphtheria toxoid. The combination of vaccines, however, usually results in no effect or a depression of the immune response to one or more components in the product. Three major mechanisms of immunologic interference have been described; (i) antigen competition; (ii) carrier induced epitope suppression, and (iii) induction of interferon.

Combination live viral vaccines can interfere with each other through local interferon production, with one virus inhibiting the replication of another. In early clinical trials with trivalent oral poliovirus vaccine, competition between strains was recognized as simultaneous replication of vaccine poliovirus in the GIT occurred.

Because the type of strain replicated faster than types 1 and 3, it induced interferon and interfered with the growth of the other two strains. To compensate, the quantity of types 1 and 3 virus was increased in the mixture. This solution was partially successful, but the administration or multiple doses of trivalent poliovirus vaccine became advised to ensure optimal take of all these serotypes. During the development of measles-mumps-rubella (MMR) vaccines, more immunogenic strains and higher viral doses were required to overcome interference with virus immunogenicity.

Influenza vaccine drug interactions have also been postulated and interference of the vaccine with the cytochrome P-450 pathway may result in decreased hepatic clearance and increased serum levels of some drugs, including theophylline and warfarin. Overall, however, the literature fails to show a constant interaction between theophylline or warfarin and influenza vaccination.

Anecdotal reports have described severe asthma exacerbations following influenza vaccination in patients with underlying reactive airway disease, but a causal relationship has not been clearly established.

Immunologic memory

Immunologic memory is not necessarily sustained throughout life. It is suggested that continuous antigenic stimulation of memory B and T cells is required to maintain long-term antibody production and, overall immune memory requires contributions from both effector B and T cells, Reinfection with virulent viruses may occur after measles, mumps, rubella or polio vaccination.

A decrease in diphtheria and tetanus titres in older adults has been reported (waning immunity in the adult population). Because memory for inactivated antigens may be shorter, booster immunization are usually recommended.

Recognition that xenobiotics can impair the function of the immune system has led to progress in immunotoxicology over the last two decades. Exposure to immunotoxic chemicals in the environment, however, may be expected to result in more subtle forms of immunosuppression that may be difficult to detect, leading to increased incidences of infections such as influenza and common cold. Studies on experimental animals and humans have shown that many environmental chemicals suppress the immune response. Immunotoxic xenobiotics are not restricted to a particular chemical class.

Compounds that adversely affect the immune system are found among drugs, pesticides solvents, halogenated and aromatic hydrocarbons, metals, etc. Therapeutic administration of immunostimulating agents can have adverse effects, and a few environmental chemicals that have immunostimulating properties (beryllium, silica, hexachlorobenzene) can have clinical consequences. Reports on the assessment of immunotoxicity in humans exposed to various agents as a part of occupational exposure are relatively scarce. Apart from various routine toxicological evaluations this is an important parameter that can provide information on body responses which may be responsible for a sequence of reactions leading to pathogenesis.

Studies have been carried out on immunological changes in various occupational exposures including pesticides such as BHC, DDT, cyfluthrin, malathion and metals such as cadmium and mercury, dust like asbestos, cotton and silica and chemicals such as methyl isocyanate (MIC).

A number of substances affect immunological parameters; these include halogenated hydrocarbons, polychlorinated dibenzoparadioxins and polychlorinated dibenzofurans; pesticides (DDT, HCH, cyfluthrin, malathion etc.); organic solvents; asbestos; silica and metals like lead, cadmium, mercury. Oxidant air pollutants like sulphur dioxide, nitrogen dioxide, ozone and air-borne dust particles may effect immune function.

Some important points regarding maintenance of vaccines

Vaccines must stay cold all the way from the manufacturer to the child. The equipment and the people that keep vaccines cold from the manufacturer to the child are together called The Cold Chain.

Arrange the vaccines correctly in the refrigerator:
- keep measles and polio vaccines on the Top shelf near the freezer.
- keep DPT, DT and typhoid vaccine on the Middle shelf.
- Keep the diluent (for measles and BCG) in the refrigerator with the vaccines (but not in the freezer).

What damages Vaccines?

A vaccine is **potent**, if it is in good condition, and able to make a child immune, if it is damaged, and unable to make a child immune, then it has *lost its potency*.

All vaccines lose their potency after a certain time, even with good care. The Expiry Date printed on vaccine vial indicates this time.

Heat, sunlight and freezing can all damage vaccines.

Keep all vaccines at the correct cold temperature, and out of the sunlight.

If a vaccine is damaged by heat or by freezing it can not be made potent again. It does not help to put it back at the correct temperature after the damage is done.

Future

The possibility of the virus causing an inapparent chronic or integrated infection as well as the potential oncogenesis and tetratogenesis can not be completely ignored. The requirement that viruses be grown in living cells also increases the risk for inadvertent contamination with unknown organisms. These esoteric concerns are far outweighed by the benefits of vaccination, but their existence emphasizes two important points : (i) active immunization should not be considered for trivial conditions and (ii) continuous diligence and study is required for all immunizing agents and procedures.

It is hoped that a vaccine specific for HIV can be developed, but this seems unlikely in the near future. Numerous problems exist, including the fact that the HIV genome is highly mutable. In addition, the accurate testing of a vaccine will be difficult because the virus is pathogenic only in primates.

The best hope for developing a vaccine against HIV lies in recombinant DNA technology.

The major disadvantages of current vaccines are that the protection they induce is less than optimal, especially in the younger age group (3-year to 5-year age group). The highest protection, on the other hand, has been reported among young adults with an efficacy of as much as 100% in decreasing infection. Due to this variability in protection. and short duration of immunity there is need for more efficacious formulations.

Future Vaccines - against many diseases are being developed, such as Leprosy, AIDS, Malaria, Syphilis, Gonorrhoea, E.coli infection etc.

STUDY QUESTIONS

1. What are the different types of immunity?
2. Compare Active and Passive Immunity.
3. Enumerate bacterial killed (inactivated) vaccines and live attenuated vaccines.
4. Enumerate Viral Killed and live attenuated vaccines.
5. Write note on mixed vaccines.
6. What are the advantages and disadvantages of combination vaccines ?
7. Describe the conditions where passive immunization is useful.
8. What are the different types of Poliovirus Vaccine ?
9. Write short notes on (i) Human Immune Sera; (ii) Animal Immune Sera and (iii) BCG Vaccine.
10. Give one official schedule of immunization in children.
11. Which bacteria produce exotoxin that are of particular importance in immunology ? What are their characteristics ?
12. Which bacteria produce endotoxin that are of interest in immunology ? What are their characteristics?
13. Discuss in short the vaccines concerning their (i) advantages; (ii) precautions; (iii) limitations and need for advances in future.
14. What is the meaning of vaccine and vaccination ? What is the difference between vaccination and immunization ?
15. What is the difference between primary and secondary immunization?
16. What are the advantages and disadvantages of live and killed vaccines?
17. What is pulse immunization schedule ?
18. Why is the immunization schedule different in different countries? Is it necessary ?
19. Describe the adverse effects of vaccines.
20. Write notes on (i) chemical interaction of vaccines, (ii) immunologic memory.
21. How important is the role of immunization in control of infectious diseases ?
22. Why should BCG vaccine be given at left upper arm only ? Can BCG be given at sites other than left upper arm ?
23. Why are vaccinations recommended mostly in early childhood ?
24. Which other vaccines are in the offing ?

GUIDE TO FURTHER READING

American Academy of Pediatrics, Committee on Infectious Disease : Varicella Vaccine Update. Pediatrics 105 : 136, 2000.

Association of American Physicians and Surgeons : Doctors call for moratorium on hepatitis B vaccine for school children citing potential deadly outcomes. Press release, July 8, 1999. Available http://www.aapsonline.org/aaps/.

Ahmed R, Gray D: Immunological memory and protective immunity: Understanding their relation. Science 272:54, 1996.

American Academy of Pediatrics Committee on Infectious Diseases : Recommended childhood immunization schedule - United States, January-December 1999. Pediatrics 103:182, 1999.

Aprile MA, Warklaw AC : Aluminum compounds as adjuvants for vaccines and toxoids in man : A review. Can J Public Health 57:343, 1966.

Blackwelder WC : Similarity/equivalence trials for combination vaccines. Ann N Y Acad Sci 754:321, 1995.

Buynak EB, Weibel RE, Whitman JE Jr, et al : Combined live measles, mumps, and rubella virus vaccines. JAMA 207:2259, 1969.

Brooks GF, Butel JS, Ornston LN: Jawetz, Melnick, & Adelberg's Medical Microbiology, 19th ed. Appleton & Lange, 1991.

Blakely, B.R. and Archer D.L., The effects of lead acetate on the immune response of mice. Toxicol Appl. Pharmacol 61:18, 1981.

Committee on Immunization, American College of Physicians: Guide for Adult Immunization. American College of Physicians, 1985.

Cremer KJ et al: Vaccinia virus recombinant expressing herpes simplex virus type 1 glycoprotein D prevents latent herpes in mice. Science 1985; 228:737.

Centers for Disease Control and Prevention : Availability of hepatitis B vaccine that does not contain thimerosal as a preservative. MMWR Morb Mortal Wkly Rep 48:780, 1999.

Committee on Infectious Diseases and Committee on Environmental Health of the American Academy of

Pediatrics : Thimerosal in vaccines : An interim report to clinicians. Pediatrics 104:570, 1999.

Dreesman GR, Bronson JG, Kennedy RC (editors): High Technology Route to Virs Vaccines. American Society for Microbiology, 1985.

Davidkin I, Valle M, Peltola H, et al : Etiology of measles- and rubella-like illnesses in measles, mumps, and rubella-vaccinated children. J Infect Dis 178:1567, 1998.

Fine PEM: Methodological issues in the evaluation and monitoring of vaccine safety. Ann N Y Acad Sci 754:300, 1995.

Germanier R (editor): Bacterial Vaccines. Beecham, 1984.

Grossman M, Cohen SN: Immunization. In: Basic & Clinical Immunology, 7th ed. Stites DP. Terr AI (editors). Appleton & Lange 1991.

Grotto I, Mandel Y, Ephros M, et al : Major adverse reactions to yeast-derived hepatitis B vaccines: A review. Vaccine 16:329, 1998.

Huang LM, Chiang BL, Lee CY, et al : Long-term response to hepatitis B vaccination and response to booster in children born to mothers with hepatitis B. Hepatology 29:954, 1999.

Immune response to exposure to occupational and environmental agents ICMR Bulletin Vol. 31, No. 6 & 7, June-July, 2001.

Karnik, A.B., Suthar, A.M., Patel, M.M. et al. Immuno-logical and biochemical studies in workers exposed to inorganic mercury in chloralkali plant. Indian J. Ind. Med. 43:4, 1997.

Langworth S., Elinder, C.G. and Sundqvist K.G. Minor effect of low exposure to inorganic mercury on the human immun system. Scand J. Work Environ Health 19:405, 1993.

Leroux-Roels G, Moreau E, Desombre I, et al: Safety and immunogenicity of a combined hepatitis A and hepatitis B vaccine in young healthy adults. Scand J Gastroenterol 31:1027, 1996.

Levine OS, Lagos R, Losonsky GA, et al: No adverse impact on protection against pertussis from combined administration of Haemophilus influenzae type b conjugate and diphtheria-tetanus toxoid-pertussis vaccines in the same syringe. J Infect Dis 174:1341, 1996.

Plotkin SA, Mortimer EA: Vaccines. Saunders, 1988.

Robbins JB, Hill JC, Sadoff JC: Bacterial Vaccines. Thieme-Stratton, 1982.

Schoenbaum SC: A perspective on the benefits, costs and risks of immunization. Chapter 9 in: Seminars in Infectious Diseases. Vol 3. Wernstein L, Fields BN (editors). Thieme-Stratton, 1980.

Scolnick EM et al: Clinical evaluation in healthy adults of a hepatitis B vaccine made by recombinant DNA. JAMA 1984; 251:2812.

Simonsen O, Kjeldsen K, Heron I: Immunity against tetanus and effect of revaccination 25-30 years after primary vaccination. Lancet 1984;2:1240.

Stiehm ER: Standard and special human immune serum globulins as therapeutic agents. Pediatrics 1979; 63:301.

Stites DP, Terr AI, Parslow TG (editors): Basic & Clinical Immunology, 8th ed. Appleton & Lange, 1994.

Tourbah A, Gout O, Liblau R, et al : Encephalitis after hepatitis B vaccination. Neurology 53:396, 1999.

Umeki S, Kusunoki Y, Cologne JB, et al: Lifespan of human memory T-cells in the absence of T-cell receptor expression. Immunol Lett 62:99, 1998.

Watson BM, Laufer DS, Kuter BJ, et al: Safety and immunogenicity of a combined live attenuated measles, mumps, rubella, and varicella vaccine (MMR-II V) in healthy children. J Infect Dis 173:731, 1996.

White CJ, Stinson D, Staehle B, et al: Measles, mumps, rubella, and varicella combination vaccine: Safety and immunogenicity alone and in combination with other vaccines given to children. Clin Infect Dis 24:925, 1997.

Woodin KA, Rodewald LE, Humiston SG, et al: Physician and parent opinions: Are children becoming pincushions from immunizations ? Arch Pediatr Adolesc Med 149:845, 1995.

World Health Organization : Lack of evidence that hepatitis B vaccine causes multiple sclerosis. Wkly Epidemiol Rec 72:149, 1997.

Yuen MF, Lim WL, Cheng CC, et al: Twelve-year follow-up of a prospective randomized trial of hepatitis B recombinant DNA vaccine. Hepatology 29:924, 1999.

Zipp F, Weil JG, Einhaupl KM : No increase in demyelinating diseases after hepatitis B vaccination. Nat Med 5:964, 1999.

Drugs Affecting Skin and Mucous Membranes

The skin is body's first line of defence against damage from infection, irritants, extremes of light and temperature and pollution. Skin's complex nervous system detects pain, touch, heat and cold. Its function also includes immune responsiveness, biochemical synthesis of Vitamin D and prevention of water loss.

Skin is the bulwark between inside and outside, but it is totally exposed and subject to problems from both within and outside. Hence, there may be dysfunction of skin's activities and an array of diseases.

An important and significant aspect of dermatological pharmacology is the accessibility of the skin for therapy. The therapeutic agents can reach epidermal keratinocytes as well as competent - immune cells in the skin that are involved in the pathogenesis of skin diseases. These agents can be employed systemically, applied topically, injected directly in the lesion (intralesionally), and through radiation (alone or in combination with oral medication).

Antibacterial, antifungal and antiviral agents are used widely both topically and systemically for the treatment of skin diseases.

In some cases, multimodel therapy is employed. For example, in the treatment of psoriasis all the therapeutic routes are used i.e. topical therapy (corticosteroids, anthralin, calcipotriene), intralesional therapy (corticosteroids), systemic therapy (methotrexate, etretinate, cyclosporin), and phototherapy (PUVA).

Topical drug delivery is very convenient and popular, however, for its effective use, the epidermal barrier and the factors that control absorption must be understood.

DERMAL PHARMACOKINETICS

Skin as a barrier

The barrier function is largely carried out by stratum corneum (outermost layer of the epidermis). The skin acts as a two-way barrier i.e. to prevent absorption or loss of water and electrolytes.

Factors that control entry of drug into the skin :

- Physicochemical nature of the drug i.e. partitioning of the drug between the vehicle and the stratum corneum.
- Type of the vehicle
- Status of the skin i.e. degree of hydration of the stratum corneum. Hydration reduces resistance to diffusion of drug.
- Rate of diffusion is proportional to the concentration of the drug in the vehicle (linear only at low drug concentration and only applies to soluble drugs in the vehicle).

Although human skin is a simple three layered structure but it offers a series of diffusion barriers.

The pharmacologic response of the drugs employed on the skin is determined by the following variables :

- **Regional variation** in drug penetration. The absorption through skin varies with site : from sole of foot and palm low, increases progressively on forearm, scalp, face until on scrotum and vulva absorption is very high. Face, axilla, scalp and scrotum are more permeable than the forearm i.e. will require less amount of drug for same effect. When skin is damaged by inflammation absorp-tion is further increased.
- **Dosage :** Skin acts as a reservoir for many

drugs (due to physical properties of the skin). Hence, once-daily application of drugs is sufficient in many conditions.

- **Concentration gradient :** Higher concentration of drug increases the mass of drug transferred per unit time.
- **Vehicles :** Ability of drug to penetrate the outer layers of the skin can be enhanced by using an appropriate vehicle. In addition, vehicles may also have their own therapeutic effects, depending on their physical properties (moistening or drying effects).
- **Occlusion :** Application of a plastic wrap to hold the drug and its vehicle in close contact with the skin is very effective in enhancing the absorption (about 10-fold) of many drugs.

Drug readily diffuses from the stratum corneum into the epidermis and then into the dermis where it enters the capillary microcirculation of the skin and thus the systemic circulation. There may be a degree of presystemic (first-pass) metabolism in the epidermis and dermis.

Transdermal delivery systems are now used (via the skin) for systemic effect (Chapter 1).

DERMATOLOGICAL VEHICLES

Consideration in the selection of vehicle :

- Solubility of the active drug in the vehicle
- Rate of release of the drug from the vehicle
- Ability of the vehicle to hydrate the stratum corneum (to enhance penetration)
- Stability of the drug in the vehicle
- Chemical and physical interactions of the vehicle, stratum corneum, and active agent

In general, vehicles are considered as inert, however, due to their physical properties many have therapeutic effects such as moistening or drying effects.

Dermatologic formulations that depend on the type of vehicle are classified as tinctures, lotions, gels, aerosols, powders, creams, pastes and ointments. In acute inflammation with oozing, vesiculation, and crusting, drying preparations such as tinctures, wet dressings, and lotions, should be applied. In chronic inflammation with xerosis and scaling, lubricating preparations such as creams and ointments should be used.

Agents for Localized Effects

Chemical agents may be applied to the skin and mucous membranes for localized effects within the skin or membrane. These are antibiotics, antiseptics, corticosteroids, antineoplastics and local anaesthetics.

These are distinct pharmacological classes which have been described in detail elsewhere in the text.

Locally acting topical agents that have limited chemical and pharmacological activity generally have a physical basis of action. This group includes protectives, adsorbents, demulcents, emollients and cleansing agents.

Topical agents that have general chemical reactivity include astringents, irritants, rubefacients, vesicants, sclerosing agents, caustics, escharotics, keratolytics (desquamating agents) and other dermatologicals including antipruritic agents and drugs affecting pigmentation.

Guidelines for topical therapy

- Vehicle : The choice of vehicle is important. Acute inflammation is treated with aqueous drying preparations. Chronic inflammation is treated with hydrating preparations. For hairy areas lotions and solutions (active drug dissolved in solvent) are ideal, creams, oil-in-water emulsions are absorbable and cosmetically acceptable. Ointments, water-in-oil emulsions are very effective hydrating agents, suitable for dry scaly eruptions, however, not so desirable being greasy.
- Hydration : Absorption of the drug is increased by hydration. It is defined as an increase in the water content of the stratum corneum produced by inhibiting loss of water. Hydration can be produced by occlusion with an impermeable film, ointments, and soaking dry skin before occlusion.
- Altered barrier function : In many skin diseases, for example, psoriasis, the stratum corneum is abnormal (barrier function is lost) and therefore topical absorption is increased resulting in

systemic toxicity. The systemic absorption of potent topical steroids may suppress hypothalamic-pituitary-adrenal axis.
- Regional anatomic variation : Penetration of drug is higher on the face and in the perineum. Hence, irritation and sensitization from steroids are more likely to develop in these areas.
- Age : Children have a greater ratio of surface area to mass than adults, hence, a given amount of topical drug is likely to produce greater effect.
- Application frequency : Generally the topical agents are applied thrice a day. Certain drugs in a large dose, applied once-daily may be as effective as more frequent applications of smaller doses.

GLUCOCORTICOIDS

The General pharmacology of these endocrine agents is discussed in Chapter 10.

Actions relevant to topical use

The clinical effectiveness of glucocorticoids is related to 4 basic properties :

1. Vasoconstriction reduces ingress of inflammatory cells.
2. Antimitotic activity suppresses proliferation of keratinocytes, fibroblasts and lymphocytes (useful in psoriasis but also produces skin thinning).
3. Anti-Inflammatory (Inhibition of formation of prostaglandins). Inflammation is suppressed particularly when there is an allergic factor.
4. Immunosuppression (immune responses are reduced).

Glucocorticoids are prescribed for :
- Immunosuppressive property
- Anti-inflammatory property

Glucocorticoids are administered locally through topical and intralesional routes, and systemically, through I.M., I.V. and oral routes.

Potency is determined by employing a vasoconstrictor assay, in which the drug is applied to skin under occlusion and the end of blanching of the skin assessed; and the psoriasis bioassay, in which the effect of the drug in psoriatic lesions is quantified. Other assays to measure the potency of steroids involve suppression of erythema and oedema following experimentally induced inflammation.

Topical Glucocorticoids

Topical glucocorticoids are grouped into 7 classes based on vasoconstriction assay in order of decreasing potency. Table 20.1 shows potency of selected topical glucocorticoids.

General principles and guidelines for the use of topical corticosteroids

- Adrenal steroids are symptomatic, and some-times curative but not for preventive treatment. They are used for symptomatic relief and never prophylactically.
- Potent preparation should be used only for severe inflammatory condition and for short duration. They are reserved for recalcitrant dermatoses, e.g. lichen simplex, lichen planus, nodular prurigo and discoid erythematosus.
- Routine use of potent steroids is not justified. Mild preparation should be used that will control the lesion.
- Corticosteroids are very useful in eczematous condition (atopic, discoid, contact and other inflammatory conditions except those due to infection).
- Topical corticosteroids are not useful for urti-carial conditions and are contraindicated in infection, e.g. fungal, herpes, impetigo, scabies, because the infection will exacerbate and spread. However, corticosteroids with antimicrobial may be used if infection is present.
- Topical corticosteroids should be applied spa-ringly. The finger tip unit should be followed. The preparation should be applied thinly on the skin.
- Appropriate potency should be selected, e.g. mild for face.
- Appropriate vehicle should be chosen i.e. water-based cream for weeping eczema, an ointment for dry scaly conditions.
- Occlusive dressing should be used for a brief period.

Table 20.1. Classes based on Vasoconstriction Assay

Class-1	
• Clobetasol propionate cream, ointment	0.05%
• Diflorasone diacetate ointment	0.05%
• Betamethasone dipropionate cream, ointment	0.05%
• Halobetasol propionate ointment	0.05%
Class-2	
• Betamethasone dipropionate ointment	0.05%
• Diflorasone diacetate ointment	0.05%
• Fluocinonide cream, ointment, gel	0.05%
• Halcinonide cream, ointment	0.1%
• Amcinonide ointment	0.1%
Class-3	
• Betamethasone dipropionate cream	0.05%
• Betamethasone valerate ointment	0.1%
• Diflorasone diacetate cream	0.05%
• Triamcinolone acetate ointment	0.1% and cream 0.5%
Class-4	
• Hydrocortisone valerate ointment	0.2%
• Triamcinolone acetonide ointment	0.1%
• Fluocinolone acetonide cream and ointment	0.025%
• Amcinonide cream	0.1%
• Fluocinolone acetonide cream	0.05%
• Desoximetasone cream	0.05%
Class-5	
• Betamethasone dipropionate lotion	0.05%
• Betamethasone valerate lotion, cream	0.1%
• Hydrocortisone valerate cream	0.2%
• Hydrocortisone butyrate cream	0.1%
• Triamcinolone acetonide lotion, cream	0.1%
• Triamcinolone acetonide cream	0.025%
Class-6	
• Aclometasone dipropionate cream, ointment	0.05%
• Betamethasone valerate lotion	0.1%
• Desonide cream	0.05%
• Fluocinolone acetonide cream, solution	0.01%
• Mometasone furoate cream, ointment	0.1%
Class-7	
• Dexamethasone sodium phosphate cream	0.1%
• Hydrocortisone cream, ointment, lotion	0.5%, 1.0%, 2.5%
• Methylprednisolone acetate ointment	1%

Class-1 = most potent; Class-7 = least potent

- Weekly quantity prescribed is 15 g for very potent, 30 g for potent and others 50 g.
- Generally 2-3 applications a day should be used. Half-life of glucocorticoids in the skin is high hence in certain conditions once-a-day application may be enough. Mild drugs are used for acute conditions, stronger ones for chronic lesions.
- Penetration of steroids is high at axilla, groin, face, scalp and scrotum; medium at limbs and trunk; low at palm, sole, elbow and knee.
- Milder agents should be used in infants and children as absorption is higher in them.
- Potent halogenated steroids should not be used on face.

Table 20.2 shows relative efficacy of some topical agents.

Therapeutic Uses

Twice-a-day application is sufficient; more frequent application does not improve response.

Intralesional injection of glucocorticoids is usually done with insoluble preparations of triamcinolone acetonide which solubilize gradually resulting in prolonged duration of action.

In general, hydrocortisone or an equivalent is the most potent steroid used on the face, axilla or groin. Tachyphylaxis can occur, hence switching to a different steroid or using the drug less frequently is helpful.

The original topical glucocorticoid was hydrocortisone. Prednisolone and methylprednisolone are as active topically as hydrocortisone. The 9 alpha fluorinated steroids dexamethasone and betamethasone do not have any advantage over hydrocortisone. However, triamcinolone and fluocinolone, the acetonide derivatives have a distinct advantage in topical therapy. Similarly, betamethasone is not very active topically, but attaching a 5-carbon valerate chain to the 17 hydroxyl position results in a compound over 300 times as active as hydrocortisone for topical use.

Corticosteroids are minimally absorbed following topical application to normal skin. However, penetration is enhanced in case occlusion with an impermeable film, such as plastic wrap is used. It produces a tenfold increase in absorption.

Table 20.2. Relative efficacy of some topical glucocorticoids

Lowest efficacy	
Hydrocortisone	0.25 - 2.5%
Methyl prednisolone acetate	0.25%
Dexamethasone	0.04%
Dexamethasone	0.1%
Methylprednisolone acetate	0.1%
Prednisolone	0.5%
Betamethasone	0.2%
Low efficacy	
Aclometasone dipropionate	0.05%
Betamethasone valerate	0.01%
Triamcinolone acetonide	0.025%
Fluocinolone acetonide	0.01%
Intermediate efficacy	
Hydrocortisone valerate	0.2%
Hydrocortisone butyrate	0.1%
Betamethasone benzoate	0.025%
Betamethasone valerate	0.1%
Triamcinolone acetonide	0.1%
Mometasone furoate	0.1%
High efficacy	
Betamethasone dipropionate	0.05%
Triamcinolone acetonide	0.5%
Amcinonide	0.1%
Desoximetasone	0.25%
Halcinonide	0.1%
Highest efficacy	
Betamethasone dipropionate	0.05%
Diflorasone diacetate	0.05%
Halobetasol propionate	0.05%
Clobetasol propionate	0.05%

There is a marked regional anatomic variation regarding corticosteroid penetration. As compared to the absorption from the forearm, hydrocortisone is absorbed 0.14 times through the planter foot, 0.03 times through the palm, 3.5 times as well through the scalp, 6 times as well through the forehead, 9 times through vulva skin and 42 times through the scrotal skin.

Penetration is increased several fold in the inflamed skin.

Single daily application may be effective in most conditions.

Ointment bases give better activity to the corticosteroids than the cream or lotion vehicles.

CHOICE

The choice of preparation relates both to the disease and the site of intended use.

High potency preparations are needed for lichen planus and discoid erythematosus.

Weaker preparations (hydrocortisone 0.5-2.5%) are good enough for eczema, on the face and in childhood.

If the skin disorder is infected, a preparation containing an antimicrobial e.g. fusidic acid or clotrimazole should be used. After the elimination of infection, the corticosteroid is to be used alone.

Intralesional agents may be required to provide local high concentration without systemic effect in chronic dermatoses, for example, hypertrophic lichen planus and discoid LE.

Table 20.3 shows dermatological diseases responsive to topical glucocorticoids.

Table 20.3. Dermatologic diseases responsive to topical glucocorticoids ranked in order of sensitivity

Very responsive
 Atopic dermatitis
 Seborrhoeic dermatitis
 Pruritus ani
 Psoriasis especially of genitalia and face
 Later phase of allergic contact dermatitis
 Later phase of irritant dermatitis

Less responsive
 Discoid lupus erythematosus
 Psoriasis of palms and soles
 Sarcoidosis
 Pemphigus
 Vitiligo

Least responsive (Intralesional injection required)
 Keloids
 Hypertrophic scars
 Alopecia areata
 Acne cysts

Uses for topical steroids

Conditions which respond well :
 Atopic eczema
 Allergic contact dermatitis
 Lichen complex
 Seborrhoeic dermatitis
 Psoriasis of face
 Varicose eczema

Conditions where potent steroids are required, and respond slowly :
 Cystic acne
 Alopecia areata
 Discoid LE
 Keloids
 Lichen planus
 Nail disorders
 Psoriasis of palm, soles, elbow, knee.

Local adverse effects of topical steroids include

- Atrophy in the form of depressed, shiny, often wrinkled "cigarette paper" appearing skin. Skin atrophy may occur within 4 weeks due to loss of connective tissue which also causes striae (irreversible). It occurs more commonly at places where dermal penetration is high i.e. face, groins, axilla.
- Steroid rosacea with persistent erythema
- Steroid acne
- Hypopigmentation
- Increased intraocular pressure
- Allergic contact dermatitis
- Thinning of epidermis
- Easy bruising
- Delayed wound healing
- Bacterial and fungal infections
- Rebound exacerbation of the diseases may occur after abrupt withdrawal of the therapy which may lead to the patient to reapply the steroid and thus create a vicious cycle.
- Systemic absorption can produce all the adverse effects of systemic corticosteroid use.

Systemic toxic effects of topical steroids

If large amounts are used repeatedly adrenal-pituitary suppression can occur (infants and children are more susceptible). Iatrogenic Cushing's syndrome may also develop.

Adverse effects due to intralesional injections

Cutaneous atrophy and hypopigmentation.

Systemic side effects

Hypothalamic-pituitary-adrenal axis suppression. However, it can be minimized if the total dose used is less than 20 mg of triamcinolone acetonide per month.

Contraindication of topical corticosteroids

Individuals who demonstrate hypersensitivity to corticosteroids.

Systemic Glucocorticoids

Therapeutic Uses

Systemic glucocorticoid therapy is employed for severe and life threatening dermatological illnesses (Table 20.4).

Table 20.4. Shows skin diseases treated with systemic glucocorticoids.

Respond to short-term therapy :
    Contact dermatitis (acute)
    Atopic dermatitis
    Exfoliative dermatitis
    Erythema nodosum
    Lichen planus
Respond to low-dose bedtime therapy :
    Acne
    Hirsutism
Require long-term therapy :
    Bullous diseases
        Pemphigus vulgaris
        Bullous pemphigoid
    Collagen vascular diseases
        Dermatomyositis
        Systemic lupus erythematosus
        Vasculitis (inflammatory)
        Eosinophilic fasciitis
        Relapsing polychondritis
    Sarcoidosis
    Pyoderma gangrenosum
    Type 1 reactive leprosy
    Capillary haemangiomas

Conditions where steroid therapy is controversial

    Erythema multiforme
    Cutaneous T-cell lymphoma
    Discoid lupus erythematosus

Toxicity

Oral glucocorticoids have several dose-dependent systemic side effects:

Psychiatric problems, cataracts, myopathy, hypertension, hyperglycaemia, seizures, acute psychosis, and sudden death. CHF and pulmonary oedema may develop.

After brief high-dose treatment is stopped, a steroid withdrawal syndrome with transient arthralgia, myalgia, and joint effusions can develop.

RETINOIDS

Retinoids include the natural compounds and synthetic derivatives of retinol that exhibit vitamin A activity.

The role of vitamin A in vision is well established and well known.

Retinoids influence a variety of biological activities, including cellular proliferation and differentiation, immune function, inflammation and sebum production. These actions are mediated through nuclear retinoic acid receptors (RARs).

Retinoids have prominent effects on epithelium and hence play an important role in dermatological therapy.

Table 20.5 shows the three generations of retinoids.

Table 20.5. Three generations of retinoids

First generation compounds
    Retinol
    Tretinoin
    Isotretinoin
Second generation compounds
    Etretinate
    Acitretin
Third generation compounds
    Arotinoid

Isotretinoin and tretinoin are approved for the treatment of acne, and etretinate for psoriasis. These drugs are also prescribed for many other skin disorders (Table 20.6)

Tretinoin (Retinoic acid)

It is used as a topical preparation in the treatment of

Table 20.6. Major retinoid responsive skin diseases

Disease	Retinoid
Acne	Isotretinoin
Disorders of keratinization	Isotretinoin, Etretinate, Tretinoin
Skin cancer	Isotretinoin, Etretinate
Psoriasis vulgaris	Etretinate
Pustular psoriasis	Etrenitate, Isotretinoin
Pustular psoriasis, palms and soles	Etretinate
Erythrodermic psoriasis	Etretinate
Psoriatic arthritis	Etretinate
Cutaneous aging	Tretinoin
Miscellaneous Discoid lupus erythematosus, warts, lichen planus, sarcoidosis etc.	

acne. The preparation contains 0.01% to 0.1% tretinoin, applied once daily before bedtime.

Adverse effects include erythema, peeling, burning, and stinging. Photosensitivity occurs resulting greater potential for sunburn.

Tretinoin given orally, is highly teratogenic.

Isotretinoin

It is taken orally, dose is 0.5 to 2mg/kg/d for 15-20 weeks for the treatment of acne. It is also used in other disorders such as gram-negative folliculitis etc.

Adverse effects include mucous membrane dryness, dry eyes, epistaxis, blepharoconjunctivitis, xerosis and enythematous eruptions. Hair loss, granular tissue formation, photosensitivity and dark adaptation dysfunction are uncommon occurrences.

Systemic side effects include hyperlipidaemia (increased TG levels, less frequently increased LDL levels and decreased HDL levels), myalgia, arthralgia, headache and depressive episodes. Long-term therapy may produce skeletal side effects including extra skeletal ossification and in children premature epiphyseal closure.

Teratogenicity is the most serious side effect. It occurs if the drug is given within the first 3 weeks of gestation. The teratogenic effects include CNS, cardiac, thymus, and craniofacial abnormalities.

Etretinate

It is an aromatic retinoid. It is very effective for the inflammatory types of psoriasis. The drug has been detected in plasma 2-3 years after cessation of therapy as the drug has high lipophilicity and is stored in the adipose tissue from where it is slowly released.

The recommended dose is 0.5 to 0.75 mg/kg per day for pustural psoriasis and the improvement takes place in 2-3 months. For erythrodermic psoriasis the dose recommended is 0.25-0.5mg/kg per day. Etretinate is less effective for the treatment of plaque psoriasis.

Adverse effects of etretinate are similar to those of isotretinoin. However, conjunctival symptoms are less common while hair loss, cutaneous exfoliation, easy bruising, sticky skin, and liver function abnormalities are more frequent with etretinate.

Etretinate in also teratogenic and hence it is contraindicated in females of child bearing potential.

Chemoprevention with Retinoids

It has been suggested that retinoids may be valuable in the treatment and prevention of cutaneous premalignant and malignant conditions. Retinoids produce reversal of oral, skin and cervical premalignancies and play role in the prevention of head and neck, lung, and skin primary tumours.

However, the benefit of long term use must be balanced by adverse effects produced.

Retinoids are photosensitizing agents, hence their use should be accompanied by protection from sun (to prevent sunburn).

β-Carotene

It is a precursor of vitamin A (present in green and yellow vegetables). It is an antioxidant and relatively benign drug that can be used as a chemopreventive agent.

Beta-carotene is used in dermatology to reduce skin photosensitivity.

Adverse effects include yellow-orange discolouration of the skin and arthralgia. Recent reports indicate that it can severely deplete vitamin E in serum and tissues. It raises a question about its long term use.

CHEMOTHERAPY FOR DETMATOLOGICAL USE

Antiseptics and Disinfectants

For skin preparation : ethanol or isopropyl alcohol.

For disinfection : chlorhexidine salts, cationic surfactants (cetrimide), soft soap, povidone-iodine (iodine complexed with polyvinylpyrollidone), phenol derivatives (hexachlorophene, triclosane) and hydrogen peroxide.

Specific antibacterials that are commonly used topically :

Against gram positive organisms

    Bacitracin, gramicidin, sodium fusidate.

Against gram negative organisms

    Polymyxin B, neomycin, gentamicin

Superficial bacterial infections e.g. impetigo, eczema are commonly staphylococcal or strepto-coccal which can be treated by a topical antimicro-bial for about 2 weeks and applied twice daily.

Topical fusidic acid and mupirocin are preferred. Framycetin and polymyxins are also used.

Neomycin can cause injury to 8th cranial nerve. It is also a contact sensitiser.

Combination of antimicrobial with a corticosteroid will be useful for secondarily infected eczema.

Deep bacterial infections e.g. boils, generally do not require antimicrobial therapy, but if they require, it should be systemic. Cellulitis requires systemic chemotherapy.

Infected burns should be treated with silver sulphadiazine and mupirocin.

Contact allergy and development of drug resis-tance are the disadvantages of topical antibacterials. However, topical antiseptics are preferred for pro-longed use as bacterial resistance is less of a problem.

Topical antibiotics used in acne

    Clindamycin

    Erythromycin

    Tetracycline

    Metronidazole

Fungal Infections : Candida infections purely involving the skin can be treated with a topical imidazole e.g. clotrimazole, miconazole. Invasion of hair or nails by a dermatophyte or a deep mycosis requires systemic therapy. Terbinafine and griseo-fulvin are ineffective against yeasts, for which itraconazole is an alternative.

Antifungal Agents

Topical Imidazoles

Clotrimazole, miconazole, sulconazole, oxiconazole, econazole, ketoconazole, tolnaftate, haloprogin.

Systemic

Griseofulvin, ketoconazole

For the treatment of cutaneous candidiasis, imida-zoles, nystatin and amphotericin B are recommended.

Nystatin and amphotericin B are effective against candidiasis and not against dermatophytosis. Griseofulvin is effective against dermatophytosis and not against candidiasis.

Adverse local reactions of topical antifungal agents include stinging, pruritus, erythema, local irritation, allergic contact dermatitis (rarely).

Ciclopirox Olamine

It is a synthetic broad-spectrum antimycotic agent.

It is available as a 1% cream for topical treatment of dermatomycosis, candidiasis, and tinea vesicolor.

Adverse effects include pruritus.

Naftifine

It is available as a 1% cream for topical treatment of dermatophytosis.

Adverse effects : Burning sensation, local irritation and erythema.

Contact with mucous membranes should be avoided.

Terbinafine

It is available as a 1% cream for the topical treatment of dermatophyte infections.

Adverse effects : Local irritation with erythema, stinging and dryness.

Contact with eyes and mucous membranes should be avoided.

Tolnaftate

It is available as a cream, solution, powder or powder

aerosol for application twice a day to infected areas.

It is well tolerated. It rarely causes irritation or allergic contact sensitization.

Haloprogin

It is available as a cream or solution.

Table 20.7 Shows cutaneous antifungal therapy.

Table 20.7. Cutaneous Antifungal Therapy

Condition	Topical Therapy	Oral Therapy
Candidiasis localized	Azoles	—
Candidiasis wide-spread and muco-cutaneous	—	Ketoconazole Itraconazole* Fluconazole*
Onchomycosis	—	Griseofulvin Terbinafine* Itraconazole* Fluconazole*
Tinea pedis	Azoles, Allylamines e.g. Naftifine	Griseofulvin Terbinafine* Itraconazole* Fluconazole*
Tinea vesicolor loca-lized	Azoles, Allylamines	—
Tinea vesicolor, wide-spread	—	Ketoconazole Itraconazole* Fluconazole*
Tinea corporis, loca-lized	Azoles, Allylamines	—
Tinea corporis, wide-spread		Griseofulvin Terbinafine* Itraconazole* Fluconazole*

* Currently experimental for the indicated condition.

Antiviral Agents

These drugs are described in Chapter 11.

Topical Antivirals

Acyclovir

Topical acyclovir is available as a 5% ointment for topical application to primary cutaneous herpes simplex infections. There is no evidence that the topical use of acyclovir is of any benefit in the treatment of recurrent disease in nonimmuno-compromised patients.

Adverse local reactions of acyclovir may include pruritus and mild pain with transient stinging or burning.

Acyclovir is used to treat cutaneous herpes simplex, herpes zoster, and chickenpox.

Famciclovir (prodrug of penciclovir) and valacyclovir (prodrug of acyclovir), may decrease the length of post therapeutic neuralgia in patients. Improvement of psoriasis in AIDS patients with oral zidovudine has been reported. It has specific antiviral effects against HSV, varicella used as 5% topically.

Idoxuridine is used as 5-15% cream locally in herpes simplex and herpes zoster.

Parasitic infection

Topical parasiticides
Ectoparasiticides

Agents used in pediculosis only

Melathion (organophosphorus ChE inhibitor) in alcohol-based lotion is applied on dry hair and scalp once to treat pediculosis capitis. After 8-12 hours shampooing is done.

Agents used in scabies only

Sulphur in ointment form is a scabicide. Due to unpleasant odour and staining of clothes, it is not commonly used now.

Crotamiton as a cream or lotion is applied twice at 24 hour intervals followed by bath 48 hours after the last application. It is applied on whole body from chin downwards.

Agents used both for pediculosis and scabies

Lindane (hexachlorocyclohexane) is used once as a shampoo in pediculosis and washed after 5 minutes. Lindane is applied once on whole body and washed after 8-12 hours in scabies.

About 10% of lindane may be absorbed which may produce neurotoxicity and haematotoxicity, hence precaution would be taken in infants, children and pregnant women. Lindane should not come in contact with eyes and mucous membranes.

Benzylbenzoate is safer than lindane when used topically, but less effective.

Permethrin cream is applied once in pediculosis

and washed after 10 minutes. It is applied once on whole body and washed after 8-12 hours in scabies.

ANTIMALARIAL DRUGS

Chloroquine, hydroxychloroquine and quinacrine are used in dermatology as antiinflammatory agents, especially in collagen, vascular and photosensitivity diseases. Hydroxychloroquine is useful in lupus.

Combination of hydroxychloroquine and quinacrine is useful in case patient does not respond to hydroxychloroquine alone. Chloroquine is also very effective for the same conditions.

The mode of action of antimalarials (though not clear) is likely to include inhibition of phospholipase A_2; inhibition of release and activity of lysomal enzymes, decreased stimulation of auto-immune CD4+T-cells, decreased cytokine release, and an antioxidant activity.

Dermatological uses of hydroxychloroquine include treatment of discoid and systemic lupus erythematosus. Other uses include cutaneous dermatomyositis, solar urticaria etc.

Hydroxychloroquine 200mg twice a day, quinacrine 100mg/day, chloroquine 250mg/day or hydroxychloroquine < 6.5mg/kg/day, chloroquine < 3mg/kg/day are recommended.

Antimalarials are drugs of choice for widespread cutaneous lupus, in conjunction with topical glucocorticoids and sunscreens.

The toxic effects of antimalarials are described in Chapter 11.

CYTOTOXIC AND IMMUNOSUPPRESSIVE DRUGS

These are used in dermatology for hyperproliferative diseases such as psoriasis and for immune diseases such as bullous dermatoses and leukocytoclastic vasculitis. These agents are also described in Chapter 11.

Antimetabolites

Methotrexate is used in highly proliferative diseases such as psoriasis, after failure of topical agents. The other diseases for which it is used as a second line treatment include pemphigus vulgaris, lupus erythematosus and chronic actinic dermatitis etc.

In treating psoriasis with methotrexate, it should not be given to patients with liver disease or alcohol abuse.

Methotrexate is used in severe psoriasis which does not respond to topical agents, and especially when psoriasis is pustular psoriasis or severe psoriatic arthritis.

Dose : Single dose weekly or split doses every 12 hours for 24 to 36 hours weekly. The initial dose is 5 or 7.5 mg and increased if necessary in 2.5 to 5 mg increments weekly (final dose 7.5 to 30 mg per week).

Azathioprine is used in dermatology as a steroid sparing agent in conditions such as pemphigus, lupus and dermatomyositis, and selected cases of psoriasis.

Dose : Initial dose is 2 mg/kg/d in single or two divided doses.

Fluorouracil (5-FU) is indicated for use in multiple actinic keratoses and superficial basal cell carcinoma not amenable to other treatment. It is used topically for 2 to 4 weeks.

It is also given by intralesional injection in conditions such as keratoacanthomas, warts, and porokeratoses.

Adverse effects of intralesional injection include burning sensation during injection and subsequent oedema, local erythema, and even ulceration.

Hydroxyurea (cytotoxic drug) and thioguanine (6-TG, antimetabolite) are indicated for psoriasis where methotrexate can not be used due to liver disease. These drugs are used in patients who do not respond to topical therapies or in whom other systemic therapies are contraindicated.

Alkylating agents

Cyclophosphamide is used for advanced cutaneous T-cell lymphoma, pemphigus in patients who are unresponsive to azathioprine.

Dose : 2 to 3mg/kg/d in divided doses or monthly I.V. cyclophosphamide, 0.5 to 1.0 g/m^2 infused over 1 hour.

Mechlorethamine hydrochloride (alkylating agent) and carmustine (bischloronitrosourea, BCNU) are used topically to treat cutaneous T-cell lymphoma, applied as a solution or as ointment. However, the solution must be made fresh daily. The solution is slightly more effective than ointment.

Adverse effects include irritant reactions, contact dermatitis, secondary cutaneous malignancies and pigmentary changes.

Cyclosporin

Cyclosporin (immunosuppressant) is used in dermatology in severe psoriasis, lichen planus, eczematous dermatitides, alopecia areata, pemphigus etc.

Dose : Initial oral dose 3-4mg/kg/d as a single daily dose or in 2 divided doses.

Cyclosporin should be reserved for severe dermatological diseases that are recalcitrant to conventional, less toxic therapies, because of potential permanent nephrotoxicity and unclear long-term safety.

Miscellaneous

Carmustine (nitrosourea) can cause more bone marrow depression than mechlorethamine.

Systemic vinblastine (vinca alkaloid) is used for advanced cutaneous T-cell lymphoma and Kaposi's sarcoma. Intralesional vinblastine is also used for this condition.

Intralesional bleomycin (antibiotic) is used for warts (has both cytotoxic and proinflammatory effects).

DAPSONE AND SULPHASALAZINE

Dapsone is used in dermatology for its antiinflammatory properties in pustular disease of the skin (in sterile noninfectious conditions), in addition its use is important in autoimmune skin diseases as it inhibits adherence of antibodies to neutrophils.

Dapsone is used in dermatitis herpetiformis, pemphigus, pemphigoid, leprosy, bullous lupus erythematosus and leukocytoclastic vasculitis etc. The dose is 50mg per day with increment 25mg per day at weekly intervals.

Sulphasalazine has antibacterial and antiinflammatory properties in treating psoriasis and pyoderma gangrenosum.

ANTIHISTAMINES

These are described in Chapter 13.

These are used in dermatology for the treatment of pruritus (due to urticaria, atopic dermatitis, contact dermatitis, psoriasis etc.).

Cutaneous injection of H_1 receptor agonists causes itching and not by H_2 agonists. However, combination of H_1 and H_2 receptor blockers is superior to H_1 blockers alone for relieving itching.

Urticaria (named after its similarity to a sting of a nettle Urtica) and angioedema can be effectively treated by H_1 antihistamines, however, severe cases respond more quickly by giving adrenaline inj. 1 mg/ml 0.1-0.3 ml. SC. In severe cases systemic corticosteroid may be needed.

Chronic urticaria usually respond to H_1-receptor antihistamines with low sedating properties e.g. cetirizine.

Newer H_1-type antihistamines such as terfenadine, astemizole, and loretadine lack anticholinergic side effects, they are nonsedating as they do not cross the blood-brain barrier.

Nonsedaling antihistamines should not be given simultaneously with drugs that inhibit cytochrome P450 activity such as ketoconazole or erythromycin (to avoid drug interactions - cardiac arrhythmias)

H_2-receptor blockers have been used to treat warts in children.

Tricyclic antidepressants act on both H_1 and H_2 receptors and have been used to treat pruritus and urticaria.

ANTIPSORIASIS DRUGS

Psoriasis is a chronic scaling-skin eruption characterized by keratinocyte hyperproliferation. There is increased (x10) epidermal undifferentiated cell proliferation and inflammation of the epidermis and dermis. The increased number of horn cells containing abnormal keratin is so much that there is no normal stratum corneum formed.

It is a disease in which the skin cells run amok. Normally skin renews itself in about 30 days - that is the time it takes for new skin cells to make their way from the innermost layer of skin to the surface. In psoriasis, cells reach the top in just about 3 days, as if the body had lost its brakes. The epidermis cells are formed and discarded too rapidly. The result is raised areas of skin called plaques, which are red and often itchy. After the cells reach the surface, they die like normal cells, but many of them in raised patches turn white with dead cells flaking off.

It has a genetic basis.

There is no cure, but for relief there are multiple therapies.

For the treatment of psoriasis, keratolysis and inhibition of cell division are the main measures followed. The routes of administration of antipsoriasis drugs are shown in Fig. 20.1.

Drugs

- Dissolve keratin (keratolysis)
- Inhibit cell division

Proliferated cells must be removed by dithranol (anthranil) ointment applied to the lesions (not on face) for one hour and removed. Start with 0.1% and increase to 1%, and to be used daily until lesions disappear.

Corticosteroids topically applied reduce epidermal cell division. Systemic corticosteroids should be avoided.

Calcipotriene, calcipotriol and tacalcitol (analogues of calcitriol) available for topical use are as effective as dithranol and corticosteroid, when used topically. They inhibit cell proliferation and encourage cell differentiation.

Etretinate (an aromatic retinoid) inhibits psoriatic hyperkeratosis. It is a prodrug, the active form is acitretin.

Psoralen followed by long-wave length UVA is used in severe cases. It inhibits DNA synthesis. The combination of UVB and dithranol is probably the safest e.g. UVB + dithranol —> PUVA + acitretin —> UVB + dithranol and so on may reduce the adverse effects of any one therapy.

Folic acid antagonist is used in life-threatening psoriasis. Its effect is temporary. Folic acid antagonist e.g. methotrexate suppresses epidermal activity (temporarily) like cyclosporin but they are very toxic to use unless psoriasis or associated arthritis are very disabling.

Anthralin

It is a synthetic compound (1, 8-dihydroxy-9-anthrone).

Its mechanism of the antipsoriasis effect is unknown.

Anthralin is unstable as it has an oxidizable centre at C10 which produces degradable products that produce violet-brown staining of the skin and clothes.

It is applied topically as 0.1% to 1.0%.

It is also available in petrolatum jelly or zinc paste with salicylic acid. Initially lower concentration (0.1%) is used for several hours and then gradually the concentration is increased. The modified treatment is application of higher concentration (0.25% or 0.5%) for 20-30 minutes. The medication must be completely removed with soap.

Adverse effects include staining of clothes and irritation of the involved skin. Systemic toxicity is not associated with anthralin.

Other uses - alopecia areata and warts.

Corticosteroids have been discussed previously.

Calcipotriene is a synthetic, 1,24-dihydroxy-vitamin D_3 analogue with a double bond and ring structure in the side chain. It is 200 times less potent than 1,25-$(OH)_2D$ in causing hypercalciuria and hypercalcaemia, whereas its affinity for the vitamin D receptor is equal to that of 1,25$(OH)_2D$.

Calcipotriene ointment is applied twice daily to plaque psoriasis, improvement is observed within 1-2 weeks and the maximum response occurs in 6-8 weeks. It is slightly more effective than betamethasone or short-contact anthralin treatment. This drug can not be used on face because of facilitated absorption resulting in irritation.

Vitamin A (retinol) has important role in epithelial function and the retinoic acid derivative acitretin (Neotigason, orally) inhibits psoriatic hyperkeratosis over 4-6 weeks. Acitretin is to be used in courses (6-9 months) with intervals of 2-6 months. It is teratogenic like other vitamin A derivatives. Precautions are needed in women of child bearing age, i.e. contraception for 2 years after cessation as the drug is stored in liver and in fat and released over many months. The plasma t-1/2 is 3 months.

Tazarotene, a topical retinol is of some benefit in mild psoriasis, but is irritant.

The role of retinoids is discussed separately. The role of psoralen and folic acid antagonist are described separately.

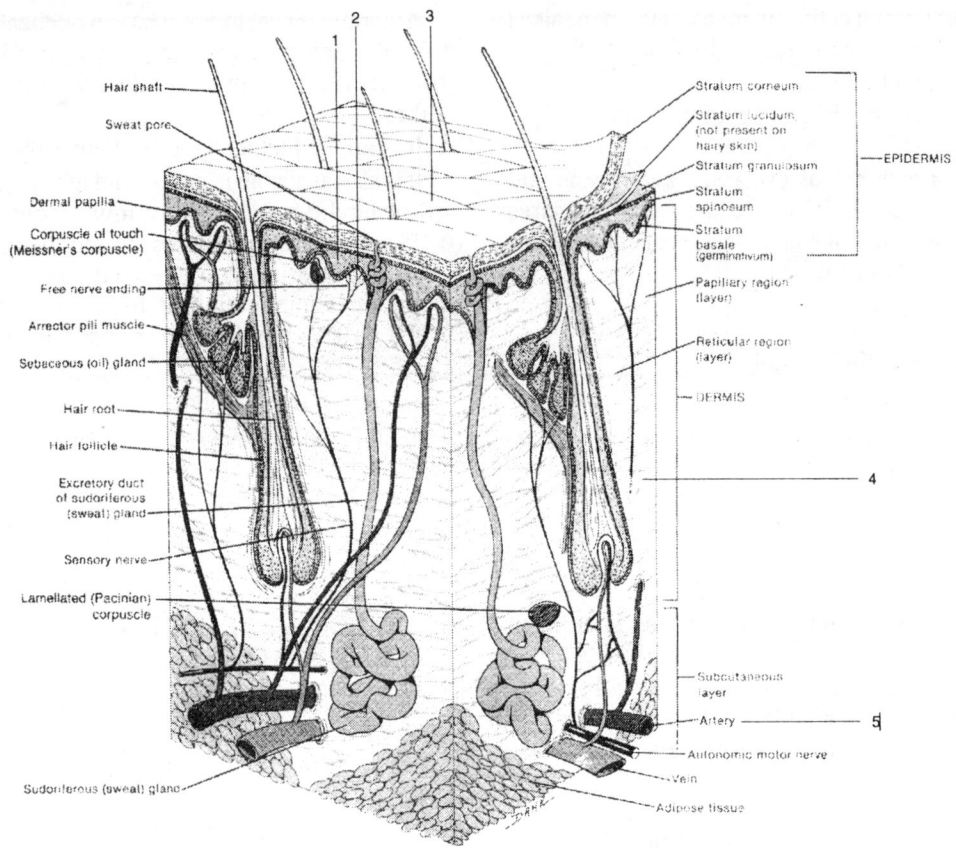

Fig. 20.1. Structure of skin, and routes of administration of antipsoriasis drugs: 1 and 2 = phototherapy; 3 = topical therapy; 4 = intralesional therapy; 5 systemic.

Box. 20.1. Antipsoriasis Drugs

- Anthranil (Dithranol) ointment applied on lesions daily and removed after an hour.
- Corticosteroids topically applied.
- Calcipotriene (analogue of calcitriol) used topically
- Etretinate (retinoic acid derivative)
- Psoralen followed by long-wave length UVA
- Folic acid antagonist used in severe life-threatening psoriasis

---

DRUGS FOR ACNE

Under androgenic stimulation in adolescent boys and girls, the sebaceous follicles of face produce excess of sebum which get colonized by bacteria (*propionibacterium acnes*) and yeast (*Pityrosporum ovale*). Bacterial lipases produce fatty acids which irritate follicular ducts, cause retention of secretions and hyperkeratosis. These may rupture causing inflammation and pusturation.

Thus acne is due to the disordered function of the pilosebaceous follicle whereby abnormal keratin and sebum form debris which plug the mouth of the follicle. Propionibacterium acnes colonises the debris. Bacterial action releases inflammatory fatty acids from the sebum.

Certain medications, for example, some types of contraceptive pills, corticosteroids, and drugs for epilepsy can make acne worse. In some women acne is a symptom of polycystic ovary syndrome, a hormonal disorder that can also cause missed periods, infertility, excess body mass and weight gain.

Measures to treat acne

- Mild keratolytic agents to unblock pilosebaceous ducts: benzyl peroxide, sulphur, salicylic acid, azelaic acid
- Systemic or topical antimicrobial therapy: tetracycline, minocycline, erythromycin, at low doses used over months. There will be suppression of bacterial lipolysis of sebum, which generates inflammatory fatty acids.
- Vitamin A (retinoic acid) derivatives reduce sebum production and keratinization. Vitamin A is a teratogen.

Tretinoin (Retin-A) is applied topically, avoided in pregnancy. Adapalene, a synthetic retinoid is better tolerated.

Isotretinoin (t1/2 15 hr) orally is highly effective in a course of 12-16 weeks. But it is a serious teratogen.

Cholesterol and triglycerides may rise, hence lipid profile should be measured before and during treatment.

Pregnancy tested before commencement in women and contraception to be used for 4 weeks before, during and for 4 weeks after cessation of therapy.

Mood change and severe depression may follow use of isotretinoin.

- Hormone therapy by using (1) oestrogen, to suppress the hypothalamic/pituitary gonadotrophin production or (2) antiandrogen (cyproterone), or both are used in females, 50 mg of ethinyloestradiol reduces sebum production by 40%.

The objective is to reduce androgen production or effect.

- Topical corticosteroid should NOT be used.

Topical Therapy

Benzoyl Peroxide

It is an effective topical agent for the treatment of acne vulgaris. It is converted metabolically to benzoic acid within the epidermis and dermis.

In the presence of water, it gradually liberates oxygen which kills bacteria (highly effective against P.acnes) and has also keratolytic property.

It is used as 5-10% cream, gel or lotion.

The adverse effects of benzoyl peroxide include dryness of skin, erythema and contact sensitization.

Its contact should be avoided with eyes, lips and denuded skin. In can bleach hair and coloured fabric.

Retinoic Acid (all-trans-retinoic acid)

It promotes lysis of keratinocytes, prevents horny cells from binding to each other. It causes peeling but has no antibacterial property.

It is used as 0.025-0.05% gel or cream.

Side effects include stinging, erythema, oedema.

Retinoic acid, known as tretinoin or all-trans-retinoic acid, is the acid form of Vitamin A.

Retinoic acid has several effects on epithelial tissues. It stabilizes lysosomes, increases ribonucleic acid polymerase activity, increases PGE_2, cAMP, and cGMP levels, and increases the incorporation of thymidine into DNA.

Retinoic acid is an effective topical treatment for acne vulgaris. Analogues of vitamin A e.g. 13-cis-retinoic acid (Isotretinoin) are effective in various dermatologic diseases when administered orally.

Retinoic acid is useful in acne as it decreases cohesion between epidermal cells and increases epidermal cell turnover, resulting in the expulsion of open comedones and the transformation of closed comedones into open ones.

Topical retinoic acid should be applied to dry skin only. It takes 8-12 weeks for optimal clinical improvement. Patients using retinoic acid are advised to avoid or minimize sun exposure and use sunscreen because animal studies suggest that it may increase the tumourigenic potential of UV radiation.

Isotretinoin

It is a synthetic retinoid. Its elimination half-life is 10-20 hours. It is indicated in the treatment of severe cystic acne. The mechanism of action is not known.

The dose is 1-2mg/kg given in 2 divided doses daily for 4-5 months.

Adverse effects resemble hypervitaminosis A, headache, corneal opacities, anorexia, alopecia, myalgia and arthralgia. These effects are reversible on discontinuation of the drug.

Women of child bearing potential must use effective form of contraception for atleast one month before, throughout isotretinoin therapy, and for one or more menstrual cycles after stopping the use of the drug. This precaution is essential due to the significant risk of teratogenicity.

Topical Antibiotics

Clindamycin 1% gel, tetracyclines, erythromycin 1-4% ointment, cream, solution, gel are less effective than benzoyl peroxide against P.acnes.

Metronidazole 0.75% gel and 1% cream is used for topical treatment of rosacea.

Keratolytics like sulphur, salicylic acid, resorcinol and anhydrotics such as zinc sulphate, aluminum chloride are less effective than benzoyl peroxide.

Azelaic acid (a natural product from Pityrosporum ovale) inhibits many aerobic and anaerobic bacteria, specially P. acnes. It is used as 10% - 20% cream. Its efficacy in acne is equivalent to that of benzoyl peroxide and retinoic acid and without producing their irritant and desquamating side effects. It is also beneficial in cutaneous malignant melanoma.

Systemic Therapy

Systemic therapy is indicated only in severe cases.

1. Antibiotics: Tetracycline, minocycline or erythromycin have been used for months. However, it should be noted that raised intracranial pressure with loss of vision has been reported by tetracycline if used for more than 2 months.
2. Oestrogens can be used only in girls above 16 years.
3. Retinoids : 13-cis retinoic acid reduces production of sebum (secondarily skin bacteria decrease). The dose is 1 mg/kg/day for 20 weeks. Side effects include dryness of skin.

Box 20.2. Measures to treat acne

- Cleansing with soap and water, or weak antiseptics
- Keratolytic agents such as salicylic acid or benzoyl peroxide
- Antibacterials such as clindamycin, erythromycin, tetracycline to suppress bacterial lipolysis
- Vitamin A derivatives such as tretinoin (topically) and isotretinoin (orally)
- Hormone therapy to reduce androgen level by using oestrogen (suppress hypothalamus-pituitary axis) and cyproterone (anti-androgen).

ANTISEBORRHOEA AGENTS

Seborrhoeic dermatitis is characterized by scaling lesions. It affects areas rich in sebaceous glands e.g. scalp, face, trunk. Dandruff is common. Pityrosporum ovale (commensal yeast) is transformed to a noninvasive pathogenic organism by various factors such as increased sweating, emotional stress etc.

For the treatment of seborrhoeic dermatitis the following drugs are used :

Selenium sulphide 2.5% lotion or shampoo. It is fungicidal to pityrosporum ovale (causal yeast). Systemic absorption may cause toxicity.

Zinc pyrithione 1% reduces dandruff.

Corticosteroids as lotion (massaged on scalp) relieve seborrhoeic dermatitis including dandruff.

Imidazole antifungals are also effective, particularly ketoconazole against P.ovale, the dose is 200 mg/d for one month. Ketoconazole has also been formulated as 2% cream/shampoo/scalp gel.

Sulphur, resorcinol, ammoniated mercury and coal tar may benefit seborrhoea by keratolytic and antiseptic actions.

Salicylic acid by removing scales (keratolytic) has mild action in seborrhoea.

PHOTOSENSITIVITY

Photosensitivity means that an adverse effect occurs as a result of drug plus light, usually sun's UV light. Table 20.8 shows drugs that can cause photosensitivity.

Photosensitivity is of 2 types. (1) Phototoxicity which stimulates sunburn with a minimal dose of sunlight. Phototoxicity is effect of too high a dose of UV in a person who has been exposed to a drug. The reaction is like a severe sunburn. The threshold returns to normal when the drug is withdrawn; (2) Photoallergy where a photochemical reaction of the drug in the skin acts as an allergen. It is a cell-mediated immunological effect that occurs only in some persons and caused by UVA in which the drug combines with tissue protein. Reactions may persist for years after the drug is withdrawn. They are usually eczematous.

PHOTOCHEMOTHERAPY

Dermatologists are concerned with the regions of

Table 20.8. Phtosensitizing drugs

Photosensitivity produced by	
Systemic use	*Topically administered drugs*
Sulphonamides	PABA and its esters
Sulphonylureas	Coaltar derivatives
Frusemide	Hexachlorophane
Thiazides	Halogenated salicylanilides
Griseofulvin	Psoralens
Tetracycline	6-Methylcoumarin (used in per-
Nalidixic acid	fumes, shaving lotions, sunscreens)
Chlordiazepoxide	
Phenothiazines	
Piroxicam	
Oral contraceptives	
Fenofibrate	
Tolbutamide	
Psoralens	
Amiodarone	
Vinblastine	
Doxycycline	
Demeclocycline	

UV radiation (UVC, 200-290 nm; UVB, 290-320 nm; and UVA, 320-400 nm) and with visible radiation (400-800 nm).

UVC is absorbed by the ozone layer and does not reach the earth at sea level. But at high altitude it can cause skin injury.

UVB is the most erythrogenic and melanogenic type of radiation that causes sunburn, suntan, skin cancer, and photoaging.

UVA is about 1000 times less erythrogenic than UVB. However, it has longer wavelength that penetrates more deeply and contributes to photosensitivity diseases and photoaging, and also increases UVB-induced erythema and the risk of UVB-induced carcinogenesis.

Visible radiation may occasionally induce photosensitive eruptions.

Despite the above side effects, nonionizing electromagnetic radiation (a form of energy defined by its wavelength) is used therapeutically in which radiation of an appropriate wavelength is used.

Prior to initiation of therapy, patients should not be taking any photosensitizing medication such as phenothiazines, thiazides, sulphonamides, sulfonylureas, tetracyclines, and benzodiazepines etc.

Chemicals used in combination with radiation in the treatment of skin disorders

Psoralens are obtained from citrus fruits and other plants, e.g. methoxsalen is used to induce photochemical reactions in the skin. After its topical or systemic administration and subsequent exposure to UVA, erythematous reaction occurs and melanocytes are activated resulting in pigmentation over the following week. This helps to repigment areas of depigmentation eg. vitiligo.

PUVA : Psoralens and UVA

Photochemotherapy with psoralen-containing plant extracts were used in India and Egypt in 1500 B.C. for the treatment of vitiligo.

PUVA promote melanogenesis in normal skin. Pigmentation results from the transfer of melanosomes from melanocytes to epidermal cells.

Psoralen interacts in the presence of UVA with DNA, thymine dimers are formed and the DNA synthesis is inhibited. Psoralen plus UVA (PUVA) is used in the treatment of psoriasis and cutaneous T-cell lymphoma.

PUVA can induce melanocyte stimulation in vitiligo resulting in repigmentation. Localized vitiligo is treated topically using 0.1% methoxsalen lotion, whereas diffuse disease is treated after systemic administration of trioxsalen or methoxsalen, the later drug is more effective.

PUVA is used 3-4 times weekly for the treatment of psoriasis.

PUVA is also used for the treatment cutaneous T-cell lymphoma, atopic dermatitis, alopecia areata, lichen planus, urticaria pigmentosa and cutaneous photosensitivity.

Methoxsalen is available in capsules. The dose is 0.5mg/kg, 1.5-2 hours before UVA exposure.

A lotion containing methoxsalen is available for topical use.

Trioxsalen can be used orally for the treatment of vitiligo. The dose is 0.2-0.5 mg/kg.

Adverse effects of PUVA therapy :

Acute side effects of PUVA include nausea, painful erythema, blistering.

Chronic effects include actinic keratoses, accelerated skin aging, increased risk of skin cancer, cancer of male genitalia, cataracts.

PHOTODYNAMIC THERAPY

Coal Tar

Coal tar is combined with UVB for the treatment of psoriasis. Little is known about its mode of action, which may be related to antimitotic effects.

Coal tar is phtotoxic in the UVA and visible ranges (action spectrum 340-430nm). In this range if the skin is exposed, erythema and smarting "Tar smarts" occur. Hence, the photodynamic potential of coal tar can not be exploited for the treatment of psoriasis.

Coal tar ointment, 2%-5% with daily UVB irradiation is an effective therapy for psoriasis.

Adverse effects : folliculitis is the primary side effect of coal tar. Irritation and allergic reaction are rare. Coal tar is a carcinogen in animal experiments, carcinoma provoked by clinical applications are rare.

Warning : There is risk of total body exfoliation if tar compounds are used in patients with erythrodermal or generalized pustular psoriasis.

SUN PROTECTIVE AGENTS

Effects of sun exposure

Acute effects of sun exposure

- Sunburn
- Drug-induced phtotoxic reactions

Chronic effects

- Photoaging
- Skin cancer

Protection from sun exposure can be done by sunscreens :

These are of two types :
1. Absorbent or chemical sunscreens
2. Reflectant or physical sunscreens (also called sunshades)

The efficacy of sunscreens is defined by their sun protection factor (SPF) which is the ratio of the dose of UVB radiation required to produce minimal erythema on sunscreen protected skin to the dose required to produce it on unprotected skin. Sunscreen with high protection factor of 15 are usually needed in fair-skinned persons, whereas in dark-skinned individuals lower protection factor 10-15 will be sufficient.

Chemical sunscreens : These are transparent. They absorb portions of UV radiation. Cinnamates, salicylates and p-aminobenzoic acid esters block UVB; benzophenones, anthranilates and particularly avobenzone are effective UVA screens. Broad-spectrum coverage can be produced by combining multiple chemical screens. In general, protection against UVB is more effective than protection against UVA.

Para - aminobenzoic acid (PABA 5% solution in alcohol, 10% cream) and its esters amyl or octyl p-dimethyl amino benzoate absorb UVB (290-320 nm). Benzophenones e.g. oxybenzone 2-6% block UVA (320-400 nm). Higher concentrations prevent tanning also.

Chemical sunscreens are used as adjuncts in vitiligo therapy, to facilitate tanning while preventing sunburn, drug induced phototoxicity. They can prevent premature aging of skin, Some evidence exists that they can prevent skin cancer.

Tables 20.9 and 20.10 show chemical sunscreen that absorb UVA and UVB radiations.

Table 20.9. UVA–Absorbing Chemical Sunscreens

Chemicals	Concentration	Spectrum
Oxybenzone	2-6%	320-360 nm
Sulisobenzone	5-10%	320-360 nm
Dioxybenzone	3.0%	320-360 nm
Methyl Anthranilate	3.0%	300-340 nm
Butylmethoxy dibenzoyl-methane (Avo benzone)	< 3%	320-400 nm

Some Examples of Sunscreens

Aminobenzoic Acid

It absorbs UV light of wavelengths in the range of 260 to 313 nm. Its molar absorptivity at 288.5nm is 18,300. However, it does not absorb throughout the near UV range so that the drug related photosensitivity and phototoxicity may not be prevented by it, but in combination with benzophenone it does prevent against some drug-induced phototoxicity. Nevertheless in the 260 to 313 nm range, it has the highest protection index of current sunscreen agents.

Table 20.10. UVB-Absorbing Chemical Sunscreen

Aminobenzoates		
PABA	5%	260-313 nm
Ethyl 4 Aminobenzoate	5%	280-330 nm
Glyceryl PABA	5%	264-315 nm
Padimate-A	4-8%	260-325 nm
Padimate-O	1.4-8%	264-320 nm
Cinnamate		
Diethanolamine p-methoxy cinnamate	8-10%	280-310nm
2-ethylhexyl p-methoxy cinnamate (Parasol)	2-7%	280-320nm
Salicylates		
2-ethylhexyl Salicylate	3.5-5%	280-320 nm
Octyl Salicylate	3-5%	280-320 nm
Triethanolamine Salicylate	5-12%	260-320 nm
Benzophenones		
Dioxybenzone	3%	260-355 nm
Sulisobenzone	5-10%	260-360 nm
Oxybenzone	2-6%	270-360 nm

Box. 20.3. Side effects of chemical sunscreens

Irritation contact dermatitis
Allergic contact dermatitis
Photocontact dermatitis
Phototoxic reactions
Comedogenicity (comedo = black head)

Cinoxate

A sunscreen that absorbs UV light at 270-328 nm. It has a relatively high molar absorptivity (19,400 at 306nm), is nonabsorbing throughout the entire range of UV light. Therefore it is used in preparations intended to promote tanning rather than to protect against photosensitivity and photoxicity.

Dioxybenzone

A sunscreen of intermediate molar absorptivity (11,950 at 282 nm) but it absorbs throughout the UV spectrum and hence affords protection not only against sunburn but also against photosensitizing and phototoxic effects of drugs. It is marketed in combination with the closely related oxybenzone.

Ethylhexyl p-methoxycinnamate

A sunscreen with a narrow absorption band of 290-320nm and a moderate molar absorptivity.

Lisadimate

A sunscreen that absorbs UV light at 264 to 315nm and has a relatively high molar absorptivity (17,197 at 295nm) but a limited spectrum, hence used primarily to promote tanning.

Oxybenzone

A sunscreen with a high molar absorptivity (20,318 at 290nm) and it absorbs both the long and short spectrum 270 to 350nm. Hence, it prevents not only sunburn but also protects against the photodynamic photosensitizing and phototoxic effects of various drugs.

Methyl Anthranilate

A sunscreen with the lowest molar absorptivity of all sunscreens (941 at 315 nm), also it does not absorb throughout the near UV range (absorption band 290 to 320 nm).

Padimate-A

A sunscreen of meoderate molar absorptivity but relatively narrow UV absorption spectrum (290 to 315 nm).

Padimate-O

Similar to Padimate-A

Roxadimate

A sunscreen with a limited spectrum (280 to 330nm), but a relatively high molar absorptivity.

Physical sunscreen or reflectant sunscreens (sunshades)

These are opaque and stop or scatter UV as well as visible light. When applied as thick lotion or cream, they prevent sunburn as well as tanning. They withhold longer wavelengths also which are involved in photoallergy.

Chemicals of physical sunscreens

Titanium Dioxide (it has a very high reflectance of visible and UV wavelenghts); **zinc oxide**.

Zinc Oxide

Advantages

(i) Low toxic potential (No evidence of phototoxic and photoallergic reactions).

(ii) High effectiveness in protecting the skin against UVB and UVA radiations.

(iii) Photostability and cost effectiveness.

Other compounds - Iron Oxide, Talc, Kaolin, Bentonite, Silica or Mica.

Sunscreens should be combined with other means of reducing or avoiding exposure of the skin to sunlight, because sunscreens allow significant UVA exposure. Sunscreens are no substitutes for proper clothing and avoidance of sun.

Photoprotection by clothing

(i) Can block 97% of harmful UV radiations.

(ii) SPF of 15-45%

(iii) Tightly woven cotton fabrics, nylon and polyester

Quick Tanning Lotions and Tanning Accelerator

Dihydroxyacetone (DHA) - induces melanoid staining of skin.

It protects mainly against UVA.

Non-classic sunscreens

Antioxidants and other agents :

Vitamin C	UVA
Vitamin E	UVB
Flavonoids	UVB
Aloe	UVB

Prostaglandin inhibitors

Aspirin and indomethacin - protect against erythema of UVB induced sunburn.

B-carotene - protects against visible radiation (400-700 nm)

AGENTS AFFECTING PIGMENTATION

Melanizing Agents (to induce repigmentation)

Melanizers are substances that promote the repigmentation of vitiliginous areas of the skin. Most

---

of them produce their effect by increasing sensitivity to solar radiation.

Psoralen (obtained from fruit of Ammi majus) stimulates melanocytes on photoactivation and induce their proliferation.

Psoralens must be phtoactivated by long-wavelength UV light (range 320-400 nm) to produce beneficial effect.

After local or systemic use of psoralen followed by exposure to UVB (290-320nm) melanocytes are activated.

Its use is in vitiligo.

Drugs are given orally but UVA is given locally.

Psoralens are furocoumarins. Psorline 5mg tablet or 0.25% solution and ointment are used.

Methoxsalen

It increases the photodynamic pigmentation of skin. It does not induce pigmentation in the absence of UV light or melanocytes. It is used in the treatment of vitiligo and to desensitize to sunlight.

The dose of methoxsalen is 10mg tablet, 1% solution.

Trioxsalen

Trioxsalen facilitates the action of near UV light to induce melanin (skin pigment) formation. It is used to cause repigmentation in idiopathic vitiligo and to increase tolerance to sunlight. The increase in dermal pigment occurs gradually over a period of several days of repeated exposures. The eyes and lips should be protected during treatment.

Children under 12 years of age should not take it.

It is contraindicated in persons with photosensitizing diseases such as infectious leukoderma, lupus erythematosus and when photosensitizing drugs are being given.

The drug may sometimes cause gastric irritation and vomiting.

The dose is 5mg tablet, 25mg dragees.

Methoxsalen and trioxsalen are synthetic psoralens, applied topically, as well as given orally.

Psoralens are also used to accelerate tanning.

Adverse effects : Mottling, blistering, burns, premature aging of skin, gastric discomfort, insomnia.

The major long-term risks of psoralen photochemotherapy are cataracts and skin cancer.

Demelanizing Agents (depigmenting agents)

These reduce hyperpigmentation areas of skin.

Hydroquinone 2-6% lotion or cream is used. It is a weak hypopigmenting agent. It decreases the formation as well as increases degradation of melanosomes. Sunscreens are usually combined.

It produces reversible depigmentation of the skin by inhibiting the enzymatic oxidation of tyrosine and also inhibiting the other melanocyte metabolic process. It is indicated for the gradual bleaching of hyperpigmented skin. As repigmentation may occur on exposure of UV radiation, hence hydroquinone is commonly combined with a broad-spectrum sunscreen. **Monobenzone** (monobenzyl ether of hydroquinone) is a potent demelanizing agent. It destroys melanocytes and interferes with the formation of melanin. It may produce permanent depigmentation.

Dose : 5% lotion or 20% ointment is applied 2-3 times daily and it takes 4-6 months for full effect. It is not effective against pigmented moles or malignant melanoma.

Topical hydroquinone results in temporary lightening, whereas monobenzone produces irreversible depigmentation.

These inhibit enzyme tyrosinase, thus interfering with the biosynthesis of melanin. Monobenzone in addition may be toxic to melanocytes that results in permanent depigmentation.

Some percutaneous absorption of these compounds may take place and for that reason monobenzone may produce hypopigmentation at sites away from the area of application.

Adverse effects of these compounds include local irritation. Allergic sensitization does occur, and it is advisable to do patch test.

Skin irritation, rashes, and allergy are possible with demelanizing agents. Their entry in eyes should be avoided.

Azelaic acid

It is a recently introduced drug effective in hyperpigmentary disorders, acts selectively on hyperactive and abnormal melanocytes. It does not cause depigmentation of normal pigmented skin; 10-20% cream is used.

Its side effect is mild and transient local irritation.

MISCELLANEOUS DERMATOLOGICALS

Minoxidil

Minoxidil may be used for the treatment of androgenic alopecia in both males and females. It should be applied topically thrice daily.

It dose not exert an antiandrogen effect. It induces proliferation of epithelial cells near the base of the hair follicle and may produce vasodilation of scalp blood vessels. The response to minoxidil is more favourable to men under the age of 40, in those who have had been bald for less than 10 years. A 2% solution is usually used.

Topical minoxidil is effective in reversing the progressive miniaturization of terminal scalp hairs associated with androgenic alopecia. Vertex balding is more responsive than frontal balding. The effect is not permanent as after 4-6 months of stopping the treatment, hair loss occurs.

Precaution should be taken in patients with cardiac disease.

Demulcents

Demulcents (L, demulcere, to soothe down). These are protective agents employd to alleviate irritation of mucous membranes or abraded tissues. They are often applied to the skin.

Examples : Gum acacia, gum tragacanth, glycyrrhiza, methylcellulose, propylene glycol, glycerin etc.

Emollients

Emollients (L., emollire, to soften). These are bland or fatty substances that may be applied locally, particularly to the skin, but also to other mucous membranes. Emollients or moisturizers increase the tissues moisture content thereby rendering the skin softer.

Emollients hydrate the skin and soothe and smooth dry scaly conditions. As their effects are short-lived, hence should be applied frequently. Various ingredients may be added to emollients, e.g. menthol, camphor, for antipruritic effect and zinc and titanium dioxide as astringetns.

The chief use of emollients or moisturizing agents beyond their therapeutic actions is to provide vehicles for lipid soluble drugs (as in ointments and liniments).

Examples : Olive oil, Lanolin, Liquid paraffin etc.

Emollients have certain disadvantages. It is now recognised that retention of perspiration below the emollient and exclusion of air render conditions favourable to the growth of anaerobic bacteria. Furthermore, rubbing and massaging during application aids in the spreading of cutaneous bacteria. Hence, the use of emollients to cover burns and abrasions is diminishing.

KERATOLYTICS (Desquamating Agents)

The epidermis consists of layers of flat cells, called stratified squamous epithelial cells which are bound together by desmosomes and penetrating tonofibrils both of which largely consist of keratin. The outer layer of the epidermis (cornified epithelium or stratum corneum is composed of the collapsed ghosts of the squamous cells).

Certain fungi, especially the dermatophytes, use keratin and, therefore reside in the stratum corneum. One way such mycoses may be suppressed is removal of the stratum corneum, a process called desquamation.

Keratolytics loosen the keratin and thus facilitate desquamation. Most keratolytics are irritant. Keratolytics dissolve the intercellular substance in the horny layer of the skin, resulting in swelling of epidermal cells which soften and desquamate.

These are used in the treatment of multiple hyperkeratotic and scaling cutaneous eruptions. Keratolytics are used in corns, warts and ringworm etc.

Keratolytic agents

Salicylic acid 10-20% solution in propylene glycol or alcohol is used for dissolving corns. Corn Cap 40% ointment in adhesive tape is effective.

Salicylic acid 3% - 6%, it solubilizes cell surface proteins leaving stratum corneum intact and leading to desquamation of keratolic debris. In concentration greater than 6%, it is destructive to tissue.

Following topical application (1g of 6% salicylic acid) the serum salicylate level is about 0.5mg/dl, whereas threshold for toxicity is 30-50 mg./dl. However, higher levels are possible in children who will develop salicylism.

Topical use may produce local irritation, acute inflammation, and even ulceration if high concentrations are used. Particular care must be taken when salicylic acid is used on extremities of diabetics or patients suffering from peripheral vascular diseases.

Salicylic acid 3-6% in used in Whitfield's ointment.

Resorcinol 3-10% is used in eczema, ringworm etc.

Benzoic acid has also keratolic action.

Keratolytic agents can produce ulceration if not used carefully.

Propylene Glycol

It has been used as a keratolytic agent in 40-70% concentration or in gel with 6% salicylic acid.

Propylene glycol is an effective keratolytic agent for the removal of hyperkeratotic debris. It is also an effective humectant and increases the water content of the stratum corneum.

Allergic contact dermatitis may occur.

Urea in cream or ointment has a softening and moisturizing effect on the stratum corneum; keratolytic effect in 20% concentration in ichthyosis, hyperkeratosis, xerosis; as a humectant it is used in 2%-20% concentration.

For softening the nail prior to avulsion 30-50% in ointment base is used.

Podophyllin is a mixture of chemicals obtained from the plant podophyllum peltatum (major constituent is podophyllotoxin). It causes mitotic arrest in metaphase. Podophyllin, 10 to 40% is applied 2 hours weekly to treat anogenital warts.

Podophyllum resin is a mixture of several substances derived from an alcoholic extract of Podophyllum peltatum. Podophyllotoxin is an active cytotoxic agent, epidermal mitosis is arrested. It is used as a 25% tincture locally and washed off after 2-3 hours. Podophyllum resin is absorbed percutaneously and as it is neurotoxic, the treatment should be changed in case no improvement occurs after 3-5 applications.

The major use of podophyllum resin is in the treatment of condyloma acuminatum.

Contraindication : During pregnancy due to possible cytotoxic effect on foetus.

Podofilox (pure podophyllotoxin) 0.5% is applied for genital condylomas.

The side effects include irritation and ulcerative local reactions, nausea, vomiting and muscle weekness. If large amounts are used on multiple lesions, serious neuropathy, coma and even death may occur.

CAUSTICS AND ESCHAROTICS

Any topical agent that causes destruction of tissues at the site of application is a caustic or corrosive.

Caustics may be used to induce desquamation of cornified epithelium (keratolytic action) e.g. to destroy warts, keratoses, certain moles and hyperplastic tissues.

If the agent also precipitates the proteins of the cell and the inflammation exudate, there is formed a scab (or eschar) which later is organized into a scar, such an agent is an escharotic (or cauterizant).

Escharotics sometimes are employed to seal cutaneous and aphthous ulcers, (ulcer on mucous membrane often covered by gray or white exudate), wounds, etc.

Agents

Trichloroacetic acid is applied as 10% by weight of water.

Silver nitrate as sticks or pencils.

Podophyllum resin 10-25% alcoholic solution or suspension in mineral oil.

Tars are mildly antiseptic, antipruritic and inhibit keratinisation, used in psoriasis. There are many preparations which usually contain other substances, e.g. coal tar and salicylic acid ointment.

Ichthanomol is a sulphurous tarry distillation product of fossilised fish, has weaker effect than coal tar.

PROTECTIVES AND ADSORBENTS

A **Protective** is any agent that isolates the exposed surface (skin or other membranes) from harmful or annoying stimuli. Substances that protect by mechanical or other means are considered to be protective, while the surface action of adsorbents and demulcents may impart some protection.

Adsorbants are inert, finely powdered and insoluble solids which have adsorbing capacity on their surface. They adsorb noxious and irritant substances. They are also protectives as they provide physical protection to skin or mucous membrane.

Magnesium stearate, zinc stearate, talc. zinc oxide, calamine, starch etc. are dermal protectives.

Dimethicone (Dimethyl polysiloxane) is a silicone polymer. It is an inert substance having water repellent and surface tension reducing actions. When topically applied it adheres and protects the skin when given orally, it may relieve flatulence due to antifoaming effect, and coat peptic ulcer providing protection from gastric hydrochloric acid.

Dusting Powders

Certain relatively inert and insoluble substances are used to cover and protect epithelical surfaces, ulcers, and wounds.

Mechanical and Chemical Protectives

Collodion, dimethicone etc. are occulsive protectives. Collodion (nitrated cellulose) in castor oil is flexible collodion which forms occlusive pellicle like coating on abraded skin. Topical medicaments may be incorporated in it.

The two principal classes of mechanical protectives are the collodions and plasters.

ASTRINGENTS AND ANTIPERSPIRANTS

Astringents are protein precipitants, used locally and have low permeability. Hence, the action is essentially limited to the cell surface and the interstitial spaces. The astringent action is accompanied by contraction and wrinkling of the tissue.

Astringents are used to treat haemorrhage by coagulating the blood (styptic action), and to check diarrhoea, reduce inflammation of the mucous membranes, promote healing, toughen the skin, or decrease sweating.

Examples of astrigents :

- Tannic acid and tannins or related polyphenolic compounds.
- Alcohol, ethanol and methanol at 50 to 90% concentration.
- Mineral astringents : Alum, aluminum hydroxychloride, zinc oxide phenolsulfonate/ sulphate.

Astringents also possess some deodorant properties by virtue of their interaction with odorous fatty acids liberated or produced by action of bacteria on lipids in sweat.

The antiperspirant effect is the result of both the closure of the sweat ducts by protein precipitation to form a plug and peritubular irritation that promotes an increase in inward pressure on the tubule.

Antiperspirants and deodorants can be applied as aerosols, sprays, pads, sticks, creams etc.

Agents commonly used as antiperspirants include aluminum chlorohydrates, aluminum chloride and buffered aluminum sulphate.

Glutaraldehyde (2-10% buffered solution), formaldehyde (5-30% solution), methanamine (5% stick or 10% solution), and scopolamine hydrobromide (0.025% solution) also are used to treat hyperhidrosis of the planar and plantar surfaces but not axillae surfaces.

Tannic acid and Tannins

Tannic acid is present in many plants, tannins are present in tea, catechu, betal nut etc. Tannins denature proteins forming protein tannate.

Uses

Tannic acid glycerin in bleeding gums, tannic acid suppository for bleeding piles. These precipitate ingested alkaloids as tannates and used in alkaloidal poisoning.

Alcohol

Ethyl alcohol and methanol at 50-90% concentrations are used as astringents, rubbed on the skin to prevent bed sores (not to be applied on the sores).

Zinc Oxide

Zinc oxide is mild astrigent, barrier and has occlusive action.

Calamine

Calamine is basic zinc carbonate, ferric oxide is a added that gives it pink colour. It has mild astrigent action, used as a dusting powder and in shake and oily lotions.

Mineral Astringents

Alum is used as a local haemostatic on minor cuts. Aluminum and zinc salts are used as antiperspirants.

Box. 20.6. Antiperspirants

1. Aluminum compounds - Aluminum chloride in solution in anhydrous ethyl alcohol (6-20%) applied for 6-8 hours.
2. Aldeydes - Gluteraldhyde 2-10%.
3. Methamine - 10% mild to moderate hyperhidrosis.
4. Formaldeyde 1-3% mild to moderate hyperhidrosis.
5. Zinc, starch and talc dusting powders.
6. Anticholinergices - Glycopyronium bromide.

IRRITANTS, RUBEFACIENTS AND VESICANTS

Irritants are drugs that act locally on the skin and mucous membranes to induce (based on irritant concentration), hyperemia, inflammation, and when the action is severe, vesication.

Agents that induce only hyperemia are known as rubefacients.

Rubefacients or Counterirritants produce soothing effect, cause vasodilation in the viscera or muscle through neuronal pathways.

Preparations contain menthol, camphor, methyl-salicylate.

Stronger irritants that induce blisters are knows as **vesicants.**

Certain irritants may be employed for counter-irritation to produce remote effect (to relieve pain and inflammation) in deeper tissues.

Drugs generally used as counterirritants are volatile oils (turpentine, clove oil, eucalyptus oil, menthol, thymol, camphor capsicum, canthridin, alcohol, methyl salicylate.

Canthridin is an irrtant isolated from cantharides (Russian or Spanish fly). Its application causes blister formation and its removal after 1-2 weeks leaves no scar. Topical use does not produce systemic toxicity. However, its systemic use is very toxic.

SCLEROSING AGENTS

A number of irritant drugs are of sufficient activity to damage cells but are not so potent to destroy large numbers of cells at the site of application. Such agents promote fibrosis, and may be used to strengthen supporting structures, close inguinal rings, etc. The intimal surface of blood vessels may break down under attack by such agents and thus initiate thrombosis (an undesirable side effect). This action is the basis of the use of scleroing agents in the reduction of varicose veins and haemorrhoids. They can be harmful if used improperly.

ANTIPRURITICS

Pruritus is common in skin diseases. If it is due to allergy, H_1-antihistamines are effective. In Pruritus due to inflammatory conditions, topical hydro-cortisone is very effective.

In generalized pruritus H_1-antihistamines, especially chlorpheniramine and hydroxyzine orally (except in urticaria) are useful.

In localized pruritus, corticosteroid preparation is useful in eczema. 0.5 - 2% menthol in aqueous cream is antipruritic probably by weak local anaesthetic action. Calamine and astrigents may help.

Besides antihistamines and corticosteroids, the other drugs useful in pruritus are naloxone, calamine, coal tar, astringents etc.

In all cases of pruritus, the aetiological factor should be found.

CAPSAICIN

Capsaicin is a naturally occurring substance derived from the plant family Solanaceae, available as a 0.025% cream and a 0.075% cream. It is applied 3-4 times daily for the relief of post herpetic neuralgia, rheumatoid arthritis, osteoarthritis and painful diabetic neuropathy.

Capsaicin causes local depletion of substance P (a neuropeptide involved in transmission of pain impulses). Its efficacy in relieving pain is debatable.

MASOPROCOL

Masoprocol is derived from a plant Larrea divaricata. It is 5-lipoxygenase inhibitor with antitumour activity. It is available as a cream, applied twice daily for about a month for the topical therapy of actinic keratoses.

Adverse effects include pruritus and redness. Some patients develop contact sensitization.

COLCHICINIE

Colchicinie is used (unapproved indication) in dermatology for treatment of cutaneous leuko-cytoclastic vasculitis and Behcet's disease.

GOLD SALTS

Gold e.g. injectable sodium thiomalate is used (unapproved second-line agent) in pemphigus vulgaris (efficacy transient) and cutaneous erythematosus (concern is development of proteinuria as it may be difficult to differentiate between gold toxicity and lupus).

Adverse effects include skin eruptions, stomatitis, pruritus, and exfoliative dermatitis. Acute hepatonecrosis can occur though rarely. Detailed description of pharmacology of gold can be found in Chapter 3.

Depilatories are sulfhydryl compounds, especially thioglycollates, which reduce the disulfide bonds of keratin, thus softening the hair to the point where it can be separated easily from the epidermis. Some of these compounds in lower concentration are used in hairwaving preparations.

Squalane is a saturated hydrocarbon insoluble in water but soluble in sebum, so penetrates the skin and is a vehicle for delivery of drugs. It is water repellent and so used for the treatement of bedsores. It appears in mixed formulations.

CLEANSING PREPARATIONS

The skin may be cleansed with detergents, solvents, or abrasives, singly or in combination.

Among detergents, soaps are commonly used more as a custom than due to special merit. The nonsoap detergents are important as household hand cleansers as well as in dermatological and surgical practice. Soap interferes with the action of many antiseptics and therefore synthetic detergents often are used in antiseptic cleansing preparations. However, synthetic detergents also interact with some antiseptics.

In case the user is allergic to soap, anionic nonsoap skin detergents are used as these rarely sensitize the skin.

Ordinary soaps are alkaline, with pH from 9.5 to 10.5. Synthetic detergents have a pH about 5.6. Neutral toilet bars contain synthetic detergents.

Shampoos are liquid soaps or detergents used to clean the hair and scalp.

Many bar soaps contain either triclosan or triclocarbon as antiseptics which suppress bacterial production of body odours but are not effectively antiseptic. Abrasive soaps contain particles of alumina, polyethylene, or sodium tetraborate deca-hydrate (borax).

It is believed (erroneously) that soap has an antiseptic action.

Soap or other anionic detergents show a negligible antiseptic action. Certain cationic detergents employed in dermatology are antiseptic.

The organic solvents to cleanse the skin are ethanol and isopropyl alcohol. Other soapless cleansers contain petrolatum, vegetable oils, lanolin, carbohydrate derivatives, oatmeal, and other ingredients.

In the skin of the eye lids cleansing agents such as benzene are suitable for only seborrhoeic

conditions, while in the dry, scaly conditions oily preparations such as olive oil are used.

Box. 20.7. Cleansing Agents

Cleansing of the skin removes environmental contaminants, sweat, sebum, desquamated cells and microorganisms.
- Soaps - Made of fatty acids and alkalies.
- Emollients - For dry and inflammatory skin.
- Synthetic detergents - Contain sodium lauryl sulphate which emulsify lipids.
- Medicated cleansers - Contain chlorhexidine and povidone - iodine.
- Swabs - of various alcohols.

SMOKING

Smoking has aging effects on skin.
- Toxins from inhaled smoke restrict the blood flow to the skin, thereby depriving it of oxygen. This reduces the ability to heal and regenerate new skin.
- After years of regular smoking, the skin may become much thinner than that of a nonsmoker, resulting in deeper wrinkles.
- Smoking reduces the collagen content of the skin so that wrinkles develop more quickly.

Box. 20.8. Miscellaneous oral medications in dermato-logical conditions

Antihistamines	Pruritus (any cause)
Antimalarials	Lupus erythematosus Photosensitization
Antimetabolites	Psoriasis, Pemphigus
Dapsone	Dermatitis herpetiformis, Erythema elevatum, Pemphigus, Bullous erythematosus
Corticosteroids	Pemphigus, Lupus erythematosus, Allergic dermatoses and certain other dermatoses

---

Table 20.11 shows choice of drugs in common skin diseases.

DERMAL ADVERSE DRUG REACTIONS

Antimicrobials, local anaesthetics, topical antihistamines, topical corticosteroid applied as cream (often due to the vehicle in which the active drug is applied) produce irritant or allergic contact dermatitis (eczematous).

Table 20.11. Choice of drugs in common skin diseases

Diseases	First Choice	Alternatives
Eczema		
acute	Calamine-aluminium acetate lotion, corticosteroids	Corticosteroids (systemic) Antimicrobials Remove cause, Antipruritic
chronic	Keratolytics (mild) Corticosteroids Moisturizing creams	
Exfoliative-dermatitis	Corticosteroids (local, systemic)	
Lichen planus	Antipruritic Corticosteroids	
Lupus erythematosus	Corticosteroids	Corticosteroids (Systemic)
Pemphigus	Corticosteroids (systemic)	Immunosuppressive
Pruritus	Antihistamines	Naloxone
Seborrheic dermatitis	Corticosteroids	Keratolytics (mild)
Urticaria	Antihistamines	H₁ + H₂ blockers, corticosteroids (systemic)
Bacterial Infections	Antibacterial agents	Combination with Corticosteroids
Pediculosis	Lindane, Melathion	Benzyl benzoate
Scabies	Benzyl benzoate Lindane	Crotamiton
Dermatophytosis	Griseofulvin (oral)	Imidazoles
Candidiasis	Nystatin, imidazoles	Hamycetin
Acne	Keratolytics (mild), Systemic antimicrobials	Isotretinoin (oral) Oestrogen, Cyproterone
Dermatitis herpetiformis	Dapsone, Sulphapyridine	
Warts, Corns	Salicylic acid, Urea	Podophyllum, Cantharidin
Psoriasis	Dithranol (Anthranil) Corticosteroids Calcipotriene	Etretinate Methoxsalen
Alopecia	Minoxidil	
Hyperhydrosis	Astringents	Antimuscarinics
Hirsutism	Contraceptive pill	Cyproterone Ethinyloestradiol
Vitiligo	Methoxsalen + UVA	
Xeroderma (ichthyosis)	Emoluments	Tretinoin
Photosensitivity sunburn	Sunscreens, Sunshades	

Systemically administered drugs produce reactions which are erythematous like those of measles, or erythema multiforme.

Local application of drugs may produce contact dermatitis. It is commonly eczematous.

Systemic drug administration may produce a variety of skin rashes (often drug specific). These are given in Table 20.12.

Table 20.12. Drug specific rashes from drugs taken systemically.

Rash	Offending drugs
Acne and pustular	Androgens, corticosteroids, penicillins, cyclosporin
Eczema	Penicillins, phenothiazines
Epidermal necrolysis	Sulphonamides, penicillins, NSAIDs, phenytoin
Erythema multiforme	Sulphonamides, barbiturates, NSAIDs, phenytoin
Erythema nodosum	Sulphonamides, oral contraceptives, prazosin
Exfoliative dermatitis and erythroderma	Penicillins, phenothiazines, gold salts, phenytoin, INH, allopurinol, neuroleptics, carbamazepine
Urticaria and angioedema	Penicillins, ACE inhibitors, gold, aspirin, codeine
Hair loss	Cytotoxic anticancer drugs, heparin, oral contraceptives, androgenic steroids (in women) sodium valproate, gold salts
Lupus erythematosus	Hydralazine, procainamide, isoniazid, phenytoin, sulphonamides, sulphasalazine
Pigmentation	Phenothiazines, oral contraceptives, heavy metals, chloroquine (pigmentation of nails and palate, depigmentation of the hair), amiodarone, minocycline
Pruritus only (unassociated with rash)	Oral contraceptives, rifampin, phenothiazines
Purpura	Quinine, sulphonamides, thiazides, sulphonylureas, aspirin induces capillaritis (pigmented purpuric dermatitis)
Serum sickness	Immunoglobulins
Scleroderma-like	Bleomycin, sodium valproate, aggravated by lithium and antimalarials.

(Contd.)

Rash	Offending drugs
Stevens-Johnson syndrome	Anticonvulsants, sulphonamides, piroxicam, allopurinol, cortico-steroids
Pemphigus	Penicillamine, captopril, penicillin, piroxicam, rifampicin
Hypertrichosis	Corticosteroids, cyclosporin, minoxidil
Lichenoid eruption	Beta-blockers, thiazides, chloro-quine, frusemide, captopril, gold, phenothiazines
Fixed eruptions (occur at same site)	Phenothiazines, sulphonamides, quinine, barbiturates, naproxen, nifedipine
Bullous pemphigoid	Frusemide, ACE inhibitors, penicillin, penicillamine, PUVA therapy
Allergic vasculitis	NSAIDs, sulphonamide, thia-zides, phenytoin, penicillin, retinoids.
Photosensitivity	Tetracyclines, phenothiazines, griseofulin, nalidixic acid, sulpho-namides, sulphonylureas, thia-zides

STUDY QUESTIONS

1. Describe the important functions of the skin.
2. Describe the variables that control absorption of drugs into the skin.
3. What do you mean by transdermal drug delivery system ?
4. Describe dermatological vehicles.
5. What are the guidelines for topical therapy?
6. Discuss topical steroids in dermatological conditions regarding their uses and adverse effects.
7. Describe the drugs used in the treatment of (a) psoriasis, (b) seborrheic dermatitis, and (c) acne
8. Describe agents affecting pigmentation (a) melanizing agents, (b) demelanizing agents
9. Comment on retinoids. List the compounds. What are their effects, uses in dermatological diseases and adverse effects ?
10. Name some important photosensitizing drugs
11. Discuss photochemotherapy
12. Describe sunscreens (chemical as well as physical).
13. Describe dermal adverse drug reactions after-(a) local application
(b) intralesional injection and (c) systemic adminis-tration.
14. Describe the following chemotherapeutic agents used topically in dermatology : (a) antiseptics (b) antibacterials, (c) antifungals, (d) antiviral agents and (e) ectoparasitocides.
15. Write short notes on : (a) cleansing agent, (b) antipruritic, (c) minoxidil, (d) keratolytic agents and (e) rubefacients.
16. Comment on the following : (a) demulcents, (b) emollients, (c) astringents, (d) antipers-pirants.

GUIDE TO FURTHER READING

Brown SK, Shalita AR Acne Vulgaris. Lancet 1998; 351: 1871-1876.

Chew A-L, Bashir ST, Maibach H_1 Treatment of head lice. Lancet 2000; 356 : 523-524.

Diffey B, Has the sun protection factor had its day? Brit Med J 2000; 320:176-177.

Franz, T.J. Kinetics of cutaneous drug penetration. Int. J. Dermatol., 1983, 22:499-505.

Fritsch, P.O. Retinoids in psoriasis and disorders of keratinization. J. Am. Acad. Dermatol., 1992, 27:S8-S14.

Gibbs S, Harvery 1, Sterling J et al Local treatments for cutaneous warts : Systematic review. BMJ 2002; 325:461-464.

Green, L.J., McCormick, A., and Weinstein, G.D. Photoaging and the skin. The effects of tretinoin. Dermatol. Clin., 1993, 11:97-105.

Gruchalla RS, Clinical assessment of drug-induced disease. Lancet 2000; 356:1505-15.

Gupta, A.K., Sauder, D.N., and Shear, N.H. Antifungal agents: An overview. Part I. J. Am. Acad. Dermatol., 1994a, 30:677-698.

Gupta, A.K., Sauder, D.N., and Shear, N.H. Antifungal agents: An overview. Part II. J. Am. Acad. Dermatol., 1994b, 30:911-933.

Harber, L.C., and Bickers, D.R. Photosensitivity Diseases. Principles of Diagnosis and Treatment, 2nd ed. B.C. Decker Inc., Philadelphia, 1989.

Kaplan KP, Chronic urticaria and angioedeonea. New Eng Journal of Medicine 2002; 346: 175-179.

Kligman, A.M., Grove, G.L., Hirose, R., and Leyden, J.J. Topical tretinoin for photoaged skin. J. Am. Acad. Dermatol., 1986, 15:836-859.

Kragballe, K. Treatment of psoriasis by the topical application of the novel cholecalciferol analog calcipotriol (MC 903). Arch. Dermatol., 1989, 125:1647-1652.

Kragballe, K. Treatment of psoriasis with calcipotriol and other vitamin D analogues. J. Am. Acad. Dermatol., 1992, 27:1001-1008.

Larsen FG et al: Pharmacokinetics and therapeutic efficacy of retinoids in skin diseases. Clin Pharmacokinetic 1992;23:42.

Layton, A.M., and Cunliffe, W.J. Guidelines for optimal use of isotretinoin in acne. J. Am. Acad. Dermatol., 1992, 27:S2-S7.

Layton, A.M., Knaggs, H., Taylor, J., and Cunliffe, W.J. Isotretinoin for acne vulgaris-10 years later : a safe and successful treatment. Br. J. Dermatol., 1993, 129:292-296.

Lever L, Marks R: Current views on the aetiology, pathogenesis, and treatment of acne vulgaris. Drugs 1990;39:681.

Leyden, J.J. Retinoids and acne. J. Am. Acad. Dermatol. 1988, 19: 164-168.

Lorette G, Valiant L : Pruritus : Current concepts in pathogenesis and treatment. Drugs 1990;39:218.

Monroe, E.W. Nonsedaling H1 antihistamines in chronic urticaria, Ann. Allergy, 1993, 71:585-591.

Pei, Y., Scholey, J.W., Katz, A., Schachter, R., Murphy, G.F., and Cattran, D. Chronic nephrotoxicity in psoriatic patients treated with low-dose cyclosporine, Am. J. Kidney Dis., 1994, 23:528-536.

Phillips TJ, Dover JS: Recent advances in dermatology. N Engl. J Med 1992;326:167.

Reichert, U., Jacques, Y., Grangeret, M., and Schmidt, R. Antirespiratory and antiproliferative activity of anthralin in cultured human keratinocytes. J. Invest. Dermatol., 1985, 84:130-134.

Roujeau JC, Stern RS Severe adverse cutaneous reactions to drugs. New England Journal of Medicine 1994; 331:1272-1285.

Savin, R.C., and Atton, A.V. Minoxidil: update on its clinical role. Dermatol. Clin., 1993, 11:55-64.

Stern RS, Psoriasis Lancet 1997; 350:349-353.

Stern, R.S., and Members of the Photochemotherapy Follow-Up Study. Genital tumors among men with psoriasis exposed to psoralens and ultraviolet A radiation (PUVA) and ultraviolet B radiation. N. Engl. J. Med., 1990, 322:1093-1097.

Thompson SC et al: Reduction of solar keratoses by regular sunscreen use. N Engl J Med 1993;329:1147.

Western, R.C., and Maibach, H.I. Percutaneous absorption of topical corticosteroids. Curr. Probl. Dermatol., 1993, 21:45-60.

Williams H, New treatments for atopic dermatitis. BMJ 2002; 324:1533-1534.

Yohn, J.J., and Weston, W.L. Topical glucocorticoids. Curr. Probl. Dermatol., 1990, 11(2):37-63.

Zachariae, H., and Thestrup-Pedersen, K. Interferon alpha and etretinate combination treatment of cutaneous T-cell lymphoma. J. Invest. Dermatol., 1990, 95:206S-208S.

Ocular Pharmacology

Certain terms associated with eye

Accommodation : The ability to change the focus of eye (by increasing the converging power of the lens) so as to see near objects clearly. The lens increases its convexity to achieve it.

Amblyopia : dimness of vision, partial loss of sight.

Astigmatism : It is a condition of unequal curvatures along the different meridians in one or more of the refractive surfaces of the eye, in consequence of which the rays from a luminous point focus at different points, producing faulty vision.

Anisocoria : Unequal pupils seen in Horner's syndrome or Aide's pupil.

Aniseikonia : Size and shape of image of both eyes unequal.

Anisometropia : Unequal refraction of the two eyes.

Anmetropia : Refractive error present.

Blepharitis : (blepharo = eyelid, itis = inflammation). Inflammation of the eyelid.

Cycloplegia : Paralysis of accommodation, loss of power in the ciliary muscle of the eye.

Cyclitis : Inflammation of ciliary body.

Cul-de-sac : A blind pouch or tubular cavity closed at one end.

Diplopia : Double vision, the condition in which a single object is perceived as two objects.

Diopters : The unit of refracting power of lenses denoting the reciprocal of the focal lengths expressed in meters.

Emmetropia : No refractive error.

Hyphema : Haemorrhage in the anterior chamber of the eye.

Hyperopia (Hypermetropia, far sightedness): The refractive state of the eye in which parallel rays of light would come to form behind the retina.

Hyperemia : Presence of increased amount of blood in a part or organ.

Keratitis : Inflammation of the cornea.

Keratomalacia : Dryness with ulceration and perforation of cornea with absence of inflammatory reaction.

Punctate keratopathy : Noninflammatory dystrophy of cornea as distinct from keratitis.

Miosis : (G. meiosis = a lessening) contraction of the pupil.

Miotic : An agent that causes the pupil to contract.

Mydriasis : Dilatation of the pupil.

Mydriatic : An agent that causes dilatation of the pupil.

Myopia : Parallel rays focus in front of the retina causing blurred distant vision. Correction by concave lens.

Nyctalopia : Night blindness

Nystagmus (G. nystagmos = a nodding) : A rhythmical rapid involuntary movement of the eye balls, either pendular or jerky.

Photophobia (photo = light, phobos = fear) : An abnormal visual intolerance to light specially of the eyes.

Presbyopia (eyesight of old age) : The near point gradually recedes the normal reading or working distance, owing to loss of elasticity of the crystalline lens. The loss is usually caused by aging.

Strabismus (G. strabismos, a squinting) : An imbalance of extrinsic eye muscles that produce squint.

Exotropia : Divergent strabismus (turning outword of the eye)

Esotropia : Convergent strabismus.

Stroma : The tissue that forms the ground substance, foundation or frame work of an organ as opposed to its functional parts.

Xerosis (xeros = dry, osis=condition) : Pathological dryness of conjunctiva.

Poliosis (polios=gray) : An absence or lessening of melanin in groups of hair of the scalp, brows or lashes.

Scotoma : An area of depressed or lost vision within the visual field.

Exophthalmos : Protrusion of the eyeballs.

Ptosis : Drooping of the eyelid.

Epiphora : Abnormal overflow of tears.

This chapter focuses on special aspects relevant to ocular pharmacology (pharmacokinetic, pharmacodynamic, and drug delivery strategies concerning ocular therapy).

Autonomic nervous system and autonomic drugs (Chapter 2) play an important role as these drugs have several uses in ophthalmology. Mydriatics, miotics, cycloplegics and anti-glaucoma drugs are discussed in detail in this chapter.

Anaesthetic agents (Chapter 3) are included as most of the ophthalmic procedures are done by using them.

Anti-inflammatory agents (chapters 3, 6) often prescribed for ophthalmic uses are also described in this chapter.

The important aspects specifically concerning the use of chemotherapeutic agents (chapter 11), vitamins (chapter 12) and immunomodulatory drugs (chapters 16) in ophthalmology are discussed in this chapter. Biological agents, hyperosmotic agents, viscoelastic agents and diagnostic dyes used in eye have been included.

This chapter also focuses on ocular toxicity due to drugs i.e. ocular manifestations of systemic medications, systemic complications following topical ocular medications, ocular manifestations following ocular topical medications and agents affecting specific ocular areas.

Classification of ophthalmic drugs

There are two main groups (convenient, but somewhat arbitrarily classified).

1. Diagnostic and prophylactic drugs :
   i. Cycloplegics : used to inhibit or paralyse the accommodation.
   ii. Mydriatics : used to produce dilatation of the pupil.
   iii. Miotics: used to constrict the pupil.
   iv. Topical local anaesthetics: drugs applied to the surface of the mucous membrane of the eye to produce local insensitivity in this area.
   v. Staining agents: used to stain corneal or conjunctival abrasions, in applanation tonometry and contact lens fitting procedures.
   vi. Decongestants: used as vasoconstrictors of congested conjunctival blood vessels.
   vii. Prophylactic anti-infective preparations: these are therapeutic anti-infective drugs used to prevent pathological conditions developing after minor abrasions of the ocular epithelial tissues, that may occur in many situations.

2. Therapeutic drugs :
   i. Anti-infective agents.
   ii. Anti-inflammatory and anti-allergic drugs.
   iii. Anti-glaucoma drugs.
   iv. Miscellaneous drugs and drugs used in surgery.

Ophthalmic preparations

These are sterile products essentially free from foreign particles, suitably corresponded and packaged for instillation into the eye.

Ophthalmic preparations include solutions, suspensions, ointments and solid dosage forms. The solutions and suspensions are, for the most part, aqueous. Ophthalmic ointments usually contain a white petrolatum-mineral oil base.

The single dominant factor characteristic of all ophthalmic products is the specification of sterility.

Several formulations that prolong the time a drug to remain on the surface of the eye include gels, ointments, solid inserts etc.

Solid inserts, such as ocusert Pilo-20 and Pilo-40 provide zero-order rate of delivery by steady-state diffusion. In zero-order delivery, a constant rate of drug is released to the precorneal tear film over a finite period of time.

Dosage forms for ophthalmic use

- Aqueous Eye Drops
- Oily Eye Drops
- Eye Ointments
- Eye Lotions
- Paper Strips
- Lamellae
- Ocuserts

Eye drops

The local or topical eye drops administration requires tolerance, tonicity, penetration, stability and sterility. The effectiveness of the drug also depends on the permeability of ocular structures. The penetration of the drug to the posterior chamber and the vitreous is poor, hence local instillations are usually ineffective.

Aqueous eye drops have the advantage of rapid absorption and effect with little or no interference with viewing the media. The effects are briefer than those of eye ointments. Aqueous eye drops carry the risk of systemic toxicity due to their absorption by the alimentary tract following drainage through the nasolacrimal duct. Oily eye drops reduce this possibility, while eye ointments allow for even less drainage.

At least 10 minutes should be allowed between drops to allow absorption.

The conjunctival sac volume is 7-10 ml, while the volume of a drop delivered by a dropper bottle is 50-70 ml (according to some normal drop size is 25-50 ml). The excess is lost mainly into the nasolacrimal system (where it poses the risk of systemic toxicity). Virtually all eye drops sting on instillation and thus cause reflex tearing, resulting in further loss of drug. Some of the compound will be absorbed by the conjunctival blood vessels and be unavailable for absorption by the cornea.

Oily eye drops can be used for three reasons; to produce an emollient effect, to protect a compound liable to hydrolysis and to obtain an enhanced effect.

Liquid paraffin and castor oil eye drops are used to form a protective film over the eye following trauma.

Some drugs such as DFP are broken down in aqueous solution and are supplied in arachis oil to prevent this.

All multi-dose drop bottles should be discarded after 28 days if used on one patient or 7 days if used on several patients.

Single use containers for unit dosing of eye drops have certain advantages: the drop is always sterile, there is no preservative so no possibility of preservative allergies; and economical as there is no need to discard a partly used container.

Eye ointments

Eye ointments have the advantage of prolonged contact with the ocular conjunctival membrane with slow but continued absorption of the medicament. This continuous absorption necessitates less frequent application. Of course, this advantage of prolonged action becomes a disadvantage when ointments are used for diagnostic purpose as opposed to their therapeutic or prophylactic use.

Table 21.1 shows differences between aqueous eye drop and eye ointment instillation.

Ocuserts

This is an elliptically shaped unit about 5.5 mm (vertical axis) by 13.5 mm (horizontal axis) by 0.3 mm thick depending on the dosage of pilocarpine enclosed in the permeable outer membrane. The former thickness represents 5 mg and the latter 11 mg of the drug, the 5 mg reservoir is possibly suitable for the patients previously on pilocarpine 1 or 2% eye drops, and the 11 mg be required for those previously on higher concentrations of the eye drops.

The slow release of pilocarpine in both strength ocuserts is by diffusion into the tears fluid over a period of 1 week after the ocusert has been placed in the lower conjunctival sac. Each individual sterile unit is replaced by the patient every 7 days.

PHARMACOKINETICS

Absorption

The rate and extent of absorption of topically applied drugs are determined by (i) time the drug remains in the cul-de-sac; (ii) elimination by nasolacrimal drainage; (iii) drug binding to tear proteins; (iv) drug metabolism by tear and tissue proteins; and (v) diffusion across the cornea and conjunctiva.

The time period between drug administration and its appearance in the aqueous humour is defined as the lag time.

Corneal absorption is much more effective than scleral or conjunctival absorption.

Many ophthalmic drugs are weak bases and are

Table 21.1. Comparison of Ophthalmic Solution and Ophthalmic Ointment

Characteristics	Aqueous eye drop	Eye ointment
Instillation	easier	more difficult
Contact time	shorter	longer (slower movement through naso-lacrimal drainage)
Irritation on instillation	frequent	rare
Discharge retention	no	yes
Skin allergic reaction	few	more frequent
Blurred vision	no	yes (film spreads over the eye)
Local symptoms (burning, stinging)	more frequent	less frequent
Readily contaminated (requires preservatives)	yes	no
Stability a problem with storage	yes	less likely

applied to the eye as aqueous solutions of their salts. The free base and the salt will be in an equilibrium which will depend on the pH and on the individual characteristics of the compound. To aid in maintaining storage, stability and solubility, the medication may be acidic at the moment of instillation but usually the neutralizing action of the lacrimal fluid will convert it rapidly to the physiological pH range (about pH 7.4) at which there will be enough free base present to begin penetration of the corneal epithelium. Once inside the epithelium the undissociated free base immediately dissociates to a degree. The dissociated moiety will then tend to penetrate the stroma because it is water soluble. Finally the dissociated drug leaves the endothelium for the aqueous humour. Here it can readily diffuse to the iris and the ciliary body.

Transcorneal drug penetration can be considered as a differential solubility process; the cornea is a trimellar fat-water-fat structure corresponding to the epithelial, stromal, and endothelial layers respectively. The epithelium and endothelium are barriers for hydrophilic substances; the stroma is a barrier for hydrophobic substances. Therefore a drug with both hydrophilic and lipophilic properties is most appropriate for transcorneal absorption. Highly water soluble drugs penetrate less readily. For example, highly water soluble steroid phosphate esters penetrate the cornea poorly. Better penetration is achieved with the poorly soluble but more lipophilic steroid acetate forms.

Several formulations prolong the time a drug remains on the surface of the eye. These are gels, ointments, solid inserts. If the time in the cul-de-sac is prolonged, it facilitates drug absorption.

Solid inserts such as Ocusert Pilo-20 and Pilo-40, produce zero-order rate of delivery by steady-state diffusion. A constant rate of drug is released over a finite period of time. for example, Pilo-20 releases pilocarpine at the rate of 20 microgram per hour.

This is a membrane-controlled drug delivery. However it has certain disadvantages, patients may have difficulty in placing and retaining the ocusert in the cul-de-sac. Inserts are also more costly than eye drops.

The possible absorption pathways of an ocular drug following topical instillation in the eye is as following:

Corneal route :
From tears to cornea → aqueous humour → iris → systemic circulation
Conjunctival/scleral route :
Tears → conjunctiva → sclera → ciliary body → systemic circulation
Tears → systemic circulation
Nasolacrimal absorption pathway :
Tears → systemic circulation

Bioavailability

Physical consideration: Under normal conditions the human tear volume averages about 7 micro litre. The estimated maximum volume of the cul-de-sac is about 30 micro litre with drainage capacity far exceeding lacrimation rate. The outflow capacity accommodates the sudden large volume resulting from the instillation of an eye drop. Most commercial eye drops range from 50 to 75 micro litre in volume, however, much in excess of 50 micro litre is probably unable to enter the cul-de-sac.

Ideally a high concentration of drug in a minimum drop volume is desirable as the bioavailability is greater due to decreased drainage loss. However, there is a practical limit or limits to the concepts of minimum dosage volume. There is difficulty in designing a dropper configuration which will deliver small volumes without overside. Secondly, the patient often cannot detect the administration of a small volume. This sensation or lack of sensation is apparent at the 5.0-7.5 microlitre dose volume range.

The following are also important factors which affect bioavailability of ocular drugs :
• pH
• Salt form of drug
• Vehicle composition
• Osmolality
• Tonicity
• Viscosity

If topical medications are used chronically, absorption from the nasal mucosa avoids the first-pass side effect (by the liver) and hence significant systemic side effects may be produced.

Distribution

Following the topical administration of a drug, it may

undergo systemic distribution via nasal mucosal absorption or local ocular transcorneal/transconjunctival absorption.

After transcorneal absorption, the aqueous humour accumulates the drug, then distributed to other intraocular structures as well as to the systemic circulation via the trabecular meshwork pathway.

Melanin binding of certain drugs is important in case of certain drugs, for example, the mydriatic effect of alpha adrenergic agonists is slower in onset in men with darkly pigmented irides compared to those with lightly pigmented irides.

Metabolism

Local tissues in the eye have a variety of enzymes, including esterases, oxidoreductases, lysosomal enzymes, peptidases, glucuronide and sulphate transferases, glutathione-conjugating enzymes, COMT, MAO and corticosteroid Beta-hdroxylase. Enzymatic biotransformation of ocular drugs may therefore be significant.

Elimination

Topically applied ocular drugs are eliminated by the liver and kidney after systemic absorption.

Blood-Ocular Barriers

The eye is a specialized sensory organ relatively secluded from systemic access by blood-ocular barriers. The retina presents a blood-retinal barrier because of tight junctions between the endothelial cells of the retinal capillaries and between the cells of the retinal pigment epithelium.

There are also tight junctions between the endothelial cells of the iris capillaries and between the non-pigmented cells of the ciliary epithelium. This constitutes blood-aqueous barrier.

The tight junctions have no clefts, gaps or pores that would allow drugs to pass unimpeded.

The tight junctions determine the blood-tissue barrier but at some places they are not as tight e.g., in choroid and ciliary processes.

ROUTES OF ADMINISTRATION

Drugs will only produce their desired effect if they are present at the site of action in appropriate quantities. Certain parts of the eye are more accessible to drugs given by one route than they would be by another. Drugs also vary in their ability to cross capillary and mucous membrane barriers.

Topical route

This is by far the most common route of administration of drugs for the eye. Topically applied agents produce effective levels mainly in the anterior segment.

Direct injection

This can be periocular (subconjunctival or retrobulbar) or intravitreal. These routes are used when large doses of drugs are required at a site very quickly. For the treatment of deep infections intravitreal injection may be the only possible route.

Subconjunctival injection : Drug is injected underneath the conjuctiva and is absorbed into the blood stream by the episcleral and conjunctival vessels by simple diffusion. If subconjunctival injection includes the underlying Tenon's capsule, effects on the ciliary body, choroid and the retina can be obtained.

Subconjunctival injections should be given if (i) there is an emergency to tackle the acute infection of the anterior chamber, and (ii) drug used has low penetrability. The most common use of subconjunctival injection is for the administration of antibiotics in infections of the anterior segment of the eye. Mydriatics and cycloplegics may also be given by this route.

Retrobulber injection : Drug is injected through the skin of the lower lid or through the lower fornix of cojunctiva, the needle emerging behind the eyeball. The retrobulbar injection is given for getting drugs in the posterior segment of the globe. In general, such injection is given for the purpose of getting medications (e.g. antibiotics, local anaethetics, enzymes with local anaethetics, steroids, vasodilators) into the posterior segment of the globe and to affect the nerves and other structures in that space.

Intracameral injection : Drugs are injected directly into the anterior chamber (certain antibiotics, steroids etc.) or directly into the vitreous chamber (amphotericin B, gentamicin, steroids).

Iontophoresis : This procedure keeps the solution in contact with the cornea by means of an eyecap bearing an electrode. Diffusion of the drug (e.g. fluorescin sodium, antibiotics, etc.) is affected by difference of electrical potential.

Intraocular injection : The dangers of this route outweigh any possible advantage. It is given in emergencies and desperate cases. It is better to give drugs by systemic administration (oral or parenteral medication).

Systemic administration

For ophthalmic treatment, drugs are given either orally or parenterally. Ophthalmologists should be conversant with all types of routes of administration. Some diseases in the posterior part or orbit can not be reached by locally applied medication, e.g. cellulitis, uveitis etc. These often require systemic medication.

Some characteristics of ocular routes are given in Table 21.2.

AUTONOMIC PHARMACOLOGY OF EYE

General aspects

Eye is a specialized sensory organ with multiple autonomic nervous system (ANS) functions, controlled by several different autonomic receptors. In the anterior chamber of the eye, there are three different muscles (pupillary dilator and constrictor muscles in the iris and the ciliary muscle) and the secretory epithelium of the ciliary body. These tissues are controlled by the autonomic nervous system (Fig. 21.1)

Muscarinic cholinomimetics induce contraction of the circular pupillary constrictor muscle pro-ducing miosis (reduction in pupil size). Contraction of ciliary muscle produces accommodation of focus for near vision. Marked contraction of the ciliary muscle is called cyclospasm. Ciliary muscle contraction also produces tension on the trabecular meshwork which results in opening its pores leading to facilitation of the outflow of the aqueous humour into the canal of Schlemm. This reduces intraocular pressure in patients with glaucoma.

Muscarinic blocking drugs such as atropine prevent or reverse the effects of muscarinic cholinomimetics.

Alpha adrenoceptors contract radially oriented pupillary dilator muscle fibres in the iris resulting in mydriasis.

Beta adrenoceptors on the ciliary epithelium facilitate the secretion of aqueous humour. Beta blocking drugs reduce the secretion of aqueous humour resulting in reduction of intraocular pressure which is useful in glaucoma.

AUTONOMIC DRUGS FOR OPHTHALMIC USE

The autonomic drugs that are commonly used in ophthalmology can be subdivided as following :
1. Parasympathomimetics (cholinergic agents):
   (i) directly acting
      acetylcholine, methacholine,
      carbachol, pilocarpine
   (ii) indirectly acting
      (a) reversible
         eserine, edrophonium
      (b) irreversible
         isofluorophate
         ecothiopate
         demecarium
Indication for use : miosis and accommodation.

Table 21.2. Some characteristics of ocular routes

Route	Absorption pattern	Special utility	Limitations and precautions
Topical	Prompt	Safe, convenient, economical	Compliance, side effects
Subconjunctival, sub-Tenon's and retrobulbar injections	Sustained	Anterior segment infections, surgical anaesthesia	Local toxicity, tissue injury
Intraocular (intracameral) injection	Prompt	Anterior segment surgery	Local toxicity
Intravitreal injection	Immediate local effect, absorption circumvented	Endophthalmitis, retinitis	Local toxicity

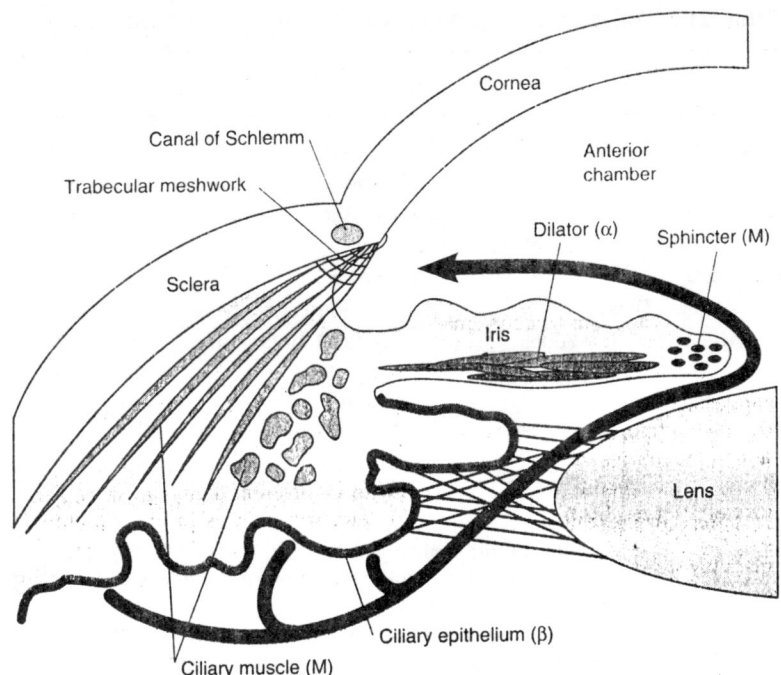

Fig. 21.1. Structure of the anterior chamber of the eye. Tissues with significant autonomic functions and the associated ANS receptors are shown in this schematic diagram. Activation of the beta adrenoceptors associated with the ciliary epithelium causes increased secretion of aqueous humour (arrow).

2. Parasympatholytics (anticholinergic or anti-muscarinic agents) Atropine, homatropine, cyclopentolate, tropicamide, eucatropine
   Indications for use : cycloplegia
3. Sympathomimetics (adrenergic agents) :
   (i) directly acting
       epinephrine
       phenylephrine
   (ii) indirectly acting
       hydroxyamphetamine
       ephedrine
   Indication for use : mydriasis
4. Sympatholytics (adrenergic antagonists)
   topical alpha - blocker
       thymoxamine
   topical beta-blockers
       non-selective
           timolol
       B_1-selective
           betaxolol

Indication for use : glaucoma

The above agents have been described separately under miotics, mydriatics, cycloplegics in this chapter.

Table 21.3 shows the autonomic pharmacology of the eye and related structures/receptors in the eye.

The formulation, uses and ocular side effects of the autonomic drugs for ophthalmic use are given in Table 21.4. They are mostly used as miotics, mydriatics and cycloplegics which are described separately.

MIOTICS

Miotics are drugs which constrict the pupil (miosis)

Ideal properties of miotics

- Quick in onset.
- Appropriate duration of action.
- An effect on the ciliary muscle which leaves the patient without cycloplegia or cyclospasm

Table 21.3. Autonomic pharmacology of the eye and related structures.

Tissue	Adrenergic subtype	Receptors response	Cholinergic subtype**	Receptors Response
Corneal epithelium	Beta$_2$	not known	undefined	unknown
Corneal endohelium	Beta$_2$	not known	undefined	unknown
Iris radial muscle	Alpha$_1$	mydriasis		
Iris sphincter muscle	Alpha & beta in equal amount		M$_3$, m$_3$	miosis
Trabecular meshwork	Beta$_2$	unknown		
Ciliary epithelium***	Alpha$_2$ /Beta$_2$	aqueous production		
Ciliary muscle	Beta$_2$ (very few Alpha)	relaxation* for far vision (slight effect)	M$_2$ for near vision (accommodation)	Contraction
Lacrimal gland	Alpha$_1$	secretion	M$_3$,M$_3$,m$_3$	secretion
Retinal pigment epithelium	Alpha$_1$ / Beta$_2$	H$_2$O transport unknown		

*   It has no significant effect on accommodation

** There are two classification systems for muscarinic cholinergic receptors, (1) based on response to agonists and antagonists and there are named M1, M2 and M3; (2) derived from molecular cloning methods and these include five distinct receptor subtypes, M1, M2, M3, M4 and M5.

*** Ciliary epithelium is also the target of carbonic anhydrase inhibitors. Carbonic anhydrase isoenzyme II is localized in ciliary epithelium (both pigmented and nonpigmented).

- An effect on the iris which allows a normal pupil light reflex.
- No other pharmacological effect
- No local or systemic toxic reactions

Indications for use

1. Principal use is in the treatment of primary open angle glaucoma.
2. To reverse the mydriasis produced by drugs such as phenylephrine and tropicamide.
3. Emergency treatment of closed angle glaucoma.

Mode of action

Miotics produce miosis either by (i) inhibiting the pupil dilator muscle (alpha blocking agents) or by (ii) stimulating the pupil sphincter muscle (parasympathomimetics or anticholinesterases).

Miotics can be classified on the basis of their mode of action :

1. Miotics inhibiting pupil dilator muscle : The dilator muscle is supplied by sympathetic innervation which is stimulatory (alpha-receptors predominate). Hence, alpha-blockers will be useful. For this purpose, only thymoxamine is available as eye drop.

2. Miotics stimulating the pupil sphincter muscle : The sphincter muscle is stimulated to contract by ACh on muscarinic receptors. Hence, drugs which mimic the action of ACh (parasympathomimetics) or by preventing the breakdown of ACh by the cholinesterases (anticholinesterases) will produce miosis.

Drug which inhibits pupil dilator muscle

Alpha-blocking agents

There are several alpha-blockers but only thymoxamine is used ophthalmically. It is effective in concentrations between 0.01% and 1.3% but is only available in single use containers as a 0.5% solution.

It produces miosis by relaxing the pupil dilator muscle. Its main indication is the reversal of mydriasis caused by sympathomimetic agents but also has some activity in overcoming the mydriasis induced by tropicamide.

Besides its use as a miotic, thymoxamine has

Table 21.4 Autonomic Drugs for Ophthalmic Use

Drug Class	Formulation	Uses	Ocular side effects
Cholinergic Agonists			
Acetylcholine	1% solution	Intraocular use for miosis in surgery	Corneal oedema
Carbachol	0.01 to 3% solution	Intraocular use for miosis in surgery, glaucoma	Corneal oedema, miosis, induced myopia, decreased vision, brow ache, retinal detachment
Pilocarpine	0.25-10% solution, 4% gel. 20, 40 µg/hr units	Glaucoma	Same as for carbachol
Anticholinesterase Agents			
Physostigmine	0.25 & 0.5% solution 0.25% ointment	Glaucoma, accommodative esotropia, louse and mite infestation of lashes	Retinal detachment, miosis, cataract, pupillary block, glaucoma, iris cysts, brow ache, punctal stenosis of the nasolacrimal system
Demecarium	0.25 & 0.5% solution	Glaucoma, accommodative esotropia	Same as for physostigmine
Ecothiopate	0.30 to 0.25% solution	Glaucoma, accommodative esotropia	Same as for physostigmine
Isoflurophate	0.025% solution	Glaucoma, accommodative esotropia	Same as for physostigmine
Muscarinic Antagonists			
Atropine	0.5-3.0% solution 0.5 & 1.0% solution	Cycloplegic retinoscopy, dilated funduscopic examination, cycloplegia	Photosensitivity, blurred vision
Homatropine	2.0 & 5.0% solution	Same as for atropine	Same as for atropine
Cyclopentolate	0.5, 1.0 & 2.0% solution	Same as for atropine	Same as for atropine
Tropicamide	0.5 & 1.0% solution	Same as for atropine	Same as for atropine
Sympathomimetic Agents			
Dipivefrin	0.1% solution	Glaucoma	Photosensitivity, conjunctival hyperemia, hypersensitivity
Epinephrine	0.5,1.0, & 2.0% solution	Glaucoma	Same as for dipivefrin
Phenylephrine	2.5 & 10% solution	Mydriasis	Same as for dipivefrin
Apraclonidine	0.5 & 1% solution	Glaucoma	Same as for dipivefrin
Cocaine	2.0-4% solution	Topical anaesthesia, evaluate anisocoria	
Hydroxyamphetamine	1.0% solution	Evaluate anisocoria	
Naphazoline	0.012 to 0.1% solution	Decongestant	Same as for dipivefrin
Tetrahydrozoline	0.05% solution	Decongestant	Same as for dipivefrin
Alpha & Beta-Adrenergic Antagonists			
Dapiprazole (Alpha)	0.5% solution	Reverse mydriasis	Conjunctival hyperemia
Betaxolol (β_1 selective)	0.25 & 0.5% solution and suspension	Glaucoma	
Carteolol (Beta)	1.0% solution	Glaucoma	
Levobunolol (Beta)	0.25 & 0.5% solution	Glaucoma	
Metipranolol (Beta)	0.3% solution	Glaucoma	
Timolol (Beta)	0.25 & 0.5% solution	Glaucoma	

been used in the treatment of exophthalmos as it paralyses the smooth muscle of the upper lid, causing a slight ptosis.

Because thymoxamine reduces pressure in closed angle but not in open angle, it can form the basis of a useful differential test.

Drugs which stimulate pupil sphincter muscle

1. Parasympathomimetic miotics (directly acting) such as pilocarpine, carbachol, bethanechol, methacholine.
2. Parasympathomimetics miotics (indirectly acting). They act by inactivating cholinesterase (also called anticholinesterases or cholinesterase inhibitors).

These are (i) reversible such as physostigmine (eserine), neostigmine, and (ii) irreversible such as ecothiopate, demecarium, isofluorophate.

Directly acting

Pilocarpine

It is obtained from the leaves of Pilocarpus microphyllus and other species of Pilocarpus.

The hydrochloride salt is preferred to the nitrate because it is compatible with a wider range of antimicrobial preservatives.

Applied locally to the eye as a 0.5-5% solution (1-2% concentration is most commonly used), miosis commences in about 10 minutes, is maximal in half an hour.

Pilocarpine is a direct acting parasympathomimetic drug. It penetrates into the eye very well. It acts by increasing the outflow facility.

The following are other parasympathomimetic miotics but they are not commonly employed.

Carbachol

It may be used as a miotic in 0.75-3% solution in the treatment of glaucoma, and is a useful alternative to pilocarpine and to other miotics where resistance or intolerance has developed.

Bethanecol chloride

It is used in a 1% solution as a miotic.

Methacholine chloride

Normal pupils require 10-20% solution to produce miosis but other miotics are generally preferred.

Indirectly acting or anticholinesterases :
1. *Reversible anticholinesterases* are short acting e.g. physostigmine and neostigmine.
2. *Irreversible anticholinesterases* are long acting e.g. di-isopropylflurophosphonate (dyflos), ecothiopate, demecarium.

Reversible anticholinesterases

Physostigmine (eserine, anti-AChE drug)

Physostigmine sulphate is preferred to the salicylate because of its greater solubility and its compatibility with a wider range of preservatives.

Solutions of physostigmine salts on exposure to light and air become pink, especially the sulphate, due to oxidation, resulting in the formation of rubreserine which is more irritating to the eye than eserine, though the miotic effect is maintained.

Strength for strength physostigmine is about twice as active as pilocarpine. Miosis commences in about 5-10 minutes, is maximal in about 30 minutes, and the effect lasts upto 12-36 hours with a 0.5% solution, and somewhat less with 0.25% solution.

Neostigmine

It is a weaker synthetic analogue of physostigmine. It is used in 3.0-5.0% strength.

Irreversible anticholinesterases

Dyflos (DFP) or di-isopropylfluoro-phosphonate or isofluorophate

It is unstable in aqueous solution, hence used 0.01-0.1% in arachis oil. It is used every 12 to 72 hours.

Miosis commences in 5-10 minutes and the effect lasts for 2-4 weeks and ciliary muscles spasm continues for 3 to 7 days. It is an extremely powerful agent employed to control the intraocular pressure if other miotics fail.

Dyflos is toxic. The adverse effects include blurring of vision, severe frontal headache and treatment with this drug carries a high risk of cataract formation. The systemic adverse effects are prolonged and similar to those produced by ecothiopate.

Ecothiopate iodide (ecothiopate iodide or phospholine iodide)

It is used in 0.06-0.25% solution mainly in the treatment of open-angle glaucoma. It is a powerful and long acting agent (days to weeks).

Ecothiopate eye drops must be freshly prepared, the drops only remaining stable if the solution is kept refrigerated. It deteriorates at room temperature.

It is toxic. The systemic adverse effects include nausea, abdominal cramps, diarrhoea, general weakness; and locally iris cysts. It may produce cataracts with prolonged usage and very rarely retinal detachment.

Demecarium is very toxic and hence rarely used. It is used when other drugs have failed. It is used in 0.125-0.25% concentration, the duration of miotic action is long (days to weeks).

Choice of miotic

If an antimuscarinic has been used then an anti-CHE is recommended because pilocarpine is insufficiently active to cause a reversal.

Pilocarpine or thymoxamine can be used after a sympathomimetic. In the reversal of phenylephrine-induced mydriasis, pilocarpine produces quicker action in onset and produce a deeper miosis than thymoxamine. Thymoxamine takes about twice as long (20 minutes or so) to return the pupil to its normal size, but is longer in action than pilocarpine, having half-life of 12 hours compared with 5 hours for pilocarpine.

Mixed miotics

The mixed miotics contain a parasympathomimetic and an anticholinesterase, e.g. pilocarpine and physostigmine, both of which are active on the sphincter.

It is more logical to mix, for example thymoxamine and pilocarpine or physostigmine in order to reverse a mixed mydriatic.

A list of miotics showing strengths of drugs used, mode of action, onset, duration and adverse reaction are given in Table 21.5.

Adverse reactions of miotics

Thymoxamine is irritant on instillation, as are some other miotics.

Spasm of accommodation is produced by miotics which mainly act on sphincter muscle.

Miotics can produce dimness of vision due to small pupil. Some patients may be allergic to pilocarpine.

Axial thicknening of the lens and decrease in anterior chamber depth in elderly patients have been reported.

Conjunctival injection due to the dilation of the blood vessels of the conjunctiva in response to parasympathomimetic agents may occur.

Following topical application of larger doses of parasympathomimetics certain systemic adverse effects may be manifested on the respiratory, cardiovascular and gastrointestinal systems.

Anti-CHEs by reducing the level of plasma CHE, produce diarrhoea.

The long acting anticholinesterases can produce side effects both locally (in the eye) and systemically.

The local effects include ocular pain due to ciliary spasm, blurred vision, cataract formation, retinal detachment and iris cysts.

The systemic effects include headache, sweating, salivation, nausea, vomiting, diarrhoea, fatigue, fall in BP and cardiac arrest. Lid twitching can be produced by anti-CHEs which have nicotinic as well as muscarinic effects.

MYDRIATICS

Mydriatics are drugs which dilate the pupil.

They are used to facilitate a more thorough examination of the fundus, lens periphery and vitreous.

The view of a fundus through a small pupil or a dilated pupil can be compared with the view of a room as seen through a keyhole or with the door open.

Adequate dilatation of the pupils reveals small details of great diagnostic significance e.g. diabetic micro-aneurisms, hypertensive arteriolar attenuation, early signs of macular degeneration, small traumatic retinal holes, etc.

Table 21.5. Miotics

Drugs	Strengths % w/v	Mode of action	Onset minutes	Duration hours	Adverse reactions
Pilocarpine	1.0, 2.0, 4.0 BD-QID	Parasympathomimetic	10	06	Ciliary spasm
Carbachol	0.75-3.0 TID	Parasympathomimetic		4-12	Ciliary spasm
Bethanechol	1.0	Parasympathomimetic			Ciliary spasm
Methacholine	5.0, 10.0 BD-QID	Parasympathomimetic			
Physostigmine (eserine)	0.25 to 1.0 QID	Reversible anti-CHE	10	12-36	Ciliary spasm
Thymoxamine	0.5	Alpha-blocking agent	30	05	
Ecothiopate iodide	0.3-0.25 OD	Irreversible anti-CHE		Days to weeks	
Demecarium bromide	0.125-0.25 OD	Irreversible anti-CHE		Days to weeks	
Isofluorophate	0.25 ointment OD	Irreversible anti-CHE		Days to weeks	

Ideal properties of mydriatics :
- Quick in onset
- Adequate duration
- Fast recovery after examination
- No cycloplegia
- No rise in IOP
- No other pharmacological effect
- No adverse reactions (local as well as systemic)

Mode of action

The pupil sphincter and dilator muscles are the two opponent muscles, hence there are 2 modes of action of mydriatics.

The sphincter pupillae muscle is innervated by the parasympathetic nervous system which can be paralysed by antimuscarinic agents (same class of drugs which cause cycloplegia), causing mydriasis. With this type of drug the pupilary light reflex is reduced or abolished.

The dilator pupillae muscle is innervated by the sympathetic nervous system and sympathomimetic drugs will cause a contraction of the dilator muscle causing mydriasis. The parasympathetic system is unaffected by such drugs and hence the pupillary light reflex remains active. Sympathomimetic drugs also have little effect on accommodation.

Therefore, mydriatics act by :
1. Dilatation of dilator pupillae muscle by stimulation of sympathetic system, sympathomimetic agents.
2. Paralysis of sphincter pupillae muscle by inhibiting the parasympathetic system by antimuscarinic agents.

DRUGS USED AS MYDRIATICS

Sympathomimetic mydriatics

- These have little effect on accommodation
- Light reflex is retained as they do not affect parasympathetic system.

Phenylephrine (Neo-synephrine)

It is the only sympathomimetic mydriatic in common use in 2.5% and 10.0% strengths. The effect commences in about 10 minutes, is maximal in 30 minutes and mydriasis lasts for several hours. The strength 2.5% is recommended for routine dilatation. In low concentrations (0.125%) it is used as a vasoconstrictor causing blanching of the conjunctival membrane.

Sympathomimetic amines produce mydriasis without cycloplegic effect.

Phenylephrine, like all sympathomimetics, is less effective in highly pigmented patients and will retain the light reflex.

The eyes of Negroes are dilated with difficulty, especially when using phenylephrine, cyclopentolate or hydroxyamphetamine as mydriatic.

Cocaine

Dilatation commences in 15-20 minutes, is maximal

in 30 minutes and may last for about 20 hours (usually around 6 hours).

Cocaine is a sympathomimetic drug. It prevents uptake of noradrenaline into storage sites in the adrenergic nerve endings. This results in an increased amount of noradrenaline for activation of the adrenergic receptors. Thus, cocaine's mydriatic effect is the result of the indirect action of a sympathomimetic drug.

Constriction of the blood vessels accompanies the mydriasis. The noradrenaline in the blood stream initiates the alpha-receptor response in the smooth muscle coat of the vessels that cause blanching of the conjunctival membrane and sclera.

Hydroxyamphetamine hydrobromide

It is not very effective as a mydriatic. It produces mydriasis slowly. When used as a mydriatic in 1-3% eye drops, maximal mydriasis occurs in 30-45 minutes and lasts for 2-3 hours. As a mydriatic it is least effective when compared with homatropine hydrobromide, phenylephrine hydrochloride and tropicamide.

Ephedrine hydrochloride

With one drop of a 4-5% solution, mydriasis commences in 10-15 minutes, is maximal in about 30 minutes and the effect lasts for several hours. Mydriasis is not as maximal as with the anti-muscarinic mydriatics. Ephedrine eye drops are often ineffective in the presence of highly pigmented irides, dark-skinned and even in dark-haired people, diabetics, and in patients over the age of 60 years.

Antimuscarinic Mydriatics (Anticholinergic mydriatics)

Tropicamide is the antimuscarinic mydriatic of choice. Its mydriatic effect is more than the cycloplegic effect.

Tropicamide is quick in onset, full mydriasis reaches in 15 minutes, short in duration (recovery occurs in 8-9 hours) and the depth of mydriasis is adequate. It is recommended that 0.5% should be used for mydriasis and 1% for cycloplegia.

Tropicamide in more effective mydriatic than phenylephrine, pupillary light reflex is abolished and rise in intraocular pressure is transient and small and not likely to cause a problem. However, diabetic patients respond poorly to tropicamide, so a combination of this agent with phenylephrine gives adequate mydriasis with minimum of accommodative paralysis.

Other antimuscarinic mydriatics include cyclopentolate, homatropine, eucatropine and atropine.

Cyclopentolate 0.1% may be used as mydriatic (for cycloplegia 0.5 and 1.0%), which commences in about 10 minutes, is maximal in about 30 minutes and effect lasts up to 24 hours. It produces similar mydriasis but more cycloplegia than homatropine.

Homatropine as 0.25% or 0.5% solution initiates mydriatic effect in 10-20 minutes, is maximal in 30-40 minutes, recovery takes same time as cyclopentolate (but may be as prolonged as 3 days).

Eucatropine instillation of a drop of 5% or 10% solution initiates mydriasis in 10-20 minutes, is maximal in about 30 minutes. At 30 minutes both light and accommodative reflexes are absent. Recovery takes about 6 hours. Unlike the other atropine-like drugs, it has little, if any, effect on accommodation, and there is little danger of increased IOP.

Atropine 1% one instillation produces mydriasis within 10-15 minutes, maximal effect reaches in 30-40 minutes and pupillary recovery occurs in 3-7 days. If it is applied twice daily for 3 days, pupillary recovery occurs after 10-14 days. A list of mydriatics showing strengths of drugs used, their onset of action, duration, agents which can reverse their mydriatic action, mode of action and adverse reactions are given in Table 21.6.

Choice of mydriatic

The probable choice is between phenylephrine and tropicamide.

Tropicamide is more effective mydriatic, especially if photography is to be done (as pupillary light reflex is abolished).

Tropicamide may cause a rise in IOP in eyes with a deep anterior chamber (however, rise is small and transient) as opposed to phenylephrine which causes a fall (like all sympathomimetics).

Table 21.6. Mydriatics

Drug	Strengths % w/v	Single dose	Mode of action	Mydriatic onset (min.)	Mydriatic duration	Reversed by	ADR	Notes
Atropine sulphate	1.0	Yes	Anti-muscarinic	40	7 days	Ecothiopate or DFP	Allergy and general anti-mscarinic effects	Too strong, rarely used
Homatropine hydrobromide	1.0 to 2.0	2.0% only	–do–	40	48 hrs.	Physostigmine	CNS effects	Rarely used
Cyclopentolate hydrobromide	0.5	Yes	–do–	30	24 hrs.	–do–	–do–	Too strong for routine examination
Tropicamide	0.5	Yes	–do–	15	8-9 hrs.	–do–	–do–	Mydriatic of choice
Eucatropine	5.0 10.0	No	–do–	30	6 hrs.	–do–	–do–	Little used
Phenylephrine	2.5 10.0	Yes	Sympatho-mimetic	30	12-24 hrs.	Thymoxamine		
Cocaine	2.5 4.0	No	–do–	30	20 hrs.			
Hydroxyamp-hetamine	1.0 to 3.0	No	–do–	45	3 hrs.			
Ephedrine	5.0	No	–do–	30	12 hrs.			

Phenylephrine can have effect on B.P. and is contraindicated in patients with cardiovascular problems.

Hence, it appears that tropicamide 0.5% is the first choice as a mydriatic. But it should be noted that diabetic patients respond poorly to tropicamide.

In such cases combination of this agent with phenylephrine is recommended to achieve adequate mydriasis.

It has also been reported that phenylephrine produces better sector pupil dilatation than tropicamide. Sector pupil dilatation in which the pupil becomes oval or pear-shaped is recommended for dilating eyes with narrow filtration angles because it reduces the risk of acute angle closure glaucoma.

Mixed mydriatics

In case sufficient depth of mydriasis is not produced by one or other of the two types of mydriatics, mixtures of sympathomimetic and antimuscarinic may be used. Some examples—tropicamide 0.5%

and phenylephrine 2.5%, cyclopentolate 0.5% and phenylephrine 2.5%

Contraindications

No mydriatic should be instilled if any of the three contraindications exist.

1. The known presence of glaucoma
2. Evidence of elevated intraocular tension
3. Presence of an abnormally shallow anterior chamber and angle.

Sympathomimetic mydriatics should not be used in patients with cardiac diseases, hypertension, aneurysms, advanced atherosclerosis and patients receiving monoamine oxidase inhibitors or tricyclic antidepressants.

Adverse effects of mydriatics

- Angle closure glaucoma. The danger will depend on the degree of dilatation, not on the mydriatic employed.

- Toxic epithelial desquamation of the cornea from topical sympathomimetic drugs.
- Liberation of iris pigment into the anterior chamber has been reported following the use of 10% phenylephrine.
- Systemic effects can be produced by sympathomimetic mydriatics. Cardiovascular system is most sensitive to their effects. Topically administered drugs may reach the vascular system either by direct absorption through the conjunctival blood vessels or via the nasolacrimal system to the alimentary tract.

CYCLOPLEGICS

Cycloplegics are drugs that paralyse the ciliary muscle by blocking the muscarinic receptors. Cycloplegia is always accompanied by mydriasis since the parasympathetic nervous system also innervates the sphincter pupillae muscle. However, mydriasis is not always accompanied by cycloplegia.

Cycloplegics are used to prevent or reduce accommodation during refraction, thus making latent refractive errors manifest.

Ideal properties of cycloplegics
- Quick in onset.
- Adequate depth of cycloplegia.
- Adequate duration of cycloplegia.
- No local or systemic adverse effect.
- Stable.
- No mydriasis (but it is not attainable).

Antimuscarinic drugs used as cycloplegics

Atropine is an alkaloid extracted from plant species such as Atropa belladonna as 1% eye drops. Because of the systemic toxic effects that can occur, the ointment form is often preferred.

The ointment is applied twice a day for 3 days prior to refraction but not on the day of refraction because the unabsorbed ointment may interfere with refractive procedures.

After one instillation with 1% concentration, mydriasis commences in 10-15 minutes, peak reaches in 30-40 minutes, recovery from mydriasis may take 3-7 days. But the recovery from mydriasis

may take from 10-14 days in children when atropine is applied twice daily for 3 days which is required for producing complete cycloplegia.

The time courses of mydriasis and cycloplegia are different. Cycloplegia commences in 30 minutes (onset of action is slow), and full ciliary muscle recovery may take 7-10 days (after the usual six application). Even with one application marked cycloplegia reaches in 1-3 hours, but is not complete, and full ciliary muscle recovery may take 3-7 days.

Due to the different time scale of mydriasis and cycloplegia, the size of the pupil is a poor indicator of cycloplegic effect.

Cyclopentolate

It is the most widely used cycloplegic. The cycloplegia (paralysis of accommodation) is not complete but achieves sufficient depth of cycloplegia for majority of cases. Many ophthalmologists consider it the cycloplegic of choice when complete cycloplegia is not required. The recovery is not as quick as that following the use of tropicamide but much quicker than after the use of atropine.

In patients up to 12 years of age, one drop of 1% solution is enough and after 40-60 minutes retinoscopic refraction is performed.

In patients aged 12 years and above, one drop of 0.5-1% solution (only repeated if within 15 minutes there is no significant effect observed) is instilled and the retinoscopic refraction is carried out in 40-60 minutes.

Time course

The mydriatic effect begins in a few minutes, peak effect reaches in 30-60 minutes (some times in 10-15 minutes) and recovery from mydriasis occurs between 24 and 48 hours.

The cycloplegic effect commences almost simultaneously with mydriasis, maximal effect reaches in 30-60 minutes. Full recovery of the accommodation occurs between 4 and 12 hours (in few cases delayed for 24 hr.)

Tropicamide

It is another rapidly acting synthetic antimuscarinic drug.

As a mydriatic, 0.5% solution is used which produces full mydriasis in 15 minutes and the pupil returns to normal in 8-9 hours.

As a cycloplegic two drops of 1% solution are instilled into the eye allowing a 5-minute interval between each drop. The full cycloplegic effect is achieved in about 30 minutes, when retinoscopy is performed. If it is delayed beyond 35 minutes a further (third) drop of 1% solution should be used. Complete recovery of the accommodation usually occurs within 6 hours, however, reading is possible after 2-4 hours from the time of the initial instillations.

Homatropine

It is a semisynthetic alkaloid prepared from atropine. Homatropine hydrobromide eye drops 0.25-0.50% are used as mydriatic and for cycloplegia 1% - 2% and 5% concentrations are employed.

Homatropine does not produce satisfactory cycloplegia in children. Its use is usually restricted to over 15 years age groups.

The conventional dosage of the eye drops is one drop of 2% solution repeated twice at 10 minute intervals i.e. total of 3 drops.

Mydriasis commences in 15 minutes and is maximal in 30-40 minutes, and recovery may take 24-48 hours.

Cycloplegia commences in 15 minutes and maximal at 45-90 minutes. Therefore, cycloplegic retinoscopic refraction should not commence until about 60 minutes after instillation. Refraction should be completed before 90 minutes have elapsed from the time of instillation of the drops. Accommodation may fully recover in 24 hours.

Hyoscine hydrobromide (scopolamine hydrobromide)

Hyoscine causes cycloplegia and mydriasis but it is not in common use as cycloplegic because it is more toxic than atropine. Giddiness, ataxia, hallucinations and psychotic disturbances have been reported.

Its antimuscarinic (anticholinergic) action in the eye is qualitatively similar to atropine but its action is more rapid and its effects are not as prolonged.

Hyoscine hydrobromide is instilled in eye drops containing 0.5%, 0.25% and upto 0.5% and in a 0.25% eye ointment.

Maximal cycloplegia is reached in 40-60 minutes. Reliability of this cycloplegic in children, as compared to atropine, is doubtful.

Hyoscine is employed in general medicine for its sedative/hypnotic properties (depression of CNS).

The strength, onset, duration and adverse reactions of some cycloplegics are given in Table 21.7.

Choice of Cycloplegics

There are many antimuscarinic agents but among them few are used to produce cyclolegia. The principle of 'as little as possible but as much as necessary' should apply to the use of drugs.

Antimuscarinic drugs can affect the whole body and stronger the cycloplegic, the stronger will be the side effects. Additionally, stronger agents will produce longer effects and cause prolonged inconvenience to the patient due to dilated pupils.

Table 21.7. Showing cycloplegics

Drug	Strength % w/v	Single dose	Cycloplegic onset	Cycloplegic duration	ADR	Notes
Atropine sulphate	1.0	Yes	36 hr	upto 7 days	Allergic reactions, general antimuscarinic side effect	Used as ointment
Cyclopentolate	0.5–1.0	Yes	60 min	24 hr	CNS effects e.g. hallucinations	
Homatropine hydrobromide	1.0–2.0	2.0% only	90 min	35 hr	As for atropine but less toxic	
Tropicamide	1.0	Yes	30 min	6 hr	Occasional hallucinations	

Adverse effects of cycloplegics

Toxic effects from topical ophthalmic use have been known for a long time.

Adverse effects of atropine eye drops: high temperature, ataxia, hallucinations, psychotic reactions, confusion, restlessness.

Patients suffering from atropine poisoning are said to be :

- blind as a bat;
- dry as a bone;
- red as a beet root;
- mad as a hatter.

Patients are as blind as a bat because of the effect on accommodation; dry as a bone because of the inhibition of the sweat glands and salivary glands (dry mouth is the earliest sign of atropine poisoning), inhibition of sweat glands deprives the body of its method of losing heat. To compensate for this there is dilatation of skin vessels which gives the appearance of 'red as a beet root'. Due to CNS effects patients become as 'mad as a hatter' (insane using abusive language).

Homatropine is less toxic than atropine. However, excessive doses can produce CNS effects such as ataxia and hallucinations.

Adverse effects following cyclopentolate :

CNS effects include confusion, difficulty in speaking, hallucinations and ataxia.

Adverse effects following tropicamide :

Tropicamide is relatively free from adverse reactions.

Allergic reactions can occur to many compounds. Of course atropine is the most notorious but cyclopentolate has also been implicated.

ANTIGLAUCOMA DRUGS

Glaucoma is a localized ocular disease characterized by (i) elevated intraocular pressure (ii) optic nerve damage and (iii) visual field loss.

Glaucoma falls into four categories

1. Primary angle-closure glaucoma.
2. Open angle, or chronic glaucoma. There is a progressive narrowing of the openings in the trabecular meshwork of the anterior chamber angle.
3. Secondary glaucoma. It can be of either the open-angle or the narrow angle type. The elevated IOP is due to some specific disease within the eye, such as iritis, or tumour, which interferes with aqueous flowing out of the eye. It may occur after trauma or may follow neovascularization in the anterior chamber, as occurs after diabetes.
4. Congenital, or infantile, glaucoma. It is rare disease. The fluid drainage system is abnormal at birth.

Some persons exhibit high IOP but do not show any change in their visual field or in their optic discs. There may be individuals who can sustain higher than normal IOP without damage. Some believe that they may be preglaucomatous. They should preferably be called ocular hypertensive. Treatment depends on the prescribed threat to vision.

Aqueous humour

Aqueous humour is produced by the ciliary processes at the rate of 2.0 to 2.5 micro litre/min., leaves by the conventional outflow pathway through the trabecular meshwork and canal of Schlemm. From the canal of Schlemm, fluid drains into an episcleral venous plexus and eventually into the systemic circulation. About 80% to 95% of the aqueous humour flow out through the conventional pathway. It is the main target for cholinergic drugs used in glaucoma therapy.

An alternative pathway is the uveoscleral route i.e. fluid flows through the ciliary muscles and into the suprachoroidal space (it holds promise for pharmacological influence by eicosanoids) to facilitate aqueous humour outflow and lower intraocular pressure.

The anterior chamber holds about 250 microlitre of aqueous humour.

The peripheral anterior chamber angle lies at the junction of the corneal endothelium and the iris root. The trabecular meshwork and canal of Schlemm are located at the apex of this angle and form the out flow pathway for aqueous humour.

Antiglaucoma Drugs

The aim is to reduce the intraocular pressure (IOP). As the level of intraocular pressure is determined by

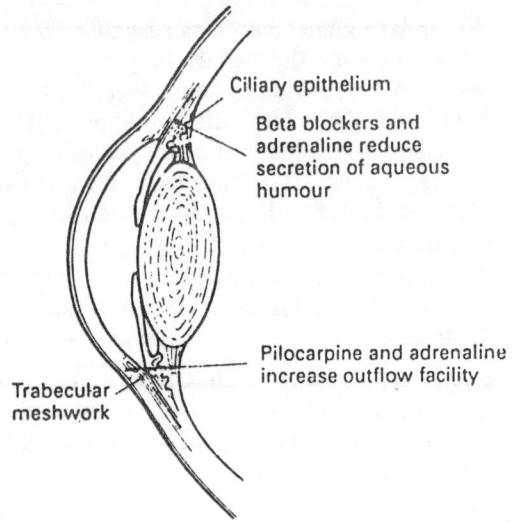

Ciliary epithelium

Beta blockers and
adrenaline reduce
secretion of aqueous
humour

Pilocarpine and adrenaline
increase outflow facility

Trabecular
meshwork

Fig. 21.2. Site of action of antiglaucoma drugs.

both the rate of production and the rate of outflow, the IOP can be reduced by reducing secretion or increasing outflow.

Of the primary glaucomas, only open angle glaucoma is amenable to chronic medical treatment.

Acute angle closure glaucoma can be relieved by a combined attack of both topical and systemic treatment, its long term relief can be from surgery. Surgical treatment of open angle glaucoma is also an option especially when medical treatment appears to be losing their effect.

Whatever be the form of treatment, it should satisfy certain criteria:

• IOP should be reduced. Glaucoma can be deemed to be 'controlled' if IOP is below 20mm Hg. It is important that the pressure should remain stable and not vary greatly during the day.

• Duration of effect should last for some hours.

• Preservation of visual field is important, the aim of treatment is that no further impairment of vision should occur.

• No loss of effect with time should occur, once a patient has been stabilized on a treatment.

• Compatibility with other treatment becomes necessary because some patients require more than one drug to be administered.

• Lack of systemic effects on topical use because a life time course of continuing therapy is required. Treatment must be easy and pleasant to use.

Anti-glaucoma treatment can be administered either topically or systemically.

The best management is early detection.

Topical treatment

The anti-glaucoma drugs fall into three principal groups (i) miotics (ii) sympathomimetics and (iii) beta-blockers. The site of action of these drugs is shown in Fig. 21.2.

Antiglaucoma medications

1. Cholinergic drugs
   Parasympathomimetic
      Pilocarpine
   Anticholinesterases
      Physostigmine
      Ecothiopate
      Isofluorophate
      Demecarium bromide
2. Adrenergic agents
   Agonists
      Epinephrine
      Dipivefrin
   Antagonists
      Timolol
      Betaxolol
      Levobunolol
3. Carbonic anhydrase inhibitors
   Acetazolamide
   Methazolamide
   Ethoxzolamide
   Dichlorphenamide
4. Hyperosmotic agents
   Oral
      Glycerol
      Isosorbide
   I.V.
      Mannitol
      Urea

Cholinergic Agonists

These contract ciliary muscle, putting tension on the trabecular meshwork, that is responsible for the increased outflow and reduced IOP. In addition the direct effects on the trabecular meshwork have also been postulated. Miosis is an important component of the drug's action if the filtration angle is narrow, but for the majority of patients, it is the cyclospam which produces the fall in intraocular pressure.

In short, all cholinergic agents increase the facility of outflow, constrict the pupil and reduce intraocular pressure (IOP). They stimulate ciliary muscles putting traction on the scleral spur and the trabecular meshwork. This action separates the trabecular sheets and the Schlemm's canal is kept open.

Uses of cholinergic drugs

1. Angle closure glaucoma. In this condition they are useful for short term management. They are used to prepare patient for surgery. They constrict the pupil, tighten the iris, decrease the volume of iris tissues at the angle and pull the iris periphery away from trabecular tissue. These changes reduce IOP by allowing aqueous humour to reach outflow channels.
2. Open-angle glaucoma. The cholinergic drugs are mainly used in the management of open-angle glaucoma and reduce IOP by increasing the outflow facility.

Acetylcholine poorly penetrates the cornea and it is rapidly destroyed (hydrolyzed) by cholinesterase enzyme. It is not used in the treatment of glaucoma.

Pilocarpine

It is the most commonly used miotic, however, it has certain disadvantages such as (i) greater possibility of allergic reactions, (ii) patient compliance is reduced as it has to be given 4 times a day and (iii) the IOP goes up and down four times a day.

To avoid the problems associated with pilocarpine, certain developments have been made.

New presentations of pilocarpine have been prepared leading to a greater effect and a more prolonged effect. They include :

(a) Viscolized solutions : Viscolizers such as hydroxyethylcellulose or polyvinyl alcohol have been added to pilocarpine which will produce more prolonged fall in IOP. However, it has been reported that following the use of such drops, the duration of effect does not seem to justify a reduction in the frequency of administration.

(b) Gels : Polymers have been developed in which pilocarpine can be incorporated and from which the drug is slowly released.

(c) Oily solution permits better absorption by the corneal epithelium but oily drops are less pleasant to use than the aqueous drops.

(d) Ocusert : This consists of viscous solution surrounded by a membrane which allows a slow conjunctival delivery of pilocarpine into the conjunctival sac. The side effects are fewer than from the drop application.

Other parasympathomimetics are also being used as antiglaucoma agents :

Aceclidine is a synthetic drug having similar efficacy and duration of action as pilocarpine and the advantage is that it can be given when pilocarpine is not tolerated.

Methacholine

Methacholine is a synthetic derivative, rarely used as it is unstable. It was used in 2% to 10% concentration.

Carbachol

Carbachol is a synthetic derivative of choline, more powerful than pilocarpine and its duration of action is more prolonged. But it penetrates cornea poorly. It is used as 0.75% to 3.0% and given 3-4 times a day.

Anticholinesterases

It is better to classify them as weak/short-acting and strong-long-acting rather than reversible and irreversible anticholinesterases.

Short acting reversible anticholinesterases :

Physostigmine (eserine) is a miotic and reduces intraocular pressure which lasts for about 12 hours. It is used every 4 to 6 hours in the concentration of

0.25% to 1%. Physostigmine solutions are unstable and decompose after exposure to sun light.

Neostigmine is a weaker, synthetic analogue of physostigmine.

Long acting irreversible anticholinesterases:

Dyflos (DFP, Isofluorphate) is administered in arachis oil as it is unstable in water.

Ecothiopate is supplied dry, and dissolved in a diluent just before use.

Demecarium bromide 0.12% to 0.25% is used every 12 to 48 hours. It is potent, stable and long acting.

The cholinergic drugs used in the treatment of glaucoma are shown in Table 21.8.

Adverse effects of cholinergic drugs

Ocular side effects

Periocular pain, lid twitching, lacrimation, conjunctival hyperaemia, irritation, allergic blepharoconjunctivitis, corneal epithelial staining and vascularization, iris cyst formation, ciliary muscle spasm, cataract formation, retinal hole, retinal detachment and vitreous haemorrhage.

The powerful miotics offer decreased frequency of administration, but have many side effects which make them undesirable unless absolutely necessary. They are contraindicated in persons who have a predisposition to retinal detachment, high myopia, or angle-closure glaucoma. They may also lead to cataract formation.

Systemic side effects

The systemic side effects include nausea, vomiting, institutional cramps, bladder cramps, sweating, salivation, lacrimation, and fatigue.

ADRENERGIC AGONISTS

Adrenaline (epinephrine) stimulates both alpha and beta receptors. It is available in 0.5%, 1.0% and 2.0% concentrations. Intraocular pressure begins to fall in 1 hour, reaches maximum in 2 to 6 hours and the effect lasts for 12 to 24 hours.

Adrenaline causes dilatation of the pupil. It will reduce pressure in the open angle glaucoma and increase it in closed angle glaucoma. Many different sympathomimetics have been tried but only adrenaline and its derivatives are used routinely.

The biochemical effect of adrenaline is the enhanced production of cyclic adenosine monophosphate from adenosine triphosphate. it produces a beta-mediated increase in secretion by stimulating chloride transport through cAMP production. This increase is more than cancelled out by the alpha-stimulated reduction. Adrenaline also causes an increase in the facility of outflow by acting on beta-receptors.

Adrenaline has been combined with guanethidine to control IOP which may be previously difficult to control. A combination of 5% guanethidine (adrenergic neuron blocker) and 1% adrenaline mixture is synergistic.

Table 21.8. Cholinergic drugs used as antiglaucoma agents

Drugs	Strength	Duration of ocular hypotensive effect	Frequency
Pilocarpine	0.25%–10%	4–8 hours	BD-QID
Methacholine	2%–20%	1–12 hours	BD-QID
Carbachol	0.75%–3%	4–12 hours	TID
Aceclidine	0.5%–4%	4–8 hours	TID
Physostigmine	0.25%–1%	4–6 hours	QID
Neostigmine	3%–5%	4–6 hours	QID
Isofluorophate	0.25% ointment	12 hrs–7 days	OD
Demecarium bromide	0.125%–0.25%	12 hrs–7 days	OD
Ecothiopate iodide	0.03%–0.25%	12 hrs–7 days	OD

The solution of adrenaline should be protected from light as the oxidized solution becomes discoloured, less effective and more irritating. The discoloured solution should be discarded.

Adrenaline is contraindicated in the presence of hypertension, cardiac diseases and thyrotoxicosis.

Adverse effects

Ocular

Hyperemia of conjunctiva, burning sensation, adrenochrome deposits in the cornea, mydriasis and angle closure, blurred vision, photophobia and iridocyclitis.

Systemic

Headache, tachycardia, palpitation, anxiety, increased B.P., cerebrovascular accident, myocardial infarction, death.

Dipiveferin (Dipivalylepinephrine)

It is a prodrug, gets converted to adrenaline by esterase enzymes in the cornea. It is highly lipid soluble. Dipiveferin 0.1% is equal to 1% adrenaline. Its side effects are less than adrenaline. The effect lasts for 12 hours. Its mode of action is shown in Fig. 21.3.

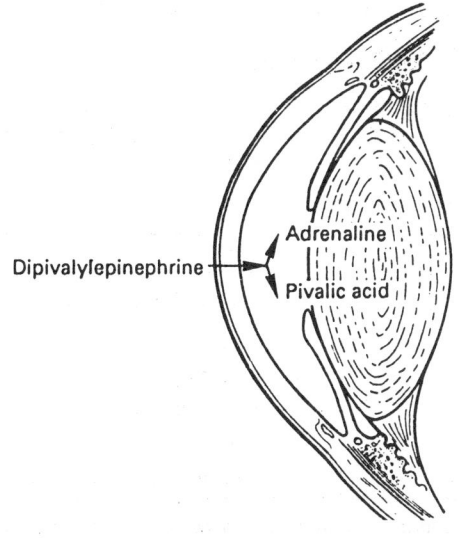

Fig. 21.3. Dipiveferin. Mode of action of prodrug.

BETA-ADRENERGIC BLOCKING AGENTS (ADRENERGIC ANTAGONISTS)

Timolol Maleate

It is a non selective beta$_1$ and beta$_2$ adrenergic antagonist. It reduces IOP in normal and glaucomatous eyes without affecting the pupillary size, accommodation and visual acuity. It is available as 0.25% and 0.5% concentrations and applied twice a day. Timolol penetrates the eye rapidly and the IOP begins to fall in 30-60 minutes and effect lasts upto 24 to 48 hours. It is more effective than pilocarpine and adrenaline.

Timolol maleate has been successfully used in the treatment for open-angle glaucoma. Solutions of 0.25% and 0.5% are used once or twice daily. Timolol produces minimal side effects. It can be used for most patients except those with asthma, and cardiopulmonary diseases.

Short term escape and long term drift

The effect of timolol diminishes over several days or weeks and this decline is called short term escape. It is probably due to increase in the number of beta adrenergic receptors in the ciliary process. Many patients maintain a reduction in intraocular pressure for months to years. Then 10% to 20% of patients show some loss of drug effect which is named as long term drift. This may be due to the time dependent decrease in cellular sensitivity to the adrenergic antagonists.

Betaxolol

It is relatively selective beta-1 adrenergic antagonist. In ciliary epithelium there are beta-2 receptors. Hence how the IOP is reduced is not clear. It may be because high concentrations that reach the ciliary epithelium beta-2 receptors are also inhibited; the other possibility is the presence of some beta-1 receptors in ciliary body. Betaxolol is available as 0.5% solution, applied twice a day.

The advantages of betaxolol are (i) more additive effect with adrenaline than timolol or levobunolol (ii) it is a better choice in patients with airway disease. CNS side effects are lesser than timolol.

The disadvantages of betaxolol are that it is less

effective and produces more burning sensation than timolol.

Levobunolol

It is a non selective adrenergic antagonist. It is available as 0.5% solution and applied every 12 to 24 hours. It can induce blepharoconjunctivitis.

Uses of beta-blockers

They are useful in all forms of glaucoma.

The dosages of beta-blockers are given in Table 21.9.

Adverse effects of beta-blockers

Ocular

Hyperemia of conjunctiva, ptosis, visual disturbances, dry eye, allergic blepharoconjunctivitis, burning sensation.

Systemic

CNS effects   depression, anxiety, hallucinations, confusion, fatigue, tinnitus.
CVS effects   hypotension, bradycardia.
Pulmonary   dyspnoea, airway obstruction
Dermatologic   alopecia, urticaria.
GI effects   nausea, vomiting, diarrhoea, abdominal cramps.

One of the troublesome side effects of beta-blockers in the treatment of glaucoma is the blocking of the effect of beta-2 stimulants used to dilate bronchi during asthma attacks, leading to aggravation of such attack.

Besides the above beta-blockers, other beta-blockers such as atenolol, carteolol, metipranolol, nadolol, pindolol, and sotalol have been tried.

Other Adrenergic Antagonists

Thymoxamine

Thymoxamine hydrochloride is a selective Alpha$_1$ blocking agent. It produces miosis by inhibiting dilator muscle. It reduces IOP after application by clearing the iris tissue from the angle in chronic angle closure glaucoma.

Guanethidine

It is a neuron blocking agent. It lowers IOP after systemic or topical administration. The application of 5% to 10% guanethidine one or four times a day also produce miosis. The side effects to topical application include conjunctival hyperemia and burning sensation.

Labetolol is a mixed alpha, beta blocker which reduces IOP in the concentration of 0.1% to 1%.

CARBONIC ANHYDRASE INHIBITORS (CAIs)

Carbonic anhydrase in the ciliary epithelium plays an important role in the formation of aqueous humour. Carbonic anhydrase inhibitors decrease the formation of aqueous humour leading to reduction in the intraocular pressure.

Drugs which inhibit carbonic anhydrase :

Acetazolamide (diamox)

It is a sulphonamide derivative, valuable in the treatment of glaucoma when used as a supplement

Table 21.9. Beta-Adrenergic Blocking Agents

Generic Name	Concentration	Doses
Timolol maleate	0.25% to 0.5%	One drop twice daily
Timolol maleate (preservative free)	0.25% to 0.5%	One drop once daily
Betaxolol hydrochloride	0.25% to 0.5%	One drop twice daily
Carteolol hydrochloride	1%	One drop twice daily
Metipranolol	0.3%	One drop twice daily
Levobunolol hydrochloride	0.25 to 0.5%	One drop one to two times a day

Note : In single drug usage the IOP is decreased by 18% to 34%. They are additive to miotics and carbonic anhydrase inhibitors. Epinephrine is poorly additive to timolol but may be added to betaxolol more effectively.

to other forms of therapy. It is of little value if used alone.

It is also beneficial when used as a preoperative drug in intraocular surgery. It decreases secretion of aqueous humour and thereby reducing the IOP.

The oral dose is 125-250mg, 1-4 times daily. The IOP is reduced in 2-4 hours and the effect lasts for about 12 hours. Sustained release tablets (500mg) are also available which act for 24 hours.

Acetazolamide can be given intravenously (500 mg ampoules) which reduce IOP within 30 minutes. This is useful in acute glaucoma.

Adverse effects include gastrointestinal upset, anorexia, ureteric colic, calculi formation.

Ethoxzolamide

It is administered orally, the dose is 125 mg given 4 times a day, effect begins after about 2 hours and lasts for about 5 hours. The side effects are similar to that of acetazolamide.

Methazolamide

Dose is 25-50mg thrice daily, effect begins within 2 hours and lasts for 4-6 hours. Adverse effects are similar to acetazolamide. But the side effects related to the CNS are more common as the drug diffuses in CNS more easily. Malaise and fatigue have been reported.

Dichlorphenamide

It is administered orally, dose is 50mg, 1-4 times daily. the time of onset of action is about 30 minutes and the effect lasts for about 6 hours.

Adverse effects are similar to acetazolamide but potassium depletion is more of a problem.

The above described carbonic anhydrase inhibitors are administered orally and are not effective on topical application.

Dorzolamide is a carbonic anhydrase inhibitor that is available as 2% eye drops.

HYPEROSMOTIC AGENTS

Hyperosmotic agents are administered systemically (orally or parenterally) to lower intraocular pressure (IOP) acutely.

Hyperosmotic agents lower IOP due to reduction of vitreous volume, lesser aqueous humour formation. There is a net movement of intraocular water from the eye (mainly from the vitreous) into the circulation via the blood vessels of the retina and uveal tract.

Oral hyperosmotics

Glycerol (Glycerin) is given orally in a dose of 1-1.5 gm/kg body weight as a 50% solution with normal saline and flavouring agent (lemon or orange juice or cola drink).

The drop in IOP starts within 15 minutes and is significant in about 30 minutes, the recovery occurs in 4-5 hours.

Glycerol produces less side effects than other osmotic agents.

The intraocular pressure reduction is due to increased osmolality which opposes the osmotic pull within the eye which is responsible for maintaining the normal pressure. Thus, the fluid is drawn out of the eye.

Adverse effects : Repeated administration may cause hyperglycaemia and glycosuria. Its use is not advisable in diabetic patients.

Nausea (due to sweet taste) in some patients and headache (due to reduced intracranial pressure) have been reported.

Isosorbide : The administration of 1.5 gm/kg body weight as 45% solution initiates decrease in IOP within 15 minutes after ingestion, is maximal in 60-90 minutes and lasts for 2-4 hours.

Isosorbide does not provide calories unlike glycerol.

No side effects other than nausea have been reported.

Ethanol : In doses of 2-3 ml/kg, 40-45% concentration, it is sufficient to lower the IOP as effectively as with other hyperosmotic agents. The administration of 0.8-1 gm/kg produces a fall of IOP 5-35 mm Hg. Maximal effect occurs in 1-2 hours and persists for 3 hours.

The effect is due to inhibition of antidiuretic hormone.

It has the same caloric value as glycerol.

Alcohol is rarely used as a hyperosmotic agent to lower IOP because of the associated undesirable side effects.

Intravenous hyperosmotic agents

Mannitol : The usual dose is 2 gm/kg of 20% or 30% solution by I.V. infusion over a period of 30 minutes (60 drops/min.)

I.V. mannitol produces a rapid fall in IOP and the effect lasts for about 6 hours.

Although the osmotic effect is some what lesser than with urea, but it is preferred due to its milder and fewer side effects. However, it is not without adverse effects.

Adverse effects include nausea, headache and dizziness. Angina like chest pain and pulmonary oedema may occur but rarely.

Urea : A rapid decrease in IOP can be obtained by I.V. administration of urea. After 30-45 minutes, marked effect is achieved, with 30% solution of urea (90-120 drops/min.), and the effect lasts for about 5-6 hours.

It is best employed as 30% solution intravenously in a dose of 2-7 ml/kg body weight.

A dose of 1-1.5 gm/kg body weight is given at the rate of 90-120 drops/min.

Adverse effects include rapid and excessive diuresis, nausea, vomiting, mental confusion, and headache (due to cerebral dehydration).

If extravasation occurs, venous thrombosis, tissue necrosis and sloughing of the skin will be produced.

Rarely hyperthermia (due to its effect on hypothalamus) may also occur.

Indications

- Acute angle-closure glaucoma
- Glaucoma secondary to hyphema
- Glaucoma secondary to inflammation
- Preparation for intraocular surgery
- Retinal detachment surgery
- Orbital surgery
- Cataract extraction
- Sickle Cell Crisis

Urea vs other hyperosmotics

Urea is considered eminently successful as an ocular hypotensive agent because -

- it has an osmotic effect more than 5 times that of sucrose

- it has low molecular weight
- it has relatively poor ocular penetration
- it has more marked and long lasting effects than mannitol. However, some prefer mannitol over urea due to its fewer side effects, and it does not cause necrosis if extravasation occurs.

Mixture of Agents

When control is not achieved with a single medication, or the effect wears off with time, it is possible to employ following combinations :

Beta-blockers and miotics;

Beta-blockers and sympathomimetics;

Miotics and sympathomimetics.

The most common combination is pilocarpine and timolol, the duration of effect is sufficient to allow twice daily administration.

Combining two agents from the same group e.g. two miotics or two beta-blockers is less successful.

It is possible to combine all four forms of medical treatment, i.e. beta-blockers, miotics, sympathomimetics and carbonic anhydrase inhibitors, but usually surgery is employed before this stage is reached.

The list of hyperosmotic agents is given in table 21.10.

CHEMOTHERAPEUTIC AGENTS

Antibacterial agents commonly used in ophthalmology

Chloramphenicol

It is by far the most commonly used topical ophthalmic agent, effective against a wide range of bacteria and other organisms such as *chlamydiae*, *rickettsiae* and *spirochaetes*. It is an excellent topical antibiotic, available as a 0.5% solution or 1% eye ointment. It penetrates easily into the cell by a process of facilitated diffusion. It has a high lipid solubility. Cross resistance is rare as it is rarely used systemically (due to incidence of aplastic anaemia).

Topical use can sometimes lead to irritation. The potential to cause blood dyscrasia is much lower from topical use compared to systemic administration.

Table 21.10. Hyperosmotic agents

Agents	Molecular weight	Dose gm/kg	Excretion	Ocular distribution	Ocular penetration	Advantages	Disadvantages
Oral agents							
Glycerol	92	1-1.5 as 50% solution	Urine and metabolised	Extra-cellular	Poor	Stable, poor ocular penetration	Nausea, vomiting, calories
Isosorbide	146	1-1.5 as 45% solution	Urine	Total body water	Good	No caloric value	Penetrates eye
Ethanol	46	0.8-1.5 as 40-50% solution	Metabolised	Total body water	Good	Hypotonic diuresis	CNS effects, penetrates eye, calories
I.V. agents							
Mannitol	182	1-2 as 20% solution	Urine	Extra-cellular	Very poor	Poor ocular penetration	large volume, dehydration
Urea	60.06	1-2 as 30% solution	Urine	Total body water	Good		

Neomycin (one of the aminoglycosides)

It is favoured, like chloramphenicol as a topical antimicrobial because of the relatively rare systemic use. It has a broad spectrum of activity, however, it is not effective against *pseudomonas aeruginosa*.

Neomycin alone as drops or ointment is used, but it is more commonly available with steroids to produce antibiotic cover while treating inflammation.

All aminoglycosides produce nephrotoxicity and ototoxicity, but not from topical use. However, keratoconjunctivitis can develop as a result of hypersensitivity to neomycin after ophthalmic use.

Gentamicin (an aminoglycoside antibiotic)

It is a potent antibacterial and also effective against many strains of *pseudomonas aeruginosa*. Gentamicin should be used for serious infections of the eye and not for trivial infections such as conjunctivitis.

Absorption across the corneal epithelium is very poor. Systemic injection does not produce sufficient ocular levels as it crosses poorly the blood-aqueous barrier.

Like other aminoglycosides it can damage ears and kidneys. Both vestibular and cochlear parts are affected, so ataxia (due to vestibular damage) and deafness (due to cochlear damage) may occur as a result of toxic doses.

Tobramycin (an aminoglycoside)

It has a better antibacterial efficacy than gentamicin. It is used in 0.3% solution. Its adverse effects (i.e. nephrotoxicity and ototoxicity) are similar to others in this group.

Tetracyclines

Tetracyclines are a group of broad spectrum antibiotics which include chlortetracycline, dimethyl chlortetracycline, oxytetracycline, tetracycline and minocycline. Among these, minocycline has a broader spectrum and more specific indications.

Tetracyclines are effective against gram positive and gram negative bacteria, spirochaetes, chlamydiae etc., but pseudomonas and proteus are resistant to them.

Penetration across the intact cornea is poor, therefore they are best used for surface infections.

Adverse effects from topical application are rare due to low dose that the patient receives in one eye drop, compared with systemic dose, for example, a drop of 1% tetracycline solution, applied four times a day for 4 months will be equivalent of one oral dose to be administered.

Topical tetracycline is useful in the treatment of trachoma (in ointment form) and is the choice for the prophylaxis of ophthalmia neonatorum.

Erythromycin

For ophthalmic use, it is well known for the effect on chlamydiae and other organisms such as Rickettsia, Treponema and Mycoplasma.

Bacitracin

It penetrates cornea poorly. It is used externally in combination with polymyxin etc. It is effective for surface infections.

Polymyxin B

It shares many properties of gentamicin. Its passage is slow across the blood-aqueous or blood-brain barriers and the intact corneal epithelium. It can damage kidneys.

It is used topically in combination with bacitracin in ointment form or trimethoprim as eye drops.

Penicillins pass across the ocular barriers very poorly. Moreover, they are notorious for hypersensitivity. They are rarely used in the treatment of ocular infections.

Table 21.11 shows topical antibacterial agents for opthalmic use.

Table 21.12 shows systemic and ophthalmic doses of certain antibacterial agents.

ANTIVIRAL AGENTS

The following four agents are in common use for topical treatment of viral infections :

Idoxuridine
Vidarabine
Trifluorothymidine
Acyclovir

Idoxuridine

It is used as 0.1% eye drops and 0.5% eye ointment. It is generally nontoxic. It must be administered intensively, i.e. every hour.

Resistant strains may develop.

Vidarabine (adenine arabinoside)

As its mode of action is different, it can be used in patients who are allergic to idoxuridine or to treat idoxuridine - resistant cases.

Used in 3% ointment form, it is better absorbed than idoxuridine and can be used topically for herpetic uveitis. Like idoxuridine it does not interfere with the healing of corneal epithelial defects, but will slow the rate of repair of stromal injuries.

Trifluorothymidine

It is a synthetic thymidine derivative. It passes into the eye more rapidly than does vidarabine and idoxuridine and produces levels in the aqueous humour which are effective against deeper viral infections.

Acyclovir

It is effective against infections with strains of herpes simplex 1 which are resistant to idoxuridine. It is more effective than the other antivirals, even on drug-sensitive strains. It does not interfere with corneal wound healing, whether epithelial or stromal.

Antiviral targets and properties of antiviral substances are given in Table 21.13. The ophthalmic uses, routes of administration and mechanism of action of some antiviral agents are given in Table 21.14. The indications, routes of administration and ocular adverse effects of antiviral agents used in ophthalmology are given in Table 21.15.

ANTIFUNGAL AGENTS

Nystatin

It is poorly absorbed by the cornea, so topical application is only effective for surface fungal infections with organisms such as candida albicans.

Amphotericin

It is poorly absorbed and its marked toxicity restricts use in topical infections.

Natamycin

It penetrates the eye very poorly, but probably one

Table 21.11. Topical Antibacterial Agents available for Ophthalmic use.

Generic name	Formulation	Indications	Toxicity
Bacitracin	500 µ/g ointment	Conjunctivitis, blepharitis	Hypersensitivity
Chloramphenicol	0.5% solution, 1% ointment	Conjunctivitis, keratitis	Hypersensitivity, blood dyscrasias
Chlortetracycline	1% ointment	Conjunctivitis, blepharitis	Hypersensitivity
Ciprofloxacin	0.3% solution	Conjunctivitis, keratitis Keratopathy	Hypersensitivity Crystalline keratopathy
Erythromycin	0.5% ointment	Conjunctivitis, blepharitis	Hypersensitivity
Gentamicin sulphate	0.3% solution, 0.3% ointment	Conjunctivitis, blepharitis, keratitis	Hypersensitivity
Norfloxacin sulphacetamide sodium	0.3% solution, 10, 15, 30% sol. 10% ointment	Conjunctivitis Conjunctivitis, blepharitis, keratitis	Hypersensitivity Hypersensitivity, blood dyscrasias
Sulphisoxazole	4% solution, 4% ointment	Conjunctivitis, blepharitis, keratitis	Hypersensitivity, blood dyscrasias
Polymyxin B Combinations (with bacitracin neomycin, or trimethoprim)	Various solutions Various ointments	Conjunctivitis, blepharitis, keratitis	Hypersensitivity, blood dyscrasias
Tetracycline Hydrochloride	1% solution	Conjunctivitis blepharitis	Hypersensitivity
Tobramycin Sulphate	0.3% solution 0.3% ointment	Conjunctivitis blepharitis, keratitis	Hypersensitivity

Table 21.12. Systemic and ophthalmic doses of certain antibacterial agents.

Agent	Topical	Subconjunctival	Intravitreal	Systemic
Penicillin G	1,00,000 units/ml	0.5-1 million units	—	1.2-2.4 million units IM.IV
Imipenem	5 mg/ml	—	—	1-4g. IV
Gentamicin	8-20 mg/ml	20 mg	100-200 mg	3-5mg/kg IM, IV
Tobramycin	8-20 mg/ml	20 mg	100-200 mg	3-5mg/kg IM, IV
Amikacin	10-50 mg/ml	25-50 mg	400 µg	15 mg/kg IM, IV
Clindamycin	10 mg/ml	15-40 mg	1.0 mg	0.6-3.6g IM, IV
Vancomycin	50 mg/ml	25 mg	1.0 mg	0.5-2g po, 2gIV
Ciprofloxacin	3 mg/ml	—	100 µg	0.5-1g po
Cefazolin	33-66 mg/ml	60-100 mg	2.25 mg	1.6g IM, IV

of the most effective ocular antifungals. It is used as eye drops, 5-10% or 1% eye ointment.

Flucytosine

It is only active against yeast, is used as 1.5% eye drops.

Clotrimazole

In eye it is used as a 1% solution.

Miconazole

It is a broad spectrum antifungal agent. Absorption takes place across the intact cornea. Antifungal agents are listed in Table 21.16.

ANTIPROTOZOAL AGENTS

The most common infection is due to toxoplasma gondii.

Table 21.13. Antiviral targets and properties of antiviral substances

Agents	Viral targets	Active against
Purine and pyrimidine analogues		
Acyclovir	DNA polymerase	Herpes simplex
Ganciclovir	DNA polymerase	Cytomegalovirus
Ribavirin	DNA polymerase	Respiratory syncytial
Vidarabine	DNA polymerase	Herpes simplex, zoster
Idoxuridine	DNA synthesis	Herpes (corneal)
Trifluridine	DNA synthesis	Herpes (corneal)
Dideoxynucleoside (AZT, ddI,ddC)	Reverse transcriptase, DNA synthesis	HIV
Other drugs		
Amantadine	Adsorption, penetration	Influenza A, rubella
Rimantadine	Adsorption, penetration	Influenza A, rubella
Foscarnet	DNA polymerase, reverse transcriptase	Cytomegalovirus, herpes simplex
Interferons	Protein synthesis	Herpes simplex and zoster, hepatitis, papilloma viruses
Gamma globulin	Adsorption, penetration	Hepatitis B, rabies, polio, papilloma,
Methisazone	Protein synthesis	Pox Viruses
Rifampin	Assembly of mature virus particle	Pox viruses

Table 21.14. Ophthalmic uses of antivirals

Ophthalmic disease	Generic name	Route of administration	Principal mechanism of action
HSV epithelial keratitis	Idoxuridine (IDU)	Topical	Abnormal base results in false mRNA and faulty viral proteins
HSV epithelial keratitis	Vidarabine (Ara-A)	Intravenous	Abnormal sugar results in premature termination of viral DNA synthesis
HSV epithelial keratitis (drug of choice)	Trifluridine (TFT)	Topical	Similar to IDU
VZV ophthalmicus Paediatric HSV epithelial	Acyclovir	Oral, intravenous	Similar to Ara-A
CMV retinitis	Ganciclovir	Intravenous, intravitreal	Similar to Ara-A
CMV retinitis	Foscarnet	Intravenous	Blocks pyrophosphate binding site of viral DNA polymerase

HSV, herpes simplex virus; VZV, varicella zoster virus; CMV, Cytomegalovirus

Table 21.15. Antiviral agents for ophthalmic use

Drug	Route of administration	Indications for use	Ocular adverse effects
Idoxuridine	Topical, 0.1% solution	herpes simplex keratitis	Punctate keratopathy, hypersensitivity
Trifluridine	Topical, 1.0% solution	herpes simplex keratitis	punctate keratopathy, hypersensitivity
Vidarabine	Topical, 3.0% ointment	herpes simplex keratitis	punctate keratopathy, hypersensitivity
Acyclovir	Oral, 200 mg tablets	herpes simplex conjunctivitis herpes zoster opthalmicus	
Foscarnet	I.V., Intravitreal	herpes simplex keratitis, cytomegalovirus retinitis	
Ganciclovir	I.V., Intravitreal	cytomegalovirus retinitis	

Table 21.16. Antifungal agents for ophthalmic use

Drug	Method of administration	Indication for use
Polyenes		
Amphoterecin B	0.1-0.5% topical solution	Fungal keratitis, endophthalmitis
	0.8-1.0 mg subconjunctival injection	
	5 μg intravitreal injection	
	5% topical suspension	
Natamycin	5% topical suspension	Fungal blepharitis, conjunctivitis, keratitis
Imidazoles		
Clotrimazole	1% topical solution and suspension	Fungal keratitis
	5-10 mg subconjunctival injection	
Econazole	1% topical suspension and ointment	Fungal keratitis
Fluconazole	2% topical suspension	Fungal keratitis
Ketoconazole	1% topical suspension	Fungal keratitis
Miconazole	1% topical solution and suspension	Fungal keratitis, endophthalmitis
	5-10 mg subconjunctival injection	
	0.25 mg intravitreal injection	
Fluorinated pyrimidine		
Flucytosine	1% topical eye drops solution	Fungal keratitis

Pyrimethamine (daraprim)

It is a folic acid antagonist, used in the treatment of toxoplasmosis. It is better to use it in combination with a sulphonamide because the combined treatment will need only 1/8 as much sulphonamide and 1/24 as much pyrimethamine as would be necessary if either is used.

Corticosteroid therapy is also simultaneously used, although its precise role is not certain.

ANTI-INFLAMMATORY AGENTS

Inflammation can be due to infection, allergy and trauma. It is characterized by reddening of the area (due to vasodilatation), oedema, loss of function and pain.

If proper steps are not taken to treat the inflammatory process in the eye, it may lead to permanent loss of vision.

Drugs

• Corticosteroids (see Chapter 10)
• NSAIDs (see Chapter 3)
• Antihistamines (see Chapter 13)
• Mast cell stabilizers (see Chapter 6)

Corticosteroids

Glucocorticoids have anti-inflammatory properties. They reduce the vasodilatation that is responsible for the redness that accompanies inflammation and stabilize mast cells, thereby reducing the release of histamine. Their use maintains the normal permeability of blood and prevents the development of oedema.

Corticosteroids also inhibit the production of prostaglandins, which mediate some of the effect of inflammation.

Corticosteroids not only provide symptomatic relief, but also prevent scar formation and loss of transparency of the cornea.

Corticosteroids are 'double-edged sword' because on the one hand they are very useful and sometimes have sight-saving effects in the treatment of inflammation, while on the other hand they may produce very serious adverse effects.

Preparations for topical application are listed in Table 21.17.

Systemic steroids are employed for the diseases of the posterior segment of the eye and acute allergic reactions of the eyelids.

Table 21.17. Preparations available for topical application

Drugs	Preparations	% concentration
Cortisone acetate	Suspension	0.5
	Ointment	1.5
Hydrocortisone acetate	Suspension	2.5
	Ointment	1.5
	Solution	0.2
Prednisolone phosphate	Solution	0.5
	Ointment	0.25
Dexamethasone	Solution	0.1
phosphate	Ointment	0.05
	Suspension	0.1
Betamethasone sodium	Solution	0.1
phosphate	Ointment	0.5
Fluorometholone (progesterone-like compound)	Suspension	0.1

Systemic Corticosteroid Preparations

Water soluble (short acting)	Dexamethasone sodium phosphate Hydrocortisone sodium succinate
Suspensions of moderately soluble compounds in polyethylene glycol (moderately acting)	Triamcinolone diacetate, Methylprednisolone acetate.
Suspension of minimal solubility (long acting)	Triamcinolone acetonide Triamcinolone acetate
Mixture of soluble and moderately soluble agents.	Betamethasone sodium phosphate Betamethasone acetate

Systemic steroids commonly used and their equivalent doses are given in Table 21.18.

The dose is decided according to the severity of inflammation. In case of mild inflammation, topical application of eye drops twice or thrice a day is quite effective. In severe cases the application may have to be every hour. In conditions like sympathetic ophthalmia, apart from topical route parenteral (ophthalmic) and systemic administration have to be added.

In the case of acute and severe disease, 60 to 80

Table 21.18. Systemic steroids commonly used and their equivalent dose

Drug	Approximate systemic equivalent dose (mg)	Approximate anti-inflammatory potency factor
Cortisone acetate	25	0.8
Hydrocortisone	20	1
Prednisone	5	4.0
Prednisolone	5	4.0
Triamcinolone	4	5.0
Methyl prednisolone	4	5.0
Dexamethasone	0.75	25.0
Betamethasone	0.6	25.0

mg prednisolone or its equivalent is advised. The dose should be tapered off gradually to prevent rebound inflammation.

No other drugs deserve the title of a "two-edged sword" as much as the corticosteroids. On the one hand they are very useful and have sight-saving effects in treatment of inflammation, for example, they reduce IOP when used to treat uveitis secondary glaucoma but can cause a rise in IOP if used topically in patients who are "steroid responders".

Although steroids are useful in a large variety of ocular conditions, they must be administered with good indications, by the proper route and under the supervision of a physician. These precautions are necessary because of the sinister complications of these agents both in the eye and in the body (see adverse effects). Patients with conditions of diabetes, hypertension, tuberculosis, peptic ulcer, if given steroid systemically, often will have an exacerbation of these diseases. The routes of steroid administration are given in Table 21.19.

Routes of Administration

A. Topical in the form of ointment and drops.
B. Parenteral routes (ophthalmic): subconjunctival, deep sub Tenon's and retrobulbar.
C. Systemic administration: Oral and Parenteral.

Topical steroids are used for disorders involving anterior segment of the eye.

Uses of corticosteroids in ophthalmology are listed in Table 21.20.

Table 21.19. Shows common routes of steroid administration for ocular inflammation

Conditions	Routes
Conjunctivitis	Topical
Blepharitis	Topical
Episcleritis	Topical
Keratitis	Topical
Scleritis	Topical and / systemic
Anterior uveitis	Topical and / or subconjunctival
Posterior uveitis	Systemic and / or depot
Endophthalmitis	Systemic / depot, intravitreal
Optic neuritis	Systemic or depot
Temporal arteritis	Systemic
Sympathetic ophthalmia	Systemic and topical

Table 21.20. Ocular indications for corticosteroid treatment.

Eyelids	Allergic blepharitis
	Contact dermatitis
	Herpes zoster
Conjunctiva	Irritant conjunctivitis
	Allergic conjunctivitis
	Herpes zoster
Sclera	Episcleritis
	Scleritis
Cornea	Acne rosacae keratitis
	Epithelial punctate keratitis
	Herpes zoster keratitis
	Superficial punctate keratitis
Uvea	Iritis, iridocyclitis
	Posterior uveitis
	Sympathetic ophthalmia
Retina	Cystoid macular oedema
	Retinal vasculitis
Optic nerve	Optic neuritis
	Traumatic optic neuropathy
Orbit	Pseudotumour of orbit
	Myasthenia gravis
Globe	Traumatic hyphema
	Endophthalmitis

Adverse effects

Due to marked side effects the use of corticosteroids must be carefully done. The adverse effects must always be balanced against their beneficial effects. For example, they inhibit wound healing and reduce the body's response to infections. If the invading organism is virus or non-pyogenic bacteria, then use antimicrobial agents at the same time, but if the infection is due to pyogenic bacteria, they will cause tissue damage and steroids will delay resolution of the infection.

Adverse effects of corticosteroids are shown in Table 21.21.

Nonsteroidal Antiinflammatory Drugs (NSAIDs)

NSAIDs are discussed in Chapter 3.

The commonly used topical NSAIDs for ocular use are :

Flubiprofen, suprofen, ketorolac, diclofenac and indomethacin.

The following are their uses in the treatment of ocular diseases :

Flubiprofen and suprofen are employed to counter unwanted intraoperative miosis during cataract surgery.

Ketorolac is used for seasonal allergic conjunctivitis.

Diclofenac is used for postoperative inflammation.

Indomethacin penetrates the cornea well. It is used in uveitis and it has also a IOP reducing property in glaucomatocyclitic iritis.

The strengths and frequency of administration are given in Table 21.22.

The NSAIDs should be used when steroids are contraindicated or as supplement to corticosteroid therapy.

IMMUNOSUPPRESSIVE AND ANTIMITOTIC AGENTS

The application of these agents in ophthalmology relates to the use of 5-fluorouracil (5-FU) and mitomycin C in corneal and glaucoma surgeries.

Both 5-FU and mitomycin C improve the success of filtration surgery by limiting the postoperative wound-healing process.

Mitomycin C is employed intraoperatively as a single subconjunctival application at the trabeculotomy site. But its intraocular penetration must be avoided as it is very toxic to the intraocular structures.

Table 21.21. Adverse effects of Corticosteroids

Ocular effects		Systemic effects
From local application	*From prolonged systemic use*	
* Glaucoma	* Decreased resistance to infection	* Water and salt retention
* Proliferation of bacteria	* Delayed wound healing	* Mental disturbance
* Overgrowth of fungi	* Papilloedema	* Wastage of skeletal muscle
* Proliferation of viruses specially herpes simplex	* Oedema of face and eyelids	* Demineralisation of bones
* Decreased wound healing	* Cataract	* Thrombophlebitis
* Cataract	* Glaucoma	* Delayed wound healing
		* Bleeding problems
		* Menstrual irregularities
		* Acne
		* Increased blood glucose level and diabetes mellitus
		* Decreased resistance to infection
		* Growth retardation in children

Table 21.22. Topical NSAIDs for ocular use

Flubiprofen solution	0.03% one drop every 30 min., two hr. preoperatively (total dose four drops)
Suprofen solution	1% two drops at 1, 2 and 3 hr. preoperatively
Ketorolac solution	0.5% tid
Diclofenac solution	0.1% qid
Indomethacin solution	0.5-1% suspension qid

Mitomycin C has been used topically after excision of pterygium (neovascular membrane that can grow on the cornea).

The currently used ophthalmic immunosuppressive and antimitotic agents are given in Table 21.23.

The major adverse reactions of immunosuppressive agents are given in Table 21.24.

MAST CELL STABILIZER

Sodium cromoglycate (cromolyn sodium)

It stabilizes the membranes of mast cells, thus preventing the release of histamine.

A topical preparation of this compound is available as a 0.2% solution or a 4% ointment for the prophylaxis of vernal conjunctivitis and other allergic reactions. It prevents the symptoms occurring but does not act as an antihistamine. Hence, it does not produce any effect once the histamine is released.

Cromolyn sodium has limited use in the treatment of conjunctivitis such as vernal conjunctivitis (thought to be allergen-mediated).

USE OF ANAESTHESIA IN OPHTHALMIC PROCEDURES

Ocular Anaesthetics

Local anaesthetics reversibly block the transmission of nerve impulses along sensory fibres. Pain, which is carried by the smallest fibres is lost first, followed by touch and temperature sensitivity. Pressure, which is carried by largest nerve fibres, is lost last, if at all.

Ideal properties of local anaesthetics

A suitable local anaesthetic should be :-
- Water soluble
- Onset of action be quick.
- Effective for a reasonable duration of time.
- No effect on pupil, accommodation or IOP.
- No effect on other drugs, e.g. mydriatics etc.
- Not interfere with the healing process.
- Non-toxic, locally as well as systemically.
- Sterilisable by heat
- Nonirritant

Indications for use

1) Foreign body removal
2) Tonometry

Table 21.23. Currently used ophthalmic immuno-suppressive and Antimitotic Agents

Drug class	Indications	Dosage	Toxic Reactions
Alkylating agents			
Cyclophosphamide	Behcet's disease, Wegener's granulomatosis, sympathetic ophthalmia	1-2 mg/kg/day po, IV	Haemorrhagic cystitis, myelosuppression, secondary malignancies, alopecia, infections.
Chlorambucil	Behcet's, disease, sympathetic ophthalmia	2-12 mg/day, po	Same as for cyclophosphamide, gonadal atrophy
Antimetabolite agents			
Azathioprine	Behcet's cicatricial pemphigoid, systemic lupus erythematosus, Wegener's rheumatoid scleritis	1-2.5 mg/kg/day, po	Myelosuppression, secondary infections nausea.
Methotrexate	Rheumatoid scleritis, (Reiter's) sympathetic ophthalmia	10-25 mg/kg in divided doses, po, IV, IM	Hepatotoxicity, mucosal ulcerations, myelosuppression
5-Fluorouracil	High-risk glaucoma at surgery	5-7.5mg SC (7-14 days)	Wound leaks, hypotony, corneal epitheliopathy
Anti-inflammatory agents			
Colchicine	Behcet's disease	0.5-0.6 g/day bid, po	Myelosupression at surgery
Antibiotics Cyclosporin A	Behcet's sympathetic ophthalmia, corneal graft rejection	5-7 mg/kg/day po, 2% topical hyperuricaemia, neurotoxicity (mild)	Nephrotoxicity, hypertension
Mitomycin C	High risk glaucoma surgery, pterygium removal	0.5mg/ml; 0.4% topical	Wound leak, hypotony scleral melting
Dapsone	Cicatricial pemphigoid	20-25 mg bid/tid, po	Hemolytic anaemia, nausea, neuropathy

Table 21.24. Major adverse reactions of immunosuppressive agents

Drug	Adverse reactions
Cyclophosphamide	Sterile haemorrhagic cystitis, myelosuppression, reversible alopecia, secondary malignancies, transient blurring of vision
Chlorambucil	Myelosuppression (moderate but rapid), gonadal dysfunction, secondary malignancies
Methotrexate	Hepatotoxicity, ulcerative stomatitis, bone marrow suppression, diarrhoea
Azathioprine	Bone marrow suppression (leukopenia), nausea, secondary infections
Cyclosporin	Nephrotoxicity, hypertension, hyperuricaemia, hyperglycaemia, hepatotoxicity, nausea, vomiting
Rapamycin	Unknown
Dapsone	Haemolytic anaemia, methaemoglobinaemia, nausea, mononucleosis like syndrome
Bromocriptine	Postural hypotension, nausea, vomiting
Ketoconazole	Hepatotoxicity, endocrine abnormalities, gastrointestinal upset
Colchicine	Nausea, vomiting, diarrhoea, bone marrow suppression

Table 21.25. Local anaesthetics

Drug	Strengths % w/v	Single dose	Onset of anaesthesia	Duration of anaesthesia
Amethocaine (tetracaine)	0.5 0.1	Yes	1 min.	20 min.
Benoxinate (oxybuprocaine)	0.4	Yes	1 min.	15 min.
Proxymetacaine (proparacaine)	0.5	Yes	1 min.	15 min.
Lignocaine (xylocaine, lidocaine)	2.1 4.0	Yes	1 min.	30 min.

3) Contact lens fitting

4) Certain diagnostic procedures

Local anaesthetics generally employed in ophthalmic practice are given in Table 21.25.

Amethocaine hydrochloride (Tetracaine hydrochloride, Pontocaine, Anethaine)

It is used in 0.25-1% solutions. It is relatively stable in solution but it is affected by light. It should be stored in an amber coloured bottle.

Benoxinate hydrochloride (oxybuprocaine hydrochloride)

It is very soluble in water, used in a 0.4% solution with characteristics similar to proxymetacaine (both causing less irritation and stinging than Amethocaine).

Benoxinate hydrochloride has an additional advantage in that it possesses bactericidal properties.

Proxymetacaine hydrochloride (Proparacaine Hydrochloride)

It has greater potency than Amethocaine.

Our drop of 0.5% solution produces anaesthesia lasting for about 15 minutes. When deep anaesthesia is required for cataract extraction, one drop every 5-10 minutes until 5 to 7 drops have been administered will be sufficient.

Proxymetacaine causes much less stinging than amethocaine.

Lignocaine hydrochloride (Lidocaine hydrochloride, xylocaine)

It is an amide type of local anaesthetic unlike amethocaine, proxymetacaine and oxybuprocaine which are

ester type. It is usually employed in 2-4% strength.

Choice of topical anaesthetics

As regards the initial stinging on instillation, the agents can be listed as :

Proxymetacaine   most comfortable
Benoxinate
Lignocaine
Amethocaine   least comfortable

The commonly used topical anaesthetics are listed in Table 21.26 and regional anaesthetics are given in Table 21.27.

Table 21.26. Topical anaesthetic agents

Drug	Conc.
Lignocaine	4%
Proparacaine	0.5%
Benoxinate	0.4%
Tetracaine hydrochloride	0.5%
Cocaine	0.25-0.15% rarely used

Adverse reactions to local anaesthetics

There is possibility of both local and systemic adverse effects.

All local anaesthetics cause delay in wound healing.

All local anaesthetics depress epithelial oxygen uptake to some extent. Repeated instillation may lead to desquamation and eventually loss of vision.

The CNS toxicity is stimulation followed by depression.

Sometimes fainting or syncope may occur : The respiratory arrest occurs at almost twice the concentration that produces unconsciousness

Table 21.27. Regional anaesthetics

Drug	Conc.	Onset min.	Duration min.	Comments
Procaine	1-4%	7-8	30-45	Short duration, poor absorption from mucous membrane
Tetracaine	0.25%	5-9	120 with epinephrine	
Lidocaine	1-2%	4-6	46-60 with epinephrine	
Mepivacaine	1-2%	3-5	120	
Prilocaine	1-2%	3-4	90-120, with epinephrine 300-600	

Currently most ophthalmic surgery is being done with local anaesthesia.

General Anaesthetics

General anaesthetics and sedation are important adjuncts for patient care for surgery and examination of the eye when one is dealing with an uncooperative patient, may be a child, a deaf person, very apprehensive patient or psychotic. Some times a combination of local anaesthesia with light general anaesthesia is the option in those cases where normal depth of general anaesthesia can not be tolerated by the patient on the grounds of health.

FLUORESCEIN AND OTHER DYES

Ideal properties of dyes (stains)

- They should be water soluble.
- They should selectively stain certain cells or structures in the eye.
- They should not stain skin, clothes, etc.
- The effect should be reversible
- They should not interfere with vision.
- They should be non-irritant and non toxic.
- They should be compatible with other stains or any other substance with which they are likely to be used.

Two stains are in regular use viz. fluorescein sodium and rose bengal.

Fluorescein sodium

Fluorescein sodium possesses fluorescent properties. It is an orange-red dye which fluoresces in high dilution. It is a dye which is water soluble and produces a green fluorescent colour in solution of pH more than 5.0. It can be detected in concen-tration as low as 1 ppm. This dye is nonirritant and nontoxic. It is a relatively inert substance.

It is used as (1) a topical stain and (2) injected for fluorescein angiography.

1. Topical application

In opthalmology a blue light (wave length range 465-490 nm) is used to illuminate the light and it is reflected back as a yellow-green light (wave length 520-530 nm).

Usually 2% fluorescein solution is used for corneal staining.

When fluorescein is topically applied the tear film appears yellow or orange coloured. If dilute solution is applied, the colour is greenish.

The intact corneal epithelium has high lipid content and so the water soluble dye does not penetrate the corneal epithelium and is not coloured by it. But in the presence of any break in the corneal epithelium the dye penetrates into the Bowman's membrane and into the corneal stroma. The dye will also penetrate into the anterior chamber if the epithelial loss is extensive. It will mix with the aqueous humour in the anterior chamber and appear as green flare biomicroscopically.

2. Fluorescein angiography

5 ml of a 10% solution or 3ml of a 25% solution is rapidly administered intravenously. The dye reaches ocular circulation in about 12 seconds and remains there for about 20 seconds.

Fluorescein angiography is very useful to study the ocular physiology as well as for the diagnosis of the diseases of choroid and retina.

Contamination

Contamination of fluorescein eye drops is a serious risk, as they are liable to become infected with bacteria, especially with *pseudomonas aeruginosa.* Phenylmercuric acetate or nitrate in 0.002% concentration is the best bactericide for preserving these eye drops and it is effective against pseudomonas. However, safest would be to use sterile single-dose units or sterile fluorescein-impregnated paper strips.

Other uses

- Contact lens fitting
- Applanation tonometry
- Corneal surgery (during anterior segment surgery to identify the raw surfaces)
- Detection of aqueous leaks
- Determination of naso-lacrimal pathway
- Antidote to poisoning by aniline dyes
- IV fluorescein (for angiography, ocular fluorophotometry and iris examination).

Contraindication

Avoid during pregnancy as teratogenic in experimental animals.

Adverse effects

Severe adverse effects are rare. However, there is possibility of vaso-vagal syncope after I.V. injection and sometimes even after topical use.

Allergic reactions have been reported.

After I.V. fluorescein administration, patients experience temporary yellow discolouration of skin and urine. In case the injection is given slowly it may produce headache, nausea and vomiting (occur 12 times more frequently if given slowly).

Extravasation of fluoroscein may produce pain at the site of injection.

The severe adverse reactions due to I.V. fluorescein administration include respiratory reactions, cardiac reactions, tonic-clonic seizures etc.

Other dyes for angiography

Indocyanine Green

It is available in a dry powder form in 25 mg and 50mg vials. It is unstable in aqueous form and must be freshly prepared and used within 10 hours of preparation. The diluent supplied with the vials should be the only one used for preparation of the solution.

Indocyanine green does not leak out of the intravascular compartments where blood-ocular barrier systems are intact. It is entirely retained in the intravascular compartments and excreted slowly by liver through biliary channels. It makes it an ideal agent to study the ocular circulatory systems and blood flow in normal and abnormal states.

The main uses of this dye are :
- In identification of occult neovascularization
- Vortex vein varices
- Central chorioretinopathy
- Pigment epithelial detachment
- Malignant melanoma of choroid

Indocyanine green 1% solution stains diseased or dead corneal epithelial cells. Hence, it is used to evaluate corneal visibility of donor. It has been found that indocyanine angiography reveals choroidal neovascular membranes better than with the use of fluorescein. Additional advantage is that nausea and vomiting does not occur at all unlike with fluorescein angiography.

Rose Bengal (dichlorotetraiodofluorescein)

It is a brownish red powder soluble in water .It is usually instilled as a 1% aqueous solution. It produces more irritation than fluorescein, but if applied via filter paper, it is less irritant.

Rose Bengal is a derivative of fluorescein but has different staining properties. It crosses the cell membrane of dead cells but not living ones.

It stains cells and their nuclei red without affecting the cells (hence called vital dye). It does not stain the normal ocular surface as the precorneal tear film blocks its effect. Mucus threads are also stained.

Indications for use

- Dendritic keratitis
- Keratoconjunctivitis sicca
- Keratitis neuroparalytica
- Exophthalmos
- Pressure areas due to contact lens wear

Mixtures of fluroescein and rose bengal

Mixed stain containing 1% fluorescein sodium and 1% rose bengal has been found better than the individual stains alone.

Triple staining i.e. alcian blue with the above mixtures has also been tried. The three dyes stain different structures - fluorescein stains epithelial lesions, rose Bengal stains degenerative cells and alcian blue, mucus.

Other stains (these are seldom used)

Alcian blue

It is a copper-containing complex compound, used in 1% solution. It is specific for staining mucus blue. The diseased epithelial cells are not stained. It is used to differentiate mucus deposits from diseased cells. Rose Bengal stain both diseased epithelial cells as well as mucus.

Trypan blue

1% solution stains mucus and dead cells.

Methylene blue

0.5% solution, 3 instillations at 5 minutes intervals stains the corneal nerves as blue filaments. The blue staining may persist for 24 hours.

It will vitally stain nerve tissue. It can outline an area of ulceration in herpetic keratitis like rose Bengal. It can artistically stain corneal ulcers when combined with fluorescein, the ulcer appears as a dark blue area with a green halo. Methylene blue is more irritating than rose Bengal.

Bromothymol blue

It stains degenerated and dead cells and mucus.

Tetrazolium and iodonitrotetrazolium

These compounds have been used for the vital staining of tumours and assessing corneal grafts. They are pro-stains. These compounds are reduced inside the cells to a red dye formazan. It takes about 4 minutes to develop colours.

Tetrazolium stains degenerated cells, not dead cells. Living healthy cells are not stained because of the impermeability of the cell membrane, and dead cells are not stained because the enzymes needed to reduce the dye to formazan are not present.

Lissamine Green

1% solution of lissamine green stains dry or devitalized corneal and conjunctival cells and therefore it may be used to detect vitamin A deficiency xerophthalmia However, this test is not popular because of high incidence of false negative results.

Argyrol

10% or 20% argyrol solution into conjunctival sac will produce dark stain of mucus strands and debris on the lid margins and the skin surface. The tissues are not stained. Argyrol is easily washed off.

The uses and adverse effects of certain dyes are given in below.

DRUGS AND BIOLOGICAL AGENTS USED IN OPHTHALMIC SURGERY

Use of Enzymes

Alpha-chymotrypsin is a proteolytic enzyme prepared from mammalian pancreas. Preparations are available in 1:5000 and 1:10000 dilution. The ophthalmic use is to produce zonulysis by applying over the cataractous lens to facilitate its removal.

The side effect of Alpha-chymotrypsin is a transient increase in IOP from digested zonular debris which may obstruct the trabecular meshwork.

Hyaluronidase enzyme is used to enhance local anaesthesia, for example, in retrobulbar optic nerve block. It depolymerizes hyaluronic acid, a mucopolysaccharide, in interstitial tissue spaces. There are no direct complications due to the use of hyaluronidase. However, retrobulbar injections of anaesthetic sometimes perforate the globe or penetrate the optic nerve and can produce CNS depression secondary to diffusion into the optic nerve sheath.

Urokinase enzyme has thrombolytic properties. It converts plasminogen to the proteolytic enzyme plasmin which degrades fibrin clots, fibrinogen and other plasma proteins.

In ophthalmology, urokinase has been tried for

Certain Dyes (stains)

Dye	Strength % w/v	Uses	Adverse reactions
Fluorescein sodium	1.0-2.0 Corneal abrasion Contact lens fitting	Tonometry Pseudomonas aeruginosa	Supports growth of
Rose Bengal	1.0	Stains dead cells, Diagnosis of dry eye	Irritant on application to dry eye
Alcian blue	1.0	Stains mucus	—
Trypan blue	1.0	Stains mucus and dead cells	—
Tetrazolium and Iodonitrotetrazolium		Stains degenerate but not dead cells	

the treatment of acute retinal artery and vein occlusion and to irrigate hyphema.

Irrigation of hyphema is done with 0.3 ml of urokinase solution containing 2,500 units/ml. For vascular occlusion, the dose is 4400 IU/Kg body weight, administered intravenously (in 10 minutes) followed by continuous infusion of 4400 IU/Kg for 12 hours.

Surgical Haemostasis and Thrombolytic Agents

In selective intraocular surgery, thrombin has a valuable role in haemostasis. Intravitreal administration of thrombin is helpful in controlling intraocular haemorrhage during vitrectomy. This coagulation factor may also be applied topically via soaked sponges to exposed conjunctiva and sclera.

Tissue plasminogen activator (t-PA) has been used during intraocular surgery to assist evacuation of a hyphema (blood in the anterior chamber), subretinal clot, or nonclearing vitreous haemorrhage. t-PA is also given sub-conjunctivally and intra-camerally (i.e. in the anterior segment) to lyse blood clots obstructing a glaucoma filtration site.

The main complication of t-PA is bleeding.

Botulinum Toxin Type A

It has been used to treat strabismus, blepharospasm and spasmodic torticolis. It causes a temporary paralysis of the locally injected muscles by preventing ACh release at the neuromuscular junction.

Complications related to this toxin include diplopia (double vision) and ptosis (lid droop).

Adhesives (surgical glues)

Adhesives provide water tight sutureless closure. Cyanoacrylate derivatives are used for this purpose. Butyl 2-cyanoacrylate is commonly used. There are hexyl, octyl and decyl derivatives which are even less irritating products.

Ocular uses of adhesives

- small corneal laceration
- blepharoplasty
- retinal detachment surgery
- muscle surgery
- orbital implant

Precautions

The surface over which adhesive is to be applied should be absolutely dry until several minutes after application. Since polymerization is immediate, no adjustments are possible after initial contact.

Minimum possible amount should be used. The thinnest possible layer gives most effective results. Moreover, the toxicity is related to the amount of the adhesive.

Metallic instruments should be avoided. Disposable polyethylene disc of required size to cover the lesion is suitable. The disc acts as a carrier for the glue which separates from the glue surface after the polymerization is over.

MISCELLANEOUS AGENTS

Antihistamines (see Chapter 13)

Histamine receptors have been divided into two types, H_1 and H_2.

H_1 receptors are found on the surface of the eye as well as other mucous membranes, e.g. nasal cavities. They are blocked by antihistamines such as antazoline.

H_2 receptors mediate gastric acid secretion and are blocked by drugs, such as cimetidine, which are used for the treatment of gastric ulcers. H_2 receptors have been found on the surface of the eye. These receptors are though to be involved in the dilatation of episcleral, conjunctival and perilimbal blood vessels.

H_1 antagonists such as antazoline (Antistine) have been used in combination with sympathomimetic vasoconstrictors, since this is more effective than each component on its own. The usual symptoms of histamine mediated allergy are lacrimation, redness, itching, pain and photophobia. Antazoline would appear to relieve the itching, while naphazoline (a vasoconstrictor) will be more effective on the blood vessels and in reducing the redness.

Topical H_1 antihistamines are the drugs most commonly used for treatment of ocular allergic conjunctivitis and are used to abate the manifestation associated with vernal keratoconjunctivitis and atopic keratoconjunctivits. These are used as eye drops 1-2 drops every 3-4 hours, atleast 4 times a day to relieve the symptoms.

H_1 antihistamines effectively reduce histamine itching, but the only antihistamine marketed that is also effective in relieving ocular redness is levo-cabastine hydrochloride. The effect is probably achieved due to blocking of H_2 receptors to such an extent that minimal effects of H_1 receptors in mediating hyperemia are eliminated.

The following H_1 antihistamines are given topically :

Levocabastine hydrochloride	0.05%
Antazoline	0.5%
Pheniramine maleate	0.3%
Naphazoline hydrochloride	0.05%, 0.025%

Ocular therapeutic uses of antihistamines :
- Allergic conjunctivitis (palliative treatment)
- Myokymia (refractory period of muscle is prolonged by antihistamines). The antihista-minic drug of choice may be given alone or together with quinine (0.32 g one to three times daily).

- Cataract surgery: Preoperative antihistamine therapy can prevent pupilloconstriction. The drug may be given orally (promethazine 25 mg 2 hours before surgery) or topically (pyrilamine maleate, 0.1% solution every 10 minutes three times).
- Histamine cephalalgia. This unusual syndrome includes excruciating unilateral headaches commonly referred to the orbit. During an attack the eye is red and congested.

On the whole topically antihistamines are associated with low incidence of systemic side effects. Rarely as with oral antihistamines, topical antihistamines may produce -

- An acute attack of angle closure glaucoma in a predisposed patient due to mydriasis
- Dryness of conjunctiva
- Ciliary muscle paresis with associated decrease in accommodation.

Oral antihistamines are ineffective against ocular disease. The piperazines (e.g. cyclizine, buclizine, meclizine) and piperidines (e.g. terfenadine, astamizole, loratadine, levocabastine) are more common in use and as they are lipid soluble, they cross the blood-ocular barriers. However, they do not attain adequate concentration in ocular tissues in doses that do not produce side effects.

VITAMINS

The general aspects and categories of vitamins along with the details about their sources, functions, preparations, doses, uses, deficiency symptoms and adverse effects are described in Chapter 12.

The functions, sources and ocular signs of deficiency of vitamins are given in Tables 21.28. and 21.29 showing ophthalmic effects of selected vitamin deficiencies and zinc deficiency.

VISCOELASTIC AGENTS

Compounds which increase viscosity are often added to ophthalmic solutions. Thickening agents or visco-elastic substances act as cushioning agent, lubricant, clinging agent and increase the contact time of drug therapy increasing therapeutic effectiveness.

Table 21.28. Showing functions, sources and ocular signs of deficiency of various vitamins.

Vitamin	Vitamin functions	Food Source	Ocular signs of deficiency
Vitamin A	Visual cycle adaptation to light and dark, tissue growth specially skin and mucous membrane. Take part in immunity	Retinol available in liver, egg, milk, cream, butter. Pro-vitamin carotine available in green and yellow vegetables and fruits	Xerophthalmia, conjunctival pigmentation, xerosis of cornea, corneal ulcer, impairment of dark adaptation, paper salt fundus.
Thiamine (B$_1$)	Normal growth coenzyme in carbohydrate metabolism, normal function of nerves and muscles	Pork, beef, grains, legumes	Corneal epithelial damage, nystagmus EOM palsy, visual loss, papilloedema, ptosis, retinal haemorrhages, red and green scotoma, nutritional amblyopia, tobacco-alcohol amblyopia.
Niacin	Coenzyme	Meat, grains	Conjunctival congestion, corneal vascularization, lenticular opacities, blepharoconjunctivitis, temporal pallor of disc, optic neuritis
Riboflavin (B$_2$)	Coenzyme in protein, energy metabolism, normal growth	Milk, liver cereals	Vascularization of cornea, cornel opacities, photophobia, lacrimation nutritional amblyopia
Pyridoxine (B$_6$)	Aminoacid metabolism	Wheat, corn, meat, liver	Seborrhoea, dermatitis of eyelid, angular conjunctivitis
Vitamin (B$_{12}$)	RBC formation, nerve function	Liver, meat, milk, egg, cheese	Retinal haemorrhages, retinal oedema, pipilloedema
Biotin	Needed in carbohydrate and fat metabolism		Keratoconjunctivitis
Vitamin C	Formation of collagen	Citrous fruits, greens	Intraocular haemorrhage, petechial haemorrhages in skin, conjunctiva, iris, retina, haemorrhages in orbit. Contraction of field for green.
Vitamin D	Teeth and bone formation	Exposure to sunlight, milk, fish	Zonular cataracts
Vitamin K	Needed in blood coagulation	Cabbage, cauliflower soyabean, spinach	Retinal haemorrhage

Table 21.29. Ophthalmic effects of selected vitamin deficiencies and zinc deficiency.

Deficiency	Effects in anterior segment	Effects in posterior segment
Vitamin A (retinol)	Conjunctiva (Bitot's spots, xerosis) Cornea (keratomalacia; punctate keratopathy)	Nyctalopia; impaired rhodopsin synthesis; retinal pigment epithelium (hypopigmentation)
B$_1$ (Thiamine)	—	Optic nerve (temporal atrophy with corresponding visual field defects)
B$_6$ (pyridoxine)	Cornea (neovascularization)	Retina (gyrate atrophy)
B$_{12}$ (cyanocobalamin)	—	Optic nerve (temporal atropy with corresponding visual field defects)
C (ascorbic acid)	Lens (? cataract formation)	—
E (tocopherol)	—	Retina and retinal pigment epithelium (macular degeneration)
K	Conjunctiva (haemorrhage)	Retina (haemorrhage)
Zinc	—	Retina and retinal pigment epithelium (? macular degeneration)

Important physical characteristics are : viscosity, elasticity, cohesiveness and coatability.

Viscoelastic Substances

* Methyl cellulose
* Hydroxyethyl cellulose
* Hydroxypropylmethyl cellulose
* Carboxymethyl cellulose
* Polyvinyl alcohol
* Polyvinyl acrylamide
* Silicone polymers
* Sodium hyaluronate
* Poloxamer

Methyl Cellulose is most commonly employed to increase viscosity in ophthalmic solutions.

0.5% methyl cellulose in buffered isotonic sodium chloride solution makes excellent artificial tears.

Methyl cellulose containing formulations remain in contact with cornea for longer time due to increased viscosity.

Methyl cellulose acts as a cushioning agent during intraocular surgery. It can be filled in the anterior chamber during surgery instead of air.

Hydroxypropylmethyl cellulose: It can be applied over IOL and injected into the anterior chamber before lens insertion. It is removed by aspiration.

Post operatively, increase in IOP with this agent is lesser than with Healon.

Corneal thickness increases initially but returns to normal.

Polyvinyl acrylamide: Its effect lasts longer than polyvinyl vehicle.

Polyvinyl Alcohol : Solution containing 1.4 to 4% polyvinyl alcohol possesses a viscosity of 440 centipoise which is less than the viscosity of methyl cellulose. Because of its low surface tension and good adhesive qualities it forms a transparent film providing greater surface contact time than methyl cellulose.

Carboxy methyl cellulose: It has been found very successful in severe keratoconjunctivitis sicca. No adverse effects have been reported. This cellulose derivative has been used in procedure like cataract extraction, corneal transplants and glaucoma procedures.

Silicone Polymers (silicone oils): These are inert protectives. Silicone oil with viscosity of 1000-8000 centistokes in commonly used during vitreous surgery.

Sodium Hyaluronate (also known as Healon) : It is a large polysaccharide molecule present in all soft connective tissue matrices of vertebrates. It functions as a natural lubricating and shock absorbing substance in musculoskeletal system and eye.

Its viscosity is about 100000-300000 centipoise.

It has been used as an adjuvant to promote tissue repair. It acts as endothelial protective. It has been successfully used in intraocular lens implantation. Diluted Sodium hyaluronate has low viscosity than Healon.

It is nontoxic and inert substance and does not adhere to intraocular surface. At the end of the surgical procedure, it is aspirated from the anterior chamber, since it blocks the trabecular meshwork.

Poloxamers: Poloxamer 407 is converted to gel at room temperature. It is similar to mucin.

Complications of viscoelastic substances are related to transient increase in IOP after surgical procedures.

Uses of viscoelastic substances

1. In cataract extraction
   * to protect the endothelium
   * to form anterior chamber
   * to cover IOL so that endothelium is not touched by IOL
   * to expand the capsular bag for IOL insertion.
2. In keratoplasty
3. In case of glaucoma surgery
   * In posterior segment surgeries
     - as a vitreous replacement substance
     - to protect the corneal endothelium
   * Miscellaneous uses include
     - Use during gonioscopic examination
     - Many ophthalmic topical preparations have methyl cellelose as a vehicle
     - Contact lens solutions contain methyl cellulose as a buffering agent
     - artificial tear drops contain methyl cellulose

Oxygen

Normal oxygen levels are essential for the function of tissues. Retina has high metabolic rate and is vulnerable to alteration in oxygen levels.

Hypoxia causes loss of function and excessive concentrations are also toxic to the eyes.

As low as 20% oxygen may be hazardous due to the increased affinity of infant's haemoglobin for oxygen. If infant is exposed for about 12 hours some degree of retinal scarring may be produced.

In normal adult volunteers, after breathing 100% oxygen after 5 minutes the retinal vessel diameter decrease by about 12%, RBC velocity by 5% and blood flow by 69%.

Hyperbaric oxygen

It is indicated in several conditions such as burns, CO poisoning, cyanide poisoning, optic neuropathy, etc.

Oxygen is even more toxic to retina under hyperbaric conditions. It should be used with great care because if used for prolonged period it may produce myopia and nuclear sclerotic cataracts.

It is known that diseased eye has reduced oxygen tolerance. Hence, hyperbaric oxygen should be used with great caution while treating various disorders.

ALCOHOL (ethanol, ethyl alcohol)

The retrobulbar injection of absolute or 95% alcohol (0.5-1 ml) has been advocated for the treatment of painful blind eyes. The procedure may have to be repeated because the sensory fibres of the ciliary nerves are capable of regeneration and pain may recur after some months.

Ethanol can counteract the visual toxicity of methanol, because ethanol has a higher affinity than methanol for alcohol dehydrogenase (enzyme responsible for oxidation of both ethanol and methanol). When due to higher affinity, this enzyme is saturated with ethyl alcohol, formate formation is reduced. The initial dose is 0.75 g/kg body weight, then doses of 0.5g/kg, 4 hourly for 2-3 days are recommended for this purpose. The eye damage may be completely prevented.

Adverse effects

Splash contact of ethyl alcohol with eye causes immediate burning and stinging, and tearing.

Industrial exposure to high concentration of alcohol vapours produce stinging and watering of the eyes.

Acute alcohol poisoning can produce a number of ocular side effects such as reduction of IOP and accommodation, diplopia, nystagmus, colour vision defect, slowed dark adaptation, prolonged recovery time from glare and transient blindness.

Chronic alcoholism may produce ocular muscle palsies, miosis and sluggish pupillary reaction to light, amblyopia (partially or completely reversible).

The ocular side effects of acute alcohol poisoning are given in Table 21.30.

Table 21.30. Ocular side effects of acute alcohol poisoning

Lowering of ocular pressure
Range of fusion decreased; exophoria for near, esophoria for distance; produces tropias
Accommodation reduced; lowering of accommodative convergence/accommodation ratio
Diplopia; impairment of binocular fusion mechanism
Nystagmus
Decreased colour vision (80% of chronic alcoholics have red-green defects)
Reduced flicker fusion frequency
Slowed dark adaptation
Prolonged recovery time from glare
Reduced visual-evoked potential
Transient blindness

Tobacco-alcohol amblyopia

It occurs in persons who smoke, drink alcohol and have poor nutrition. There is a progressive bilateral optic neuropathy.

Methyl alcohol

3g/kg body weight produces mild intoxication

6g/kg body weight produces semicoma, followed by respiratory failure and death.

The acute toxicity of methanol is somewhat less than that of ethanol.

Methanol produces formaldehyde which is further oxidized to formic acid which produces intense acidosis.

Formation of formaldehyde in the retina is responsible for the main ocular toxic effects including blindness.

Quinine

The status of quinine as an antimalarial drug is discussed in Chapter 11.

Quinine has limited value in the treatment of myokymia due to its curare-like effect. Oral administration of 0.32 g repeated several times a day relieves twitching of the orbicularis muscle. However, quinine produces several ocular adverse effects including blurred vision, constricted visual field, scotomas, disturbed colour vision and even amblyopia (it may be sudden).

Quinine is of ophthalmic interest because of its characteristic ocular toxicity. The adverse effects of quinine include blurred vision, constricted visual field, scotomas, disturbed colour vision and even blindness.

Quinine poisoning, if it persists for about 2 weeks there is retinal swelling and cherry red macula (same appearance as produced by bilateral acute occlusion of the central retinal artery).

Quinine amblyopia

It is a toxic effect acting directly on the ganglion cells. The swelling of this layer of the retina resembles occlusion of the central retinal artery. As the cause of visual loss is severe vasoconstriction, vasodilator therapy has been advised (which does not appear rational if the primary toxic effect is directly on the ganglion cells).

There is hardly any drug known that benefits amblyopia.

The onset of quinine amblyopia may be sudden and spontaneous partial recovery frequently occurs.

Quinine in large doses can also damage iris resulting in a dilated irregular pupil with poor light reaction.

Chloroquine

It is a useful antimalarial drug, possesses slight quinidine like effect as well as anti-inflammatory property (useful in the treatment of rheumatoid arthritis). It is also a useful drug for the treatment of amoebiasis and giardiasis. The status of chloroquine in the treatment of these conditions has been discussed in Chapter 11.

The *adverse effects* of chloroquine are of interest in ophthalmology. The ocular toxicity includes blurring of vision, visual disturbances and severe (and often permanent) retinal eye damage due to prolonged administration of chloroquine in high doses.

About 10 to 30% of patients taking large doses of chloroquine develop corneal deposits (usually symptomless) which always regress when chloroquine is discontinued. However, if high daily doses (more than 250 mg) are administered for the treatment of diseases other than malaria it can result in irreversible ototoxicity and retinopathy.

Besides ocular toxicity, there are several other side effects which are described in Chapter 11.

OCULAR TOXICITY DUE TO DRUGS

The list of drugs toxic to the eye is long. However, the list of "worst offenders" would include : anti-inflammatory agents of the aminoquinoline family e.g. chloroquine, phenothiazine tranquillizers (e.g. chlorpromazine, thioridazine) and corticosteroids. Certain other drugs such as chloramphenicol, ethambutol and anti-cholinergics can also produce ocular adverse effects.

Drugs applied topically in the eye as well as certain drugs administered for the treatment of various systemic diseases e.g. diabetes mellitus, hypertension etc. may produce, ocular adverse effects.

The factors which influence the occurrence of adverse reactions are :

Age : The metabolism in children and elderly persons is different to that of adults and therefore they are more susceptible to adverse drug reactions.

Sex : Many middle-aged women have a tendency to become more tear deficient than men.

Weight : Variation in fat/water ratio is more likely to occur in obese persons.

General state of health : The rate of elimination of drugs is reduced in the presence of liver and kidney dysfunction.

Ophthalmic state of health : A patient with a narrow anterior chamber angle closure may occur in case of dilated pupil. In a patient with slightly constricted pupil, miosis will be a great problem.

Concurrent medication : Drug-drug interaction may occur when two or more drugs are administered together.

Contact lenses : If the tear film is reduced, the patient may have problems in wearing the contact lenses.

TOXICITY DUE TO DRUGS ON DIFFERENT SYSTEMS

Drugs acting on the alimentary tract: Drugs such as Dicyclomine, Hyoscine and Probanthine can produce mydriasis and cycloplegia (mild and transitory).

Drugs acting on cardiovascular system: Cardiotonic drugs, diuretics, anti-arrhythmics, beta-blockers, antihypertensives and anticoagulants can directly affect the ocular tissues as well as indirectly by producing fluctuations in blood pressure and blood flow.

Cardiotonics mainly cardiac glycosides may produce ocular adverse effects including disturbance in colour vision and a glare phenomonon (objects appear to be surrounded by a white halo). Visual field may be affected. Digitalis may reduce IOP which is not significant.

Diuretics such as acetazolamide, thiazides, spironolactone, triameterene (potassium sparing) may produce slight myopia which also regresses spontaneously.

Anti-arrhythmic drugs such as amiodarone and disopyramide can produce certain ocular adverse effects.

Amiodarone produces in cornea yellow-brown deposits which disappear slowly after discontinuation of the drug. Vision can also be blurred.

Disopyramide may produce mydriasis and blurred vision due to its anticholinergic effect. The beta-blockers e.g. atenolol, labetalol, metoprolol, oxprenolol, propranolol etc. are safe and ocular adverse effects are mild and transient.

Antihypertensives such as clonidine may produce retinal changes, resulting in visual loss; methyldopa affects the anterior eye; hydralazine may produce bilateral retinal vasculitis.

Drugs acting on the respiratory system: These are usually corticosteroids, antihistamines and bronchodilators.

A well-documented adverse effect of topically administered anti-inflammatory corticosteroids is their potential for increasing intraocular pressure. Intraocular pressure may also be increased after systemic therapy, but this effect is much less common. Pressure increases occur in a matter of weeks after topical administration whereas they occur in a matter of months after systemic therapy. The increase in pressure reverses in most cases on withdrawing the drug. However, if the pressure increases go unrecognized, irreversible damage can occur.

The increase in intraocular pressure is due to reduction in the outflow caused by an accumulation of insoluble polymerized acid mucopolysaccharides leading to water retention.

Increased resistance to outflow of aqeous humour is probably the mechanism by which corticosteroids produce pressure rises.

Posterior subcapsular cataract formation is a known complication of long-term high-dose systemic administration of corticosteroids. Generally, high doses for a period of one year or more are required for cataract production. Vision is not usually impaired initially. Regression of the cataract is not always noted when therapy is discontinued.

Corticosteroids such as betamethasone, dexamethasone, prednisolone, fludrocortisone, triamcinolone and methyl prednisolone are notorious for producing a number of unwanted effects.

Systemic use of corticosteroids can produce cataract in about 30% patients, the cataract is situated below the posterior capsule and occurs after a year's treatment. Cataract is rarely produced by topical application.

Antihistamines such as chlorpheniramine, promethazine, terfenadine etc. can produce slight mydriasis and cycloplegia, depressed secretion of tears.

Bronchodilators such as ephedrine, orciprenaline, pseudoephedrine, salbutamol, terbutaline can produce slight mydriasis. Large doses of ephedrine can lead to visual hallucinations.

Drugs Acting on Nervous System

Phenothiazine antipsychotic medications may produce ocular side effects including diplopia, myopia, and oculogyric crisis. These effects are dose-dependent and rapidly reverse on discontinuing therapy.

Corneal and lens opacities have been observed in patients receiving usually over 300 mg of chlorpromazine daily for periods of 3 years or more years. In few cases chlorpromazine produces retinal toxic effect if about 2.5g daily is taken for 2 or more years.

Thioridazine is associated with significant retinotoxicity. Doses of thioridazine below 800 mg daily are considered low enough to avoid irreversible retinal toxicity.

Phenothiazine derivatives accumulate in the choroid and retina. Conjunctival pigmentation in the form of grayish brown discolouration is a dose-related adverse effect seen in conjunction with other phototoxic effects of phenothiazines.

Patient with narrow filtration angles i.e. those with a predisposition for an attack of acute glaucoma may have an attack of acute angle closure glaucoma precipitated by doses of anticholinergic medications which are large enough to produce sustained wide mydriasis.

Systemically administered antichlolinergics have little effect on IOP in the nondiseased eye. In patients with open-angle glaucoma, rises in IOP are seen when patients ingest anticholinergics while not taking topical glaucoma medications.

Antipsychotic agents

Antipsychotic agents or neuroleptics such as chlorpromazine, promazine, trifluoroperazine, thioridazine and haloperidol (these are phenothiazine derivatives, with the exception of haloperidol), if used for longer period can produce ocular adverse effects. These drugs have antimuscarinic effects. They affect the iris and ciliary muscles resulting in loss of accommodation and mydriasis.

The long term use of large doses of chlorpromazine can produce pigmentary deposits, appearing first on the lens surface, in the pupillary area, then affecting Descemet's membrane.

Phenothiazines may produce retinopathy resulting in visual problems.

Haloperidol (a butyrophenone) may cause mydriasis.

Anxiolytic agents

Anxiolytic drugs such as diazepam, lorazepam and a number of other benzodiazepines if used for a longer period produce few ocular adverse reactions which are reversible, including decreased accommodation and a reduction in corneal reflex. Patients who are allergic develop allergic conjunctivitis.

Hypnotics and sedatives

Barbiturate addicts may develop decreased convergence or nystagmus due to the effect on extraocular muscles.

Benzodiazepines produce few ocular adverse effects such as blurred vision (due to loss of accommodation or abnormal extraocular movements).

Antiparkinsonism agents

Amantadine may produce visual hallucinations. Benzhexol due to antimuscarinic effect may produce loss of accommodation and mydriasis. The dopaminergic drugs such as levodopa produces initial mydriasis followed by persistent miosis.

Antiepileptic drugs such as ethosuximide, phenytoin and sodium valproate may produce nystagmus and diplopia. Phenytoin has been reported to produce Stevens-Johnson syndrome.

Antidepressants

Among the tricyclic antidepressants, amitriptyline can produce marked sedation. The other antidepressants of the same class eg. imipramine is much less sedative.

Regarding the ocular adverse effects, all tricyclic antidepressants can cause mydriasis and cycloplegia as they possess anticholinergic properties. These effects are reversible.

Anti-infective agents

Chloramphenicol can produce optic neuritis. Acute bilateral loss of visual acuity, with field constriction, are early symptoms. Progress for return of normal visual function is variable on discontinuation of therapy.

Sulphonamides may cause keratoconjunctivitis. Tetracyclines may produce transient myopia, colour vision defects, as well as certain ocular effects such as papilloedema and diplopia which are due to the penetration of tetracyclines into the cerebrospinal fluid. Besides these adverse effects, tetracyclines can be secreted in tears and stain soft contact lenses.

Some **antibiotics, particularly penicillin** may produce allergic reactions which may involve eyes.

Urinary antiseptics

Ocular irritation and profuse lacrimation can be produced by nitrofurantoin which regress when the drug is discontinued. Nalidixic acid can produce disturbances in colour vision and glare, which regress on discontinuation of the drug.

Antimalarials

Antimalarials such as chloroquine, hydroxychloroquine and quinine can cause several ocular adverse effects. These can affect both retina and cornea. Effects on the cornea include deposits in the superficial cornea and sub-epithelial layers. Pigmentary changes occur in the retina giving rise to the well-known 'bull's eye maculopathy'.

A few months of **chloroquine** therapy may produce deposits in the superficial cornea and sub-epithelial layers which appear greyish white. Patients who have visual complaints may see halos around lights or experience photophobia. Some may have corneal deposits which completely disappear after the drug is stopped.

Chloroquine - retinopathy is the most severe manifestation of ocular toxicity induced by this agent and unless diagnosed in the earliest stages it is not reversible. In some cases retinopathy is delayed and occurs after the drug is discontinued. It is estimated that a total dose of more than 100 gm during a period of one year must be taken for retinopathy to develop.

The adverse effects include pigmentary changes in retina giving rise to the well known 'bull's eye maculopathy', constricted visual fields and scotomata. These effects are dose dependent and unfortunately continue to develop even when the drug is stopped.

Quinine amblyopia may be due to a direct effect of over dosage of quinine on the ganglion cells.

Anthelminthic drugs like piperazine can produce ocular adverse effects such as cycloplegia and extraocular muscle paralysis.

Antituberculosis drugs

Ethambutol can produce optic neuritis which regresses slowly in some cases but in some other cases it is permanent. The optic neuritis may take two forms, an axial and a paraxial form. The central fibres of the optic nerve when involved (axial form) will result in changes in colour vision, loss of central visual acuity and macular degeneration. In case of paraxial form, central acuity and colour vision are not affected but visual field defects occur. Toxic effects on optic nerve can also be produced by isoniazid and streptomycin. Rifampicin produces a pink coloured by-product which can be excreted in tears and will colour soft contact lenses. It can also cause conjunctivitis.

Ethambutol can produce optic neuritis and atrophy. Decrease in visual acuity, central scotoma, and green-colour blindness is seen at high doses, e.g. 25mg/kg/day.

Anti-inflammatory drugs

Non-steroidal anti-inflammatory drugs (NSAIDs): The nonsteroidal anti-inflammatory drugs such as ibuprofen, indomethacin, ketoprofen, naproxen and others can produce ocular adverse effects including reduced colour vision and visual acuity. Indomethacin can induce retinopathy, similar to that produced by chloroquine. There is contraction of the visual field and a granular appearance of the fundus and diplopia. The effects are transitory. Blurred vision can be produced by ibuprofen.

Drugs acting on the blood

Desferrioxamine can produce minor changes in the retinal function.

Drugs acting on the endocrine system

Antidiabetic drugs

Chlorpropamide may produce toxic amblyopia, and other adverse effects such as diplopia.

Corticosteroids

Corticosteroids are very notorious for the adverse effects they produce. Systemic uses can produce cataract after a year's treatment. Topical use rarely leads to cataract formation.

Topical ophthalmic use of corticosteroids increase intraocular pressure. It may affect one eye only in which the drug has been used topically. If a patient receiving corticosteroid develops IOP greater than 21 mmHg, subsequent corticosteroid therapy should be under strict supervision.

Oral contraceptives

So far as the ocular adverse effects are concerned with the use of oral contraceptives, there are certain reports which indicate the possible incompatibility between the pill and wearing of contact lenses but the problem may be due to overwear, humidity changes and infection and not due to the pill.

For ready reference, the following Tables 21.31 to 21.34 list the adverse effects produced by certain commonly used drugs. In majority of cases these unwanted effects are produced due to over dosage and long term use. In many cases the adverse effects are reversible.

Ocular adverse effects are summarized in the following tables :

Table 21.31 Ocular adverse effects following systemic medication.

Table 21.32 Systemic adverse effects following topical ocular medication.

Table 21.33 Ocular adverse effects following topical ocular medication.

Table 21.34 Agents affecting specific ocular area.

Table 21.31. Ocular adverse effects following systemic medication

Medication	Adverse effects
Alimentary tract	
Probanthine	mydriasis, cycloplegia
Cardiovascular system	
Digitalis	colour distortions, blurred vision
Quinidine	toxic amblyobia
Amiodarone	corneal deposit, lens opacities
Oxprenolol	dry eyes, scaring of conjunctiva and cornea
Propranolol	visual hallucinations
Hydralazine	bilateral retinal vasculitis
Respiratory system	
Corticosteroids	posterior subcapsular cataracts, increased IOP, aggravations of herpes simplex keratitis, ptosis, papilloedema
Antihistamines	mydriasis, cycloplegia, reduced tear flow
Bronchodilators	mild mydriasis, hallucinations with ephedrine
Nervous system	
Antipsychotic agents	
Chlorpromazine	pigment deposition in anterior portion of lens,
Prochlorperazine	rolling up of eyes,
Thioridazine	pigmentary retinopathy
Anxiolytic agents	
Diazepam	Allergic conjunctivitis
Antiparkinsonism drugs	
Amantadine	visual hallucinations
Benztropine	blurring of vision, mydriasis, cyclopegia
Levodopa	initial mydriasis followed by miosis, ptosis, blepharospasm
Antiepileptics	
Phenytoin	nystagmus, diplopia, weakness of convergence and of accommodation
Antidepressants	
Lithium carbonate	blurred vision, accommodative weakness

(Contd.)

Medication	Adverse effects
Monoamine Oxidase inhibitors (MAOIs)	mydriasis, papilloedema, optic atrophy
Tricylic antidepressants	increased IOP, accommodation impaired

Anti-infective agents

Antimicrobials

Penicillin	allergic reactions
Chloramphenicol	optic neuritis, central scotoma, toxic amblyopia
Tetracylines	blurred vision, diplopia, papilloedema
Streptomycin	optic neuritis,
Sulphonamides	conjunctival and corneal scarring, Stevens-Johnson syndrome

Antitubercular drugs

Ethambutol	opitc neuritis,
Rifampicin	conjunctival hyperemia and lacrimation,
Isoniazid	optic neuritis, optic atrophy

Urinary antiseptics

Nalidixic acid	colour vision defects and glare,
Nitrofurantoin	ocular irritation, profuse lacrimation

Antiparasitic drugs

Chloroquine	corneal deposit, bilateral macular degeneration,
Quinine	toxic amblyopia

Antineoplastic drugs

Adriamycin	lacrimation, conjunctivitis,
Busulfan	cataracts,
Chlorambucil	keratitis, retinal haemorrhage,
5-FU	lacrimation, conjunctivitis,
Methotrexate	cataract, photophobia,
Vincristine	ptosis, diplopia,
Cyclophosphamide	dry eye

Anti-inflammatory drugs (Non-steroidal)

Ibuprofen	blurred vision, colour vision defect, optic neuritis,
Indomethacin	corneal deposits, mydriasis, diplopia, retinopathy,
Phenylbutazone	conjunctival and corneal scarring, Steven-Johnson syndrome,
Oxyphenbutazone	
Naproxen	scotomas, blurring of vision, cataract, optic neuritis

Medication	Adverse effects
Drugs acting on the blood	
Desferrioxamine	retrobulbar neuritis
Anticoagulants	intraocular haemorrhage
Endocrine system	
Antidiabetic drugs	
Chlorpropamide	toxic amblyopia
Oral contraceptives	occlusion of retinal arteries and veins, retinal haemorrhages, corneal oedema, nystagmus, contact lens intolerance (rare)
Miscellaneous	
Tobacco	toxic amblyopia, colour vision defect, central scotomas,
Nicotinic acid	reduced vision due to maculopathy,
Vitamin A	blurred vision due to papilloedema
Vitamin D	conjunctival opacities, corneal calcification,
Oxygen	retrolental fibroplasia

Table 21.32. Systemic adverse effects following topical ocular medication

Medication	Adverse effects
Local Anaesthetics	
Benoxinate	allergic reactions, hypotension
Tetracaine	same as benoxinate
Antimicrobials	
Sulphacetamide	photosensitivity, Steven-Johnson syndrome,
Chloramphenicol	allergic reactions, bone marrow depression,
Tetracycline	photosensitivity, skin discolouration
Anticholinergics	
Atropine	dry mouth, fever, thirst, tachycardia, confusion, dermatitis, psychosis
Cyclopentolate	disorientation, psychosis, hallucinations, amnesia
Homatropine, Scopolamine	same as atropine
Tropicamide	same as cyclopentolate
Long acting anticholinesterase	
Demecarium	nausea, abdominal pain, rhinorrhoea

(Contd.)

Medication	Adverse effects
Short acting anticholinesterases	
Neostigmine	abdominal cramps, nausea, vomiting,
Physostigmine	diarrhoea
Adrenoceptor Beta-blocker	
Timolol	hallucinations, psychosis, confusion, dizziness, depression, arrhythmia, bradycardia
Parasympathomimetics	
Carbachol	diarrhoea, hypotension, increased salivation, nausea, vomiting, rhinorrhoea, abdominal cramps
Pilocarpine	same as carbachol
Sympathomimetics	
Epinephrine	cardiac arrhythmia, palpitation, tachycardia
Ephedrine	same as epinephrine, and hallucinations
Phenylepherine	same as epinephrine

Table 21.33. Ocular adverse effects following ocular topical medication

Medication	Adverse effects
Epinephrine	discolouration of conjunctiva, cornea, and soft contact lens, decreased lacrimal out flow
Pilocarpine	myopia, retinal detachment, accommodative spams
Timolol	dry eyes, diplopia, ptosis, keratitis
Idoxuridine, Vidarabine	keratitis, lacrimal outflow obstruction
Corticosteroids	cataracts, corneal thinning, decreased corneal wound healing, infection, increased IOP
Chlortetracyline	allergic reactions, corneal
Tetracycline	discolouration
Neomycin	allergic reactions, conjunctivitis, keratitis

CONTACT LENS CARE

General Guidelines

- Hands to be cleaned before insertion or removal
- Lens should be cleaned with normal saline before insertion

Table 21.34. Agents affecting specific ocular areas.

Agents	Specific areas
Corticosteroids, miotics, busulfan	Cataract
Ethambulol, INH, methanol, lead, sulphonamides, streptomycin	optic neuritis
Chloramphenicol, ethambulol, dicoumarol	Retinal haemorrhages
Acetazolamide, urea	Anterior chamber shallowing
Carbon monoxide, isoniazid, methanol	Optic atrophy
Copper, iron, mercury, silver after local penetration; siver, chlorpromazine, silver, copper, mercury after systemic use	Lens deposits and discolouration
Digitalis, ethambutol, INS, nicotinic acid tolbutamide, chlorpropamide, tobacco smoking	Retro bulbar neuritis
	Eye and Lid movement disturbances
Barbiturates diazepam, phenytoin ethanol, streptomycin	Nystagmus
Haloperidol, Phenothiazine derivatives	Oculogyric crisis
Diazepam, ethanol, lidocaine, phenytoin, imipramine	Diplopia
Barbiturates, curare, reserpine	Ptosis of eyelids
Adrenaline	Pigmentation
Thio-tepa, Physostigmine	Depigmentation
Spinal anaesthesia, barbiturates, curare, ethanol, streptomycin	Paralysis of extraocular muscles
Chloral hydrate, hydralazine (systemic use)	Lid oedema
Reserpine, guanethidine, vincristine	Eyelid, eyelash, eyebrow disturbances
Chloroquine	Poliosis
Actinomycin D, vitamin A, nicotinic acid, tolbutamide, tobacco, smoking	Alopecia

- Store lens in air tight case, fully immersed in multipurpose solution. Never let lens dry.
- Solution in case should be replaced every 2-3 days
- Never boil lens
- Solutions using benzalkonium chloride

preservative should never be used with soft lens.
- Thiomersal containing solutions cause toxic reactions to the eye.
- Do not sleep with lenses on.

An ideal contact lens solution should possess the following qualities:
- Should be non-toxic
- Non-irritant
- Non-allergenic
- Stable

Solutions employed in the care and use of contact lenses (CL) may be **categorized** as follows :
1. Wetting Solutions
2. Cleaning Solutions
3. Soaking Solutions
4. Combination Purpose Solutions

The **prerequisites** of all contact lens solutions are :
- They must be sterile, stable and transparent
- All solutions must be harmless to the eye if instilled undiluted
- They must not have adverse effects on the contact lens material
- They must be compatible with all other solutions used for the same lens material.
- In addition to being sterile; if presented in multipurpose form, all solutions should be self-sustaining.

Adverse Reactions of Solution

- Discomfort on insertion
- Photophobia
- Epiphora
- Conjunctival hyperemia
- Decreased wearing time
- Possible mild diffuse superficial punctate keratitis
- Possible intraepithelial microcytes and/or perilimbal infiltrates if the condition has been present for some time.

Cleaning Methods

Surfactant Cleaners (Surface active agents) :
- Lower surface tension of oil or solid-water surfaces (emulsify lipids).

- Help remove lipids (emulsify lipids), mascara, lip sticks, facial make-up, calcium salts before deposition, and protein before it becomes denatured. They solubilise debris and remove accumulated contaminants most favourably in an alkaline (pH 7.4 & above) environment.
- Improve wettability of a lens.
- Break up and disperse particles that adhere to its surface.

Surfactants

Although anionic, non-anionic and amphoteric (balanced positive and negative constituents) surfactants are used in contact lens cleaning products, preference seems to favour non-ionic cleaners, because non-ionic surfactants e.g. polysorbates are :
- More chemically compatible
- More stable
- Lens toxic

Anionic surfactant consists of carboxylate, sulphonate, sulphate ions e.g. soap

Cationic e.g. benzalkonium chloride used more as preservative rather than surfactant.

Amphoteric, e.g. lecithins.

Household detergents such as soaps, dish cleaners and shampoos are not recommended. They contain strong ionic detergents. They produce harsh action on the lens surface or potential damage to cornea. They interact with cationic preservatives such as benzalkonium, chlorhexidine and cetyl pyridinium resulting in deposition of water-insoluble film on the lens.

Cleaning and Wetting

Common solution for cleaning and wetting is termed Multipurpose Solution. It usually contains :
- Sodium borate (maintains neutral pH).
- Sodium chloride (makes the solution isotonic).
- Poloxamine (a non-ionic surfactant, removes lipids).
- Disodium edetate (chelating agent), removes loosely bound proteins, calcium and other deposits.
- Dymed (polyamino - propyl biguanide (anti-microbial agent, non-toxic to ocular tissue).

Some cleaning solutions contain thiomersal (banned in Japan and Canada), and benzalkonium chloride (usually do not have neutral pH). Chlorhexidine is antimicrobial but less than dymed and has tendency to bind to lens material and to protein deposits on lens surface. It can also cause more irritation and sensitization.

DEPOSITS OF CONTACT LENSES AND THEIR MANAGEMENT

Types of Deposits

- Protein
- Lipid
- Mucin
- Inorganic
- Environmental
- Cosmetic factors influencing lens deposits

Factors influencing lens deposits

1. Lens material. Lipid deposits are more commonly formed on hard lenses, whereas protein deposits are more common on soft lens material.
2. Patient variation. Environmental and climatic factors influence the tear quality which in turn results in variation of deposits in individual patients.
3. The frequency of protein deposits is reduced if proper cleaning in clean water and enzymatic cleaning at recommended intervals is done. Thermal disinfection systems accelerate protein deposition on soft lenses.
4. Environmental factors. Factors like heat, dust, smoke, pollens, and cosmetics influence deposits. Dry climate leads to lipid deposits.

Lens deposits produce symptoms such as foreign body sensation, photophobia, red eye, reduced visual acuity and discomfort. Lens wettability is reduced and there is risk of infection. Giant papillary conjunctivitis may also be produced.

LENS DEPOSITS

Protein Deposits

Protein is a natural component of human tears. In time this protein or mucin secreted by the glands of the eyelid and found in the tears will have a tendency to stick to the surface of the soft lens and coat it. Protein deposits are resistant to prophylactic cleaning regimen.

Protein deposits develop from the interaction of the contact lens with proteins in the aqueous tear film layer. The tear protein lysozyme has a strong affinity for most soft lens material. Lysozyme is a positively charged small size protein and hence it binds strongly. The bond between lysozyme and lens material is referred to as ionic bond. The deposited proteins get denatured which gives more symptoms. Hence, the longer the time interval of protein deposits, more the denaturation and more symptoms.

Most common type of protein film is white, partially opaque.

Enzymatic Cleaners for Protein Deposits

They remove protein deposits and have no direct effect on other types of deposits like lipids. Ca, environmental or cosmetics.

An enzyme is a protein with active sites. These active sites enable the enzyme to perform specific chemical reactions. These work to break chemical bonds of the protein deposits primary structure i.e. amino acid sequence. The broken protein fragments are readily removed by the post cleaning rinse step.

The enzyme works differently from a detergent. Enzyme breaks down proteinaceous deposits whereas detergent can remove only loosely deposited matter.

- Chemical disinfection is better than heat
- Use proteolytic enzyme weekly.

Preparations used

1. Papain enzyme tablet degrades protein into proteases and peptones. After weekly papain treatment incidence of deposit is significantly reduced.

   Disadvantage of papain is that some patients experience discomfort or mild conjunctival hyperemia. It is essential that lenses are not soaked for more than 2-3 hours in enzyme solution and careful surfactant cleaning is carried out after the treatment.

   Lenses must be disinfected with hydrogen peroxide following enzymatic cleaning to destroy any residual enzyme that might cause damage to the corneal epithelium.

2. Pancreatin tablets contain trypsin, chymotrypsin and carboxy peptidase as proteases; amylase to break down polysaccharides (mucins); deoxyribonuclease; lipase. The current name of lipase is glycerol ester hydrolase.

3. Pronase tablets contain 3 enzymes - a bacterial protease (subtilisin) isolated from bacillus subtilis; a lipase isolated from Rhizopus and pronase a proteolytic enzyme obtained from streptomyces griseus which removes mucus. The efficacy of subtilisin is greater than papain and pancreatin due to its less specific binding characteristics. It breaks most protein bonds into fragments.

These are basically aimed to remove protein deposits. They do not have any direct effect on deposits like lipid, Ca, cosmetics.

Lipid Deposits

Lipid appears as greasy deposit on the lens surface. Lipid may also be present from meibomian glands and by finger contacts.

Lipids from tear-film, cosmetics, skin lotions can bind to lens material. Since lipids are hydrophobic, they reduce the wettability of the lens material resulting in patient discomfort.

Some times lipid deposits combine with protein and calcium to form jelly bump-deposits which may bore a hole into the lens.

Lipid appears as greasy deposit on the lens surface.

Caution and cleaners for lipid deposits

• Avoid chlorhexidine - preserved solutions because this increases surface hydrophobicity and allows lipid adhesion.
• Use specific lipase cleaners.
• Lipids and mucin are easily removed by surfactants cleaning but the white calculi on lens surface are stubborn which can not be removed either by surfactant or enzymatic cleaning.

Calcium Deposits

The main cause appears to be precipitation and growth of calcium phosphate from tears. Calcium phosphate may form as a result of interaction between free Ca ions in the tears and phosphate buffers used in certain solution, the resulting phosphate is insoluble and precipitated out in lens matrix.

Ca salts may be deposited from lacrimal fluid. Calcium salts form a hazy white surface layer often resembling protein. The presence of protein films may also predispose the ions to the build up of inorganic materials because protein-covered lens surface becomes hydrophobic.

There is alternate layer of protein and Ca so that cleaner for both types of deposits are necessary.

Caution and cleaners for calcium deposits

• Less with thermal disinfection
• Use hydrogen peroxide (low pH dissolves)
• Use protective enzyme weekly
• Use Ca deposit preventor

Preventor contains a heat-activated chelating agent (sodium hexameta-phosphate).

It removes Ca ions present in or on lens matrix.

Sodium edetate 0.1% solution (EDTA, Ethylene-diamine tetra acetic acid) is a chelating agent which removes Ca ions. It has synergistic action with benzalkonium chloride, antagonizes action of thiomersal.

Calculi

Lens Calculi (jelly bumps, mulberry-like growth) appear as small white elevations on the lens surface. These deposits are an annulus, the central 'hole' is filled with mucus. The outer annulus is mainly lipid on which secondary calcium salts have deposited.

Cleaners for Calculi

• Use lipid solvent cleaner
• Use lipase containing enzyme
• Use weekly intensive surfactant cleaner

Pigment deposits

Pigment deposits in soft lenses are usually yellow to brown. They are made up of a melanin-like polymer derived from the polymerization of aromatic compounds in the tears. Because melanin is formed by oxidative polymerization, the rate of melanin formation may be increased by thermal disinfection procedures.

Stains

These are often caused by a change in the polymer itself which no chemical treatment will remove. Hence, the use of stain removers and neutralizing solutions should not be attempted by the wearer.

Cosmetic Deposits

Cosmetics such as kajal, eye shadow, mascara and hair sprays are other sources of lens contamination. Hand lotions often contain lipids which may be transferred to the lens during handling.

Environmental Deposits

Dust, dirt, smoke, chemical fumes can be deposited which cause discomfort and conjunctivitis. Nicotine from cigar and cigarette smoke can be deposited which may appear as brownish colouration throughout the lens.

STUDY QUESTIONS

1. Write short notes on (i) fluorescein sodium, (ii) Rose Bengal, (iii) ocusert, (iv) blood-ocular barriers, (v) hyperosmotic agents, (vi) visco-elastic agents (vii) adverse effects of quinine and chloroquine, (viii) Drugs and biological agents used in ophthalmic surgery.

2. Describe the factors which affect transcorneal absorption of drugs.

3. Describe routes of administration of drugs for ocular therapy.

4. Discuss anti-glaucoma drugs regarding their efficacy, mode of action and adverse drug reactions.

5. Describe the possible absorption pathways of an ocular drug following topical instillation in the eye.

6. How are drugs distributed after transcorneal absorptions ? How are they metabolized and excreted?

7. Describe the role of autonomic nervous system in eye. Name important autonomic drugs which act as adrenergic agonists, adrenergic antagonists, cholinergic agonists and cholinergic antagonists, used in ophthalmology.

8. Describe the ideal properties of mydriatics. How is mydriasis produced by different group of drugs? What are their uses and adverse effects?

9. Describe the ideal properties of miotics. Describe the source, preparations, mode of action, uses and adverse effects of pilocarpine.

10. Describe the ideal properties of cycloplegics. Name the drugs that produce cycloplegia. Discuss choice of cycloplegic drugs.

11. Give a list of topically used antibacterial, antifungal, and antiviral agents, along with their concentrations.

12. Which are the currently used ophthalmic immunosuppressive and antimitotic agents? What are their uses and adverse reactions?

13. Mention the ophthalmic effects of vitamin deficiencies in a tabulated form.

14. Describe the ocular indications for corticosteroids. What are their contraindications? Describe their ocular adverse effects, from local application as well as from prolonged systemic use.

15. Name the non-steroidal anti-inflammatory agents commonly employed in eye.

16. Discuss the merits and demerits of local anaesthetics employed in ophthalmic procedures.

17. Write short notes on (i) enzymatic cleaners for contact lens protein, lipid and calcium deposits, and (ii) surfactant cleaners.

18. What are the toxic effects of (i) chloroquine, (ii) quinine, (iii) ethambutol, (iv) phenothiazine derivatives, (v) pilocarpine and (vi) tobacco.

GUIDE TO FURTHER READING

Barnes PJ, Adcock I. (1993) Anti-inflammatory actions of steroids : molecular mechanisms. Trends Pharmacol Sci 172:436-441.

Behlau, I., and Baker, A.S. Fungal infections and the eye. In, Principles and Practice of Ophthalmology, Vol. 5. (Albert, D.M., and Jakobiec, F.A., eds.) W.B. Saunders Co., Philadelphia, 1994, pp. 3030-3064.

Bodor N. (1994) Designing softer ophthalmic drugs by soft drug approaches. J Ocul Pharmacol Ther 10:3-15.

Chylak, L.T. Medical treatment of cataract. In, Principles and Practice of Ophthalmology, Basic Sciences. (Albert, D.M., and Jakobiec, F.A., eds.) W.B. Saunders Co., Philadelphia, 1994, pp. 1107-1111.

DeSantis, L.M., and Patil, P.N. Pharmacokinetics. In, Havener's Ocular Pharmacology, 6th ed. (Mauger, T.F., and Craig, E.L., eds.) Mosby Year Book, Inc., St. Louis, 1994, pp. 22-52.

Duffner L.R., Pflugfelder S.C. (1990) Mandelbaum S et al : Potential bacterial contamination in fluorescein - anaesthetic solutions, Am J Ophthalmol 110:199.

Emest Jm. (1992) Topical antifungal agents. Obstet Gynecol Clin North Am 19:587-607.

Feenstra R.P., Scheffer C.G. Tseng C.G: (1992) What is actually stained by rose bengal ? Arch Ophthalmol 110:984.

Field, A.K. et al (1994) : Combination and monotherapy with zidovudine and zalcitabine in patients with advanced HIV disease. Ann. Intern. Med., 122:24-32.

Fraunfelder, F.T., and Meyer, S.M. Drug-Induced Ocular Side Effects and Drug Interactions, 3rd ed. Lea and Febiger,Philadelphia, 1989.

Fry LL. (1995) Efficacy of diclofenac sodium solution in reducing discomfort after cataract surgery. J Cataract Refract Surg 21:187-190.

Ginsburg AP, Chetham JK, DeGryse RE, Abelson M. (1995) Effects of flurbiprofen and indomethacin on acute cystoid macular edema after cataract surgery : functional vision and contrast sensitivity. J Cataract Refract Surg 21:82-92.

Hersh P.S. et al (1990) : Topical nonsteroidal agents and corneal wound healing, Arch Ophthalmol, 108:577-583.

Jankovic, J., and Hallett, M., eds. Therapy with Botulinum Toxin. Marcel Dekker, Inc., New York, 1994.

Kyncl J.J. et al (1993): Pharmacology of terazosin: an alphal-selective blocker J Clin Pharmacol., 33:878-883.

Liesegang, T.J. Viscoelastic substances in ophthalmology. Surv. Ophthal., 1990, 34:268-293.

Lonnquist, F. et al (1993): Evidence for a functional Beta3-adrenoceptor in man. Br. J. Pharmacol 110:929-936.

Mitra, A.K., ed. Ophthalmic Drug Delivery Systems. Marcel Dekker, Inc., New York, 1993.

O'Brien TP, Green WR. Fungus infections of the eye and periocular tissues. In: Garner A, Klintworth GK, eds. Pathobiology of ocular disease: a dynamic approach, part A, 2nd ed. New York: Marcel Dekker, 1994; 299-333.

Osako, M Keltner J.L. (1991) : Botulinum A toxin (Oculinum) in ophthalmology, Surv Ophthalmol, 36:28.

Physicians' Desk Reference for Ophthalmology, 23rd ed. Medical Economics Data Production Co., Montvale, NJ, 1995.

Polansky J.R. et al : (1990) Beta-adrenergic therapy for glaucoma, Int. Ophthalmol Clin, 30:219.

Robinson, J.C. Ocular anatomy and physiology relevant to ocular drug delivery. In, Ophthalmic Drug Delivery Systems. (Mitra, A.K., ed.) Marcel Dekker, Inc., New York, 1993, pp. 29-58.

Salminen L (1990) Review : Systemic absorption of topically applied ocular drugs in humans, J Ocul Pharmacol 6:243.

Schaffer D.B. et al (1985) : Vitamin E and retinopathy of prematurity, Ophthalmology, 92:1005.

Schoenwad RD : Ocular pharmacokinetics pharmaco-dynamics. In Mitra AK, (editor) Ophthalmic drug delivery systems, Marcel Dekker, New York, 1993.

Sommer A (1983): Effects of vitamin A deficiency on the ocular surface, Ophthalmology, 90 : 592.

Van Buskirk E.M. et al (1980) : Adverse reactions from timolol administration, Ophthalmology, 87:447.

Varma S.D (1991) : Scientific basis for medical therapy of cataracts by anti-oxidants. Am J Clin Nutr 53: 3358.

Vogel R. et al : The effect of timolol, betaxolol, and placebo on corneal sensitivity in healthy volunteers, J Ocular Pharmacol (1990) 6:85.

Weissman S.S. et al (1992) : Effects of topical timolol (0.5%) and betaxolol (0.5%) on corneal sensitivity, Br J Ophthalmol, 74:409.

West S et al (1994) : Are antioxidants or supplements protective for age-related macular degeneration? Arch Ophthalmol, 112:222-227.

Pharmacovigilance

PHARMACOVIGILANCE

GENERAL ASPECTS

What is pharmacovigilance?

- Collection & collation of data related to the detection, assessment, understanding, and prevention of adverse events.
- Identifying new information relating to hazards associated with medicines in an attempt to prevent harm to patients.
- Post-marketing surveillance.

WHO's definition: "Pharmacovigilance is the science and activities relating to the detection, assessment, understanding and prevention of adverse effects or any other drug related problems".

The ethynological roots of the word pharmacovigilance are pharmakon (Greek), 'drug' and vigilare (Latin), 'to keep awake, or alert, to keep watch'.

Being 'vigilant regarding medicines' is essential because of (i) high usage of medicines; (ii) increasing complexity of medicines; (iii) polypharmacy; (iv) population growth and diversity.

Pharmacovigilance is therefore an Awakening of Drug Monitoring System.

Concern

Pharmacovigilance is concerned with identifying, validating, quantifying and evaluating adverse reactions associated with the use of drugs.

Pharmacovigilance concerns standard medicines, medication errors, lack of efficacy reports, use of medicines for indications that are not approved and for which there is inadequate scientific basis, case reports of acute and chronic poisoning, assessment of drug-related mortality, use and misuse of medicines and food. Recently, the concerns of pharmacovigilance have been widened to include herbals, traditional and complementary medicines, blood products, biologicals, medical devices and vaccines. Pharmacovigilance is a demanding science offering great opportunities in reducing harm to patients.

Role

- To identify, quantify and document drug-related problems.
- To reduce the risk of drug-related problems.
- To increase knowledge of factors responsible for drug-related injury.

Hence, it makes an important contribution to the health of the nation.

Importance

Pharmacovigilance is an important system because:
- Every patient who is taking a drug is at risk for developing adverse drug reactions (ADRs).
- World statistics show that 5-10% hospital admissions are due to ADRs and 0.3% are fatal in nature.
- ADRs increase human suffering.
- ADRs enhance healthcare cost.
- Medicine is evaluated for toxicity in a limited group of patients before marketing (during clinical trials).
- Much may be known about the efficacy of medicine, while little may be known about its safety.
- The tunnel vision of drug development focuses to identify drug effects on single biological process.

Hence, information about new drug's safety is incomplete, and there is need for pharmacovigilance.

Pharmacovigilance acts as a tool for prophylaxis of adverse drug reactions. Pitfalls are due to inadequate pharmacovigilance.

The ultimate goal of pharmacovigilance

- The rational and safe use of medicines.
- The assessment and communication of the risks and benefits of drugs on the market.
- Educating and informing of patients.

Major aims of pharmacovigilance

- Early detection of hitherto unknown adverse reactions and interactions.
- Detection of increase in frequency of (known) adverse reactions.
- Estimation of quantitative aspects of benefits/risk analysis and dissemination of information needed to improve drug prescribing and regulation.
- Improve patient care and safety related to the use of medicines and all medical and paramedical interventions.
- Promote understanding, education and clinical training in pharmacovigilance and its effective communication to the public.

Concepts/Basics of pharmacovigilance

- Collecting new information from reliable sources (healthcare professionals, consumers, literature, etc.).
- Analyzing the above information.
- Continuous monitoring of the safety of medicines.
- Identification of the patients at particular risk (e.g. elderly, children, hepatic and renal compromised patients and terminally ill patients).
- Understanding the mechanism by which the particular medicine produces ADR.
- Providing information to users.
- Monitoring the impact of any action taken.

Milestones of Pharmacovigilance

- *Short-term objectives:* To foster a culture of notification.
- *Medium-term objectives:* To engage several healthcare professionals in the drug monitoring and information dissemination processes.
- *Long-term objectives:* To achieve such operational efficiencies that would make

Pharmacovigilance Programme a benchmark for global drug monitoring endeavours.

Pharmacovigilance is a dynamic and scientific discipline because it:

- Improves communication between health professionals and the public.
- Educates health professionals to understand the effectiveness/risk of medicines that they prescribe.
- Plays critical role in meeting the challenges posed by the ever increasing range and potency of medicines.
- Provides regulators with the necessary information.
- Promotes rational use of medicines.
- Identifies gaps in our understanding and drug - related ADRs.
- Ensures the safe use of medicines.

Box 22.1. For effective Pharmacovigilance (responsibility lies on three players)

- Health care professionals

    Role in reporting ADRs is the starting point of collecting data
- Pharmaceutical companies

    They are obligated by regulations to ensure reporting ADRs to the regulators in a time bound manner
- Government Agencies (regulatory authorities) in India:

    Central Drugs Standards Control Organization (CDSCO)

    National Pharmacovigilance Centre operating at CDSCO (H.Q.)

Box 22.2. Success factors for Pharmacovigilance system

- Public awareness on need to report ADRs
- Government support
- Trained healthcare workers
- Quality control of laboratories
- Free communication between public and policy makers
- Ability to have free flow of information
- Understanding and tackling the constraints (including training resources) which are an essential prerequisite for development of the science and practice of pharmacovigilance.
- Removal of ambiguity and confusion.

WHY PHARMACOVIGILANCE IS NEEDED?

Phase IV of the evaluation of the drugs starts when the marketing license is granted and extends over many years. It consists of pharmacoepidemiological studies to evaluate the effectiveness, safety, and utilization of the drug in large populations, under real-life conditions. The results confirm or disprove the effectiveness of the drug in clinical practice to determine whether approved uses should be expanded or restricted.

As the newer and newer drugs hit the market, the need for Pharmacovigilance grows more than ever before.

Once put into the market, a medicine leaves the secure and protected scientific environment of clinical trials and is legally set free for consumption by the general population. At this point, most medicines would only have been tested for short-term safety and efficacy on a limited number of carefully selected individuals, in some cases as few as 500 subjects, and rarely more than 5000, would have received the product prior to its release (Table 22.1).

Table 22.1. Phases in clinical trials.

Phase-I	20-50 healthy volunteers to gather preliminary data.
Phase-II	150-350 subjects with disease to determine safety and dosage recommendations.
Phase-III	250-4000 more varied patient groups – to determine short-term safety and efficacy.
Phase-IV	Post-approval phase, drug is released for marketing after phase-III clinical trials.

For good reason, therefore, it is essential that new medicines are monitored for their effectiveness and safety under real-life conditions. More information is generally needed about use in specific population groups notably children, pregnant women and the elderly, and about the efficacy and safety of chronic use, especially in combination with other medicines. Experience has shown that many adverse effects, interactions (with food or other medicines) and risk factors come to light only during the years after the release of medicine. Some examples are given in Table 22.2.

Table 22.2. Classical examples of serious and unexpected adverse reactions.

Medicine	Adverse reaction
Aminophenazone (amidopyrine)	Agranulocytosis
Chloramphenicol	Aplastic anaemia
Clioquinol	Myelooptic neuropathy
Erythromycin estolate	Cholestatic hepatitis
Fluothane	Hepatocellular hepatitis
Methyldopa	Haemolytic anaemia
Oral contraceptives	Thromboembolism
Practolol	Sclerosing peritonitis
Reserpine	Depression
Statine	Rhabdomyolysis
Thalidomide	Congenital malformations

Many times a large number of patients is required to detect adverse reactions (Table 22.3).

Table 22.3. Number of patients required to be 95% certain of detecting one, two and three cases of an adverse reaction.

Incidence of adverse reactions	Number of patients required for reactions detecting one, two, and three cases of ADRs		
	One case	Two cases	Three cases
1 in 100	300	480	650
1 in 200	600	960	1300
1 in 1,000	3000	4800	6500
1 in 2,000	6000	9600	13000
1 in 10,000	30000	48000	65000

COMMONLY USED TERMS IN DRUG SAFETY

Benefits are the proven therapeutic good of a product, but should also include patient's subjective assessment of its effects.

Risk is the probability of occurrence, of harm being caused.

Harm is the actual damage that could be caused. It should not be confused with risk.

Efficacy is used to express the extent to which a drug works under ideal circumstances (i.e. in clinical trials).

Effectiveness is used to express the extent to which a drug works in clinical practice (not clinical trials).

Adverse Event (AE)/Adverse experience is any unfavourable and unintended sign, symptom, or disease temporarily associated with the use of a medicinal product, whether or not considered related to the medicinal product. Adverse events (AEs) also include post treatment complications that occur as a result of protocol-mandated procedures. Pre-existing events that increase in severity during or as a consequence of the use of a medicinal product in a human clinical trial are also considered AEs.

An AE does not include the following:

- Medical or surgical procedures (e.g. endoscopy, tooth extraction, transfusion): the condition that necessitates the procedures is an AE.
- Any pre-existing disease or condition or laboratory abnormality present or detected prior to the start of the study treatment regimen that does not worsen.
- Situation where an untoward occurrence has not occurred (e.g. hospitalization for selective surgery or admission for convenience).
- Laboratory test abnormalities, without clinical manifestations which do not require medical intervention, or that do not result in termination or delay.

Side effect is an old term and is broad enough to include both positive and negative effects of a drug apart from its main properties or indications. Side effect is any unintended effect of a pharmaceutical product occurring at doses normally used in humans which is related to the pharmacological properties of the drug. Some use the term as synonymous with 'adverse reaction', but the proposed definition of ADR will improve clarity of the use of this term.

Side effects are due to the actions on organ systems other than on the desired system in therapeutic doses and usually do not necessitate stopping of treatment. For example, phenobarbitone when used as an antiepileptic, produces drowsiness as a side effect. In most cases side effects are not desirable but in few cases the side effects may be desirable e.g. reserpine as antihypertensive, the side effect such as bradycardia, calmness and laxative effects are beneficial.

Toxic effect (overdose effect) is due to the exaggerated undesirable pharmacological effect.

Adverse reactions: Possible causes

- Intrinsic factors of the drug
  - Idiosyncrasy
  - Carcinogenicity, Mutagenicity
  - Teratogenicity
- Extrinsic factors
  - Adulterants
  - Contamination
- Underlying medical conditions
- Interactions
- Wrong usage

Adverse Drug Reactions (ADRs) are considered as one among the leading causes of morbidity and mortality.

Adverse Drug Reaction (ADR) may be defined as an apparently harmful or unpleasant reaction, resulting from an intervention related to the use of a medicinal product. It predicts hazard from future administration and warrants prevention or specific treatment, or alteration of the dosage regimens, or withdrawal of the product.

ADR has to be contrasted with the term adverse drug event, which refers to untoward occurrences following drug exposure but not necessarily caused by the medicine.

ADR is a response to a drug which is noxious and unintended, and which occurs at doses normally used in humans for the prophylaxis, diagnosis, or therapy of disease, or for the restoration, correction or modification of physiological function.

This basic definition includes all doses prescribed clinically, but is intended to exclude accidental or deliberate overdose.

The ADRs may range from minor reactions to serious events. Reactions may occur within minutes or years after exposure to the product.

The **classification** and characteristics of types A and B ADRs is shown in Table 22.4. The adverse reaction grading scale is given in Table 22.5, the direct and indirect effects of ADRs are shown in Table 22.6 and estimates of frequency of ADRs are given in Table 22.7.

Classification of ADRs

There are many different classifications of ADRs. The original classification proposed by Rawlins and Thompson (1991) divided ADRs into two types, type A (pharmacological) and type B (idiosyncratic) (Table 22.4).

Table 22.4. Characteristics of types A and B ADRs.

Characteristic	Type A	Type B
Dose dependency	Usually shows a good relationship	No simple relationship
Predictable from known Pharmacology	Yes	Not usually
Host factors	Genetic factors may be important	Dependent on (usually uncharacterized) host factors
Frequency	Common	Uncommon
Severity	Variable but usually mild	Variable, proportionately more severe than type A
Morbidity	High	High
Mortality	Low	High
Overall proportion of ADRs	80%	20%
First detection	Phases I-III	Usually phase-IV, occasionally Phase-III.
Mechanism	Usually because of parent drug or stable metabolite	May be because of parent drug or stable metabolite
Animal models	Usually reproducible in animals	Very few reproducible in animal models.

Table 22.5. Adverse Reaction Grading (Severity) Scale

Severity	Definition
Mild	Symptom(s) usually transient in nature, causing no limitation of usual activities, patient may experience slight discomfort. Prescription drugs are not ordinarily needed for relief of symptoms.
Moderate	Causing some limitation of usual activities, patient may experience annoying discomfort. Treatment of symptom(s) is needed.
Severe	Causing inability to carry out usual activities, patient may experience intolerable discomfort. Severity may cause cessation of treatment with the drug. Treatment of symptom(s) is needed.

Table 22.6. The direct and indirect effects of ADRs

Cause admission to hospitals or attendance in primary care

Responsible for deaths

Increase length of hospital stay

Increase cost of patient care

Adversely affect patient's quality of life

Cause patients to lose confidence in their doctors

Mimic disease and result in unnecessary investigations and/or delay treatment

Table 22.7. The recommended estimate of frequency of adverse drug reactions.

Very common	$\geq 1/10$	$\geq 10\%$
Common (frequent)	$\geq 1/100$ and $< 1/10$	$\geq 1\%$ and $< 10\%$
Uncommon (infrequent)	$\geq 1/1,000$ and $< 1/100$	$\geq 0.1\%$ and $< 1\%$
Rare	$\geq 1/10,000$ and $< 1,000$	$\geq 0.01\%$ and $< 0.1\%$
Very rare	$< 1/10,000$	$(< 0.01\%)$

ADR or Medication Error?

The relationship between medication errors and Adverse Drug Events/Reactions may be complex, with medication errors being generally more common than ADRs. About a third to a half of ADEs are typically associated with medication errors; of course, not all ADRs necessarily spring from medication errors. The close intersection of medication error and ADEs demands careful attention in pharmaco-vigilance.

When does a side effect of a drug become an ADE, an ADR or a medication-related error? Different players in the healthcare system will have different perception on this point.

Medication errors can be categorized as 'mistakes' and 'slips' or 'lapses'.

Mistakes occur when something is wrong with the premise on which an action is based. Example of a reported case - while doing carotid angiography staff failed to recognize that no contrast medium (a clear, colourless liquid) had been loaded into the syringe, and therefore a bolus of air, instead of contrast, was injected into the right carotid artery. The patient died inspite of emergency treatment of air embolism.

Slip or Laps: Example of a reported case - A woman with suspected tuberculosis was injected with 100000 units of tuberculin purified protein derivative (PPD) intradermally, a 1000-fold overdose. She developed pulmonary fibrosis and died. Such errors may happen when there are two formulations of the same product that differ enormously in concentration.

Serious Adverse Event (SAE) or reaction is any untoward medical occurrence that at any dose:

- Results in death.
- Requires inpatient hospitalization or prolongation of existing hospitalization.
- Results in persistent or significant disability/incapacity.
- Is life-threatening (that is at immediate risk of dying).
- Results in anomaly/birth defect in the offspring of a subject who received treatment.
- Jeopardise the subject sufficiently that medical or surgical intervention may be required.
- Examples may include, but are not limited to:
  - Intensive treatment in emergency room or at home for allergic bronchospasm.
  - Blood dyscrasias that do not result in hospitalization.
  - Seizures that do not result in hospitalization.

Note: The term "life-threatening" in the definition of "serious" refers to an event in which the patient was at risk of death at the time of the event; it does not refer to an event which hypothetically might have caused death if it was more severe.

Serious vs Severe adverse event

The term 'severe' indicates the intensity (severity) of a specific event (as in mild, moderate or severe MI), the event itself may be of minor significance (such as severe headache).

The term 'serious' is based on subject/event outcome or action criteria usually that poses a threat to a subject's life or functioning.

Severity is not equivalent to event seriousness.

Unexpected Adverse Reaction means an adverse reaction, the nature, severity or outcome of which is inconsistent with the summary of product characteristics of the drug.

Abuse of medicinal products means regular or sporadic intentional use of medicinal products which is accompanied by harmful physical or psychological reactions.

Causality Assessment terms (relationship of AE or SAE to the drug):

Certain/Definite: A reaction that follows a reasonable temporal sequence from administration of the drug or in which the drug level has been established in body fluids or tissue, that follows a known or expected response pattern to the suspected drug, and that is confirmed by improvement of stopping or reducing the dosage of the drug, and reappearance of the reaction on repeated exposure.

Probable/Likely: A reaction that follows a reasonable temporal sequence from administration, that follows a known or expected response pattern to the suspected drug, that is confirmed by stopping or reducing the dosage of the drug. Rechallenge information is not required to fulfill this definition.

Possible: A clinical event, including laboratory test abnormality, with a reasonable time sequence to administration of the drug, but which could also be explained by concurrent diseases or other drugs or chemicals. Information on drug withdrawal may be lacking or unclear.

This definition is used when drug causality is one of the other possible causes for the described clinical event.

Unlikely: A clinical event, including laboratory test abnormality, with a temporal relationship to drug

administration which makes a causal relationship improbable, and in which other drugs, chemicals or underlying disease provide plausible explanation.

This definition is used when the exclusion of drug causality of a clinical event seems most plausible.

Conditional/Unclassified: A clinical event, including laboratory test abnormality, reported as an adverse reaction, about which more data is essential for a proper assessment or the additional data are under examination.

Unassessible/Unclassifiable: A report suggesting an adverse reaction which cannot be judged because information is insufficient or contradictory, and which can not be supplemented or verified.

Not related: Any event that is judged clearly that the event is due to causes other than the treatment.

Unknown: A reaction that follows a reasonable temporal sequence from administration of the drug, but that can not be assessed based on the known or expected response pattern of the suspected drug.

Note: When an AE has been assessed and the causal relation to the drug is established (definite, probable, possible) it must be referred to as an **adverse drug reaction.**

Various causality terms are in use but the terms described above are used most widely. Some, however, do not use all the terms. Many do not believe that a 'certain' classification is possible for a single report. Some make no distinction between 'probable' and 'possible'. Whilst 'conditional/unclassified' and 'unassessible/unclassifiable' are not causality terms, they describe the status of adverse reaction reports and therefore allow for practical communication about ADR issues.

GOOD PHARMACOVIGILANCE PRACTICE (GPvP)

Good pharmacovigilance is linked with:
- **Identification of the drug-related problems:**
  - Lack of effect, counterfeiting
  - Resistance
  - Interaction
  - Dependence and abuse

  These should be monitored and reported under pharmacovigilance.
- **Identification of patients at particular risk,** e.g., elderly, children, pregnant women, hepatic

and renal compromised patients and terminally ill patients.

- **Signal detection: What constitutes a signal?**

The WHO has defined a signal as: 'Reported information on a possible causal relationship between an adverse event and a drug, the relationship being unknown or incompletely documented previously'.

An additional note says: 'Usually more than one report is required to generate a signal, depending on the seriousness of the event and the quality of the information'.

Signal describes the first alert or expression that something might be wrong with a drug which is not regarded as definite but indicates need for further enquiry or action. Usually more than one signal is required to generate a signal, however, depending on the seriousness of the event and the quality of the information even a single well-documented case report may be viewed as a signal.

Pre-clinical findings or experiences with other products in the class may be sufficient to generate a signal even in the absence of case reports in patients.

Both quantitative and qualitative factors come into the decision of whether something is a signal or not.

Signal detection is traditionally focused on phase-IV (post-approval or marketing surveillance). Now its place is also emphasized during clinical trials. Both clinical trial safety and post-marketing pharmacovigilance are critical throughout the product life cycle.

In practice, some have used simply the number of reports for a particular reaction/drug combination as a cut-off. This cut-off has been, for example, two or more, or three or more reports.

The primary objective of any reporting system is to generate a signal: An early indication or warning of a potential problem. This may be compared to a fire-watcher, who looks for smoke and if he thinks he spots it, must then determine whether there is indeed a fire and where that fire is located.

Signal detection is one of the most important objectives of pharmacovigilance because the process of risk/benefit evaluation depends on effective statistical signal detection (Fig. 22.1).

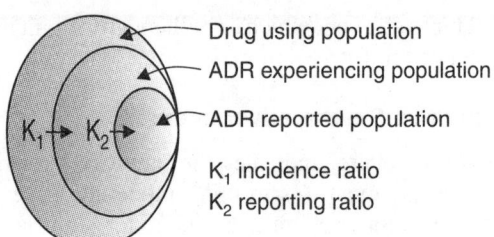

Fig. 22.1. Statistical signal detection

The methods of signal detection include:
- Observation by clinicians and patients.
- Case reports in literature.
- Data from formal studies e.g., clinical studies, epidemiological studies like cohort studies.

Detection of signals requires clinical assessment assisted by epidemiological and statistical analysis.

The absence of a signal does not rule out a safety problem. Similarly, the presence of a signal is not a proof of a causal relationship, between a drug and an adverse event. Therefore, review of the cases is critical to the evaluation of positional identity through data mining.

Signals of potential harmful effects may arise from literature reports, observational epidemiological studies, randomized trials and spontaneous reports of suspected ADRs.

'Data mining' is a technique for extracting meaningful, organized information from large complex databases and has been used to identify hidden patterns of associations or unexpected occurrences (signals) in spontaneous reporting system database. If this can be religiously achieved, data mining serves as a potentially useful adjunct to traditional pharmacovigilance practices.

Importantly data mining *cannot* prove or refute causal associations between drugs and events. Data mining simply identifies – disproportionality of drug-event reporting pattern in databases. Results obtained from data mining technique should be interpreted with caution and with the knowledge of the weakness of the spontaneous reporting system.

Spontaneous reporting is the core data-generating system of international pharmacovigilance, relying on healthcare professionals and in some places consumers to identify and report any suspected adverse drug reaction to their national pharmaco-vigilance centre or to the manufacturer. Spontaneous reports are almost always submitted voluntarily. However, one of this system's major weaknesses is under-reporting.

The overworked medical personnel do not always see reporting as a priority. If the symptoms are not serious, they may not notice them at all. And even if the symptoms are serious, they may not be recognised as the effect of a particular drug. Even so, spontaneous reports are a crucial element in the worldwide enterprise of pharmacovigilance and form the core of the WHO database, which includes around 3.7 million reports (September 2006), growing annually by about 2,50,000.

Pharmacoepidemiology is study of utilization and effects of drugs in large number of people. It complements pharmacovigilance as both go hand-in-hand. Pharmacovigilance is a branch of pharmaco-epidemiology but is restricted to the study, on an epidemiological scale, of drug events, or adverse reactions. It also helps in detecting adverse drug reactions sooner and decreasing the time to removal of drugs that are causing problem. Indeed, it is a bridge science spanning both clinical pharmacology and epidemiology (Fig. 22.2).

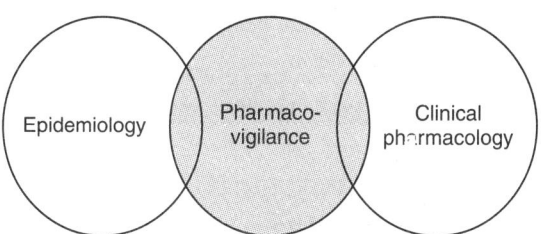

Fig. 22.2. Position of pharmacovigilance.

- Continuous monitoring of the safety of medicines during the use and also to ensure that their risks and benefits remain acceptable.
- Understanding the mechanism by which the particular product produces adverse drug reaction.
- Providing information to users through news-letters, medical journals, websites, patient information leaflets, media statements etc.
- Monitoring the impact of any action taken.

- Ethics of reporting i.e. report any time and every time an ADR occurs, report all suspected ADRs both serious and others. ADR reporting should be mandatory, rather than voluntary.
- Cooperation and integration among national and international bodies.

  Close and effective collaboration is essential to meet challenges so that this discipline continues to develop and flourish.
- Removal of obstructive and interfering challenges.

  One of the main challenge is that there is no data on ADRs that may occur due to the interaction between the established medicines, traditional and herbal medicines. The available reports are negligible. There are multiple herbal and herb-mineral fixed dose combinations being consumed at the same time. Patients often use drugs from different systems of medicine concomitantly. This leads to difficulties in making definite causality assessment virtually impossible. There is need for pharmacovigilance in Ayurvedic and Unani system. There is a popular misconception that Ayurvedic and Unani medicines are devoid of ADRs. The pharmaceutical industries manufacturing these medicines are not adequately motivated to focus on pharmaco-vigilance, safety data - either before or after marketing of the formulations.

Another important challenge is lack of proper education in the field of pharmacovigilance.

Obviously, learning about pharmacovigilance should start early in professional training by healthcare students. Without proper educatio-nal training in the field of pharmacovigilance it is difficult to understand the various problems. Although, there is need for pharma-covigilance training but so far it is not an academic specialism. Specific courses in this field are offered by very few universities in the world. It is difficult to fit the spans of large range of subjects required for pharmaco-vigilance teaching (pharmacology, epidemio-logy, clinical medicine, data management, drug legislation and communication, etc.) in any one particular course. Hence, specialized training courses in pharmacovigilance should be regularly arranged. The International Society of Pharmacovigilance (ISoP) provides specialized adhoc training courses in pharmacovigilance. The Indian chapter, the Society of Pharmacovigilance in India (SoPI) can provide regular pharmacovigilance training.

Pharmacovigilance training programme may include the following topics:

Historical development of pharmacovigilance, terminologies, need for and aims of pharmacovigilance, clinical manifestation of ADRs, signal detection, epidemiological methods, regulatory requirements, benefit/risk assessment, communication skills, preventing drug related problems, rational and safe use of medicines, good pharmacovigilance practice, literature sources for drug safety information, ethics in pharmacovigilance, reporting ADRs, causality assessment criteria (definite, probable, possible, etc.), respect for privacy laws in pharmacovigilance, role of pharmaceutical companies for effective pharmacovigilance.

In due course of time, it may be possible to include pharmacovigilance as a regular subject (theory as well as practical) in pharmacology teaching syllabus.

- Correct, unbiased and updated communication. Patient information leaflets are promoted by some authorities. These moves seem reasonable, but there must be a review of their effectiveness.

Box 22.3. Ambiguity leads to unanswered questions

"And/or when the number of patients to be included in the study will add significantly to existing safety data for the products".

- How large is large enough, 1,000; 2,000; 10,000 patients?
- Should threshold size vary with therapeutic area and the safety experience to data on the product?
- How to assess whether risks undermine benefits?

No simple formula compares risks to benefits.

Risk and benefit numbers, types, measures, vary.

Box 22.4. Confusion reigns!!

- **Under-reporting:**
  inadequate company oversight
  non-inclusion of relevant study updates and reports
- **Over-reporting:**
  inclusion of every post-marketing study
  generation reporting of data irrelevant to safety
  significant unnecessary work for competent authorities

Box 22.5. Benefit to Risk Analysis

The debate about comparative benefit and risk is bedeviled by failures of logic and definition (e.g. clearly differentiating between 'harm' and 'risk'). Methods have been promoted that will enhance more rigorous benefit-risk analysis, for example:

- Comparing like with like.
- Use of best-case and worst-case analysis for uncertain safety information.
- To determine reasons for differences in reporting ADR.

Box 22.6. Communicating the outcome of pharmaco-vigilance

It is not sufficient for the experts to be satisfied with the safety evidence for a given medicine. The public perception of the hazards associated with medicines is an equally important factor. How safe is safe enough? Which risks are acceptable? These are critical questions that providers of medicines need to consider when communicating with patients and the general public. The pharmacovigilance system has a duty to build public trust through effective communication.

RESPECT OF CONFIDENTIALITY IN PHARMACOVIGILANCE

It is always in the patients' interest that healthcare personnel should have access to information from patients who have been exposed to the drug. Only by encouraging reporting can regulatory agencies and manufacturers take responsibility for the safety, efficacy and quality of the drugs they have approved or marketed for public consumption.

However, the processing of personal data and the free movement of such data should be such that the individual should feel protected and respected. Physicians have a duty to protect the use of information from treatment only in relation to that patients' care, unless they are permitted otherwise by prior informed consent. It is essential that healthcare personnel should obtain the consent of the patient when identity is disclosed on an adverse drug reaction form or in a drug surveillance study. However, these rights and duties are not absolute. In some instances, the needs of public health may override those of the individual patient for protection of confidentiality. Public health requirements such as mandatory notification of certain diseases may justify disclosure of patient information. But even when such disclosure is required in terms of public health need, it remains the responsibility of the health worker to protect patient's confidentiality as far as possible.

National centres have to maintain high standards of data protection when information has been received on patients who have not given their informed consent. Patients should also be helped to understand that the information they provide is likely to contribute to an international understanding of drug safety.

PHARMACEUTICAL COMPANIES AND PHARMACOVIGILANCE

Pharmaceutical companies face consumers who know and care more about drug safety; regulators are setting higher standards in drug safety and are increasingly vigilant about it. Globalization is demanding a need for real-time safety reporting, ICH (International Conference on Harmonisation of Technical Requirements for Registration of Pharmaceuticals for Human Use) and other efforts to harmonize international safety data and AEs reporting require companies to increase reporting standardization. AE data volume is being driven skyward by the growth of clinical trials and greater number of approved drugs must be tracked. Pharmacovigilance pressures are increasing day-by-day.

Failure to effectively manage drug safety data and pharmacovigilance process can affect patient well-being, jeopardize a company's reputation, and create a regulatory disaster. And if a post-approval drug is withdrawn the potential legal expenses and the negative impact result in huge losses.

The pharmaceutical companies realize that 'data

agility' is needed for their survival as well as to assure both regulators and consumers regarding efficacy and safety of drugs. They are responsible to establish a reliable and transparent pharmacovigilance system with continual monitoring of drug safety – prompt reporting to the competent authorities (within 15 days of receipt of information), detection of signals with a timely initiation of a risk management plan.

For the pharmaceutical industries, pharmacovigilance has been the post-marketing surveillances of the safety of authorized medicinal products during their life on the market. It includes safety monitoring and re-evaluation of suspected adverse drug reactions from phase-IV clinical trials, observational non-interventional studies e.g., post-marketing surveillance studies, pharmacoepidemiologic studies, solicited reports from survey registries, patient diaries etc. but now the pharmaceutical industries know that they have prime responsibility for the safety of medicines, from the *start of drug development (i.e. clinical trials) and thereafter throughout the life time of the drug.*

Pharmacovigilance in clinical trials phase-I to III covers drug safety monitoring and evaluation of all adverse events with or without a causal relationship to the investigational medicinal product and any adverse reaction to concomitant medication.

Drug safety monitoring in clinical trials ensures the safety of the participants and a continual assessment of the risk and benefit. Even in oncology clinical trials, often with patients with unfavourable progress where emphasis is placed on survival, a risk benefit assessment is essential.

Adverse event documentation and reporting in clinical trials has been harmonized. Time limits for reporting serious unexpected suspected adverse reactions (SUSAR) from clinical trials to competent authorities and ethics committees have been enforced. All the relevant information about SUSAR that are fatal or life threatening is reported as soon as possible but and in any case not later than 7 days after first knowledge by the sponsor of such a case, and 15 days for all others.

In addition, adverse drug reactions associated with concomitant medication administered in clinical trials, where the sponsor is not the marketing authorization holder should be reported either directly to competent authorities or to the marketing authorization holder of the concomitant medication, so that regulatory requirements can be met and the serious drug reactions can be reported to the competent authorities within 15 days.

In India, the pharmaceutical companies holding the marketing license should ensure that they have adequate pharmacovigilance system working in place to ensure the responsibility and reliability of their marketed products, as specified in Schedule Y.

The recent introduction of a legal requirement (Schedule Y amendment) for pharmaceutical companies to submit suspected ADRs from clinical trials performed in India to the regulatory authority has created a new demand for pharmacovigilance.

Pharmaceutical companies are doing their best efforts as fast as they can in managing safety data through their own pharmacovigilance built-in system.

Many companies have developed innovative and efficient monitoring systems that have contributed to the detection of new safety signals.

PHARMACOVIGILANCE AND RATIONAL USE OF MEDICINE

Pharmacovigilance plays an important role in the rational use of medicines by providing information about ADRs.

Challenges are posed by the ever increasing range and potency of medicines, all of which carry an inevitable and sometimes unpredictable potential for harm. For all medicines there is a trade-off between benefits and the potential for harm. The harm can be minimized by ensuring that medicines of good quality, safety and efficacy are used rationally, and that the expectations and concerns of the patients are taken into account. For this, the following aspects are important:

- Serve public health and to foster a sense of trust among patients in the medicines they use that would extend to confidence in the health service in general.
- Ensure that risks in drug use are anticipated and managed.
- Provide regulators with the necessary information to amend the recommendations on the use of the medicines.
- Improve communication between the health professionals and the public.

- Educate health professionals to understand the effectiveness/risk of medicines that they prescribe.

In view of the importance and significance of pharmacovigilance and its role in promoting rational use of drugs, it is essential that medical, dental, pharmacy students should be taught pharmacovigilance. The objective should be to create awareness among students so that in their future practice they should be able to do the needful. At least a few lectures and practical exercises (relating to safety of drugs and assessment of causality etc.) should be included in the pharmacovigilance teaching programme at the time of professional courses. This programme should also be evaluated. The theoretical aspect can be assessed using short answer type questions and multiple choice questions. Designing the ADR reporting form, causality and severity assessment of the ADR can be done through practical examination.

This will equip the students adequately to detect, understand, evaluate and report ADRs when they practice as professionals. This will ensure safety in the use of medicines.

PHARMACOVIGILANCE IN THE REGULATION OF MEDICINES

Strong regulatory arrangements provide the foundation for a national ethos of medicines safety, and for public confidence in medicines. To be effective, the regulatory authorities need to go further than the approval of new medicines to encompass a wider range of issues relating to the safety of medicines.

In order to achieve these objectives relating to the safety of medicines, pharmacovigilance programme and drug regulatory authority must be mutually supporting. On the one hand pharmacovigilance programme needs to maintain strong links with the drug regulatory authorities to ensure that the latter are well briefed on safety issues. On the other, regulators need to understand the specialized and pivotal role that pharmacovigilance plays in ensuring the ongoing safety of medicinal products.

PHARMACOVIGILANCE IN CLINICAL PRACTICE

Safety monitoring of medicines in common use

should be an integral part of clinical practice. The degree to which clinicians are informed about the principles of pharmacovigilance has a large impact on the quality of healthcare.

Education and training of health professionals regarding safety of medicines, exchange of informations between national pharmacovigilance centres, the coordination of such exchange, and the linking of clinical experience of medicines safety with research and health policy, all serve to enhance effective patient care.

National pharmacovigilance programmes are ideally placed to identify gaps in understanding of medicine induced adverse reactions.

PHARMACOVIGILANCE AND DISEASES CONTROL PUBLIC HEALTH PROGRAMMES

There are situations that involve the use of medicines in specific communities e.g. for the treatment of tropical diseases and for the treatment of HIV/AIDS and Tuberculosis.

In some settings, several disease control initiatives involving the administration of medicines to large communities are being implemented with little knowledge of, or regards to how, these various medicines could interact with each other.

Pharmacovigilance is of great value for every country in planning public health disease control programmes.

PHARMACOVIGILANCE PROGRAMME ACROSS THE GLOBE

Although many drugs have been extensively used and studied in developed countries, their safety profile can not necessarily be generalized to developing countries. Every country needs to have its own Pharmacovigilance Programme because of the following differences:

- Pattern presentation, incidence and severity of Adverse Drug Reactions.
- Diseases and prescribing practices.
- Genetic composition of the population.
- Diet and traditions of the people.

Almost all the countries have a pharmacovigilance center or a unit carrying out the activities related to ADR monitoring. The following brief description

is regarding WHO programme and the systems prevalent in some selected countries.

Historical Background of Pharmacovigilance

From mid 19th Century to mid 20th Century, emphasis was only designing and synthesizing drugs, and there was no awareness of their darker side i.e. adverse drug reactions. People lost their near and dear ones without knowing cause or reason.

Several disasters led to the awareness that drugs not only can heal but also can harm. Some such disasters include sudden death caused by chloroform anaesthesia in 1877 and fatal hepatic necrosis due to arsenicals in 1922. In 1930s in USA a tragic mistake in the formulation of a children's syrup was the trigger for setting up the product authorization system under the Food and Drug Administration (FDA). FDA had the authority to review new drugs for safety. Child deaths, after diethylenglycol was mistakenly used to solubilise sulphanilamide in 1937, led to the first enactment of legislation on adverse reactions (FDA and Cosmetic Act, 1938). Following 100 deaths in France in 1952 which occurred after diethyl tin diodide, and thalidomide tragedy in 1960s in England and Germany, there was a rapid increase in laws, regulations and guidelines for reporting and evaluating the data on safety, quality, and efficacy of new medicinal products.

Thalidomide was introduced in 1957 and widely prescribed as an allegedly harmless hypnotic for the treatment of morning sickness and nausea. By 1965, this drug was removed from the market in most countries as it was soon linked to a congenital abnormality which caused severe birth defects (phocomelia and micromelia) in children of women who had been prescribed this medicine during pregnancy. During 1969 and 1995 several cases of thalidomide embryopathy were registered.

The thalidomide disaster awakened a need to regulate pharmacovigilance not only by the national regulatory authorities but also over and above this at an international level. The Sixteenth World Health Assembly in 1963 adopted a resolution in regard to rapid dissemination of information on ADRs and led to initiation of the WHO Pilot Research Project for International Drug Monitoring in 1968. The purpose of this was to develop a system applicable internationally, for detecting adverse effects of medicines, to improve the safe and cost effective use of medicines by avoiding further disasters in both developed and developing countries in the interests of improved public health.

In 1962 a new bill amended 1938 Food, Drug and Cosmetic Act, the Kefauver-Harris Amendment gave the FDA the power to approve or disallow the introduction of new drugs and the continual marketing of established compounds based on substantial evidence of their therapeutic efficacy as well as safety. Around 1980 it became compulsory to record side effects (adverse drug reactions) by the regulatory authorities in many countries to allow for a continual monitoring of the risk and benefit of products both in the investigational phase before authorization and as post-marketing surveillance when the product is commercialized as an authorized product.

In the early 1980s, in close collaboration with the WHO, the Council for International Organizations of Medical Sciences (CIOMS) launched its programme on drug development and use. The recommendation of CIOMS by the International Conference on Harmonization (ICH) in the 1990s has made notable impact on international drug regulation.

The creation of the International Society of Pharmacoepidemiology (ISPE) in 1984 and of the European Society of Pharmacovigilance (ESoP – later ISoP – the International Society) in 1992 marked the introduction of pharmacovigilance formally into the research and academic world and its increasing integration into clinical practice.

The consequences of this are that over the last three decades there have been continued instances of drug recalls or warning due to the discovery of potential hazards during their use. Some more notable examples are: practolol induced mucocutaneous syndrome, benoxaprofen caused hepatic disorders/ deaths in the elderly, temafloxacin resulted in haemolytic anaemia, fenfluramine/phentermine produced valvulopathy or pulmonary hypertension, terfenadine or cisapride was cause of potential cardiac arrhythmias, cerivastatin induced rhabdomyolysis, Vioxx increased risk of cardiovascular events.

When crises arise, whether real or suspected, regulatory authorities are expected to deal them efficiently. They have powers to suspend registration, impose certain conditions, or restrict their use. These decisions are communicated by drug alerts, letters to doctors and pharmacists, press statements, through websites, news letters and publications in journals. However, there must be clear procedures as undue caution may result in removal of a product from the market even when there may be no justification for it.

WHO Programme for International Drug Monitoring

As a means of pooling existing data on ADRs, WHO's programme was established in 1968 as a pilot project with the participation of 10 countries that had organized national pharmacovigilance system at the time. The intent was to record ADRs not revealed during clinical trials. The international drug monitoring centre was moved from the WHO headquarters in Geneva, Switzerland to a WHO Collaborating Center for International Drug Monitoring in Uppsala, Sweden in 1978. The WHO collaborating Center is often referred to as the Uppsala Monitoring Centre (UMC). The number of national centres which are active members of the WHO programme has increased to more than 80 countries.

Current work

- Identification and analysis of new adverse reaction signal.
- The database of the WHO programme is a unique reference source.
- The UMC has an important role as a communication centre – a clearing house for information on drug safety at the service of drug regulatory agencies, pharmaceutical industry, researchers and other groups in need of drug safety information.
- The UMC organizes training courses to foster education and communication in pharmacovigilance.
- The UMC has been active in refining the concept of benefit-harm analysis for drugs safety: we need to know what are the benefits and their chance of occurring (benefit and effectiveness);

and what is the harm and its chances of occurring (harm and risk).

- It has become increasingly clear that adverse reaction monitoring must be extended to herbal remedies.
- Development of pharmacovigilance as a science.

International collaboration

At the global level, the WHO programme for international drug monitoring at the Uppsala Monitoring Centre collates ADR reports via the national pharmacovigilance centres of the 81 member countries (www.who-umc.org). Currently only six sub-Saharan African Countries (South Africa, Zimbabwe, Tanzania, Mozambique, Nigeria, and Ghana) are full members of the programme. Infact, less than 27% of lower middle income and low income economies have national pharmacovigilance systems registered with the WHO programme. The main reasons for this are lack of resources, infrastructure, and expertise.

What can be done to improve drug safety-monitoring in such developing countries where health resources are limited? No easy answers are available. However, WHO alongwith funding agencies provide significant support for pharmacovigilance activities in developing countries. This problem is further tackled through developing exchange programmes with the major regulatory agencies and sharing of best practices.

The principle of international collaboration in the field of pharmacovigilance is the principal basis for the WHO International Drug Monitoring Programme, through which over 80 member nations have systems in place which encourage healthcare personnel to record and report adverse effects of drugs in their patients. These reports are assessed locally and may lead to action within the country. Through membership of the WHO programme one country can know if similar reports are being made elsewhere.

Member countries send their reports to the Uppsala Monitoring Centre where they are processed, evaluated and entered into the WHO International Database. When there are several reports of adverse reactions to a particular drug this process may lead to the detection of a signal – an alert about a possible hazard communicated to

members countries. This happens only after detailed evaluation and expert review.

Pharmacovigilance Programme in India

Pharmacovigilance is not new in India, it has been going on from 1998 when India decided to join the Uppsala Centre for Adverse Event Monitoring.

However, in the wake of new patent regime, efficient viable and vibrant pharmacovigilance system has become the need of the hour in India. India has emerged as a global hub for clinical research because it is a vast country with multiethnic population.

Standard Control Organization (CDSCO) launched the National Pharmacovigilance Program (NPP) in November 2004 under the aegis of Directorate General of Health Services, Union Ministry of Health and Family Welfare. The basic purpose of this program is to collate, analyze and archive adverse drug reaction data for making regulatory decisions regarding drugs marketed in India. The National Pharmacovigilance Program will have the following goals:

- To foster a culture of notification.
- To engage several healthcare professionals and NGOs in the drug monitoring and information dissemination processes.
- To achieve such operational efficiencies that would make Indian National Pharmacovigilance Program a benchmark of global drug monitoring endeavours.
- All adverse events suspected to have been caused by new drug and 'Drugs of current interest' (List to be published by CDSCO from time-to-time).
- Reactions to any other drugs which are suspected of significantly affecting a patient's management.

Specific objectives of the programme

- To create an ADR database for the Indian population.
- To create awareness of ADR monitoring among people.
- To ensure optimum safety of drug products in Indian market.
- To create infrastructure for ongoing regulatory

review of PSURs (periodic safety update reports).

This programme is ramified into 3 blocks
(Fig. 22.3)

- Zonal Centres, situated in Mumbai and Delhi; for causality analysis of the reported AE and to provide training.
- Regional centres, to collate and scrutinize data received from peripheral centres.
- Primary peripheral centres, for recording AE.
- The National Pharmacovigilance Advisory Committee (NPAC) oversees the various zonal, regional and peripheral pharmacovigilance centres and recommends possible regulatory measures. It also oversees collection, assessment and interpretation of data.

The programme recommends mandatory reporting of ADRs/AE.

ADVICE ABOUT REPORTING ADR/AE

When it is suspected that the patient has experienced an Adverse Drug Reaction, report without any delay.

Patients' reports have certain advantages:

- Patient often provide more detailed information
- Information on actual drug use, also on OTC
- ADR is reported without a medical filter

Report adverse experiences with medications

Report serious adverse reactions. A reaction is serious when the patient outcome is:

- Death
- Life-threatening (real risk of dying)
- Hospitalization (initial or prolonged)
- Disability (significant, persistent or permanent)
- Congenital anomaly

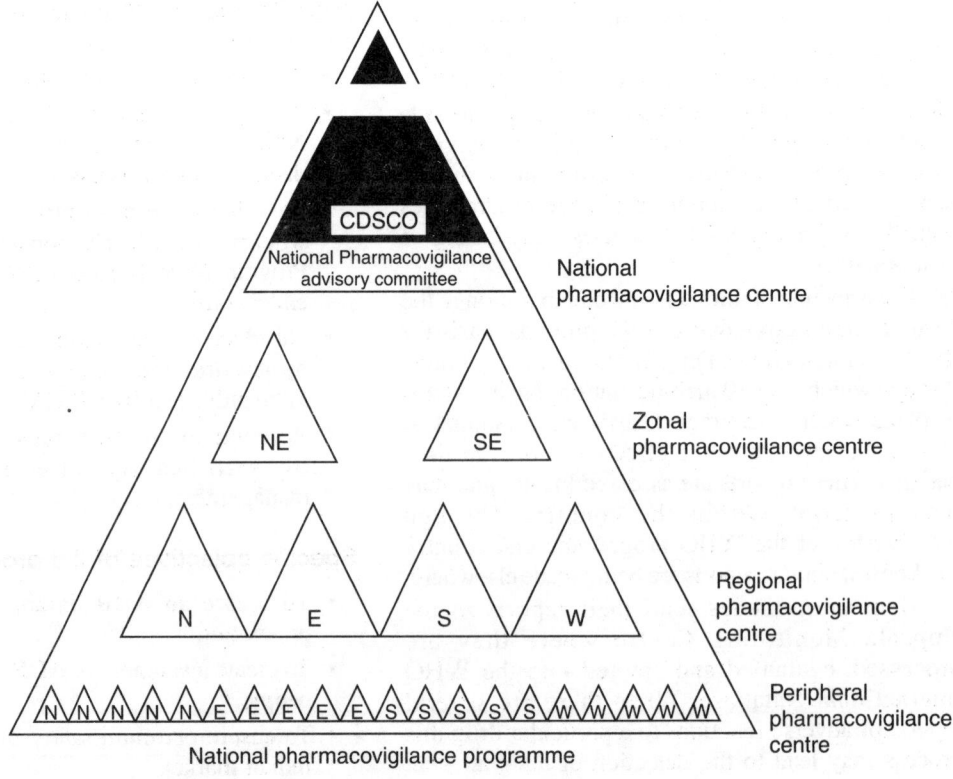

National pharmacovigilance programme

Fig. 22.3. Pharmacovigilance system in India

- Required intervention to prevent permanent impairment or damage

Report even if:

- It is not certain that the product caused adverse reaction
- All the details in the form may not be available, but the following information is essentially required: Patient identifier initials, date of reaction started (day/month/year), description of reaction or problem, information about suspected medication (brand and/or generic name), dose and route used, reason for use, frequency, concomitant medical products including self-medication and herbal remedies, outcomes, name and professional address – speciality, signature, date of this report.

The ADR report has four main elements:

Patient, drug, ADR and *reporter.*

Who can report:

- Any health care professional (doctors including dentists, nurses and pharmacists)

Where to report:

- After completing, the form should be returned to the same pharmacovigilance centre from where it was received.
- A list of countrywide pharmacovigilance centres is available at: www.cdsco.nic.in
- Reporting can be done to any pharmacovigilance centre nearest to the reporter. The form may also be sent (in case of doubt) to the National Pharmacovigilance Centre at CDSCO, DGHS, Ministry of Health and Family Welfare, Nirman Bhawan, New Delhi 110 011

What happens to the submitted information:

- Information provided in this form is handled in strict confidence. Peripheral Pharmacovigilance Centres forward this form to the Regional Pharmacovigilance Centres, where the causality analysis is carried out and the information is forwarded to the Zonal Pharmacovigilance Centres. The final report based on the analyzed data is reviewed by the National Pharmacovigilance Advisory Committee constituted by the Ministry of Health and Family Welfare. The Committee is entrusted with the responsibility to review and suggest any regulatory interventions that may be required with respect to the drug / drugs or class of drugs. The data is statistically analyzed and forwarded to the global pharmacovigilance database managed by WHO, Uppsala Monitoring Centre in Sweden.

Confidentiality:

The patient's identity is held in strict confidence and protected to the fullest extent. Programme staff is not expected to and will not disclose the reporter's identity in response to a request from the public.

Submission of a report does not constitute an admission that medical personnel or manufacturer or product caused or contributed to the reaction. The prescribed Suspected Adverse Drug Reaction Reporting Form is used for the purpose of National Pharmacovigilance Programme (NPP).

PHARMACOVIGILANCE IN SOME OTHER SELECTED COUNTRIES

Pharmacovigilance in USA

- The **US FDA** is responsible for assuring the safety and efficacy of all regulated marketed medical products.
- **MedWatch,** FDA safety information and Adverse Event Reporting programme serves both healthcare professionals and the public using medical products.
- Important and timely clinical information is provided about safety issues involving prescription and over-the-counter drugs, biologics, radiation-emitting devices, dietary supplements and infant formulae.

Pharmacovigilance in U.K.

- Committee on Safety of Medicines (CSM) runs the UK's spontaneous adverse drug reaction reporting scheme – called the *Yellow Card* Scheme.
- CSM receives reports of adverse drug reactions from health professionals and patients.

SUSPECTED ADVERSE DRUG REACTION REPORTING FORM
CDSCO
Central Drugs Standard Control Organization

Directorate General of Health Services, Ministry of Health & Family Welfare Government of India, Nirman Bhawan, New Delhi – 110011 www.cdsco.nic.in	**For VOLUNTARY reporting of Adverse Drug Reactions** by health care professionals	Report# To be filled in by Pharmacovigilance centres receiving the form.

A. Patient information

1. Patient identifier initials _____ In confidence	2. Age at time of event: _____ or _____ Date of Birth	3. Sex ☐ M ☐ F _____ 4. Weight __ Kgs

B. Suspected Adverse Reaction

5. Date of reaction started (dd/mm/yy):

6. Date of recovery (dd/mm/yy)

7. Describe reaction or problem

12. Relevant tests / laboratory data, including dates.

13. Other relevant history, including pre-existing medical conditions (e.g., allergies, race, pregnancy, smoking, alcohol use, hepatic/ renal dysfunction, etc.)

14. Seriousness of the reaction
☐ Death (dd/mm/yy)   ☐ Congenital anomaly
☐ Life threatening   ☐ Required intervention
☐ Hospitalization-initial   to prevent permanent
   or prolonged   impairment/damage
☐ Disability   ☐ Other (specify)____

15. Outcomes
☐ Fatal   ☐ Recovering   ☐ Unknown
☐ Continuing ☐ Recovered   ☐ Other (specify)

C. Suspected medication(s)

S. No.	8. Name (brand and/ or generic name)	Manufact urer (if known)	Batch No./ Lot No. (if known)	Exp. Date (If known)	Dose used	Route used	Frequency	Therapy dates (if unknown, give duration) Date started	Date stopped	Reason for use or prescribed for

S. No. As per C	9. Reaction abated after drug stopped or dose reduced					10. Reaction reappeared after reintroduction				
	Yes	No	Unknown	NA	Reduced dose	Yes	No	Unknown	NA	If reintroduced, dose

11. Concomitant medical products and therapy was including self medication and herbal remedies (exclude those used to treat reaction)

D. Reporter

16.   Name and Professional Address: _____
_____
_____

Pin code: _____ E-mail: _____
Cell No. / Tel No. with STD Code: _____

Speciality: _____   Signature:

17. Occupation	18. Date of this report (dd/mm/yy)

Pharmacovigilance in Europe

The pharmacovigilance effort in Europe is coordinated by the European Medicines Agency (EMEA) and conducted by the national competent medicines authorities (NCA). The main responsibility of the EMEA is to maintain and develop the pharmacovigilance database consisting of all suspected serious adverse reactions to medicines observed in the European community. The system is called Eudra Vigilance and contains separate but similar databases of human and veterinary reactions.

Pharmacovigilance in Canada

- Health Canada is responsible for approving drugs for marketing in Canada.
- Canadian Adverse Drug Reaction Monitoring Programme (CADRMP) monitors all adverse drug reactions reported.
- ADR reports are submitted voluntarily directly by health professionals and consumers to ADR centres as well as to the national centre in Ottawa.
- It is mandatory for manufacturers to report serious ADRs.
- ADR reports are reviewed, and entered into the Canadian Adverse Drug Reaction Information System.

The French pharmacovigilance system

The French pharmacovigilance system has a number of features that make it stand out: It is based on a number of specificities which have proven successful.

- The existence of real network, where alert investigation is done in the Regional Centres.
- The use of common procedures, to ensure quality of data, including the use of causality method.
- The integration of the center in clinical pharmacology department within university hospitals.
- The emphasis of the drug information function as a continuing source of education

Pharmacovigilance in the Netherlands

Following the thalidomide affair of the late 1950s and early 1960s, the Netherlands decided to adopt a more systematic approach to the safety of prescription medicines. The Dutch Medicines Evaluation Board was founded in 1963. The Medicines Evaluation Board plays a central coordinating role and makes the final decisions regarding marketing authorization of the Netherlands. The Medicines Evaluation Board includes a pharmacovigilance department primarily concerned with ADRs and with maintaining international contents in the field. Many decisions are taken at European level by the European medicines agency (EMEA).

The Netherlands Pharmacovigilance Center Lareb has extensive network of doctors and pharmacists. In the context of pharmaceutical patient care pharmacists in the Netherlands are highly involved in ensuring the safe and responsible use of medicines.

Lareb maintains the spontaneous reporting system for the Netherlands

Lareb is an independent organization working on behalf of the Government. Reports are forwarded to the Medicines Evaluation Board Agency weekly.

Pharmacovigilance in New Zealand

PEM (Prescription Event Monitoring) in New Zealand like PEM in the U.K. is a valuable method of post-marketing surveillance. The value of data collected in PEM studies is that it is derived from 'real-life' use of medicines. The populations used are more representative of normal clinical practice without exclusion criteria of pre-marketing clinical trials. The NZ IMMP (Intensive Medicines Monitoring Programme) has enhanced PEM to perform many different pharmacoepidemiology studies.

Pharmacovigilance in Japan

Pharmacovigilance in Japan has traditionally been characterized by a small no. of spontaneous reports of suspected adverse drug reactions (ADRs). The Japanese SRS was created in 1967. The no. of ADR reports increased with the increase in the no. of 'designated medical institutions' and 'designated pharmacists'. After further expansion of the system in 1997, the Ministry of Health and Welfare (MHW) renamed the Ministry of Health and Labour Welfare (MHLW) in 2000 received around 5000 reports per annum from health professionals. Since 1997 the MHLW has received ADR reports sent via drug companies, as well as reports directly from the doctors.

Under the strict and somewhat intricate regulations concerned with post-approval safety, pharmacovigilance is generally regarded as the activity performed almost exclusively by the regulatory body in Japan.

TEACHING AND LEARNING PHARMACO-VIGILANCE

The educational need associated with the field of pharmacovigilance has two dimensions. The principal primary dimension is that of the clinical practitioner who needs knowledge, understanding and wisdom about effects of medicines in his day-to-day practice. The secondary dimension is that of professionals in the field who must amass and evaluate emerging evidence from broad populations exposed to pharmacotherapies.

On the one hand, the health care practitioner needs to learn to continually discriminate benefits and risks associated with the pharmacotherapies they are supervising. On the other hand, the professional pharmacovigilist needs to develop and maintain the same fundamental clinical knowledge and discriminatory skill as well as mastery of increasingly complex systems of signal generation, effective communication back to the public and healthcare practitioners. There are learners and teachers of pharmacovigilance.

Teaching Pharmacovigilance

At undergraduate levels

Pharmacotherapeutics education needs to be solidly grounded on principles of benefit and risk from drug therapies. The concept of benefit/risk management is fundamental to sound preparation for practice in any of the disciplines that are involved in pharmacotherapy processes.

The undergraduate health professional needs to be instructed at the outset in the realities of both error and uncertainty in health care.

Building on this approach of pharmacotherapy, at the undergraduate level, pharmacovigilance and continually refreshed knowledge of benefits and risks from pharmacotherapy can become central to the experience of all health care clinicians.

At postgraduate levels

The International Society of Pharmacovigilance (ISOP: http:// www. isoponline.org) is a non-profit organization whose aims are to foster pharmacovigilance both scientifically and educationally and enhance all aspects of safe and proper use of medicines, in all countries.

Another organization is International Society for Pharmacoepidemiology (ISPE: http://www.pharmacoepi.org). It is an international organization dedicated to advancing the health of the public by providing a forum for the open exchange of scientific information and for the development of policy; education; and advocacy for the field of pharmacoepidemiology and therapeutic risk management.

Some other authorities also provide this discipline for professionals who work specifically in the fields of pharmacovigilance and therapeutic risk management. For example, the Drug Information Association (DIA: http://www.diahome.org); The United Kingdom Drug Safety-Research Unit and the London School of Hygiene and Tropical Medicine; the European Agency for the Evaluation of Medicinal Products (EMEA: http://eudravigilance.emea.eu.int) in collaboration with the DIA are providing training for pharmacovigilance professionals.

Uppsala Monitoring Centre (WHO Collaborating Centre for International Drug Monitoring http://www.who-umc.org) has developed the training programme. The main content is given in Table 22.8.

Table 22.8. The main content of Uppsala Monitoring Centre for providing training.

The aims and content of pharmacovigilance

Clinical aspects, pharmacology and epidemiology of ADRs

The practice of spontaneous reporting and running a pharmacovigilance centre, use of the WHO data base

Connection of drug regulation, International harmonization and standardization

Principles of pharmacoepidemiology and methods of research

Special fields such as vaccines, herbal remedies, dependence and quality defects

Literature sources benefits/harm assessment

Communication

Crisis management

STUDY QUESTIONS

1. What is Pharmacovigilance? Mention its specific aims.

2. Why Pharmacovigilance is needed?

3. Why should Pharmacovigilance be developed in every country?

4. Describe the National Pharmacovigilance System in India.

5. Describe WHO Programme for International Drug Monitoring.

6. Define: i) Adverse drug reaction, (ii) Serious Adverse Event (SAE).

7. Write short notes on: i) Respect of privacy in pharmacovigilance, ii) Signal detection methods, iii) Pharmacoepidemiology.

8. Describe the responsibility of pharmaceutical companies to pharmacovigilance programme.

9. Describe the information which helps to assess the drug causality to adverse clinical event, whether the relationship is definite, probable, possible or unlikely.

10. Discuss Good Pharmacovigilance Practices.

11. What are the main elements in ADR report. Describe: i) What to report, ii) Who can report, iii) Where to report and iv) What happens to the information submitted?

12. Discuss the need for proper educational training in the field of pharmacovigilance. Also list ten important topics which should be covered in the training programme.

13. Explain: (i) Role of pharmacovigilance in rational use of medicines. (ii) How pharmacovigilance is useful in public health disease control programmes.

14. Describe briefly the pharmacovigilance systems in (i) UK; (ii) USA; and (iii) Canada.

GUIDE TO FURTHER READINGS

Academia Industry Synergy Continuum: Symposium on Promotion of Pharmacovigilance in India. Organized by Dept. of Pharmacology, AIIMS, New Delhi on March 15, 2007.

Bahri P, Tsintis P, Pharmacovigilance related topics at the level of the International Conference on Harmonisation (ICH) Pharmacoepidemiology and Drug Safety 2005; 14: 377-387.

Bates DW, Spell N, Cullen DJ *et al.* The costs of adverse drug reactions in hospitalized patients. JAMA. 1997; 277:301-7.

Bavdekar Sandeep B, Karande S. National Pharmacovigilance Program. Indian Pediatrics. 2006; 43:27-32.

Bhatt HA, Gogtay NJ, Dalavi SS, Shirsagar NA. The international journal of risk and safety in medicine 2004, 16: 73-82.

Biswas P, Biswas A.K. Setting standards for proactive pharmacovigilance in India. Indian J. Pharmacol, 2007; 39:124-8.

Central Drugs Standard Control Organization. Available from: http:/www.cdsco.

Detailed guidance on the collection, verification and presentation of adverse reaction reports arising from clinical trials on medicinal products for human use April 2003 Brussels. ENTR/F2/BL D(2003).

Epstem M (2005) Guidelines for good pharmacoepidemiology practices (GPP) Pharmacoepidemiol Drug Saf, 14, 589-95.

FDA Guidance for industry. Good pharmacovigilance practices and pharmacoepidemiologic assessment. March, 2005.

Gogtay NJ, Dalavi SS, Shirsagar NA. Safety monitoring an Indian perspective. The International Journal of Risk and Safety in Medicine 2003, 16: 21-30.

Lazarou J, Pomeranz B, Corey PN. Incidence of adverse drug reactions in hospitalized patients: A meta-analysis of prospective studies. JAMA. 1988; 279:1200-05.

LL Leape. Errors in medicine. JAMA. 1994; 272:1851-7.

Mc Whinney IR (1997) A textbook of family medicine, Oxford University Press New York; London. P. 129.

Montastruca Jean, Agnes S, Lacroixa Isabelle, Oliviera Pascale. Pharmacovigilance for evaluating adverse drug reactions: value, organization, and methods. Joint Bone Spine. 2006; 73:629-32.

National Health Surveillance Agency. Available from: http:/www.anvisa.gov.br.

Panos Tsintis P, Lal Mache E CIOMS and ICH Initiatives in Pharmacovigilance and Risk Management Overview and Implications European Agency for the Evaluation of Medicinal Products. London, United Kingdom Drug Safety 2004; 27(8): 509-517.

Prakash S. Pharmacovigilance in India. Indian J Pharmaco 2007, 29:123. Available at: www.ijp-online.com, Indian Journal of Pharmacology vol. 40, Feb. 2008 supplement/Review articles on pharmacovigilance.

Protocol for National Pharmacovigilance Program. CDSCO, Ministry of Health and Family Welfare, Government of India, November, 2004.

Rules Governing Medicinal Products in the European Union – Volume-9 Pharmacovigilance and the Guideline Post-Approval Safety Data Management –

Definitions and Standards for Expedited Reporting (CPMP/ICH/3945/03).

Scobie S, Thomson R, Cook A et al. (2005) Building a memory: preventing harm, reducing risks and improving patient safety. The National Patient Safety Agency, London.

Snyder C, Anderson G (2005) Do quality improvement organizations improve the quality of hospital care for Medicare beneficiaries? JAMA, 293, 2900-7.

Therapeutic Goods Administration. Available from: http:/www.tga.gov.au.

WHO. Dialogue in pharmacovigilance – more effective communication. Uppsala, World Health Organization Collaborating Centre for International Drug Monitoring, 2002.

WHO. Expecting the worst. Anticipating, preventing and managing medicinal product crises. Uppsala. World Health Organization Collaborating Centre for International Drug Monitoring, 2002.

WHO. Safety monitoring of medicinal products. The importance of pharmacovigilance. Geneva, World Health Organization, 2002.

WHO. The World Health Organization Collaborating Centre for International Drug Monitoring (website). The World Health Organization Collaborating Centre for International Drug Monitoring. Uppsala (http://www.who-umc.org. accessed 15 October, 2004.

Stem Cells: Basics and Potential Uses

STEM CELL BASICS

Introduction:

Stem cells are potentially immortal cells capable of self-renewal and also give rise to differentiated cells.

No area of research except gene therapy has evolved so much enthusiasm and hope as stem cells. Most medical experts view stem cell research as the new frontier in medicine, a huge breakthrough that could save millions of lives.

Medicines today are based on drug therapy dominated by antibiotics, chemotherapy and other pharmaceuticals. Medicine of future will be based on cell therapies, focused on repair of tissues/organs by cell transplants i.e. instead of drugs to prevent malfunction or death, diseased cells will be replaced by healthy differentiated stem cells.

What are stem cells?

The classical definition of stem cells requires that they possess three unique general properties (regardless of their source of origin) that distinguish them from other types of cells - 1. Self-renewal, 2. unspecialized nature, and 3. Potency. Self-renewal and differentiation is shown in figure 23.1. The characteristics are described below:

1. **Stem cells are capable of dividing and renewing themselves for long periods:** Self-renewal is an ability to go through numerous cycles of cell division while maintaining the undifferential state i.e. stem cells are potentially immortal cells. Unlike muscle cells, blood cells or nerve cells – which do not normally replicate themselves – stem cells may replicate many times over (it is called proliferation). A starting population of stem cells that proliferates for

many months in the laboratory can yield millions of cells. If the resulting cells continue to be unspecialized, like the parent stem cells, the cells are said to be capable of long-term self-renewal.

2. **Stem cells are unspecialized:** One of the fundamental properties of a stem cell is that it does not have any tissue-specific structure that allows it to perform specialized functions. A stem cell can not work with its neighbours to pump blood (like a heart muscle cell); it cannot carry molecules of oxygen in the bloodstream (like a red blood cell); and it can not fire electrochemical signals to or other cells that allow the body to move or speak (like a nerve cell). However, unspecialized stem cells can give rise to specialized cells, including heart muscle cells, blood cells, or nerve cells.

3. **Potency: Stem cells can give rise to specialized cells:** When unspecialized stem cells give rise to specialized cells, the process is called differentiation. Potency refers to the potential to differentiate into any specialized cell type of the mature stem cell.

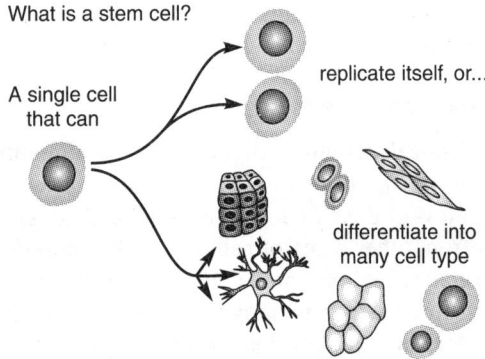

Fig. 23.1. Self-renewal and differentiation.

Potency signifies the differentiation potential i.e. the potential to differentiate into **different cell types:**

- *Totipotent* stem cells are produced from the fusion of an egg and sperm cell. Cells produced by the first few divisions of the fertilized egg are totipotent. These cells can differentiate into embryonic and non-embryonic cell types.

At 2 or 3 days after fertilization, an embryo consists of identical cells which are totipotent.

That is to say that each cell could give rise to an embryo on its own producing, for example, identical twins or quadruplets. They are totally unspecialized and have the capacity to differentiate into any of the cells, which will constitute the foetus as well as the placenta and membranes around the foetus.

- *Pluripotent:* Embryonic stem cells are the descendents of totipotent cells and can differentiate into cells derived from any of the three germ layers (mesoderm, endoderm and ectoderm) but can not develop into an embryo on its own.

Pluripotent adult stem cells are rare and generally small in number but can be found in a number of tissues including umbilical blood.

- *Multipotent* stem cells are those which are capable of giving rise to several different types of specialized cells constituting a specific tissue or organ. They produce only cells of a closely related family of cells e.g. haemopoietic stem cells differentiate into red blood cells, white blood cells and platelets.

- *Unipotent* stem cells can produce only one cell type, but have the property of self-renewal.

The relationship amongst various types of stem cells is shown in Fig. 23.2.

Types of stem cells (Fig. 23.3)

There are two broad types of mammalian stem cells:

1. Embryonic stem cells that are derived from blastocysts.
2. Adult stem cells (somatic) that are derived from foetal or adult tissues or organs, including umbilical cord blood/placenta.

1. Embryonic stem cells

Within about eight days after fertilization, the totipotent stem cells divide, mature, and give rise to more restricted cells called "pluripotent" stem cells. These cells can self-renew and can give rise to any cell of the body. However, pluripotent cells lose the potential to form an organ and certainly cannot form a fully developed organism. This complex cellular

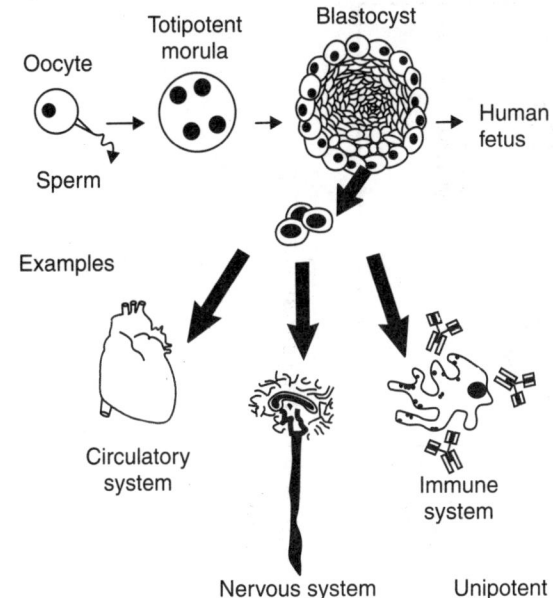

Fig. 23.2. Relationship amongst various types of stem cells.

development takes place before organs begin to form in the embryo or even before the embryo leaves the fallopian tube and implants in the uterus.

These more restricted pluripotent cells are called embryonic stem (ES) cells. These cells can divide indefinitely and may be able to be used to replace missing, damaged, or dying cells in any organ of the developing and adult body. Certain diseases, in which specific types of cells are damaged, as in diabetes, Parkinson's disease, heart disease, and cancers, are likely to be the first targets for such therapeutic applications.

These pluripotent cells are thought to be the most versatile type of stem cells, as they can develop into any type of cell in the body. Stem cells can be sourced from leftover embryos stored at fertility clinics, unused by couples to have children, or aborted foetuses in their early development. Also, special purpose embryos can be created by in vitro fertilization for the sole purpose of extracting their stem cells.

Before organs are formed, embryos are comprised of a collection of cells with potential to give rise to many different organs and tissues. These stem cells

are first derived from inner cell mass of the 3-5 days old developing embryo at the blastocyst stage. They divide endlessly in laboratory culture dishes and maintain the ability to differentiate into numerous types of unipotent cells when exposed to the appropriate growth factors e.g., nerve growth factor. Their removable plasticity makes them as excellent candidates for use in major therapies. The embryonic stem cells are though flexible, immortal and easily available, but could involve ethical controversies and transplant rejections in the recipient patient.

2. Adult Stem Cells

Adult stem cells are stem cells derived from the tissues or organs of an organism after birth.

The term adult stem cell refers to any cell which is found in a developed organism that has two properties: the ability to divide and create another cell like itself and also divide and create a cell more differentiated than itself.

An adult stem cell is an undifferentiated cell found among differentiated cells in a tissue or organ, can renew itself, and can differentiate to yield the major specialized cell types of the tissue or organ.

Most adult stem cells are lineage – restricted (multipotent) and are generally referred to by their tissue origin (mesenchymal stem cell, adipose-derived stem cell, endothelial stem cell, hair stem cells, tooth stem cells, neural stem cells, endometrial stem cells etc.) (Fig. 23.4).

Lineage – to ensure self-renewal stem cells undergo two types of cell division. Symmetric division gives rise to two identical daughter cells both endowed with stem cell properties. Asymmetric division, on the other hand, produces only one stem cell and a progenitor cell with limited self-renewal potential. Progenitor can go through several rounds of cell division before terminally differentiating into mature cell.

In 1960s, researchers discovered that the bone marrow contains at least two kinds of stem cells – haematopoietic stem cells (which form all the types of blood cells in the body; bone marrow stromal cells (which are a mixed cell population that generates bone, cartilage, fat and fibrous connective tissue).

It was in 1990s that scientists agreed that the adult brain does contain stem cells that are able to generate

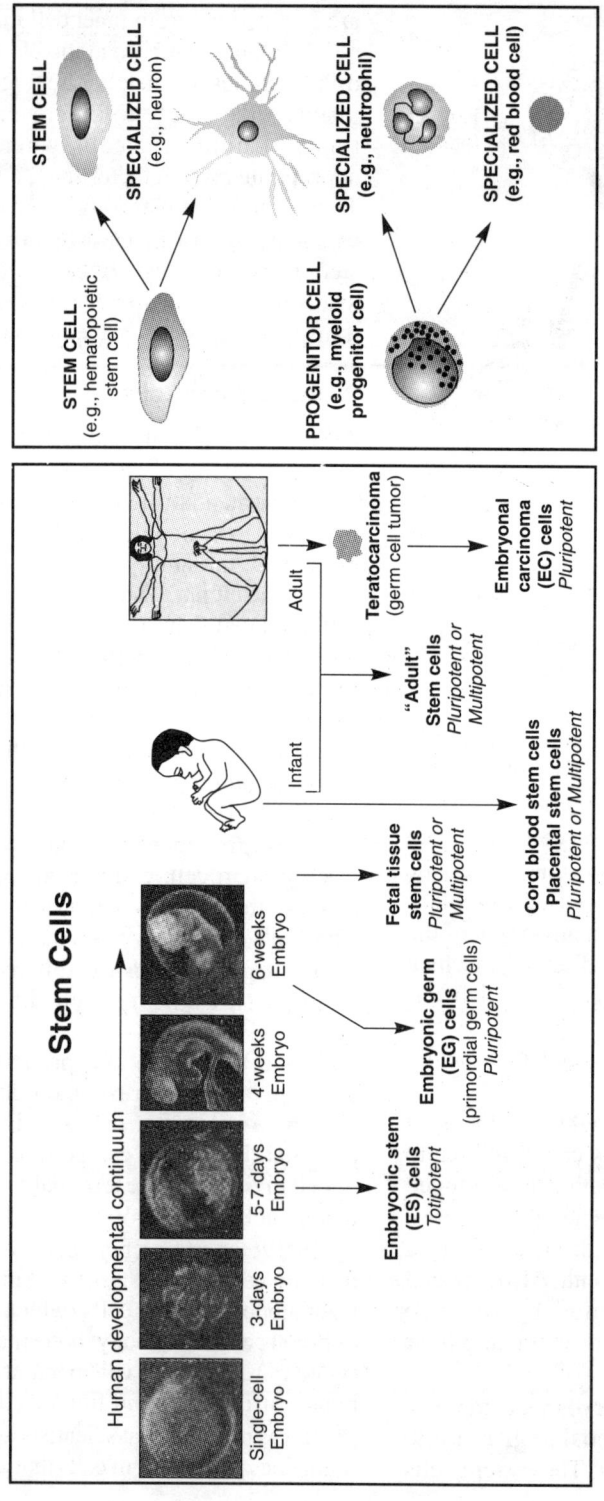

Fig. 23.3. Types of stem cells – Embryonic & Adult.

Adult stem cell-marrow, skin, liver, bone, brain, GIT (*0.05-5% of all cells*)

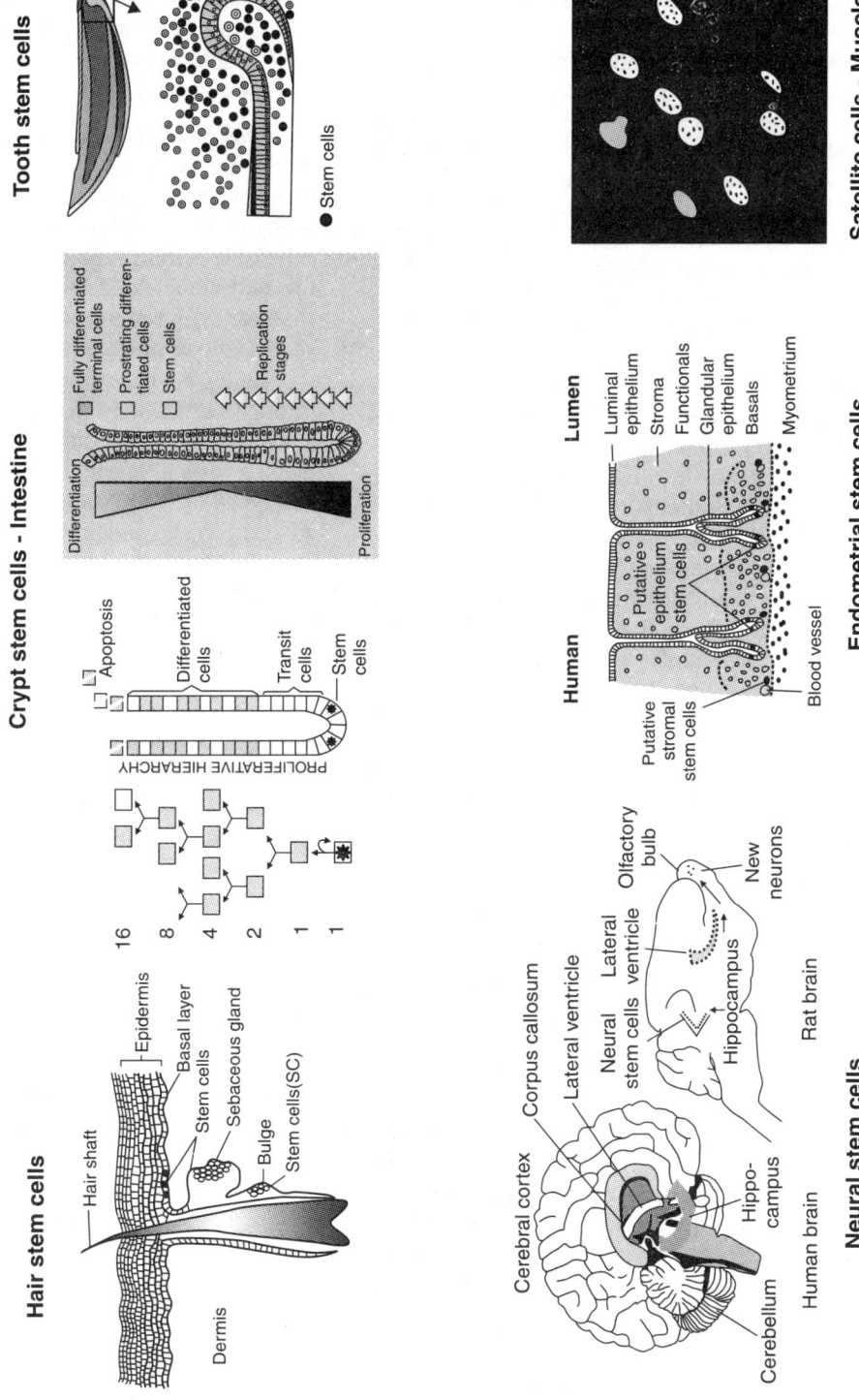

Fig. 23.4. Types of adult stem cells.

the brain's three major cell types – astrocytes and oligodendrocytes (non-neuronal cells) and neurons, or nerve cells.

Adult stem cells typically generate the cell types of the tissue in which they reside. A blood-forming adult stem cell in the bone marrow normally gives rise to the many types of blood cells such as red blood cells, white blood cells and platelets. Until recently, it had been thought that a blood-forming cell in the bone marrow (called haematopoietic stem cell) could not give rise to the cells of a different tissue. However, a number of experiments over the last few years have raised the possibility that stem cells from one tissue may be able to give rise to cell types of completely different tissues, a phenomenon known as plasticity, e.g. blood cells becoming neurons, liver cells can be made to produce insulin, and haematopoietic stem cells can develop into heart muscle. Therefore, exploring the possibility of using adult stem cells for cell-based therapies has become a very active area of investigation by researchers.

Adult stem cells occur in many tissues and they enter normal differential pathways to form the specialized cell types of other tissues, which is known as transdifferential or plasticity.

The following are examples of normal differential pathways of adult stem cells:

- Haematopoietic stem cells give rise to all types of blood cells: red blood cells, B lymphocytes, T lymphocytes, natural killer cells, neutrophils, basophils, eosinophils, monocytes, macrophages, and platelets.
- Bone marrow stromal cells (mesenchymal stem cells) give rise to a variety of cell types: bone cells (osteocytes), cartilage cells (chondrocytes), fat cells (adipocytes), and other kinds of connective tissue cells such as those in tendons.
- Neural stem cells in the brain give rise to its three major cell types: nerve cells (neurons) and two categories of non-neuronal cells- astrocytes and oligodendrocytes.
- Epithelial stem cells in the lining of the digestive tract occur in deep crypts and give rise to several cell types: absorptive cells, goblet cells, enteroendocrine cells.
- Skin stem cells occur in the basal layer of the epidermis and at the base of hair follicles. The epidermal stem cells give rise to keratinocytes, which migrate to the surface of the skin and form a protective layer. The follicular stem cells can give rise to both the hair follicle and to the epidermis.

Adult stem cells are obtained from the tissue or organs of living adults during surgery. There are many different types of multipotent adult stem cells, each of which is responsible for developing into the cells of a certain type of tissue, with their natural fate to become blood and immune cells. Multipotent stem cells can be found in some types of adult tissue such as blood stem cells.

Adult stem cells are undifferentiated cells found throughout the body that divide to replenish dying cells and regenerate damaged tissues. These renew themselves and become specialized to yield all the cell types of the tissue from which it was isolated. Also known as somatic stem cells, they can be found in children, as well as adults. Many adult stem cells have been classified as progenitor cells due to their limited capacity for cellular differentiation. Earlier thought to be restricted to produce differentiated cells specific to the organ from which they were isolated, adult stem cells have recently been found to transdifferentiate (i.e., induce to form other cell types) too, e.g., neural stem cells (NSC) to blood and skeletal muscle, and bone marrow cells to muscle, liver cells, and astrocytes.

The multipotent bone marrow stem cells can give rise to fully differentiated connective tissue, including cartilage, bone, adipose tissue, fibrous tissue and myelosupportive stromal cell. Perhaps the best-known stem cell therapy to date is the bone marrow transplant used primarily to treat leukemias and lymphomas.

While most blood stem cells reside in the bone marrow, a small number are present in the bloodstream too. These multipotent peripheral blood stem cells (PBSCs) can be used just like bone marrow stem cells to treat various malignant blood disorders. Bone marrow adult stem cells have also been used with fruition for other types of cancer and various blood disorders. Since they can be obtained from drawn blood, PBSCs are easier to collect than bone marrow stem cells, which must be extracted from within bones. This makes PBSCs a less invasive treatment option than bone marrow stem cells. PBSCs are sparse in the blood stream. However, with use of various growth factors (G-CSF, GM-CSF), enough PBSCs can be collected to perform a transplant.

There are several advantages of using adult stem cells, as one can isolate them from the patients and cajole them to divide, direct their specialization and even fortify them with the therapeutic drugs and then transplant them back to the patient. Neither these adult cells have the plausibility of getting rejected, nor becoming target for ethical consideration. Adult stem cells are also immune-hardy, i.e., the recipients receiving the products of their own stem cells will hardly experience immune rejection, thus circumventing the use of immunosuppressive drugs.

Umbilical Cord Blood Stem Cells

The umbilical cord, connecting the foetus with the mother is cut at the time of delivery and discarded. Cord blood (the remaining blood in the umbilical cord) is full of 'stem cells' which is the origin of the body's immune system.

In the 1970s, medical researchers discovered that human umbilical cord blood contained the same kind of stem cells found in bone marrow. Because stem cells from bone marrow had already been used to treat patients suffering from diseases like leukaemia and other immune system disorders, researchers believed that they could also use stem cells from umbilical cord blood to save patients.

Umbilical cord blood stem cells hold immense promise as availability of donor is not a hiccup. Cord blood stem cell transplants are less prone to rejection than either bone marrow or peripheral blood stem cells. This is ostensibly because the cells have not yet developed the features that can be recognized and attacked by the recipient's immune system. Also, as umbilical cord blood lacks well-developed immune cells, there is less plausibility that the transplanted cells will trigger a common life-threatening problem called graft-versus-host disease. The versatility and availability of umbilical cord blood stem cells make them a potent resource for transplant therapies. New research shows that as the umbilical cord cells proliferate rapidly, they can

indeed replace bone marrow and other sources of stem cells to treat adults.

More than 45 diseases have now been treated using cord blood cells. These include malignant diseases like leukaemia, lymphoma, neuroblastoma and retinoblastoma, and several other non-malignant diseases as well. The non-malignant diseases are primarily inherited disorders of the blood and immune systems, or genetic diseases affecting metabolism.

Research is also going on to treat diseases like stroke, Alzheimer's disease, multiple sclerosis, lupus and diabetes by transplanting cord blood stem cells.

Placental Stem Cells

Recently, the researchers have discovered that one type of cell in the human placenta has characteristics strikingly similar to embryonic stem cells in their ability to regenerate a wide variety of tissues. The cells, called amniotic epithelial cells, could potentially be used to produce new liver cells to treat liver failure, or new pancreatic islet cells to cure diabetes or new neurons to treat Parkinson's disease. Unlike embryonic stem cells, obtained only by destroying human embryos, these cells can be extracted from the placentas that are routinely discarded after birth. Like cord cells, placental cells could also be a non-controversial alternative to embryonic stem cells. The stem cells in the placenta hold huge promise as remarkable healers, as their yield seems to exceed any other tissue place known before and immuno-rejection is hardly a concern. Like cord cells, placental cells from newborns are unlikely to contain viruses.

Similarities and differences between embryonic and adult stem cells

Adult and embryonic stem cells differ in the number and type of differentiated cell types they can become.

- Embryonic stem cells can become all cell types of the body because they are pluripotent.
- Adult stem cells are generally limited to differentiating into different cell types of their tissue of origin. However, adult stem cell plasticity may exist, increasing the number of cell types a given adult stem cell can become.

- Large number of embryonic stem cells can be grown in culture, while adult stem cells are rare in mature tissues and methods of expending their numbers in cell culture have not yet been worked out. This is an important distinction, as large numbers of cells are needed for stem cell replacement therapies.
- A potential advantage of using stem cells from an adult is that the patient's own cells could be expanded in culture and then reintroduced into the patient. In this case, cells would not be rejected by the immune system
- Adult stem cells are already specialized; their potential to regenerate damaged tissue is very limited. Skin cells will only become skin, and cartilage cells will only become cartilage.
- Adults do not have stem cells in many vital organs, so when these tissues are damaged, scar tissue develops. Only embryonic stem cells, which have the capacity to become any kind of human tissue, have the potential to repair vital organs.
- Another limitation of adult stem cells is their inability to proliferate in culture, unlike embryonic stem cells, which have a capacity to reproduce indefinitely in the laboratory. Adult stem cells are difficult to grow in the laboratory

Sources of stem cells

Table 23.1. Stem cells obtained from various body organs.

Source	Types of stem cells	Potential
Adult	Cord blood stem cells	Multipotent and
	Liver stem cells	unipotent
	Epithelial stem cells	
	Neuronal stem cells	
	Pancreatic stem cells	
	Spermatogonial stem cells	
Embryo	Trophoectodermal stem cells	Totipotent or
	Embryonic stem cells	pluripotent
	Morula stem cells	
Foetus	Foetal germ stem cells	Pluripotent
	Foetal germ carcinoma cells	

and their potential to reproduce diminishes with age. Therefore, obtaining significant amounts of adult stem cells may prove to be difficult.

Intrinsic and extrinsic properties of stem cells

There are signals inside and outside cells that trigger stem cell differentiation. The internal signs are controlled by cell's genes and mediated through metabolically active enzymes and receptors. The external signals for cell differentiation include chemicals secreted by other cells, physical contact with neighbouring 'stromal' cells, blood vessels and micro-environment (Table 23.2).

Table 23.2. Unique features of stem cells

• Self-renewal cells	• Intrinsic properties
• Asymmetric DNA segregation	– Metabolically active
	– Enzymes
• Low mitotic activity	– Receptors
• Error-free proliferation	– Genes
• Poor differentiation	• Extrinsic properties "Niche"
• Quiescence	– Blood vessels
• Special anatomical protection	– Basement membrane
	– Stroma

Plasticity of stem cells

Stem cells are the body's "master" cells. They can renew themselves indefinitely and differentiate into any of a number of cell types, such as muscle, nerve, organ, bone, blood and so on. These properties make stem cells different from the body's other mature cells, which are permanently committed to their fate – for example, a skin cell can only divide and generate new skin cells.

This attribute of stem cells is called plasticity, i.e., to give rise to cell types of a completely different tissue from one tissue, e.g., blood cells becoming neurons, liver cells producing insulin like pancreas, haematopoietic cells developing into heart muscle, etc.

Adult stem cell plasticity (Transdifferentiation): Certain adult stem cell types are pluripotent. This ability to differentiate into multiple cell types is called plasticity or Transdifferentiation (Fig. 23.5). The following are examples of adult stem cell plasticity:

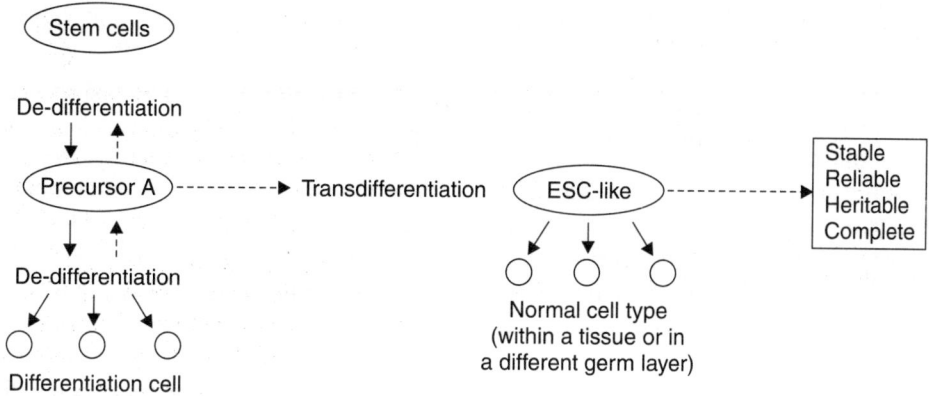

Fig. 23.5. Stem cell plasticity or transdifferentiation

- Haematopoietic stem cells may differentiate into three major types of brain cells (neuron, oligodendrocytes, and astrocytes); skeletal muscle cells; cardiac muscle cells; and liver cells.
- Bone marrow stromal stem cells may differentiate into cardiac muscle cell and skeletal muscle cell.
- Brain stem cells may differentiate into blood cells and skeletal muscle cells.

The process of manipulating autologous adult stem cells, some of which are present in sufficient numbers in the adult for therapeutic purposes (e.g. MSC, HSC) to obtain the desired differentiated cell or stem cell is termed trans-differentiation or de-differentiation.

In recent times, cord blood stem cells are being investigated for their ability to de-differentiate or transdifferentiate into desired differentiated cells. There is some emerging evidence that cord blood transplants may work not just for haemotopoietic system or mesenchymal system disorders but may also be in correcting other multisystem disorders by providing a useful delivery vehicle via the macrophages and microglia that differentiate from HSC and are present throughout the body. Indeed, a possibility has been used to treat lysosomal storage diseases.

The current understanding of the process and control of transdifferentiation is still in its infancy and at present, one cannot apply this to clinical treatment.

Importance of stem cells for living organisms

Stem cells are formed at conception and specialize to become the various tissues of the growing embryo. After birth the body retains stem cell reserves in various organs and, throughout life, those reserves help to repair and replace injured or diseased tissues. Unfortunately, the stem cell reserves are finite and, when they become depleted, it results in a variety of disorders and ravages of aging. Thus, stem cell therapy offers the potential to replenish the reserves.

Stem cells have the remarkable potential to develop into many different cell types in the body. Serving as a sort of repair system in the body, they can theoretically divide without limit to replenish other cells as long as the person or animal is alive. When a stem cell divides, each new cell has the potential to either remain a stem cell, or become another type of cell with a more specialized function, such as a muscle cell, a red blood cell, or a brain cell.

In some adult tissues, such as bone marrow, muscle, and brain, discrete populations of adult stem cells generate replacements for cells that are lost through normal wear and tear, injury or disease.

The primary roles of adult stem cells in a living organism are to maintain and repair the tissue in which they are found. Some scientists now use the term somatic stem cell instead of adult stem cell. Unlike embryonic stem cells, which are defined by their origin (the inner cell mass of the blastocyst), the origin of adults stem cells in mature tissues is unknown.

The adult tissues reported to contain stem cells are brain, bone marrow, peripheral blood, blood vessels, skeletal muscle, skin and liver. There are a very small number of stem cells in each tissue. Stem cells are thought to reside in a specific area of each tissue where they remain non-dividing for long periods (many years) until they are activated by disease or tissue injury. Some examples are given below:

Distinct stem cell types have been established from embryos and identified in the foetal tissues and umbilical cord blood (UCB) as well as in specific niches in many adult mammalian tissues and organs, such as bone marrow (BM), brain, skin, eyes, heart, kidneys, lungs, gastrointestinal tract, pancreas, liver, breast, ovaries, prostate, and testis. All stem cells are undifferentiated cells that exhibit unlimited self-renewal and can generate multiple cell lineages or more restricted progenitor populations that can contribute to tissue homeostasis by replenishment of cells or regeneration of tissue after injury.

Embryonic Stem Cells: Several mammalian pluripotent embryonic stem cell (ESC) lines derived from blastocyst early-stage embryos have been established. More specifically, human embryonic stem cell (hESC) lines express many markers that are common to pluripotent and undifferentiated cells.

Amniotic Epithelial Cells: Amniotic epithelial cells (AECs) derived from the amniotic membrane in human term placenta also express the markers that are present on pluripotent ESCs and EGCs.

Foetal Stem Cells: Multipotent foetal stem cells (FSCs) are generally more tissue-specific than CSCs. Therefore, FSCs are able to generate a more limited number of progenitor types. One of the particular therapeutic advantages of FSCs as compared with ESCs is the fact that FSCs do not form teratomas in vivo.

Umbilical Cord Stem Cells: Umbilical cord epithelium (UCE), which appears to derive from amniotic membrane epithelium, and UCB represent other sources of multipotent stem cells that might be used for generating diverse differentiated cell types.

Stromal Stem Cells: The BM stroma is a highly vascularized, complex structure containing mesenchymal stem cells and extracellular matrix elements supporting for haematopoiesis. Mesenchymal stem cell populations from BM stroma, which can give rise to stromal mature mesenchymal cells and regenerate the BM microenvironment, have been identified in a perivascular region in BM tissue.

Cardiac Stem Cells: The clusters of multipotent cardiac stem cells have recently been identified and localized throughout the myocardium, and more particularly, at the atria and lower region of the left ventricle of the heart, termed apex. CSCs possess the ability to self-renew and differentiate into three major cell types of the myocardium: myocytes, smooth muscle cells, and endothelial cells. In fact, CSCs appear to be involved in maintenance of heart homeostasis and repair of myocardial tissue after injury.

Neural Stem Cells: During prenatal development of the mammalian CNS, the neural stem cells (NSCs) and their progenitors may expand and give rise to the functional neurons and glial cells that constitute the growing brain. Similarly, in the adult CNS of mammals, a small number of NSCs, which possess astrocytic morphology and high telomerase levels, are also able to self-renew and generate different neural cell lineages. NSCs appear to be principally localized in two regions in adult mammalian CNS. More specifically, one population of NSCs resides in the subventricular zone (SVZ) around the lateral ventricle in the forebrain and can differentiate into neurons and glia. The other populations, which is localized in the subgranular cells layer of hippocampus in a region termed dentate gyrus, may give rise to granule cell projection neurons. NSCs are also localized in close proximity to a perivascular basal lamina (BL) within the SVZ, which is composed of laminin, collagen-1, fibroblasts, and macrophages and appears to assume a critical function for the maintenance of NSC homing. In fact, NSCs might expand with these niches and give rise to more differentiated progenitors that, in turn, may migrate to distinct distant sites. Although, several reports revealed that neural crest stem-derived progenitors may migrate from SVZ into the olfactory bulb in the rodent brain, no available evidence suggests that this could also be prevalent in the human brain. Hence, the generation of new differentiated neural cells from adult neural stem cells in the specific brain regions during a lifespan might assume the maintenance of CNS homeostasis and functions, particularly for learning and memory.

Skin Stem Cells: In adult mammalian skin, the epithelial compartment consists of the interfollicular epidermis (IFE) and its related appendages, such as the hair follicles and sebaceous glands. Numerous studies have revealed that the upper region of hair follicles, the bulge area, constitutes the principal niche of multipotent stem cells, which are responsible for the long-term growth of the hair follicles and epidermis regeneration after injury.

The bulge area in adult mammalian hair follicle also contains a pluripotent epidermal neural crest stem cell (eNCSCs) population that shows several properties similar to embryonic neural crest stem cells.

Ocular Stem Cells: The human surface epithelium includes the corneal, limbal, and conjunctival stratified epithelia. Several recent lines of evidence have revealed that the corneal epithelial stem cells (CESCs) are localized at the basal cell layer of the peripheral cornea, and particularly at the limbus within the limbal epithelial crypts. Furthermore, the conjunctival epithelial stem cells appear to be enriched in the bulbar and forniceal conjunctiva. More specifically, CESCs can give rise to the progenitors that are able to migrate at the corneal epithelium. These corneal cell progenitors show a rate of proliferation inferior to that of CESCs *in vitro.*

Bone Marrow Stromal Stem Cells: There is considerable evidence indicating that bone marrow stromal cells (MSCs) contain multipotent stem cells that can be induced to differentiate into cells of various phenotypes including myocardiocytes, both *in vitro* and *in vivo.* Following acute MI, experimental and early clinical studies reveal that these cells can survive and engraft into the peri-infarcted myocardium where they can differentiate to participate in the repair process.

Human embryonic stem cells: Opportunities and challenges

Although, stem cell therapy has been used successfully in the past, particularly in bone marrow transplants for leukemia, it is only in the last 5-7 years that human embryonic stem cells have been successfully isolated, cultured and somatic cell nuclear-transfer technology pioneered.

Human embryonic stem (hES) cells are derived from the inner cell mass of the mammalian blastocyst. These cells are pluripotent in nature and are capable of indefinite proliferation *in vitro* in an undifferentiated state. They maintain a normal karyotype through prolonged culture to exhibit potential to differentiate into derivatives of all 3 embryonic germ layers.

Human embryonic stem (hES) cells hold tremendous promise for future use in developmental biology and cell-based therapies. Replacement of non-functional cells using hES cell-derived cells can offer a permanent treatment in cases of debilitating diseases like Parkinson's diseases, Alzheimer's diseases, multiple sclerosis, stroke, cardiac ischemia, hepatic failure, juvenile-onset diabetes mellitus etc.

However, rapid as the program has been in this fascinating area of research, numerable challenges remain to be addressed before therapeutic application of hES cells become a reality. For embryonic stem cell research, development in transplantation analogy in animal models have raised the expectation for the treatment of degenerating diseases, yet the supply of tissues has not kept pace with demand and immuno-suppression remain a problem. Understanding this is the key to allogenic stem cell product development.

Further, developmental biology is yet to fully comprehend the manner of stem cell differentiation. ES cells are also known to cause tumor formation, if not properly differentiated before transplantation. Yet another challenge in clinical practice is to establish dosages as measured by counts of specific stem cell marker based population, for different types of transplantation and patient constitution. The number of stem cells that survive and get grafted soon after transplantation is yet another imponderable. The route of administration is also a subject of several studies especially in cardiology. And, then, there are the questions of ethic and regulation. In this regard,

Dept. of Biotechnology (DBT) and ICMR have recently drafted guidelines to ensure a proper regulatory environment to conduct stem cell research in India.

How stem cells work?

These cells are capable of performing three important functions with unique abilities:

- Plasticity: Potential to change into other cell types like nerve cells
- Homing: To travel to the site of tissue damage
- Engraftment: To unite with other tissues

This means that, if specific stem cell is injected into a patient who has a nerve disorder, that cell should migrate to the site of injury attracted by specific chemicals released by the damaged tissue. The cell, by homing to the damaged area will fuse with the damaged tissue by the process of engraftment and become the same tissue by displaying the property of plasticity. In this instance, the stem cell should, for example, become a nerve cell.

Immediately after the cells are injected, the body secretes numerous chemicals called cytokines. They can cause the remarkable effects sometimes seen immediately after treatment, but are usually transitory, although these effects have persisted on occasion.

The rest of the injected cells, which have not migrated or engrafted, will travel to the bone marrow where they will be stored with the body's blood cells until needed. They can still respond, from the bone marrow, to signals from damaged tissue elsewhere in the body and migrate to that site. This is why responses are sometimes not noted until a few months after treatment.

ACTIVE RESEARCHES IN THE FIELD OF STEM CELLS

There are many questions about stem cell differentiation, for example, are the internal and external signals similar for all kinds of stem cells? Can specific sets of signals be identified that promote differentiation into specific cell types? The answers to these questions may lead to scientists to find new ways of controlling stem cell differentiation in the laboratory, thereby growing cell or tissues that can be used for specific purposes including cell based therapies.

Scientists are intensively studying the fundamental properties of stem cells, which include:

1. Determining precisely how stem cells remain unspecialized and self-renewing for many years;
2. Identifying the signals that cause stem cells to become specialized cells.

Scientists are trying to understand two fundamental properties of stem cells that relate to their long-term self-renewal.

1. Why can embryonic stem cells proliferate for a year or more in the laboratory without differentiating but most adult stem cells can not?
2. What are the factors in living organisms that normally regulate stem cell proliferation and self-renewal?

The answer to these questions will clarify how cell proliferation is regulated during normal embryonic development or during the abnormal cell division that leads to cancer.

No doubt, the promise of stem cell therapies is an exciting one, but significant technical hurdles remain that will only be overcome through years of intensive research.

Certain key questions about adult stem cells remain unanswered:

- How many kinds of adult stem cells exist and in which tissues they exist?
- What are the sources of adult stem cells in the body?
- Are they 'leftover' embryonic stem cells or do they arise in some other way?
- Why do they remain in an undifferentiated state when all the cells around them have differentiated?
- Do adult stem cells normally exhibit plasticity or do they only transdifferentiate when the researchers manipulate them experimentally?
- What are the signals that regulate the proliferation and differentiation of stem cells that show plasticity?

- What are the factors that stimulate stem cells to relocate to sites of injury or damage?

In recent years, high profile and provocative publications have made extraordinary claims of stem cell plasticity at both nuclear and cellular levels. These include the ability of a stem cell to 'dedifferentiate' to a more primitive state and to 'transdifferentiate' from tissues such as bone marrow or tooth pulp into neurons, as well as the capacity to home exclusively to sites of injury and undergo targeted repair in disease models.

Scientists want to study stem cells in the laboratory so that they can learn about their essential properties and what makes them different from specialized cell types. As scientists learn more about stem cells, it may become possible to use the cells not just in cell-based therapies, but also for screening new drugs and toxins and understanding birth defects.

The Indian Council of Medical Research (ICMR) has submitted the final guidelines for stem cell research regulation in the country prescribing strict procedures for the use of stem cells by research institutions.

The ICMR guidelines on stem cells hold significance as stem cell research raises many ethical, legal, scientific, and policy issues that are of concern to the policy makers and public at large. Like any other scientific advances, it also raises questions about balancing the promises offered by stem cell therapy against its potential harm for appropriate application.

Guidelines for stem cell research and therapy have been prepared for adult, cord blood and embryonic stem cells to facilitate stem cell research in India so as to improve understanding of human health and disease, and evolve strategies to treat serious diseases.

Box. 23.1. ICMR guidelines: Salient features

- Permissible areas of research
- Restricted areas of research
- Prohibited areas of research
- Research using umbilical cord blood stem cells
- Research using foetal stem cells / placenta
- Responsibilities of investigators and institutions.

Box. 23.2. Stem cell therapy

- As of date in India there is no approved indication for stem cell therapy as a part of routine medical practice, other than "Bone Marrow Transplantation (BMT)".
- All stem cell therapy other than BMT shall be treated as experimental.
- It should be conducted only as a clinical trial after approval of the institutional ethics committee (IEC), Institutional Committee – Stem Cell Research and Therapy (IC-SCRT) and DCGI.
- All such trials shall be registered with the National Apex Committee – Stem Cell Research and Therapy (NAC-SCRT).

Possible Stem Cell Deferences

Unquestionably, stem cells are one of the most fascinating areas of biology today. And stem therapy has the potential to radically change the approach to battle against a wide variety of serious degenerative diseases including cancer.

Certainly, stem cells are not panacea to all ailments. Like many expanding fields of scientific inquiry, research on stem cells raises scientific questions as rapidly as it generates new discoveries.

Replacing the failed, missing or damaged tissue with those grown from embryonic stem cells has created a moral and ethical debate about stem cell research. Some religious groups believe it is not the right of medical practitioners and scientists to "play God" by experimenting with stem cells. Some pro-life activists argue that an embryo which represents a human life is destroyed in the cell harvesting process and should not be condoned. Meanwhile, others try and rationalize with the idea that any advancement in medical technology should be used for saving lives or improving the quality of living for those suffering with disease. Stem cell research has offered insight on how diseases can be treated or even cured. However, there are various moral and ethical concerns.

Widespread controversies, ethical, legal, religious, and scientific, exist over the techniques used in the creation and usage of stem cell especially on human embryo research. Some consider that an embryo is a human being entitled to dignity even if legally slated for destruction. The ensuing debate has prompted the political and regulatory frameworks across the world. It has highlighted that stem cell research represents a social and ethical challenge.

STEM CELL PHARMACOLOGY

The domain of medicine is moving rapidly towards the development of more effective cures for a host of diseases. In the past, the science of pharmacotherapeutics aimed to treat only the symptoms of disease, rarely addressing its cause(s) or mechanism(s). The advances in medicine, nevertheless, tend to follow the advances in biology. Accordingly, many cures being developed by scientists are currently based upon the sophisticated techniques capable to target the cause or mechanisms of a disease rather than simply treating its symptoms. This new and rational way of thinking about treating a disease has brought one of the frontiers in biomedical research, viz. "stem cells" to the vanguard. Stem cells have led scientists to investigate the possibility of cell-based therapies to treat diseases, a domain often referred to as regenerative or reparative medicine. The vast therapeutic potential of the stem cell therapy, though still in its formative years, is likely to be the major focus of the Pharma industry in the coming years.

Stem cells, owing to their inimitable abilities for therapeutic intervention, have virtually become a buzz word in biomedical research today. After moving from lab to the clinic, the domain of stem cell therapy seems poised to revolutionize, the way a degenerative disease is treated. Medical and pharmaceutical sciences being interwoven and complementary to each other, the area of stem cell has lately gained significant imperative pharmaceutical significance too. Stem cells are the fundamental building blocks that function as a normal reservoir for new cells, needed to replace damaged or dying cells. Various types of stem cells, obtained from diverse biological tissues, have enormous potential in curing a vast number of diseases including, oncological, neurological, endocrine, cardiac, dermatological, genetic, ophthalmic disorders, to name a few. As they are being used to treat a diseased state, they can be safely regarded as drugs.

Stem Cells as Drugs

As a "drug" is a substance, natural, synthetic or semi-synthetic, used for diagnosis, treatment, mitigation or prevention of a disease, stem cells can rationally and safely be regarded as drugs. Drug discovery and development for today and in future would navigate primarily towards stem cell usage for this purpose as an emerging major field in the pharmaceutical research. The cause of various diseases can broadly be categorized among three problems at the cellular level, i.e., too much cell division, too little cell division and defective cell function. Too much cell division results in tumors are sometimes cancerous, too little cell division results in the inability to repair damaged tissues and organs (e.g., severed spinal cords, weak heart muscle, etc.), whereas defective cell function results in diseases like heamophilia, diabetes mellitus, etc. The plausibility of unlimited supply, of these cells capable of generating any tissue of the human body has led to the development and use of drugs in the cure of various disease(s).

Stem Cells in Drug Discovery

Besides their tremendous potential in regenerative medicine, the stem cells have numerous applications in drug discovery too. Stem cells are also a valuable tool in drug discovery, high-content screening assays, and toxicology studies. The benefits that stem cell technology offers involve understanding of the disease mechanisms and identifying the targets.

Stem cells will help in the better comprehension of action of existing drugs and would aid in the discovery of new drugs for many debilitating diseases. They are important for understanding differentiation pathways, identifying factors needed to manipulate cell lineages, improving screening assays, and identifying disease targets. The production of stem-cell-derived human hepatocytes, for instance, has an immediate impact on toxicology and metabolism studies. Another approach that would be a road map to drug development involves the use of differentiated engineered stem cells to have specific disease characteristics allowing drug testing on those cells, e.g., cancer cell lines. However, to screen drugs effectively, the conditions must be identical while comparing different drugs.

Stem Cells in Drug Delivery

This unique type of drug delivery approach ensures that any therapy for diseases, e.g., Parkinson's disease and other neurodegenerative disorders are reaching the right place in the brain.

Therapeutic Potential (Fig. 23.6)

The significance of stem cell therapy in modern medicine is that it offers hope in the treatment of incurable diseases such as spinal cord injuries, muscular disorders, leukemia and heart ailments. The process of stem cell treatment is relatively simple. Stem cells are extracted from an embryo, an umbilical cord, blood or even bone marrow. They are then replicated in a cell culture. These new cells are then transplanted to the problem area in the patient to help repair damaged tissue. Embryonic stem cells are the viable option because at such an early age in the life cycle, they can be artificially altered into whatever specialized cells that are required.

The promise of stem cell therapies is an exciting one, but technical hurdles remain. Through intensive research, stem cell therapeutics can be nurtured safely and methodically to provide tangible benefit to the patients. The procedure needs to be refined such that its rewards outweigh the risks.

Stem cells open the prospect of treatment for a number of diseases and injuries and, at the same time, raise a number of crucial questions. How realistic are these expectations? What are the ethical and social implications? How do we decide whether or not to use this technology? Who can make that decision?

As of date, there is no approved indication for stem cell therapy as a part of routine medical practice, other than Bone Marrow Transplantation (BMT). Accordingly all stem cell therapy other than BMT (for accepted indications) shall be treated as experimental. It should be conducted only as a clinical trial after approval of the Institutional Ethics Committee (IEC), Institutional Committee – Stem Cell Research and Therapy (IC-SCRT) and DCGI. All such trials shall be registered with the National Apex Committee – Stem Cell Research and Therapy (NAC-SCRT).

Stem cells, directed to differentiate into specific cell types, offer the possibility to treat a myriad of diseased states. Of the numerous diseases, where stem cells have found tremendous promise, the noteworthy are being discussed briefly as under:

Cardiac Disorders

Heart ailments account for maximum number of fatalities in the world including in India. Even in the best-case scenarios, cardiologists are usually only able to save about 60% of cardiac muscle following a heart attack. It implies that for millions of cardiac patients, there has been no way to restore their damaged hearts and their function. But now after years of promising basic science research, early clinical trials hint that stem cells may be able to regenerate damaged heart tissue in humans just as it has been shown to do in animal models.

Dermatological disorders

The knowledge of stem cells has made it possible for scientists to grow skin from a patient's plucked hair. Skin (keratinocyte) stem cells reside in the hair follicle and can be removed when a hair is plucked. These cells can be cultured to form an epidermal equivalent of the patients own skin and provides tissue for an autologous graft, bypassing the problem of rejection. It is presently being studied in clinical trials as an alternative to surgical grafts used for venous ulcers and burn victims.

Nervous System Disorders & Spinal Cord Injuries

There are a variety of nervous system disorders. While these conditions differ in their cause, symptoms and course, most involve a degeneration of nerve tissue. Common disorders include:

- Spinal cord injuries involving a break in the spinal cord prevent the brain from transmitting signals to nerves branching from below the break in the spinal cord. The higher the break in the spinal cord, the greater the loss of body function and control.
- Stroke involves the death of nerve cells in the brain due to a lack of oxygen. This is caused by the blockage (ischaemic stroke, often due to a blood clot), or rupturing (haemorrhagic stroke) of one or more blood vessel in the brain.

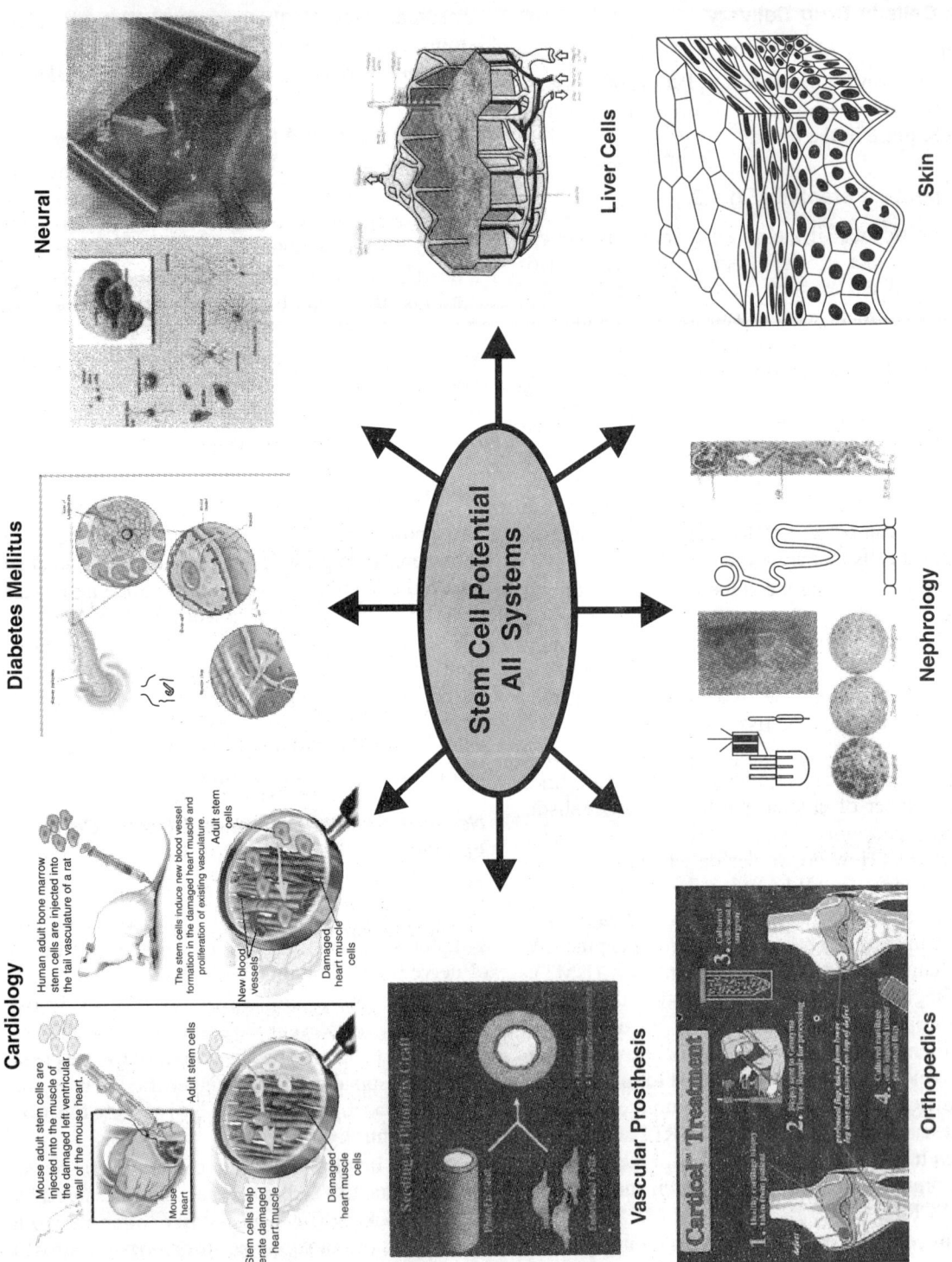

Fig. 23.6 Therapeutic potential of stem cell.

Depending on the area of the brain that is damaged, a stroke can cause death, coma, paralysis, speech problems and/or memory loss.

- Multiple Sclerosis (MS) is caused by the body's immune system attacking and damaging the outer covering of nerve cells (myelin) in the brain and spinal cord, resulting in decreased nerve functioning. This leads to the progressive loss of motor control, sensation, and several autonomic nervous functions, eventually resulting in death.
- Parkinson's disease is caused by progressive deterioration of the nerve cells in the part of the brain that controls muscle movement. Dopamine, one of the substances used to transmit signals from nerve to nerve, is normally produced in this area. The nerve deterioration caused by Parkinson's disease reduces the amount of dopamine available, resulting in symptoms such as shaking (tremor) and difficulty with walking, movement, and coordination.
- Alzheimer's disease is a progressive, degenerative brain disease in which the accumulation of abnormal structures such as dead and dying nerve cells and senile plaques cause nerve cell death. This results in impaired memory and cognitive function, as well as abnormal behavior (dementia).

How stem cell transplant therapy helps

Although, research is still underway, stem cells and stem cell treatment show promise in the treatment of a variety of central nervous system disorders. The Institute for Regenerative Medicine (IRM) has successfully used foetal-derived neuronal cell (FNC) stem cells to treat a range of neurological disorders. In most cases, the IRM Stem Cell Complex is administered via intravenous infusion.

Where the condition is caused by a localized deterioration of nerve cell bundles, the treatment may serve to elicit regeneration at the site of damage. In cases where damage is widespread, the treatment seems to act systemically. Thus far, IRM's stem cell treatment has often proved highly effective. However, overall results have been mixed, depending on the specific condition and individual patient.

Diabetes

How stem cell transplant therapy helps

Research suggests that stem cell therapy can be beneficial for those suffering from diabetes. This is based upon indications that foetal-derived cell (FLC) stem cells may transform into insulin-producing pancreas cells, assisting in the maintenance of normal blood sugar levels for extended periods of time.

Although, stem cell therapy has been shown to be effective (see below), the exact mechanism of action for diabetes is not completely understood. It is possible that stem cells help regenerate the defective insulin-producing pancreas cells, and/or somehow improve the body's insulin sensitivity. The beneficial effect of reversing the complications is particularly exciting, because such complications (e.g., blindness, limb amputations, heart disease and kidney disease) can be devastating, and no other currently available therapies for diabetes have been shown to have such beneficial effects.

Blood disorders

There are three main blood cell types in the human body: red blood cells, white blood cells, and platelets. All of these are made primarily in the bone marrow from stem cells known as haematopoietic stem cells. This process can be disrupted at many different possible points, leading to a variety of diseases and disorders. For example:

- **Aplastic Anemia:** Exposure to certain drugs, radiation or toxins can halt the production of red and white blood cells, a condition known as aplastic anemia.
- **Thrombocytopenia:** This condition can result if similar assaults stop the production of platelets.
- **Leukemias:** These conditions are the result of abnormally high production of white blood cells.
- **Lymphomas:** These cancers involve abnormal production of white blood cell types known as B cells or T cells.
- **Immune Deficiencies:** Primary immune deficiencies occur when there is defective production of white blood cells due to a genetic defect.

How stem cell transplant therapy helps

Because all blood cells originate from stem cells. Stem cell transplant therapy is a logical and promising treatment for blood and immune system disorders. Indeed, over the last 30 years in the United States and Europe, foetal-derived liver cell (FLC) stem cells have been used to treat many such disorders, even to treat infants in the womb and shortly after birth.

Diseases and Disorders of the Eye

The vast majority of all vision disorders are caused by one of two degenerative conditions:

Macular Degeneration (MD) is a degenerative condition of the macula (the central retina).

Diabetic Retinopathy is damage to the eye caused by the progression of diabetes.

How stem cell transplant therapy helps

Several patients suffering from macular degeneration have shown significant improvement after treatment by the Institute for Regenerative Medicine. For those with macular degeneration. It is believed that the stem cells target the damaged retinal tissue and induce regeneration. In patients with diabetic retinopathy, the cells not only target damaged ocular tissue, but may also help to resolve the underlying diabetes.

Arthritis

There are two major types of arthritis: Rheumatoid arthritis and Osteoarthritis.

How stem cell transplant therapy helps

Because both Osteoarthritis and Rheumatoid arthritis involve destruction of cartilage around joints, stem cell therapy has the potential to help treat the disease by restoring some of the lost tissue.

Liver Disease

Among diseases of the liver, hepatitis and liver cirrhosis are among the most difficult to treat.

Current mainstream treatment options

Unfortunately, the efficacy of even the most advanced current therapies for chronic viral hepatitis is low.

Unfortunately, the great discrepancy between the availability of healthy, viable organs and the large number of patients needing a liver transplant puts this option out of reach for most patients. Socio-medical problems related to liver transplantation – currently the only treatment for patients at the terminal phase of illness – are well known. For example, because of the shortage of donated livers, over 50 percent of patients on the waiting list die while waiting for transplantation surgery.

How stem cell transplant therapy helps

Therapy with foetal liver stem cells (FLC) has potential to help regenerate liver function in patients with liver disorders.

The ability of FLC transplant to cause tissue regeneration in the liver may extend the life of the patient long enough for a transplant to become available, in effect, saving the life of the patient.

Age reversal therapy

The Institute for Regenerative Medicine is the world leader in providing stem cell treatment therapies as a remedy for aging. These therapies are based on 30 years of research during which the evidences below have been observed and documented. As we age, the stem cell reserves we are born with decline. Our cells diminish in their ability to regenerate and repair tissue. Age-related changes occur in the skin, organs, sex glands, immune system, blood-forming system, muscles and other systems. These changes are all due to the decrease in the robustness of the cells and loss of stem cells.

How stem cell transplant therapy helps

Although, an exact mechanism of action for the anti-aging effects of IRM's stem cell therapy are still being studied, one thing is certain: cells become progressively weaker over time and die. Thus, replacing aging cells with new ones, which stem cell therapy accomplishes, effectively remediates aging. This is the promise of stem cell therapy.

PARADIGM SHIFTS THAT HAVE OCCURRED DUE TO STEM CELL RESEARCH

Cancer Stem Cells

Recently, it has been shown that all kinds of cancers are stem cell diseases. Even after extensive research, it appears that current approaches to cure cancer are targeting wrong cells. New treatment modalities need to target cancer stem cells, which form a very small fraction of cells within the tumor. This has resulted in a conceptual paradigm shift of how tumors are formed, spread and are treated. Recurrence of cancer is now understood to be because conventional cancer therapies target majority of cells in the tumor and the cancer stem cells escape the treatment. These immature stem cells are more resistant to chemotherapy and radiotherapy than the mature cancer cells and result in recurrence.

Studies have shown that cancer stem cells are the only cells present in different kind of cancers including solid tumors (breast cancer, brain tumor) that have the capacity to keep the tumors growing. To cure the cancer, it will ideal to devise therapies that will target cancer stem cells.

Stem Cell in Ovaries

It has been demonstrated that proliferative germ cells exist in the surface epithelial cell layer of mice ovary which keep replenishing the oocytes pool in the postnatal life. Similar evidence has also been generated in human ovaries. These results have significant clinical implication related to the therapeutic expansion of the follicular reserve as a means to postpone normal and premature ovarian failure.

STEM CELL RESEARCH IN INDIA

Developments so far Basic research

In India, both basic and clinical research are being promoted by several science agencies of the Government in various institutions and hospitals. The programmes have been identified and implemented on various aspects of both embryonic and adult stem cells such as limbal, haematopoietic, embryonic, pancreatic, neural, cardiac stem cells, generation of human embryonic stem cells lines, use of banana lectins for stem cell preservation, haematopoietic stem cells (HSC) for haplo-identical HSC transplantation, use of limbal stem cells for ocular surface disorders, isolation and characterization of mesenchymal and liver stem cells, *in vitro* differentiation of human embryonic stem cells to neural and non-neural lineages, etc. City cluster programmes have been implemented at Pune and

Vellore by involving basic researchers and clinicians. This includes sharing of information, explore collaboration with clinicians and discuss emerging policy issues in this area, etc. In 2003, a separate Task Force on "Stem Cell Biology and Regenerative Medicine" was constituted to consider new projects, monitor the progress of ongoing projects, discuss the priority areas and other issues related to stem cells.

Major research leads

- Use of limbal stem cells to repair corneal surface disorders caused by limbal stem cell deficiencies. So far, more than 300 patients have been treated at LV Prasad Eye Institute (LVPEI), Hyderabed.
- A technology has been established at Christian Medical College (CMC), Vellore for collection, isolation and purification of HSCs for haplo-identical haematopoietic stem cell transplantation.
- Banana lectins have been isolated and purified showing stem cell preservation activities.
- Indigenous human embryonic stem cell lines are being generated at few institutions in the country.

Clinical research system established

Clinical research is an integral part of stem cell science. The ultimate outcome of the research in this field is for the welfare of the human kind. Thorough clinical research for determining the safety and efficacy of stem cells initially in animal and then in human is constituting four separate committees. They are:

- "Human Studies Committee" for evaluation and guidance of clinical research particularly for development of clinical research protocols;
- National Bioethics Committee" to ascertain rigid ethical guidelines being followed while conducting research on human beings;
- "Task Force on Stem Cells and Regenerative Medicine" to evaluate basic research and also recommend funding for clinical research based on the evaluation of the above committees and
- "Programme Advisory Committee" to consider the proposals of Centre of Excellence and infrastructure.

Clinical research

Following this system and based on the thorough review of literature, multi-centric phase-I clinical study has been implemented at five hospitals to determine the safety and efficacy of bone marrow mononuclear cells in acute myocardial infarction. The pilot study on acute stroke bone marrow mononuclear cells has also been implemented initially at one centre and based on the results of the pilot study the main study would be designed. The multi-centric phase-I proposal on limb is ischemia is under active consideration. Efforts are being made to generate more proposals on clinical research based on the well-established animal data in the field.

Stem Cell Centres and Institutes

The science of stem cell is complex and extensive research is required to understand how these cells work and how the potential of these cells may be harnessed for therapeutic applications. Keeping in view major consensus, it was felt that there should be a dedicated research centre completely focused on stem cells and cell developmental science. Therefore, concerted efforts were made to establish "CMC-DBT Centre for Stem Cell Research" at CMC, Vellore to carry out basic and translational stem cell research. It was further realized that only a "Centre" may not be sufficient for stem cell research in the country like India. It was felt that there is a need for a full fledged institution for stem cell research in the country which has been started at NCBS, Bangalore.

Facilities to handle stem cells

Though some of the institutions in the country initiated stem cell research few years ago, facilities were limited and were not adequate for taking up challenges coming continuously in this area as this is a comparatively new field of life sciences. Realizing the need to establish clean room facilities to handle stem cells and also carry out research in this field, a number of facilities have been created. These facilities have been established mainly in hospital set up because hospitals are the main source for providing these cells and no facilities were available to handle stem cells in their set up. Therefore the facilities have been created at Post Graduate Institute of Medical Education and Research (PGIMER), Chandigarh; Sanjay Gandhi

Post Graduate Institute of Medical Sciences (SGPGIMS), Lucknow; LVPEI, Hyderabad and KEM Hospital, Mumbai (Table 23.3).

Table 23.3. List of some of the institutions and hospitals supported by DBT.

CMC-DBT Centre for Cell Research	Christian Medical College, Vellore
Establishment of cGMP facility	
Network programmes	CMC, Vellore
	SGPGIMS, Lucknow
	PGIMER, Chandigarh;
	All India Institute of Medical Sciences (AIIMS), New Delhi
	R&R Centre, New Delhi
	National Centre for Cell Science (NCCS), Pune and
	National Brain Research Centre (NBRC), Manesar
Stem cell research facilities	PGIMER, Chandigarh
	SGPGIMS, Lucknow
	KEM Hospital, Mumbai and
	LVPEI, Hyderabad
Embryonic stem cell research	National Institute for Research in Reproductive Health (NIRRH), Mumbai
	National Centre for Biological Sciences (NCBS), Bangalore;
	National Centre for Cell Science (NCCS), Pune; National Brain Research Centre (NBRC), Manesar and
	Jawaharlal Nehru Centre for Advanced Scientific Research (JNCASR), Bangalore
Limbal stem cells	LVPEI, Hyderabad
	R.P. Centre for Ophthalmic Sciences, AIIMS, New Delhi and Regional Institute of Ophthalmology, Kolkata
Neural stem cells	National Brain Research Centre (NBRC), Manesar
	National Institute of Mental Health and Neurosciences (NIMHANS), Bangalore and

(Contd.)

Table 23.3. Contd.

	NCCS, Pune and University of Hyderabad, Hyderabad
Mesenchymal stem cells	CMC, Vellore; SGPGIMS, Lucknow and Manipal Hospital, Bangalore
Pancreatic progenitor cells	National Institute of Nutrition (NIN), Hyderabad and NCCS, Pune
Cardiac stem cells	Sree Chitra Tirunal Institute for Medical Sciences and Technology (SCTIMST), Thiruvananthapuram and AIIMS, New Delhi
Cancer stem cells	Indian Institute of Science (IISc), Bangalore

Efforts made for Human Resource Development

Creation of human resource of desired expertise is the most critical component of stem cell research. In order to train young researchers in both embryonic as well as adult stem cells, a training proposal has been implemented jointly at NCBS and JNCASR, Bangalore. Efforts have also been made to bring clinicians and basic researchers together for close interaction by organizing a number of clinical research workshops, extensive training programmes, brainstorming sessions, etc. in addition, the training programmes have been formulated to support long and short-term overseas training in niche areas of biotechnology including stem cell research. The need was also felt for a regular discussion on the subject among the research. The need was also felt for a regular discussion on the subject among the researchers in the country especially the new developments that are taking place globally in this area. In order to provide an opportunity for close interaction to the researchers, a "Stem Cell Research Forum of India" has been created. The "Forum" will provide a platform to the scientists and clinicians for close interaction for discussion and to share the achievements of their efforts.

Draft guidelines for stem cell research

Draft guidelines for stem cell researches in the country have been formulated jointly by the Department of Biotechnology under Ministry of Science and Indian Council for Medical Research. Draft document was discussed jointly by both the Committees to finalize this document (guidelines are available). As per the guidelines, stem cell research has been classified under permissible, restricted and prohibited categories. The research pertaining to adult and umbilical cord blood stem cells would be classified as permissible. It would require approval from Institutional committee. However, embryonic stem cells research falls under restricted category. It can be carried out with the approval of Institutional Committees and National Apex Committee. Research pertaining to reproductive cloning, introducing animal embryos in human, etc. has been categorized as prohibited.

FUTURE OUTLOOK OF STEM CELLS

Stem cells have come a long way and are with us to stay. But lot of hurdles need to be overcome and methodologies need to be refined before they can be incorporated in clinical settings. Technologies have to be developed to control their differentiation into pure cell populations in large numbers. The availability of a homogenous cell population will enable stem cell transplantation to replace diseased cells possible in future. Secondly, there is a need to achieve 100% differentiation of these cells, since even a single undifferentiated cell may lead to teratoma formation. Therapeutic cloning protocols need to be developed with fair success rate to avoid immune rejection at time of cell therapy. Finally, there is a need to produce large number of ESC lines and make them available for research purposes. Extensive research needs to be carried out to elucidate the mechanism of stem cell lineage specific differentiation. They are like a wild horse, which has to be tamed before being used to its full potential.

Extensive work on embryos will help to understand some of the secrets of how early cells are controlled. What makes a cell committed or how they get out of control to form tumor are some basic questions that will be answered in near future.

STUDY QUESTIONS

1. Define (a) totipotent stem cells, (b) pluripotent stem cells, (c) multipotent and (d) unipotent stem cells.

2. How stem cells differ from other types of cells?

3. How stem cells work?

4. How stem cells are important for living organisms?

5. What are the main types of stem cells?

6. Describe the differences between embryonic and adult types of stem cells.

7. Describe the potential clinical uses of stem cells.

8. Why stem cells can be considered as drugs?

9. How stem cells have application in (a) drug discovery, (b) drug delivery approach?

10. Comment on (a) umbilical cord stem cells, (b) bone marrow stem cells, (c) embryonic stem cells and (d) adult stem cells.

11. How stem cells transplant therapy helps in (a) diabetes, (b) Parkinson's disease, (c) heart diseases?

GUIDE TO FURTHER READINGS

1. Abbott et al (2006). The lure of stem-cell lines. Nature 442 : 336-337.

2. Finkel (2005). Stem Cells: Controversy at the frontiers of science. (ABC Books). p. 85.

3. Vogel (2005). Ready or not? Human ES cells head towards the clinic. Science 308 : 1534-1538.

4. Berns A. Stem cells for lung cancer? Cell 2005; 121:811-813.

5. Galderisi U, Cipollaro M, Giordano A. Stem cells and brain cancer. Cell Death Differ 2006; 13:5-11.

6. M.V. Padma Srivastava, Stem Cell Therapy in Stroke, Ann Natl Acad Med. Sci. (India), 44(1): 47-56, 2008.

7. Foudi, A. et al. Analysis of histone 2B-GFP retention reveals slowly cycling hematopoietic stem cells. Nature Biotechnol. 27, 84-90 (2009).

8. Welt FG, Losordo DW. Cell therapy for acute myocardial infarction: curb your enthusiasm? Circulation, 2006;113:1272-1274.

9. Vogel G. International standards proposed for stem cell work, Science, 2006;313:26.

10. Shaw G (2007). Can Stem Cells Repair a Broken Heart? PharmaAsia, 2:12-15.

11. Das MC, De B, Debnath, M (2006). Stem cell therapy, Pharma Times, 38:24-26.

12. http://en.wikipedia.org/wiki/Stem_cell_therapy, June 21, 2007.

13. Michael R. Rosen, Are Stem Cells Drugs, Circulation, 2006; 114:1992-2000.

14. Liu Y & Rao MS. Transdifferentiation: factor artifact. J cell Prochem 2003; 88(1): 29-40.

KEY STEM CELL RESEARCH EVENTS

- **1908** - The term "stem cell" was proposed for scientific use by the Russian histologist Alexander Maksimov (1874-1928) at congress of hematologic society in Berlin. It postulated existence of haematopoietic stem cells.

- **1960s** - Joseph Altman and Gopal Das presented scientific evidence of adult neurogenesis, ongoing stem cell activity in the brain; their reports contradict Cajal's "no new neurons" dogma and are largely ignored.

- **1963** - McCulloch and Till illustrated the presence of self-renewing cells in mouse bone marrow.

- **1968** - Bone marrow transplant between two siblings successfully treated SCID.

- **1978** - Haematopoietic stem cells were discovered in human cord blood.

- **1981** - Mouse embryonic stem cells were derived from the inner cell mass by scientists Martin Evans, Matthew Kaufman, and Gail R. Martin. Gail Martin is attributed for coining the term "Embryonic Stem Cell".

- **1992** - Neural stem cells were cultured *in vitro* as neurospheres.

- **1997** - Leukemia was shown to originate from a haematopoietic stem cell, the first direct evidence for cancer stem cells.

- **1998** - James Thomson and co-workers derived the first human embryonic stem cell line at the University of Wisconsin-Madison.

- **2000s** - Several reports of adult stem cell plasticity were published.

- **2001** - Scientists at Advanced Cell Technology clone first early (four- to six-cell stage) human embryos for the purpose of generating embryonic stem cells.

- **2003** - Dr. Songtao Shi of NIH discovered new source of adult stem cells in children's primary teeth.

- **2004-2005** - Korean researcher Hwang Woo-Suk claimed to have created several human embryonic stem cell lines from unfertilised human oocytes. The lines were later shown to be fabricated.

- **2005** - Researchers at Kingston University in England claimed to have discovered a third category of stem cell, dubbed cord-blood-derived embryonic-like stem cells (CBEs), derived from umbilical cord blood. The group claimed these cells are able to differentiate into more types of tissue than adult stem cells.

- **August 2006 - Rat Induced pluripotent stem cells**: The journal *Cell* published Kazutoshi Takahashi and Shinya Yamanaka, "Induction of Pluripotent Stem Cells from Mouse Embryonic and Adult Fibroblast Cultures by Defined Factors".

- **October 2006** - Scientists at Newcastle University in England created the first ever artificial liver cells using umbilical cord blood stem cells.

- **January 2007** - Scientists at Wake Forest University led by Dr. Anthony Atala and Harvard University reported discovery of a new type of stem cell in amniotic fluid. This may potentially provide an alternative to embryonic stem cells for use in research and therapy.

- **June 2007** - Research reported by three different groups shows that normal skin cells can be reprogrammed to an embryonic state in mice. In the same month, scientist Shoukhrat Mitalipov reported the first successful creation of a primate stem cell line through somatic cell nuclear transfer.

- **October 2007** - Mario Capecchi, Martin Evans, and Oliver Smithies won the 2007 Nobel Prize for Physiology or Medicine for their work on embryonic stem cells from mice using gene targeting strategies producing genetically engineered mice (known as knockout mice) for gene research.

- **November 2007 - Human Induced pluripotent stem cells**: Two similar papers released by their respective journals prior to formal publication: in *Cell* by Kazutoshi Takahashi and Shinya Yamanaka, "Induction of Pluripotent Stem Cells

from Adult Human Fibroblasts by Defined Factors", and in *Science* by Junying Yu, et al., from the research group of James Thomson, "Induced Pluripotent Stem Cell Lines Derived from Human Somatic Cells": pluripotent stem cells generated from mature human fibroblasts. It is possible now to produce a stem cell from almost any other human cell instead of using embryos as needed previously, albeit the risk of tumorigenesis due to c-myc and retroviral gene transfer remains to be determined.

- **January 2008** - Robert Lanza and colleagues at Advanced Cell Technology and UCSF created the first human embryonic stem cells without destruction of the embryo.

- **January 2008** - Development of human cloned blastocysts following somatic cell nuclear transfer with adult fibroblasts.

- **February 2008** - Generation of Pluripotent Stem Cells from Adult Mouse Liver and Stomach: these iPS cells seemed to be more similar to embryonic stem cells than the previous developed iPS cells and not tumorigenic, moreover genes that are required for iPS cells do not need to be inserted into specific sites, which encourages the development of non-viral reprogramming techniques.

- **March 2008** - The first published study of successful cartilage regeneration in the human knee using autologous adult mesenchymal stem cells was published by Clinicians from Regenerative Sciences.

- **October 2008** - Sabine Conrad and colleagues at Tübingen, Germany generated pluripotent stem cells from spermatogonial cells of adult human testis by culturing the cells *in vitro* under leukemia inhibitory factor (LIF) supplementation.

- **30 October 2008** - Embryonic-like stem cells from a single human hair.

- **1 March 2009** - Andras Nagy, Keisuke Kaji, et al. discovered a way to produce embryonic-like stem cells from normal adult cells by using a novel "wrapping" procedure to deliver specific genes to adult cells to reprogram them into stem cells without the risks of using a virus to make the change. The use of electroporation is said to allow for the temporary insertion of genes into the cell.

- **28 May 2009** - Kim et al. announced that they had devised a way to manipulate skin cells to create patient specific "induced pluripotent stem cells" (iPS), claiming it to be the 'ultimate stem cell solution'.
- **11 October 2010** - First trial of embryonic stem cells in humans.
- **2 October 2010** - Ishikawa et al. wrote in the Journal of Experimental Medicine that research shows that transplanted cells that contain their new host's nuclear DNA could still be rejected by the individual's immune system due to foreign mitochondrial DNA. Tissue made from a person's stem cell could therefore be rejected, because mitochondrial genomes tend to accumulate mutations.
- **2011** - Israeli scientist Inbar Friedrich Ben-Nun led a team which produced the first stem cells from endangered species, a breakthrough that could save animals in danger of extinction.
- **2012** - Katsuhiko Hayashi et al. reported in the Journal Science that they used mouse skin cells to create stem cells and then used these stem cells to create mouse eggs. These eggs were then fertilized and produced healthy baby offspring. These latter mice were able to have their own babies.
- **8 October 2012** - The Nobel Prize in Physiology or Medicine 2012 was awarded jointly to John B. Gurdon and Shinya Yamanaka for the discovery that mature cells can be reprogrammed to become pluripotent.

GLOSSARY

Adult stem cell: A stem cell derived from the tissues or organs of an organism after birth (in contrast to embryonic or foetal stem cells).

Blastocyst: A hollow ball of 50-100 cells reached after about 5 days of embryonic development. It consists of a sphere made up of an outer layer of cells (the trophoectoderm), a fluid-filled cavity (the blastocoele), and a cluster of cells in the interior (the inner cell mass).

Cell line: Cells of common descent continuously cultured in the laboratory is referred to as a cell line.

Cell nuclear replacement (CNR): The transfer of an adult cell nucleus into an oocyte that has had its nucleus removed to asexually create an embryo without the fusion of sperm and oocyte. **It is also known as Somatic Cell Nuclear Transfer (SCNT).**

Clone: A cell or organism derived from, and genetically identical to another cell or organism.

Clonal: Derived from a single cell.

Cloning: Creating an organism that is genetically identical to another organism, or a cell that is genetically identical to another cell provided that the so-called mother and daughter cells are subsequently separated (see also reproductive and therapeutic cloning).

Cloning by somatic cell nuclear transfer: Involves replacing an oocyte's nucleus with the nucleus of the adult cell to be cloned (or from an embryo or foetus) and then activating oocyte's further development without fertilization. The oocyte genetically reprogramme the transferred nucleus, enabling it to direct development of a whole new organism.

Reproductive cloning: The embryo developed after Somatic Cell Nuclear Transfer (SCNT) is implanted into the uterus (of the donor of the ovum or a surrogate recipient) and allowed to develop into a foetus and whole organism. The organism so developed is genetically identical to the donor of the somatic cell nucleus.

Therapeutic cloning: The development of the embryo after Somatic Cell Nuclear Transfer (SCNT) is stopped at the blastocyst stage and embryonic stem cells are derived from the inner cell mass. These stem cells could be differentiated into desired tissue using a cocktail of growth and differentiation factors. The generated tissue/cells could then be transplanted into the original donor of the nucleus avoiding rejection.

Consent: The voluntary consent is given by a patient (or their next of kin-legal heir) to participate in a study (which may include donating of tissue) after being informed of its purpose, method of treatment, and procedure for assignment to treatment, benefits and risks associated with participation, and required data collection procedures and schedule. *The consent besides being voluntary and informed has to be without any coercion or inducement. It can be withheld, or even withdrawn at any time, without giving any reason or prejudice to present or future treatment of the individual.*

Cord blood stem cell: Stem cells collected from the umbilical cord at birth that can produce all of the blood cells in the body (hematopoietic). Cord blood is currently used to treat patients who have undergone chemotherapy to destroy their bone marrow due to cancer or other blood-related disorders.

Embryo: In humans is the developing stage from the time of fertilization until the end of the eighth week of gestation, when it becomes known as a foetus.

Early embryo: The term "early embryo" covers stages of development up to the appearance of primitive streak i.e., until 14 days after fertilization.

Embryonic germ cell: Embryonic germ cells are primordial germ cells isolated from the gonadal ridge of 5-10 weeks foetus.

Embryonic stem cell: Embryonic stem cells are derived from the inner cell mass up to the stage of blastocysts. These cells can be cultured indefinitely under in vitro conditions that allow proliferation without differentiation, but have the potential of differentiating into any cell of the body.

Feeder layer: Cells used in co-culture to maintain pluripotent nature of the stem cells.

Foetus: In humans, it is a developing stage from eight weeks after conception to birth.

Foetal stem cell: A stem cell derived from foetal tissue, including placenta. A distinction is drawn between the foetal germ cells, from which the

gametes develop, and foetal somatic cells, from which rest of the organism develops.

Gamete: The male sperm or female oocyte.

Germ cells: Ova and sperm, and their precursors.

Implantation: The embedding of a blastocyst in the wall of uterus. In humans implantation takes place between 7-14 days after fertilization.

***In vitro* and *in vivo*:** Outside and inside the body; *in vitro* (literally, in glass) generally means in the laboratory.

Mesenchymal stem cells: Stem cells present in human bone marrow and umbilical cord that have been shown to differentiate into a variety of cell types.

Multipotent: Multipotent stem cells are those which are capable of giving rise to several different types of specialized cells constituting a specific tissue or organ.

Pluripotent stem cell: Has the ability to give rise to various types of cells that develop from the three germ layers (mesoderm, endoderm and ectoderm). Pluripotent stem cell has the potential to generate into every cell type in the body, but cannot develop into an embryo on its own.

Primitive streak: A collection of cells, which appears at about 14 days after fertilization from which the foetal body plan develops.

Somatic cell: Cell of the body other than oocyte or sperm.

Somatic stem cell: An undifferentiated cell found among differentiated cells in a tissue or organ, which can renew itself and can differentiate to yield the major specialized cell types of the tissue or organ.

Somatic cell nuclear transfer: The transfer of a cell nucleus to an oocyte (or another cell) from which the nucleus has been removed.

Stem cells: Cells capable of self-replication, proliferation and differentiation.

Stem cell Bank: A facility that is responsible for accessing, processing, packaging, labeling, storage and delivery of a finished stem cell line issued under its name. It is required to characterize the cells, provide quality assurance and meet the laid down standards and procedures.

Supernumerary embryo or spare embryo: An embryo created by means of *in vitro* fertilization (IVF) for the purpose of assisted reproduction but subsequently not used for it.

Totipotent: At two to three days after fertilization, an embryo consists of identical cells, which are **totipotent.** That is to say that each cell could give rise to an embryo on its own producing for example identical twins or quadruplets. They are totally unspecialized and have the capacity to differentiate into any of the cells, which will constitute the foetus as well as the placenta and membranes around the foetus.

Appendices

APPENDIX 1

WEIGHT, MEASURES AND CONCENTRATION EXPRESSIONS

METRIC SYSTEM

1 kilogram	= 1000 gms
1 mg	= 0.001 gram
1 microgram	= 0.000,001 gram
1 nanogram	= 1×10^{-9} g
a decilitre	= 0.1 L
1 millilitre	= 0.001 L

DOMESTIC (HOME) MEASURES

1 drop	= 0.06 ml
1 teaspoonful	= 5 ml
1 dessertspoonful	= 8 ml
1 tablespoonful	= 15 ml
1 teacupful	= 120 ml
1 tumblerful	= 240 ml

Conversion of Milligrams to Milliequivalents per Litre or to Millimoles per Litre

$$mEq/L = \frac{mg/L}{equivalent\ weight}$$

$$Equivalent\ Weight = \frac{atomic\ weight}{valence\ of\ element}$$

$$mM/L\ (millimoles\ per\ litre) = \frac{mg/L}{molecular\ weight}$$

Prefixes and Multiples

Prefix	Symbol	Power	Multiple or Portion of a Multiple
deci	d	10^{-1}	0.1
centi	c	10^{-2}	0.01
milli	m	10^{-3}	0.001
micro	u	10^{-6}	0.000001
nano	n	10^{-9}	0.000000001
pico	p	10^{-12}	0.000000000001
femto	f	10^{-15}	0.000000000000001
atto	a	10^{-18}	0.000000000000000001

CONCENTRATION EXPRESSION

- Percent by weight (% w/w) is the number of grams of solute per 100 gm of solution.
- Percent weight in volume (% w/v) is the number of grams of solute per 100 ml of solution.
- Percent by volume (% v/v) is the number of millilitres of solute in 100 ml of solution, referring to solutions of liquids in liquids.
- Molality is the number of moles of solute in 1000 grams of solvent.
- Normality refers to the gram equivalents of solute dissolved in 1000 ml of solution.

APPENDIX 2

THE PRESCRIPTION WRITING

A prescription is a written order for medication issued by a physician, dentist, veterinarian or any other registered/licensed medical practitioner for the patient. It is an important therapeutic transaction between physician and patient. Prescriptions designate a specific medication and dosage to be administered at a specific time or time interval to a specific patient. Earlier, when compounded prescriptions were common, prescriptions also contained the directions for the pharmacist regarding the type and quantity of preparation to be made.

At present, the practice of writing complex prescription order containing many active ingredients, adjuvants, correctives and elegant vehicles has been abandoned in favour of single drugs and mixtures of drugs compounded by pharmaceutical companies. The precompounded prescriptions have brought in the convenience of ready availability of medications saving the patients's waiting time during compounding. But, at the same time, it is not free from drawbacks. Many phyicians now rely upon fixed dose combinations available, rather than adjust the doses of the drugs according to the needs of the patient. More than a fourth of the commonly prescribed drugs are combination products.

The requirements of a prescription are that it should state : (i) when it is prescribed; (ii) to whom it is given; (iii) what is to be given; (iv) how much, how often, by what route and for how long the drug is required to be administered. Thus, the first four elements of the prescription establish the identity of the doctor : name, professional degree, address, telephone number and the date when the prescription is written, the identity of patient by name, age and address; the body of the prescription specify the medication, dose and directions for use. The symbol R_x (not R and x separately but cut R) or superscription is an abbreviation for Latin word, recipe, meaning "take thou"". The body of the prescription order i.e. drug ir mixture of drugs supplied by pharmaceutical company, or compounded (extemporaneous) which the pharmacist prepares as desired by the physician.

The directions to the pharmacist or subscription are abbreviated as Mix meaning "make a solution" for two or more drugs; for single drug prescription order it consists of "Dispense .... tablets".

The instructions to the patient in the portion of the prescription called signatura or signa or sig (meaning 'mark thou') contain direction as to amount of drug to be taken, frequency and route of administration.

Instructions such as "take as directed" or "take as necessary" should be avoided. It is better to use the word 'take' for drugs meant for internal use; word 'apply' for ointment or lotion; 'insert' for suppositories and drops for conjunctival sac; and 'place' for ear and nose.

The instructions should have brevity, clarity and accuracy. There should be a balance between the unintelligibly short and the inconvenient long. All the details necessary for the patient to know how, with what, when, and for how long to continue the therapy should be included in the prescription order.

At the end of the prescription order the physician/prescriber should put his signature, the last name in full with ink.

Prescriptions are usually written on printed forms having blank spaces for required information. These forms are known as prescription blanks and supplied in the form of a pad. It is a common practice to have the prescriber's name, address, telephone number, office hours, registration number and other pertinent informations imprinted on the prescription order blank for convenience. Since prescriptions are medicolegal documents, informations like date, particulars of the patient, medications prescribed, signature of the prescriber, etc. should be written with ink. This practice is compulsory for controlled substances in Schedule II. However, imprinted prescription blank is not a legal requirement, any paper or other writing material may be used.

A MODEL PRESCRIPTION

```
┌─────────────────────────────────────────────────────────────────────────┐
│  Dr. ..........................................M.D.      Add ............................  │
│                                                          ............................  │
│                                                          ............................  │
│  Regd. No.................                               Telephones :              │
│                                                          Clinic ...........................  │
│                                                          Residence ......................  │
│                                                                                    │
│  For (Name of patient)                                   Age ............................  │
│  Add. : ..............................................   Date ............................  │
│                                                                                    │
│      R_x                                                                           │
│                                                                                    │
│      Codeine Linctus                                                               │
│                                                                                    │
│      Mix Send 60 ml                                                                │
│      Take 5 ml twice a day and at bed time                                         │
│                                                          Signature of doctor       │
└─────────────────────────────────────────────────────────────────────────┘
```

Some examples for poor prescription writing are given below:

Prescribing errors

Illegible handwriting can result in serious mistakes when drugs with similar names but very different effects are available e.g. acetazolamide and acetohexamide, apresoline and priscoline, digitoxin and digotin, prednisone and prednisolone, lasix and losec. The error can be avoided by noting the indication for the drug.

Generic names are generally not likely to be confused with other classes of drugs.

The decimal point may be displaced or may be ambiguous e.g. ".1" may be misread as "1." (a tenfold overdose) or "1.0 mg" may be misread as "10 mg" in place of "1 mg", the use of U for unit say "10 U" may be misread as "100" hence the word units should be written and not the abbreviation letter U for units. Similarly the abbreviated form "mcg" can be misread as milligram, that means 1000 fold overdose.

Ordering "one ampoule" is not proper because the drug may be available in ampoules that contain 20, 40 or 100 mg of the drug.

Omission of information

Regarding dose, frequency of administration and the duration of drug therapy or just mentioning as needed without telling which condition will justify the need.

Inappropriate drug prescriptions

(i) Failure to recognize contraindications imposed by the presence of other diseases in the patient or other drugs that the patients may be taking including over the counter drugs.

(ii) Failure to recognize the possible physiochemical incompatibilities.

(iii) Even the most carefully written prescription may become therapeutically useless, unless it communicates clearly with the pharmacist and properly instructs the patient on how to take the medication.

Reading and checking the prescription

The prescription order first should be completely and carefully read in the privacy of the prescription department. There should be no doubt as to the ingredients or quantities prescribed. If something is illegible or if it appears that an error has been made, the pharmacist should consult another pharmacist or the prescriber. The pharmacist has justifiably earned the reputation of being able to read the handwriting of physicians. It is essential, however, that he never allows his pride in this reputation to prevent his admitting an inability to decipher a prescription. He should never guess at the meaning of an indistinct word or unrecognized abbreviation. There is no "official" or standard list of prescription abbreviations. Many are recognized as given below; however, many others may be simply shorthand creations of the individual prescriber. Anyone who has the opportunity to inspect medical prescriptions may conclude that if doctors wrote their personal bank cheques as badly as they write prescriptions, they would be in financial trouble and will surely change their ways.

The use of Latin words, phrases, and abbreviations in prescriptions is a carry-over from the time that Latin was considered the international language of medicine. Latin was used extensively in writing prescription orders until the early part of the 20th century. Although its use has gradually diminished, it is still widely used, in the form of abbreviations, in the subscription and signa portions of prescriptions. Some abbreviations are given below :

Pharmacoeconomics

Four economic concepts are important in relation to health care resources :

1. Opportunity cost means that which has to be sacrificed to carry out a certain course of action, i.e. costs are benefits foregone elsewhere
2. Cost effectiveness analysis is concerned with how to get a given objective at the minimum cost.
3. Cost benefit analysis is concerned with issues of whether to persue objectives.
4. Cost-utility analysis is concerned with comparisons between programmes
   Cost-minimisation analysis finds the least costly programme among those shown to be of equal benefit when both quantity and quality of life be measured.

Examples of Latin and English prescription abbreviations

Word or phrase	Abbreviation	Meaning	Word or phrase	Abbreviation	Meaning
Ad	Ad	To, up to	Gram	g, gm or gm	gram
Ad libitum	Ad lib	At pleasure, freely	Gutta	gtt	A drop
Ante cibum	ac	Before meals	Hora	h	An hour
Ante meridien	am	Before noon, morning	Hora somni	hs	At bedtime
Aqua	Aq	Water	Injectio	inj	An injection
Bis in die	bid/bd	Twice a day	Intramuscular	im	By intramuscular injection
Bolus	bol	A large pill			
	BP	British Pharmacopoeia	Intravenous	iv	By intravenous injection
	BPC	British Pharmaceutical Codex		IP	Indian Pharmacopoeia
Capsula	caps	Capsule		IU	International units
Collunarium	collun	A nose wash	Laevo	L	Left
Collutorium	collut	A mouth wash	Linimentum	lin	Liniment
Collyrium	collyr	An eye wash	Liquor	liq	Solution
Compositus	comp	Compounded	Microgram	mcg	One-millionth gram
Cum	c with bar	With	Milligram	mg	One-thousandth gram

Word or phrase	Abbreviation	Meaning
Millilitre	ml	One-thousandth litre
Misce	m	Mix
Mistura	mist	Mixture
Nebula	nebul	A spray
Omni die	od	Every day
Omni mane	om	Every morning
Omni nocte	on	Every night
Per os	po	By mouth
Post cibum	pc	After meals
Post peridien	pm	After noon- evening
Pro re nata	prn	As required (where many repetitions are required, max, frequency of repetition should be added)
PR		Per rectum
Pulvis	pulv	A powder
PV	per vaginam	By vaginal route
Quantum sufficiat	qs	As much as is sufficient
Quantum sufficiat ad	qs ad	A sufficient quantity of prepare
Quarter die sumendus	qid/qds	Four times a day

Word or phrase	Abbreviation	Meaning
Quaque	q or qq	Every, e.g. qq 6h (6 hours)
Quarta quake hora	qqh	Every four hours
Recipe	R_x	(You) Take
Repetatur	Rep	Let it be repeated e.g. rep mist (ura), repeat the mixture
Semis	ss	One-half
Si opus sit	sos	If necessary, to be repeated once only, and use prn in case many repetitions are intended
Signa	sig	You write
Sine	s with bar	Without
Solutio	sol	Solution
Statim	stat	Immediately
Subcutaneous	sc	By subcutaneous injection
Tabella	tab	Tablet
Ter in die	tid	Three times a day
Tablespoon	tbsp	Tablespoon
Teaspoon	tsp	Teaspoon
Unguentum	ung	Ointment
	USP	United States Pharmacopoeia

APPENDIX 3

PATIENT COMPLIANCE WITH PRESCRIBED MEDICATION

Compliance is the extent to which patients follow instructions. Educational, economic, ethnic, and personality factors influence patient compliance. However, the role of interacton between physician/pharmacist and patient is also very important. The most important thing is that the patient must clearly understand the instructions and also know the consequences of noncompliance.

Compliance may be defined as the extent to which an individual's behaviour coincides with medical or health advice. The term adherence can also be used for compliance.

Patient noncompliance suggests that the patient is at fault for inappropriate use of medicine. It is often correct. But in some cases the responsibility for noncompliance can be directed at the physician and/or pharmacist for failing to give the patient adequate instructions or not presenting them in a manner he understands.

As a consequence of noncompliance, problems may develop, for example, noncompliance by a hypertensive patient, physician fells that more dose of the drug is required. This may produce toxic effect. In a patient of tuberculosis noncompliance results in relapse.

The underutilization of one drug may result in excessive response to other concurrently used drugs e.g. digoxin and KCl, if he stops KCl heart becomes more sensitive to digoxin.

The overutilization is also bad, the patient forgets one dose and doubles the next dose.

Factors that lead to poor patient compliance or noncompliance

- Taking a medicine several times a day i.e. multiple medications, frequent dose regimens i.e. frequency and complexity of drug regimen.
- Various social or personal beliefs about the use of medications may be barriers to compliance.
- Certain diseases like hypertension and diabetes have no symptoms to remind them to take their medication.
- Some patients especially suffering from severe pain such as arthritis frequently alter the medication in the hope of finding a better drug, if the necessity to continue the therapy for the prescribed period after the acute symptoms have subsided is not explained to the patient by the physician/pharmacist.
- Common errors of compliances may be of omission, dosage, timing, adding medications not prescribed, or premature termination of drug therapy (may be due to relief of symptoms or cost). It may also be due to lack of information.
- On appearance of minor side effects the drug may be discontinued if the patient has already not been told that these are common and not to be feared.
- Errors and noncompliance occur more frequently at the extremes of age and in patients who live alone. It may be due to forgetfulness (unintentional noncompliance).
- Poor patient-doctor relationship (patient dissatisfaction with the doctor).

Patient compliance can be improved by :

- Giving psychological support "putting the ill at ease".
- Development of a routine for taking drug e.g. at meal times.
- Providing "information and education".
- Patient's active participation in the treatment.
- The importance of compliance, in other words the consequences of noncompliance, should be explained. The undesirable effects produced by underutilization as well as overutilization should be explained.
- Presenting instructions in a manner patient understands.
- Enhanced communication between the patient and doctor or pharmacist.
- Patient noncompliance (failure to adhere to the drug regimen) is a major cause of treatment failure.

APPENDIX 4

IRRATIONAL COMBINATIONS AND BANNED DRUGS

More than 60,000 branded formulations are available in India. These preparations contain either single drug or drugs in fixed dose combination (FDC). All formulations are used for treatment or prevention of diseases. Out of it only few drugs are lifesaving and essential drugs, otherwise maximum of them are available as alternative or substitute to each other.

At the same time it is clinically proved that almost all the drugs have side effect at therapeutic level besides toxic effect. The unwanted side effect is referred to as adverse drug reaction (ADR). Hence a drug is used or prescribed by physician on seeing risk-benefit ratio.

Though the drug is approved by the Drugs Controller General India (DCGI) for manufacturing and marketing in country only after consideration of all aspects such as therapeutic effect, side effect, toxic effect etc; the physician has to follow rational prescription practice in consideration of drugs available in the market.

It is a fact that on seeing serious hazardous effect of drug Thalidomide in 1960 in UK, the FDA of all the countries gave a thought on banning of drugs. Accordingly in our country, after amendment of Drugs Act in 1982, Government has acquired the power to prohibit the manufacture and sale of drugs and fixed dose combinations of irrational drugs. The government, subsequently, issued a first gazette notification in July 1983 banning several drugs and their Fixed Dose Combinations (FDC) after due consideration. A ban or restricted use order is being issued on a continuous basis on seeing ADR on Indian patients. This is being done in the interest of common people of India and also to safeguard their health from menace of ADR of drugs.

Till date the Indian government has banned several FDCs and imposed restriction on many drugs and their combinations with other drugs for its manufacturing and marketing in India. Following is the list :

1. Amidopyrine
2. Phenacetin
3. Sulphanilamide
4. Practolol
5. Methapyrilene and its salts
6. Penicillin skin/eye ointment
7. Tetracycline liquid
8. Oxytetracycline liquid oral preparation
9. Demeclocycline liquid oral preparation
10. Methaqualone
11. FDC of chloramiphericol with other drugs for internal use
12. FDC of Ergot with any drugs
13. FDC of Vitamins with anti-inflammatory agents and tranquilisers
14. FDC of Atropine with analgesics and antipyretics
15. FDC of Yohimbine and strychnine with Testosterone and vitamins.
16. FDC of iron with Strychnine, Arsenic and Yohimbine.
17. Chloral hydrate
18. FDC of sodium bromide with other drugs.
19. FDC of Tetracycline with vitamin C.
20. FDC of antihistamines with antidiarrhoeals.
21. FDC of Penicillins with Sulfonamides

22. FDC of vitamins with analgesics
23. FDC of prophylactic vitamins with Anti TB drugs except isoniazid with Pyridoxine Hydrochloride (Vitamin B_6).
24. FDC of Strychnine and Caffeine in Tonic.
25. FDC of Hydroxy Quinolines groups of drugs with other drugs and liquid oral antidiarroheal or any other dosage form for paediatric use except for external use.
26. FDC of corticosteroid for internal use
27. FDC of Anabolic steroid with other drugs.
28. Combination of high dose of Estrogen and Progesterone (low dose combination is allowed for its use as contraceptive)
29. FDC of Sedatives/ hypnotics/ anxiolytics with analegesic and antipyretics.
30. FDC of anti-TB drugs except the under-stated combinations.
    I II
    (a) (i) Pyrizinamide 1000mg; 1500mg
         (ii) Rifampicin 450mg; 600mg
         (iii) Isoniazid 300mg; 300mg
    (b) (i) Ethambutol 600mg; 800mg
         (ii) Isoniazid 200mg; 300mg.
31. FDC of Histamin H_2 receptor antagonists with antacid except any combination approved by DCGI.
32. Patent and proprietary medicines having alcohol more than 20% except preparation listed in IP.
33. All preparations containing chloroform exceeding 0.5% w/w or v/v whichever is appropriate.
34. FDC of anthelmintics with cathartics or purgatives except for piperazine.
35. FDC containing more than one antihistaminic drug.
36. FDC of Salbutamol or any other bronchodilator with central acting antitussives and/ or antihistamines.
37. FDC of Laxatives and/ or antispasmodic drugs in enzyme preparations.
38. FDC if metoclopramide with other drugs except with Aspirin/ Paracetamol.
39. FDC of centrally acting antitussives with antihistamin as having atropine like activity in expectorent.
40. Preparations claiming to combat cough associated with asthma that contain a centrally acting antitusive and/ or antihistamine.
41. Liquid oral tonic having glycercl phosphates and other phosphates and/ or CNS stimulants and such preparations having alcohol more than 20%.
42. FDC containing Pectin and/ or Kaolin with any drug which is systemically absorbed through GI tract.
43. Toothpaste/ toothpowder containing tobacco.
44. Dovers powder IP Dovers Powder IP Tablets.
45. Antidiarrhoeal preparations containing kaolin/ pectin/ attapulgite/ activated charcoal.
46. Antidiarrhoeal preparations having phthalye sulphathiozole, Sulphaguinidine, succinic sulphathiozole, Neomycin, streptromycin, dihydro streptomycin or their salt.
47. Antidiarrhoeal formulation in any form for Pediatric use containing Diphenoxylate or Loperamide or Atropine or belladonna including their salts, esters or metabolites or their extracts or alkaloids.
48. FDC of antidiarrhoeals with electrolytes,
49. Oral Rehydration salts (ORS)-other than conforming to WHO formula or Pharmacapoeial preparation.
50. FDC of Analgin with any other drugs.
51. FDC of Dextropropoxyphene with any other drug except with antispasmodics and or NSAID

52. FDC of Phenylbutazone or Oxyphenbutazone with other drugs.
53. FDC of allopathic drugs with Ayurvedic, Siddha or Unani drugs.
54. Mepacrine Hydrochloride (Quina-crine and its salts) in any dosage form for use for female sterilization or contraception.
55. Fenfluramine and Dexfenfluramine.
56. FDC of streptomycin with penicillin.
57. FDC of Vitamin B1, B6 & B12.
58. Fixed dose combination of Nitrofuratoin and Trimethoprim.
59. Fixed dose combination of Phenobarbitone with any antiasthamatic drugs.
60. Fixed dose combination of Phenobarbitone with Hyoscin and/or Hyoscyamine.
61. Fixed dose combination of Phenobarbitone with Ergotamine and/or Belladona.
62. Fixed dose combination of Haloperidol with any anti-cholinergic agent including Propentheline Bromide.
63. Fixed dose combination of Nalidixic acid with any antiramoebics including Metronidazole.
64. Fixed dose combination of Loperamide Hydrochloride with Furazolidone.
65. Fixed dose combination of Cyproheptadine with Lysine or Peptone.
66. Fixed dose combination of Diazepam and Diphenhydramine Hydrochloride.
67. Cisapride- Only qualified gastro-enterologists such as super specilists holding DM in gastro-enterology are permitted to prescribe cisapride.
68. Astemizole
69. Terfenadine
70. Sildenafil citrate. To be prescribed by endocrinologists, Urologists and Psychiatrist only.

The safety of health of a patient from drug is a vital aspect during treatment. The health professionals -- physicians, pharmacists and nurses have to prescribe, handle and administer the medicines respectively. So it is imperative for them to acquaint themselves with the above list. In addition to it, they should also go through the notification issued time to time by DCGI. This helps them to use proper medicines only and also to save patients from unsafe drug. Further it is also imperative for the industrial pharmacists and marketing professionals to keep themselves abreast with list of banned drugs, drugs of restricted use and banned FDCs. This ultimately helps them in formulating right products mix and a proper marketing strategy. Lastly it saves the Indian patients from hazardous drugs.

APPENDIX 5

RATIONAL USE OF DRUGS

Rational use of drugs requires that patients receive medications appropriate to their clinical needs, in doses that meet their own requirements, for an adequate period of time, and the reasonable cost to them.

Rational use of drug is based on rule of right : the right drug given to the right patient at the right time with the right dosages. They should also fulfill such criteria : safety, affordability, need and efficacy. Rational prescribing, therefore, involves a right decision of the prescribers. This will eventually encourage the patients to take the medication and comply the prescription served by the prescribers to them.

Drugs can cure ailments when used rationally. On the other hand, they may become harmful and can even threaten life when used irrationally. Irrational drug use includes overuse, underuse and inappropriate use.

Rational Prescribing

Teaching medical students and doctors to prescribe rationally has a strong impact on the quality of future health care. This is true also in situations where doctors are not only prescribers, as it has strong influence on other health workers and on the prescribed value of specific treatment within the community.

Guide to good prescribing - a new WHO training manual is an example of one such approach i.e. teaching skills to the students to learn how to develop a set of first choice of drugs, drawing on a wide range of authoritative drug information. Students not only learn how to use drugs rationally but how to consult, understand and use existing treatment guidelines intelligently and where necessary to adapt them to the individual patient.

Criteria for rational prescribing

Rational prescribing should meet the certain criteria such as appropriate diagnosis, indication, drug, patient, dosage, duration, route of administration, information and monitoring.

Appropriate diagnosis

To achieve correct diagnosis one has to depend on the clinical features and laboratory investigations. Clinical feature is the most important criterion, specially when facility for laboratory investigations is seldom available as in the rural areas. However, sometimes laboratory investigation may confuse making accurate diagnosis. So, if some one knows the clinical features of a disease then he can easily diagnose and treat the cases rationally and thereby avoid the misuse of money, time and labour.

Appropriate indication

It is necessary to know whether drug is actually necessary or not. The decision to prescribe drug is entirely based on medical rationale and that drug therapy is an effective and safe treatment, for example, most of the diarrhoea in children are self limiting and there is no rationale for the use of any drug in most cases. The WHO guidelines suggest the use of ORS in acute non-specific diarrhoea.

Appropriate drug

The selection of drug is based on efficacy, safety, suitability, cost considerations, and easy availability. For example, a child suffering from cholera may be treated with erythromycin, which is safe and effective. Here, tetracycline although indicated should be avoided because the patient is a child.

Appropriate patient

While considering the patient, one should consider about any history of sensitivity to drug, as well as other considerations e.g. geriatric and paediatric age group must be prescribed with caution; pregnant and lactating women must be administered life saving drugs, but little else.

Appropriate dosage

Consideration of doses is important specially when the patient is either a child, geriatric, or having a history of concomitant diseases such as hepatic or renal impairment. For example, digoxin must be administered at a loading dose when the plasma concentration of free drug is very low for therapeutic response in usual dosage as it is highly protein bound drug.

Appropriate route of administration

When the oral route is appropriate for a patient, then intravenous route should be avoided as it is expensive, having more adverse effects, and irrational. In many occasions, diazepam is given parenterally (i.m.) but oral drug is indicated because of better bioavailability.

Appropriate information

The patient should be informed with relevant, accurate, important, and clear information regarding his/her condition and the medications that are prescribed.

Appropriate monitoring

The anticipated and unexpected effects of medications should be appropriately monitored. For example, in case of tissue transplantation the monitoring of cyclosporin is vital for the effectiveness of treatment, trough level should be less than 200 mg/ml.

Irrational Prescribing

Common pattern of irrational prescribing may be manifested in the following forms (a) unnecessary use of drugs when not indicated e.g. antibiotic for viral upper respiratory tract infections; (b) use of wrong drug for the specific condition requiring drug therapy, e.g. tetracycline in childhood diarrhea requiring ORS; (c) the use of drug with doubtful / unproven efficacy, e.g. the use of antimotility agents such as loparamide in acute diarrhea; (d) use of drugs having uncertain safety status, e.g. the use of dipyrone to relieve visceral pain; (e) failure to provide available safe and effective drugs, e.g. the failure to vaccinate against measles or tetanus, failure to prescribe ORS for acute diarrhoea (f) use of correct drugs with incorrect administration, dosage and duration, e.g. the use of intravenous metronidzole when suppository or oral formulation would be appropriate ; (g)the use of effective drug but one which has higher level of potential toxicity, e.g. injection kanamycin / gentamicin : (h) prescribing new costly drugs even when an alternative cheaper drug of equal efficacy is available e.g. prescribing more costly NSAIDS in place of aspirin which is cheap and efficacious with very similar risks of side effects for the relief of somatic pains and inflammation. (i) overuse and misuse of antibiotics cause drug resistance, adverse reactions, super - infection and excessive cost.

Prevention of irrational prescribing

To prevent irrational prescribing the following measures should be taken -
- making correct diagnosis
- limiting the number of drugs
- encouraging the availability of essential drugs

- providing adequate training, drug information and standard treatment guidelines to the prescribers through continuing education and incorporating the concept of essential drugs.
- teaching of rational prescribing into the curricula of medicine, pharmacy, dentistry and nursing
- providing effective education to the consumers and to the public.

Rational use of drugs can be improved if the physician is aware of the cost of drugs, prescribes the cheapest preparation without compromising on the quality or the efficacy of the medicine, and prescribes only the minimum number of drugs particularly from the Essential Drug List.

Criteria for Rational Prescribing

- Appropriate diagnosis
- Appropriate indication
- Appropriate drug
- Appropriate patient
- Appropriate dosage
- Appropriate duration
- Appropriate route of administration
- Appropriate information
- Appropriate monitoring

Irrational Prescribing

- Overdue of antibiotics
- Indiscriminate use of injection
- Polypharmacy
- Excessive use of drug
- Anabolic steroid for growth
- Tonics and multivitamins for malnutrition

APPENDIX 6

Orphan drugs

When a drug is not developed because the developer will not recover the costs, then it is known as an orphan drug.

Drugs for rare diseases must be licensed on less than ideal amounts of clinical evidence.

The cost of treating a rare genetic Gaucher's liposome storage disease with genetically engineered enzyme will cost US $ 145000 to 400000 per year. Who can and will pay ?

Official recognition of orphan drug status in USA is accorded (population 240 million) where the relevant disease affects fewer than 200000 people; in Japan (population 121 million) for fewer than 50000 people.

The remedy with regard to orphan drug lies with the government who should offer incentives, e.g. tax relief, subsidies, exclusive marketing rights to pharmaceutical companies, and in case of poor countries, international aid programmes.

Biological agents as weapons (bioterrorism)

The following are the candidates among the pathogens which can be employed as biological weapons against people.
- Bacillus anthracis (the causal agent of anthrax)
- Brucella (brucellosis)
- Clostridium botulinum (botulism)
- Franeisella tularensis (tularaemia)
- Yersinia pestis (plague)
- Variola virus (smallpox)

Incapacitating agents (harassing, disabling, antiriot agents)

These are chemical agents that are capable of rapidly causing a temporary disablement that lasts for little longer than the period of exposure when used in field conditions.
- Dibenzoxazepine has the usual properties (above) and in addition induce a rise in IOP. Its solubility allows its use in water 'cannons'.
- Chlorobenzylidine malononitrile (CS) a tear 'gas'. It is not a gas. It is a solid that is disseminated as an aerosol (particles of 1 micron diameter).
  It gives slight pricking or peppery sensation in the eyes and nose, spasm of eyelids, profuse salivation and lacrimations, sometimes vomiting, cough and gripping pain in the chest.
  The symptoms appear immediately on exposure and they disappear dramatically.
- Chloroacetophenone, a tear gas (CN) used as a solid aerosol or smoke.

Drugs used for torture, interrogation and judicial execution

Suxamethonium, hallucinogens, thiopentone, neuroleptics, amphetamines, apomorphine and cyclophosphamide.

These substances have been used to hurt, frighten, confuse or debilitate.

According to some, it is justifiable to use drugs to protect society against serious crimes such as murder. But there is no such thing as 'truth-drug' in the sense that it guarantees the truth of what the subject says. There is always uncertainty of the truth of evidence obtained with drugs, e.g. thiopentone.

In some countries, drugs are used for judicial execution, e.g. combinations of thiopentone, potassium, curare, given intravenously.

APPENDIX 7

WHO ESSENTIAL DRUGS

Essential drugs are those that satisfy health care needs of the majority of population; they should therefore be available at all times in adequate amounts and in appropriate dosage forms.

For making optimal use of limited resources, the choice of such drugs depends on many factors such as the pattern of prevalent diseases, the treatment facilities; the training and experience of available personnel; the financial resources, and genetic, demographic and environmental factors. Only those drugs should be selected for which sound and adequate data on efficacy and safety are available from adequate studies and for which evidence of performance in general use in a variety of medical settings has been obtained.

In the great majority of cases essential drugs should be formulated as single compounds. Fixed ratio combinations products are acceptable only when the dosage of each ingredient meets the requirements of a defined population group and when combination provides a proven advantage over single compounds administered separately in therapeutic effect, safety or compliance.

Preparing a rational list of essential / restricted drugs has several advantages: Medical, Economic, Social and Administrative.

World Health Organization has provided guidelines for establishing a list of Essential Drugs.

- Each country should appoint a committee to establish a list of essential drugs.
- Drug selection should be based on the results of benefit and safety evaluations obtained in controlled clinical trials and/or epidemiological studies.
- International nonproprietary (Generic) names should be used.
- Selected drugs should meet Quality Control Standards including stability and when necessary, bioavailability.
- Cost of treatment must be considered.
- Influence of local diseases or conditions on pharmacokinetic and pharmacodynamic parameters should be considered in making the selection e.g. malnutrition, kidney and liver diseases.
- Fixed ratio combinations are acceptable only when :
  1. Clinical documentation justifies concomitant use of more than one drug.
  2. Therapeutic effect is greater than the sum of the effect of each.
  3. Cost of combination product is less than the sum of individual products.
  4. Compliance is improved.

Acetazolamide
Acetylsalicylic acid
Albendazole
Albumin, human
Alcuronium
Allopurinol
Aluminium diacetate
Aluminium hydroxide
Amidotrizoate
Amiloride
p-Aminobenzoic acid
Aminophylline
Amitriptyline
Amoxicillin
Amphotericin B

Ampicillin
Anti-D immunoglobulin (human)
Antihaemophilic fraction (see Factor VIII concentrate)
Antihaemorrhoidal preparation : Local anaesthetic, astringent drug
Antiscorpion sera
Antitetanus immunoglobulin (human)
Antivenom sera
Ascorbic acid
Asparaginase
Atenolol
Atropine
Azathioprine

Bacitracin + neomycin
Barium sulfate
BCG vaccine (dried)
Beclomethasone
Benzathine
Benznidazole
Benzoic acid + salicylic acid
Benzophenones
Benzoyl peroxide
Benzyl benzoate
Benzylpenicillin dithranol
Betamethasone
Biperiden
Bupivacaine

Calamine lotion
Calcium folinate
Calcium gluconate
Calcium hypochloride
Captopril
Carbamazepine
Carbidopa + levodopa
Charcoal, activated
Chloral hydrate
Chloramphenicol
Chlorhexidine
Chloroquine
Chlorphenamine
Chlorpromazine
Cyclosporin
Cimetidine
Cirpofloxacin
Cisplatin
Clindamycin
Clofazimine
Clomifene
Cloxacillin
Coal tar
Codeine
Colchicine
Condoms
Copper-containing intrauterine device
Cromoglicic acid
Cyclophosphamide
Cytarabine

Decarbazine
Dactinomycin
Dapsone
Deferoxamine
Desmopressin
Dexamethasone
Dextran 70
Diaphragms
Diazepam
Diethylcarbamazine
Diethyltoluamide
Digitoxin
Diloxanide
Dimercaprol
Diphtheria antixocin
Diphtheria-pertussis-tetanus vaccine

Diphtheria-tetanus vaccine
Dopamine
Doxorubicin
Doxycycline

Eflorinthine
Ephedrine
Epinephrine
Ergocalciferol
Ergometrine
Ergotamine
Erythromycin
Ethambutol
Ether; anaesthetic
Ethinylestradiol
Ethinylestradiol + levonorgestrel
Ethinylestradiol + norethisterone
Ethosuximide
Etoposide

Factor VIII concentrate
Factor IX complex (coagulation Factors II, VII, IX, X) concentrate ferrous salt
Ferrus salt + folic acid
Flucytosine
Fludrocortisone
Fluorescein
Fluorouracil
Fluphenazine
Folic acid
Folic acid + ferrous salt
Furosemide (frusemide)

Gentamicin
Gentian violet (see Methylrosanilinium chloride)
Glucose
Glucose with sodium chloride
Glutaral, activated
Glycdryl trinitrate
Griseofulvin

Haloperidol
Halothane
Heparin
Hepatitis B vaccine
Hydralazine
Hydrochlorothiazide

Hydrocortisone
Hydrogen peroxide
Hydrooxocobalamin

Ibuprofen
Idoxuridine
Immunoglobulin, human normal
Indomethacin
Influenza vaccine
Insulin injection, soluble
Insulin, intermediate-acting
Intraperitoneal dialysis solution
Iodine
Iopanoic acid
Iotroxate (see meglumine iotroxate)
Ipecac
Iron dextran
Isoniazid
Isoniazid + rifampicin
Isoniazid + thioacetazone
Isosorbide dinitrate
Ivermectin

Ketamine
Ketoconazole

Levamisole
Levodopa + carbidopa
Levonorgestrel + ethinylestradiol
Levothyroxine
Lidocaine
Lithium carbonate

Magnesium hydroxide
Mannitol
Measles caccine
Measles-mumps-rubella vaccine
Mebendazole
Medroxyprogesterone acetate (depot)
Mefloquine
Meglumine antimoniate
Meglumine iotroxate
Melarsoprol
Meningococcal vaccine
Mercaptopurine
DL-Methionine
Methyldopa
Methylene blue (see Methylthioninium chloride)

Methylrosanilinium chloride (gentian violet)
Methylthionium chloride (methylene blue)
Metoclopramide
Metrifonate
Metronidazole
Miconazole
Morphine
Mustine (see Chlormethine)

Nalidixic acid
Naloxone
Neomycin + bacitracin
Neostigmine
Niclosamide
Nicotinamide
Nifedipine
Nifurtimox
Nitrofurantoin
Nitrous oxide
Nonoxinol
Norethisterone
Norethisterone enantate
Norethisterone + ethinylestradiol
Nystatin

Oral rehydration salts (for glucose-electrolyte solution)
Oxamniquine
Oxygen
Oxytocin

Paracetamol
Penicillamine
Pentamidine sodium chloride
Permethrin
Pethidine
Phenobarbital
Phenoxymethylpenicillin
Phenytoin
Phytomenadione
Pilocarpine
Piperacillin
Piperazine
Podophyllum resin
Poliomyelitis vaccine
Polygeline
Polyvidone iodine

Potassium chloride
Potassium ferric hexacyanoferrate (II) $2H_2O$ (Prussian blue)
Potassium iodide
Praziquantel
Prednisolone
Primaquine
Procainamide
Procaine benzylpenicillin
Procarbazine
Proguanil
Promethazine
Propranolol
Propyliodone
Propylthiouracil
Protamine sulfate
Prussian blue (see Potassium ferric hexacyanoferrate (II) $2H_2O$)
Pyrantel
Pyrazinamide
Pyridostigmine
Pyridoxine
Pyrimethamine
Pyrimethamine + sulfadoxine

Quinidine
Quinine

Rabies immunoglobulin
Rabies vaccine
Reserpine
Retinol
Riboflavin
Rifampicin
Rifampicin + isoniazid
Rubella vaccine

Salbutamol
Salicylic acid
Salicylic acid + benzoic acid
Selenium sulfide
Senna
Silver nitrate
Silver sulfadiazine
Sodium bicarbonate (see Sodium hydrogen carbonate)
Sodium calcium edetate
Sodium chloride with glucose

Sodium fluoride
Sodium hydrogen carbonate
Sodium lactate, compound solution
Sodium nitrite
Sodium nitroprusside
Sodium thiosulfate
Spectinomycin
Spironolactone
Streptokinase
Streptomycin
Sulfadimidine
Sulfadoxine
Sulfamethoxazole + trimethoprim
Sulfasalazine
Suramin sodium
Suxamethonium

Tamoxifen
Testosterone
Tetanus vaccine
Tetracaine
Tetracycline
Thiamine
Thioacetazone + isoniazid
Thiopental
Thiabendazole
Timolol
Tolbutamide
Trimethoprim
Trimethoprim + sulfamethoxazole
Tropicamide
Tuberculin, purified protein derivative (PPD)
Typhoid vaccine

Valproic acid
Vecuronium bromide
Verapamil
Vinblastine
Vincristine

Warfarin
Water for injection

Yellow fever vaccine

Zinc oxide

APPENDIX 8

DRUGS USED FOR ERECTILE DYSFUNCTION

Sildenafil Citrate (Viagra)

It is the first orally administered treatment of proven efficacy for erectile dysfunction. Detumescence is associated with catabolism of cyclic guanosine monophosphate (cGMP) by type 5, phosphodiestrase. Sildenafil acts by blocking the latter enzyme resulting in prolonging the life of cGMP. This causes relaxation of smooth muscle in corpus cavernosum and vasodilation, which produces engorgement of corpus cavernosum and penile erection and as a result increases both the number and duration of erections in men with erectile dysfunction.

For maximum effectiveness, sildenafil should be taken orally about one hour before sexual activity. The initial dose should be 50 mg, and it should be reduced to 25 mg if side effects occur.

Side effects associated with sildenafil are related to its vasodilatory properties and are similar to those induced by nitrates. These include headache, lightheadedness, dizziness, flushing, distorted vision (transient blue haze or increased brightness) and in some cases syncope. Possible tachyphylaxis has been reported.

Sildenafil is contraindicated in patients taking nitrates of any form, regularly or intermittently. If a man who has taken sildenafil has an acute ischaemic syndrome, nitrates should not be prescribed within 24 hours or longer in patients with renal or hepatic dysfunction.

In summary there are no clinical data on the safety and efficacy of slidenafil in the following groups :
1. Men who have had a myocardial infarction, stroke, or life-threatening arrhythmia within the last six months.
2. Men with resting hypotension (<90, 50 mmHg) or hypertension (>170/110 mmHg).
3. Men with cardiac failure or coronary artery disease causing unstable angina.
4. Men with retinitis pigmentosa.

Tadalafil

Tadalafil is a selective inhibitor of phosphodiestrase type 5 (PDE5). An initial dose of 10 mg is recommended prior to sexual activity. Depending on efficacy, the dose may be decreased to 5 mg or increased to 20 mg. Dosing adjustments are required in patients with renal and/or hepatic dysfunction. Peak plasma levels occur 2 hours after a 20 mg oral dose. Metabolism is predominantly by CPY3A4 and excretion (as metabolites) is mainly in the faeces (61% of dose) and to a lesser extent in the urine (36% of a dose). An elimination half-life is about 18 hours which is substantially longer than that of sildenafil or vardenafil. The long duration of action of this agent (upto 36 hours) is an advantage over sildenafil and vardenafil.

Adverse effects include headache, back pain, dyspepsia, myalgia. Changes in colour vision have been reported rarely.

Vardenafil

Vardenafil is a phosphodiestrase type 5 inhibitor with actions and uses similar to sildenafil.

The initial dose is 10 mg taken orally prior to sexual activity. A lower 5 mg dose is recommended in the elderly and in patients with moderate hepatic dysfunction.

Peak plasma levels occur 30 to 120 minute after oral administration.

Vardenafil is metabolized in the liver with 1 active metabolite. It is excreted as metabolites primarily in the faeces and has a half-life of 4 to 5 hours.

Adverse effects include headache, flushing, rhinitis, dyspepsia, nausea, visual effects (e.g., light sensitivity, changes in colour vision). It is unclear if hypotensive effects will be less with vardenafil compared to sildenafil. Priapsim has also been reported (rarely).

APPENDIX 9

OVERVIEW OF PHARMIONICS

One can redefine the biopharmaceutical sciences as being comprised by the following three sub-disciplines: a) pharmacokinetics (what the patient's body does to the drug); b) pharmacodynamics (what the drug does to the patient's body); and c) pharmionics (what the patients do with the prescribed medicines). In presently available knowledge, pharmacokinetic information vastly exceeds pharmacodynamic information. Pharmionics information is in its infancy. However, it points to critical gaps in pharmacodynamic information that need to be filled for efficient drug regimens, for understanding, how common variations in drug dosing patterns may create adverse drug reactions and for intervening efficiently to minimize efficacy – and safety – compromising errors in ambulatory patients' use of prescription drugs.

Pharmionics concerns itself with learning what patients actually do with prescribed drugs and analyzing the clinical and economic consequences of drug exposure that arise from patient's variable adherence to prescribed drug dosing patterns.

Three basic patterns characterize the main deviations:

- Some patients (5% –10%), but sometimes more or sometime less – never start the prescribed course of drug dosing. This pattern is known as "nonacceptance."
- There are patients who never start the dosing regimen, though have enrolled in the treatment programme. They may take an initial dose or two but most of them take none.
- Once the patient engages with the drug dosing regimen the question arises about the quality of patient's execution of that regimen – 'how much drug adherence is enough'? It is the degree of "forgiveness" that each medicine produces.

There are examples of 'forgiveness' regarding drug regimens. One extreme example of 'forgiveness' is bendroflumethiazide (a diuretic used as antihypertensive drug) which has a once – daily dosing regimen, though it is able to maintain anti-hypertensive action for over 6 days after a missed dose. The 'unforgiving' extreme example is that of combined estrogen /progestin oral contraceptive. Taking the once – daily "pill" more than 12 hours late increases the risk of breakthrough ovulation and conception during the part of the monthly cycle in which ovulation is most likely and correspondingly high likelihood of unwanted conception, even though 100% of prescribed doses have been taken.

The main errors in the execution are to delay or omit doses. Occasionally some patient takes extra doses but missed doses generally out number extra doses by 4:1.

There is also what is called 'drug holidays' which means abrupt cessation and resumption of dosing.

This general topic of pharmionics is very old. Hippocrates is said to have complained that some of his patients did not take the medicines he prescribed and then blamed for a poor outcome. At that time many medicines were not very effective or free from toxicity. Thus, the patients who declined to take his prescribed medicine(s) were perhaps making a better choice.

The situation today is radically different. The pharmaceutical products of increasing therapeutic and prophylactic power and economic cost has led to the formation of new sub-discipline called pharmionics.

The pharmionics field is just the beginning of systematic work with very few published studies of satisfactory design and analysis, however, the study showed clear-cut benefits of measurement-guided medication managements.

Lessons learned

The first lesson is that continuity of exposure to most drugs results in a substantially greater effectiveness, relative to what can be achieved in the setting of 'usual' or typical care.

A second lesson is that the vagaries in ambulatory patients' adherence to prescribed drug dosing regimens and some of their clinical and economic consequences are important which affect pharmacotherapy.

The third lesson is that the 'unforgiving' drugs can provide full effectiveness only for the 15-20% of patients who are strictly punctual in their re-medication.

A fourth lesson is that implants or depot injections, if properly designed and developed, can provide continuity of drug exposure throughout the interval between placement and replacement of the implant, or during the interval between successive depot injections.

A fifth lesson is that it appears to be possible for certain patterns of on-off-on dosing to cause hazardous rebound effects or recurrent first-dose effects.

A sixth lesson is the need to have reliable, quantitative pharmionics data so that it is clear what role under-usage of prescription drugs plays in failed therapy, thus also clearly distinguishing failures of pharmacological origin from failures of pharmionic origin.

A seventh lesson is the crucial role that erratic dosing appears to play in the emergence of drug resistance in the treatment of infectious and parasitic diseases. On a worldwide basis, this lesson is probably the most important of all because of the leading role that infectious diseases play in morbidity and mortality.

APPENDIX 10

OVERVIEW OF PHARMACOEPIDEMIOLOGY

The appropriate use of medications is an important central aspect of health care. Every year, basic science research and biotechnology produce new treatments which hold the promise of major clinical benefit. However, these medications also carry risks which must be rigorously measured and evaluated against the efficacy of the treatment.

What is Pharmacoepidemiology?

Pharmacoepidemiology is the study of the use and effects of drugs in large group of people. It is a relatively new and evolving science that attempts to quantify (i) mainly adverse drug events and (ii) patterns of drug use in a large population. To accomplish this study, pharmacoepidemiology borrows from both clinical pharmacology and epidemiology. Clinical pharmacology is the study of effects of drugs in humans. Epidemiology is the study of the distribution and determinants of diseases in populations. Thus, pharmacoepidemiology is considered a bridge science spanning both clinical pharmacology and epidemiology.

Epidemiological studies can be *categorised* into two main types (i) descriptive epidemiology and (ii) analytic epidemiology.

   (i) *Descriptive epidemiology* describes disease and/or exposure and may consist of calculating rates, for example, incidence and prevalence. Such descriptive studies do not use control groups and can only generate hypotheses. Studies of drug use would generally fall under descriptive studies.

   (ii) *Analytic epidemiology* includes two types of studies: observational studies, such as case-control and cohort studies, and experimental studies which would include clinical trials such as randomised clinical trials. The analytic studies compare an exposed group with a control group and are usually designed as hypotheses testing studies.

Significance of pharmacoepidemiology

Pharmacoepidemiology is being used increasingly to evaluate health care systems, interventions, and health-related behaviours. Pharmacoepidemiology is the scientific backbone of therapeutic risk management—the process of assessing a product's benefits and risks, and developing, implementing, and evaluating strategies to enhance the overall balance of such benefits and risks.

Pharmacoepidemiology has also certain unique areas, such as pharmacovigilance. Pharmacovigilance is a type of continual monitoring for unwanted effects and other safety-related aspects of drugs that are already on the market. The strength of pharmacoepidemiology over randomized trials is the ability to quantify rare adverse events that may occur over long periods. Recently, discordance in the results of pharmacoepidemiologic studies has made it difficult for clinicians and policy makers to make informed drug-therapy decisions. For example, in USA the antidiabetic drug called Rezulin was found associated with a risk of liver damage. The US FDA and manufacturer sent four separate warning letters to doctors, asking them to watch out for the problem and order liver tests for their patients on Rezulin. Less than half of patients got the recommended liver tests and, though liver monitoring was to be done monthly, only 5% of doctors were regularly testing the liver function of patients on the drug 5 months after the warnings. Finally, Rezulin was withdrawn from the market.

This example addresses the strength of pharmacoepidemiology and the advances in the methodology of pharmacoepidemiologic studies over the years. This also focuses on emphasis of potential problem of discordant results and urge pharmacoepidemiologists to develop good practice guidelines for the conduct of pharmacoepidemiologic studies which will provide valuable information about the effects of healthcare products.

International Society of Epidemiology (ISPE)

The ISPE Guidelines for Good Pharmacoepidemiology Practices (GPP) are intended to assist investigators with issues pertaining to the planning, conduct, and evaluation of pharmacoepidemiologic research. The Guidelines for Good Pharmacoepidemiology Practices (GPP) have been adapted from a document prepared by the Chemical Manufacturer's Association Epidemiology Task Group. The first revision done in 2004, revised and superseded the Guidelines for Good Epidemiologic Practice (GEP) developed in 1996.The focus of the revision was, the scope of the guidelines shall be broadened geographically and conceptually, to reflect ISPE's international membership, to include risk management and pharmacoeconomic activities, and to address more clearly the role of epidemiologic studies from industry and regulatory perspectives. Thus, the 2004 revision provided guidance on regulatory reporting requirements as they relate both to individual cases and to aggregate data. The second revision has been done to emphasise on the use and communication of statistical measures and to add clarification to specific items throughout the document.

The goal of GPP is to provide minimum practices and procedures that should be considered to help ensure the quality and integrity of pharmacoepidemiologic research, and to provide adequate documentation of research methods and results. The GPP are intended to apply broadly to all types of pharmacoepidemiologic research, including feasibility studies, validation studies, descriptive studies, as well as etiologic investigations, and all of their related activities from design through publication. As such, the GPP also support risk management activities.

The GPP address the following areas:
- Protocol Development
- Responsibilities, Personnel, Facilities, Resource Commitment, and Contractors
- Study Conduct
- Communication
- Adverse Event Reporting
- Archiving

ISPE recognizes that pharmacoepidemiologic research which is the study of the use and effects of healthcare products (including pharmaceuticals, devices and vaccines), has expanded to include clinical, economic and other health outcomes, requiring study methods that were not covered in previous guidelines. These guidelines are intended to address these activities and other pharmacoepidemiologic studies.

Increasingly, automated databases are being used by universities, pharmaceutical companies, and other commercial enterprises to evaluate the relationship between exposure to a healthcare product and adverse effects. Aggregate analysis of database studies can identify an unexpected increase in risk associated with a particular exposure. Formal studies conducted using these databases should adhere to GPP guidelines.

In addition to such studies, drug utilization research and pharmacoepidemiology are indispensable for the development of a structured programme to link drug use data to other medical service data. Hence, attention is required to the assessment of therapeutic results on the level of the individual patient as well as on the level of the community. This is how one can evaluate the quality of services by reviewing the results of the treatment programme.

APPENDIX 11

OVERVIEW OF PHARMACOECONOMICS

Pharmacoeconomics refers to the scientific discipline that compares the value of one pharmaceutical drug or drug therapy to another. It is a sub-discipline of health economics. Economics is about trade-off's and choices between wants, needs and the security of resources to fulfill these wants. Pharmacoeconomics has been defined as "the description and analysis of the costs of drug therapy to health care systems and society."A pharmacoeconomic study evaluates the cost and effects of a pharmaceutical product. Prescribing doctors, who have a duty to the community as well as to individual patients, cannot escape involvement with pharmacoeconomics.

The inroad of Economics into medical territory has proved beneficial. The two disciplines have mutually enriched their research methodologies.

$$\text{Pharmacoeconomics}$$
$$\text{INPUT COSTS} \longrightarrow \text{HEALTH CARE} \longrightarrow \text{OUTCOMES}$$

Importance of pharmacoeconomics

- Pharmacoeconomics may be a guide on resource allocation for decision makers. Pharmacoeconomics provide an assistance in the planning process and help in assigning the priorities.
- Pharmacoeconomic studies serve to guide optimal healthcare resource allocation, in a standardized and scientifically grounded manner.
- Pharmacoeconomics and outcome research can enhance the quality of the practice of healthcare professionals by strengthening the evaluation process and increasing the probability that one deliver better value in patient care.
- Clinical trials, decision analytic models, and observational studies can be used to support messages about value for the cost. Cutting edge evaluation of the value for the cost is supported by an evaluation from a randomized trial that include economic outcomes as primary or secondary endpoints of the trial. Short-term economic impacts can be directly observed while long term impacts are potentially projected by use of decision analysis. Reported results include point estimates and confidence intervals for estimates of incremental costs, outcomes, and comparison of costs and effects.

Types of pharmacoeconomic analysis

- Cost-minimization analysis (CMA) - It estimates costs of an intervention, but not the benefits that can be obtained. It is appropriate when two drugs of equal efficacy and equal tolerability are compared.
- Cost-effectiveness analysis (CEA) - It estimates costs and outcomes of intervention, but the two are measured in different units. CEA compares the relative expenditure (costs) and outcomes (effects) of two or more courses of action.
- Cost-benefit analysis (CBA) - It estimates costs and benefits in the same units (usually monetary units). CBA is a formal discipline used to help appraise, or assess, the case for a project or proposal and/or an informal approach to making decisions of any kind.
- Cost utility analysis (CUA) – It is used to guide procurement decisions. In CUA, outcome is measured in terms of utility.

Objective of pharmacoeconomics

The objective of pharmacoeconomics is to examine the impact of pharmaceutical services and products on patients' quality of life and healthcare outcomes through cost-effectiveness, cost-benefit, cost-utility, and cost-minimization analyses. Time and money can only be spent once - choice is inevitable, whether done unconsciously or with a consistent process. Health care professionals are constantly evaluating patient care choices and acting on them.

Drugs are a growing component of health care expenditures, and more attention is being drawn to the relation between the costs of medication and their benefits. It is anticipated that international pharmaceutical companies will increasingly invest in pharmacoeconomics while government staff will become more experienced, thus resulting in an upward momentum in the quality and usability of pharmacoeconomic data.

As there is growing pressure on healthcare budgets, justification of current expenditures and future investments in public healthcare are becoming increasingly important. Cost-effectiveness analysis is one means of justifying these expenditures. Justification often depends on demonstration that the value for the cost falls below a maximum acceptable cost-effectiveness ratio. Decision makers may also be interested in one's confidence level that the therapy represents. Confidence intervals for cost-effectiveness ratios, confidence intervals for net monetary benefits, and acceptability all provide information about these confidence levels.

Relevance of pharmacoeconomics to the pharmaceutical industry

Pharmaceutical companies have been quick to recognize the relevance of pharmacoeconomic analysis to strategic planning, both in early drug development and in determining the probable prices of the drugs in future. Principles of pharmacoeconomics assist in making informed clinical decisions by providing information about costs and consequences of alternative methods of treatment. Health related quality of life (HRQOL) is an outcome measure in pharmacoeconomics analyses as it examines health status and allows comparisons of treatments of different conditions. In 1994, the Department of Health, UK issued guidelines for pharmacoeconomics evaluations in joined working with Association of British Pharmaceutical Industry. These guidelines on good practices in the conduct of economic evaluation of medicines included, demographic characteristics of the population group, treatment paths of the option being compared and identifying the impact on all parts of society including patients.

The relationship between pharmacoepidemiology and pharmacoeconomics is important, as pharmacoeconomics relies heavily on good clinical and epidemiological data. The pharmacoepidemiology databases provide an invaluable component in pharmacoeconomic analysis, like assessing cost effectiveness of the treatment.

Future of pharmacoeconomics

The development of pharmacoeconomics from health economics provides a sound theoretical structure that is in turn based on knowledge derived from the evolution of economics. This is the right time to test this theoretical base in control clinical trials. The challenge for future research is to examine the links between pricing and efficiency. This can be achieved by the evolution of managed care systems. The future confront is to show that pharmacoeconomic analysis increases the efficiency of allocation of healthcare resources. This will only be managed by integration of health economics into the different disciplinary structure of health services research.

Index